HANDBOOK OF STATISTICS
VOLUME 27

Handbook of Statistics

VOLUME 27

General Editor

C.R. Rao

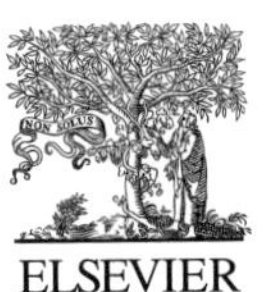

Amsterdam • Boston • Heidelberg • London • New York • Oxford
Paris • San Diego • San Francisco • Singapore • Sydney • Tokyo

Epidemiology and Medical Statistics

Edited by

C.R. Rao
Center for Multivariate Analysis
Department of Statistics, The Pennsylvania State University
University Park, PA, USA

J.P. Miller
Division of Biostatistics
School of Medicine, Washington University in St. Louis
St. Louis, MO, USA

D.C. Rao
Division of Biostatistics
School of Medicine, Washington University in St. Louis
St. Louis, MO, USA

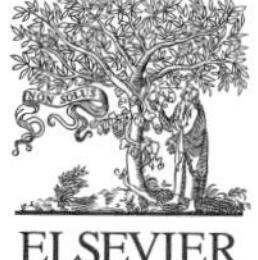

Amsterdam • Boston • Heidelberg • London • New York • Oxford
Paris • San Diego • San Francisco • Singapore • Sydney • Tokyo
North-Holland is an imprint of Elsevier

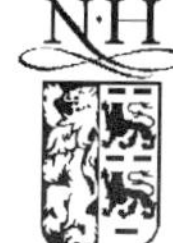

North-Holland is an imprint of Elsevier
Radarweg 29, PO Box 211, 1000 AE Amsterdam, The Netherlands
Linacre House, Jordan Hill, Oxford OX2 8DP, UK

First edition 2008

British Library Cataloguing in Publication Data
A catalogue record for this book is available from the British Library

Library of Congress Cataloging-in-Publication Data
A catalog record for this book is available from the Library of Congress

ISBN: 978-0-444-52801-8
ISSN: 0169-7161

For information on all North-Holland publications
visit our website at books.elsevier.com

Printed and bound in The Netherlands

08 09 10 11 12 10 9 8 7 6 5 4 3 2 1

Table of contents

Preface xiii

Contributors xv

Ch. 1. Statistical Methods and Challenges in Epidemiology and Biomedical Research 1
Ross L. Prentice

1. Introduction 1
2. Characterizing the study cohort 3
3. Observational study methods and challenges 6
4. Randomized controlled trials 12
5. Intermediate, surrogate, and auxiliary outcomes 17
6. Multiple testing issues and high-dimensional biomarkers 18
7. Further discussion and the Women's Health Initiative example 21
References 22

Ch. 2. Statistical Inference for Causal Effects, With Emphasis on Applications in Epidemiology and Medical Statistics 28
Donald B. Rubin

1. Causal inference primitives 28
2. The assignment mechanism 36
3. Assignment-based modes of causal inference 41
4. Posterior predictive causal inference 47
5. Complications 55
References 58

Ch. 3. Epidemiologic Study Designs 64
Kenneth J. Rothman, Sander Greenland and Timothy L. Lash

1. Introduction 64
2. Experimental studies 65
3. Nonexperimental studies 73
4. Cohort studies 73

5. Case-control studies 84
6. Variants of the case-control design 97
7. Conclusion 104
References 104

Ch. 4. Statistical Methods for Assessing Biomarkers and Analyzing Biomarker Data 109
Stephen W. Looney and Joseph L. Hagan

1. Introduction 109
2. Statistical methods for assessing biomarkers 110
3. Statistical methods for analyzing biomarker data 126
4. Concluding remarks 143
References 144

Ch. 5. Linear and Non-Linear Regression Methods in Epidemiology and Biostatistics 148
Eric Vittinghoff, Charles E. McCulloch, David V. Glidden and Stephen C. Shiboski

1. Introduction 148
2. Linear models 151
3. Non-linear models 167
4. Special topics 176
References 182

Ch. 6. Logistic Regression 187
Edward L. Spitznagel Jr.

1. Introduction 187
2. Estimation of a simple logistic regression model 188
3. Two measures of model fit 191
4. Multiple logistic regression 192
5. Testing for interaction 194
6. Testing goodness of fit: Two measures for lack of fit 195
7. Exact logistic regression 196
8. Ordinal logistic regression 201
9. Multinomial logistic regression 204
10. Probit regression 206
11. Logistic regression in case–control studies 207
References 209

Ch. 7. Count Response Regression Models 210
Joseph M. Hilbe and William H. Greene

1. Introduction 210
2. The Poisson regression model 212
3. Heterogeneity and overdispersion 224
4. Important extensions of the models for counts 230

5. Software 247
6. Summary and conclusions 250
References 251

Ch. 8. Mixed Models 253
Matthew J. Gurka and Lloyd J. Edwards

1. Introduction 253
2. Estimation for the linear mixed model 259
3. Inference for the mixed model 261
4. Selecting the best mixed model 264
5. Diagnostics for the mixed model 268
6. Outliers 270
7. Missing data 270
8. Power and sample size 272
9. Generalized linear mixed models 273
10. Nonlinear mixed models 274
11. Mixed models for survival data 275
12. Software 276
13. Conclusions 276
References 277

Ch. 9. Survival Analysis 281
John P. Klein and Mei-Jie Zhang

1. Introduction 281
2. Univariate analysis 282
3. Hypothesis testing 288
4. Regression models 295
5. Regression models for competing risks 310
References 317

Ch. 10. A Review of Statistical Analyses for Competing Risks 321
Melvin L. Moeschberger, Kevin P. Tordoff and Nidhi Kochar

1. Introduction 321
2. Approaches to the statistical analysis of competing risks 324
3. Example 327
4. Conclusion 339
References 340

Ch. 11. Cluster Analysis 342
William D. Shannon

1. Introduction 342
2. Proximity measures 344
3. Hierarchical clustering 350
4. Partitioning 355
5. Ordination (scaling) 358

6. How many clusters? 361
7. Applications in medicine 364
8. Conclusion 364
References 365

Ch. 12. Factor Analysis and Related Methods 367
Carol M. Woods and Michael C. Edwards

1. Introduction 367
2. Exploratory factor analysis (EFA) 368
3. Principle components analysis (PCA) 375
4. Confirmatory factor analysis (CFA) 375
5. FA with non-normal continuous variables 379
6. FA with categorical variables 380
7. Sample size in FA 382
8. Examples of EFA and CFA 383
9. Additional resources 389
Appendix A 391
Appendix B 391
References 391

Ch. 13. Structural Equation Modeling 395
Kentaro Hayashi, Peter M. Bentler and Ke-Hai Yuan

1. Models and identification 395
2. Estimation and evaluation 399
3. Extensions of SEM 410
4. Some practical issues 415
References 418

Ch. 14. Statistical Modeling in Biomedical Research: Longitudinal Data Analysis 429
Chengjie Xiong, Kejun Zhu, Kai Yu and J. Philip Miller

1. Introduction 429
2. Analysis of longitudinal data 431
3. Design issues of a longitudinal study 456
References 460

Ch. 15. Design and Analysis of Cross-Over Trials 464
Michael G. Kenward and Byron Jones

1. Introduction 464
2. The two-period two-treatment cross-over trial 467
3. Higher-order designs 476
4. Analysis with non-normal data 482
5. Other application areas 485
6. Computer software 488
References 489

Ch. 16. Sequential and Group Sequential Designs in Clinical Trials: Guidelines for Practitioners 491
Madhu Mazumdar and Heejung Bang

1. Introduction 492
2. Historical background of sequential procedures 493
3. Group sequential procedures for randomized trials 494
4. Steps for GSD design and analysis 507
5. Discussion 508
References 509

Ch. 17. Early Phase Clinical Trials: Phases I and II 513
Feng Gao, Kathryn Trinkaus and J. Philip Miller

1. Introduction 513
2. Phase I designs 514
3. Phase II designs 526
4. Summary 539
References 541

Ch. 18. Definitive Phase III and Phase IV Clinical Trials 546
Barry R. Davis and Sarah Baraniuk

1. Introduction 546
2. Questions 548
3. Randomization 550
4. Recruitment 551
5. Adherence/sample size/power 552
6. Data analysis 554
7. Data quality and control/data management 558
8. Data monitoring 558
9. Phase IV trials 563
10. Dissemination – trial reporting and beyond 564
11. Conclusions 565
References 565

Ch. 19. Incomplete Data in Epidemiology and Medical Statistics 569
Susanne Rässler, Donald B. Rubin and Elizabeth R. Zell

1. Introduction 569
2. Missing-data mechanisms and ignorability 571
3. Simple approaches to handling missing data 573
4. Single imputation 574
5. Multiple imputation 578
6. Direct analysis using model-based procedures 581
7. Examples 584
8. Literature review for epidemiology and medical studies 586
9. Summary and discussion 587
Appendix A 588
Appendix B 592
References 598

Ch. 20. Meta-Analysis 602
Edward L. Spitznagel Jr.

1. Introduction 602
2. History 603
3. The Cochran–Mantel–Haenszel test 604
4. Glass's proposal for meta-analysis 606
5. Random effects models 607
6. The forest plot 609
7. Publication bias 610
8. The Cochrane Collaboration 614
References 614

Ch. 21. The Multiple Comparison Issue in Health Care Research 616
Lemuel A. Moyé

1. Introduction 616
2. Concerns for significance testing 617
3. Appropriate use of significance testing 618
4. Definition of multiple comparisons 619
5. Rational for multiple comparisons 620
6. Multiple comparisons and analysis triage 621
7. Significance testing and multiple comparisons 623
8. Familywise error rate 625
9. The Bonferroni inequality 626
10. Alternative approaches 629
11. Dependent testing 631
12. Multiple comparisons and combined endpoints 635
13. Multiple comparisons and subgroup analyses 641
14. Data dredging 651
References 651

Ch. 22. Power: Establishing the Optimum Sample Size 656
Richard A. Zeller and Yan Yan

1. Introduction 656
2. Illustrating power 658
3. Comparing simulation and software approaches to power 663
4. Using power to decrease sample size 672
5. Discussion 677
References 677

Ch. 23. Statistical Learning in Medical Data Analysis 679
Grace Wahba

1. Introduction 679
2. Risk factor estimation: penalized likelihood estimates 681
3. Risk factor estimation: likelihood basis pursuit and the LASSO 690

4. Classification: support vector machines and related estimates 693
5. Dissimilarity data and kernel estimates 700
6. Tuning methods 704
7. Regularization, empirical Bayes, Gaussian processes priors, and reproducing kernels 707
References 708

Ch. 24. Evidence Based Medicine and Medical Decision Making 712
Dan Mayer

1. The definition and history of evidence based medicine 712
2. Sources and levels of evidence 715
3. The five stage process of EBM 717
4. The hierarchy of evidence: study design and minimizing bias 718
5. Assessing the significance or impact of study results: Statistical significance and confidence intervals 721
6. Meta-analysis and systematic reviews 722
7. The value of clinical information and assessing the usefulness of a diagnostic test 722
8. Expected values decision making and the threshold approach to diagnostic testing 726
9. Summary 727
10. Basic principles 727
References 728

Ch. 25. Estimation of Marginal Regression Models with Multiple Source Predictors 730
Heather J. Litman, Nicholas J. Horton, Bernardo Hernández and Nan M. Laird

1. Introduction 730
2. Review of the generalized estimating equations approach 732
3. Maximum likelihood estimation 735
4. Simulations 737
5. Efficiency calculations 740
6. Illustration 741
7. Conclusion 743
References 745

Ch. 26. Difference Equations with Public Health Applications 747
Asha Seth Kapadia and Lemuel A. Moyé

1. Introduction 747
2. Generating functions 748
3. Second-order nonhomogeneous equations and generating functions 750
4. Example in rhythm disturbances 752
5. Follow-up losses in clinical trials 758
6. Applications in epidemiology 765
References 773

Ch. 27. The Bayesian Approach to Experimental Data Analysis 775
Bruno Lecoutre

Preamble: and if you were a Bayesian without knowing it? 775
1. Introduction 776
2. Frequentist and Bayesian inference 778
3. An illustrative example 783
4. Other examples of inferences about proportions 795
5. Concluding remarks and some further topics 803
References 808

Subject Index 813

Handbook of Statistics Contents of Previous Volumes 823

Preface

The history of statistics suggests two important lessons. First and foremost, methodological research flourished in the hands of those who were not only highly focused on problems arising from real data, but who were themselves immersed in generating highly valuable data, like the late Sir Ronald A. Fisher. Second, although theoretical statistics research can be nurtured in isolation, only an applied orientation has made it possible for such efforts to reach new heights. Throughout the history of statistics, the most innovative and path breaking methodological advances have come out when brilliant statisticians have confronted the practical challenges arising from real data. The computational revolution has certainly made many of the most difficult computational algorithms readily available for common use, which in turn made the data-centric approach to methodological innovation sustainable. That the data-centric approach enriched statistics itself is amply demonstrated by the varied applications of statistical methods in epidemiology and medical studies.

This volume presents a collection of chapters that focus on applications of statistical methods in epidemiology and medical statistics. Some of them are time tested and proven methods with long-track records while others bring the latest methodologies where their promise and relevance compensate for their relatively short-track records. This volume includes 27 chapters. In Chapter 1, Prentice addresses methodological challenges in epidemiology and biomedical research in general. Conceptually, the remaining 26 chapters may be divided into three categories: standard and traditional methods, relatively more advanced methods, and recent methods. These less traditional methods generally provide models with greater fidelity to the underlying data generation mechanisms at the expense of more computational complexity.

The first category includes 10 chapters. Chapter 3 by Rothman et al. discusses epidemiological study designs. Chapter 5 by Vittinghoff et al. discusses linear and non-linear regression methods. Spitznagel discusses logistic regression methods in Chapter 6. In Chapter 8, Gurka and Edwards review mixed models. In Chapter 11, Shannon discusses cluster analysis. Woods and Edwards discuss factor analysis in Chapter 12. A few chapters are devoted to clinical trials. Chapter 15 by Kenward and Jones discusses design and analysis of cross-over trials, Chapter 17 by Gao et al. discusses early phase clinical trials (I and II), and Chapter 18 by Davis and Baraniuk discusses definitive phases III and IV clinical trials. In Chapter 22, Zeller and Yan discuss the sample size and power issues.

The second category of advanced topics includes 9 chapters. Chapter 2 by Rubin discusses statistical inference for causal effects. Chapter 9 by Klein and Zhang discusses survival analysis. Chapter 13 by Hayashi et al. discusses structural equations modeling. In Chapter 14, Xiong et al. discuss statistical modeling of longitudinal data. In Chapter 16, Mazumdar and Bang discuss sequential and group sequential designs in clinical trials. Chapter 19 by Rässler et al. discusses incomplete data in epidemiology and medical statistics. Chapter 20 by Spitznagel reviews meta-analysis. Chapter 21 by Moyé discusses the multiple comparisons issue. And, in Chapter 25, Litman et al. discuss estimation of marginal regression models with multiple source predictors.

Finally, the third category of relatively recent methods includes 7 chapters. Chapter 4 by Looney and Hagan discusses statistical methods for assessing and analysis of biomarkers. In Chapter 7, Hilbe and Greene discuss count response regression models. In Chapter 10, Moeschberger et al. review statistical analysis of competing risks. In Chapter 23, Wahba discusses statistical learning in medical data analysis. In Chapter 24, Mayer discusses evidence-based medicine and medical decision-making. Chapter 26 by Kapadia and Moyé discusses difference equations with public health applications. And, Chapter 27 by Lecoutre discusses the Bayesian approach to experimental data analysis.

The editors sincerely hope that this combination of topics will be found useful by statisticians of all walks of life, notably by theoretical and applied statisticians at pharmaceutical companies, statisticians in the FDA, EPA, and other regulatory agencies and, most notably, by those who are working at the forefront of biomedical research enterprise.

C.R. Rao
J. Philip Miller
D.C. Rao

Contributors

Bang, Heejung, *Division of Biostatistics and Epidemiology, Department of Public Health, Weill Medical College of Cornell University, New York, NY 10021*; *e-mail: heb2013@med.cornell.edu* (Ch. 16).

Baraniuk, Sarah, *The University of Texas Health Science Center at Houston, 1200 Herman Pressler, RAS-E835, Houston, TX 77030*; *e-mail: mary.baraniuk@uth.tmc.edu* (Ch. 18).

Bentler, Peter M., *University of California, Los Angeles, UCLA Psych-Measurement, Box 951563, 4627 FH, Los Angeles, CA 90095-1563*; *e-mail: bentler@ucla.edu* (Ch. 13).

Davis, Barry R., *Coordinating Center for Clinical Trials, The University of Texas Health Science Center at Houston, School of Public Health, 1200 Herman Pressler, Houston, TX 77030*; *e-mail: barry.r.davis@uth.tmc.edu* (Ch. 18).

Edwards, Lloyd J., *Department of Biostatistics, CB #7420, University of North Carolina, Chapel Hill, NC 27599-7420*; *e-mail: lloyd_edwards@unc.edu* (Ch. 8).

Edwards, Michael C., *The Ohio State University, 1827 Neil Ave, Columbus, OH 43210*; *e-mail: edwards.134@osu.edu* (Ch. 12).

Gao, Feng, *Division of Biostatistics, Campus Box 8067, Washington University School of Medicine, 660 S. Euclid Ave, St. Louis, MO 63110-1093*; *e-mail: feng@wustl.edu* (Ch. 17).

Glidden, David V., *Division of Biostatistics, Department of Epidemiology and Biostatistics, University of California, San Francisco, 185 Berry Street, 5700, San Francisco, CA 94143*; *e-mail: dave@biostat.ucsf.edu* (Ch. 5).

Greene, William H., *New York University, Henry Kaufman Mgmt Ctr, 44 West 4 Street, 7-78, New York City, NY 10012, NYU Mail Code: 0251*; *e-mail: wgreene@stern.nyu.edu* (Ch. 7).

Greenland, Sander, *Department of Epidemiology, UCLA School of Public Health, Room # 73-315 CHS, Los Angeles, CA 90095*; *e-mail: lesdomes@ucla.edu* (Ch. 3).

Gurka, Matthew J., *Division of Biostatistics and Epidemiology, Department of Public Health Sciences, School of Medicine, University of Virginia, Charlottesville, VA 22908-0717*; *e-mail: mgurka@virginia.edu* (Ch. 8).

Hagan, Joseph L., *Biostatistics Program, School of Public Health, Louisiana State University Health Sciences Center, 2021 Lakeshore Dr., Suite 210, New Orleans, LA 70122*; *e-mail: jhagan@lsuhsc.edu* (Ch. 4).

Hayashi, Kentaro, *Department of Psychology, University of Hawaii at Manoa, 2430 Campus Drive, Honolulu, HI 96822*; *e-mail: hayashik@hawaii.edu* (Ch. 13).

Hernández, Bernardo, *Direccion de Salud Reproductiva Centro de Investigacion en Salud Poblacional, Instituto Nacional de Salud Publica, Cuernavaca, Morelos, Mexico 62508*; *e-mail: bhernand@insp.mx* (Ch. 25).

Hilbe, Joseph M., *School of Social and Family Dynamics, Arizona State University, Tempe, AZ 85232*; *e-mail: hilbe@asu.edu* (Ch. 7).

Horton, Nicholas J., *Department of Mathematics and Statistics, Smith College, Burton Hall 314, Northampton, MA 01063*; *e-mail: nhorton@email.smith.edu* (Ch. 25).

Jones, Byron, *IPC 001, Pfizer Global Research & Development, Ramsgate Road, Sandwich, Kent, CT13 9NJ, UK*; *e-mail: byron.jones@pfizer.com* (Ch. 15).

Kapadia, Asha S., *Division of Biostatistics, University of Texas School of Public Health, 1200 Herman Pressler Drive, Houston, TX 77030*; *e-mail: asha.s.kapadia@uth.tmc.edu* (Ch. 26).

Kenward, Michael G., *Medical Statistics Unit, London School of Hygiene & Tropical Medicine, Keppel Street, London, WCIE 7HT, UK*; *e-mail: mike.kenward@lshtm.ac.uk* (Ch. 15).

Klein, John P., *Division of Biostatistics, Department of Population Health, Medical College of Wisconsin, 8701 Watertown Plank Road, Milwaukee, WI 53226*; *e-mail: klein@mcw.edu* (Ch. 9).

Kochar, Nidhi, *Division of Biostatistics, College of Public Health, The Ohio State University, 320 West 10th Avenue, Columbus, OH 43210*; *e-mail: nidhi.kochar@gmail.com* (Ch. 10).

Laird, Nan M., *Department of Biostatistics, Harvard School of Public Health, Bldg 2, 4th FL, 655 Huntington Ave, Boston, MA 02115*; *e-mail: laird@biostat.harvard.edu* (Ch. 25).

Lash, Timothy L., *Department of Epidemiology, Boston University School of Public Health, 715 Albany St, T, Boston, MA 02118*; *e-mail: tlash@bu.edu* (Ch. 3).

Lecoutre, Bruno, *ERIS, Laboratoire de Mathématiques Raphael Salem, UMR 6085 C.N.R.S. and Université de Rouen, Avenue de l'Université, BP 12, 76801 Saint-Etienne-du-Rouvray (France)*; *e-mail: bruno.lecoutre@univ-rouen.fr* (Ch. 27).

Litman, Heather J., *New England Research Institutes, 9 Galen Street, Watertown, MA 02472*; *e-mail: litmanh@yahoo.com* (Ch. 25).

Looney, Stephen W., *Department of Biostatistics, Medical College of Georgia, 1120 15th Street, AE-3020, Augusta, GA 30912-4900*; *e-mail: slooney@mcg.edu* (Ch. 4).

Mayer, Dan, *Albany Medical College, Mail Code 34, 47 New Scotland Ave, Albany, NY 12208*; *e-mail: mayerd@mail.amc.edu* (Ch. 24).

Mazumdar, Madhu, *Division of Biostatistics and Epidemiology, Department of Public Health, Weill Medical College of Cornell University, 411 East 69th Street, New York, NY 10021*; *e-mail: mam2073@med.cornell.edu* (Ch. 16).

McCulloch, Charles E., *Division of Biostatistics, Department of Epidemiology and Biostatistics, University of California, San Francisco, 185 Berry Street, 5700, San Francisco, CA 94143*; *e-mail: cmcculloch@epi-ucsf.org* (Ch. 5).

Miller, J. Philip, *Division of Biostatistics, Campus Box 8067, Washington University School of Medicine, 660 S. Euclid Ave, St. Louis, MO 63110-1093*; *e-mail: jphilipmiller@wustl.edu* (Chs. 14, 17).

Moeschberger, Melvin L., *Division of Biostatistics, College of Public Health, The Ohio State University, 320 West 10th Avenue, Columbus, OH 43210*; *e-mail: moeschberger.1@osu.edu* (Ch. 10).

Moyé, Lemuel A., *University of Texas School of Public Health, Coordinating Center for Clinical Trials, 1200 Herman Pressler Drive, E815, Houston, TX 77030*; *e-mail: lemuel.a.moye@uth.tmc.edu* (Chs. 21, 26).

Prentice, Ross L., *Division of Public Health Sciences, Fred Hutchinson Cancer Research Center, 1100 Fairview Avenue North, Seattle, WA 98109-1024*; *e-mail: rprentic@fhcrc.org* (Ch. 1).

Rässler, Susanne, *Institute for Employment Research and Federal Employment Agency, Weddigenstr. 20-22, 90478 Nuremberg, Germany*; *e-mail: susanne.rassler@iab.de* (Ch. 19).

Rothman, Kenneth J., *328 Country Club Road, Newton, MA 02459*; *e-mail: krothman@rti.org* (Ch. 3).

Rubin, Donald B., *Department of Statistics, Harvard University, 1 Oxford Street, Cambridge, MA 02318*; *e-mail: rubin@stat.harvard.edu* (Chs. 2, 19).

Shannon, William D., *Department of Medicine and Division of Biostatistics, Washington University School of Medicine, 660 S. Euclid Ave, Campus Box 8005, St. Louis, MO 63110*; *e-mail: wshannon@wustl.edu* (Ch. 11).

Shiboski, Stephen C., *Division of Biostatistics, Department of Epidemiology and Biostatistics, University of California, San Francisco, 185 Berry Street, 5700, San Francisco, CA 94143*; *e-mail: steve@biostat.ucsf.edu* (Ch. 5).

Spitznagel, Edward L., *Department of Mathematics, Washington University, One Brookings Drive, St. Louis, MO 63130*; *e-mail: ed@wustl.edu* (Chs. 6, 20).

Tordoff, Kevin P., *The Ohio State University, 320 West 10th Avenue, Columbus, OH 43210*; *e-mail: tordoff.1@osu.edu* (Ch. 10).

Trinkaus, Kathryn, *Division of Biostatistics, Campus Box 8067, Washington University School of Medicine, 660 S. Euclid Ave, St. Louis, MO 63110-1093*; *e-mail: kimt@wubios.wustl.edu* (Ch. 17).

Vittinghoff, Eric, *Division of Biostatistics, Department of Epidemiology and Biostatistics, University of California, San Francisco, 185 Berry Street, 5700, San Francisco, CA 94143*; *e-mail: eric@biostat.ucsf.edu* (Ch. 5).

Wahba, Grace, *Department of Statistics, University of Wisconsin-Madison, 1300 University Avenue, Madison, WI 53706*; *e-mail: wahba@stat.wisc.edu* (Ch. 23).

Woods, Carol M., *Psychology Department, Washington University in St. Louis, Campus Box 1125, St. Louis, MO 63130*; *e-mail: cwoods@artsci.wustl.edu* (Ch. 12).

Xiong, Chengjie, *Division of Biostatistics, Campus Box 8067, Washington University School of Medicine, 660 S. Euclid Ave, St. Louis, MO 63110-1093*; *e-mail: chengjie@wubios.wustl.edu* (Ch. 14).

Yan, Yan, *Washington University, Campus Box 8242, 4960 Children's Place, St. Louis, MO 63110*; *e-mail: yany@wustl.edu* (Ch. 22).

Yu, Kai, *Biostatistics Branch, Division of Cancer Epidemiology and Genetics National Cancer Institute Executive Plaza South, Room 8050 Bethesda, MD 20892*; *e-mail: yuka@mail.nih.gov* (Ch. 14).

Yuan, Ke-Hai, *University of Notre Dame, 105 Haggar Hall, Notre Dame, IN 46556*; *e-mail: ke-hai.yuan.5@nd.edu* (Ch. 13).

Zell, Elizabeth R., *Centers for Disease Control and Prevention, 1600 Clifton Rd NE, MS-C09, Atlanta, GA 30329-4018*; *e-mail: ezell@cdc.gov* (Ch. 19).

Zeller, Richard A., *College of Nursing, Kent State University, Kent, OH 44242*; *e-mail: rzeller@tusc.kent.edu* (Ch. 22).

Zhang, Mei-Jie, *Medical College of Wisconsin, 8701 Watertown Plank Rd., Milwaukee, WI 53226*; *e-mail: meijie@mcw.edu* (Ch. 9).

Zhu, Kejun, *School of Management, China University of Geosciences, Wuhan, PRC 4330074*; *e-mail: zhubingl@public.wh.hb.cn* (Ch. 14).

Handbook of Statistics, Vol. 27
ISSN: 0169-7161

DOI: 10.1016/S0169-7161(07)27001-4

1

Statistical Methods and Challenges in Epidemiology and Biomedical Research

Ross L. Prentice

Abstract

This chapter provides an introduction to the role, and use, of statistics in epidemiology and in biomedical research. The presentation focuses on the assessment and understanding of health-related associations in a study cohort. The principal context considered is estimation of the risk of health events in relation to individual study subject characteristics, exposures, or treatments, generically referred to as 'covariates'. Descriptive models that focus on relative and absolute risks in relation to preceding covariate histories will be described, along with potential sources of bias in estimation and testing. The role, design, and conduct of randomized controlled trials will also be described in this prevention research context, as well as in therapeutic research. Some aspects of the sources and initial evaluation of ideas and concepts for preventive and therapeutic interventions will be discussed. This leads naturally to a discussion of the role and potential of biomarkers in biomedical research, for such purposes as exposure assessment, early disease diagnosis, or for the evaluation of preventive or therapeutic interventions. Recently available biomarkers, including high-dimensional genomic and proteomic markers, have potential to add much knowledge about disease processes and to add specificity to intervention development and evaluation. These data sources are attended by many interesting statistical design and analysis challenges. A brief discussion of ongoing analytic and explanatory analyses in the Women's Health Initiative concludes the presentation.

1. Introduction

The topic of this chapter is too broad to allow an in-depth coverage of its many important aspects. The goal, rather, will be to provide an introduction to some specific topics, many of which will be covered in later chapters, while attempting to provide a unifying framework to motivate statistical issues that arise in biomedical research, and to motivate some of the models and methods used to address these issues.

Much of epidemiology, and biomedical research more generally, involves following a set of study 'subjects', often referred to as the study cohort. Much valuable basic biological research involves the study of lower life forms. Such studies are often attended by substantial homogeneity among study subjects, and relatively short life spans. Here, instead, the presentation will focus on a cohort of humans, in spite of the attendant greater heterogeneity and statistical challenges. For research purposes the individuals in a cohort are of interest through their ability to yield health-related information pertinent to a larger population. Such a larger population may, for example, include persons residing in the geographic areas from which cohort members are drawn, who meet certain eligibility and exclusionary criteria. The ability to infer health-related information about the larger population involves assumptions about the representativeness of the cohort for the 'target' population. This typically requires a careful characterization of the cohort so that the generalizability of study findings can be defined. The target population is often somewhat conceptual, and is usually taken to be practically infinite in size. The major long-term goal of biomedical research is to decrease the burden of premature disease morbidity and mortality, and to extend the period of time that members of target populations live without major health-related restrictions.

The principal focus of epidemiologic research is understanding the determinants of disease risk among healthy persons, with a particular interest in modifiable risk factors, such as dietary or physical activity patterns, or environmental exposures. There is a long history of epidemiologic methods development, much of which is highly statistical, whose aim is to enhance the likelihood that associations between study subject characteristics or exposures and disease risk are causal, thereby providing reliable concepts for disease prevention.

The availability of disease screening programs or services, and the health care-seeking behavior of cohort members, have potential to affect the timing of disease diagnosis. Early disease detection may allow the disease course to be interrupted or altered in a manner that is beneficial to the individual. Disease screening research has its own set of methodologic challenges, and is currently the target of intensive efforts to discover and validate early detection 'biomarkers'.

Much biomedical research is directed to the study of cohorts of person having a defined disease diagnosis, with emphasis on the characterization of prognosis and, especially, on the development of treatments that can eradicate the disease or can facilitate disease management, while avoiding undue adverse effects.

The ultimate products of biomedical research are interventions, biomarkers, or treatments that can be used to prevent, diagnose, or treat disease. Additionally, the knowledge of the biology of various life forms and the methodologic knowledge that underlies the requisite research agenda, constitutes important and durable contributions from biomedical research. These developments are necessarily highly interdisciplinary, and involve a wide spectrum of disciplines. Participating scientists may include, for example, molecular geneticists studying biological processes in yeast; technologists developing ways to assess a person's genome or proteome in a rapid and reliable fashion; population scientists studying disease-occurrence patterns in large human cohorts; and expert panels and government regulators synthesizing research developments and providing recommendations and regulations for consumption by the general population.

Statisticians and other quantitative scientists have important roles to fulfill throughout this research spectrum. Issues of study design, quality control, data analysis, and reporting are important in each biomedical research sector, and resolving methodologic challenges is crucial to progress in some areas. The biomedical research enterprise includes natural tensions, for example, basic versus applied research; in-depth mechanistic research versus testing of current concepts; and independent versus collaborative research. Statisticians can have a unifying role across related cultural research norms, through the opportunity to bring ideas and motivations from one component of this research community to another in a non-threatening manner, while simultaneously applying critical statistical thinking and methods to the research at hand.

2. Characterizing the study cohort

A general regression notation can be used to represent a set of exposures and characteristics to be ascertained in a cohort under study. Let $z(u)' = \{z_1(u), z_2(u), \ldots\}$ be a set of numerically coded variables that describe an individual's exposures and characteristics at 'time' u, where, to be specific, u can be defined as time from selection into the cohort, and a prime ($'$) denotes vector transpose. Let $Z(t) = \{z(u), u<t\}$ denote the history of each covariate at times less than t. The 'baseline' covariate history $Z(0)$ may include information that pertains to time periods prior to selection into the cohort.

Denote by $\lambda\{t, Z(t)\}$ the occurrence rate for a health event of interest in the targeted population at cohort follow-up time t, among persons having a preceding covariate history $Z(t)$. A typical cohort study goal is to assess the relationship between aspects of $Z(t)$ and the corresponding disease rate $\lambda\{t; Z(t)\}$. Doing so involves recording over time the pertinent covariate histories and health event histories for cohort members, whether the cohort is comprised of healthy individuals as in an epidemiologic cohort study or disease prevention trial, or persons having a defined disease in a therapeutic context. The notation $Z(t)$ is intended to encompass evolving, time-varying covariates, but also to include more restrictive specifications in which, for example, only baseline covariate information is included.

A cohort available for study will typically have features that distinguish it from the target population to which study results may be applied. For example, an epidemiologic cohort study may enroll persons who are expected to continue living in the same geographic area for some years, or who are expected to be able and willing to participate in research project activities. A therapeutic cohort may have characteristics that depend on institutional referral patterns and clinical investigator experience and expertise. Hence, absolute health event (hereafter 'disease') occurrence rates may be less pertinent and transferable to the target population, than are relative rates that contrast disease rates among persons receiving different treatments or having different exposures.

The hazard ratio regression model of Cox (1972) captures this relative risk notion, without imposing further restrictions on corresponding absolute rates. It can be written

$$\lambda\{t; Z(t)\} = \lambda_0(t) \exp\{x(t)'\beta\}, \tag{1}$$

where $x(t)' = \{x_1(t), \ldots, x_p(t)\}$ is a modeled regression p-vector formed from $Z(t)$ and product (interaction) terms with t, $\beta' = (\beta_1, \ldots, \beta_p)$ is a corresponding hazard ratio, or relative risk, parameter to be estimated, and $\lambda_0(\cdot)$ is an unrestricted 'baseline' hazard function corresponding to $x(t) \equiv 0$. For example, $x(t) \equiv x_1$ may be an indicator variable for active versus placebo treatment in a prevention trial, or an indicator for test versus the standard treatment in a therapeutic trial, in which case e^{β_1} is the ratio of hazard rates for the test versus the control group, and there may be special interest in testing $\beta_1 = 0$ ($e^{\beta_1} = 1$). Such a constant hazard ratio model can be relaxed, for example, to $x(t) = \{x_1, x_1 \log t\}$ in which case the 'treatment' hazard ratio function becomes $e^{\beta_1} t^{\beta_2}$, which varies in a smooth manner with 'follow-up time' t. Alternatively, one may define $x(t)$ to include a quantitative summary of a study subject's prior exposure to an environmental or lifestyle factor in an epidemiologic context.

Let T be the time to occurrence of a disease under study in a cohort. Typically some, and perhaps most, of cohort members will not have experienced the disease at the time of data analysis. Such a cohort member yields a 'censored disease event time' that is known to exceed the follow-up time for the individual. Let Y be a process that takes value $Y(t) = 1$ if a subject is 'at risk' (i.e., without prior censoring or disease occurrence) for a disease event at follow-up time t, and $Y(t) = 0$ otherwise. Then a basic independent censoring assumption requires

$$\lambda\{t; Z(t),\ Y(u) = 1,\ u < t\} = \lambda\{t; Z(t)\},$$

so that the set of individuals under active follow-up is assumed to have a disease rate that is representative for the cohort given $Z(t)$, at each follow-up time t. The hazard ratio parameter β in (1) is readily estimated by maximizing the so-called partial likelihood function (Cox, 1975)

$$L(\beta) = \prod_{i=1}^{k} \left[\frac{\exp\{x_i(t_i)'\beta\}}{\sum_{l \varepsilon R(t_i)} \exp\{x_l(t_i)'\beta\}} \right], \tag{2}$$

where $t_1, \ldots, t_k$ are the distinct disease occurrence times in the cohort and $R(t)$ denotes the set of cohort members at risk (having $Y(t) = 1$) at follow-up time t. Standard likelihood procedures apply to (2) for testing and estimation on β, and convenient semiparametric estimators of the cumulative baseline hazard function $\Omega_0(t) = \int_0^t \lambda_0(u)\, du$ are also available (e.g., Andersen and Gill, 1982) thereby also providing absolute disease rate estimators.

The score test $\partial \log L(\beta)/\partial\beta$ for $\beta = 0$ is referred to as the logrank test in the special case in which $x(t) \equiv x$ is comprised of indicator variables for p of $p+1$ groups, for which disease rates are to be compared. A simple, but practically useful refinement of (1) replaces the baseline hazard rate $\lambda_0(t)$ by $\lambda_{0s}(t)$ thereby allowing the baseline rates to differ arbitrarily among strata $s = 1, 2, \ldots$ that may be time-dependent. This refinement allows a more flexible modeling of disease rates on stratification factors, formed from $\{Z(t), t\}$, than would conveniently be possible through hazard ratio regression modeling. The partial likelihood function under a stratified Cox model is simply the product of terms (2) formed from the stratum-specific disease occurrence and covariate data. Other modifications are needed to accommodate tied disease occurrence times, and for more complex disease occurrence time data as may arise with specialized censoring schemes or with recurrent or correlated disease occurrence times. The Cox regression method has been arguably the major statistical advance relative to epidemiology and biomedical research of the past 50 years. Detailed accounts of its characteristics and extensions have been given various places (e.g., Andersen et al., 1993; Kalbfleisch and Prentice, 2002).

The Cox model provides a powerful and convenient descriptive tool for assessing relative associations with disease incidence. There are other descriptive models, such as accelerated failure time models

$$\lambda\{t, Z(t)\} = \lambda_0\left(\int_0^t e^{x(u)'\beta} du\right) e^{x(t)'\beta},$$

for which the regression parameter may have a more useful interpretation in some contexts. This model tends to be rather difficult to apply, however, though workable implementations have been developed, with efficiency properties dependent on the choice of model for $\lambda_0(\cdot)$ that is used to generate estimating functions (e.g., Jin et al., 2003).

In some settings mechanistic or biologically-based disease occurrence rate models are available (e.g., Moolgavkar and Knudson, 1981). The parameters in such models may characterize aspects of the disease process, or provide specific targets for treatments or interventions that allow them to valuably complement descriptive modeling approaches. Biologically based models with this type of potential also tend to be more challenging to apply, but the payoff may sometimes justify the effort. Of course, it is useful to be able to examine a cohort dataset from more than a single modeling framework, to assure robustness of principal findings, and to garner maximal information.

The statistical issues in study design, conduct, and analysis differ somewhat between the epidemiologic, early detection, and therapeutic contexts, according to differences in disease outcome rates and outcome ascertainment issues, and according to covariate definition and measurement issues. However, there are also some important commonalities; for example, issues of multiple hypothesis testing, especially in relation to high-dimensional covariate data and study monitoring procedures, arise in each context. We will proceed by describing some of the context-specific statistical issues first, and subsequently include a discussion of shared statistical issues.

3. Observational study methods and challenges

3.1. Epidemiologic risk factor identification

3.1.1. Sampling strategies

Cohort studies provide a mainstay epidemiologic approach to the identification of disease risk factors. A single cohort study has potential to examine the associations between multiple exposures, behaviors or characteristics and the risk of various diseases, and has potential to examine both short- and long-term associations. A distinguishing feature of the epidemiologic cohort study is the typical low incidence rates for the diseases under study. Even such prominent chronic diseases as coronary heart disease or lung cancer typically occur at a rate of 1% or less per year among ostensibly healthy persons. It follows that epidemiologic cohorts may need to be quite large, often in the range of tens of thousands to more than 100,000, depending on the age distribution and on the frequencies of 'exposures' of interest in the cohort, to provide precise estimates on association parameters of interest in a practical time frame. Well-characterized cohorts tend to be followed for substantial periods of time, as their value typically increases as more disease events accrue, and marginal costs for additional years of follow-up tend to diminish.

The rare disease aspect of epidemiologic cohort studies opens the way to various design and analysis simplifications. For example, the partial likelihood-based estimating function for β from (2) can be written

$$\partial \log L(\beta)/\partial \beta' = \sum_{i=1}^{k} \left\{ x_i(t_i) - \frac{\sum_{l \varepsilon R(t_i)} x_l(t_i) W_{il}(\beta)}{\sum_{l \varepsilon R(t_i)} W_{il}(\beta)} \right\}, \tag{3}$$

where $W_{il}(\beta) = \exp\{x_l(t_i)'\beta\}$, which contrasts the modeled regression vector for the individual developing disease at time t_i (the case), to a suitably weighted average of the regression vectors, $x_l(t_i)$, for cohort members at risk at t_i (the controls). Most of the variance in this comparison derives from the 'case' regression vector, and the summations over the 'risk set' at t_i can be replaced by a summation over a few randomly selected controls from this risk set with little loss of estimating efficiency. This 'nested case–control' (Liddell et al., 1977; Prentice and Breslow, 1978) approach to estimation is attractive if the determination of some components of $x(t)$ is expensive. Often only one, or possibly two or three, controls will be 'time-matched' to the corresponding case. Depending somewhat on the covariate distribution and hazard ratio magnitude, the efficiency reduction for a nested case–control versus a full-cohort analysis is typically modest if, say, five or more controls are selected per case. With large cohorts, it is often possible to additionally match on other factors (e.g., baseline, age, cohort enrollment date, gender) to further standardize the case versus control comparison. Another within-cohort sampling strategy selects a random subcohort, or a stratified random subcohort, for use as the comparison group for the case at each t_i, instead of the entire risk set $R(t_i)$ in (3). If some care is taken to ensure that the subcohort is well aligned with the case group, there will be little to choose between this case–cohort (e.g., Prentice, 1986) estimation approach and the nested case–control approach, and there may be value in having covariate data determination on a random subcohort. Within-cohort sampling strategies of this type are widely used in epidemiology when the focus is on blood or urine biomarkers for which determinations on the entire cohort may be prohibitively expensive, and has application also to the analysis and extraction of information from stored records, for example, nutrient consumption estimates from food records, or occupational exposure estimates from employer records.

In a large cohort with only a small fraction experiencing disease one can, with little concern about bias, select a distinct comparison group to replace $R(t_i)$ in (3) for the case occurring at t_i, for each $i = 1, 2, \ldots$. The estimating equation (3) is then formally that for a conditional logistic regression of case versus control status at t_i on the corresponding regression vectors $x(t)$. In fact, since most association information for baseline risk factors derives from whether or not disease occurs during cohort follow-up, rather than from the timing of case occurrence, it is often convenient to pool the case and the control data and analyze using unconditional logistic regression, perhaps including follow-up duration and other matching characteristics as control variable in the regression model. The estimates and interpretation of odds ratios from such a logistic regression analysis will typically differ little from that for hazard ratios defined above. Breslow and Day (1987) provide a detailed account of the design and analysis of these types of case–control studies.

Note that the case–control analyses just described do not require a cohort roster to be available. Rather, one needs to be able to ascertain representative cases and controls from the underlying cohort, and ascertain their covariate histories in a reliable fashion. In fact, the classic case–control study in the context of a population-based disease register proceeds by randomly sampling cases occurring during a defined accrual period along with suitably matched controls, and subsequently ascertains their covariate histories. The challenges with this study design include avoiding selection bias as may arise if the cases and controls enrolled are not representative of cases and controls in the cohort, and especially, avoiding 'recall bias', as persons who have recently experienced a disease may recall exposures and other characteristics differently than do continuing healthy persons. The classic case–control study may be the only practical study design for rare diseases, but in recent years, as several large cohort studies have matured, this design has been somewhat overtaken by cohort studies having a defined roster of members and prospective assessment of covariate histories and health events.

3.1.2. Confounding

The identification of associations that are causal for the study disease represents a major challenge for cohort studies and other observational study (OS) designs.

The association of a disease incidence rate at time t with a covariate history $Z_1(t)$ may well depend on the histories $Z_2(t)$ of other factors. One can then model the hazard rate $\lambda\{t; Z(t)\}$, where $Z(t) = \{Z_1(t), Z_2(t)\}$ and examine the association between λ and $Z_1(t)$ in this model, that has now 'controlled' for factors $Z_2(t)$ that may otherwise 'confound' the association. Unfortunately, there is no objective means of knowing when the efforts to control confounding are sufficient, so that one can only argue toward causation in an OS context. An argument of causation requires a substantial knowledge of the disease processes and disease determinants. The choices of confounding factors to control through regression modeling or through stratification can be far from straightforward. For example, factors that are time-dependent may offer greater confounding control (e.g., Robins, 1987), but if such 'factors are on a causal pathway' between Z, and disease risk, they may 'overcontrol'. Some factors may both confound and mediate, and specialized modeling techniques have been proposed to address this complex issue (e.g., Hernan et al., 2001). Randomized controlled trials provide the ability to substantially address this confounding issue. However, randomized prevention trials having disease outcomes tend to be very expensive and logistically difficult, so that for many important prevention topics one must rely strongly on observational associations. OS findings that are consistent across multiple populations may provide some reassurance concerning confounding, but it may be unclear whether the same sources of confounding could be operative across populations or whether other biases, such as may arise if common measurement instruments are used across studies, are present.

3.1.3. Covariate measurement error

The issue of measurement error in covariate data is one of the most important and least developed statistical topics in observational epidemiology. Suppose that some elements of $Z(t)$, and hence of the modeled regression vector $x(t)$ in (2) are not precisely measured. How might tests and estimation on β be affected? Some of the statistical literature on covariate measurement error assumes that $x(t)$ is precisely measured in a subset of the cohort, a so-called validation subsample, while some estimate, say $w(t)$ of $x(t)$ is available on the remainder of the cohort. The hazard rate at time t induced from (1) in the non-validation part of the cohort is then

$$\lambda_0(t)E\{\exp\{x(t)'\beta\}|w(t),\ Y(t) = 1\}. \qquad (4)$$

The expectation in (4) can be estimated using the validation sample data on $\{x(t), w(t)\}$ and consistent non-parametric estimates of β are available (Pepe and Fleming, 1991; Carroll and Wand, 1991) with the measurement error simply reducing estimating efficiency.

Frequently in epidemiologic contexts, however, the 'true' covariate history is unascertainable for any study subjects, and only one or more estimates thereof will be available. Important examples arise in nutritional and physical activity epidemiology where $Z(t)$ may include the history of consumption of certain nutrients over preceding years, or aspects of lifetime physical activity patterns.

A classical measurement model, ubiquitous in the statistical measurement error literature, assumes that available measurements $w_1(t)$, $w_2(t)$, … of $x(t)$ are the sum of $x(t)$ plus error that is independent across replicates for an individual, and that is independent of $x(t)$ and of other study subject characteristics. A variety of hazard ratio estimators are available from this type of reliability data including regression calibration (Carroll et al., 1995), risk set regression calibration (Xie et al., 2001), conditional score (Tsiatis and Davidian, 2001), and non-parametric corrected score procedures (Huang and Wang, 2000; Song and Huang, 2005). These modeling assumptions and estimation procedures may be sufficient for objectively assessed covariates (e.g., certain exposure biomarkers), but the classical measurement model may be inadequate for many self-reported exposures. For example, the relationship between the consumption of fat, carbohydrate, and total energy (calories) to the risk of chronic disease has been the subject of continuing cohort and case–control study research for some decades. Almost all of this work has involved asking cohort members to self-report their dietary patterns, most often in the form of the frequency and portion size of consumption of each element of a list of foods and drinks. For certain nutrients, including short-term total energy and protein energy, there are objective consumption markers that plausibly adhere to a classical measurement model. Though published data on the relationship of such markers to corresponding self-reported consumption remains fairly sparse, it is already evident, for example for total energy, that the measurement error properties may depend on such individual characteristics as body mass (e.g., Heitmann and Lissner, 1995), age, and certain behavioral characteristics, and that replicate measurements have measurement errors that tend to be positively correlated (e.g., Kipnis et al., 2003). This work underscores the need for more flexible and realistic models (e.g., Carroll et al., 1998; Prentice et al., 2002) for certain exposure assessments in epidemiologic cohort settings, and for the development of additional objective (biomarker) measures of exposure in nutritional and physical activity epidemiology. Typically, it will not be practical to obtain such objective measures for the entire epidemiologic cohort, nor can some key biomarkers be obtained from stored specimens. Hence, the practical way forward appears to be to use the biomarker data on a random subsample to calibrate (correct) the self-report data for the entire cohort prior to hazard ratio estimation or odds ratio estimation (e.g., Sugar et al., 2006). This is a fertile area for further data gathering and methods development, and one where statisticians have a central role to fulfill.

3.1.4. Outcome data ascertainment

A cohort study needs to include a system for regularly updating disease event information. This may involve asking study subjects to periodically self-report any of a list of diagnoses and to report all hospitalizations. Hospital discharge summaries may then be examined for diagnoses of interest with confirmation by other medical and laboratory records. Sometimes outcomes are actively ascertained as a part of the study protocol; for example, electrocardiographic tracings for coronary heart disease or mammograms for breast cancer. Diagnoses that require considerable judgment may be adjudicated by a committee of experts, toward standardizing the accuracy and timing of disease event diagnoses. Disease incidence or mortality registers can sometimes provide efficient outcome ascertainment, or can supplement other ascertainment approaches.

Unbiased ascertainment of the fact and timing of disease events relative to the elements of $Z(t)$ under study is needed for valid hazard ratio estimation. Valid absolute risk estimation has the more stringent requirement of comprehensive disease event ascertainment. For example, a recent NIH workshop assessed the state-of-the science in the topic of multivitamin and multimineral (MVM) supplements and chronic disease risk. MVM users tend to have many characteristics (e.g., highly educated, infrequent smoking, regular exercise, low-fat and high-fruit and vegetable dietary habits) that could confound a disease association, but also MVM user engage more frequently in such disease-screening activities as mammography or prostate-specific antigen testing (e.g., White et al., 2004). Hence, for example, a benefit of MVMs for breast or prostate cancer could be masked by earlier or more complete outcome ascertainment among users. Careful standardization for disease screening and diagnosis practices, at the design or analysis stages, may be an important element of cohort study conduct. Similarly, differential lags in the reporting or adjudication of disease events can be a source of bias, particularly toward the upper end of the distribution of follow-up time for the cohort.

3.2. Observational studies in treatment research

Observational approaches are not used commonly for the evaluation of a treatment for a disease. Instead, the evaluation of treatments aimed at managing disease, or reducing disease recurrence or death rates, rely primarily on randomized controlled trials, typically comparing a new treatment or regimen to a current standard of care. Because of the typical higher rate of the outcome events under study, compared to studies of disease occurrence among healthy persons, therapeutic studies can often be carried out with adequate precision with at most a few hundred patients. Also, the process for deciding a treatment course for a patient is frequently complex, often involving information and assumption related to patient prognosis. Hence, the therapeutic context is one where it may be difficult or impossible to adequately control for selection factors, confounding and other biases using an OS design.

Observational studies do, however, fulfill other useful roles in disease-treatment research. These include the use of data on cohorts of persons having a defined diagnosis to classify patients into prognostic categories within which tailored treatments may be appropriate, and supportive care measures may need to be standardized. For example, classification and regression trees (e.g., LeBlanc and Tibshirani, 1996), as well as other explanatory and graphical procedures, are used by cooperative oncology and other research groups. Also, observational studies in patient cohorts, often under the label 'correlationals studies' are frequently used as a part of the treatment development enterprise. For example, observational comparisons, between persons with or without recurrent disease, of gene expression patterns in pre-treatment tissue specimens may provide important insights into the 'environment' that allows a disease to progress, and may suggest therapeutic targets to interrupt disease progression and improve prognosis.

3.3. Observational studies in disease-screening research

Disease-screening research aims to identify sensitive and specific means of diagnosing disease prior to its clinical surfacing. In conjunction with effective means of disease treatment, such screening programs can reduce disease-related mortality, and can reduce morbidity that accompanies advanced stage disease. For similar reasons to the therapeutic area, observational studies to evaluate screening programs are most challenging, and randomized controlled trials offer important advantages.

At present, substantial efforts are underway to discover biomarkers for the early detection of various cancers. These research efforts can be expected to identify a number of novel early detection markers in upcoming years. The cost and duration of disease-screening trials encourage additional research to enhance the reliability of observational evaluations in this setting, including the possibility of joint analyses of observational and randomized trial data.

Observational studies play a crucial role in the identification of disease-screening biomarkers and modalities. For example, a current concept in the early detection of cancer is that, early in their disease course, malignant tumors may shed minute amounts of novel proteins into the blood stream, whence the presence of, or an elevated concentration of, the protein could trigger biopsy or other diagnostic work-up. For such a protein to yield a test of sufficient sensitivity and specificity to be useful as a screening tool, corresponding hazard ratios need to be considerably larger than is the case for typical epidemiologic risk factors. Hence, stored blood specimens from rather modest numbers of cases and controls (e.g., 100 of each) from an epidemiologic cohort may be sufficient to allow identification of a biomarker that would satisfy demanding diagnostic test criteria.

In terms of the notation of Section 2, the principal covariate in the diagnostic test setting is a binary variable that specifies whether or not the test is positive (e.g., prostate-specific antigen concentration, or change in concentration, above a certain value), so that the issue of converting a quantitative variable (e.g., PSA concentration) to a binary variate is important in this context.

This leads to a focus on receiver-operator characteristic (ROC) curves from case–control data, with test evaluation based in part on 'area under' the ROC 'curve' (AUC), or partial AUC if one chooses to focus on a range of acceptable specificities. A focus on the predictiveness of a diagnostic marker, typically using a logistic regression version of (3), is also important in this context and requires a linkage of the case–control data to absolute risks in the target population. This too is an active and important statistical research area. See Pepe (2003) and Baker et al. (2006) for accounts of the key concepts and approaches in evaluating diagnostic tests. Issues requiring further development include study design and analysis methods with high-dimensional markers, and methods for the effective combination of several screening tests (e.g., McIntosh and Pepe, 2002).

3.4. Family-based cohort studies in genetic epidemiology

There is a long history of using follow-up studies among family members to study genetic aspects of disease risk. For example, one could compare the dependence patterns among times to disease occurrence in a follow-up study of monozygotic and dizygotic twins having shared environments to assess whether there is a genetic component to disease risk. The so-called frailty models that allow family members to share a random multiplicative hazard rate factor are often used for this type of analysis (e.g., Hougaard, 2000). Such models have also been adapted to case–control family studies in which one compares the disease-occurrence patterns of family members of persons affected by a disease under study to corresponding patterns for unaffected persons (e.g., Hsu et al., 1999).

Often the ascertainment schemes in family-based studies are complex, as families having a strong history of the study disease are selected to increase the probability of harboring putative disease genes. Linkage analysis has been a major approach to the mapping of genes that may be related to disease risk. Such analyses proceed by determining the genotype of family members for a panel of genetic markers, and assessing whether one or more such markers co-segregate with disease among family members. This approach makes use of the fact that segments of the chromosome are inherited intact so that markers over some distance on a chromosome from a disease gene can be expected to associate with disease risk. There are many possible variations in ascertainment schemes and analysis procedures that may differ in efficiency and robustness properties (e.g., Ott, 1991; Thomas, 2004). Following the identification of a linkage signal, some form of finer mapping is needed to close in on disease-related loci.

Markers that are sufficiently close on the genome tend to be correlated, depending somewhat on a person's evolutionary history (e.g., Felsenstein, 1992). Hence, if a dense set of genetic markers is available across the genome, linkage analysis may give way to linkage-disequilibrium (LD) analyses. Genome-wide association studies with several hundred thousand single-nucleotide polymorphism (SNP) markers have only recently become possible due to efficient high-throughput SNP genotyping. High-dimensional SNP panels can be applied in family study contexts, or can be applied to unrelated cases and controls. There are many interesting statistical questions that attend these study designs (Risch and Merikangas, 1996; Schork et al., 2001), including the choice of SNPs for a given study population, and the avoidance of the so-called population stratification wherein correlations with disease may be confounded by ethnicity or other aspects of evolutionary history. Some further aspects of high-dimensional SNP studies will be discussed below.

4. Randomized controlled trials

4.1. General considerations

Compared to purely observational approaches, the randomized controlled trial (RCT) has the crucial advantage of ensuring that the intervention or treatment assignment is statistically independent of all pre-randomization confounding factors, regardless of whether or not such factors can be accurately measured and modeled, or are even recognized. The randomization assignment is also independent of the pre-randomization disease-screening patterns of enrollees. Hence, if outcomes of interest during trial follow-up are equally ascertained, tests to compare outcome rates among randomized groups represent fair comparisons, and a causal interpretation can be ascribed to observed differences. Such tests are often referred to as 'intention-to-treat (ITT)' tests, since the comparisons is among the entire randomized groups, without regard to the extent to which the assigned intervention or treatment was adhered to by trial enrollees. Note that the validity of comparisons in RCTs depends on the equality of outcome ascertainment (e.g., disease-occurrence times) between randomization groups. This implies an important role for an outcome ascertainment process that is blinded to randomization group, and implies the need for a protocol that standardizes all aspects of the outcome identification and adjudication. The RCT often provides a clinical context, which makes such unbiased outcome data ascertainment practical.

4.2. Prevention trials

For the reasons just noted, RCTs have some major advantages compared to observational studies for the evaluation of preventive interventions. The major limitations of the RCT design in this context are the typical large sample sizes, challenging logistics, and very substantial costs. For example, a simple sample size formula based on the approximate normality of the logarithm of the odds ratio indicates that a trial cohort sample size must be at least

$$n = \{p_2(1-p_2)\}^{-1}(\log \lambda)^{-2}Q, \tag{5}$$

for a trial having active and control groups, assigned with probabilities γ and $1-\gamma$ that have corresponding outcome event probabilities of p_1 and p_2 over trial follow-up. In this expression $\lambda = p_1(1-p_2)/\{p_2(1-p_1)\}$ is the active versus control group odds ratio, and

$$Q = \{\gamma(1-\gamma)\}^{-1}[W_{\alpha/2} - W_{1-\eta}\{\gamma + \lambda^{-1}(1-p_2+\lambda p_2)^2(1-\gamma)\}^{1/2}]^2,$$

is a rather slowly varying function of λ and p_2 at specified test size (type I error rate) α and power η, while $W_{\alpha/2}$ and $W_{1-\eta}$ are the upper $\alpha/2$ and $1-\eta$ percentiles of the standard normal distribution. The above formula also allows calculation of study power at a specified trial sample size. For example, that a trial of size 10,000 study subjects with randomization fraction $\gamma = 0.50$, control group incidence rate of 0.30% per year, and an odds ratio of 0.67, would have power of about 61% over an average 6-year follow-up period, and of 79% over an average 9-year follow-up period. Although more sophisticated power and sample size formulas are available (e.g., Self et al., 1992), the simple formula (5) illustrates the sensitivity to the magnitude of the intervention effect, and secondarily to the control group incidence rate. Primarily because of cost, it is common to design prevention trials with power that is just adequate under design assumptions, for the overall ITT comparison. It follows that trial power may be less than desirable if the intervention effect is somewhat less than designed. Often there will not be firm preliminary information on the magnitude, or especially the time course, of intervention effects and less than designed adherence to the assigned interventions or treatments can reduce the trial odds ratio. Less than expected control group outcome rates (p_2) also reduces trial power, as may occur if extensive eligibility or exclusionary criteria are applied in trial recruitment, or because volunteers for a prevention trial, that may be time consuming and of long duration, have distinctive biobehavioral characteristics that are related to the outcome of interest. Also, there may be substantive questions of intervention benefits and risks in relation to important subsets of trial enrollees, but power may be marginal for such subset intervention comparisons and for related interaction tests. In summary, sample size and power is an important topic for RCTs in the prevention area, particularly since such full-scale trials typically have little chance of being repeated. Additional statistical work on design procedures to ensure sufficient robustness of study power would be desirable.

On the topic of intervention effects within subsets, the typical low hazard rates in prevention trials implies a role for 'case–only' analyses (e.g., Vittinghoff and Bauer, 2006). Let $s = 1, 2, \ldots$ denote strata formed by baseline characteristics in a prevention trial, and let $x(t) \equiv x$ take values 1 and 0 in the active and control groups. A simple calculation under a stratified Cox model

$$\lambda_s(t; x) = \lambda_{0s}(t) \exp(x\beta_s)$$

gives

$$p(x = 1|s, T = t) = \frac{\exp \beta_s p(s,t)/\{1 - p(s,t)\}}{1 + \exp \beta_s p(s,t)/\{1 - p(s,t)\}}, \tag{6}$$

where $p(s,t) = p(x = 1|s, T \geq t)$. If outcome and censoring rates are low during trial follow-up, then $p(s,t)$ is very close to γ, the active group randomization fraction, and (6) is approximately

$$\frac{\{\gamma/(1-\gamma)\}e^{\beta_s}}{1 + \{\gamma/(1-\gamma)\}e^{\beta_s}}.$$

Hence, logistic regression methods can be applied for estimation and testing on $\beta_1, \beta_2, \ldots$. This type of analysis evidently has efficiency very similar to a 'full-cohort' analysis under this stratified Cox model, and hence may be more efficient than case–control or case–cohort estimation for this specific purpose. The case–only analyses may provide valuable cost saving if the baseline factors to be examined in relation to the hazard ratio involve expensive extraction of information from stored materials.

Ensuring adequate adherence to intervention goals can be a substantial challenge in prevention trials, as such trials are typically conducted in free living, ostensibly healthy, persons who have many other priorities, and may have other major life events occur during a possible lengthy trial intervention period. Various types of communications, incentives, and adherence initiatives may help maintain adherence to intervention goals, for either pill taking or behavioral interventions. If the adherence to intervention goals is less than desirable, there is a natural desire to try to estimate the intervention effects that may have arisen had there been full adherence to intervention goals. An interesting approach to such estimation (Robins and Finkelstein, 2000) involves censoring the follow-up times for study subjects when they are no longer adherent to their assigned intervention and weighting the contributions of each individual in the risk set $R(t)$ by the inverse of the estimated adherence probability at time t. Following the development of a model for time to non-adherence, perhaps using another Cox model, these weights can be estimated, thereby allowing the continuing adherent study subjects, in a sense, to 'represent' those with the same risk factors for non-adherence in the overall trial cohort. This approach has considerable appeal, but it is important to remember that the validity of the 'full adherence' comparison among randomization groups is dependent on the development of an adequate adherence rate model, and that one never knows whether or not residual confounding attends any such adherence model specification.

Most chronic disease-prevention trials to date have involved pill-taking interventions, with tamoxifen for breast cancer prevention (Fisher et al., 1998), statins for heart disease prevention (Shepherd et al., 1995), and alendronate for fracture prevention (Cummings et al., 1998) providing examples of important advances. Behavioral and lifestyle interventions arguably provide the desirable long-term targets for chronic prevention and for public health recommendation. There have been fewer such trials, with the Diabetes Prevention Program trial of a combination of a dietary pattern change and physical activity increase standing out as providing impressive findings (Diabetes Prevention Program Research Group, 2002). An analytic challenge in this type of 'lifestyle' trial is the estimation of the contributions of the various components of a multi-faceted intervention to the overall trial result. Usually, it will not be practical to blind study participants to a behavioral intervention assignment, so that unintended, as well as intended, differences in behaviors between intervention groups may need to be considered in evaluating and interpreting trial results. These are complex modeling issues where further statistical methodology research is needed.

4.3. Therapeutic trials

As noted above, RCTs provide the central research design for the evaluation and comparison of treatment regimens for a defined population of patients. Compared to prevention trials, therapeutic trials are typically smaller in size and of shorter duration though, depending on the disease being treated and the interventions being compared may require a few hundred, or even a few thousand, patients followed for some years.

For some diseases, such as coronary disease or osteoporosis, there is an underlying disease process that may be underway for some years or decades and intervention concepts arising, for example, in risk factor epidemiology might logically apply to either primary prevention or recurrence prevention. Because of sample size and cost issues, it may often be reasonable to study the intervention first in a therapeutic setting, perhaps using trial results to help decide whether a subsequent primary prevention trial is justified. The above examples of tamoxifen, statins, and alendronate each followed this pattern, as is also the case for ongoing trials of estrogen deprivation agents (aromatase inhibitors) for breast cancer treatment and prevention.

Therapeutic interventions may particularly target diseased tissue or organs. Surgical interventions to remove cancerous or damaged tissue, or to arrest the progression of an infectious disease, provide a classic example. Other therapeutic interventions for cancer may, for example, restrict the blood supply to tumor tissue (angiogenesis inhibitors), induce cancerous cells to self-destruct (apoptosis inducers), or interfere with signal transduction or other biological processes relevant to tumor progression. Some such interventions have potential for adverse effects during an early intensive treatment phase followed by longer-term benefit. Statistical tools of the type already described are useful for trial evaluation. Further developments would be useful in relation to hazard ratio models that reflect time-dependent treatment effects, and in relation to summary measures that can bring together such time-to-response outcomes as time to disease response to treatment, disease-free survival time, and overall survival toward a comparative summary of treatment benefits and risks. The development and evaluation of a therapeutic intervention is typically a multiphase process, and important statistical issues attend study design and analyses at each phase, including methods for deciding which treatments move on for testing in subsequent phases.

4.4. Disease-screening trials

There have been rather few RCTs of interventions for the early detection of disease, with mortality outcomes. As an exception there have been several trials of mammography, or of mammography in conjunction with other breast-screening modalities, for the reduction in breast cancer mortality, including the classic New York Health Insurance Plan breast-screening trial (Shapiro, 1977), which is often credited with establishing the value of mammography screening among older women, the Canadian National Breast Screening Study (Miller et al., 1992a, 1992b), and several group randomized trials in Europe. The latter pose some interesting analytic challenges as persons randomized in the same group to active screening or control tend to have correlated mortality times that give rise to inflation in the variance of test statistics, like the logrank test from (3), that need to be acknowledged. Such acknowledgement can take place by allowing a robust variance estimator (Wei et al., 1989) for the logrank test from (3), or by adopting a permutation approach to testing with the randomized group as the unit of analysis (Gail et al., 1996; Feng et al., 1999).

Another special feature of a screening trial with disease outcomes is the presence of a strong correlate of the primary outcome, disease-specific mortality. Specifically one observes the occurrence of the targeted disease during the course of the trial, and disease occurrence is a strong risk factor for the corresponding mortality. A statistical challenge is to use the disease incidence data in a manner that strengthens mortality comparisons relative to analyses based on the mortality data alone. To do so without making additional modeling assumptions requires a nonparametric estimator of the bivariate survivor function that can improve upon the efficiency of the Kaplan–Meier estimator, for separate application in each randomization group. Such estimation is known to be possible asymptotically (Van der Laan, 1996), but estimation procedures that can make practical improvements to the KM estimator with a moderate number (e.g., a few hundred) of disease events have yet to be developed. This 'auxiliary data' problem is one of a range of statistical challenges related to the use of intermediate outcomes and biomarkers.

5. Intermediate, surrogate, and auxiliary outcomes

The cost and duration of RCTs in the treatment area, and especially in the disease prevention and screening areas, naturally raises questions about whether some more frequently occurring or proximate outcome can suffice for the evaluation of an intervention. Alternatively, there may be a battery of intermediate outcomes that together convey most information concerning intervention benefits and risks.

On the contrary, it is clear that there are often readily available intermediate outcomes that are highly relevant to intervention effects. The effects of statin family drugs on blood lipids and lipoproteins, is undoubtedly a major aspect of the associated heart disease risk reduction, and the effects of the bone-preserving agent alendronate on bone mass and bone mineral density is likely an important determinant of fracture risk reduction. But one is typically not in a position to know whether or not such intermediate outcomes are comprehensive in respect to pathways relevant to the targeted disease, or are comprehensive in relation to unrecognized adverse effects. Recent controversy surrounding the use of the Cox-2 inhibitor VIOXX for colorectal adenoma recurrence prevention and an unexpected increase in cardiovascular disease risk illustrate the latter point (Bresalier et al., 2005). See Lagakos (2006) for a discussion of related interpretational issues. On the data analysis side, we often lack indices that bring together data on several pertinent intermediate outcomes for a meaningful projection of benefits versus risks for a disease outcome of interest, so that intermediate outcome trials typically play the roles of refinement and initial testing of an intervention, rather than of definitive testing in relation to a subsequent 'hard' endpoint.

In some circumstances, however, one may ask whether there is an intermediate outcome that so completely captures the effect of an intervention of interest on a 'true' outcome, that treatment decisions can be based on the intermediate outcome alone – the so-called surrogate outcome problem. Unfortunately, such circumstances are likely to be quite rare unless one defines a surrogate that is so proximate as to be tantamount to the true outcome. Specifically, the conditions for a test of the null hypothesis of no relationship between an intervention and intermediate outcome to be a valid test for the null hypothesis concerning the treatment and a true outcome require the surrogate to fully mediate the intervention effect on the time outcome (Prentice, 1989). This assumption is very restrictive, and one can never establish full mediation empirically. Nevertheless, the lack of evidence against such mediation in sizeable data sets is sometimes used to argue the practical surrogacy of certain intermediate outcomes, as in recent analysis of prostate-specific antigen 'velocity' as a surrogate for prostate cancer recurrence for the evaluation of certain types of treatments (D'Amico et al., 2003).

A rather different 'meta-analytic' approach to this issue of replacing a true outcome by a suitable intermediate outcome arises by modeling joint treatment effect parameters for the intermediate and true outcome in trials of similar interventions to that under study, and assuming some aspects of this joint distribution to apply to a subsequent trial in which only the intermediate ('surrogate') is observed (e.g., Burzykowski et al., 2005). It is not clear how often one would be in a position to have sufficient prior trial data available to apply this concept, and the issues of how one decides which treatments or interventions are close enough to the test treatment to support this type of approach also appears to be challenging.

The approaches described thus far in this section may not often allow a definitive evaluation of a treatment effect on a clinical outcome, such as disease incidence or mortality. The auxiliary data idea mentioned in Section 4.4 may have potential to streamline a definitive intervention evaluation, without making additional strong assumptions, if short-term and frequent outcomes exist that correlate strongly with the clinical outcome of interest. Essentially, the short-term outcome data provide dependent censorship information for the true clinical outcome, which may be able to add precision to comparative analysis of the clinical outcome data. High-dimensional short-term outcome data (e.g., changes in the proteome following treatment initiation) may offer particular opportunities, but, as noted previously, the requisite statistical methodology has yet to be developed.

In some circumstances, available data sources will have established an adverse effect of an exposure on disease risk. Cigarette smoking in relation to lung cancer or heart disease, occupational asbestos exposure and mesothelioma and lung cancer, human papilloma virus exposure and cervical cancer, provide important examples. RCTs in such contexts may be aimed at finding effective ways of reducing the exposures in question, for example, through smoking cessation or prevention educational approaches, through protective strategies in the workplace, or through safe-sex practices. Related dissemination research projects fulfill an important role in the overall epidemiology and biomedical research enterprise.

6. Multiple testing issues and high-dimensional biomarkers

6.1. Study monitoring and reporting

It is well recognized that Type I error rates may be inflated if trial data are analyzed periodically with analytic results having potential to alter trial conduct or to trigger trial reporting. Monitoring methods that preserve the size of tests to compare randomized group disease rates (e.g., Jennison and Turnbull, 2000) are widely used in RCT settings. These methods tend to depend strongly on proportional hazards assumptions. Settings in which the intervention may plausibly affect multiple clinical outcomes, either beneficially or adversely, present participation challenges in trial monitoring. For example, Freedman et al. (1996) propose a global index that is defined as the time to the earliest of a set of outcomes that may be affected by an intervention, and propose a monitoring process that first examines designated primary outcomes for the trial, but also examines at the global index to determine whether early trial stopping should be considered. Special efforts are required to estimate treatment effect parameters in the presence of sequential monitoring (Jennison and Turnbull, 2000). Conditional power calculations that make use of the data in hand in projecting study power also have value for trial monitoring.

It is interesting that most attention to the specification of testing procedures that acknowledge multiplicity of tests occurs in the RCT setting; where this is typically a well-defined treatment or intervention, a specified primary outcome, a specified test statistic for intervention group comparisons, and a trial monitoring plan. In contrast multiple testing issues are often not formally addressed in OS settings where there may be multiple covariate and covariate modeling specifications, multiple possible outcome definitions, multiple association test statistics, and where associations may be repeatedly examined in an ad hoc fashion. See Ioannidis (2005) for an assertion that 'most published findings are false', as a result of these types of multiple testing issues, and other sources of bias. The development of testing procedures that can avoid error rate inflation as a result of this array of multiplicities could add substantial strength to observational epidemiologic studies.

6.2. High-dimensional biomarker data

The development of high-dimensional biologic data of various types has greatly stimulated the biomedical research enterprise in recent years. One example is the identification of several million SNPs across the human genome (e.g., Hinds et al., 2005) and the identification of tag SNP subsets that convey most genotype information as a result of linkage disequilibrium among neighboring SNPs. Tag SNP sets in the 100,000 to 500,000 range, developed in part using the publicly funded HapMap project (The International HapMap Consortium, 2003), have recently become commercially available for use in a sufficiently high-throughput fashion that hundreds, or even thousands, of cases and controls can be tested in a research project. The photolithographic assessment methods used for high-dimensional SNP studies can also be used to generate comparative gene expression (transcript) assessments for cases versus controls, or for treated versus untreated study subjects, for thousands of genes simultaneously, also in a high-throughput fashion. There are also intensive technology developments underway to assess the concentrations of the several thousands of proteins that may be expressed in specific tissues, or may be circulating in blood serum or plasma. The genomic and transcriptomic methods rely on the chemical coupling of DNA or RNA in target tissue with labeled probes having a specified sequence. This same approach is not available for studying the proteome, and current technologies mainly rely on separation techniques followed by tandem mass spectrometry in subfractions for comparative proteomic assessments (e.g., Wang et al., 2005a). Antibody arrays involving a substantial number of proteins are also beginning to emerge as a useful proteomic platform (e.g., Wang et al., 2005b). Technologies for interrogating the metabolome (small molecules) are also under intensive investigation (e.g., Shurubor et al., 2005). High-dimensional data sources also include various other types of scans and images that may be of interest as risk factors, as early detection markers, or as outcomes (e.g., PET scans for neurologic disease progression) in RCTs.

High-dimensional genomic, transcriptomic, or proteomic data, or combinations thereof, even on a modest number of persons, may provide valuable insights into biological processes and networks, or intervention mechanisms that can lead to the development of novel treatments or interventions. Evaluation of the relationship of high-dimensional data to disease rates, however, can be expected to require large sample sizes to identify associations of moderate strength and to control for various sources of heterogeneity and bias. In fact, these studies may require sample sizes much larger than the corresponding low-dimensional problems, or a multistage design, to eliminate most false positive findings. For example, 1000 cases and 1000 controls from a study cohort may yield an association test of acceptable power for a 0.01 level test of association for a candidate SNP. Testing at this significance level for 500,000 SNPs would be expected to yield 5000 false positives under the global null hypothesis. A test at the 0.00001 (10 in a million) level would reduce this expected false positive number to 5, but corresponding study power would be greatly reduced.

A multistage design in which only markers satisfying statistical criteria for association with disease move on to a subsequent stage can yield important cost savings, as less promising markers are eliminated early. In the case of SNP association tests, pooled DNA provides the opportunity for much additional cost saving, but there are important trade-offs to consider (Downes et al., 2004; Prentice and Qi, 2006).

Proteomic markers in blood may have particular potential as early detection biomarkers. Special efforts may be needed to ensure equivalent handling of serum or plasma specimens between cases of the study disease and matched controls. Specimens that are stored prior to diagnosis are much to be preferred in this context, even for biomarker discovery. For cancer early detection markers, controls having benign versions of the disease under study may be needed to identify markers having acceptable specificity. Multistage designs again may be needed if a large number of proteins are being investigated (e.g., Feng et al., 2004).

Proteomic approaches also provide an opportunity for more targeted preventive intervention development, which heretofore has relied mainly on leads from observational epidemiology, or from therapeutic trials. For example, there is potential to examine the effects of an intervention on the plasma proteome, in conjunction with knowledge of proteomic changes in relation to disease risk, as a means for the development and initial testing of biobehavioral interventions.

Much additional research is needed to identify study designs that make good use of these types of emerging high-dimensional data. The high-dimensionality also opens the way to some novel empirical testing procedures (Efron, 2004), that may provide valuable robustness compared to standard tests that assume a theoretical null distribution. Also, false discovery rate procedures (Benjamini and Hochberg, 1995) provide a useful alternative to controlling experiment-wise Type I error rates in these contexts. Additional statistical research is needed on parameter estimation, and simultaneous confidence interval specification, in the context of multistage designs in which the biomarkers of interest satisfy a series of selection criteria (e.g., Benjamini and Yekutieli, 2005).

7. Further discussion and the Women's Health Initiative example

The Women's Health Initiative (WHI) clinical trial (CT) and OS in which the author has been engaged since its inception in 1992, provides a context for illustrating a number of the points raised above. The WHI is conducted among postmenopausal women, in the age range 50–79 when enrolled during 1993–1998 at one of 40 clinical centers in the United States. The CT is conducted among 68,132 such women and evaluates four interventions in a randomized, controlled fashion in a partial factorial design (WHI Study Group, 1998). Two CT components involve postmenopausal hormone therapy, either conjugated equine estrogen alone (E-alone) among women who were post-hysterectomy at enrollment, or the same estrogen plus medroxyprogesterone acetate (E + P) among women with a uterus. The E + P trial among 16,608 women ended early in 2002 (Writing Group for the WHI, 2002) when an elevated risk of breast cancer was observed, and the 'global index' was also elevated, in part because of an unexpected increase in the designated primary outcome, coronary heart disease, as well as increases in stroke and venous thromboembolism. The E-alone trial among 10,739 women also ended early in 2004 (WHI Steering Committee, 2004) largely because of a stroke elevation, along with little potential for showing a heart disease benefit by the planned completion date in 2005.

The WHI OS includes 93,676 women recruited from the same populations, over the same time period, with much common covariate data collection, and with similar outcome ascertainment procedures. Comparison of study findings between the CT and OS provides a particular opportunity to identify sources of bias and to improve study design and analysis procedures. In the case of hormone therapy and cardiovascular disease joint analyses of the two cohorts using Cox models that stratify on cohort and baseline age reveal that careful control for confounding and for time from hormone therapy initiation provide an explanation for substantially different hazard ratio functions in the two cohorts (Prentice et al., 2005a; Prentice et al., 2006b). Corresponding unpublished breast cancer analyses draw attention to the need to carefully control for mammography patterns in outcome ascertainment, and also raise thorny issues of assessment when the intervention has potential to affect outcome ascertainment.

A series of case–control studies are underway using candidate biomarkers to elucidate hormone therapy effects on cardiovascular disease, breast cancer, and fractures. For example, the cardiovascular disease studies focus on blood-based markers of inflammation, coagulation, lipids, and candidate gene polymorphisms. A genome-wide association study involving 360,000 tag SNPs is also underway in collaboration with Perlegen Sciences to identify genetic risk factors for coronary heart disease, stroke, and breast cancer, and to elucidate hormone therapy effects in these three diseases (e.g., Prentice and Qi, 2006).

The WHI specimen repository also serves as a resource for a wide range of biomarker studies by the scientific community. A novel ongoing example aims to identify colon cancer early detection markers by studying prediagnostic stored plasma from 100 colon cancer cases and matched controls. A total of 10 labs across the United States are applying various proteomic platforms for shared discovery analyses, under the auspices of the NCI's Early Detection Research Network and WHI.

The other two CT components involve a low-fat dietary pattern for cancer prevention (48,835 women) and calcium and vitamin D supplementation for fracture prevention (36,282 women). Initial reports from these trials have recently been presented (Prentice et al., 2006a, 2006b; Beresford et al., 2006; Howard et al., 2006, for the low-fat trial; Jackson et al., 2006; Wactawski-Wende et al., 2006, for the calcium and vitamin D trial), with much further analytic work, and explanatory analyses underway. Biomarker studies are underway in both the dietary modification trial cohort and the OS to examine the measurement properties of frequencies, records, and recalls for self-reporting both dietary consumption and physical activity patterns. These same biomarkers will be used to calibrate the self-report data for a variety of disease association studies in WHI cohorts. See Prentice et al. (2005b) for a detailed discussion of statistical issues arising in the WHI, and for commentary by several knowledgeable epidemiologists and biostatisticians.

In summary, epidemiology and biomedical research settings are replete with important statistical issues. The population science and prevention areas have attracted the energies of relatively few statistically trained persons, even though the public health implications are great, and methodologic topics often stand as barriers to progress. These and other biomedical research areas can be recommended as stimulating settings for statistical scientists at any career stage.

Acknowledgement

This work was supported by grants CA 53996, CA86368, and CA106320.

References

Andersen, P.K., Borgan, D., Gill, R.D., Keiding, N. (1993). *Statistical Models Based on Counting Processes*. Springer, New York.

Andersen, P.K., Gill, R.D. (1982). Cox's regression model for counting processes: A large sample study. *The Annals of Statistics* **10**, 1100–1120.

Baker, S.G., Kramer, B.S., McIntosh, M., Patterson, B.H., Shyr, Y., Skates, S. (2006). Evaluating markers for the early detection of cancer: Overview of study designs and methods. *Clinical Trials* **3**, 43–56.

Benjamini, Y., Hochberg, Y. (1995). Controlling false discovery rate: A practical and powerful approach to multiple testing. *Journal of the Royal Statistical Society. Series B* **57**, 289–300.

Benjamini, Y., Yekutieli, D. (2005). False discovery rate-adjusted multiple confidence intervals for selected parameters (with discussion). *Journal of the American Statistical Association* **100**, 71–93.

Beresford, S.A., Johnson, K.C., Ritenbaugh, C., Lasser, N.L., Snetselaar, L.G., Black, H.R., Anderson, G.L., Assaf, A.R., Bassford, T., Bowen, D., Brunner, R.L., Brzyski, R.G., Caan, B., Chlebowski, R.T., Gass, M., Harrigan, R.C., Hays, J., Heber, D., Heiss, G., Hendrix, S.L., Howard, B.V., Hsia, J., Hubbell, F.A., Jackson, R.D., Kotchen, J.M., Kuller, L.H., LaCroix, A.Z., Lane, D.S., Langer, R.D., Lewis, C.E., Manson, J.E., Margolis, K.L., Mossavar-Rahmani, Y., Ockene, J.K., Parker, L.M., Perri, M.G., Phillips, L., Prentice, R.L., Robbins, J., Rossouw, J.E., Sarto, G.E., Stefanick, M.L., Van Horn, L., Vitolins, M.Z., Wactawski-Wende, J., Wallace, R.B., Whitlock, E. (2006). Low-fat dietary pattern and risk of colorectal cancer: The Women's Health Initiative randomized controlled dietary modification trial. *The Journal of the American Medical Association* **295**, 643–654.

Bresalier, R.S., Sandler, R.S., Quan, H., Bolognese, J.A., Oxenius, B., Horgan, K., Lines, C., Riddell, R., Morton, D., Lanas, A., Konstam, M.A., Baron, J.A., Adenomatous Polyp Prevention on Vioxx (APPROVe) Trial Investigators. (2005). Cardiovascular events associated with rofecoxib in a colorectal cancer chemoprevention trial. *The New England Journal of Medicine* **352**, 1092–1102.

Breslow, N.E., Day, N.E. (1987). Statistical methods in cancer research, Vol. 2. The Design and Analysis of Cohort Studies. IARC Scientific Publications No. 82, International Agency for Research on Cancer, Lyon, France.

Burzykowski, T., Molenberghs, G., Buyse, M. (2005). *The Evaluation of Surrogate Endpoints*. Springer, New York.

Carroll, R.J., Freedman, L., Kipnis, V., Li, L. (1998). A new class of measurement error models, with application to dietary data. *Canadian Journal of Statistics* **26**, 467–477.

Carroll, R.J., Ruppert, D., Stefanski, L.A. (1995). *Measurement Error in Nonlinear Models*. Chapman & Hall, London.

Carroll, R.J., Wand, M.P. (1991). Semiparametric estimation in logistic measurement error models. *Journal of Royal Statistical Society. Series B* **53**, 573–585.

Cox, D.R. (1972). Regression models and life tables (with discussion). *Journal of Royal Statistical Society. Series B* **34**, 187–220.

Cox, D.R. (1975). Partial likelihood. *Biometrika* **62**, 269–276.

Cummings, S.R., Black, D.M., Thompson, D.E., Applegate, W.B., Barrett-Connor, E., Musliner, T.A., Palermo, L., Prineas, R., Rubin, S.M., Scott, J.C., Vogt, T., Wallace, R., Yates, A.J., LaCroix, A.Z. (1998). Effect of alendronate on risk of fracture in women with low bone density but without vertebral fractures. *The Journal of the American Medical Association* **280**, 2077–2082.

D'Amico, A.V., Moul, J.W., Carroll, P.R., Sun, L., Lubeck, D., Chen, M.H. (2003). Surrogate endpoint for prostate cancer-specific mortality after radical prostatectomy or radiation therapy. *Journal of the National Cancer Institute* **95**, 1376–1383.

Diabetes Prevention Program Research Group (2002). Reduction in the incidence of Type 2 diabetes with lifestyle intervention or metformin. *The New England Journal of Medicine* **346**, 393–403.

Downes, K., Barratt, B.J., Akan, P., Bumpstead, S.J., Taylor, S.D., Clayton, D.G., Deloukas, P. (2004). SNP allele frequency estimation in DNA pools and variance component analysis. *BioTechniques* **36**, 840–845.

Efron, B. (2004). Large-scale simultaneous hypothesis testing: The choice of a null hypothesis. *Journal of the American Statistical Association* **99**, 96–104.

Felsenstein, J. (1992). *Theoretical Evolutionary Genetics*. University of Washington/ASUW Publishing, Seattle, WA.

Feng, Z., Diehr, P., Yasui, Y., Evans, B., Beresford, S., Koepsell, T. (1999). Explaining community-level variance in group randomized trials. *Statistics in Medicine* **18**, 539–556.

Feng, Z., Prentice, R.L., Srivastava, S. (2004). Research issues and strategies for genomic and proteomic biomarker discovery and validation: A statistical perspective. *Pharmacogenomics* **5**, 709–719.

Fisher, B., Costantino, F.P., Wickerham, J.L., Redmond, C.K., Kavanah, M., Cronin, W.M., Vogel, V., Robidoux, A., Dimitrov, N., Atkins, J., Daly, M., Wieand, S., Tan-Chiu, E., Ford, L., Wolmark, N. (1998). Tamoxifen for prevention of breast cancer: Report of the National Surgical Adjuvant Breast and Bowel Project P-1 study. *Journal of the National Cancer Institute* **90**, 1371–1388.

Freedman, L., Anderson, G., Kipnis, V., Prentice, R., Wang, C.Y., Rossouw, J., Wittes, J., DeMets, D. (1996). Approaches to monitoring the results of long-term disease prevention trials: Examples from the Women's Health Initiative. *Controlled Clinical Trials* **17**, 509–525.

Gail, M.H., Mark, S.D., Carroll, R.J., Green, S.B., Pee, D. (1996). On design considerations and randomization-based inference for community intervention trials. *Statistics in Medicine* **15**, 1069–1092.

Heitmann, B.L., Lissner, L. (1995). Dietary underreporting by obese individuals – is it specific or non-specific? *British Medical Journal* **311**, 986–989.

Hernan, M.A., Brumback, B., Robins, J.M. (2001). Marginal structural models to estimate the joint causal effect of nonrandomized treatments. *Journal of the American Statistical Association* **96**, 440–448.

Hinds, D.A., Stuve, L.L., Nilsen, G.B., Halperin, E., Eskin, E., Ballinger, D.G., Frazer, K.A., Cox, D.R. (2005). Whole-genome patterns of common DNA variation in three human populations. *Science* **307**, 1072–1079.

Hougaard, P. (2000). *Analysis of Multivariate Survival Data*. Springer, New York.

Howard, B.V., Van Horn, L., Hsia, J., Manson, J.E., Stefanick, M.L., Wassertheil-Smoller, S., Kuller, L.H., LaCroix, A.Z., Langer, R.D., Lasser, N.L., Lewis, C.E., Limacher, M.C., Margolis, K.L., Mysiw, W.J., Ockene, J.K., Parker, L.M., Perri, M.G., Phillips, L., Prentice, R.L., Robbins, J., Rossouw, J.E., Sarto, G.E., Schatz, I.J., Snetselaar, L.G., Stevens, V.J., Tinker, L.F., Trevisan, M., Vitolins, M.Z., Anderson, G.L., Assaf, A.R., Bassford, T., Beresford, S.A., Black, H.R., Brunner, R.L., Brzyski, R.G., Caan, B., Chlebowski, R.T., Gass, M., Granek, I., Greenland, P., Hays, J., Heber, D., Heiss, G., Hendrix, S.L., Hubbell, F.A., Johnson, K.C., Kotchen, J.M. (2006). Low-fat dietary pattern and risk of cardiovascular disease: The Women's Health Initiative randomized controlled dietary modification trial. *The Journal of the American Medical Association* **295**, 655–666.

Hsu, L., Prentice, R.L., Zhao, L.P., Fan, J.J. (1999). On dependence estimation using correlated failure time data from case–control family studies. *Biometrika* **86**, 743–753.

Huang, Y., Wang, C.Y. (2000). Cox regression with accurate covariate unascertainable: A nonparametric correction approach. *Journal of the American Statistical Association* **45**, 1209–1219.

Ioannidis, J.P.A. (2005). Why most published findings are false. *PLoS Medicine* **2**(8), e124.

Jackson, R.D., LaCroix, A.Z., Gass, M., Wallace, R.B., Robbins, J., Lewis, C.E., Bassford, T., Beresford, S.A., Black, H.R., Blanchette, P., Bonds, D.E., Brunner, R.L., Brzyski, R.G., Caan, B., Cauley, J.A., Chlebowski, R.T., Cummings, S.R., Granek, I., Hays, J., Heiss, G., Hendrix, S.L., Howard, B.V., Hsia, J., Hubbell, F.A., Johnson, K.C., Judd, H., Kotchen, J.M., Kuller, L.H., Langer, R.D., Lasser, N.L., Limacher, M.C., Ludlam, S., Manson, J.E., Margolis, K.L., McGowan, J., Ockene, J.K., O'Sullivan, M.J., Phillips, L., Prentice, R.L., Sarto, G.E., Stefanick, M.L., Van Horn, L., Wactawski-Wende, J., Whitlock, E., Anderson, G.L., Assaf, A.R., Barad, D., Women's Health Initiative Investigators. (2006). Calcium plus vitamin D supplementation and the risk of fractures. *The New England Journal of Medicine* **354**, 669–683.

Jennison, C., Turnbull, B.W. (2000). *Group Sequential Methods with Application to Clinical Trials*. Chapman & Hall/CRC, Boca Raton, LA.

Jin, Z., Lin, D.Y., Wei, L.J., Ying, Z. (2003). Risk-based inference for the accelerated failure time model. *Biometrika* **90**, 341–353.

Kalbfleisch, J.D., Prentice, R.L. (2002). *The Statistical Analysis of Failure Time Data*, 2nd ed. Wiley, New York.

Kipnis, V., Subar, A.F., Midthune, D., Freedman, L.S., Ballard-Barbash, R., Troiano, R.P., Bingham, S., Schoeller, D.A., Schatzkin, A., Carroll, R.J. (2003). Structure of dietary measurement error: Results of the OPEN biomarker study. *American Journal of Epidemiology* **158**, 14–21.

Lagakos, S. (2006). Time-to-event analyses for long-term treatments in the APPROVE trial. *The New England Journal of Medicine* **355**, 113–117.

LeBlanc, M., Tibshirani, R. (1996). Combining estimates in regression and classification. *Journal of the American Statistical Association* **91**, 1641–1650.

Liddell, F.D.K., McDonald, J.C., Thomas, D.C. (1977). Methods for cohort analysis: Appraisal by application to asbestos mining. *Journal of Royal Statistical Society Series A* **140**, 469–490.

McIntosh, M., Pepe, M.S. (2002). Combining several screening tools: Optionality of the risk score. *Biometrics* **58**, 657–664.

Miller, A.B., Baines, C.J., To, T., Wall, C. (1992a). Canadian National Breast Screening Study. I. Breast cancer detection and death rates among women aged 40–49 years. *Canadian Medical Association Journal* **147**, 1459–1476.

Miller, A.B., Baines, C.J., To, T., Wall, C. (1992b). Canadian National Breast Screening Study. 2. Breast cancer detection and death rates among women aged 50–59 years. *Canadian Medical Association Journal* **147**, 1477–1488.

Moolgavkar, S.H., Knudson Jr., A.G. (1981). Mutation and cancer: A model for human carcinogenesis. *Journal of the National Cancer Institute* **66**, 1037–1052.

Ott, J. (1991). *Analysis of Human Genetic Linkage*. Johns Hopkins University Press, Baltimore, MD.

Pepe, M.S. (2003). *The Statistical Evaluation of Medical Tests for Classification and Production*. Oxford University Press, London.

Pepe, M., Fleming, T.R. (1991). A nonparametric method for dealing with mis-measured covariate data. *Journal of the American Statistical Association* **86**, 108–113.

Prentice, R.L. (1986). A case–cohort design for epidemiologic cohort studies and disease prevention trials. *Biometrika* **73**, 1–11.

Prentice, R.L. (1989). Surrogate endpoints in clinical trials: Discussion, definition and operational criteria. *Statistics in Medicine* **8**, 431–440.

Prentice, R.L., Breslow, N.E. (1978). Retrospective studies and failure time models. *Biometrika* **65**, 153–158.

Prentice, R.L., Caan, B., Chlebowski, R.T., Patterson, R., Kuller, L.H., Ockene, J.K., Margolis, K.L., Limacher, M.C., Manson, J.E., Parker, L.M., Paskett, E., Phillips, L., Robbins, J., Rossouw, J.E., Sarto, G.E., Shikany, J.M., Stefanick, M.L., Thomson, C.A., Van Horn, L., Vitolins, M.Z., Wactawski-Wende, J., Wallace, R.B., Wassertheil-Smoller, S., Whitlock, E., Yano, K., Adams-Campbell, L., Anderson, G.L., Assaf, A.R., Beresford, S.A., Black, H.R., Brunner, R.L., Brzyski, R.G., Ford, L., Gass, M., Hays, J., Heber, D., Heiss, G., Hendrix, S.L., Hsia, J., Hubbell, F.A., Jackson, R.D., Johnson, K.C., Kotchen, J.M., LaCroix, A.Z., Lane, D.S., Langer, R.D., Lasser, N.L., Henderson, M.M. (2006a). Low-fat dietary pattern and risk of invasive breast cancer: The Women's Health Initiative randomized controlled dietary modification trial. *The Journal of the American Medical Association* **295**, 629–642.

Prentice, R.L., Langer, R., Stefanick, M.L., Howard, B.V., Pettinger, M., Anderson, G., Barad, D., Curb, J.D., Kotchen, J., Kuller, L., Limacher, M., Wactawski-Wende, J., for the Women's Health Initiative Investigators. (2005a). Combined postmenopausal hormone therapy and cardiovascular disease: Toward resolving the discrepancy between Women's Health Initiative clinical trial and observational study results. *American Journal of Epidemiology* **162**, 404–414.

Prentice, R.L., Langer, R.D., Stefanick, M.L., Howard, B.V., Pettinger, M., Anderson, G.L., Barad, D., Curb, J.D., Kotchen, J., Kuller, L., Limacher, M., Wactawski-Wende, J., for the Women's Health Initiative Investigators. (2006b). Combined analysis of Women's Health Initiative observational and clinical trial data on postmenopausal hormone treatment and cardiovascular disease. *American Journal of Epidemiology* **163**, 589–599.

Prentice, R.L., Pettinger, M., Anderson, G.L. (2005a). Statistical issues arising in the Women's Health Initiative (with discussion). *Biometrics* **61**, 899–941.

Prentice, R.L., Qi, L. (2006). Aspects of the design and analysis of high-dimensional SNP studies for disease risk estimation. *Biostatistics* **7**, 339–354.

Prentice, R.L., Sugar, E., Wang, C.Y., Neuhouser, M., Peterson, R. (2002). Research strategies and the use of nutrient biomarkers in studies of diet and chronic disease. *Public Health Nutrition* **5**, 977–984.

Risch, N., Merikangas, K. (1996). The future of genetic studies of complex human diseases. *Science* **273**, 1516–1517.

Robins, J. (1987). A graphical approach to the identification and estimation of causal parameters in mortality studies with sustained exposure periods. *Journal of Chronic Diseases* **2**, 139–161.

Robins, J.M., Finkelstein, D.M. (2000). Correcting for noncompliance and dependent censoring in an AIDS clinical trial with inverse probability of censoring weighted (IPCW) log-rank tests. *Biometrics* **56**, 779–781.

Schork, N.J., Fallin, D., Thiel, B., Xu, X., Broeckel, U., Jacob, H.J., Cohen, D. (2001). The future of genetic case–control studies. *Advances in Genetics* **42**, 191–212.

Self, S.G., Mauritsen, R.H., Ohara, J. (1992). Power calculations for likelihood ratio tests in generalized linear models. *Biometrics* **48**, 31–39.

Shapiro, S. (1977). Evidence of screening for breast cancer from a randomized trial. *Cancer* **39**, 2772–2782.

Shepherd, J., Cobbe, S.M., Ford, I., Isles, C.G., Lorimer, A.R., MacFarlane, P.W., McKillop, J.H., Packard, C.J. (1995). Prevention of coronary heart disease with pravastatin in men with hypercholesterolemia. West of Scotland Coronary Prevention Study Group. *The New England Journal of Medicine* **333**, 1301–1307.

Shurubor, Y.I., Matson, W.R., Martin, R.J., Kristal, B.S. (2005). Relative contribution of specific sources of systematic errors and analytic imprecision to metabolite analysis by HPLC-ECD. *Metabolomics: Official Journal of the Metabolomic Society* **1**, 159–168.

Song, X., Huang, Y. (2005). On corrected score approach to proportional hazards model with covariate measurement error. *Biometrics* **61**, 702–714.

Sugar, E.A., Wang, C.Y., Prentice, R.L. (2007). Logistic regression with exposure biomarkers and flexible measurement error. *Biometrics* **63**, 143–151.

The International HapMap Consortium (2003). The International HapMap Project. *Nature* **426**, 789–796.

Thomas, D.C. (2004). *Statistical Methods in Genetic Epidemiology*. Oxford University Press, London.

Tsiatis, A.A., Davidian, M. (2001). A semiparametric estimator for the proportional hazards model with longitudinal covariates measured with error. *Biometrika* **88**, 447–458.

Van der Laan, M.J. (1996). Efficient estimation in the bivariate censoring model and repaired NPMLE. *The Annals of Statistics* **24**, 596–627.

Vittinghoff, E., Bauer, D. (2006). Case–only analysis of treatment-covariate interactions in clinical trials. *Biometrics* **62**, 769–776.

Wactawski-Wende, J., Kotchen, J.M., Anderson, G.L., Assaf, A.R., Brunner, R.L., O'Sullivan, M.J., Margolis, K.L., Ockene, J.K., Phillips, L., Pottern, L., Prentice, R.L., Robbins, J., Rohan, T.E., Sarto, G.E., Sharma, S., Stefanick, M.L., Van Horn, L., Wallace, R.B., Whitlock, E., Bassford, T., Beresford, S.A., Black, H.R., Bonds, D.E., Brzyski, R.G., Caan, B., Chlebowski, R.T., Cochrane, B., Garland, C., Gass, M., Hays, J., Heiss, G., Hendrix, S.L., Howard, B.V., Hsia, J., Hubbell, F.A., Jackson, R.D., Johnson, K.C., Judd, H., Kooperberg, C.L., Kuller, L.H., LaCroix, A.Z., Lane, D.S., Langer, R.D., Lasser, N.L., Lewis, C.E., Limacher, M.C., Manson, J.E., Women's Health Initiative Investigators. (2006). Calcium plus vitamin D supplementation and the risk of colorectal cancer. *The New England Journal of Medicine* **354**, 684–696.

Wang, H., Clouthier, S.G., Galchev, V., Misek, D.E., Duffner, U., Min, C.K., Zhao, R., Tra, J., Omenn, G.S., Ferrara, J.L., Hanash, S.M. (2005a). Intact-protein-based high-resolution three-dimensional quantitative analysis system for proteome profiling of biological fluids. *Molecular and Cellular Proteomics* **4**, 618–625.

Wang, X., Yu, J., Sreekumar, A., Varambally, S., Shen, R., Giacherio, D., Mehra, R., Montie, J.E., Pienta, K.J., Sanda, M.G., Kantoff, P.W., Rubin, M.A., Wei, J.T., Ghosh, D., Chinnaiyan, A.M. (2005b). Autoantibody signatures in prostate cancer. *The New England Journal of Medicine* **353**, 1224–1235.

Wei, L.J., Lin, D.Y., Weissfeld, L. (1989). Regression analysis of multivariate incomplete failure time data by modeling marginal distributions. *Journal of the American Statistical Association* **84**, 1065–1073.

White, E., Patterson, R.E., Kristal, A.R., Thornquist, M., King, I., Shattuck, A.L., Evans, I., Satia-Abouta, J., Littman, A.J., Potter, J.D. (2004). Vitamins and lifestyle cohort study: Study design and characteristics of supplement users. *American Journal of Epidemiology* **159**, 83–93.

Women's Health Initiative (WHI) Steering Committee (2004). Effects of conjugated equine estrogen in postmenopausal women with hysterectomy. *The Journal of the American Medical Association* **291**, 1701–1712.

Women's Health Initiative Study Group (1998). Design of the Women's Health Initiative clinical trial and observational study. *Controlled Clinical Trials* **19**, 61–109.

Writing Group for the Women's Health Initiative (WHI) Investigators (2002). Risks and benefits of estrogen plus progestin in healthy postmenopausal women: Principal results from the Women's Health Initiative randomized controlled trial. *The Journal of the American Medical Association* **288**, 321–333.

Xie, S., Wang, C.Y., Prentice, R.L. (2001). A risk set calibration method for failure time regression by using a covariate reliability sample. *Journal of Royal Statistical Society. Series B* **63**, 855–870.

Handbook of Statistics, Vol. 27
ISSN: 0169-7161

DOI: 10.1016/S0169-7161(07)27002-6

2

Statistical Inference for Causal Effects, With Emphasis on Applications in Epidemiology and Medical Statistics ☆

Donald B. Rubin

Abstract

A central problem in epidemiology and medical statistics is how to draw inferences about the causal effects of treatments (i.e., interventions) from randomized and nonrandomized data. For example, does the new drug really reduce heart disease, or does exposure to that chemical in drinking water increase cancer rates relative to drinking water without that chemical? This chapter provides an overview of the approach to the estimation of such causal effects based on the concept of potential outcomes. We discuss randomization-based approaches and the Bayesian posterior predictive approach.

1. Causal inference primitives

We present here a framework for causal inference that is now commonly referred to as "Rubin's Causal Model" (RCM, Holland, 1986), for a series of articles written in the 1970s (Rubin, 1974, 1975, 1976a, 1977, 1978, 1979a, 1980). The framework has two essential parts and one optional part. The first part of the RCM defines causal effects through potential outcomes, and is the theme of Section 1. The second part of this framework for causal inference concerns the assignment mechanism, and this is developed in Section 2. In Section 3, the classical use of the framework in randomized experiments, due to Neyman (1923) and Fisher (1925), is described, and then extended to nonrandomized observational studies. The third part of the RCM, which is optional, is the use of Bayesian posterior predictive inference for causal effects, as developed in Rubin (1975, 1978), and this perspective is presented in Section 4. The remaining Section 5 discusses some extensions and complications. Other approaches to causal inference, such as graphical ones (e.g., Pearl, 2000), I find conceptually less

☆ This chapter is a revision and expansion of the analogous chapter in Rao and Sinharay (2006).

satisfying, for reasons discussed, for instance, in Rubin (2004a, 2005). The presentation here is essentially a compact version of the perspective more fully developed in the text by Imbens and Rubin (2007a).

1.1. Units, treatments, potential outcomes

For causal inference, there are several primitives – concepts that are basic and on which we must build. A "unit" is a physical object, e.g., a person, at a particular point in time. A "treatment" is an action that can be applied or withheld from that unit. We focus on the case of two treatments, although the extension to more than two treatments is simple in principle although not necessarily so with real data.

Associated with each unit are two "potential outcomes": the value of an outcome variable Y at a point in time after the active treatment is applied and the value of that outcome variable at the *same* point in time when the active treatment is withheld. The objective is to learn about the causal effect of the application of the active treatment relative to the control treatment (when the active treatment is withheld) on the variable Y.

For example, the unit could be "you now" with your headache, the active treatment could be taking aspirin for your headache, and the control treatment could be not taking aspirin (as in Rubin, 1974, p. 489). The outcome Y could be the intensity of your headache pain in two hours, with the potential outcomes being the headache intensity if you take aspirin and if you do not take aspirin.

Notationally, let W indicate which treatment the unit, you, received: $W = 1$ for the active treatment, $W = 0$ for the control treatment. Also let $Y(1)$ be the value of the potential outcome if the unit received the active version, and $Y(0)$ the value if the unit received the control version. The causal effect of the active treatment relative to its control version is the comparison of $Y(1)$ and $Y(0)$ – typically the difference, $Y(1) - Y(0)$, or perhaps the difference in logs, $\log[Y(1)] - \log[Y(0)]$, or some other comparison, possibly the ratio.

We can observe only one or the other of $Y(W)$ as indicated by W. The key problem for causal inference is that, for any individual unit, we observe the value of the potential outcome under only one of the possible treatments, namely the treatment actually assigned, and the potential outcome under the other treatment is missing. Thus, inference for causal effects is a missing-data problem – the "other" value is missing. For example, your reduction in blood pressure one week after taking a drug measures a change in time, in particular, a change from before taking the drug to after taking the drug, and so is not a causal effect without additional assumptions. The comparison of your blood pressure after taking the drug with what it would have been at the same point in time without taking the drug is a causal effect.

1.2. Relating this definition of causal effect to common usage

The definition of a causal effect provided so far may appear a bit formal and the discussion a bit ponderous, but the presentation is simply intended to capture the way we use the concept in everyday life. Also this definition of causal effect as the comparison of potential outcomes is frequently used in contemporary culture, for example, as revealed by movies. Let us consider some movie plots to illustrate this point.

Most of us have probably seen parts of "It's a Wonderful Life" with Jimmy Stewart as George Bailey more times than we can remember (around Christmas time). In this movie, at one point in George's life, he becomes very depressed and sincerely wishes he had never been born. At the appropriate moment, a wingless angel named Clarence shows him exactly what the world he knows would be like if, contrary to fact, he had not been born.

The actual world is the real observed potential outcome, but Clarence reveals to George the other potential outcome, the counterfactual one, and George experiences this other world as a real phenomenon, just as real as his actual world. Not only are there obvious consequences, like his own children not existing, but there are many other untoward events. For example, his younger brother, Harry, who was, in the actual world, a World War II hero, in the counterfactual world drowned in a skating accident at age eight, because George was never born and thus was not there to save Harry as he did in the actual world. And there was the pharmacist, Mr. Gower, who filled the wrong prescription and was convicted of manslaughter because George was not there to catch the error as he did in the actual world.

The causal effect of George not being born is the comparison of (a) the entire stream of events in the actual world with him in it, to (b) the entire stream of events in the counterfactual world without him in it. Fortunately for George, he has Clarence to show him both potential outcomes, and George regrets ever having wished he had never been born, and he returns to the actual world.

Another movie often shown around Christmas time is based on Dickens' classic novel "A Christmas Carol". Here, the wealthy and miserly Ebenezer Scrooge is fortunate enough to have a visit from a trio of ghosts on Christmas Eve. Although the first two ghosts make Scrooge feel guilty about things he has done in the distant and recent past, the third ghost, the most frightening of all, the Ghost of Christmas Future, is the most effective. The ghost reveals to Ebenezer the potential outcome that will occur if Ebenezer continues his current mean-spirited ways. Not surprisingly, Scrooge does not want to live this potential outcome, and because it is the future, he can reject it in favor of the other potential outcome, by altering his behavior. Neither outcome was counterfactual at the time of the third ghost's visit, but one was by the end of the movie.

These and modern movies with similar themes clearly indicate that the causal effects of actions or treatments are the comparison of potential outcomes under alternative actions. A current list includes, among others, "Sliding Doors", "The Family Man" and "Mr. Destiny". Sometimes one of the potential outcomes is clearly counterfactual, as in "It's a Wonderful Life", sometimes the revealed potential outcomes are not yet counterfactual because they are in the future, as in "A Christmas Carol". Sometimes the movie is not clear about whether one of the potential outcomes is counterfactual or not. But, invariably, the causal effect of actions involves the comparison of potential outcomes, which are the stream of events at the same times but after different actions.

1.3. Relationship to the "but-for" concept in legal damages settings

Probably the setting outside science where causal effects are most seriously considered is in law. Suppose you committed an action that you should not have, *and as a result of that action* someone else suffered damages. That is, the causal effect of your action relative to the absence of that action is the comparison of potential outcomes, the first the actual, the second the counterfactual. For example, let us suppose that because you were driving and talking on a cell phone, you ran a stop sign and hit another car. "But for" your negligence, the other car would not have been involved in any accident. The causal effect of your negligence is the amount of damage in this accident.

One of the more interesting and expensive recent examples of trying to assess causal effects in a legal damages setting has revolved around the alleged misconduct of the tobacco industry (e.g., lying about the health risks of smoking) in the United States and other countries. Here, the world with the alleged misconduct is the actual world, with its cigarette smoking and health-care expenditures. The other potential outcome, the counterfactual one, is the world without the alleged misconduct and, according to the plaintiffs, with reduced cigarette smoking, and different amounts and kinds of health-care expenditures. One cannot simply assume the complete absence of cigarette smoking in a counterfactual world without the alleged misconduct of the tobacco industry, and so only a fraction of all expenditures that may be attributable to smoking are the causal effect of the alleged misconduct.

This point has been made repeatedly in the tobacco litigation by both plaintiffs' experts and defendants' experts (including me) in both their reports and their testimony. For example, the well-known economist, Franklin Fisher (1999), in an expert witness report for the plaintiffs, (p. 2, item #6) wrote:

> It is necessary to generate a stream of damages taking into account that not all smoking-related expenditures result from the alleged behavior of the defendants. Thus, the smoking-related expenditures estimated by Glenn Harrison and Wendy Max, and Henry Miller [experts for the plaintiffs] need to be adjusted by what Jeffrey Harris [expert for the plaintiffs] has calculated to be the proportion of total smoking-attributable expenditures caused by defendants' improper conduct. The monetary amount of damage resulting from the defendants' alleged behavior in each past and future year is thus calculated by multiplying the annual smoking related expenditures by the proportion caused by defendants' improper conduct.

Also, the September 22, 1999, news conference held to announce the United States filing of its lawsuit against the tobacco industry, Assistant Attorney General Ogden (1999) stated:

> The number that's in the complaint is not a number that reflects a particular demand for payment. What we've alleged is that each year the federal government expends in excess of 20 billion on *tobacco* related medical costs. What we would actually recover would be our portion of that annual toll that is

> the result of the illegal conduct that we allege occurred, and it simply will be a matter or proof for the court, which will be developed through the course of discovery, what that amount will be. So, we have not put out a specific figure and we'll simply have to develop that as the case goes forward.

These positions are supported by the Federal Judicial Center's (2000, p. 284):

> The first step in a damages study is the translation of the legal theory of the harmful event into an analysis of the economic impact of that event. In most cases, the analysis considers the difference between the plaintiff's economic position if the harmful event had not occurred and the plaintiff's actual economic position. The damages study restates the plaintiff's position "but for" the harmful event; this part is often called the *but-for analysis*. Damages are the difference between the but-for value an the actual value.

The "but-for" analysis compares the observed actual world potential outcome with the alleged misconduct to the counterfactual world potential outcome without the alleged misconduct. The difference between the monetary values in these worlds is the basis for calculating damages. This is not necessarily an easy quantity to estimate in the tobacco litigation, but it is the relevant causal estimand (i.e., the causal quantity to be estimated).

1.4. Learning about causal effects: Replication and the stable unit treatment value assumption – SUTVA

How do we learn about causal effects? The answer is replication, more units. The way we personally learn from our own experience is replication involving the same physical object (e.g., you) with more units in time. That is, if I want to learn about the effect of taking aspirin on headaches for me, I learn from replications in time when I do and do not take aspirin to relieve my headache, thereby having some observations of $Y(1)$ and some of $Y(0)$. When we want to generalize to units other than ourselves, we typically use more objects; that is what is done in epidemiology and medical experiments, for example, when studying the causal effects of hormone replacement therapy on post-menopausal women (e.g., Piantadosi, 2003; Whittemore and McGuire, 2003).

Suppose instead of only one unit we have two. Now in general we have at least four potential outcomes for each unit: the outcome for unit 1 if both unit 1 and unit 2 received control, $Y_1(0,0)$; the outcome for unit 1 if both units received the active treatment, $Y_1(1,1)$; the outcome for unit 1 if unit 1 received control and unit 2 active, $Y_1(0,1)$, and the outcome for unit 1 if unit 1 received active and unit 2 received control, $Y_1(1,0)$; and analogously for unit 2 with values $Y_2(0,0)$, etc. In fact, there are even more potential outcomes because there have to be at least two "doses" of the active treatment available to contemplate all assignments, and it could make a difference which one was taken. For example, in the aspirin case, one tablet may be very effective and the other quite ineffective.

Clearly, replication does not help unless we can restrict the explosion of potential outcomes. As in all theoretical work with applied value, simplifying assumptions are crucial. The most straightforward assumption to make is the "stable unit treatment value assumption" (SUTVA – Rubin, 1980, 1990a) under which the potential outcomes for the *i*th unit just depend on the treatment the *i*th unit received. That is, there is "no interference between units" (Cox, 1958) and there are "no unrepresented treatments for any unit". Then, all potential outcomes for N units with two possible treatments can be represented by an array with N rows and two columns, the *i*th unit having a row with two potential outcomes, $Y_i(0)$ and $Y_i(1)$.

Obviously, SUTVA is a major assumption. But there is no assumption-free causal inference, and nothing is wrong with this. It is the quality of the assumptions that matters, not their existence or even their absolute correctness. Good researchers attempt to make such assumptions plausible by the design of their studies. For example, SUTVA becomes more plausible when units are isolated from each other in the schools. For example, when studying an intervention such as a smoking prevention program (e.g., see Peterson et al., 2000), define the units to be intact schools rather than individual students or classes in the schools.

The stability assumption (SUTVA) is very commonly made, even though it is not always appropriate. For example, consider a study of the effect of vaccination on a contagious disease. The greater the proportion of the population that gets vaccinated, the less any unit's chance of contracting the disease, even if not vaccinated—an example of interference. Throughout this chapter, we assume SUTVA, although there are other assumptions that could be made to restrict the exploding number of potential outcomes with replication and no assumptions.

In general, some of the N units may receive neither the active treatment $W_i = 1$ nor the control treatment $W_i = 0$. For example, some of the units may be in the future, as when we want to generalize to a future population. Then formally W_i must take on a third value, $W_i = *$ representing neither 1 nor 0; we often avoid this extra notation here.

1.5. Covariates

In addition to (1) the vector indicator of the treatment for each unit in the study, $W_i = \{W_i\}$, (2) the array of potential outcomes when exposed to the treatment, $Y(1) = \{Y_i(1)\}$, and (3) the array of potential outcomes when not exposed, $Y(0) = \{Y_i(0)\}$, we have (4) an array of covariates $X = \{X_i\}$, which are, by definition, unaffected by treatment, such as pretreatment baseline blood pressure. All causal estimands involve comparisons of $Y_i(0)$ and $Y_i(1)$ on either all N units, or a common subset of units; for example, the average causal effect across all units that are female as indicated by their X_i, or the median causal effect for units with X_i indicating male and $Y_i(0)$ indicating unacceptably high blood pressure after exposure to the control treatment.

Thus, under SUTVA, all causal estimands can be calculated from the matrix of "scientific values" with *i*th row: $(X_i, Y_i(0), Y_i(0))$. By definition, all relevant information is encoded in X_i, $Y_i(0)$, $Y_i(1)$ and so the labeling of the N rows is a random permutation of 1, ..., N. In other words, the N-row array

$$(X,\ Y(0),\ Y(1)) = \begin{bmatrix} X_1 & Y_1(0) & Y_1(1) \\ & \vdots & \\ X_i & Y_i(0) & Y_i(1) \\ & \vdots & \\ X_N & Y_N(0) & Y_N(1) \end{bmatrix}$$

is row exchangeable. We call this array "the Science" because its values are beyond our control; by changing treatments, we get to change which values are actually observed, but not the values themselves. That is, the observed values of Y are $Y_{obs} = \{Y_{obs,i}\}$, where $Y_{obs,i} = Y_i(1)W_i + Y_i(0)(1-W_i)$.

Covariates (such as age, race and sex) play a particularly important role in observational studies for causal effects where they are often known as possible "confounders" or "risk factors" in epidemiology and medical statistics. In some studies, the units exposed to the active treatment differ on their distribution of covariates in important ways from the units not exposed. To see how this issue influences our formal framework, we must define the "assignment mechanism", the probabilistic mechanism that determines which units get the active version of the treatment and which units get the control version. The assignment mechanism is the topic of Section 2.

1.6. A brief history of the potential outcomes framework

The basic idea that causal effects are the comparisons of potential outcomes seems so direct that it must have ancient roots, and we can find elements of this definition of causal effects among both experimenters and philosophers. See, for example, the philosopher John Stuart Mill, who, when discussing Hume's views, offers (Mill, 1973, p. 327):

> If a person eats of a particular dish, and dies in consequence, that is, would not have died if he had not eaten of it, people would be apt to say that eating of that dish was the source of his death.

And Fisher (1918, p. 214) wrote:

> If we say, "This boy has grown tall because he has been well fed," we are not merely tracing out the cause and effect in an individual instance; we are suggesting that he might quite probably have been worse fed, and that in this case he would have been shorter.

Despite the insights evident in these quotations, apparently there was no formal notation for potential outcomes until Neyman (1923), which appears to have been the first place where a mathematical analysis is written for a randomized experiment with explicit notation for the potential outcomes. This notation became standard for work in randomized experiments from the randomization-based perspective (e.g., Pitman, 1937; Welch, 1937; McCarthy, 1939; Anscombe, 1948; Kempthorne, 1952; Cox, 1958; Hodges and Lehmann, 1970, Section 9.4; Brillinger et al., 1978). Neyman's formalism was a major advance because it allowed explicit frequentist probabilistic causal inferences to be drawn from data obtained by a randomized experiment, an approach discussed in Section 3.

Independently and nearly simultaneously, Fisher (1925) created a somewhat different method of inference for randomized experiments, also based on the special class of randomized assignment mechanisms; Fisher's approach is also discussed in Section 3. The notion of the central role of randomized experiments seems to have been "in the air" in the 1920s, but Fisher was apparently the first to recommend the actual physical randomization of treatments to units and then use this randomization to justify theoretically an analysis of the resultant data, a point emphasized by Neyman (1935, p. 109; also see Reid, 1982, p. 45).

Despite the almost immediate acceptance in the late 1920s of Fisher's proposal for randomized experiments and Neyman's notation for potential outcomes in randomized experiments, this same framework was not used outside randomized experiments for a half century thereafter, apparently not until Rubin (1974), and these insights therefore were entirely limited to randomization-based frequency inference.

The approach used in nonrandomized settings during the half century following the introduction of Neyman's seminal notation for randomized experiments was based on mathematical models relating the observed value of the outcome variable $Y_{\text{obs},i}$ to covariates and indicators for the treatment received, and then to define causal effects as parameters in these models. This approach is illustrated by the Lord's Paradox example in Section 2.2. The same statistician would simultaneously use Neyman's potential outcomes to define causal effects in randomized experiments and the observed outcome setup in observational studies. This led to substantial confusion because the role of randomization cannot even be stated using the observed outcome notation.

The framework that we describe here that uses potential outcomes to define causal effects in general is the first part of the RCM. This perspective conceives of all problems of statistical inference for causal effects as missing data problems with a mechanism for creating missing data in the potential outcomes (Rubin, 1976a). Of course, there were seeds of the RCM before 1974, including the aforementioned Neyman (1923), but also Tinbergen (1930), Haavelmo (1944) and Hurwicz (1962) in economics. Also see Imbens and Rubin (2007b) for further discussion.

The potential outcomes framework seems to have been basically accepted and adopted by most workers by the end of the twentieth century. Sometimes the move was made explicitly, as with Pratt and Schlaifer (1984) who moved from the "observed outcome" to the potential outcomes framework in Pratt and Schlaifer (1988). Sometimes it was made less explicitly as with those who were still trying to make a version of the observed outcome notation work in the late 1980s (e.g., see Heckman and Hotz, 1989), before fully accepting the RCM in subsequent work (e.g., Heckman, 1989, after discussion by Holland, 1989).

The movement to use potential outcomes to define causal inference problems seems to be the dominant one at the start of the 21st century, especially in epidemiology and medical statistics, as well as in the behavioral sciences. See for example, Baker (1998), Dempster (1990), Efron and Feldman (1991), Gelman and King (1991), Greenland and Poole (1988), Greenland et al. (1999), Holland (1988a, 1988b), Kadane and Seidenfeld (1990), Robins (1989), Rosenbaum (1987, 2002), Smith and Sugden (1988), Sobel (1990, 1995, 1996), Sugden (1988) and their references. A recent article exploring whether the full potential outcomes framework can be avoided when conducting causal inference is Dawid (2000) with discussion. Also see Cox (1992) and Rubin (2005) on this perspective and other perspectives.

2. The assignment mechanism

Even with SUTVA, inference for causal effects requires the specification of an assignment mechanism: a probabilistic model for how some units were selected to receive the active treatment and how other units were selected to receive the control treatment. We first illustrate this model in two trivial artificial examples, and then present formal notation for this model. The formalization of the assignment mechanism is the second part of the RCM.

2.1. Illustrating the criticality of the assignment mechanism

Consider a doctor who is considering one of two medical operations to apply to each of her eight patients, a standard one and a new one. This doctor is a great doctor: she chooses the treatment that is best for each patient! When they are equally effective, she effectively tosses a fair coin. Table 1 gives the hypothetical potential outcomes in years lived post-operation under each treatment for these eight patients, and so also gives their individual causal effects. The column

Table 1
Perfect doctor example

	Potential Outcomes		Observed Data		
	$Y(0)$	$Y(1)$	W	$Y(0)$	$Y(1)$
	13	14	1	?	14
	6	0	0	6	?
	4	1	0	4	?
	5	2	0	5	?
	6	3	0	6	?
	6	1	0	6	?
	8	10	1	?	10
	8	9	1	?	9
True averages	7	5	Observed averages	5.4	11

labelled "*W*" shows which treatment each patient received, $W_i = 0$ or $W_i = 1$ for the *i*th patient, and the final columns show the observed potential outcomes.

Notice that the averages of the $Y_i(0)$ and $Y_i(1)$ potential outcomes indicate that the typical patient will do better with the standard operation: the average causal effect is two years of life in favor of the standard. But the doctor, who is conducting ideal medical practice for the benefit of her patients, reaches the opposite conclusion from an examination of the observed data: the patients assigned the new operation live, on average, twice as long as the patients assigned the standard operation, with absolutely no overlap in their distributions! Moreover, if the doctor now applies the new treatment to all patients in a population of patients who are just like the eight in the study, she will be disappointed: the average life span post-operation will be closer to five years under the new operation rather than the eleven years seen in this study.

What is wrong? The simple comparison of observed results assumes that treatments were *randomly assigned*, rather than as they were, to provide maximal benefit to the patients. We will have more to say about randomized experiments, but the point here is simply that the assignment mechanism is crucial to valid inference about causal effects, and the doctor used a "nonignorable" assignment mechanism (formally defined in Section 2.4). With a posited assignment mechanism, it is possible to draw causal inferences; without one, it is impossible. It is in this sense that, when drawing inferences, a model for the assignment mechanism is more fundamental than a "scientific" model for the potential outcomes: Without positing an assignment mechanism, we basically cannot draw causal inferences.

More precisely, notice that the doctor, by comparing observed means, is using the three observed values of $Y_i(1)$ to represent the five missing values of $Y_i(1)$, effectively imputing, or filling in, the mean observed $Y_i(1)$, $\bar{y}_1$, for the five $Y_i(1)$ question marks, and analogously effectively filling in $\bar{y}_0$ for the three $Y_i(0)$ question marks. This process makes sense for point estimation if the three observed values of $Y_i(1)$ were randomly chosen from the eight values of $Y_i(1)$, and the five observed values of $Y_i(0)$ were randomly chose from the eight values of $Y_i(0)$. But under the actual assignment mechanism, it does not. It would obviously make much more sense under the actual assignment mechanism to impute the missing potential outcome for each patient to be less than or equal to that patient's observed potential outcome.

2.2. Lord's paradox

We now consider a "paradox" in causal inference that is easily resolved with the simple ideas we have already presented, despite the controversy that it engendered in some literatures. This example illustrates how important it is to keep this perspective clearly in mind when thinking about causal effects of interventions and when reading the remainder of this chapter. Lord (1967) proposed the following example:

> A large university is interested in investigating the effects on the students of the diet provided in the university dining halls and any sex differences in these

> effects. Various types of data are gathered. In particular, the weight of each student at the time of arrival in September and the following June are recorded.

The result of the study for the males is that their average weight is identical at the end of the school year to what it was at the beginning; in fact, the whole distribution of weights is unchanged, although some males lost weight and some males gained weight – the gains and losses exactly balance. The same thing is true for the females. The only difference is that the females started and ended the year lighter on average than the males. On average, there is no weight gain or weight loss for either males or females. From Lord's description of the problem quoted above, the quantity to be estimated, the estimand, is the difference between the causal effect of the university diet on males and the causal effect of the university diet on females. That is, the causal estimand is the difference between the causal effects for males and females, the "differential" causal effect.

The paradox is generated by considering the contradictory conclusions of two statisticians asked to comment on the data. Statistician 1 *observes* that there are no differences between the September and June weight distributions for either males or females. Thus, Statistician 1 concludes that

> as far as these data are concerned, there is no evidence of any interesting effect of diet (or of anything else) on student weight. In particular, there is no evidence of any differential effect on the two sexes, since neither group shows any systematic change. (p. 305).

Statistician 2 looks at the data in a more "sophisticated" way. Effectively, he examines males and females with about the same initial weight in September, say a subgroup of "overweight" females (meaning simply above-average-weight females) and a subgroup of "underweight" males (analogously defined). He notices that these males tended to gain weight on average and these females tended to lose weight on average. He also notices that this result is true no matter what group of initial weights he focuses on. (Actually, Lord's Statistician 2 used covariance adjustment, i.e., regression adjustment.) His conclusion, therefore, is that after "controlling for" initial weight, the diet has a differential positive effect on males relative to females because for males and females with the same initial weight, on average the males gain more than the females.

Who's right? Statistician 1 or Statistician 2? Notice the focus of both statisticians on gain scores and recall that gain scores are not causal effects because they do not compare potential outcomes. If both statisticians confined their comments to *describing* the data, both would be correct, but for causal inference, both are wrong because these data cannot support any causal conclusions about the effect of the diet without making some very strong assumptions.

Back to the basics. The units are obviously the students, and the time of application of treatment (the university diet) is clearly September and the time of the recording of the outcome Y is clearly June; accept the stability assumption. Now, what are the potential outcomes and what is the assignment mechanism? Notice that Lord's statement of the problem has reverted to the already criticized observed outcome notation, Y_{obs}, rather than the potential outcome notation being advocated here.

The potential outcomes are June weight under the university diet $Y_i(1)$ and under the "control" diet $Y_i(0)$. The covariates are sex of students, male versus female, and September weight. But the assignment mechanism has assigned everyone to the active treatment! There is no one, male or female, who is assigned to the control treatment. Hence, there is absolutely no purely empirical basis on which to compare the effects, either raw or differential, of the university diet with the control diet. By making the problem complicated with the introduction of the covariates "male/female" and "initial weight", Lord has created partial confusion. For more statistical details of the resolution of this paradox, see Holland and Rubin (1983), and for earlier related discussion, see for example, Lindley and Novick (1981) or Cox and McCullagh (1982). But the point here is that the "paradox" is immediately resolved through the explicit use of potential outcomes. Either statistician's answer could be correct for causal inference depending on what we are willing to assume about the potential outcomes under the control diet, which are entirely missing.

2.3. Unconfounded and strongly ignorable assignment mechanisms

We have seen that a model for the assignment mechanism is needed for statistical inference for causal effects. The assignment mechanism gives the conditional probability of each vector of assignments given the covariates and potential outcomes:

$$\Pr(W|X, Y(0), Y(1)). \tag{1}$$

Here W is a N by 1 vector and, as earlier, X, $Y(1)$ and $Y(0)$ are all matrices with N rows. A specific example of an assignment mechanism is a completely randomized experiment with N units, where $n<N$ are assigned to the active treatment, and $N-n$ to the control treatment:

$$\Pr(W|X, Y(0), Y(1)) = \begin{array}{ll} 1/C_n^N & \text{if } \Sigma W_i = n \\ 0 & \text{otherwise.} \end{array} \tag{2}$$

An "unconfounded assignment mechanism" (Rubin, 1990b) is free of dependence on either $Y(0)$ or $Y(1)$:

$$\Pr(W|X, Y(0), Y(1)) = \Pr(W|X). \tag{3}$$

The assignment mechanism is "probabilistic" if each unit has a positive probability of receiving either treatment:

$$0<\Pr(W_i = 1|X, Y(0), Y(1))<1. \tag{4}$$

If the assignment mechanism is unconfounded and probabilistic, it is called "strongly ignorable" (Rosenbaum and Rubin, 1983a), a stronger version of ignorable, defined in Section 2.4.

The assignment mechanism is fundamental to causal inference because it tells us how we got to see what we saw. Because causal inference is basically a missing data problem with at least half of the potential outcomes missing, when we have no understanding of the process that creates missing data, we have no hope of inferring anything about the missing values. That is, without a stochastic model for how treatments are assigned to individuals, formal causal inference, at least using probabilistic statements, is impossible. This statement does not mean that we need to know the assignment mechanism, but rather that without positing one, we cannot make any statistical claims about causal effects, such as unbiased estimation or the coverage of confidence intervals or the coverage of Bayesian posterior intervals, all defined in Sections 3 and 4.

Strongly ignorable assignment mechanisms often allow particularly straightforward estimation of causal effects from all perspectives, as we see shortly. Therefore, these assignment mechanisms form the basis for inference for causal effects in more complicated situations, such as when assignment probabilities depend on covariates in unknown ways, or when there is noncompliance with the assigned treatment. Strongly ignorable (i.e., probabilistic unconfounded) assignment mechanisms, which essentially are collections of separate completely randomized experiments at each value of X_i with a distinct probability of treatment assignment, form the basis for the analysis of observational nonrandomized studies, as we see in Section 3.

2.4. *Confounded and ignorable assignment mechanisms*

A confounded assignment mechanism is one that depends on the potential outcomes:

$$\Pr(W|X, Y(0), Y(1)) \neq \Pr(W|X). \tag{5}$$

A special class of possibly confounded assignment mechanisms is particularly important to Bayesian inference: ignorable assignment mechanisms (Rubin, 1978). Ignorable assignment mechanisms are defined by their freedom from dependence on any *missing* potential outcomes:

$$\Pr(W|X, Y(0), Y(1)) = \Pr(W|X, Y_{\text{obs}}). \tag{6}$$

Ignorable confounded assignment mechanisms arise in practice, especially in sequential experiments. Here, the next unit's probability of being exposed to the active treatment depends on the observed outcomes of those previously exposed to the active treatment versus the observed outcomes of those exposed to the control treatment, as in "play-the-winner" sequential designs (e.g., see Chernoff, 1959): expose the next patient with higher probability to whichever treatment appears to be more successful, as in the initial extracorporeal membrane oxygenation (ECMO) experiment (e.g., Ware, 1989).

All unconfounded assignment mechanisms are ignorable, but not all ignorable assignment mechanisms are unconfounded (e.g., play-the-winner designs). Seeing why ignorable and strongly ignorable assignment mechanisms play critical roles in causal inference is easily seen in the two trivial examples in

Sections 2.1 and 2.2: The first, "the perfect doctor", involved a nonignorable treatment assignment mechanism, and the second, "Lord's paradox", involved an unconfounded but nonprobabilistic assignment mechanism, and so was not strongly ignorable.

3. Assignment-based modes of causal inference

Fundamentally, there are three formal statistical modes of causal inference; one is Bayesian, discussed in Section 4, which treats the potential outcomes as random variables, and two are based only on the assignment mechanism, which treat the potential outcomes as fixed but unknown quantities. Rubin (1990b) describes these three as well as a combination, which is fundamentally not as conceptually tight, and so is not discussed here as a distinct mode. Of the two distinct forms of assignment-based inference, one is due to Neyman (1923) and the other is due to Fisher (1925). Both will first be described in the absence of covariates, X. The assignment-based modes as developed by Fisher and Neyman were randomization-based modes of inference because they both assumed randomized experiments. Our presentation is a generalization of those randomization-based modes.

3.1. Fisherian randomization-based inference

Fisher's approach is the more direct conceptually and is therefore introduced first. It is closely related to the mathematical idea of proof by contradiction. It basically is a "stochastic proof by contradiction" giving the significance level (or p-value) – really, the plausibility – of the "null hypothesis", which often is that there is absolutely no treatment effect whatsoever. Fisher's method only works for the set of units with $W_i = 1$ or 0, and not for units with $W_i = *$, so in this subsection, we assume that all units are exposed to either the active treatment or the control treatment.

The first element in Fisher's mode of inference is the null hypothesis, which is usually that $Y_i(1) \equiv Y_i(0)$ for all units: the treatment has absolutely no effect on the potential outcomes. Under this null hypothesis, all potential outcomes are known from the observed values of the potential outcomes, Y_{obs}, because $Y(1) \equiv Y(0) \equiv Y_{\text{obs}}$. It follows that, under this null hypothesis, the value of any statistic, S, such as the difference of the observed averages for units exposed to treatment 1 and units exposed to treatment 0, $\bar{y}_1 - \bar{y}_0$, is known, not only for the observed assignment, but for all possible assignments W.

Suppose we choose a statistic, S such as $\bar{y}_1 - \bar{y}_0$, and calculate its value under each possible assignment (assuming the null hypothesis) and also calculate the probability of each assignment under the randomized assignment mechanism. In many classical experiments, these probabilities are either zero or a common value for all possible assignments. For example, in a completely randomized experiment with $N = 2n$ units, n are randomly chosen to receive treatment 1 and n to receive treatment 0. Then any assignment W that has n 1's and n 0's has probability $1/C_n^N$, and all other Ws have zero probability. Knowing the value of S

for each W and its probability, we can then calculate the probability (under the assignment mechanism and the null hypothesis) that we would observe a value of S as "unusual" as, or more unusual than, the observed value of S, S_{obs}. "Unusual" is defined *a priori*, typically by how discrepant S_{obs} is from zero. This probability is the plausibility (p-value or significance level) of the observed value of the statistic S under the null hypothesis: the probability of a result (represented by the value S_{obs} of the statistic, S) as rare, or more rare, than the actual observed result if the null hypothesis were true, where the probability is over the distribution induced by the assignment mechanism.

This form of inference is elegant: Unless the data suggest that the null hypothesis of absolutely no treatment effect is false (for an appropriate choice of statistic, S), it is not easy to claim evidence for differing efficacies of the active and control treatments.

Fisher's approach can be extended to other "sharp" null hypotheses, that is, a null hypothesis such that from knowledge of Y_{obs}, the values of $Y(1)$ and $Y(0)$ are known; e.g., an additive null, which asserts that for each unit, $Y_i(1)-Y_i(0)$ is a specified constant, e.g., 3. The collection of such null hypotheses that do not lead to an extreme p-value can be used to create interval estimates of the causal effect assuming additivity. Extensions to other statistics and other fully specified assignment mechanisms, including unconfounded and even nonignorable ones, are immediate, because all potential outcomes are known from Y_{obs}, and thus the probabilities of any assignment are known; Fisher, however, never discussed such extensions. Notice that Fisher's perspective provides no ability to generalize beyond the units in the experiment, nor to consider "nuisance" null hypotheses when there are multiple treatments, as in factorial designs (e.g., Cochran and Cox, 1957). These limitations are not present in Neyman's approach.

3.2. *Neymanian randomization-based inference*

Neyman's form of randomization-based inference can be viewed as drawing inferences by evaluating the expectations of statistics over the distribution induced by the assignment mechanism in order to calculate a confidence interval for the typical causal effect. The essential idea is the same as in Neyman's (1934) classic article on randomization-based (now often called "designed-based") inference in surveys. Typically, an unbiased estimator of the causal estimand (the typical causal effect, e.g., the average, the median) is created. Second, an unbiased, or upwardly biased, estimator of the variance of that unbiased estimator is found (bias and variance both defined with respect to the randomization distribution). Then, an appeal is made to the central limit theorem for the normality of the estimator over its randomization distribution, whence a confidence interval for the causal estimand is obtained.

To be more explicit, the causal estimand is typically the average causal effect $\overline{Y(1)} - \overline{Y(0)}$, where the averages are over all units in the population being studied, and the traditional statistic for estimating this effect is the difference in observed sample averages for the two groups, $\bar{y}_1 - \bar{y}_0$, which can be shown to be unbiased for $\overline{Y(1)} - \overline{Y(0)}$ in a completely randomized design. A common choice for estimating the variance of $\bar{y}_1 - \bar{y}_0$ over its randomization distribution, in completely randomized experiments with $N = n_1 + n_0$ units, is $se^2 = s_1^2/n_1 + s_0^2/n_0$, where s_1^2, s_0^2, n_1 and n_0 are the observed sample variances and sample sizes in the two treatment groups. Neyman (1923) showed that se^2 overestimates the actual variance of $\bar{y}_1 - \bar{y}_0$, unless additivity holds (i.e., unless all individual causal effects are constant), in which case se^2 is unbiased for the variance of $\bar{y}_1 - \bar{y}_0$. The standard 95% confidence interval for $\overline{Y(1)} - \overline{Y(0)}$ is $\bar{y}_1 - \bar{y}_0 \pm 1.96\, se$, which, in large enough samples, includes $\overline{Y(1)} - \overline{Y(0)}$ in at least 95% of the possible random assignments.

Neyman's form of inference is less direct than Fisher's. It is really aimed at evaluations of procedures: In repeated applications, how often does the interval $\bar{y}_1 - \bar{y}_0 \pm 1.96\, se$ include $\overline{Y(1)} - \overline{Y(0)}$? Nevertheless, it forms the theoretical foundation for much of what is done in important areas of application, including in medical experiments. However, Neyman's approach is not prescriptive in the sense of telling us what to do to create an inferential procedure, but rather it tells us how to evaluate a proposed procedure for drawing causal inferences. Thus, it really is not well suited to deal with complicated problems except in the sense of telling us how to evaluate proposed answers that are obtained by insight or another method. Fisher's approach also suffers from this disadvantage of lack of prescription, in fact, more so, because there is little guidance in Fisher's approach for which test statistics to use or how to define "more unusual".

3.3. *The role for covariates in randomized experiments*

As stated earlier, covariates are variables whose values are not affected by the treatment assignment, for example, variables where values are determined before randomization into treatment groups (e.g., year of birth, baseline blood pressure or cholesterol). In classical randomized experiments, if a covariate is used in the assignment mechanism, as with a blocking variable in a randomized block design, that covariate must be reflected in the analysis because it affects the randomization distribution induced by the assignment mechanism. Also, covariates can be used to increase efficiency of estimation, even when not used in the assignment mechanism.

The point about efficiency gains can be seen in the context of a completely randomized experiment in medicine with X = baseline cholesterol and Y post-treatment cholesteroll. From either the Fisherian or Neymanian perspectives, we can use covariates to define a new statistic to estimate causal estimands. For example, one can use the difference in average observed cholesterol reduction, $(\bar{y}_1 - \bar{x}_1) - (\bar{y}_0 - \bar{x}_0)$ – where $\bar{x}_1$ and $\bar{x}_0$ are the average observed X values for those exposed to $W = 1$ and $W = 0$, respectively – rather than the difference in average Y values, $\bar{y}_1 - \bar{y}_0$, to estimate $\overline{Y(1)} - \overline{Y(0)}$. Suppose X and Y are correlated, which is to be expected for baseline and post-treatment cholesterol. From the Neymanian perspective, the variance of the difference in average $Y{-}X$ change should be less than the variance of the difference in average Y values, which translates into smaller estimated variances and therefore shorter confidence intervals. From the Fisherian perspective, this reduced variance translates into more significant p-values when the null hypothesis is false.

This point is easily seen in examples. Suppose as an extreme case, the new treatment subtracts essentially 10 points from everyone's baseline cholesterol, whereas the old treatment does nothing. The observed $Y-X$ changes have essentially zero variance in each treatment group, whereas the Y values have the same variances in each treatment group as the X values. This result means that the Neymanian confidence interval for the treatment effect based on the average treated minus control difference in $Y-X$ changes is much shorter than the corresponding interval based on Y values. Also, the observed value of the difference of $Y-X$ changes is the most extreme value that can be observed under Fisher's null hypothesis, and so the observed result with $Y-X$ changes is as significant as possible, which is not true for the difference in Y values.

3.4. Propensity scores

Suppose that the assignment mechanism is unconfounded:

$$\Pr(W|X(1), Y(0)) = \Pr(W|X),$$

(e.g., older males have probability .8 of being assigned the new treatment; younger males, .6; older females, .5; and younger females, .2), and that for some $W \in \mathscr{W}$, $\Pr(W|X) > 0$ and for all other $W \in \mathscr{W}$, $\Pr(W|X) = 0$, for example in completely randomized experiments with $N = 2\,\mathrm{n}$ units, $\mathscr{W}$ includes W such that $\Sigma_1^N W_i = n$. Because of the random indexing of units, by appealing to de Finetti's theorem (1963), we can write $\Pr(W|X)$ as

$$\Pr(W|X) \propto \int \prod_1^N e(X_i|\phi)\pi(\phi)\mathrm{d}\phi, \quad \text{for } W \in \mathscr{W}, \tag{7}$$

where the function $e(X_i|\phi)$ gives the probability that a unit with value X_i of the covariate has $W_i = 1$ as a function of the parameter ϕ with prior (or marginal) probability density function $\pi(\phi)$.

Assignment mechanisms for which the representation in Eq. (7) is true have $0 < e(X_i|\phi) < 1$ (for all X_i,ϕ) and are called "regular", whether or not the functions $e(\cdot \mid \phi)$ and $\pi(\phi)$ are known, and are strongly ignorable. The unit-level assignment probabilities, $e_i = e(X_i|\phi)$, are called propensity scores (Rosenbaum and Rubin, 1983a). Regular designs are the major template for the analysis of observational, nonrandomized studies, and propensity scores are the key ingredients of regular designs. That is, even with an observational data set, we try to structure the problem so that we can conceptualize at least some of the data as having arisen from an underlying regular assignment mechanism. Three situations need to be distinguished when this assumption is accepted for some set of units: (1) The propensity scores are known, that is, the function $\pi(\phi)$ and the parameter ϕ are known; (2) the functional form $e(X_i|\phi)$ is known, but ϕ is not; and (3) the functional form, $e(X_i|\phi)$, is unknown. When the assignment mechanism is not known to be unconfounded, we typically begin by assuming that (7) holds for some set of units, if this assumption is at all plausible.

3.5. Known propensity scores

When the propensity scores are known, the assignment mechanism is known except for the set $\mathcal{W}$. As a result, simple generalizations of Fisherian and Neymanian modes of inference can be applied, for example, by considering the number of treated ΣW_i and number of controls $\Sigma(1-W_i)$ to be fixed by design, thereby determining $\mathcal{W}$. In particular, Horvitz–Thompson (1952) estimation (or ratio-adjusted versions, see Cochran, 1963), where observations are weighted by the inverse probabilities of their being observed, play an important role for both randomization-based modes of inference because the resulting estimates are unbiased for average treatment effects over the randomization distribution with no modeling assumptions. As the overlap in propensity scores in the treatment and control groups becomes more limited (i.e., as propensity scores approach zero or one), the Neymanian variance of the estimator for the average causal effect increases, with the result that confidence intervals become wider, and the Fisherian randomization distribution has more of its probability mass on the observed randomization, with the result that it becomes more difficult to get a "significant" p-value. If there is no, or little, overlap of the propensity scores in the treatment groups, no sharp causal inference is possible using the basic Fisherian or Neymanian perspectives. This is a critical issue that researchers must appreciate, no matter what their field is.

In general, with the assignment-based modes of inference and known propensity scores that take many values, it is often acceptable to create several (e.g., 5–10) subclasses of propensity scores to approximate a randomized block experiment (i.e., a series of completely randomized experiments with different propensities across them). This conclusion is based on Cochran's (1968) basic investigation, but more subclasses should be used with larger samples. Alternatively, pairs of treatment-control units can be created that are matched on the propensity scores, thereby approximating a paired comparison experiment.

3.6. Unknown propensity scores, but regular design

When the propensity scores are unknown, but the function $e(X_i|\phi)$ is known, the obvious first step is to estimate them, i.e., estimate ϕ, and thereby e_i, typically using maximum likelihood estimates of ϕ. When the function $e(X_i|\phi)$ is not known, various methods can be used to estimate propensity scores (e.g., discriminant analysis, logistic regression, probit regression). In either case, typically, estimated propensity scores are used as if they were known, and often this leads to more precision than using true propensity scores (Rubin and Thomas, 1992a).

Generally, with a design that is known to be regular, the issues that arise with estimated propensity scores are the same as with known ones, and the reduction to a paired-comparison or randomized-block design is acceptable when there is enough overlap in the estimated propensity scores. A common technique is the use of matched sampling to create treated-control pairs whose values of X are "close". Typically, each treated unit is matched to one "close" control unit, and the unused control units are discarded, thereby accepting (7) for the set of matched units. Various definitions of "close" can be formulated: there are techniques for scalar X (Rubin, 1973); ones for multivariate X summarized by the scalar (estimated) propensity score or best linear discriminant (Cochran and Rubin, 1973; Rosenbaum and Rubin, 1983a), or using multivariate metrics, such as the Mahalanobis metric (Rubin, 1976b, 1976c, 1979b); or methods can be combined, such as Mahalanobis metric matching within propensity score calipers (Rosenbaum and Rubin, 1985; Rubin and Thomas, 1996).

The closely related technique of subclassification is also commonly used when no control units are to be discarded, as discussed years ago in Cochran (1968). Subclassification is used to reconstruct an underlying, hypothetical, randomized block design, sometimes after discarding some units so that (7) is acceptable for the remaining units.

Some theoretical results, for instance, concerning "Equal Percent Bias Reducing" (EPBR, Rubin, 1976b, 1976c) matching methods are important, as are extensions involving affinely invariant matching methods with ellipsoidal distributions (Rubin and Thomas, 1992b) and further extensions involving discriminant mixtures of ellipsoidal distributions (Rubin and Stuart, 2006). Much of this previous work is collected in Rubin (2006c). Other important work involves consideration of optimal matching and full matching (Gu and Rosenbaum, 1993; Ming and Rosenbaum, 2000; Rosenbaum, 1989, 1991, 1995, 2002). Much work is currently taking place on theoretical and computational aspects of matching algorithms, much of it in social science, including economics (e.g., see page 1 of Rubin, 2006b, for a list of some references).

3.7. *Observational studies – possibly confounded*

To draw statistical inferences in observational studies, a model for the assignment mechanism is needed, and this defines the template into which we can map the data from an observational study. That is, we need to posit a particular form for the assignment mechanism, and the major template that we try to use is the class of complicated randomized experiments, i.e., regular designs. Although designs that are known to be regular but that have unknown propensity scores are not that common in practice (because of the need to know all covariates used in the assignment mechanism), they are the most critical template for inference for causal effects from observational data. That is, we attempt to assemble data with enough covariates that it becomes plausible (or initially arguable) that the unknown assignment mechanism is unconfounded given these covariates. Then an observational study can be analyzed using the techniques for a regular design with unknown propensity scores. The resulting causal inferences will be valid under the assumption of strong ignorability given the observed covariates.

That is, we begin by estimating propensity scores. If there is little or no overlap in the distributions of the estimated propensity scores in the treatment and control groups, the data appear to arise from a nonprobabilistic assignment mechanism, and there is no hope for drawing valid causal inferences from these data without making strong external assumptions (i.e., questionable modeling assumptions on the science). The message that sometimes a data set cannot support a decent causal inference is very important for all researchers to understand and accept.

The desirability of discarding irrelevant units from the control group is also an important point to recognize. For example, in the tobacco litigation (Rubin, 2002), nonsmokers who have characteristics not matching any smokers were discarded. Sometimes it may even be necessary to discard some treated units as "unmatchable", and then their characteristics should be carefully described because of the limitations on generalization of results. A recent example of the discarding of some treated patients is Karkouti et al. (2006), which presents an observational study comparing the use of "aprotinin" with "tranexamic acid" during coronary bypass surgery. Here, 10,870 patients were available for analysis: 586 treated with aprotinin, and the remaining 10,284 controls treated with tranexamic acid. After propensity score matching on a variety of important pre-operation background variables, 137 aprotinin patients were considered unmatchable despite the 20:1 ratio of controls to treated.

Sometimes subclassification can be used. The example in Rubin (1997) on treatments for breast cancer compares results from randomized experiments and an observational study based on subclassification, and suggests that this approach can work well in practice in certain situations. Also, see Dehijia and Wahba (1999) and Shadish and Clark (2006) for further support for this assertion in the context of examples from economics and education, respectively.

A key idea is that, like good experiments, good observational studies are designed, not simply "found". When designing an experiment, we do not have any outcome data, but we plan the collection, organization and analysis of the data to improve our chances of obtaining valid, reliable and precise causal answers. The same exercise should be done in an observational study: Even if outcome data are available at the design stage, they should be put aside. This theme is emphasized in Rubin (2007) and applied in Langenskold and Rubin (2008).

Because observational studies are rarely known to be unconfounded, we are concerned with sensitivity of answers to unobserved covariates. Because in my view, this and other complications are better dealt with from the model-based perspective, these are addressed after discussing Bayesian methods, although methods for sensitivity analyses described by Rosenbaum (2002) are appropriate from the randomization-based perspective.

4. Posterior predictive causal inference

Bayesian inference for causal effects requires a model for the underlying data, $\Pr(X, Y(0), Y(1))$, and this is where "science" enters, and is the third, and optional, part of the RCM. A virtue of the RCM framework is that it separates science – a model for the underlying data, from what we do to learn about science – the assignment mechanism, $\Pr(W|X, Y(0), Y(1))$. Notice that together, these two models specify a joint distribution for all observables, an approach commonly called Bayesian.

4.1. The posterior predictive distribution of causal effects

Bayesian inference for causal effects directly and explicitly confronts the missing potential outcomes, $Y_{\text{mis}} = \{Y_{\text{mis},i}\}$, where $Y_{\text{mis},i} = W_i Y_i(0) + (1 - W_i) Y_i(1)$. The perspective takes the specification for the assignment mechanism and the specification for the underlying data, and derives the posterior predictive distribution of Y_{mis}, that is, the distribution of Y_{mis} given all observed values:

$$\Pr(Y_{\text{mis}} | X, Y_{\text{obs}}, W). \tag{8}$$

This distribution is posterior because it is conditional on all observed values (X, Y_{obs}, W) and predictive because it predicts (stochastically) the missing potential outcomes. From (a) this distribution, (b) the observed values of the potential outcomes, Y_{obs}, (c) the observed assignments, W, and (d) the observed covariates, X, the posterior distribution of any causal effect can, in principle, be calculated.

This conclusion is immediate if we view the posterior predictive distribution in Eq. (8) as specifying how to take a random draw of Y_{mis}. Once a value of Y_{mis} is drawn, any causal effect can be directly calculated from the drawn value of Y_{mis} and the observed values of X and Y_{obs}, e.g., the median causal effect for males: $\text{med}\{Y_i(1) - Y_i(0) | X_i \text{ indicate males}\}$. Repeatedly drawing values of Y_{mis} and calculating the causal effect for each draw generates the posterior distribution of the desired causal effect. Thus, we can view causal inference entirely as a missing data problem, where we multiply impute (Rubin, 1987, 2004b) the missing potential outcomes to generate a posterior distribution for the causal effects. We now describe how to generate these imputations. A great advantage of this general approach is that we can model the data on one scale (e.g., log (income) is normal), impute on that scale, but transform the imputations before drawing inferences on another scale (e.g., raw dollars).

4.2. The posterior predictive distribution of Y_{mis} under ignorable treatment assignment

First consider how to create the posterior predictive distribution of Y_{mis} when the treatment assignment mechanism is ignorable (i.e., when Eq. (6) holds). In general:

$$\Pr(Y_{\text{mis}} | X, Y_{\text{obs}}, W) = \frac{\Pr(X, Y(0), Y(1)) \Pr(W | X, Y(0), Y(1))}{\int \Pr(X, Y(0), Y(1)) \Pr(W | X, Y(0), Y(1)) \mathrm{d} Y_{\text{mis}}}. \tag{9}$$

With ignorable treatment assignment, Eq. (9) becomes:

$$\Pr(Y_{\text{mis}} | X, Y_{\text{obs}}, W) = \frac{\Pr(X, Y(0), Y(1))}{\int \Pr(X, Y(0), X(1)) \mathrm{d} Y_{\text{mis}}}. \tag{10}$$

Equation (10) reveals that, under ignorability, all that we need model is the science $\Pr(X, Y(0), Y(1))$.

4.3. de Finetti's theorem applied to model the data

Because all information is in the underlying data, the unit labels are effectively just random numbers, and hence the array $(X, Y(0), Y(1))$ is row exchangeable. With essentially no loss of generality, therefore, by de Finetti's (1963) theorem, we have that the distribution of $(X, Y(0), Y(1))$ may be taken to be iid (independent and identically distributed) given some parameter θ, with prior distribution $p(\theta)$:

$$\Pr(X, Y(0), Y(1)) = \int \left[\prod_{i=1}^{N} f(X_i, Y_i(0), Y_i(1)|\theta) \right] p(\theta)\mathrm{d}(\theta). \tag{11}$$

Equation (11) provides the bridge between fundamental theory and the common practice of using iid models. Of course, there remains the critical point that the functions $f(\cdot \mid \theta)$ and $p(\theta)$ are rarely, if ever known, and this limitation will haunt this form of inference despite its great flexibility. We nevertheless proceed with this approach with completely general $f(\cdot \mid \theta)$ and $p(\theta)$.

4.4. Assumption: Parametric irrelevance of marginal distribution of X

Without loss of generality, we can factor $f(X_i, Y_i(0), Y_i(1)|\theta)$ into:

$$f(Y_i(0), Y_i(1)|X_i, \theta_{y \cdot x}) f(X_i|\theta_x),$$

where $\theta_{y \cdot x} = \theta_{y \cdot x}(\theta)$ is the parameter governing the conditional distribution of $Y_i(0)$, $Y_i(1)$ given X_i, and analogously, $\theta_x = \theta_x(\theta)$ is the parameter governing the marginal distribution of X. The reason for doing this factorization is that we are assuming X is fully observed, and so we wish to predict the missing potential outcomes Y_{mis} from X and the observed potential outcomes, Y_{obs}, and therefore must use $f(Y_i(0), Y_i(1)|X_i, \theta_{y \cdot x})$.

To do this, we factor $f(Y_i(0), Y_i(1)|X_i, \theta_{y \cdot x})$ into either

$$f(Y_i(0)|X_i, Y_i(1), \theta_{0 \cdot x1}) f(Y_i(1)|X_i, \theta_{1 \cdot x})$$

when $Y_i(0)$ is missing, or

$$f(Y_i(1)|X_i, Y_i(0), \theta_{1 \cdot x0}) f(Y_i(0)|X_i, \theta_{0 \cdot x})$$

when $Y_i(1)$ is missing; here the various subscripted θs are all functions of θ governing the appropriate distributions in an obvious notation.

These factorizations allow us to write Eq. (11) as

$$\int \prod_{i \in S_1} f(Y_i(0)|X_i, Y_i(1), \theta_{0 \cdot x1}) \prod_{i \in S_1} f(Y_i(1)|X_i, \theta_{1 \cdot x}) \tag{12a}$$

$$\times \prod_{i \in S_0} f(Y_i(1)|X_i, Y_i(0), \theta_{1 \cdot x0}) \prod_{i \in S_0} f(Y_i(0)|X_i, \theta_{0 \cdot x}) \tag{12b}$$

$$\times \prod_{i \in S_*} f(Y_i(0), Y_i(1)|X_i, \theta_{y \cdot x}) \tag{12c}$$

$$\times \prod_{i=1}^{N} f(X_i|\theta_x) p(\theta) \mathrm{d}\theta, \tag{12d}$$

where $S_0 = \{i|W_i = 0\}$, $S_1 = \{i|W_i = 1\}$ and $S_* = \{i|W_i = *\}$.

Notice that the first factor in Eq. (12a), times the first factor in Eq. (12b), times Eq. (12c) is proportional to the posterior predictive distribution of Y_{mis} given θ (i.e., given X, Y_{obs} and θ), $\Pr(Y_{\text{mis}}|X, Y_{\text{obs}}, \theta)$. Also notice that the remaining factors in Eq. (12), that is the second factor in Eq. (12a) times the second factor in Eq. (12b) times Eq. (12d), is proportional to the posterior distribution of θ, $\Pr(\theta|X, Y_{\text{obs}})$, which is equal to the likelihood of θ, $L(\theta|X, Y_{\text{obs}})$, times the prior distribution of θ, $p(\theta)$.

Let us now assume that θ_{yx} and θ_x are *a priori* independent:

$$p(\theta) = p(\theta_{y \cdot x}) p(\theta_x). \tag{13}$$

This assumption is not innocuous, but it is useful and is standard in many prediction environments. For an example of a situation where it might not be reasonable, suppose X includes many baseline measurements of cholesterol going back many years; the relationships among previous X values may provide useful information for predicting $Y(0)$ (i.e., Y without intervention), from X, using, for example, a time-series model (e.g., Box and Jenkins, 1970).

For simplicity in the presentation here, we make assumption Eq. (13), although, as with all such assumptions, it should be carefully considered. Then the integral over θ_x in Eq. (12) passes through all the products in Eqs (12a), (12b) and (12c), and we are left with the integral over Eq. (12d); Eq. (12d) after this integration is proportional to $p(\theta_{y \cdot x}) \mathrm{d}\theta_{y \cdot x}$.

As a consequence, Eq. (12) becomes

$$\int \Pr(Y_{\text{mis}}|X, Y_{\text{obs}}, \theta_{y \cdot x}) \Pr(\theta_{y \cdot x}|X, Y_{\text{obs}}) \mathrm{d}\theta_{y \cdot x}, \tag{14}$$

where the second factor in Eq. (14) is proportional to the product of the second factors in Eqs (12a) and (12b), and the first factor in Eq. (14) is, as before, proportional to the product of the first factors of Eqs (12a) and (12b) times (12c).

4.5. *Assumption: No contamination of imputations across treatments*

We now make an assumption that is sometimes implicitly made and sometimes explicitly *not* made, which is the case discussed in Section 3. Specifically, we now assume that entirely separate activities are to be used to impute the missing $Y_i(0)$ and the missing $Y_i(1)$. This is accomplished with two formal assumptions:

$$f(Y_i(0), Y_i(1)|X_i, \theta_{y \cdot x}) = f(Y_i(0)|X_i, \theta_{0 \cdot x}) f(Y_i(1)|X_i, \theta_{1 \cdot x}) \tag{15}$$

and

$$p(\theta_{y\cdot x}) = p(\theta_{0\cdot x})p(\theta_{1\cdot x}). \tag{16}$$

Thus, in Eq. (15) we assume $Y_i(0)$ and $Y_i(1)$ are conditionally independent given X_i and $\theta_{y\cdot x}$, and in Eq. (16), that the parameters governing these conditional distributions are *a priori* independent. Consequently, $f(Y_i(0)|\ X_i, Y_i(1), \theta_{0\cdot x1}) = f(Y_i(0)|X_i, \theta_{0\cdot x})$, and $f(Y_i(1)|X_i, Y_i(0), \theta_{1\cdot 0x}) = f(Y_i(1)|X_i, \theta_{1\cdot x})$. Thus, Eq. (12) or (14) can be written in four distinct parts with associated activities as follows.

1. Using the control units, obtain the posterior distribution of $\theta_{0\cdot x}$:

$$\begin{aligned} p(\theta_{0\cdot x}|X, Y_{\text{obs}}) &\propto L(\theta_{0\cdot x}|X, Y_{\text{obs}})p(\theta_{0\cdot x}) \\ &\propto \prod_{i\in S_0} p(Y_i(0)|X_i, \theta_{0\cdot x})p(\theta_{0\cdot x}). \end{aligned}$$

2. Using $\theta_{0\cdot x}$, obtain the conditional posterior predictive distribution of the missing $Y_i(0)$:

$$\prod_{i\in S_1\cup S_*} \Pr(Y_i(0)|X_i, \theta_{0\cdot x}).$$

3. Using the treated units, obtain the posterior distribution of $\theta_{1\cdot x}$:

$$\begin{aligned} \Pr(\theta_{1\cdot x}|X, Y_{\text{obs}}) &\propto L(\theta_{1\cdot x}|X, Y_{\text{obs}})p(\theta_{1\cdot x}) \\ &\propto \prod_{i\in S_1} \Pr(Y_i(1)|X_i, \theta_{1\cdot x})p(\theta_{1\cdot x}). \end{aligned}$$

4. Using $\theta_{1\cdot x}$, obtain the conditional posterior predictive distribution of the missing $Y_i(1)$:

$$\prod_{i\in S_0\cup S_*} \Pr(Y_i(1)|X_i, \theta_{1\cdot x}).$$

For simulation, perform steps 1–4 repeatedly with random draws, thereby multiply imputing Y_{mis}.

4.6. *Simple normal example illustrating the four steps*

To illustrate the idea of imputing the missing potential outcomes, suppose $f(\cdot|\theta)$ is normal with means (μ_0, μ_1), variances (σ_0^2, σ_1^2) and zero correlation.

The units with $W_i = 1$ (i.e., $i\in S_1$) have $Y_i(1)$ observed and are missing $Y_i(0)$, and so their $Y_i(0)$ values need to be imputed. To impute $Y_i(0)$ values for them, intuitively we need to find units with $Y_i(0)$ observed who are exchangeable with the $W_i = 1$ units, but these units must have $W_i = 0$ (i.e., $i \in S_0$). Therefore, we estimate (in a Bayesian way) the distribution of $Y_i(0)$ from the units with $W_i = 0$, and use this estimated distribution to impute $Y_i(0)$ for the units missing $Y_i(0)$.

Because the n_0 observed values of $Y_i(0)$ are a simple random sample of the N values of $Y(0)$, and are normally distributed with mean μ_0 and variance σ_0^2, with the standard independent non-informative prior distributions on (μ_0, σ_0^2), we have for the posterior distribution of σ_0^2:

$$\sigma_0^2/s_0^2 \sim \text{inverted } \chi^2_{n_0-1}/(n_0 - 1);$$

and for the posterior distribution of μ_0 given σ_0:

$$\mu_0 \sim N(\bar{y}_0, s_0^2/n_0);$$

and for the missing $Y_i(0)$ given μ_0 and σ_0:

$$Y_i(0) \ni W_i \neq 0 \overset{\text{iid}}{\sim} N(\mu_0, s_0^2).$$

The missing values of $Y_i(1)$ are analogously imputed using the observed values of $Y_i(1)$.

When there are covariates observed, these are used to help predict the missing potential outcomes using, for example, one regression model for the observed $Y_i(1)$ given the covariates, and another regression model for the observed $Y_i(0)$ given the covariates.

4.7. Simple normal example with covariate – numerical example

For a specific example with a covariate, suppose we have a large population of patients with a covariate X_i indicating baseline health, which is dichotomous, *HI* versus *LO*, with a 50%/50% mixture in the population. Suppose that a random sample of 100 with $X_i = HI$ is taken, and 10 are randomly assigned to the control treatment, and 90 are randomly assigned to the active treatment. Further suppose that a random sample of 100 with $X_i = LO$ is taken, and 90 are randomly assigned to the control treatment and 10 are assigned to the active treatment. The outcome Y is cholesterol level a year after randomization, with $Y_{i,\text{obs}}$ and X_i observed for all 200 units; X_i is effectively observed in the population because we know the proportions of X_i that are *HI* and *LO* in the full population.

Suppose the hypothetical observed data are as displayed in Table 2, Then the inferences based on the normal-model are as follows in Table 3.

Table 2
Observed data in artificial example

X	$\bar{y}_0$	n_0	s_0	$\bar{y}_1$	n_1	s_1
HI	400	10	60	300	90	60
LO	200	90	60	100	10	60

Table 3
Causal inferences for example in Table 2

	$X = HI$	$X = LO$	Population $= \frac{1}{2}HI + \frac{1}{2}LO$
$E(\bar{Y}_1 - \bar{Y}_0 \mid X, Y_{\text{obs}}, W)$	−100	−100	−100
$V(\bar{Y}_1 - \bar{Y}_0 \mid X, Y_{\text{obs}}, W)^{1/2}$	20	20	$10\sqrt{2}$

The obvious conclusion in this artificial example is that the treatment leads to cholesterol reduction relative to control for both those with *HI* and *LO* baseline health by about 100 points, and thus for the population, which is a 50%/50% mixture of these two subpopulations. In this sort of situation, the final inference is insensitive to the assumed normality of $Y_i(1)$ given X_i and of $Y_i(0)$ given X_i; see Pratt (1965) or Rubin (1987, 2004b, Section 2.5) for the argument. But, in general, this is not so.

4.8. Dangers of model-based extrapolations with some regular designs

A great strength of the model-based approach is that it allows us to conduct causal inference by predicting all of the missing potential outcomes from observed values. The problem with this approach is the need to specify the distributions $f(\cdot|\theta)$ and $p(\theta)$, which sometimes can implicitly involve extrapolations that are extremely unreliable. This situation can be easily conveyed by a simple example based on the one in Section 4.7.

Suppose that the half of units with *LO* baseline health are *POOR* and half are *FAIR*, and further suppose that the 10 with *LO* assigned the active treatment all are *FAIR*; the 90 with *LO* assigned the control treatment are 50 *POOR* and 40 *FAIR*. Now, although the comparison of treatment versus control for $X_i = HI$ is unaffected, the comparison of treatment versus control for the $X = POOR$ group is entirely dependent on our model specifications. That is, there are no $X = POOR$ units in the active treatment condition, and so to impute $Y_i(1)$ values for the $X_i = POOR$ control units, we must rely entirely on some external information.

For example, suppose we associate *POOR* with $X_i = 0$, *FAIR* with $X_i = 1$, and *HI* with $X_i = 2$, and claim that $Y_i(1)$ is linearly related to X_i (given θ). In the control group, we can then impute the missing $Y_i(1)$ for units with $X_i = POOR$ even though there are no units with $X_i = POOR$ and $Y_i(1)$ observed, based on the assumed linear relationship between $Y_i(1)$ and X_i estimated from the 10 treatment units with $X_i = 1$ and the 90 with $X_i = 2$. Moreover, as the sample sizes get bigger and bigger, the posterior variance of the estimated average causal effect shrinks to zero under this linear model, so we appear to be certain of our answer for the $X_i = POOR$ causal effect, even though it is reliant on an assumption that may be only implicitly recognized: the linear relationships between the treatment potential outcomes and the covariate, which allows the extrapolation to take place.

Because of the issues of model-based extrapolation, propensity score methods (i.e., based on matching or subclassification) are highly relevant to the application of Bayesian methods to causal inference. For example, it is always a good idea to examine the overlap in multivariate X distributions between treatment and control groups, and, by design, to create treated and control units with very similar distributions of X. Then, formal model-based imputations that rely on interpolation can be made within these samples, thereby avoiding extrapolation. This approach is illustrated in a psychological/medical study in Reinisch et al. (1995), where matching was used to select a subset of controls, and linear model adjustments were made in the resulting samples. Objective design is critical for all researchers, a point emphasized in Rubin (2007).

4.9. Nonignorable treatment assignment mechanisms

With nonignorable treatment assignment, the simplifications in previous sections, which follow from ignoring the specification for $\Pr(W|X, Y(0), Y(1))$, do not follow in general, and valid analysis typically becomes far more difficult and uncertain. As a simple illustration, take the example in Section 4.7 and assume that everything is the same except that only Y_{obs} is recorded, so that we do not know whether X_i is *HI* or *LO* for anyone. The actual assignment mechanism is now

$$\Pr(W|Y(0), Y(1)) = \int \Pr(W|X, Y(0), Y(1))\mathrm{d}P(X)$$

because X itself is missing, and so treatment assignment depends explicitly on the potential outcomes, both observed and missing, which are generally both correlated with the missing X_i.

Inference for causal effects, assuming the identical model for the science, now depends on the implied normal mixture model for the observed Y data within each treatment arm, because the population is a 50%/50% mixture of those with *LO* and *HI* baseline health, and these subpopulations have different probabilities of treatment assignment. Here the inference for causal effects is sensitive to the propriety of the assumed normality and/or the assumption of a 50%/50% mixture, as well as to the prior distributions on μ_0, μ_1, σ_0 and σ_1.

If we mistakenly ignore the nonignorable treatment assignment and simply compare the sample means of all treated with all controls, for example, using the simple model of Section 4.6, we have $\bar{y}_1 = .9(300) + .1(100) = 280$ versus $\bar{y}_0 = .1(400) + .9(200) = 220$; doing so, we reach the incorrect conclusion that the active treatment hurts cholesterol reduction relative to control in the population. This sort of example is known as "Simpson's Paradox" (Simpson, 1951) and can easily arise with incorrect analyses of nonignorable treatment assignment mechanisms, and thus indicates why such assignment mechanisms are to be avoided whenever possible. Randomized experiments are the most direct way of avoiding nonignorable treatment assignments. Other alternatives are ignorable designs with nonprobabilistic features so that all units with some specific value of covariates are assigned the same treatment, like the extreme example in Section 4.8 or "regression discontinuity" designs (Shadish, Cook and Campbell, 2002). In practice, the analyses of observational studies proceeds as if they were ignorable, as discussed previously. Then, to assess the consequences of this assumption, sensitivity analyses can be conducted under various hypothetical situations.

Typically sensitivity analyses utilize the idea of a fully missing covariate, U, such that treatment assignment is ignorable given U but not given the observed data. The relationships between U and W, and between U, $Y(0)$, and $Y(1)$, all given X, are then varied. See for example Rosenbaum and Rubin (1983b) and Cornfield et al. (1959). Extreme versions of sensitivity analyses examine bounds (e.g., see Imbens and Manski, 2004). Bounds on point estimates examine estimates that would be obtained over extreme distributions of the unobserved covariate U. Although often very broad, such bounds can play an important role in informing us about the sources of sharpness in inferences. Some relevant references for this approach include Manski et al. (1992), Manski and Nagin (1998) and Horowitz and Manski (2000).

Related techniques for assessing nonignorable designs include the formal role of a second control group (Rosenbaum, 1987) and tests of unconfoundedness (Rosenbaum, 1984). Generally I prefer to use evidence to produce better estimates rather than to test assumptions. That is, if there is evidence in the data available to test an assumption, then there is evidence for how to generalize the questionable assumption, and thereby improve the estimation of causal effects.

5. Complications

There are many complications that occur in real world studies for causal effects, many of which can be handled much more flexibly with the Bayesian approach than with assignment-based methods. Of course, the models involved, including the associated prior distributions, can be very demanding to formulate in a practically reliable manner. Also, Neymanian evaluations are still important. Here I simply list some of these complications with some admittedly idiosyncratically personal references to current work from the Bayesian perspective.

5.1. Multiple treatments

When there are more than two treatments, the notation becomes more complex but is still straightforward under SUTVA. Without SUTVA, however, both the notation and the analysis can become very involved. The exploding number of potential outcomes can become an especially serious issue in studies where the units are exposed to a sequence of repeated treatments in time, each distinct sequence corresponding to a possibly distinct treatment. Most of the field of classical experiment design is devoted to issues that arise with more than two treatment conditions (e.g., Kempthorne, 1952; Cochran and Cox, 1957; Cox, 1958), although sequential designs are certainly challenging.

5.2. Unintended missing data

Missing data, due perhaps to unit dropout or machine failure, can complicated analyses more than one would expect based on a cursory examination of the problem. Fortunately, Bayesian/likelihood tools for addressing missing data, such as multiple imputation (Rubin, 1987, 2004b) or the EM algorithm (Dempster et al., 1977) and its relatives, including data augmentation (Tanner and Wong, 1987) and the Gibbs sampler (Geman and Geman, 1984) are fully compatible with the Bayesian approach to causal inference outlined in Section 4. Gelman et al. (2003), Parts III and IV, provide guidance on many of these issues from the Bayesian perspective.

5.3. *Noncompliance with assigned treatment*

Another complication, common when the units are people, is noncompliance. For example, some of the subjects assigned to take the active treatment take the control treatment instead, and some assigned to take the control manage to take the active treatment. A nice example of this in the context of a medical experiment is given in Sommer and Zeger (1991). Initial interest focuses on the effect of the treatment for the subset of people who will comply with their treatment assignments. Early work related to this issue can be found in economics (e.g., Tinbergen, 1930; Haavelmo, 1944) and elsewhere (e.g., Zelen, 1979; Bloom, 1984). Much progress has been made on this topic in the last decade (e.g., Baker, 1998; Baker and Lindeman, 1994; Goetghebeur and Molenberghs, 1996; Angrist et al., 1996; Imbens and Rubin, 1997; Little and Yau, 1998; Hirano et al., 2000; Jin and Rubin, 2007, 2008). In this case, sensitivity of inference to prior assumptions can be severe, and the Bayesian approach is well suited, not only to revealing this sensitivity, but also to formulating reasonable prior restrictions.

5.4. *Truncation of outcomes due to death*

In other cases, the unit may "die" before the final outcome can be measured. For example, in an experiment with new fertilizers, a plant may die before the crops are harvested and interest may focus on both the effect of the fertilizer on plant survival and the effect of the fertilizer on plant yield when the plant survives. Or with a medical intervention designed to improve quality of life, patients who die before quality of life can be measured, effectively have their data "truncated due to death". This problem is far more subtle than it may at first appear to be, and valid approaches to it have only recently been formulated (Rubin, 2000; Zhang and Rubin, 2003). Surprisingly, the models also have applications in economics (Zhang, Rubin and Mealli, 2007) and the evaluation of job-training programs. A recent article on the quality of life situation with discussion is Rubin (2006a).

5.5. *Direct and indirect causal effects*

Another topic that is far more subtle than it first appears to be is the one involving direct and indirect causal effects. For example, the separation of the "direct" effect of a vaccination on disease from the "indirect" effect of the vaccination that is due solely to its effect on blood antibodies and the "direct" effect of the antibodies on disease. This language turns out to be too imprecise to be useful within our formal causal effect framework. This problem is ripe for Bayesian modeling as briefly outlined in Rubin (2004a). This topic is one on which Fisher gave flawed advice, as discussed in Rubin (2005), possibly because he eschewed the use of Neyman's potential outcomes.

5.6. Principal stratification

All the examples in Sections 5.3–5.5 can be viewed as special cases of "principal stratification" (Frangakis and Rubin, 2002), where the principal strata are defined by partially unobserved intermediate potential outcomes, namely in our examples: compliance behavior under both treatment assignments, survival under both treatment assignments, and antibody level under both treatment assignments. This appears to be an extremely fertile area for research and application of Bayesian methods for causal inference, especially using modern simulation methods such as MCMC (Markov Chain Monte Carlo); see, for example, Gilks et al. (1995), and more recently, Liu (2001).

5.7. Combinations of complications

In the real world, such complications typically do not appear simply one at a time. For example, the massive randomized experiment in medicine evaluating hormone replacement therapy for post-menopausal women suffered from missing data in both covariates and longitudinal outcomes; also, the outcome was multicomponent as each point in time; in addition, it suffered from noncompliance, and moreover, had censoring due to death for some outcomes (e.g., five-year cancer-free survival). Some of these combinations of complications are discussed in Barnard et al. (2003) in the context of a school choice example, and in Mealli and Rubin (2003) in the context of a medical experiment.

Despite the fact that Bayesian analysis is quite difficult when confronted with these combinations of complications, I believe that it is still a far more satisfactory attack on the real scientific problems of causal inference than the vast majority of ad hoc frequentist approaches commonly in use today.

5.8. More missing data

The problem of missing data, both in covariates and outcomes, is very common in practice. Standard methods (e.g., as in Little and Rubin, 2002) are highly valuable here, and special methods, for instance, for dealing with missing covariates in propensity score analyses (D'Agostino and Rubin, 1999) are also relevant. Outcomes that are censored, e.g., survival data, can be viewed as a special but important case of coarsened data (Heitjan and Rubin, 1991). Moreover, dealing with combined complications, such as missing outcomes with noncompliance (Frangakis and Rubin, 1999), is important, as is clustering in design issues (Frangakis et al., 2002). These topics create a superb area for research, with immediate applications to epidemiology and medical experiments.

References

Angrist, J.D., Imbens, G.W., Rubin, D.B. (1996). Identification of causal effects using instrumental variables. *Journal of the American Statistical Association* **91**, 444–472, as applications invited discussion article with discussion and rejoinder.

Anscombe, F.J. (1948). The validity of comparative experiments. *Journal of the Royal Statistical Society. Series A* **61**, 181–211.

Baker, S.G. (1998). Analysis of survival data from a randomized trial with all-or-none compliance: Estimating the cost-effectiveness of a cancer screening program. *Journal of the American Statistical Association* **93**, 929–934.

Baker, S.G., Lindeman, K.S. (1994). The paired availability design: A proposal for evaluating epidural analgesia during labor. *Statistics in Medicine* **13**, 2269–2278.

Barnard, J., Hill, J., Frangakis, C., Rubin, D. (2003). School choice in NY city: A Bayesian analysis of an imperfect randomized experiment. In: Gatsonis, C., Carlin, B., Carriquiry, A. (Eds.),**Vol. V** *Case Studies in Bayesian Statistics*. Springer, New York.

Bloom, H.S. (1984). Accounting for no-shows in experimental evaluation designs. *Evaluation Review* **8**, 225–246.

Box, G.E.P., Jenkins, G.M. (1970). *Time Series Analysis: Forecasting and Controls*. Holden-Day, San Francisco.

Brillinger, D.R., Jones, L.V., Tukey, J.W. (1978). Report of the statistical task force for the weather modification advisory board. *The Management of Western Resources*, Vol. II: *The Role of Statistics on Weather Resources Management*. Stock No. 003-018-00091-1, Government Printing Office, Washington, DC.

Chernoff, H. (1959). Sequential design of experiments. *Annals of Statistics* **30**, 755–765.

Cochran, W.G. (1963). *Sampling Techniques*, 2nd ed. Wiley, New York.

Cochran, W.G. (1968). The effectiveness of adjustment by subclassification in removing bias in observational studies. *Biometrics* **24**, 295–313.

Cochran, W.G., Cox, G.M. (1957). *Experimental Designs*, 2nd ed. Wiley, New York, Reprinted as a "Wiley Classic" (1992).

Cochran, W.G., Rubin, D.B. (1973). Controlling bias in observational studies: A review. *Sankhyā. Series A* **35**, 417–446.

Cornfield, J., Haenszel, W., Hammond, E.C., Lilienfeld, A.M., Shimkin, M.B., Wynder, E.L. (1959). Smoking and lung cancer; recent evidence and a discussion of some questions. *Journal of the National Cancer Institute* **22**, 173–203.

Cox, D.R. (1958). *The Planning of Experiments*. Wiley, New York.

Cox, D.R. (1992). Causality: Some statistical aspects. *Journal of the Royal Statistical Society. Series A* **155**, 291–301.

Cox, D.R., McCullagh, P. (1982). Some aspects of covariance. *Biometrics* **38**, 541–561, (with discussion).

D'Agostino Jr., R., Rubin, D.B. (1999). Estimation and use of propensity scores with incomplete data. *Journal of the American Statistical Association* **95**, 749–759.

Dawid, A.P. (2000). Causal inference without counterfactuals. *Journal of the American Statistical Association* **95**, 407–424, (with discussion).

de Finetti, B. (1963). Foresight: Its logical laws, its subjective sources. In: Kyburg, H.E., Smokler, H.E. (Eds.), *Studies in Subjective Probability*. Wiley, New York.

Dehijia, R.H., Wahba, S. (1999). Causal effects in nonexperimental studies: Reevaluating the evaluation of training programs. *Journal of the American Statistical Association* **94**, 1053–1062.

Dempster, A.P. (1990). Causality and statistics. *Journal of Statistical Planning and Inference* **25**, 261–278.

Dempster, A.P., Laird, N., Rubin, D.B. (1977). Maximum likelihood from incomplete data via the EM algorithm. *Journal of the Royal Statistical Society. Series B* **39**, 1–38, (with discussion and reply).

Efron, B., Feldman, D. (1991). Compliance as an explanatory variable in clinical trials. *Journal of the American Statistical Association* **86**, 9–17.

Federal Judicial Center (2000). *Reference Manual on Scientific Evidence*, 2nd ed. Federal Judicial Center, Washington, DC.

Fisher, F. (1999). Expert Witness Report for the Plaintiffs, U.S. vs. Tobacco Industry.

Fisher, R.A. (1918). The causes of human variability. *The Eugenics Review* **10**, 213–220.
Fisher, R.A. (1925). *Statistical Methods for Research Workers*. Oliver and Boyd, Edinburgh.
Frangakis, C., Rubin, D.B. (1999). Addressing complications of intention-to-treat analysis in the combined presence of all-or-none treatment-noncompliance and subsequent missing outcomes. *Biometrika* **86**, 366–379.
Frangakis, C.E., Rubin, D.B. (2002). Principal stratification in causal inference. *Biometrics* **58**, 21–29.
Frangakis, C., Rubin, D.B., Zhou, X.-H. (2002). Clustered encouragement designs with individual noncompliance: Bayesian inference with randomization, and application to advance directive forms. *Biostatistics* **3**, 147–177, (with discussion and rejoinder).
Geman, S., Geman, D. (1984). Stochastic relaxation: Gibbs distributions, and the Bayesian restoration of images. *IEEE Transactions on Pattern Analysis and Machine Intelligence* **6**, 721–741.
Gelman, A., Carlin, J., Stern, H., Rubin, D. (2003). *Bayesian Data Analysis*, 2nd ed. CRC Press, New York.
Gelman, A., King, G. (1991). Estimating incumbency advantage without bias. *American Journal of Political Science* **34**, 1142–1164.
Gilks, W.R., Richardson, S., Spiegelhalter, D.J. (1995). *Markov Chain Monte Carlo in Practice*. CRC Press, New York.
Goetghebeur, E., Molenberghs, G. (1996). Causal inference in a placebo-controlled clinical trial with binary outcome and ordered compliance. *Journal of the American Statistical Association* **91**, 928–934.
Greenland, S., Poole, C. (1988). Invariants and noninvariants in the concept of interdependent effects. *Scandinavian Journal of Work, Environment & Health* **14**, 125–129.
Greenland, S., Robins, J.M., Pearl, J. (1999). Confounding and collapsibility in causal inference. *Statistical Science* **14**, 29–46.
Gu, X.S., Rosenbaum, P.R. (1993). Comparison of multivariate matching methods: Structures, distances, and algorithms. *Journal of Computational and Graphical Statistics* **2**, 405–420.
Haavelmo, T. (1944). The probability approach in econometrics. *Econometrica* **15**, 413–419.
Heckman, J.J. (1989). Causal inference and nonrandom samples. *Journal of Educational Statistics* **14**, 159–168.
Heckman, J.J., Hotz, J. (1989). Alternative methods for evaluating the impact of training programs. *Journal of the American Statistical Association* **84**, 862–874, (with discussion).
Heitjan, D., Rubin, D.B. (1991). Ignorability and coarse data. *Annals of Statistics* **19**, 2244–2253.
Hirano, K., Imbens, G., Rubin, D.B., Zhou, X. (2000). Assessing the effect of an influenza vaccine in an encouragement design. *Biostatistics* **1**, 69–88.
Hodges, J.L., Lehmann, E. (1970). *Basic Concepts of Probability and Statistics*, 2nd ed. Holden-Day, San Francisco.
Holland, P.W. (1986). Statistics and causal inference. *Journal of the American Statistical Association* **81**, 945–970.
Holland, P.W. (1988a). Causal inference, path analysis, and recursive structural equation models. *Sociological Methodology*, 449–484.
Holland, P.W. (1988b). Comment on "Employment discrimination and statistical science" by A.P. Dempster. *Statistical Science* **3**, 186–188.
Holland, P.W. (1989). It's very clear. Comment on "Choosing among alternative nonexperimental methods for estimating the impact of social programs: The case of manpower training" by J. Heckman and V. Hotz. *Journal of the American Statistical Association* **84**, 875–877.
Holland, P.W., Rubin, D.B. (1983). On Lord's paradox. In: Wainer, M. (Ed.), *Principals of Modern Psychological Measurement: A Festschrift for Frederic M. Lord*. Earlbaum, Hillsdale, NJ.
Horowitz, J.L., Manski, C.F. (2000). Nonparametric analysis of randomized experiments with missing covariates and outcome data. *Journal of the American Statistical Association* **95**, 77–84.
Horvitz, D.G., Thompson, D.J. (1952). A generalization of sampling without replacement from a finite population. *Journal of the American Statistical Association* **47**, 663–685.
Hurwicz, L. (1962). On the structural form of interdependent systems. In: Nagel, E., Suppes, P., Tarski, A. (Eds.), *Logic, Methodology, and Philosophy of Science. Proceedings of the 1960 International Congress*. Stanford, CA: Stanford University Press.

Imbens, G.W., Manski, C.F. (2004). Confidence intervals for partially identified parameters. *Econometrica* **72**, 1845–1857.
Imbens, G.W., Rubin, D.B. (1997). Bayesian inference for causal effects in randomized experiments with noncompliance. *Annals of Statistics* **25**, 305–327.
Imbens, G.W., Rubin, D.B. (2007a). *Causal Inference in Statistics and the Medical and Social Sciences.* Cambridge University Press, Cambridge U.K.
Imbens, G.W., Rubin, D.B. (2007b). Rubin causal model. Entry to appear in *The New Palgrave Dictionary of Economics*, 2nd ed. Palgrave MacMillan, New York.
Jin, H., Rubin, D.B. (2007). "Principal Stratification for Causal Inference with Extended Partial Compliance: Application to Efron-Feldman Data." To appear in *The Journal of the American Statistical Association.*
Jin, H., Rubin, D.B. (2008). "Public Schools Versus Private Schools: Causal Inference with Extended Partial Compliance." To appear in *The Journal of Educational and Behavioral Statistics.*
Kadane, J.B., Seidenfeld, T. (2007b). Randomization in a Bayesian perspective. *Journal of Statistical Planning and Inference* **25**, 329–346.
Karkouti, K., Beattie, W.S., Dattilo, K.M., McCluskey, S.A., Ghannam, M., Hamdy, A., Wijeysundera, D.N., Fedorko, L., Yau, T.M. (2006). Blood conservation and transfusion alternatives: A propensity score case-control comparison of aprotinin and tranexamic acid in high-transfusion-risk cardiac surgery. *Transfusion* **46**, 327–338.
Kempthorne, O. (1952). *The Design and Analysis of Experiments.* Wiley, New York.
Langenskold, S., Rubin, D.B. (2008). Outcome-free design of observational studies with application to investigating peer effects on college freshman smoking behaviors. *Les Annales d'Economie et de Statistique.*
Lindley, D.V., Novick, M.R. (1981). The role of exchangeability in inference. *Annals of Statistics* **9**, 45–58.
Little, R.J.A., Rubin, D.B. (2002). *Statistical Analysis with Missing Data*, 2nd ed. Wiley, New York.
Little, R.J., Yau, L. (1998). Statistical techniques for analyzing data from prevention trials: Treatment of no-shows using Rubin's causal model. *Psychological Methods* **3**, 147–159.
Liu, J.S. (2001). *Monte Carlo Strategies in Scientific Computing.* Springer, New York.
Lord, F.M. (1967). A paradox in the interpretation of group comparisons. *Psychological Bulletin* **68**, 304–305.
Manski, C. (1992). Alternative estimates of the effect of family structure during adolescence on high school. *Journal of the American Statistical Association* **87**, 25–37.
Manski, C.F., Nagin, D.S. (1998). Bounding disagreements about treatment effects: A study of sentencing and recidivism. *Sociological Methodology* **28**, 99–137.
McCarthy, M.D. (1939). On the application of the z-test to randomized blocks. *Annals of Mathematical Statistics* **10**, 337.
Mealli, F., Rubin, D.B. (2003). Assumptions when analyzing randomized experiments with noncompliance and missing outcomes. *Health Services & Outcomes Research Methodology*, 2–8.
Mill, J.S. (Ed.) (1973). A system of logic. *Collected Works of John Stuart Mill*, vol. 7. University of Toronto Press, Toronto.
Ming, K., Rosenbaum, P. (2000). Substantial gains in bias reduction from matching with a variable number of controls. *Biometrics* **42**, 109–143.
Neyman, J. (1923). On the application of probability theory to agricultural experiments: Essay on principles, section 9. Translated in *Statistical Science* **5**, 465–480, 1990.
Neyman, J. (1934). On the two different aspects of the representative method: The method of stratified sampling and the method of purposive selection. *Journal of the Royal Statistical Society. Series A* **97**, 558–606.
Neyman, J., with cooperation of K. Iwaskiewicz and St. Kolopdziejczyk (1935). Statistical problems in agricultural experimentation (with discussion). Supplement to the *Journal of the Royal Statistical Society. Series B* **2**, 107–180.
Ogden, D.W. (Acting Assistant Attorney General). (1999). News Conference (Sept. 22), http://www.usdoj.gov/archive/ag/speeches/1999/tobaccopc92299.htm.
Pearl, J. (2000). *Causality: Models, Reasoning and Inference.* Cambridge University Press, Cambridge, UK.

Peterson, A.V., Kealey, K.A., Mann, S.L., Marek, P.M., Sarason, I.G. (2000). Hutchinson smoking prevention project: Long-term randomized trial in school-based tobacco use prevention – results on smoking. *Journal of the National Cancer Institute* **92**, 1979–1991.

Piantadosi, S. (2003). Larger lessons from the women's health initiative. *Epidemiology* **14**, 6–7.

Pitman, E.J.G. (1937). Significance tests which can be applied to samples from any population. III. The analysis of variance test. *Biometrika* **29**, 322–335.

Pratt, J.W. (1965). Bayesian interpretation of standard inference statements. *Journal of the Royal Statistical Society. Series B* **27**, 169–203, (with discussion).

Pratt, J.W., Schlaifer, R. (1984). On the nature and discovery of structure. *Journal of the American Statistical Association* **79**, 9–33, (with discussion).

Pratt, J.W., Schlaifer, R. (1988). On the interpretation and observation of laws. *Journal of Econometrics* **39**, 23–52.

Rao, C.R., Sinharay, S. (Eds.). (2006). Statistical inference for causal effects, with emphasis on applications in psychometrics and education. *Handbook of Statistics Volume 26 Psychometrics*. Elsevier, The Netherlands, 769–800.

Reid, C. (1982). *Neyman from Life*. Springer, New York.

Reinisch, J. (1995). In utero exposure to phenobarbital and intelligence deficits in adult men. *Journal of the American Medical Association* **27**, 1518–1525.

Robins, J.M. (1989). The control of confounding by intermediate variables. *Statistics in Medicine* **8**, 679–701.

Rosenbaum, P.R. (1984). From association to causation in observational studies: The role of tests of strongly ignorable treatment assignment. *Journal of the American Statistical Association* **79**, 41–48.

Rosenbaum, P.R. (1987). The role of a second control group in an observational study. *Statistical Science* **2**, 292–316, (with discussion).

Rosenbaum, P.R. (1989). Optimal matching for observational studies. *Journal of the American Statistical Association* **84**, 1024–1032.

Rosenbaum, P.R. (1991). A characterization of optimal designs for observational studies. *Journal of the Royal Statistical Society. Series B* **53**, 597–610.

Rosenbaum, P.R. (1995). *Observational Studies*. Springer, New York.

Rosenbaum, P.R. (2002). *Observational Studies*, 2nd ed. Springer, New York.

Rosenbaum, P.R., Rubin, D.B. (1983a). The central role of the propensity score in observational studies for causal effects. *Biometrika* **70**, 41–55.

Rosenbaum, P.R., Rubin, D.B. (1983b). Assessing sensitivity to an unobserved binary covariate in an observational study with binary outcome. *Journal of the Royal Statistical Society. Series B* **45**, 212–218.

Rosenbaum, P.R., Rubin, D.B. (1985). Constructing a control group using multivariate matched sampling incorporating the propensity score. *The American Statistician* **39**, 33–38.

Rubin, D.B. (1973). Matching to remove bias in observational studies. *Biometrics* **29**, 159–183. Printer's correction note **30**, 728.

Rubin, D.B. (1974). Estimating causal effects of treatments in randomized and nonrandomized studies. *Journal of Educational Psychology* **66**, 688–701.

Rubin, D.B. (1975). Bayesian inference for causality: The importance of randomization. In: *Proceedings of the Social Statistics Section*, American Statistical Association, Alexandria, VA, pp. 233–239.

Rubin, D.B. (1976a). Inference and missing data. *Biometrika* **63**, 581–592.

Rubin, D.B. (1976b). Multivariate matching methods that are equal percent bias reducing, I: Some examples. *Biometrics* **32**, 109–120, Printer's correction note p. 955.

Rubin, D.B. (1976c). Multivariate matching methods that are equal percent bias reducing, II: Maximums on bias reduction for fixed sample sizes. *Biometrics* **32**, 121–132, Printer's correction note p. 955.

Rubin, D.B. (1977). Assignment of treatment group on the basis of a covariate. *Journal of Educational Statistics* **2**, 1–26.

Rubin, D.B. (1978). Bayesian inference for causal effects: The role of randomization. *Annals of Statistics* **7**, 34–58.

Rubin, D.B. (1979a). Discussion of "Conditional independence in statistical theory" by A.P. Dawid. *Journal of the Royal Statistical Society. Series B* **41**, 27–28.
Rubin, D.B. (1979b). Using multivariate matched sampling and regression adjustment to control bias in observational studies. *Journal of the American Statistical Association* **74**, 318–328.
Rubin, D.B. (1980). Comment on "Randomization analysis of experimental data: The Fisher randomization test" by D. Basu. *Journal of the American Statistical Association* **75**, 591–593.
Rubin, D.B. (1987). *Multiple Imputation for Nonresponse in Surveys*. Wiley, New York.
Rubin, D.B. (1990a). Comment: Neyman (1923) and causal inference in experiments and observational studies. *Statistical Science* **5**, 472–480.
Rubin, D.B. (1990b). Formal modes of statistical inference for causal effects. *Journal of Statistical Planning and Inference* **25**, 279–292.
Rubin, D.B. (1997). Estimating causal effects from large data sets using propensity scores. *Annals of Internal Medicine* **127**, 757–763.
Rubin, D.B. (2000). The utility of counterfactuals for causal inference. Comment on A.P. Dawid, 'Causal inference without counterfactuals'. *Journal of the American Statistical Association* **95**, 435–438.
Rubin, D.B. (2002). Using propensity scores to help design observational studies: Application to the tobacco litigation. *Health Services & Outcomes Research Methodology* **2**, 169–188.
Rubin, D.B. (2004a). Direct and indirect causal effects via potential outcomes. *Scandinavian Journal of Statistics* **31**, 161–170, (with discussion and reply).
Rubin, D.B. (2004b). *Multiple Imputation for Nonresponse in Surveys*. Wiley, New York, Reprinted with new appendices as a "Wiley Classic."
Rubin, D.B. (2005). Causal inference using potential outcomes: Design, modeling, decisions. 2004 Fisher Lecture. *Journal of the American Statistical Association* **100**, 322–331.
Rubin, D.B. (2006). *Matched Sampling for Causal Inference*. Cambridge University Press, New York.
Rubin, D.B. (2007). The design versus the analysis of observational studies for causal effects: Parallels with the design of randomized trials. *Statistics in Medicine* **26**(1), 20–30.
Rubin, D.B., Stuart, E.A. (2006). Affinely invariant matching methods with discriminant mixtures of ellipsoidally symmetric distributions. *Annals of Statistics* **34**(4), 1814–1826.
Rubin, D.B., Thomas, N. (1992a). Characterizing the effect of matching using linear propensity score methods with normal covariates. *Biometrika* **79**, 797–809.
Rubin, D.B., Thomas, N. (1992b). Affinely invariant matching methods with ellipsoidal distributions. *Annals of Statistics* **52**, 1079–1093.
Rubin, D.B., Thomas, N. (1996). Matching using estimated propensity scores: Relating theory to practice. *Biometrics*, 249–264.
Shadish, W.R., Clark, M.H. (2006). A randomized experiment comparing random to nonrandom assignment. Unpublished paper, University of California, Merced, CA.
Shadish, W.R., Cook, T.D., Campbell, D.T. (2002). *Experimental and Quasi-Experimental Designs for Generalized Causal Inference*. Houghton Mifflin, Boston.
Simpson, E.H. (1951). The interpretation of interaction in contingency tables. *Journal of the Royal Statistical Society. Series B* **13**, 238–241.
Smith, T.M.F., Sugden, R.A. (1988). Sampling and assignment mechanisms in experiments, surveys and observational studies. *International Statistical Review* **56**, 165–180.
Sobel, M.E. (1990). Effect analysis and causation in linear structural equation models. *Psychometrika* **55**, 495–515.
Sobel, M.E. (1995). Causal inference in the social and behavioral sciences. In: Arminger, G., Clogg, C.C., Sobel, M.E. (Eds.), *Handbook of Statistical Modeling for the Social and Behavioral Sciences*. Plenuum, New York.
Sobel, M.E. (1996). An introduction to causal inference. *Sociological Methods & Research* **24**, 353–379.
Sommer, A., Zeger, S. (1991). On estimating efficacy from clinical trials. *Statistics in Medicine*, 45–52.
Sugden, R.A. (1988). The 22 table in observational studies. In: Bernardo, J.M., DeGroot, M.H., Lindley, D.V., Smith, A.F.M. (Eds.), *Bayesian Statistics 3*. Oxford University Press, New York.
Tanner, M.A., Wong, W.H. (1987). The calculation of posterior distributions by data augmentation. *Journal of the American Statistical Association* **82**, 528–550, (with discussion).

Tinbergen, J. (1930). Determination and interpretation of supply curves: An example [Zeitschrift fur Nationalokonomie], reprinted in: Henry, Morgan (Eds.), *The Foundations of Economics.*

Ware, J. (1989). Investigating therapies of potentially great benefit: ECMO. *Statistical Science* **4**, 298–306.

Welch, B.L. (1937). On the z test in randomized blocks and Latin squares. *Biometrika* **29**, 21–52.

Whittemore, A.S., McGuire, V. (2003). Observational studies and randomized trials of hormone replacement therapy: What can we learn from them? *Epidemiology* **14**, 8–10.

Zelen, M. (1979). A new design for randomized clinical trials. *The New England Journal of Medicine* **300**, 1242–1245.

Zhang, J., Rubin, D.B. (2003). Estimation of causal effects via principal stratification when some outcomes are truncated by 'death'. *Journal of Educational and Behavioral Statistics* **28**, 353–368.

Zhang, J., Rubin, D., Mealli, F. (2007). Evaluating the effects of training programs with experimental data. Submitted to *Journal of the American Statistical Association.*

Handbook of Statistics, Vol. 27
ISSN: 0169-7161

DOI: 10.1016/S0169-7161(07)27003-8

3

Epidemiologic Study Designs

Kenneth J. Rothman, Sander Greenland and Timothy L. Lash

Abstract

In this chapter, we present an overview of the primary types of epidemiologic study designs addressing both experimental and nonexperimental designs. For experimental studies, we describe the role of randomization and the ethical concerns of conducting experiments with human subjects, as well as the distinctions between clinical trials, field trials, and community intervention trials. For nonexperimental studies, we describe the design principles for cohort and case-control studies; the selection of subjects, including control selection in case-control studies; and several variants of the case-control design, including proportional-mortality, case-crossover, case-specular, and two-stage studies.

1. Introduction

Epidemiologic study designs comprise both experimental and nonexperimental studies. The experiment is emblematic of scientific activity. But what constitutes an experiment? In common parlance, an experiment refers to any trial or test. For example, a professor might introduce new teaching methods as an experiment. For many scientists, however, the term has a more specific meaning: An experiment is a set of observations, conducted under controlled circumstances, in which the scientist manipulates the conditions to ascertain what effect such manipulation has on the observations. For epidemiologists, the word experiment usually implies that the investigator manipulates the exposure assigned to participants in the study. Experimental epidemiologic studies are therefore limited at a minimum to topics for which the exposure condition can be manipulated and for which all exposure assignments are expected to cause no harm.

When epidemiologic experiments are feasible and ethical, they should be designed to reduce variation in the outcome attributable to extraneous factors and to account for the remaining extraneous variation. In epidemiologic experiments, participants receive an intervention that is assigned to them by the researcher. There are generally two or more forms of the intervention. Intervention assignments are ordinarily determined by the researcher by applying a randomized allocation scheme. The purpose of random allocation is to create groups that differ only randomly at the time of allocation with regard to the prospective occurrence of the study outcome. Epidemiologic experiments include clinical trials (with patients as subjects), field trials (with interventions assigned to individual community members), and community intervention trials (with interventions assigned to whole communities).

When experiments are infeasible or unethical, epidemiologists design nonexperimental (also known as observational) studies in an attempt to simulate what might have been learned had an experiment been conducted. In nonexperimental studies, the researcher is an observer rather than an agent who assigns interventions. The four main types of nonexperimental epidemiologic studies are cohort studies – in which all subjects in a source population are classified according to their exposure status and followed over time to ascertain disease incidence; case-control studies – in which cases arising from a source population and a sample of the source population are classified according to their exposure history; cross-sectional studies, including prevalence studies – in which one ascertains exposure and disease status as of a particular time; and ecologic studies – in which the units of observation are groups of people. We will discuss cohort and case-control designs in some detail, including in the latter proportional-mortality, case-crossover, case-specular, and two-stage studies. The material is adapted from Chapters 5–7 of the third edition of *Modern Epidemiology*, to which we refer the interested reader for more comprehensive discussion. For details of ecologic studies see Greenland (2001, 2002, 2004) and Morgenstern (2008).

2. Experimental studies

A typical experiment on human subjects creates experimental groups that are exposed to different treatments or agents. In a simple two-group experiment, one group receives a treatment and the other does not. Ideally, the experimental groups are identical with respect to extraneous factors that affect the outcome of interest, so that if the treatment had no effect, identical outcomes would be observed across the groups. This objective could be achieved if one could control all the relevant conditions that might affect the outcome under study. In the biologic sciences, however, the conditions affecting most outcomes are so complex and extensive that they are mostly unknown and thus cannot be made uniform. Hence there will be variation in the outcome even in the absence of a treatment effect. In the study of the causes of cancer, for example, it is impossible to create conditions that will invariably give rise to cancer after a fixed time interval, even if the population is a group of cloned laboratory mice. Inevitably, there will be what is called "biologic variation," which reflects variation in the set of conditions that produces the effect.

Thus, in biologic experimentation, one cannot create groups across which only the study treatment varies. Instead, the experimenter may settle for creating groups in which the net effect of extraneous factors is expected to be small. For example, it may be impossible to make all animals in an experiment eat exactly the same amount of food. Variation in food consumption could pose a problem if it affected the outcome under study. If this variation could be kept small, however, it might contribute little to variation in the outcome across the groups.

The investigator would usually be satisfied if the net effect of extraneous factors across the groups were substantially less than the expected effect of the study treatment. Often not even that can be achieved, however. In that case, the experiment must be designed so that the variation in outcome due to extraneous factors can be accurately measured and thus accounted for in comparisons across the treatment groups.

2.1. Randomization

In the early 20th century, R.A. Fisher and others developed a practical basis for experimental designs that accurately accounts for extraneous variability across experimental units (whether the units are objects, animals, people, or communities). This basis is called *randomization* (random allocation) of treatments or exposures among the units: each unit is assigned treatment using a random assignment mechanism such as a coin toss. Such a mechanism is unrelated to the extraneous factors that affect the outcome, so any association between the treatment allocation it produces and those extraneous factors will be random. The variation in the outcome across treatment groups that is not due to treatment effects can thus be ascribed to these random associations, and hence can be justifiably called chance variation.

A hypothesis about the size of the treatment effect, such as the null hypothesis, corresponds to a specific probability distribution for the potential outcomes under that hypothesis. This probability distribution can be compared with the observed association between treatment and outcomes. The comparison links statistics and inference, which explains why many statistical methods, such as analysis of variance, estimate random outcome variation within and across treatment groups. A study with random treatment assignment allows one to compute the probability of the observed association under various hypotheses about how treatment assignment affects outcome. In particular, if assignment is random and has no effect on the outcome except through treatment, any systematic (nonrandom) variation in outcome with assignment must be attributable to a treatment effect, provided that the study implements design strategies, such as concealment of the random assignment, that prevent biases from affecting the estimate of effect. Without randomization, systematic variation is a composite of all uncontrolled sources of variation – including any treatment effect – but also including confounding factors and other sources of systematic error. As a result, in studies without randomization, the systematic variation estimated by standard statistical methods is not readily attributable to treatment effects, nor can it be reliably compared with the variation expected to occur by chance. Separation of treatment effects from the mixture of uncontrolled systematic variation in nonrandomized studies (or in randomized studies with noncompliance) requires additional hypotheses about the sources of systematic error. In nonexperimental studies, these hypotheses are usually no more than speculations, although they can be incorporated into the analysis as parameter settings in a sensitivity analysis or as prior distributions in Bayesian analysis. In this sense, causal inference in the absence of randomization is largely speculative. The validity of such inference depends on how well the speculations about the effect of systematic errors correspond with their true effect.

2.2. Validity versus ethical considerations in experiments on human subjects

In an experiment, those who are exposed to an experimental treatment are exposed only because the investigator has assigned the exposure to the subject. Because the goals of the study, rather than the subject's needs, determine the exposure assignment, ethical constraints limit severely the circumstances in which valid experiments on humans are feasible. Experiments on human subjects are ethically permissible only when adherence to the scientific protocol does not conflict with the subject's best interests. Specifically, there should be reasonable assurance that there is no known and feasible way a participating subject could be treated better than with the treatment possibilities that the protocol provides. From this requirement comes the constraint that any exposures or treatments given to subjects should be limited to potential preventives of disease or disease consequences. This limitation alone confines most etiologic research to the non-experimental variety.

Among the more specific implications is that subjects admitted to the study should not be thereby deprived of some preferable form of treatment or preventive that is not included in the study. This requirement implies that best available therapy should be included to provide a reference (comparison) for any new treatment. Another implication, known as the equipoise requirement, is that the treatment possibilities included in the trial must be equally acceptable given current knowledge. This requirement severely restricts use of placebos: the Declaration of Helsinki states that it is unethical to include a placebo therapy as one of the arms of a clinical trial if an accepted remedy or preventive of the outcome already exists (World Medical Association: http://www.wma.net/e/policy/b3.htm; Rothman and Michels, 2002).

Even with these limitations, many epidemiologic experiments are conducted. Most fall into the specialized area of clinical trials, which are epidemiologic studies evaluating treatments for patients who already have acquired disease (trial is used as a synonym for experiment). Epidemiologic experiments that aim to evaluate primary preventives (agents intended to prevent disease onset in the first place) among the healthy are less common than clinical trials; these studies are either field trials or community intervention trials.

2.3. Clinical trials

A clinical trial is an experiment with patients as subjects. The goal of most clinical trials is either to evaluate a potential cure for a disease or to find a preventive of disease sequelae such as death, disability, or a decline in the quality of life. The exposures in such trials are not primary preventives, since they do not prevent occurrence of the initial disease, but they are preventives of the sequelae of the initial disease. For example, a modified diet after an individual suffers a myocardial infarction may prevent a second infarction and subsequent death, chemotherapeutic agents given to cancer patients may prevent recurrence of cancer, and immunosuppressive drugs given to transplant patients may prevent transplant rejection. Subjects in clinical trials of sequelae prevention must be diagnosed as having the disease in question and should be admitted to the study soon enough following diagnosis to permit the treatment assignment to occur in a timely fashion.

It is desirable to assign treatments in clinical trials in a way that allows one to account for possible differences among treatment groups with respect to unmeasured "baseline" characteristics. As part of this goal, the assignment mechanism should deter manipulation of assignments that is not part of the protocol. It is almost universally agreed that randomization is the best way to deal with concerns about confounding by unmeasured baseline characteristics and by personnel manipulation of treatment assignment (Byar et al., 1976; Peto et al., 1976; Gelman et al., 2003). The validity of the trial depends strongly on the extent to which the random assignment protocol is the sole determinant of the treatments received. When this condition is satisfied, confounding due to unmeasured factors can be regarded as random, is accounted for by standard statistical procedures, and diminishes in likely magnitude as the number randomized increases (Greenland and Robins, 1986; Greenland, 1990). When the condition is not satisfied, however, unmeasured confounders may bias the statistics, just as in observational studies. Even when the condition is satisfied, the *generalizability* of trial results may be affected by selective enrollment. Trial participants do not often reflect the distribution of sex, age, race, and ethnicity of the target patient population (Murthy et al., 2004; Heiat et al., 2002). When treatment efficacy is modified by sex, age, race, ethnicity, or other factors, however, and the study population differs from the population that would be receiving the treatment with respect to these variables, then the average study effect will differ from the average effect among those who would receive treatment. In these circumstances, extrapolation of the study results is tenuous or unwarranted, and one may have to restrict the inferences to specific subgroups, if the size of those subgroups permits.

Given that treatment depends on random allocation, rather than patient and physician treatment decision-making, patients' enrollment into a trial requires their informed consent. At a minimum, informed consent requires that participants understand (a) that they are participating in a research study of a stated duration, (b) the purpose of the research, the procedures that will be followed, and which procedures are experimental, (c) that their participation is voluntary and that they can withdraw at any time, and (d) the potential risks and benefits associated with their participation.

Although randomization methods often assign subjects to treatments in approximately equal proportions, this equality is not always optimal. True equipoise provides a rationale for equal assignment proportions, but often one treatment is expected to be more effective based on a biologic rationale, earlier studies, or even preliminary data from the same study. In these circumstances, equal assignment probabilities may be a barrier to enrollment and may even become unethical. Adaptive randomization (Armitage, 1985) or imbalanced assignment (Avins, 1998) allows more subjects in the trial to receive the treatment expected to be more effective with little reduction in power.

Whenever feasible, clinical trials should attempt to employ blinding with respect to the treatment assignment. Ideally, the individual who makes the assignment, the patient, and the assessor of the outcome should all be ignorant of the treatment assignment. Blinding prevents certain biases that could affect assignment, assessment, or compliance. Most important is to keep the assessor blind, especially if the outcome assessment is subjective, as with a clinical diagnosis. (Some outcomes, such as death, will be relatively insusceptible to bias in assessment.) Patient knowledge of treatment assignment can affect compliance with the treatment regime and can bias perceptions of symptoms that might affect the outcome assessment. Studies in which both the assessor and the patient are blinded as to the treatment assignment are known as *double-blind studies*. A study in which the individual who makes the assignment is unaware which treatment is which (such as might occur if the treatments are coded pills and the assigner does not know the code) may be described as *triple-blind*, though this term is used more often to imply that the data analyst (in addition to the patient and the assessor) does not know which group of patients in the analysis received which treatment.

Depending on the nature of the intervention, it may not be possible or practical to keep knowledge of the assignment from all of these parties. For example, a treatment may have well-known side effects that allow the patients to identify the treatment. The investigator needs to be aware of and to report these possibilities, so that readers can assess whether all or part of any reported association might be attributable to the lack of blinding.

If there is no accepted treatment for the condition being studied, it may be useful to employ a placebo as the comparison treatment, when ethical constraints allow it. *Placebos* are inert treatments intended to have no effect other than the psychologic benefit of receiving a treatment, which itself can have a powerful effect. This psychologic benefit is called a *placebo response*, even if it occurs among patients receiving active treatment. By employing a placebo, an investigator may be able to control for the psychologic component of receiving treatment and study the nonpsychologic benefits of a new intervention. In addition, employing a placebo facilitates blinding if there would otherwise be no comparison treatment. These benefits may be incomplete, however, if noticeable side effects of the active treatment inform the subject that he or she has been randomized to the active treatment. This information may enhance the placebo response – that is, the psychologic component of treatment – by encouraging the expectation that the therapy should have a positive effect.

Placebos are not necessary when the objective of the trial is solely to compare different treatments with one another. In such settings, however, one should be alert to the possibility of enhanced placebo effect or compliance differences due to differences in noticeable side effects.

Noncompliance with assigned treatment results in a discrepancy between treatment assigned and actual treatment received by trial participants. Standard practice bases all comparisons on treatment assignment rather than on treatment received. This practice is called the intent-to-treat principle, because the analysis is based on the intended treatment, not the received treatment. Although this principle helps preserve the validity of tests for treatment effects, in typical applications it biases estimates of treatment effect toward the null. Hence, alternative analytic methods have been developed (Goetghebeur and Van Houwelingen, 1998). Compliance may sometimes be measured by directly querying subjects about their compliance, by obtaining relevant data (e.g., by asking that unused pills be returned), or by biochemical measurements. These compliance measures can then be used to adjust estimates of treatment effects using special methods (Sommer and Zeger, 1991; Angrist et al., 1996; Greenland, 2000).

Most trials are monitored while they are being conducted by a Data and Safety Monitoring Committee or Board (DSMB). The primary objective of these committees is to ensure the safety of the trial participants (Wilhelmsen, 2002). The committee reviews study results, including estimates of the main treatment effects and the occurrence of adverse events, to determine whether the trial ought to be stopped before its scheduled completion. The rationale for early stopping might be (a) the appearance of an effect favoring one treatment that is so strong that it would no longer be ethical to randomize new patients to the alternative treatment or to deny enrolled patients access to the favored treatment, (b) the occurrence of adverse events at rates considered to be unacceptable, given the expected benefit of the treatment or trial results, or (c) the determination that the reasonably expected results are no longer of sufficient value to continue the trial. The deliberations of DSMB involve weighing issues of medicine, ethics, law, statistics, and costs to arrive at a decision about whether to continue a trial. Given the complexity of the issues, the membership of DSMB must comprise a diverse range of training and experiences, and thus often includes clinicians, statisticians, and ethicists, none of whom have a material interest in the trial's result.

The frequentist statistical rules commonly used by DSMB to determine whether to stop a trial were developed to ensure that the chance of Type I error (incorrect rejection of the main null hypothesis of no treatment effect) would not exceed a prespecified level (the alpha level) during the planned interim analyses (Armitage et al., 1969). Despite these goals, DSMB members may misinterpret interim results (George et al., 2004) and strict adherence to these stopping rules may yield spurious results (Wheatley and Clayton, 2003). Stopping a trial early because of the appearance of an effect favoring one treatment will often result in an overestimate of the true benefit of the treatment (Pocock and Hughes, 1989). Furthermore, trials stopped early may not allow sufficient follow-up to observe adverse events associated with the favored treatment (Cannistra, 2004), particularly if those events are chronic sequelae. Bayesian alternatives have been suggested to ameliorate many of these shortcomings (Berry, 1993; Carlin and Sargent, 1996; Spielgelhalter et al., 2004).

2.4. Field trials

Field trials differ from clinical trials in that their subjects are not defined by presence of disease or by presentation for clinical care; instead the focus is on the initial occurrence of disease. Patients in a clinical trial may face the complications of their disease with high probability during a relatively short time. In contrast, the risk of incident disease among free-living subjects is typically much lower. Consequently, field trials usually require a much larger number of subjects than clinical trials and are usually much more expensive. Furthermore, since the subjects are not under active health care, and thus do not come to a central location for treatment, a field trial often requires visiting subjects at work, home, school, or establishing centers from which the study can be conducted and to which subjects are urged to report. These design features add to the cost.

The expense of field trials limits their use to the study of preventives of either extremely common or extremely serious diseases. Several field trials were conducted to determine the efficacy of large doses of vitamin C in preventing the common cold (Karlowski et al., 1975; Dykes and Meier, 1975). Poliomyelitis, a rare but serious illness, was a sufficient public health concern to warrant what may have been the largest formal human experiment ever attempted, the Salk vaccine trial, in which the vaccine or a placebo was administered to hundreds of thousands of school children (Francis et al., 1955). When the disease outcome occurs rarely, it is more efficient to study subjects thought to be at higher risk. Thus, the trial of hepatitis B vaccine was carried out in a population of New York City male homosexuals, among whom hepatitis B infection occurs with much greater frequency than is usual among New Yorkers (Szmuness, 1980). Similarly, the effect of cessation of douching on the risk of pelvic inflammatory disease was studied in women with a history of recent sexually transmitted disease, a strong risk factor for pelvic inflammatory disease (Rothman et al., 2003).

Analogous reasoning is often applied to the design of clinical trials, which may concentrate on patients at high risk of adverse outcomes. Because patients who had already experienced a myocardial infarction are at high risk for a second infarction, several clinical trials of the effect of lowering serum cholesterol levels on the risk of myocardial infarction were undertaken on such patients (Leren, 1966; Detre and Shaw, 1974). It is much more costly to conduct a trial designed to study the effect of lowering serum cholesterol on the first occurrence of a myocardial infarction, because many more subjects must be included to provide a reasonable number of outcome events to study. The Multiple Risk Factor Intervention Trial (MRFIT) was a field trial of several primary preventives of myocardial infarction, including diet. Although it admitted only high-risk individuals and endeavored to reduce risk through several simultaneous interventions, the study involved 12,866 subjects and cost \$115 million (more than half a billion 2008 dollars) (Kolata, 1982).

As in clinical trials, exposures in field trials should be assigned according to a protocol that minimizes extraneous variation across the groups, e.g., by removing any discretion in assignment from the study's staff. A random assignment scheme is again an ideal choice, but the difficulties of implementing such a scheme in a large-scale field trial can outweigh the advantages. For example, it may be convenient to distribute vaccinations to groups in batches that are handled identically, especially if storage and transport of the vaccine is difficult. Such practicalities may dictate use of modified randomization protocols such as cluster randomization (explained below). Because such modifications can seriously affect the informativeness and interpretation of experimental findings, the advantages and disadvantages need to be carefully weighed.

2.5. Community intervention and cluster randomized trials

The community intervention trial is an extension of the field trial that involves intervention on a community-wide basis. Conceptually, the distinction hinges on whether or not the intervention is implemented separately for each individual. Whereas a vaccine is ordinarily administered singly to individual people, water fluoridation to prevent dental caries is ordinarily administered to individual water supplies. Consequently, water fluoridation was evaluated by community intervention trials in which entire communities were selected and exposure (water treatment) was assigned on a community basis. Other examples of preventives that might be implemented on a community-wide basis include fast-response emergency resuscitation programs and educational programs conducted using mass media, such as Project Burn Prevention in Massachusetts (MacKay and Rothman, 1982).

Some interventions are implemented most conveniently with groups of subjects smaller than entire communities. Dietary intervention may be made most conveniently by family or household. Environmental interventions may affect an entire office, factory, or residential building. Protective sports equipment may have to be assigned to an entire team or league. Intervention groups may be army units, classrooms, vehicle occupants, or any other group whose members are simultaneously exposed to the intervention. The scientific foundation of experiments using such interventions is identical to that of community intervention trials. What sets all these studies apart from field trials is that the interventions are assigned to groups rather than to individuals.

Field trials in which the treatment is assigned randomly to groups of participants are said to be cluster randomized. The larger the size of the group to be randomized relative to the total study size, the less that is accomplished by random assignment. If only two communities are involved in a study, one of which will receive the intervention and the other will not, such as in the Newburgh–Kingston water fluoridation trial (Ast et al., 1956), it cannot matter whether the community that receives the fluoride is assigned randomly or not. Differences in baseline (extraneous) characteristics will have the same magnitude and the same effect whatever the method of assignment – only the direction of the differences will be affected. It is only when the numbers of groups randomized to each intervention are large that randomization is likely to produce similar distributions of baseline characteristics among the intervention groups. Analysis of cluster randomized trials should thus involve methods that take account of the clustering (Omar and Thompson, 2000; Turner et al., 2001; Spiegelhalter, 2001), which are essential to properly estimate the amount of variability introduced by the randomization (given a hypothesis about the size of the treatment effects).

3. Nonexperimental studies

The limitations imposed by ethics and costs restrict most epidemiologic research to nonexperimental studies. While it is unethical for an investigator to expose a person to a potential cause of disease simply to learn about etiology, people often willingly or unwillingly expose themselves to many potentially harmful factors. People in industrialized nations expose themselves, among other things, to tobacco, to a range of exercise regimens from sedentary to grueling, to diets ranging from vegan to those derived almost entirely from animal protein, and to medical interventions for diverse conditions. Each of these exposures may have intended and unintended consequences that can be investigated by observational epidemiology.

Ideally, we would want the strength of evidence from nonexperimental research to be as high as that obtainable from a well-designed experiment, had one been possible. In an experiment, however, the investigator has the power to assign exposures in a way that enhances the validity of the study, whereas in nonexperimental research the investigator cannot control the circumstances of exposure. If those who happen to be exposed have a greater or lesser risk for the disease than those who are not exposed, a simple comparison between exposed and unexposed will be confounded by this difference and thus not reflect validly the sole effect of the exposure. The comparison will be confounded by the extraneous differences in risk across the exposure groups (i.e., differences that are not attributable to the exposure under study).

Because the investigator cannot assign exposure in nonexperimental studies, he or she must rely heavily on the primary source of discretion that remains: the selection of subjects. There are two primary types of nonexperimental studies in epidemiology. The first, the *cohort study* (also called the "follow-up study" or "incidence study"), is a direct analogue of the experiment. Different exposure groups are compared, but the investigator only selects subjects to observe, and only classifies these subjects by exposure status rather than assigning them to exposure groups. The second, the *incident case-control study*, or simply the *case-control study*, employs an extra step of sampling from the source population for cases. Whereas a cohort study would include all persons in the population giving rise to the study cases, a case-control study selects only a sample of those persons and chooses who to include in part based on their disease status. This extra sampling step can make a case-control study much more efficient than a cohort study of the same population, but it introduces a number of subtleties and avenues for bias that are absent in typical cohort studies.

4. Cohort studies

The goal of a cohort study is to measure and usually to compare the incidence of disease in one or more study cohorts. In epidemiology, the word *cohort* often designates a group of people who share a common experience or condition. For example, a birth cohort shares the same year or period of birth, a cohort of smokers has the experience of smoking in common, and a cohort of vegetarians share their dietary habit. Often, if there are two cohorts in the study, one of them is described as the exposed cohort – those individuals who have experienced a putative causal event or condition – and the other is thought of as the unexposed, or reference, cohort. If there are more than two cohorts, each may be characterized by a different level or type of exposure.

4.1. Definition of cohorts and exposure groups

In principle, a cohort study could be used to estimate average risks, rates, or occurrence times. Except in certain situations, however, average risks and occurrence times cannot be measured directly from the experience of a cohort. Observation of average risks or times of specific events requires that the whole cohort remain at risk and under observation for the entire follow-up period. Loss of subjects during the study period prevents direct measurements of these averages, since the outcome of lost subjects is unknown. Subjects who die from competing risks (outcomes other than the one of interest) likewise prevent the investigator from estimating conditional risks (risk of a specific outcome conditional on not getting other outcomes) directly. Thus, the only situation in which it is feasible to measure average risks and occurrence times directly is in a cohort study in which there is little or no loss to follow-up and little competing risk. While some clinical trials provide these conditions, many epidemiologic studies do not. When losses and competing risks do occur, one may still directly estimate the incidence rate, whereas average risk and occurrence time must be estimated using survival (life-table) methods.

Unlike average risks, which are measured with individuals as the unit in the denominator, incidence rates have person-time as the unit of measure. The accumulation of time rather than individuals in the denominator of rates allows flexibility in the analysis of cohort studies. Whereas studies that estimate risk directly are conceptually tied to the identification of specific cohorts of individuals, studies measuring incidence rates can, with certain assumptions, define the comparison groups in terms of person-time units that do not correspond to specific cohorts of individuals. A given individual can contribute person-time to one, two, or more exposure groups in a given study, because each unit of person-time contributed to follow-up by a given individual possesses its own classification with respect to exposure. Thus, an individual whose exposure experience changes with time can, depending on details of the study hypothesis, contribute follow-up time to several different exposure-specific rates. In such a study, the definition of each exposure group corresponds to the definition of person-time eligibility for each level of exposure.

As a result of this focus on person-time, it does not always make sense to refer to the members of an exposure group within a cohort study as if the same set of individuals were exposed at all points in time. The terms *open* or *dynamic population* describe a population in which the person-time experience can accrue from a changing roster of individuals. (Sometimes the terms *open cohort* or *dynamic cohort* are used, but this usage conflicts with other usage in which a cohort is a fixed roster of individuals.) For example, the incidence rates of cancer reported by the Connecticut Cancer Registry come from the experience of an open population. Since the population of residents of Connecticut is always changing, the individuals who contribute to these rates are not a specific set of people who are followed through time.

When the exposure groups in a cohort study represent groups that are defined at the start of follow-up, with no movement of individuals between exposure groups during the follow-up, the exposure groups are sometimes called *fixed cohorts*. The groups defined by treatment allocation in clinical trials are examples of fixed cohorts. If the follow-up of fixed cohorts suffers from losses to follow-up or competing risks, incidence rates can still be directly measured and used to estimate average risks and incidence times. If no losses occur from a fixed cohort, the cohort satisfies the definition of a *closed population*, so is then called *a closed cohort*. In such cohorts, unconditional risks (which include the effect of competing risks) and average survival times can be directly measured.

It is tempting to think of the identification of study cohorts as simply a process of identifying and classifying individuals as to their exposure status. The process can be complicated, however, by the need to classify the experience of a single individual in different exposure categories at different times. If the exposure can vary over time, at a minimum the investigator needs to allow for the time experienced by each study subject in each category of exposure in the definition of the study cohorts. The sequence or timing of exposure could also be important. If there can be many possible exposure sequences, each individual could have a unique sequence of exposure levels and so define a unique exposure cohort containing only that individual.

A simplifying assumption common in epidemiologic analysis is that the only aspect of exposure determining current risk is some simple numeric summary of exposure history. Typical summaries include current level of exposure, average exposure, or cumulative exposure, that is, the sum of each exposure level multiplied by the time spent at that level. Often, exposure is *lagged* in the summary, which means that only exposure at or up to some specified time before the current time is counted. Although one has enormous flexibility in defining exposure summaries, methods based on assuming that only a single summary is relevant can be severely biased under certain conditions (Robins, 1987). For now, we will assume that a single summary is an adequate measure of exposure. With this assumption, cohort studies may be analyzed by defining the cohorts based on person-time rather than on persons, so that a person may be a member of different exposure cohorts at different times. We nevertheless caution the reader to bear in mind the single-summary assumption when interpreting such analyses.

The time that an individual contributes to the denominator of one or more of the incidence rates in a cohort study is sometimes called the *time at risk*, in the sense of being at risk for development of the disease. Some people and, consequently, all their person-time are not at risk for a given disease because they are immune or they lack the target organ for the study disease. For example, women who have had a hysterectomy and all men are by definition not at risk for uterine cancer, because they have no uterus.

4.2. Classifying person-time

The main guide to the classification of persons or person-time is the study hypothesis, which should be defined in as much detail as possible. If the study addresses the question of the extent to which eating carrots will reduce the subsequent risk of lung cancer, the study hypothesis is best stated in terms of what quantity of carrots consumed over what period of time will prevent lung cancer. Furthermore, the study hypothesis should specify an induction time between the consumption of a given amount of carrots and the subsequent effect: The effect of the carrot consumption could take place immediately, begin gradually, or only begin after a delay, and it could extend beyond the time that an individual might cease eating carrots (Rothman, 1981).

In studies with chronic exposures (i.e., exposures that persist over an extended period of time), it is easy to confuse the time during which exposure occurs with the time at risk of exposure effects. For example, in occupational studies, time of employment is sometimes confused with time at risk for exposure effects. The time of employment is a time during which exposure accumulates. In contrast, the time at risk for exposure effects must logically come after the accumulation of a specific amount of exposure, because only after that time disease can be caused or prevented by that amount of exposure. The lengths of these two time periods have no constant relation to one another. The time at risk of effects might well extend beyond the end of employment. It is only the time at risk of effects that should be tallied in the denominator of incidence rates for that amount of exposure.

How should the investigator study hypotheses that do not specify induction times? For these, the appropriate time periods on which to stratify the incidence rates are unclear. There is no way to estimate exposure effects, however, without making some assumption, implicitly or explicitly, about the induction time. The decision about what time to include for a given individual in the denominator of the rate corresponds to the assumption about induction time. But what if the investigator does not have any basis for hypothesizing a specific induction period? It is possible to learn about the period by estimating effects according to categories of time since exposure. For example, the incidence rate of leukemia among atomic bomb survivors relative to that among those who were distant from the bomb at the time of the explosion can be examined according to years since the explosion. In an unbiased study, we would expect the effect estimates to rise above the null value when the minimum induction period has passed. This procedure works best when the exposure itself occurs at a point or narrow interval of time, but it can be used even if the exposure is chronic, as long as there is a way to define when a certain hypothesized accumulation of exposure has occurred.

The definition of chronic exposure based on anticipated effects is more complicated than when exposure occurs only at a point in time. We may conceptualize a period during which the exposure accumulates to a sufficient extent to trigger a step in the causal process. This accumulation of exposure experience may be a complex function of the intensity of the exposure and time. The induction period begins only after the exposure has reached this hypothetical triggering point, and that point will likely vary across individuals. Occupational epidemiologists have often measured the induction time for occupational exposure from the time of first exposure, but this procedure involves the extreme assumption that the first contact with the exposure can be sufficient to produce disease. Whatever assumption is adopted, it should be made an explicit part of the definition of the cohort and the period of follow-up.

4.3. Nonexposed time in exposed subjects

What happens to the time experienced by exposed subjects that does not meet the definition of time at risk of exposure effects according to the study hypothesis? Specifically, what happens to the time after the exposed subjects become exposed and before the minimum induction has elapsed, or after a maximum induction time has passed? Two choices are reasonable for handling this experience. One possibility is to consider any time that is not related to exposure as unexposed time and to apportion that time to the study cohort that represents no exposure. Possible objections to this approach would be that the study hypothesis may be based on guesses about the threshold for exposure effects and the induction period and that time during the exposure accumulation or induction periods may in fact be at risk of exposure effects. To treat the latter experience as not at risk of exposure effects may then lead to an underestimate of the effect of exposure. Alternatively, one may simply omit from the study the experience of exposed subjects that is not at risk of exposure effects according to the study hypothesis. For this alternative to be practical, there must be a reasonably large number of cases observed among subjects with no exposure.

For example, suppose a 10-year minimum induction time is hypothesized. For individuals followed from start of exposure, this hypothesis implies that no exposure effect can occur within the first 10 years of follow-up. Only after the first 10 years of follow-up an individual can experience disease due to exposure. Therefore, under the hypothesis, only person-time occurring after 10 years of exposure should contribute to the denominator of the rate among exposed. If the hypothesis were correct, we should assign the first 10 years of follow-up to the denominator of the unexposed rate. Suppose, however, that the hypothesis were wrong and exposure could produce cases in less than 10 years. Then, if the cases and person-time from the first 10 years of follow-up were added to the unexposed cases and person-time, the resulting rate would be biased toward the rate in the exposed, thus reducing the apparent differences between the exposed and unexposed rates. If computation of the unexposed rate were limited to truly unexposed cases and person-time, this problem would be avoided.

The price of avoidance, however, would be reduced precision in estimating the rate among the unexposed. In some studies, the number of truly unexposed cases is too small to produce a stable comparison and thus the early experience of exposed persons is too valuable to discard. In general, the best procedure in a given situation would depend on the decrease in precision produced by excluding the early experience of exposed persons and the amount of bias that is introduced by treating the early experience of exposed persons as if it were equivalent to that of people who were never exposed. An alternative that attempts to address both problems is to treat the induction time as a continuous variable rather than a fixed time, and model exposure effects as depending on the times of exposure (Thomas, 1983, 1988). This approach is arguably more realistic insofar as the induction time varies across individuals.

Similar issues arise if the exposure status can change from exposed to unexposed. If the exposure ceases but the effects of exposure are thought to continue, it would not make sense to put the experience of a formerly exposed individual in the unexposed category. On the other hand, if exposure effects are thought to be approximately contemporaneous with the exposure, which is to say that the induction period is near zero, then changes in exposure status should lead to corresponding changes in how the accumulating experience is classified with respect to exposure.

4.4. Categorizing exposure

Another problem to consider is that the study hypothesis may not provide reasonable guidance on where to draw the boundary between exposed and unexposed. If the exposure is continuous, it is not necessary to draw boundaries at all. Instead one may use the quantitative information from each individual fully either by using some type of smoothing method, such as moving averages, or by putting the exposure variable into a regression model as a continuous term. Of course, the latter approach depends on the validity of the model used for estimation. Special care must be taken with models of repeatedly measured exposures and confounders, which are sometimes called longitudinal-data models.

The simpler approach of calculating rates directly will require a reasonably sized population within categories of exposure if it is to provide a statistically stable result. To get incidence rates, then, we need to group the experience of individuals into relatively large categories for which we can calculate the incidence rates. In principle, it should be possible to form several cohorts that correspond to various levels of exposure. For a cumulative measure of exposure, however, categorization may introduce additional difficulties for the cohort definition. An individual who passes through one level of exposure along the way to a higher level would later have time at risk for disease that theoretically might meet the definition for more than one category of exposure.

For example, suppose we define moderate smoking as having smoked 50,000 cigarettes (equivalent to about 7 pack-years), and we define heavy smoking as having smoked 150,000 cigarettes (about 21 pack-years). Suppose a man smoked his 50,000th cigarette in 1970 and his 150,000th in 1980. After allowing for a 5-year minimum induction period, we would classify his time as moderate smoking beginning in 1975. By 1980 he has become a heavy smoker, but the 5-year induction period for heavy smoking has not elapsed. Thus, from 1980 to 1985, his experience is still classified as moderate smoking, but from 1985 onward his experience is classified as heavy smoking. Usually, the time is allocated only to the highest category of exposure that applies. This example illustrates the complexity of the cohort definition with a hypothesis that takes into account both the cumulative amount of exposure and a minimum induction time. Other apportionment schemes could be devised based on other hypotheses about exposure action, including hypotheses that allowed induction time to vary with exposure history.

One invalid allocation scheme would apportion to the denominator of the exposed incidence rate the unexposed experience of an individual who eventually became exposed. For example, suppose that in an occupational study, exposure is categorized according to duration of employment in a particular job, with the highest exposure category being at least 20 years of employment. Suppose a worker is employed at that job for 30 years. It is a mistake to assign the 30 years of experience for that employee to the exposure category of 20 or more years of employment. The worker only reached that category of exposure after 20 years on the job, and only the last 10 years of his or her experience is relevant to the highest category of exposure. Note that if the worker had died after 10 years of employment, the death could not have been assigned to the 20-years-of-employment category, because the worker would have only had 10 years of employment.

A useful rule to remember is that the event and the person-time that is being accumulated at the moment of the event should both be assigned to the same category of exposure. Thus, once the person-time spent at each category of exposure has been determined for each study subject, the classification of the disease events (cases) follows the same rules. The exposure category to which an event is assigned is the same exposure category in which the person-time for that individual was accruing at the instant in which the event occurred. The same rule – that the classification of the event follows the classification of the person-time – also applies with respect to other study variables that may be used to stratify the data. For example, person-time will be allocated into different age categories as an individual ages. The age category to which an event is assigned should be the same age category in which the individual's person-time was accumulating at the time of the event.

4.5. Average intensity and alternatives

One can also define current exposure according to the average (arithmetic or geometric mean) intensity or level of exposure up to the current time, rather than by a cumulative measure. In the occupational setting, the average concentration of an agent in the ambient air would be an example of exposure intensity, although one would also have to take into account any protective gear that might affect the individual's exposure to the agent. Intensity of exposure is a concept that applies to a point in time, and intensity typically will vary over time. Studies that measure exposure intensity might use a time-weighted average of intensity, which would require multiple measurements of exposure over time. The amount of time that an individual is exposed to each intensity would provide its weight in the computation of the average.

An alternative to the average intensity is to classify exposure according to the maximum intensity, median intensity, minimum intensity, or some other function of the exposure history. The follow-up time that an individual spends at a given exposure intensity could begin to accumulate as soon as that level of intensity is reached. Induction time must also be taken into account. Ideally, the study hypothesis will specify a minimum induction time for exposure effects, which in turn will imply an appropriate lag period to be used in classifying individual experience.

4.6. Immortal person-time

Occasionally, a cohort's definition will require that everyone meeting the definition must have survived for a specified period. Typically, this period of immortality comes about because one of the entry criteria into the cohort is dependent on survival. For example, an occupational cohort might be defined as all workers who have been employed at a specific factory for at least 5 years. There are certain problems with such an entry criterion, among them that these will guarantee that the study will miss effects among short-term workers who may be assigned more highly exposed jobs than regular long-term employees, may include persons more susceptible to exposure effects, and may quit early because of those effects. Let us assume, however, that only long-term workers are of interest for the study and that all relevant exposures (including those during the initial 5 years of employment) are taken into account in the analysis.

The 5-year entry criterion will guarantee that all of the workers in the study cohort survived their first 5 years of employment, since those who died would never meet the entry criterion and so would be excluded. It follows that mortality analysis of such workers should exclude the first 5 years of employment for each worker. This period of time is referred to as *immortal person-time.* The workers at the plant were not immortal during this time, of course, since they could have died. The subset of workers that satisfy the cohort definition, however, is identified after the fact as those who have survived this period.

The correct approach to handling immortal person-time in a study is to exclude it from any denominator, even if the analysis does not focus on mortality. This approach is correct because including immortal person-time will downwardly bias estimated disease rates and, consequently, bias effect estimates obtained from internal comparisons. To avoid this bias, if a study has a criterion for a minimum amount of time before a subject is eligible to be in a study, the time during which the eligibility criterion is met should be excluded from the calculation of incidence rates. More generally, the follow-up time allocated to a specific exposure category should exclude time during which the exposure-category definition is being met.

4.7. Postexposure events

Allocation of follow-up time to specific categories should not depend on events that occur after the follow-up time in question has accrued. For example, consider a study in which a group of smokers is advised to quit smoking with the objective of estimating the effect on mortality rates of quitting versus continuing to smoke. For a subject who smokes for a while after the advice is given and then quits later, the follow-up time as a quitter should only begin at the time of quitting not at the time of giving the advice, because it is the effect of quitting that is being studied not the effect of advice (were the effect of advice under study, follow-up time would begin with the advice). But how should a subject be treated who quits for a while and then later takes up smoking again?

When this question arose in an actual study of this problem, the investigators excluded anyone from the study who switched back to smoking. Their decision was wrong, because if the subject had died before switching back to smoking, the death would have counted in the study and the subject would not have been excluded. A subject's follow-up time was excluded if the subject switched back to smoking, something that occurred only *after* the subject had accrued time in the quit-smoking cohort. A proper analysis should include the experience of those who switched back to smoking up until the time that they switched back. If the propensity to switch back was unassociated with risk, their experience subsequent to switching back could be excluded without introducing bias. The incidence rate among the person-years while having quit could then be compared with the rate among those who never quit.

As another example, suppose that the investigators wanted to examine the effect of being an ex-smoker for at least 5 years, relative to being an ongoing smoker. Then, anyone who returned to smoking within 5 years of quitting would be excluded. The person-time experience for each subject during the first 5 years after quitting should also be excluded, since it would be immortal person-time.

4.8. Timing of outcome events

As may be apparent from earlier discussion, the time at which an outcome event occurs can be a major determinant of the amount of person-time contributed by a subject to each exposure category. It is therefore important to define and determine the time of the event as unambiguously and precisely as possible. For some events, such as death, neither task presents any difficulty. For other outcomes, such as human immunodeficiency virus (HIV) seroconversion, the time of the event can be defined in a reasonably precise manner (the appearance of HIV antibodies in the bloodstream), but measurement of the time is difficult. For others, such as multiple sclerosis and atherosclerosis, the very definition of the onset time can be ambiguous, even when the presence of the disease can be unambiguously determined. Likewise, time of loss to follow-up and other censoring events can be difficult to define and determine. Determining whether an event occurred by a given time is a special case of determining when an event occurred, because knowing that the event occurred by the given time requires knowing that the time it occurred was before the given time.

Addressing the aforementioned problems depends heavily on the details of available data and the current state of knowledge about the study outcome. In all situations, we recommend that one start with at least one written protocol to classify subjects based on available information. For example, seroconversion time may be measured as the midpoint between time of last negative and first positive test. For unambiguously defined events, any deviation of actual times from the protocol determination can be viewed as measurement error. Ambiguously timed diseases, such as cancers or vascular conditions, are often taken as occurring at diagnosis time, but the use of a minimum lag period is advisable whenever a long latent (undiagnosed or prodromal) period is inevitable. It may sometimes be possible to interview cases about the earliest onset of symptoms, but such recollections and symptoms can be subject to considerable error and between-person variability.

Some ambiguously timed events are dealt with by standard, if somewhat arbitrary, definitions. For example, in 1993, AIDS onset was redefined as occurrence of any AIDS-defining illnesses or clinical event (e.g., CD4 count $<200/\mu L$). As a second example, time of loss to follow-up is conventionally taken as midway between the last successful attempt to contact and the first unsuccessful attempt to contact. Any difficulty in determining an arbitrarily defined time of an event is then treated as a measurement problem. One should recognize, however, that the arbitrariness of the definition for the time of an event represents another source of measurement error.

4.9. Expense

Cohort studies are usually large enterprises. Most diseases affect only a small proportion of a population, even if the population is followed for many years. To obtain stable estimates of incidence requires a substantial number of cases of disease, and therefore the person-time giving rise to the cases must also be substantial. Sufficient person-time can be accumulated by following cohorts for a long span of time. Some cohorts with special exposures (e.g., Japanese victims of atomic bombs (Beebe, 1979)) or with detailed medical and personal histories (e.g., the Framingham, Massachusetts, study cohort (Kannel and Abbott, 1984)) have indeed been followed for decades. If a study is intended to provide more timely results, the requisite person-time can be attained by increasing the size of the cohorts. If exposure accumulation is time dependent and the disease induction time is lengthy (Rothman, 1981), either a lengthy study or obtaining some information retrospectively may be necessary. Of course, lengthy studies of large populations are expensive. It is not uncommon for cohort studies to cost millions of dollars, and expenses in excess of $100 million have occurred. Most of the expense derives from the need to establish a continuing system for monitoring disease occurrence in a large population.

The expense of cohort studies often limits feasibility. The lower the disease incidence, the poorer the feasibility of a cohort study. Feasibility is further handicapped by a long induction period between the hypothesized cause and its effect. A long induction time contributes to a low overall incidence because of the additional follow-up time required to obtain exposure-related cases. To detect any effect, the study must span an interval at least as long as, and in practice considerably longer than, the minimum induction period. Cohort studies are poorly suited to study the effect of exposures that are hypothesized to cause rare diseases with long induction periods. Such cohort studies are expensive in relation to the amount of information returned, which is to say that they are not efficient.

The expense of cohort studies can be reduced in a variety of ways. One way is to use an existing system for monitoring disease occurrence. For example, a regional cancer registry may be used to ascertain cancer occurrence among cohort members. If the expense of case ascertainment is already being borne by the registry, the study will be considerably cheaper.

Another way to reduce cost is to rely on historical cohorts. Rather than identifying cohort members concurrently with the initiation of the study and planning to have the follow-up period occur during the study, the investigator may choose to identify cohort members based on records of previous exposure. The follow-up period until the occurrence of disease may be wholly or partially in the past. To ascertain cases occurring in the past, the investigators must rely on records to ascertain disease in cohort members. If the follow-up period begins before the period during which the study is conducted but extends into the study period, then active surveillance or a new monitoring system to ascertain new cases of disease can be devised.

To the extent that subject selection occurs after the follow-up period under observation (sometimes called retrospective), the study will generally cost less than an equivalent study in which subject selection occurs before the follow-up period (sometimes called prospective). A drawback of retrospective cohort studies is their dependence on records, which may suffer from missing or poorly recorded information. Another drawback is that entire subject records may be missing. When such "missingness" is related to the variables under study, the study may suffer from selection biases similar to those that can occur in case-control studies (see below). For example, if records are systematically deleted upon the death of a cohort member, then all of the retrospective person-time will be immortal, and should therefore be excluded.

A third way to reduce cost is to replace one of the cohorts, specifically the unexposed cohort, with general population information. Rather than collecting new information on a large unexposed population, existing data on a general population is used for comparison. This procedure has several drawbacks. For one, it is reasonable only if there is some assurance that only a small proportion of the general population is exposed to the agent under study, as is often the case with occupational exposures. To the extent that part of the general population is exposed, there is misclassification error that will introduce a bias into the comparison in the direction of underestimating the effect. Another problem is that information obtained for the exposed cohort may differ in quality from the existing data for the general population. If mortality data are used, the death certificate is often the only source of information for the general population. If additional medical information were used to classify deaths in an exposed cohort, the data thus obtained would not be comparable with the general population data. This noncomparability may reduce or increase bias in the resulting comparisons (Greenland and Robins, 1985a). Finally, another problem is the high likelihood that the exposed cohort will differ from the general population in many ways that are not measured, thus leading to uncontrollable confounding in the comparison. The classical "healthy worker effect" is one example of this problem, in which confounding arises because workers must meet a minimal standard of health (they must be able to work) that the general population does not.

A fourth way to reduce the cost of a cohort study is to conduct a case-control study within the cohort rather than including the entire cohort population in the study. Such "nested" case-control studies can often be conducted at a fraction of the cost of a cohort study and yet produce the same findings with nearly the same level of precision.

4.10. Special-exposure and general-population cohorts

An attractive feature of cohort studies is the capability they provide to study a range of possible health effects stemming from a single exposure. A mortality follow-up can be accomplished just as easily for all causes of death as for any specific cause. Health surveillance for one disease endpoint can sometimes be expanded to include many or all endpoints without much additional work. A cohort study can provide a comprehensive picture of the health effect of a given exposure. Attempts to derive such comprehensive information about exposures motivate the identification of "special-exposure" cohorts, which are identifiable groups with exposure to agents of interest. Examples of such special-exposure cohorts include occupational cohorts exposed to workplace exposures, studies of fishermen or farmers exposed chronically to solar radiation, atomic bomb victims and the population around Chernobyl exposed to ionizing radiation, the population around Seveso, Italy exposed to environmental dioxin contamination, Seventh Day Adventists who are "exposed" to vegetarian diets, and populations who are exposed to stress through natural calamities, such as earthquakes. These exposures are not common and require the identification of exposed cohorts to provide enough information for study.

Common exposures are sometimes studied through cohort studies that survey a segment of the population that is identified without regard to exposure status. Such "general-population" cohorts have been used to study the effects of smoking, oral contraceptives, diet, and hypertension. It is most efficient to limit a general-population cohort study to exposures that a substantial proportion of people have experienced; otherwise, the unexposed cohort will be inefficiently large relative to the exposed cohort. A surveyed population can be classified according to smoking, alcoholic beverage consumption, diet, drug use, medical history, and many other factors of potential interest. A disadvantage is that usually the exposure information must be obtained by interviews with each subject, as opposed to obtaining information from records, as is often done with special-exposure cohorts.

5. Case-control studies

Conventional wisdom about case-control studies is that they do not yield estimates of effect that are as valid as measures obtained from cohort studies.

This thinking may reflect common misunderstandings in conceptualizing case-control studies, which is clarified below, but it also reflects concern about quality of exposure information and biases in case or control selection. For example, if exposure information comes from interviews, then cases will have usually reported the exposure information after learning of their diagnosis, which can lead to errors in the responses that are related to the disease (recall bias). While it is true that recall bias does not occur in prospective cohort studies, neither does it occur in all case-control studies. Exposure information that is taken from records will not be subject to recall bias. Similarly, while a cohort study may log information on exposure for an entire source population at the outset of the study, it still requires tracing of subjects to ascertain exposure variation and outcomes, and the success of this tracing may be related to exposure. These concerns are analogous to case-control problems of loss of subjects with unknown exposure and to biased selection of controls and cases. Each study, whether cohort or case-control, must be considered on its own merits.

Conventional wisdom also holds that cohort studies are useful for evaluating the range of effects related to a single exposure, while case-control studies provide information only about the one disease that afflicts the cases. This thinking conflicts with the idea that case-control studies can be viewed simply as more efficient cohort studies. Just as one can choose to measure more than one disease outcome in a cohort study, it is possible to conduct a set of case-control studies nested within the same population using several disease outcomes as the case series. The case-cohort study (see below) is particularly well suited to this task, allowing one control group to be compared with several series of cases. Whether or not the case-cohort design is the form of case-control study that is used, case-control studies do not have to be characterized as being limited with respect to the number of disease outcomes that can be studied.

For diseases that are sufficiently rare, cohort studies become impractical, and case-control studies become the only useful alternative. On the other hand, if exposure is rare, ordinary case-control studies are inefficient, and one must use methods that selectively recruit additional exposed subjects, such as special cohort studies or two-stage designs. If both the exposure and the outcome are rare, two-stage designs may be the only informative option, as they employ oversampling of both exposed and diseased subjects.

Ideally, a case-control study can be conceptualized as a more efficient version of a corresponding cohort study. Under this conceptualization, the cases in the case-control study are the same cases as would ordinarily be included in the cohort study. Rather than including all of the experience of the source population that gave rise to the cases (the study base), as would be the usual practice in a cohort design, controls are selected from the source population. The sampling of controls from the population that gave rise to the cases affords the efficiency gain of a case-control design over a cohort design. The controls provide an estimate of the prevalence of the exposure and covariates in the source population. When controls are selected from members of the population who were at risk for disease at the beginning of the study's follow-up period, the case-control odds ratio estimates the risk ratio that would be obtained from a cohort design. When controls are selected from members of the population who were noncases at the times that each case occurs, or otherwise in proportion to the person-time accumulated by the cohort, the case-control odds ratio estimates the rate ratio that would be obtained from a cohort design. Finally, when controls are selected from members of the population who were noncases at the end of the study's follow-up period, the case-control odds ratio estimates the incidence odds ratio that would be obtained from a cohort design. With each control selection strategy, the odds ratio calculation is the same, but the measure of effect estimated by the odds ratio differs. Study designs that implement each of these control selection paradigms will be discussed after topics that are common to all designs.

5.1. *Common elements of case-control studies*

In a cohort study, the numerator and denominator of each disease frequency (incidence proportion, incidence rate, or incidence odds) are measured, which requires enumerating the entire population and keeping it under surveillance. A case-control study attempts to observe the population more efficiently by using a control series in place of complete assessment of the denominators of the disease frequencies. The cases in a case-control study should be the same people who would be considered cases in a cohort study of the same population.

5.2. *Pseudo-frequencies and the odds ratio*

The primary goal for control selection is that the exposure distribution among controls be the same as it is in the source population of cases. The rationale for this goal is that, if it is met, we can use the control series in place of the denominator information in measures of disease frequency to determine the ratio of the disease frequency in exposed people relative to that among unexposed people. This goal will be met if we can sample controls from the source population such that the ratio of the number of exposed controls (B_1) to the total exposed experience of the source population is the same as the ratio of the number of unexposed controls (B_0) to the unexposed experience of the source population, apart from sampling error. For most purposes, this goal need only be followed within strata of factors that will be used for stratification in the analysis, such as factors used for restriction or matching.

Using person-time to illustrate, the goal requires that B_1 has the same ratio to the amount of exposed person-time (T_1) as B_0 has to the amount of unexposed person-time (T_0):

$$\frac{B_1}{T_1} = \frac{B_0}{T_0}$$

Here B_1/T_1 and B_0/T_0 are the control-sampling rates – that is, the number of controls selected per unit of person-time. Suppose A_1 exposed cases and A_0 unexposed cases occur over the study period. The exposed and unexposed rates are then

$$I_1 = \frac{A_1}{T_1} \quad \text{and} \quad I_0 = \frac{A_0}{T_0}$$

We can use the frequencies of exposed and unexposed controls as substitutes for the actual denominators of the rates to obtain exposure-specific case-control ratios, or *pseudo-rates*:

$$\text{Pseudo-rate}_1 = \frac{A_1}{B_1}$$

and

$$\text{Pseudo-rate}_0 = \frac{A_0}{B_0}$$

These pseudo-rates have no epidemiologic interpretation by themselves. Suppose, however, that the control-sampling rates B_1/T_1 and B_0/T_0 are equal to the same value r, as would be expected if controls are selected independently of exposure. If this common sampling rate r is known, the actual incidence rates can be calculated by simple algebra, since apart from sampling error, B_1/r should equal the amount of exposed person-time in the source population and B_0/r should equal the amount of unexposed person-time in the source population: $B_1/r = B_1/(B_1/T_1) = T_1$ and $B_0/r = B_0/(B_0/T_0) = T_0$. To get the incidence rates, we need only to multiply each pseudo-rate by the common sampling rate, r.

If the common sampling rate is not known, which is often the case, we can still compare the sizes of the pseudo-rates by division. Specifically, if we divide the pseudo-rate for exposed by the pseudo-rate for unexposed, we obtain

$$\frac{\text{Pseudo-rate}_1}{\text{Pseudo-rate}_0} = \frac{A_1/B_1}{A_0/B_0} = \frac{A_1/[(B_1/T_1)T_1]}{A_0/[(B_0/T_0)T_0]} = \frac{A_1/(r \cdot T_1)}{A_0/(r \cdot T_0)} = \frac{A_1/T_1}{A_0/T_0}$$

In other words, the ratio of the pseudo-rates for the exposed and unexposed is an estimate of the ratio of the incidence rates in the source population, provided that the control-sampling rate is independent of exposure. Thus, using the case-control study design, one can estimate the incidence rate ratio in a population without obtaining information on every subject in the population. Similar derivations in the section below on variants of case-control designs show that one can estimate the risk ratio by sampling controls from those at risk for disease at the beginning of the follow-up period (case-cohort design) and that one can estimate the incidence odds ratio by sampling controls from the noncases at the end of the follow-up period (cumulative case-control design). With these designs, the pseudo-frequencies correspond to the incidence proportions and incidence odds, respectively, multiplied by common sampling rates.

There is a statistical penalty for using a sample of the denominators rather than measuring the person-time experience for the entire source population: The precision of the estimates of the incidence rate ratio from a case-control study is less than the precision from a cohort study of the entire population that gave rise to the cases (the source population). Nevertheless, the loss of precision that stems from sampling controls will be small if the number of controls selected per case is large. Furthermore, the loss is balanced by the cost savings of not having to obtain information on everyone in the source population. The cost savings might allow the epidemiologist to enlarge the source population and so obtain more cases resulting in a better overall estimate of the incidence rate ratio, statistically and otherwise, than would be possible using the same expenditures to conduct a cohort study.

The ratio of the two pseudo-rates in a case-control study is usually written as A_1B_0/A_0B_1 and is sometimes called the *cross-product ratio*. The cross-product ratio in a case-control study can be viewed as the ratio of cases to controls among the exposed subjects (A_1/B_1) divided by the ratio of cases to controls among the unexposed subjects (A_0/B_0). This ratio can also be viewed as the odds of being exposed among cases (A_1/A_0) divided by the odds of being exposed among controls (B_1/B_0) in which case it is termed the *exposure odds ratio*. While either interpretation will give the same result, viewing this odds ratio as the ratio of case-control ratios shows more directly how the control group substitutes for the denominator information in a cohort study and how the ratio of pseudo-frequencies gives the same result as the ratio of the incidence rates, incidence proportion, or incidence odds in the source population, if sampling is independent of exposure.

5.3. Defining the source population

If the cases are a representative sample of all cases in a precisely defined and identified population and the controls are sampled directly from this source population, the study is said to be *population based* or a *primary* base study. For a population-based case-control study, random sampling of controls may be feasible if a population registry exists or can be compiled. When random sampling from the source population of cases is feasible, it is usually the most desirable option.

Random sampling of controls does not necessarily mean that every person should have an equal probability of being selected to be a control. As explained above, if the aim is to estimate the incidence rate ratio, then we would employ longitudinal (density) sampling, in which a person's control selection probability is proportional to the person's time at risk. For example, in a case-control study nested within an occupational cohort, workers on an employee roster will have been followed for varying lengths of time, and a random sampling scheme should reflect this varying time to estimate the incidence rate ratio.

When it is not possible to identify the source population explicitly, simple random sampling is not feasible and other methods of control selection must be used. Such studies are sometimes called studies of *secondary* bases, because the source population is identified secondarily to the definition of a case-finding mechanism. A secondary source population or *secondary* base is therefore a source population that is defined from (secondary to) a given case series.

Consider a case-control study in which the cases are patients treated for severe psoriasis at the Mayo Clinic. These patients come to the Mayo Clinic from all corners of the world. What is the specific source population that gives rise to these cases? To answer this question, we would have to know exactly who would go to the Mayo Clinic if he or she had severe psoriasis. We cannot enumerate this source population because many people in it do not know themselves that they would go to the Mayo Clinic for severe psoriasis, unless they actually developed severe psoriasis. This secondary source might be defined as a population spread around the world that constitutes those people who would go to the Mayo Clinic if they developed severe psoriasis. It is this secondary source from which the control series for the study would ideally be drawn. The challenge to the investigator is to apply eligibility criteria to the cases and controls so that there is good correspondence between the controls and this source population. For example, cases of severe psoriasis and controls might be restricted to those in counties within a certain distance of the Mayo Clinic, so that at least a geographic correspondence between the controls and the secondary source population can be assured. This restriction might however leave very few cases for study.

Unfortunately, the concept of a secondary base is often tenuously connected to underlying realities, and can be highly ambiguous. For the psoriasis example, whether a person would go to the Mayo Clinic depends on many factors that vary over time, such as whether the person is encouraged to go by their regular physicians and whether the person can afford to go. It is not clear, then, how or even whether one could precisely define let alone sample from the secondary base, and thus it is not clear one could ensure that controls were members of the base at the time of sampling. We therefore prefer to conceptualize and conduct case-control studies as starting with a well-defined source population and then identify and recruit cases and controls to represent the disease and exposure experience of that population. When one instead takes a case series as a starting point, it is incumbent upon the investigator to demonstrate that a source population can be operationally defined to allow the study to be recast and evaluated relative to this source. Similar considerations apply when one takes a control series as a starting point, as is sometimes done (Greenland, 1985).

5.4. Case selection

Ideally, case selection will amount to a direct sampling of cases within a source population. Therefore, apart from random sampling, all people in the source population who develop the disease of interest are presumed to be included as cases in the case-control study. It is not always necessary, however, to include all cases from the source population. Cases, like controls, can be randomly sampled for inclusion in the case-control study, so long as this sampling is independent of the exposure under study within strata of factors that will be used for stratification in the analysis. Of course, if fewer than all cases are sampled, the study precision will be lower in proportion to the sampling fraction.

The cases identified in a single clinic or treated by a single medical practitioner are possible case series for case-control studies. The corresponding source population for the cases treated in a clinic is all people who would attend that clinic and be recorded with the diagnosis of interest if they had the disease in question.

It is important to specify "if they had the disease in question" because clinics serve different populations for different diseases, depending on referral patterns and the reputation of the clinic in specific specialty areas. As noted above, without a precisely identified source population, it may be difficult or impossible to select controls in an unbiased fashion.

5.5. Control selection

The definition of the source population determines the population from which controls are sampled. Ideally, control selection will amount to a direct sampling of people within the source population. Based on the principles explained above regarding the role of the control series, many general rules for control selection can be formulated. Two basic rules are that: (1) Controls should be selected from the same population – the source population – that gives rise to the study cases. If this rule cannot be followed, there needs to be solid evidence that the population supplying controls has an exposure distribution identical to that of the population that is the source of cases, which is a very stringent demand that is rarely demonstrable. (2) Within strata of factors that will be used for stratification in the analysis, controls should be selected independently of their exposure status, in that the sampling rate for controls (r in the above discussion) should not vary with exposure.

If these rules and the corresponding case rule are met, then the ratio of pseudo-frequencies will, apart from sampling error, equal the ratio of the corresponding measure of disease frequency in the source population. If the sampling rate is known, then the actual measures of disease frequency can also be calculated (see Chapter 21 of Rothman and Greenland, 1998). For a more detailed discussion of the principles of control selection in case-control studies, see Wacholder et al. (1992a, 1992b, 1992c).

When one wishes controls to represent person-time, sampling of the person-time should be constant across exposure levels. This requirement implies that the sampling *probability* of any person as a control should be proportional to the amount of person-time that person spends at risk of disease in the source population. For example, if in the source population one person contributes twice as much person-time during the study period as another person, the first person should have twice the probability of the second of being selected as a control.

This difference in probability of selection is automatically induced by sampling controls at a steady rate per unit time over the period in which cases occur (longitudinal, or density sampling), rather than by sampling all controls at a point in time (such as the start or end of the study). With longitudinal sampling of controls, a population member present for twice as long as another will have twice the chance of being selected.

If the objective of the study is to estimate a risk or rate ratio, it should be possible for a person to be selected as a control and yet remain eligible to become a case, so that person might appear in the study as both a control and a case. This possibility may sound paradoxical or wrong, but is nevertheless correct. It corresponds to the fact that in a cohort study, a case contributes to both the numerator and the denominator of the estimated incidence. If the controls are intended to represent person-time and are selected longitudinally, similar arguments show that a person selected as a control should remain eligible to be selected as a control again, and thus might be included in the analysis repeatedly as a control (Lubin and Gail, 1984; Robins et al., 1986).

5.6. Common fallacies in control selection

In cohort studies, the study population is restricted to people at risk for the disease. Because they viewed case-control studies as if they were cohort studies done backwards, some authors argued that case-control studies ought to be restricted to those at risk for exposure (i.e., those with exposure opportunity). Excluding sterile women from a case-control study of an adverse effect of oral contraceptives and matching for duration of employment in an occupational study are examples of attempts to control for exposure opportunity. Such restrictions do not directly address validity issues and can ultimately harm study precision by reducing the number of unexposed subjects available for study (Poole, 1986). If the factor used for restriction (e.g., sterility) is unrelated to the disease, it will not be a confounder, and hence the restriction will yield no benefit to the validity of the estimate of effect. Furthermore, if the restriction reduces the study size, the precision of the estimate of effect will be reduced.

Another principle sometimes been used in cohort studies is that the study cohort should be "clean" at start of follow-up, including only people who have never had the disease. Misapplying this principle to case-control design suggests that the control group ought to be "clean," including only people who are healthy, for example. Illness arising after the start of the follow-up period is not reason to exclude subjects from a cohort analysis, and such exclusion can lead to bias; similarly controls with illness that arose after exposure should not be removed from the control series. Nonetheless, in studies of the relation between cigarette smoking and colorectal cancer, certain authors recommended that the control group should exclude people with colon polyps, because colon polyps are associated with smoking and are precursors of colorectal cancer (Terry and Neugut, 1998). But such an exclusion reduces the prevalence of the exposure in the controls below that in the actual source population of cases, and hence biases the effect estimates upward (Poole, 1999).

5.7. Sources for control series

The methods suggested below for control sampling apply when the source population cannot be explicitly enumerated, so random sampling is not possible. All these methods should only be implemented subject to the reservations about secondary bases described above.

5.7.1. Neighborhood controls

If the source population cannot be enumerated, it may be possible to select controls through sampling of residences. This method is not straightforward. Usually, a geographic roster of residences is not available, so a scheme must be devised to sample residences without enumerating them all. For convenience, investigators may sample controls who are individually matched to cases from the same neighborhood. That is, after a case is identified, one or more controls residing in the same neighborhood as that case are identified and recruited into the study. If neighborhood is related to exposure, the matching should be taken into account in the analysis.

Neighborhood controls are often used when the cases are recruited from a convenient source, such as a clinic or hospital. Such usage can introduce bias, however, for the neighbors selected as controls may not be in the source population of the cases. For example, if the cases are from a particular hospital, neighborhood controls may include people who would not have been treated at the same hospital had they developed the disease. If being treated at the hospital from which cases are identified is related to the exposure under study, then using neighborhood controls would introduce a bias. For any given study, the suitability of using neighborhood controls needs to be evaluated with regard to the study variables on which the research focuses.

5.7.2. Random digit dialing

Sampling of households based on random selection of telephone numbers is intended to simulate sampling randomly from the source population. *Random digit dialing*, as this method has been called (Waksberg, 1978), offers the advantage of approaching all households with a wired telephone in a designated area. The method requires considerable attention to details, however, and carries no guarantee of unbiased selection.

First, case eligibility should include residence in a house that has a telephone, so that cases and controls come from the same source population. Second, even if the investigator can implement a sampling method so that every telephone has the same probability of being called, there will not necessarily be the same probability of contacting each eligible control subject, because households vary in the number of people who reside in them, the amount of time someone is at home, and the number of operating phones. Third, making contact with a household may require many calls at various times of day and various days of the week, demanding considerable labor; to obtain a control subject meeting specific eligibility characteristics can require many dozens of telephone calls on average (Wacholder et al., 1992b). Fourth, some households use answering machines, voicemail, or caller identification to screen calls, and may not answer or return unsolicited calls. Fifth, the substitution of mobile telephones for landlines by some households further undermines the assumption that population members can be selected randomly by random digit dialing. Finally, it may be impossible to distinguish accurately business from residential telephone numbers, a distinction required to calculate the proportion of nonresponders.

Random-digit-dialing controls are usually matched to cases on area code (in the U.S., the first three digits of the telephone number) and exchange (the three digits following the area code). In the past, area code and prefix were related to residence location and telephone type (landline or mobile service). Thus, if geographic location or participation in mobile telephone plans was likely related to exposure, then the matching should be taken into account in the analysis. More recently, telephone companies in the U.S. have assigned overlaying area codes and have allowed subscribers to retain their telephone number when they move within the region, so the correspondence between assigned telephone numbers and geographic location has diminished. Furthermore, the increasing use of mobile telephones and caller identification continues to diminish the utility of this method.

5.7.3. Hospital- or clinic-based controls

As noted above, the source population for hospital- or clinic-based case-control studies is not often identifiable, since it represents a group of people who would be treated in a given clinic or hospital if they developed the disease in question. In such situations, a random sample of the general population will not necessarily correspond to a random sample of the source population. If the hospitals or clinics that provide the cases for the study only treat a small proportion of cases in the geographic area, then referral patterns to the hospital or clinic are important to take into account in the sampling of controls. For these studies, a control series comprising patients from the same hospitals or clinics as the cases may provide a less-biased estimate of effect than general-population controls (such as those obtained from case neighborhoods or by random-digit dialing). The source population does not correspond to the population of the geographic area, but rather to those people who would seek treatment at the hospital or clinic if they developed the disease under study. While the latter population may be difficult or impossible to enumerate or even define very clearly, it seems reasonable to expect that other hospital or clinic patients will represent this source population better than general-population controls. The major problem with any nonrandom sampling of controls is the possibility that they are not selected independently of exposure in the source population. Patients hospitalized with other diseases, for example, may be unrepresentative of the exposure distribution in the source population either because exposure is associated with hospitalization, or because the exposure is associated with the other diseases, or both. For example, suppose the study aims to evaluate the relation between tobacco smoking and leukemia using hospitalized cases. If controls are people hospitalized with other conditions, many of them will have been hospitalized for conditions associated with smoking. A variety of other cancers, as well as cardiovascular diseases and respiratory diseases, are related to smoking. Thus, a control series of people hospitalized for diseases other than leukemia would include a higher proportion of smokers than would the source population of the leukemia cases.

Limiting the diagnoses for controls to conditions for which there is no prior indication of an association with the exposure improves the control series. For example, in a study of smoking and hospitalized leukemia cases, one could exclude from the control series anyone who was hospitalized with a disease known to be related to smoking. Such an exclusion policy may exclude most of the potential controls, since cardiovascular disease by itself would represent a large proportion of hospitalized patients. Nevertheless, even a few common diagnostic categories should suffice to find enough control subjects, so that the exclusions will not harm the study by limiting the size of the control series. Indeed, in limiting the scope of eligibility criteria, it is reasonable to exclude categories of potential controls even on the suspicion that a given category might be related to the exposure. If wrong, the cost of the exclusion is that the control series becomes more homogeneous with respect to diagnosis and perhaps a little smaller. But if right, then the exclusion is important to the ultimate validity of the study.

On the other hand, an investigator can rarely be sure that an exposure is not related to a disease or to hospitalization for a specific diagnosis. Consequently, it would be imprudent to use only a single diagnostic category as a source of controls. Using a variety of diagnoses has the advantage of potentially diluting the biasing effects of including a specific diagnostic group that is related to the exposure.

Excluding a diagnostic category from the list of eligibility criteria for identifying controls is intended simply to improve the representativeness of the control series with respect to the source population. Such an exclusion criterion does not imply that there should be exclusions based on disease history (Lubin and Hartge, 1984). For example, in a case-control study of smoking and hospitalized leukemia patients, one might use hospitalized controls but exclude any who are hospitalized because of cardiovascular disease. This exclusion criterion for controls does not imply that leukemia cases who have had cardiovascular disease should be excluded; only if the cardiovascular disease was a cause of the hospitalization should the case be excluded. For controls, the exclusion criterion should only apply to the cause of the hospitalization used to identify the study subject. A person who was hospitalized because of a traumatic injury and who is thus eligible to be a control would not be excluded if he or she had previously been hospitalized for cardiovascular disease. The source population includes people who have had cardiovascular disease, and they should be included in the control series. Excluding such people would lead to an underrepresentation of smoking relative to the source population and produce an upward bias in the effect estimates.

If exposure directly affects hospitalization (for example, if the decision to hospitalize is in part based on exposure history), the resulting bias cannot be remedied without knowing the hospitalization rates, even if the exposure is unrelated to the study disease or the control diseases. This problem was in fact one of the first problems of hospital-based studies to receive detailed analysis (Berkson, 1946), and is often called Berksonian bias.

5.7.4. Other diseases

In many settings, especially in populations with established disease registries or insurance-claims databases, it may be most convenient to choose controls from people who are diagnosed with other diseases. The considerations needed for valid control selection from other diagnoses parallel those just discussed for hospital controls. It is essential to exclude any diagnoses known or suspected to be related to exposure, and better still to include only diagnoses for which there is some evidence to indicate they are unrelated to exposure. These exclusion and inclusion criteria apply only to the diagnosis that brought the person into the registry or database from which controls are selected. The history of an exposure-related disease should not be a basis for exclusion. If however the exposure directly affects the chance of entering the registry or database, the study will be subject to the Berksonian bias mentioned earlier for hospital studies.

5.7.5. Friend controls

Choosing friends of cases as controls, like using neighborhood controls, is a design that inherently uses individual matching and needs to be evaluated with regard to the advantages and disadvantages of such matching. Aside from the complications of individual matching, there are further concerns stemming from use of friend controls. First, being named as a friend by the case may be related to the exposure status of the potential control (Flanders and Austin, 1986). For example, cases might preferentially name as friends their acquaintances with whom they engage in specific activities that might relate to the exposure. Physical activity, alcoholic beverage consumption, and sun exposure are examples of such exposures. People who are more reclusive may be less likely to be named as friends, so their exposure patterns will be underrepresented among a control series of friends. Exposures more common to extroverted people may become overrepresented among friend controls. This type of bias was suspected in a study of insulin-dependent diabetes mellitus in which the parents of cases identified the controls. The cases had fewer friends than controls, had more learning problems, and were more likely to dislike school. Using friend controls could explain these findings (Siemiatycki, 1989).

5.7.6. Dead controls

A dead control cannot be a member of the source population for cases, since death precludes the occurrence of any new disease. Suppose, however, that the cases are dead. Does the need for comparability argue in favor of using dead controls? While certain types of comparability are important, choosing dead controls will misrepresent the exposure distribution in the source population if the exposure causes or prevents death in a substantial proportion of people or if it is associated with an uncontrolled factor that does. If interviews are needed and some cases are dead, it will be necessary to use proxy respondents for the dead cases. To enhance comparability of information while avoiding the problems of taking dead controls, proxy respondents can also be used for those live controls matched to dead cases (Wacholder et al., 1992b). The main justification for using dead controls is convenience, such as in studies based entirely on deaths (see the discussion of proportional-mortality studies below).

5.8. Other considerations for subject selection

5.8.1. Representativeness

Some textbooks have stressed the need for representativeness in the selection of cases and controls. The advice has been that cases should be representative of all people with the disease and that controls should be representative of the entire nondiseased population. Such advice can be misleading. A case-control study may be restricted to any type of case that may be of interest: female cases, old cases, severely ill cases, cases that died soon after disease onset, mild cases, cases from Philadelphia, cases among factory workers, and so on. In none of these examples the cases would be representative of all people with the disease, yet in each one perfectly valid case-control studies are possible (Cole, 1979). The definition of a case can be virtually anything that the investigator wishes.

Ordinarily, controls should represent the source population for cases, rather than the entire nondiseased population. The latter may differ vastly from the source population for the cases by age, race, sex (e.g., if the cases come from a Veterans Administration hospital), socioeconomic status, occupation, and so on – including the exposure of interest. One of the reasons for emphasizing the similarities rather than the differences between cohort and case-control studies is that numerous principles apply to both types of study but are more evident in the context of cohort studies. In particular, many principles relating to subject selection apply identically to both types of study. For example, it is widely appreciated that cohort studies can be based on special cohorts rather than on the general population. It follows that case-control studies can be conducted by sampling cases and controls from within those special cohorts. The resulting controls should represent the distribution of exposure across those cohorts, rather than the general population, reflecting the more general rule that controls should represent the source population of the cases in the study, not the general population.

5.8.2. Comparability of information

Many authors discuss a general principle that information obtained from cases and controls should be of comparable accuracy (e.g., Wacholder et al., 1992a). The rationale for this principle is the notion that nondifferential exposure measurement error biases the observed odds ratio toward the null. This rationale underlies the argument that bias in studies with comparably accurate case and control information is more predictable than in studies without such comparability.

The comparability-of-information principle is often used to guide selection of controls and collection of data. For example, it is the basis for using proxy respondents instead of direct interviews for living controls whenever case information is obtained from proxy respondents. Unfortunately, in most settings, the arguments for the principle are logically unsound. For example, in a study that used proxy respondents for cases, use of proxy respondents for the controls might lead to greater bias than use of direct interviews with controls, even if measurement error is differential. The comparability-of-information principle is therefore applicable only under very limited conditions. In particular, it would seem to be useful only when confounders and effect modifiers are measured with negligible error and when measurement error is reduced by using comparable sources of information. Otherwise, the effect of forcing comparability of information may be as unpredictable as the effect of using noncomparable information.

5.8.3. *Timing of classification and diagnosis*

The principles for classifying persons, cases, and person-time units in cohort studies according to exposure status also apply to cases and controls in case-control studies. If the controls are intended to represent person-time (rather than persons) in the source population, one should apply principles for classifying person-time to the classification of controls. In particular, principles of person-time classification lead to the rule that controls should be classified by their exposure status as of their selection time. Exposures accrued after that time should be ignored. The rule necessitates that information (such as exposure history) be obtained in a manner that allows one to ignore exposures accrued after the selection time. In a similar manner, cases should be classified as of time of diagnosis or disease onset, accounting for any built-in lag periods or induction-period hypotheses. Determining the occurrence time of cases can involve all the problems and ambiguities discussed earlier for cohort studies and needs to be resolved by study protocol before classifications can be made.

6. Variants of the case-control design

6.1. *Nested case-control studies*

Epidemiologists sometimes refer to specific case-control studies as *nested* case-control studies when the population within which the study is conducted is a fully enumerated cohort, which allows formal random sampling of cases and controls to be carried out. The term is usually used in reference to a case-control study conducted within a cohort study, in which further information (perhaps from expensive tests) is obtained on most or all cases, but for economy is obtained from only a fraction of the remaining cohort members (the controls). Nonetheless, many population-based case-control studies can be thought of as nested within an enumerated source population.

6.2. *Case-cohort studies*

The *case-cohort study* is a case-control study in which the source population is a cohort and (within sampling or matching strata) every person in this cohort has an equal chance of being included in the study as a control, regardless of how much time that person has contributed to the person-time experience of the cohort or whether the person developed the study disease. This is a logical way to conduct a case-control study when the effect measure of interest is the ratio of incidence proportions rather than a rate ratio, as is common in perinatal studies. The average risk (or incidence proportion) of falling ill during a specified period may be written as

$$R_1 = \frac{A_1}{N_1}$$

for the exposed subcohort and

$$R_0 = \frac{A_0}{N_0}$$

for the unexposed subcohort, where R_1 and R_0 are the incidence proportions among the exposed and unexposed, respectively, and N_1 and N_0 are the initial sizes of the exposed and unexposed subcohorts. (This discussion applies equally well to exposure variables with several levels, but for simplicity we will consider only a dichotomous exposure.) Controls should be selected such that the exposure distribution among them will estimate without bias the exposure distribution in the source population. In a case-cohort study, the distribution we wish to estimate is among the N_1+N_0 cohort members, not among their person-time experience (Thomas, 1972; Kupper et al., 1975; Miettinen, 1982).

The objective is to select controls from the source cohort such that the ratio of the number of exposed controls (B_1) to the number of exposed cohort members (N_1) is the same as ratio of the number of unexposed controls (B_0) to the number of unexposed cohort members (N_0), apart from sampling error:

$$\frac{B_1}{N_1} = \frac{B_0}{N_0}$$

Here, B_1/N_1 and B_0/N_0 are the control-sampling fractions (the number of controls selected per cohort member). Apart from random error, these sampling fractions will be equal if controls have been selected independently of exposure.

We can use the frequencies of exposed and unexposed controls as substitutes for the actual denominators of the incidence proportions to obtain "pseudo-risks":

$$\text{Pseudo-risk}_1 = \frac{A_1}{B_1}$$

and

$$\text{Pseudo-risk}_0 = \frac{A_0}{B_0}$$

These pseudo-risks have no epidemiologic interpretation by themselves. Suppose, however, that the control-sampling fractions are equal to the same fraction, f. Then, apart from sampling error, B_1/f should equal N_1, the size of the exposed subcohort; and B_0/f should equal N_0, the size of the unexposed subcohort: $B_1/f = B_1/(B_1/N_1) = N_1$ and $B_0/f = B_0/(B_0/N_0) = N_0$. Thus, to get the incidence proportions, we need only to multiply each pseudo-risk by the common sampling fraction, f. If this fraction is not known, we can still compare the sizes of the pseudo-risks by division:

$$\frac{\text{Pseudo-risk}_1}{\text{Pseudo-risk}_0} = \frac{A_1/B_1}{A_0/B_0} = \frac{A_1/[(B_1/N_1)N_1]}{A_0/[(B_0/N_0)N_0]} = \frac{A_1/fN_1}{A_0/fN_0} = \frac{A_1/N_1}{A_0/N_0}$$

In other words, the ratio of pseudo-risks is an estimate of the ratio of incidence proportions (risk ratio) in the source cohort if control sampling is independent of exposure. Thus, using a case-cohort design, one can estimate the risk ratio in a cohort without obtaining information on every cohort member.

Thus far, we have implicitly assumed that there is no loss to follow-up or competing risks in the underlying cohort. If there are such problems, it is still possible to estimate risk or rate ratios from a case-cohort study provided that we have data on the time spent at risk by the sampled subjects or we use certain sampling modifications (Flanders et al., 1990). These procedures require the usual assumptions for rate-ratio estimation in cohort studies, namely, that loss-to-follow-up and competing risks are either not associated with exposure or not associated with disease risk.

An advantage of the case-cohort design is that it facilitates conduct of a set of case-control studies from a single cohort, all of which use the same control group. Just as one can measure the incidence rate of a variety of diseases within a single cohort, one can conduct a set of simultaneous case-control studies using a single control group. A sample from the cohort is the control group needed to compare with any number of case groups. If matched controls are selected from people at risk at the time a case occurs (as in risk-set sampling, which is described below), the control series must be tailored to a specific group of cases. To have a single control series serve many case groups, another sampling scheme must be used. The case-cohort approach is a good choice in such a situation.

Wacholder (1991) has discussed the advantages and disadvantages of the case-cohort design relative to the usual type of case-control study. One point to note is that, because of the overlap of membership in the case and control groups (controls who are selected may also develop disease and enter the study as cases), one will need to select more controls in a case-cohort study than in an ordinary case-control study with the same number of cases, if one is to achieve the same amount of statistical precision. Extra controls are needed because the statistical precision of a study is strongly determined by the numbers of distinct cases and noncases. Thus, if 20% of the source cohort members will become cases, and all cases will be included in the study, one will have to select 1.25 times as many controls as cases in a case-cohort study to insure that there will be as many controls who never become cases in the study. On average, only 80% of the controls in such a situation will remain noncases; the other 20% will become cases. Of course, if the disease is uncommon, the number of extra controls needed for a case-cohort study will be small.

6.3. Density case-control studies

Earlier, we described how case-control odds ratios will estimate rate ratios if the control series is selected so that the ratio of the person-time denominators T_1/T_0 is validly estimated by the ratio of exposed to unexposed controls B_1/B_0. That is, to estimate rate ratios, controls should be selected so that the exposure distribution among them is, apart from random error, the same as it is among the person-time in the source population. Such control selection is called density sampling because it provides for estimation of relations among incidence rates, which have been called "incidence densities."

If a subject's exposure may vary over time, then a case's exposure history is evaluated up to the time the disease occurred. A control's exposure history is evaluated up to an analogous index time, usually taken as the time of sampling; exposure after the time of selection must be ignored. This rule helps to ensure that the number of exposed and unexposed controls will be in proportion to the amount of exposed and unexposed person-time in the source population.

The time during which a subject is eligible to be a control should be the time in which that person is also eligible to become a case, if the disease should occur. Thus, a person in whom the disease has already developed or who has died is no longer eligible to be selected as a control. This rule corresponds to the treatment of subjects in cohort studies. Every case that is tallied in the numerator of a cohort study contributes to the denominator of the rate until the time that the person becomes a case, when the contribution to the denominator ceases. One way to implement this rule is to choose controls from the set of people in the source population who are at risk of becoming a case at the time that the case is diagnosed. This set is sometimes referred to as the *risk set* for the case, and this type of control sampling is sometimes called *risk-set sampling*. Controls sampled in this manner are matched to the case with respect to sampling time; thus, if time is related to exposure, the resulting data should be analyzed as matched data (Greenland and Thomas, 1982). It is also possible to conduct unmatched density sampling using probability sampling methods if one knows the time interval at risk for each population member. One then selects a control by sampling members with probability proportional to time at risk and then randomly samples a time to measure exposure within the interval at risk.

As mentioned earlier, a person selected as a control who remains in the study population at risk after selection should remain eligible to be selected once again as a control. Thus, although unlikely in typical studies, the same person may appear in the control group two or more times. Note, however, that including the same person at different times does not necessarily lead to exposure (or confounder) information being repeated, because this information may change with time. For example, in a case-control study of an acute epidemic of intestinal illness, one might ask about food ingested within the previous day or days. If a contaminated food item was a cause of the illness for some cases, then the exposure status of a case or control chosen 5 days into the study might well differ from what it would have been 2 days into the study when the subject might also have been included as a control.

6.4. Cumulative ("epidemic") case-control studies

In some research settings, case-control studies may address a risk that ends before subject selection begins. For example, a case-control study of an epidemic of diarrheal illness after a social gathering may begin after all the potential cases have occurred (because the maximum induction time has elapsed). In such a situation, an investigator might select controls from that portion of the population that remains after eliminating the accumulated cases; that is, one selects controls from among noncases (those who remain noncases at the end of the epidemic follow-up).

Suppose that the source population is a cohort and that a fraction f of both exposed and unexposed noncases are selected to be controls. Then the ratio of pseudo-frequencies will be

$$\frac{A_1/B_1}{A_0/B_0} = \frac{A_1/f(N_1 - A_1)}{A_0/f(N_0 - A_0)} = \frac{A_1/(N_1 - A_1)}{A_0/(N_0 - A_0)}$$

which is the incidence odds ratio for the cohort. The latter ratio will provide a reasonable approximation to the rate ratio, provided that the proportions falling ill in each exposure group during the risk period are low, that is, less than about 20%, and that the prevalence of exposure remains reasonably steady during the study period. If the investigator prefers to estimate the risk ratio rather than the incidence rate ratio, the study odds ratio can still be used (Cornfield, 1951), but the accuracy of this approximation is only about half as good as that of the odds ratio approximation to the rate ratio (Greenland, 1987a). The use of this approximation in the cumulative design is the basis for the common and mistaken teaching that a rare-disease assumption is needed to estimate risk ratios in all case-control studies.

Prior to the 1970s, the standard conceptualization of case-control studies involved the cumulative design, in which controls are selected from noncases at the end of a follow-up period. As discussed by numerous authors (Sheehe, 1962; Miettinen, 1976a; Greenland and Thomas, 1982), density designs and case-cohort designs have several advantages outside of the acute epidemic setting, including potentially much less sensitivity to bias from exposure-related loss-to-follow-up.

6.5. Case-only studies

There are a number of situations in which cases are the only subjects used to estimate or test hypotheses about effects. For example, it is sometimes possible to employ theoretical considerations to construct a prior distribution of exposure in the source population, and use this distribution in place of an observed control series. Such situations naturally arise in genetic studies, in which basic laws of inheritance may be combined with certain assumptions to derive a population or parental-specific distribution of genotypes (Self et al., 1991). It is also possible to study certain aspects of joint effects (interactions) of genetic and environmental factors without using control subjects (Khoury and Flanders, 1996).

6.6. Case-specular and case-crossover studies

When the exposure under study is defined by proximity to an environmental source (e.g., a power line), it may be possible to construct a *specular* (hypothetical) control for each case by conducting a "thought experiment." Either the case or the exposure source is imaginarily moved to another location that would be equally likely were there is no exposure effect; the case exposure level under this hypothetical configuration is then treated as the (matched) "control" exposure for the case (Zaffanella et al., 1998). When the specular control arises by examining the exposure experience of the case outside of the time in which exposure could be related to disease occurrence, the result is called a *case-crossover study*.

The classic *crossover* study is a type of experiment in which two (or more) treatments are compared, as in any experimental study. In a crossover study, however, each subject receives both treatments, with one following the other. Preferably, the order in which the two treatments are applied is randomly chosen for each subject. Enough time should be allocated between the two administrations so that the effect of each treatment can be measured and can subside before the other treatment is given. A persistent effect of the first intervention is called a *carryover effect*. A crossover study is only valid to study treatments for which effects occur within a short induction period and do not persist, i.e., carryover effects must be absent, so that the effect of the second intervention is not intermingled with the effect of the first.

The *case-crossover* study is a case-control analogue of the crossover study (Maclure, 1991). For each case, one or more predisease or postdisease time periods are selected as matched "control" periods for the case. The exposure status of the case at the time of the disease onset is compared with the distribution of exposure status for that same person in the control periods. Such a comparison depends on the assumption that neither exposure nor confounders are changing over time in a systematic way. There are a number of ways to select control time periods under a case-crossover design, each with different analytic consequences. See Vines and Farrington (2001), Navidi and Weinhandl (2002), and Janes et al. (2005) for details.

Only a limited set of research topics are amenable to the case-crossover design. The exposure must vary over time within individuals rather than stay constant. If the exposure does not vary within a person, then there is no basis for comparing exposed and unexposed time periods of risk within the person. Like the crossover study, the exposure must also have a short induction time and a transient effect; otherwise, exposures in the distant past could be the cause of a recent disease onset (a carryover effect).

Maclure (1991) used the case-crossover design to study the effect of sexual activity on incident myocardial infarction. This topic is well suited to a case-crossover design because the exposure is intermittent and is presumed to have a short induction period for the hypothesized effect. Any increase in risk for a myocardial infarction from sexual activity is presumed to be confined to a short time following the activity. A myocardial infarction is an outcome well suited to this type of study because it is thought to be triggered by events close in time.

Each case and its control in a case-crossover study is automatically matched on all characteristics (e.g., sex and birth date) that do not change within individuals. Matched analysis of case-crossover data controls for all such fixed confounders, whether or not they are measured. Control for measured time-varying confounders is possible using modeling methods for matched data. It is also possible to adjust case-crossover estimates for bias due to time trends in exposure through use of longitudinal data from a nondiseased control group (case-time controls) (Suissa, 1995). Nonetheless, these trend adjustments themselves depend on additional no-confounding assumptions and may introduce bias if those assumptions are not met (Greenland, 1996b).

6.7. *Two-stage sampling*

Another variant of the case-control study uses two-stage or two-phase sampling (Walker, 1982; White, 1982). In this type of study, the control series comprises a relatively large number of people (possibly everyone in the source population), from whom exposure information or perhaps some limited amount of information on other relevant variables is obtained. Then, for only a subsample of the controls, more detailed information is obtained on exposure or on other study variables that may need to be controlled in the analysis. More detailed information may also be limited to a subsample of cases. This two-stage approach is useful when it is relatively inexpensive to obtain the exposure information (e.g., by telephone interview), but the covariate information is more expensive to obtain (say, by laboratory analysis). It is also useful when exposure information already has been collected on the entire population (e.g., job histories for an occupational cohort), but covariate information is needed (e.g., genotype). This situation arises in cohort studies when more information is required than was gathered at baseline. This type of study requires special analytic methods to take full advantage of the information collected at both stages.

6.8. *Proportional-mortality studies*

In proportional-mortality studies, the cases are deaths occurring within the source population. Controls are not selected directly from the source population, which consists of living people, but are taken from other deaths within the source population. This control series is acceptable if the exposure distribution within this group is similar to that of the source population. Consequently, the control series should be restricted to categories of death that are not related to the exposure. These studies should be analyzed as ordinary case-control studies, with the odds ratio as the effect measure, instead of using the proportional-mortality ratio, a biased measure of the mortality rate ratio (Miettinen and Wang, 1981).

6.9. *Case-control studies with prevalent cases*

Case-control studies are sometimes based on prevalent cases rather than incident cases. When it is impractical to include only incident cases, it may still be possible to select existing cases of illness at a point in time. If the prevalence odds ratio in the population is equal to the incidence rate ratio, then the odds ratio from a case-control study based on prevalent cases can unbiasedly estimate the rate ratio. The conditions required for the prevalence odds ratio to equal the rate ratio are very strong, however, and a simple relation does not exist for age-specific ratios. If exposure is associated with duration of illness or migration out of the prevalence pool, then a case-control study based on prevalent cases cannot by itself distinguish exposure effects on disease incidence from the exposure association with disease duration or migration, unless the strengths of the latter associations are known. If the size of the exposed or the unexposed population changes with time or there is migration into the prevalence pool, the prevalence odds ratio may be further removed from the rate ratio. Consequently, it is always preferable to select incident rather than prevalent cases when studying disease etiology.

Prevalent cases are usually drawn in studies of congenital malformations. In such studies, cases ascertained at birth are prevalent because they have survived with the malformation from the time of its occurrence until birth. It would be etiologically more useful to ascertain all incident cases, including affected abortuses that do not survive until birth. Many of these, however, do not survive until ascertainment is feasible, and thus it is virtually inevitable that case-control studies of congenital malformations are based on prevalent cases. In this example, the source population comprises all conceptuses, and miscarriage and induced abortion represent emigration before the ascertainment date. Although an exposure will not affect duration of a malformation, it may very well affect risks of miscarriage and abortion.

Other situations in which prevalent cases are commonly used are studies of chronic conditions with ill-defined onset times and limited effects on mortality, such as obesity and multiple sclerosis, and studies of health services utilization.

7. Conclusion

Epidemiologic research employs a range of study designs, including both experimental and nonexperimental studies. No epidemiologic study is perfect, and this caution applies to experimental as well as nonexperimental studies. A clear understanding of the principles of study design is essential for valid study design, conduct, and analysis, and for proper interpretation of results.

References

Angrist, J.D., Imbens, G.W., Rubin, D.B. (1996). Identification of causal effects using instrumental variables (with discussion). *Journal of the American Statistical Association* **91**, 444–472.

Armitage, P. (1985). The search for optimality in clinical trials. *International Statistical Review* **53**, 1–13.

Armitage, P., McPherson, C.K., Rowe, B.C. (1969). Repeated significance tests on accumulating data. *Journal of the Royal Statistical Society. Series A* **132**, 235–244.

Ast, D.B., Smith, D.J., Wachs, B., Cantwell, K.T. (1956). Newburgh-Kingston caries-fluorine study. XIV. Combined clinical and roentgenographic dental findings after ten years of fluoride experience. *The Journal of the American Dental Association* **52**, 314–325.

Avins, A.L. (1998). Can equal be more fair? Ethics, subject allocation, and randomized clinical trials. *Journal of Medical Ethics* **24**, 401–408.

Beebe, G.W. (1979). Reflections on the work of the Atomic Bomb Casualty Commission in Japan. *Epidemiologic Reviews* **1**, 184–210.
Berkson, J. (1946). Limitations of the application of 4-fold tables to hospital data. *Biometrics Bulletin* **2**, 47–53.
Berry, D.A. (1993). A case for Bayesianism in clinical trials. *Statistics in Medicine* **12**, 1377–1393.
Byar, D.P., Simon, R.M., Friedewald, W.T., Schlesselman, J.J., DeMets, D.L., Ellengerg, J.H. et al. (1976). Randomized clinical trials: Perspectives on some recent ideas. *New England Journal of Medicine* **295**, 74–80.
Cannistra, S.A. (2004). The ethics of early stopping rules: Who is protecting whom? *Journal of Clinical Oncology* **22**, 1542–1545.
Carlin, B.P., Sargent, D.J. (1996). Robust Bayesian approaches for clinical trial monitoring. *Statistics in Medicine* **15**, 1093–1106.
Cole, P. (1979). The evolving case-control study. *Journal of Chronic Diseases* **32**, 15–27.
Cornfield, J. (1951). A method of estimating comparative rates from clinical data: Application to cancer of the lung, breast and cervix. *Journal of the National Cancer Institute* **11**, 1269–1275.
Detre, K.M., Shaw, L. (1974). Long-term changes of serum cholesterol with cholesterol-altering drugs in patients with coronary heart disease. *Circulation* **50**, 998–1005.
Dykes, M.H.M., Meier, P. (1975). Ascorbic acid and the common cold: Evaluation of its efficacy and toxicity. *Journal of the American Medical Association* **231**, 1073–1079.
Flanders, W.D., Austin, H. (1986). Possibility of selection bias in matched case-control studies using friend controls. *American Journal of Epidemiology* **124**, 150–153.
Flanders, W.D., DerSimonian, R., Rhodes, P. (1990). Estimation of risk ratios in case-base studies with competing risks. *Statistics in Medicine* **9**, 423–435.
Francis, T. Jr., Korns, R.F., Voight, R.B., Hemphill, F.M., Boisen, M., Tolchinsky, E., Napier, J.A., Johnson, M.M., Wenner, H.A., Seibert, R.H., Diamond, E.L., Tumbusch, J.J. (1955). An evaluation of the 1954 poliomyelitis vaccine trials. *American Journal of Public Health* **45**(May), 1–63.
Gelman, A., Carlin, J.B., Stern, H.S., Rubin, D.B. (2003). *Bayesian Data Analysis*, 2nd ed. Chapman and Hall/CRC, New York.
George, S.L., Freidlin, B., Korn, E.L. (2004). Strength of accumulating evidence and data monitoring committee decision making. *Statistics in Medicine* **23**, 2659–2672.
Goetghebeur, E., Van Houwelingen (Eds.) (1998). Analyzing non-compliance in clinical trials (special issue). *Statistics in Medicine* **17**(3), 247–393.
Greenland, S. (1987). Interpretation and choice of effect measures in epidemiologic analysis. *American Journal of Epidemiology* **125**, 761–768.
Greenland, S. (1990). Randomization, statistics, and causal inference. *Epidemiology* **1**, 421–429.
Greenland, S. (1996). Confounding and exposure trends in case-crossover and case-time-control designs. *Epidemiology* **7**, 231–239.
Greenland, S. (2000). An introduction to instrumental variables for epidemiologists. *International Journal of Epidemiology* **29**, 722–729, (Erratum: 2000, **29**, 1102).
Greenland, S. (2001). Ecologic versus individual-level sources of confounding in ecologic estimates of contextual health effects. *International Journal of Epidemiology* **30**, 1343–1350.
Greenland, S. (2002). A review of multilevel theory for ecologic analyses. *Statistics in Medicine* **21**, 389–395.
Greenland, S. (2004). Ecologic inference problems in studies based on surveillance data. In: Stroup, D.F., Brookmeyer, R. (Eds.), *Monitoring the Health of Populations: Statistical Principles and Methods for Public Health Surveillance*. Oxford University Press, New York, pp. 315–340.
Greenland, S. (1985). Control-initiated case-control studies. *International Journal of Epidemiology* **14**, 130–134.
Greenland, S., Robins, J.M. (1985). Confounding and misclassification. *American Journal of Epidemiology* **122**, 495–506.
Greenland, S., Robins, J.M. (1986). Identifiability, exchangeability and epidemiologic confounding. *International Journal of Epidemiology* **15**, 413–419.

Greenland, S., Thomas, D.C. (1982). On the need for the rare disease assumption in case-control studies. *American Journal of Epidemiology* **116**, 547–553.

Heiat, A., Gross, C.P., Krumholz, H.M. (2002). Representation of the elderly, women, and minorities in heart failure clinical trials. *Archives of Internal Medicine* **162**, 1682–1688.

Janes, H., Sheppard, L., Lumley, T. (2005). Case-crossover analyses of air pollution exposure data: Referent selection strategies and their implications for bias. *Epidemiology* **16**, 717–726.

Kannel, W.B., Abbott, R.D. (1984). Incidence and prognosis of unrecognized myocardial infarction: An update on the Framingham study. *New England Journal of Medicine* **311**, 1144–1147.

Karlowski, T.R., Chalmers, T.C., Frenkel, L.D. et al. (1975). Ascorbic acid for the common cold: A prophylactic and therapeutic trial. *JAMA* **231**, 1038–1042.

Khoury, M.J., Flanders, W.D. (1996). Nontraditional epidemiologic approaches in the analysis of gene-environment interactions: Case-control studies with no controls!. *American Journal of Epidemiology* **144**, 207–213.

Kolata, G. (1982). Heart study produces a surprise result. *Science* **218**, 31–32.

Kupper, L.L., McMichael, A.J., Spirtas, R. (1975). A hybrid epidemiologic design useful in estimating relative risk. *Journal of the American Statistical Association* **70**, 524–528.

Leren, P. (1966). The effect of plasma cholesterol lowering diet in male survivors of myocardial infarction. *Acta medica Scandinavica Supplementum* **466**, 5–92.

Lubin, J.H., Gail, M.H. (1984). Biased selection of controls for case-control analyses of cohort studies. *Biometrics* **40**, 63–75.

Lubin, J.H., Hartge, P. (1984). Excluding controls: Misapplications in case-control studies. *American Journal of Epidemiology* **120**, 791–793.

MacKay, A.M., Rothman, K.J. (1982). The incidence and severity of burn injuries following Project Burn Prevention. *American Journal of Public Health* **72**, 248–252.

Maclure, M. (1991). The case-crossover design: A method for studying transient effects on the risk of acute events. *American Journal of Epidemiology* **133**, 144–153.

Miettinen, O.S. (1976). Estimability and estimation in case-referent studies. *American Journal of Epidemiology* **103**, 226–235.

Miettinen, O.S. (1982). Design options in epidemiologic research: An update. *Scandinavian Journal of Work, Environment & Health* **8**(suppl 1), 7–14.

Miettinen, O.S., Wang, J.-D. (1981). An alternative to the proportionate mortality ratio. *American Journal of Epidemiology* **114**, 144–148.

Morgenstern, H. (2008). Ecologic studies. In: Rothman, K.J., Greenland, S., Lash, T.L. (Eds.), *Modern Epidemiology (3rd ed)*. Lippincott, Philadelphia, PA.

Murthy, V.H., Krumholz, H.M., Gross, C.P. (2004). Participation in cancer clinical trials: Race, sex, and age-based disparities. *Journal of the American Medical Association* **291**, 2720–2726.

Navidi, W., Weinhandl, E. (2002). Risk set sampling for case-crossover designs. *Epidemiology* **13**, 100–105.

Omar, R.Z., Thompson, S.G. (2000). Analysis of a cluster randomized trial with binary outcome data using a multi-level method. *Statistics in Medicine* **19**, 2675–2688.

Peto, R., Pike, M.C., Armitage, P., Breslow, N.E., Cox, D.R., Howard, S.V., Mantel, N., McPherson, K., Peto, J., Smith, P.G. (1976). Design and analysis of randomized clinical trials requiring prolonged observation of each patient. I. Introduction and design. *British Journal of Cancer* **34**, 585–612.

Pocock, S.J., Hughes, M.D. (1989). Practical problems in interim analyses, with particular regard to estimation. *Controlled Clinical Trials* **10**(Suppl.), 209S–221S.

Poole, C. (1986). Exposure opportunity in case-control studies. *American Journal of Epidemiology* **123**, 352–358.

Poole, C. (1999). Controls who experienced hypothetical causal intermediates should not be excluded from case-control studies. *American Journal of Epidemiology* **150**, 547–551.

Robins, J.M., Gail, M.H., Lubin, J.H. (1986). More on biased selection of controls for case-control analyses of cohort studies. *Biometrics* **42**, 293–299.

Robins, J.M. (1987). A graphical approach to the identification and estimation of causal parameters in mortality studies with sustained exposure periods. *Journal of Chronic Diseases* **40**(Suppl. 2), 139s–161s.

Rothman, K.J. (1981). Induction and latent periods. *American Journal of Epidemiology* **114**, 253–259.

Rothman, K.J., Funch, D.P., Alfredson, T., Brady, J., Dreyer, N.A. (2003). Randomized field trial of vaginal douching, pelvic inflammatory disease, and pregnancy. *Epidemiology* **14**, 340–348.

Rothman, K.J., Greenland, S. (1998). *Modern Epidemiology*, 2nd ed. Lippincott, Philadelphia.

Rothman, K.J., Michels, K.B. (2002). When is it appropriate to use a placebo arm in a trial? In: Guess, H.A., Kleinman, A., Kusek, J.W., Engel, L.W. (Eds.), *The Science of the Placebo: Toward an Interdisciplinary Research Agenda*. BMJ Books, London.

Self, S.G., Longton, G., Kopecky, K.J., Liang, K.Y. (1991). On estimating HLA/disease association with application to a study of aplastic anemia. *Biometrics* **47**, 53–61.

Sheehe, P.R. (1962). Dynamic risk analysis in retrospective matched-pair studies of disease. *Biometrics* **18**, 323–341.

Siemiatycki, J. (1989). Friendly control bias. *Journal of Clinical Epidemiology* **42**, 687–688.

Sommer, A., Zeger, S.L. (1991). On estimating efficacy from clinical trials. *Statistics in Medicine* **10**, 45–52.

Spiegelhalter, D.J. (2001). Bayesian methods for cluster randomized trials with continuous responses. *Statistics in Medicine* **20**, 435–452.

Spielgelhalter, D.J., Abrams, K.R., Myles, J.P. (2004). *Bayesian Approaches to Clinical Trials and Health-Care Assessment*. John Wiley and Sons, London.

Suissa, S. (1995). The case-time-control design. *Epidemiology* **6**, 248–253.

Szmuness, W. (1980). Hepatitis B vaccine. Demonstration of efficacy in a controlled clinical trial in a high-risk population in the United States. *New England Journal of Medicine* **303**, 833–841.

Terry, M.B., Neugut, A.L. (1998). Cigarette smoking and the colorectal adenoma-carcinoma sequence: A hypothesis to explain the paradox. *American Journal of Epidemiology* **147**, 903–910.

Thomas, D.B. (1972). Relationship of oral contraceptives to cervical carcinogenesis. *Obstetrics and gynecology* **40**, 508–518.

Thomas, D.C. (1983). Statistical methods for analyzing effects of temporal patterns of exposure on cancer risks. *Scandinavian Journal of Work, Environment & Health* **9**, 353–366.

Thomas, D.C. (1988). Models for exposure-time-response relationships with applications to cancer epidemiology. *Annual Review of Public Health* **9**, 451–482.

Turner, R.M., Omar, R.Z., Thompson, S.G. (2001). Bayesian methods of analysis for cluster randomized trials with binary outcome data. *Statistics in Medicine* **20**, 453–472.

Wacholder, S. (1991). Practical considerations in choosing between the case-cohort and nested case-control design. *Epidemiology* **2**, 155–158.

Wacholder, S., McLaughlin, J.K., Silverman, D.T., Mandel, J.S. (1992a). Selection of controls in case-control studies: I. Principles. *American Journal of Epidemiology* **135**, 1019–1028.

Wacholder, S., Silverman, D.T., McLaughlin, J.K., Mandel, J.S. (1992b). Selection of controls in case-control studies: II. Types of controls. *American Journal of Epidemiology* **135**, 1029–1041.

Wacholder, S., Silverman, D.T., McLaughlin, J.K., Mandel, J.S. (1992c). Selection of controls in case-control studies: III. Design options. *American Journal of Epidemiology* **135**, 1042–1050.

Waksberg, J. (1978). Sampling methods for random digit dialing. *Journal of the American Statistical Association* **73**, 40–46.

Walker, A.M. (1982). Anamorphic analysis: Sampling and estimation for confounder effects when both exposure and disease are known. *Biometrics* **38**, 1025–1032.

Wheatley, K., Clayton, D. (2003). Be skeptical about unexpected large apparent treatment effects: The case of an MRC AML12 randomization. *Controlled Clinical Trials* **24**, 660.

White, J.E. (1982). A two stage design for the study of the relationship between a rare exposure and a rare disease. *American Journal of Epidemiology* **115**, 119–128.

Wilhelmsen, L. (2002). Role of the data and safety monitoring committee. *Statistics in Medicine* **21**, 2823–2829.

Zaffanella, L.E., Savitz, D.A., Greenland, S., Ebi, K.L. (1998). The residential case-specular method to study wire codes, magnetic fields, and disease. *Epidemiology* **9**, 16–20.

Handbook of Statistics, Vol. 27
ISSN: 0169-7161

DOI: 10.1016/S0169-7161(07)27004-X

Statistical Methods for Assessing Biomarkers and Analyzing Biomarker Data

Stephen W. Looney and Joseph L. Hagan

Abstract

The analysis of biomarker data often requires the proper application of statistical methods that are typically not covered in introductory statistics textbooks. In this chapter, we use examples from the biomarker literature to illustrate some of the challenges faced in handling data from biomarker studies and describe methods for the appropriate analysis and interpretation of these data.

1. Introduction

According to the *Dictionary of Epidemiology*, a *biomarker* is "a cellular or molecular indicator of exposure, health effects, or susceptibility" (Last, 1995, p. 17). Our primary focus here will be on markers of exposure, although the techniques we describe can be applied to any type of biomarker.

In this chapter, we provide descriptions and illustrations of many of the statistical methods that we have found useful in the analysis of biomarker data. It is often the case that data collected in studies involving biomarkers require "non-standard" analyses because of the presence of such characteristics as non-normality, heterogeneity, dependence, censoring, etc. In addition, sample sizes in biomarker studies can be rather small, so that large-sample approximations to the null distributions of test statistics are no longer valid. For these reasons, we have emphasized using exact methods whenever possible, and have recommended distribution-free and robust methods in many situations. In some instances, we have illustrated improper applications of "standard" statistical analyses by citing articles from the biomarker literature. It is not our intention to be overly critical of the authors of these articles, but rather to demonstrate that many of the published accounts of biomarker data analyses have not made proper use of the methods included in this chapter. It is often the case that the statistical analyses that appear in print represent the best that could be done at the time of publication due to unavoidable limitations on time, personnel, or resources, and that more thorough analyses could have been performed under different circumstances. It is hoped, however, that those who read this chapter will be better able to assess the quality of a biomarker and to conduct proper analyses of biomarker data in their future research endeavors.

It should also be noted that our discussion of the statistical analysis of biomarker data is not intended to be comprehensive. We have attempted instead to offer practical advice on the appropriate methods to use when analyzing biomarker data and we hope that our recommendations will be helpful to those who perform statistical analyses of these data on a regular basis. To the greatest extent possible, we have based our recommendations on the published advice of recognized authorities in the field. Our emphasis is on statistical methods and procedures that can be implemented using widely available statistical software, and we have indicated how commonly used statistical packages (primarily StatXact (Cytel Inc., Cambridge, MA) and SAS (SAS Institute Inc., Cary, NC)) can be used to carry out the recommended analyses. However, since statistics is a dynamic field, many of the recommendations contained in this chapter may soon prove to be obsolete because of new developments in the discipline and/or new advances in statistical software.

2. Statistical methods for assessing biomarkers

2.1. Validation of biomarkers

The proper statistical analysis of biomarker data cannot proceed unless it has been established that the biomarker has been *validated*; i.e., that it is known to be both valid and reliable. *Reliability* refers to "the degree to which the results obtained by a measurement procedure can be replicated" (Last, 1995). The reliability of a measurement process is most often described in terms of intra-rater and inter-rater reliability. *Intra-rater reliability* refers to the agreement between two different determinations made by the same individual and *inter-rater reliability* refers to the agreement between the determinations made by two different individuals. A reliable biomarker must exhibit adequate levels of both types of reliability. *The reliability of a biomarker must be established before validity can be examined*; if the biomarker cannot be assumed to provide an equivalent result upon repeated determinations on the same biological material, it will not be useful for practical application.

The *validity* of a biomarker is defined to be the extent to which it measures what it is intended to measure. For example, Qiao et al. (1997) proposed that the expression of a tumor-associated antigen by exfoliated sputum epithelial cells could be used as a biomarker in the detection of preclinical, localized lung cancer. For their biomarker to be valid, there must be close agreement between the classification of a patient (cancer/no cancer) using the biomarker and the diagnosis of lung cancer using the gold standard (in this case, consensus diagnosis using "best information"). As another example, body-fluid levels of cotinine have been proposed for use as biomarkers of environmental tobacco smoke exposure (Benowitz, 1999). For cotinine level to be a valid biomarker of tobacco exposure, it must be the case that high levels of cotinine consistently correspond to high levels of tobacco exposure and low levels of cotinine consistently correspond to low levels of exposure.

The appropriate statistical methods for assessing the reliability and validity of a biomarker are discussed in detail in Looney (2001) and therefore will not be treated fully in this chapter. However, there are two types of statistical analyses involving biomarker comparisons that are typically part of the validation process for a biomarker that we feel are worthy of consideration here. These analyses are discussed in Sections 2.2 and 2.3.

2.2. Comparing biomarkers with other diagnostic tests in terms of accuracy

It is often of interest to compare the accuracies of two or more biomarkers or to compare the accuracy of a biomarker with those of other diagnostic tests. One may wish to determine which of several newly proposed biomarkers is the most accurate, or to compare one or more newly proposed biomarkers to an existing measure of exposure or disease. For example, Qiao et al. (1997) used the "paired χ^2 test" to compare the accuracy of a new biomarker they were proposing with two "routine clinical detection methods" for lung cancer (sputum cytology and chest X-ray). When analyzing paired data of this type, the appropriate method for comparing two biomarkers in terms of accuracy is McNemar's test (Conover, 1999, pp. 166–170). There is no statistical method that is commonly known as the "paired χ^2 test." Although a χ^2 approximation is available for McNemar's test, it is preferable to use the exact version of the test (Siegel and Castellan, 1988, pp. 78–79; Suissa and Shuster, 1991). When comparing the accuracies of three or more biomarkers (as in the Qiao et al. study), the preferred method to use is the Cochran Q test (Lehmann, 1975, pp. 267–270).

2.2.1. McNemar test

Qiao et al. (1997) did not present sufficient data in their article for us to be able to perform the exact version of McNemar's test. A hypothetical 2×2 table for the comparison of their biomarker with chest X-ray based on the assumption that their biomarker agreed with the result of the chest X-ray on all true cases of the disease is given in Table 1.

To perform McNemar's test, let n_{ij} = # of subjects in the (i,j) cell of Table 1. Let π_{ij} = true probability that a subject falls into cell (i,j) in Table 1. Then the true probabilities of accurate lung cancer diagnoses by the two methods are given by π_{1+} and π_{+1}, respectively. When $\pi_{1+} = \pi_{+1}$, we say that *marginal homogeneity* is present. Since $\pi_{1+} - \pi_{+1} = \pi_{12} - \pi_{21}$, marginal homogeneity in a 2×2 table is equivalent to equality of the "off-diagonal" probabilities, i.e., $\pi_{12} = \pi_{21}$. Let $n^* = n_{12} + n_{21}$ denote the total count in the two off-diagonal cells. Conditional on the value of n^*, the allocation of the n^* observations to one of the two off-diagonal cells is a binomial random variable (RV) with n^* trials and probability of "success" π. Under the null hypothesis H_0: $\pi_{12} = \pi_{21}$, each of the n^*

Table 1
Hypothetical 2 × 2 table for comparison of accuracy of a new biomarker for lung cancer vs. chest X-ray

Biomarker	Chest X-Ray Positive	Chest X-Ray Negative	Total
Positive	24	41	65
Negative	7	61	68
Total	31	102	133

observations has probability 1/2 of being in cell (1,2) and probability 1/2 of being in cell (2,1). So, n_{12} and n_{21} are the number of "successes" and "failures" for a binomial RV having n^* trials and probability of success 1/2. Thus, a conditional test of H_0: $\pi_{12} = \pi_{21}$ can be performed using the binomial distribution to calculate the exact p-value. First, consider the one-sided alternative hypothesis H_a: $\pi_{1+} > \pi_{+1}$ or, equivalently, H_a: $\pi_{12} > \pi_{21}$. From Table 1, $n_{12} = 41$, $n_{21} = 7$, and $n^* = 48$. The reference distribution (conditional on the value of n^*) is a binomial with $n^* = 48$ and $\pi = 0.5$. The p-value for the one-sided alternative above is then Pr $(n_{12} \geqslant 41 | n^* = 48,\ \pi = 0.5) = 0.0000003$. For the two-sided alternative H_a: $\pi_{1+} \neq \pi_{+1}$, the two-tailed p-value would be twice the upper-tailed p-value, or 0.0000006. Thus, there is very strong evidence of a difference in diagnostic accuracy between the new biomarker and chest X-ray.

2.2.2. *Cochran Q test*

Let n denote the number of biological specimens under study, and let k denote the number of biomarkers being compared. Let y_{ij} denote the determination (usually "positive" or "negative") based on the jth biomarker for the ith specimen, where $y_{ij} = 1$ for "positive" and $y_{ij} = 0$ for "negative," and let

$$y_{i.} = \sum_{j=1}^{k} y_{ij}$$

denote the total number of positive findings for the ith specimen. Similarly, let

$$y_{.j} = \sum_{i=1}^{n} y_{ij}$$

denote the total number of specimens that are classified as positive by the jth biomarker.

The test statistic for Cochran's Q test is

$$Q = \frac{k(k-1)\sum_{j=1}^{k}\left(y_{.j} - (y_{..}/k)\right)^2}{k y_{..} - \sum_{i=1}^{n} y_{i.}^2}, \tag{1}$$

Table 2
Data layout for hypothetical agreement among three diagnostic tests for lung cancer

Pattern of Agreement[a]	Frequency
Cases	
1 1 1	12
1 0 1	12
0 0 1	18
0 0 0	15
Controls	
1 1 1	0
1 0 0	7
0 0 1	16
0 0 0	53

[a] The first value in each pattern indicates the result for sputum cytology, the second value indicates the result for chest X-ray, and the third value indicates the result of the new biomarker. The pattern 1 0 1, for example, indicates that sputum cytology classified the specimen as positive, the chest X-ray classified the specimen as negative, and the new biomarker classified the specimen as positive.

where $y_{..}$ denotes the total number of specimens that are classified as positive by any biomarker. The test statistic Q is asymptotically distributed as χ^2_{k-1}, so an approximate two-sided p-value is given by $p = \Pr(Q \geq Q_{\text{cal}})$, where Q_{cal} is the observed value of the test statistic given by (1) above. The exact two-sided p-value for Cochran's Q test can be obtained using the permutation approach, as described by Mehta and Patel (2005, p. 227).

Qiao et al. (1997) did not present sufficient data in their article for us to perform Cochran's test. A hypothetical data set for the comparison of their biomarker with sputum cytology and chest X-ray was generated based on the assumption that their biomarker agreed with the sputum cytology and X-ray results on all true cases of the disease. This hypothetical data set is given in Table 2.

The value of Cochran's Q for the data in Table 2 is 122.43 and with df $= 2$, the χ^2 asymptotic p-value is < 0.001. The exact p-value, approximated by StatXact using simulation, is also < 0.001. Thus, there is strong evidence to indicate that there is a difference in the accuracies of the three classifiers.

2.3. Measuring agreement among biomarkers

2.3.1. Dichotomous biomarkers

Tockman et al. (1988) examined the use of murine monoclonal antibodies to a glycolipid antigen of human lung cancer as a biomarker in the detection of early lung cancer. As part of their assessment of the inter-rater reliability of scoring stained specimens, they compared the results obtained on 123 slides read by both a pathologist and a cytotechnologist (Table 3). The authors stated that they used McNemar's test to test for "significant agreement ($P = 1.000$)" between the readers. However, what they really did was to test for a significant difference in

Table 3
2 × 2 Table showing agreement between a pathologist and a cytotechnologist when scoring the same stained specimen

Pathologist's Reading	Cytotechnologist's Reading	
	Positive	Negative
Positive	31	1
Negative	0	91

Source: Reprinted from Table 4 of Tockman et al. (1988) with permission from the American Society of Clinical Oncology.

Table 4
2 × 2 Table showing agreement between two dichotomous variables

Variable A	Variable B		
	Positive	Negative	Total
Positive	n_{11}	n_{12}	$n_{1.}$
Negative	n_{21}	n_{22}	$n_{2.}$
Total	$n_{.1}$	$n_{.2}$	n

classification accuracy between the two readers. While such a test is often informative, one should also measure the degree of agreement between the readers (Kraemer, 1980). The generally accepted method for assessing agreement between two dichotomous biomarkers, neither of which can be assumed to be the gold standard, is Cohen's kappa, although alternative measures are also available (see Section 2.3.1.1). When measuring agreement among three or more dichotomous biomarkers, we recommend the method of Fleiss (1971), which is described in Section 2.3.1.2.

2.3.1.1. Cohen's kappa and alternatives (two dichotomous biomarkers). Consider the general 2 × 2 table showing agreement between two dichotomous variables A and B given in Table 4. The two most commonly used measures of agreement between two dichotomous variables are the *Index of Crude Agreement*, given by

$$p_0 = \frac{n_{11} + n_{22}}{n}, \tag{2}$$

and *Cohen's kappa*, given by

$$\hat{\kappa} = \frac{p_0 - \hat{p}_e}{1 - \hat{p}_e},$$

where p_e is the percentage agreement between the two variables that "can be attributed to chance" (Cohen, 1960). This degree of agreement is estimated by

$$\hat{p}_e = p_{1.}p_{.1} + p_{2.}p_{.2},$$

where $p_{1.} = n_{1.}/n$, $p_{.1} = n_{.1}/n$, $p_{2.} = 1 - p_{1.}$, and $p_{.2} = 1 - p_{.1}$. The formula for Cohen's kappa now becomes

$$\hat{\kappa} = \frac{2(n_{11}n_{22} - n_{12}n_{21})}{n^2(p_{1.}p_{.2} + p_{.1}p_{2.})}. \tag{3}$$

The approximate variance of $\hat{\kappa}$ is given by

$$\widehat{\mathrm{Var}}(\hat{\kappa}) = \frac{1}{n(1-\hat{p}_e)^2} \times \left(\sum_{i=1}^{2} p_{ii}\{1 - (p_{i.} + p_{.i})(1 - \hat{\kappa})\}^2 + (1-\hat{\kappa})^2 \sum_{i \neq j} p_{ij}(p_{i.} + p_{.j})^2 - \{\hat{\kappa} - \hat{p}_e(1-\hat{\kappa})\}^2 \right), \tag{4}$$

where n is the number of subjects being rated by the two raters, and $p_{ij} = n_{ij}/n$, $i = 1, 2$; $j = 1, 2$.

Approximate $100(1-\alpha)\%$ confidence limits for κ are given by $\hat{\kappa} \pm z_{\alpha/2}\sqrt{\widehat{\mathrm{Var}}(\hat{\kappa})}$. For the data given in Table 3, we obtain $\hat{\kappa} = 0.98$ using Eq. (3) and $\widehat{\mathrm{Var}}(\hat{\kappa}) = 0.0004494$ using (4).

This yields an approximate 95% confidence interval (CI) for κ of (0.94, 1.00). These results indicate excellent inter-rater reliability for the biomarker proposed by Tockman et al. (1988).

Cohen's kappa is the generally accepted method for assessing agreement between two dichotomous variables, neither of which can be assumed to be the gold standard (Bartko, 1991), but several deficiencies have been noted (Feinstein and Cicchetti, 1990, p. 545; Byrt et al., 1993, p. 425). These deficiencies include: (i) If either method classifies no subjects into one of the two categories, $\hat{\kappa} = 0$. (ii) If there are no agreements for one of the two categories, $\hat{\kappa} < 0$. (iii) The value of $\hat{\kappa}$ is affected by the difference in the relative frequency of "disease" and "no disease" in the sample. The higher the discrepancy, the larger the value of $\hat{p}_e$ and the smaller the value of $\hat{\kappa}$. (iv) The value of $\hat{\kappa}$ is affected by any discrepancy between the relative frequency of "disease" for Method A and the relative frequency of "disease" for Method B. The greater the discrepancy, the smaller the expected agreement, and the larger the value of $\hat{\kappa}$.

To adjust for these deficiencies, Byrt et al. (1993) propose that, in addition to $\hat{\kappa}$, one also reports the prevalence-adjusted and bias-adjusted kappa (*PABAK*),

$$\mathrm{PABAK} = \frac{(n_{11} + n_{22}) - (n_{12} + n_{21})}{n} = 2p_0 - 1,$$

where p_0 is the index of crude agreement given in Eq. (2). (Note that *PABAK* is equivalent to the proportion of "agreements" between the variables minus the proportion of "disagreements.") The approximate variance of PABAK is given

Table 5
Hypothetical 2 × 2 table showing agreement between two dichotomous biomarkers

Biomarker *A*	Biomarker *B* Positive	Negative	Total
Positive	80	15	95
Negative	5	0	5
Total	85	15	100

by $\widehat{\text{Var}}(\text{PABAK}) = 4p_0(1 - p_0)/n$ and approximate 100(1−α)% confidence limits for the true value of PABAK are given by

$$\text{PABAK} \pm z_{\alpha/2}\sqrt{\widehat{\text{Var}}(\text{PABAK})}.$$

As an illustration of some of the deficiencies of $\hat{\kappa}$, consider the hypothetical data on the agreement between two dichotomous biomarkers given in Table 5. Even though the two biomarkers agree on 80% of the specimens, the value of $\hat{\kappa}$ is −0.08, indicating poor agreement (Landis and Koch, 1977, p. 165). Two of the previously mentioned deficiencies are at work here. First, since the two biomarkers did not agree on any of the subjects who were classified as "negative," $\hat{\kappa}<0$. Second, the value of $\hat{\kappa}$ is adversely affected by the difference in the relative frequencies of "disease" (90%) and "no disease" (10%) in the sample. The *PABAK* coefficient, which adjusts for both of these shortcomings, has the value $2p_0-1 = 2(0.80)-1 = 0.60$, with an approximate 95% CI for the true value of PABAK of (0.44, 0.76). We contend that the PABAK coefficient is a much more accurate measure than $\hat{\kappa}$ of the agreement between the two biomarkers suggested by Table 5.

In addition to using $\hat{\kappa}$ and the *PABAK* coefficient to measure overall agreement, it is also advisable to describe the agreement separately in terms of those specimens that appear to be positive and those that appear to be negative. Using measures of positive agreement and negative agreement in assessing reliability is analogous to using sensitivity and specificity in assessing validity in the presence of a gold standard. Such measures can be used to help diagnose the type(s) of disagreement that may be present.

Cicchetti and Feinstein (1990) proposed indices of *average positive agreement* (p_{pos}) and *average negative agreement* (p_{neg}) for this purpose:

$$p_{\text{pos}} = \frac{n_{11}}{(n_{1.} + n_{.1})/2}$$

and

$$p_{\text{neg}} = \frac{n_{22}}{(n_{2.} + n_{.2})/2}$$

Note that the denominators of p_{pos} and p_{neg} are the average number of subjects which the two methods classify as positive and negative, respectively.

Following Graham and Bull (1998), let

$$\phi_{11} = 2/(2p_{11} + p_{12} + p_{21}) - 4p_{11}/(2p_{11} + p_{12} + p_{21})^2,$$

$$\phi_{12} = \phi_{21} = -2p_{11}/(2p_{11} + p_{12} + p_{21})^2,$$

and

$$\phi_{22} = 0.$$

Then the variance of p_{pos} can be estimated using

$$\widehat{\text{Var}}(p_{\text{pos}}) = \frac{1}{n}\left(\sum_{i=1}^{2}\sum_{j=1}^{2}\phi_{ij}^2 p_{ij} - \left(\sum_{i=1}^{2}\sum_{j=1}^{2}\phi_{ij}p_{ij}\right)^2\right).$$

Similarly, let

$$\gamma_{11} = 0,$$

$$\gamma_{12} = \gamma_{21} = -2p_{22}/(2p_{22} + p_{12} + p_{21})^2,$$

and

$$\gamma_{22} = 2/(2p_{22} + p_{12} + p_{21}) - 4p_{22}/(2p_{22} + p_{12} + p_{21})^2.$$

Then the variance of p_{neg} can be estimated using

$$\widehat{\text{Var}}(p_{\text{neg}}) = \frac{1}{n}\left(\sum_{i=1}^{2}\sum_{j=1}^{2}\gamma_{ij}^2 p_{ij} - \left(\sum_{i=1}^{2}\sum_{j=1}^{2}\gamma_{ij}p_{ij}\right)^2\right). \tag{5}$$

Approximate $100(1-\alpha)\%$ confidence intervals (CIs) for the true values of p_{pos} and p_{neg} are given by $p_{\text{pos}} \pm z_{\alpha/2}\sqrt{\widehat{\text{Var}}(p_{\text{pos}})}$ and $p_{\text{neg}} \pm z_{\alpha/2}\sqrt{\widehat{\text{Var}}(p_{\text{neg}})}$, respectively. Simulation results due to Graham and Bull (1998) suggest that these approximate CIs provide adequate coverage for $n > 200$. For smaller n, they recommend that a bootstrap or Bayesian procedure be used to construct the CI. However, they do not provide software for implementing either of these approaches, both of which require rather extensive computer programming.

For the data in Table 5, $p_{\text{pos}} = 80/\big((95+85)/2\big) = 88.9\%$ and $p_{\text{neg}} = 0/\big((5+15)/2\big) = 0.0\%$. Thus, there is moderate overall agreement between the two observers (as measured by the *PABAK* coefficient of 0.60), "almost perfect agreement" on specimens that appear to be positive, and no agreement on specimens that appear to be negative. Hence, efforts to improve the biomarker determination process should be targeted toward those specimens that are negative.

Using the formulas given above, we obtain an approximate 95% CI for the true value of p_{pos} of $p_{\text{pos}} \pm z_{\alpha/2}\sqrt{\widehat{\text{Var}}(p_{\text{pos}})} = (84.0\%,\ 94.7\%)$. Of course, this interval may be inaccurate since $n < 200$ (Graham and Bull, 1998). In terms of a CI for the true value of p_{neg}, note that if $p_{22} = 0$ as in Table 5, $\widehat{\text{Var}}(p_{\text{neg}}) = 0$ using Eq. (5). Therefore, the asymptotic approach does not yield a meaningful CI for the true value of p_{neg} in this case.

2.3.1.2. More than two dichotomous biomarkers. The method of Fleiss (1971) can be used to calculate an overall measure of agreement among $k \geqslant 2$ dichotomous biomarkers. As described in Section 2.2.2, Cochran's Q test could also be used to test for significant disagreement among the biomarkers (what Shoukri (2004, pp. 49–51) refers to as "inter-rater bias"). Let n denote the number of biological specimens under study, and let k denote the number of biomarkers being compared. Let y_{ij} denote the determination (usually "positive" or "negative") based on the jth biomarker for the ith specimen, where $y_{ij} = 1$ for "positive" and $y_{ij} = 0$ for "negative," and let

$$y_i = \sum_{j=1}^{k} y_{ij}$$

denote the number of positive ratings on the ith specimen. Fleiss (1971) generalized Cohen's kappa to a new measure, $\hat{\kappa}_{\text{f}}$ as follows:

$$\hat{\kappa}_{\text{f}} = \frac{p_0 - \hat{p}_{\text{e}}}{1 - \hat{p}_{\text{e}}},$$

where

$$p_0 = 1 - \frac{2}{n}\sum_{i=1}^{n} \frac{y_i(k - y_i)}{k(k-1)},$$

$$\hat{p}_{\text{e}} = 1 - 2\hat{\pi}(1 - \hat{\pi}),$$

and

$$\hat{\pi} = \frac{\sum_{i=1}^{n} y_i}{nk}.$$

For the hypothetical data in Table 2, $\hat{\pi} = 0.2531, \hat{p}_{\text{e}} = 0.6219$, $p_0 = 0.7343$, and $\hat{\kappa}_{\text{f}} = 0.30$, indicating "fair" agreement of the new biomarker with sputum cytology and chest X-ray. Of course, Cohen's kappa (or the *PABAK* coefficient) could also be used to describe the agreement between the new biomarker and either sputum cytology or chest X-ray.

2.3.2. Continuous biomarkers

Bartczak et al. (1994) compared a high-pressure liquid chromatography (HPLC)-based assay and a gas chromatography (GC)-based assay for urinary muconic acid, both of which have been used as biomarkers to assess exposure to benzene. Their data, after omitting an outlier due to an unresolved chromatogram peak,

Table 6
Data on comparison of determinations of muconic acid (ng/ml) in human urine by HPLC–diode array and GC–MS analysis

Specimen Number	HPLC (X_1)	GC–MS (X_2)	X_1–X_2	$(X_1 + X_2)/2$
1	139	151	−12.00	145.00
2	120	93	27.00	106.50
3	143	145	−2.00	144.00
4	496	443	53.00	469.50
5	149	153	−4.00	151.00
6	52	58	−6.00	55.00
7	184	239	−55.00	211.50
8	190	256	−66.00	223.00
9	32	69	−37.00	50.50
10	312	321	−9.00	316.50
11	19	8	11.00	13.50
12	321	364	−43.00	342.50

Source: Copyright (1994) from "Evaluation of Assays for the Identification and Quantitation of Muconic Acid, a Benzene Metabolite in Human Urine," Journal of Toxicology and Environmental Health, by A. Bartczak et al. Reproduced by permission of Taylor & Francis Group, LLC., http://www.taylorandfrancis.com.

are given in Table 6. They used Pearson's correlation coefficient r in their assessment of the agreement between the two methods (p. 255). However, at least as far back as 1973, it was recognized that r is not appropriate for assessing agreement in what are typically called "method comparison studies," i.e., studies in which neither method of measurement can be considered to be the gold standard (Westgard and Hunt, 1973). In fact, Westgard and Hunt go so far as to state that "the correlation coefficient ... is of no practical use in the statistical analysis of comparison data" (1973, p. 53).

Despite the general agreement among statisticians that r is not an acceptable measure of agreement in method comparison studies, its use in this context is still quite prevalent. Hagan and Looney (2004) found that r was used in 28% (53/189) of the method comparison studies published in the clinical research literature in 2001. The prevalence of the use of r in method comparison studies involving biomarkers was not examined separately in their study, but it is unlikely that it differed substantially from that found in the clinical research literature as a whole.

Acceptable alternatives to Pearson's r that are recommended for assessing agreement between continuous biomarkers include the coefficient of concordance (Lin, 1989, 2000), the Bland–Altman method (Altman and Bland, 1983; Bland and Altman, 1986), and Deming regression (Strike, 1996). Each of these is discussed in the sections that follow. It is interesting to note, however, that these methods are rarely used even today in method comparison studies published in the clinical research literature: Hagan and Looney (2004) found that Deming regression was used in none of the 189 method comparison studies published in 2001 and Lin's coefficient was used in only one. The Bland–Altman method was used in only 25 of the published studies (13.2%). The most commonly used method was the intra-class correlation coefficient (ICC), appearing in 118 (62.4%) of the published studies. However, the use of the ICC in method comparison studies has been criticized by several authors (e.g., Bartko, 1994; Bland and Altman, 1990; Lin, 1989; Looney, 2001) and its general use for this purpose is not recommended.

2.3.2.1. Lin's coefficient of concordance. An alternative to r that is often useful in evaluating agreement between continuous biomarkers is the *coefficient of concordance* proposed by Lin (1989, 2000). In general, to calculate the agreement between two continuous measurements X_1 and X_2, one calculates the sample version of Lin's coefficient, denoted by r_c:

$$r_c = \frac{2s_{12}}{s_1^2 + s_2^2 + (\bar{x}_1 - \bar{x}_2)^2}, \tag{6}$$

where s_{12} is the sample covariance of X_1 and X_2, $\bar{x}_1$ the sample mean of X_1, $\bar{x}_2$ the sample mean of X_2, s_1^2 the sample variance of X_1, and s_2^2 the sample variance of X_2.

It can be shown that $r_c = 1$ if there is perfect agreement between the sample values of X_1 and X_2, $r_c = -1$ if there is perfect disagreement, and $-1 < r_c < 1$ otherwise.

The approximate standard error (SE) of Lin's coefficient is given by

$$\widehat{\text{se}}(r_c) = \sqrt{\frac{1}{n-2}\left[\left(\frac{1-r^2}{r^2} r_c^2 (1 - r_c^2)\right) + \left(2r_c^3(1 - r_c)\frac{(\bar{x}_1 - \bar{x}_2)^2}{s_1 s_2 r}\right) - r_c^4 \frac{(\bar{x}_1 - \bar{x}_2)^4}{2s_1^2 s_2^2 r^2}\right]}, \tag{7}$$

where r is the Pearson correlation coefficient for X_1 and X_2 and n the number of samples for which paired observations for X_1 and X_2 are obtained.

When $n \geqslant 30$, an approximate $100(1-\alpha)\%$ CI for the population value of Lin's coefficient, denoted by ρ_c, can be obtained using $r_c \pm z_{\alpha/2}\widehat{\text{se}}(r_c)$. When $n < 30$, an approximate CI based on a bootstrap approach is recommended. SAS code for calculating the bootstrap CI and the interval based on $\widehat{\text{se}}(r_c)$ can be found at http://www.ucsf.edu/cando/resources/software/linscon.sas. See Cheng and Gansky (2006) for more details.

For the data given in Table 6, $n = 12$, $\bar{x}_1 = 179.75$, $\bar{x}_2 = 191.67$, $s_1 = 137.87$, $s_2 = 134.06$, $s_{12} = 17{,}906.5455$, and $r = 0.969$. Therefore, from Eqs (6) and (7),

$$r_c = \frac{2s_{12}}{s_1^2 + s_2^2 + (\bar{x}_1 - \bar{x}_2)^2} = \frac{2(17{,}906.5455)}{(137.87)^2 + (134.06)^2 + (179.75 - 191.67)^2}$$
$$= 0.965$$

and $\widehat{\text{se}}(r_c) = 0.022$. An approximate 95% CI for ρ_c based on 1,000 bootstrap samples is given by (0.879, 0.985).

2.3.2.2. The Bland–Altman method. An alternative method for measuring agreement between two biomarkers X_1 and X_2 in which both biomarker determinations are in the same units is to apply the methodology proposed by Altman and Bland

(Altman and Bland, 1983; Bland and Altman, 1986). The steps involved in this approach are as follows:

(1) Construct a scatterplot and superimpose the line $X_2 = X_1$.
(2) Plot the difference between X_1 and X_2 (denoted by d) vs. the mean of X_1 and X_2 for each subject.
(3) Perform a visual check to make sure that the within-subject repeatability is not associated with the size of the measurement, i.e., that the bias (as measured by $(X_1–X_2)$) does not increase (or decrease) systematically as $(X_1+X_2)/2$ increases.
(4) Perform a formal test to confirm the visual check in Step (3) by testing the hypothesis H_0: $\rho = 0$, where ρ is the true correlation between $(X_1–X_2)$ and $(X_1+X_2)/2$.
(5) If there is no association between the size of the measurement and the bias, then proceed to Step (6) below. If there does appear to be significant association, then an attempt should be made to find a transformation of X_1, X_2, or both, so that the transformed data do not exhibit any association. This can be accomplished by repeating Steps (2)–(4) for the transformed data. The logarithmic transformation has been found to be most useful for this purpose. [If no transformation can be found, Altman and Bland (1983) recommend describing the differences between the methods by regressing $(X_1–X_2)$ on $(X_1+X_2)/2$.]
(6) Calculate the "limits of agreement": $\bar{d} - 2s_d$ to $\bar{d} + 2s_d$, where $\bar{d}$ is the mean difference between X_1 and X_2 and s_d the standard deviation of the differences.
(7) Approximately 95% of the differences should fall within the limits in Step (6) (assuming a normal distribution). If the differences within these limits are not clinically relevant, then the two methods can be used interchangeably. However, it is important to note that this method is applicable *only* if both measurements are made in the same units.

Figure 1 shows the scatterplot of X_2 vs. X_1 with the line $X_2 = X_1$ superimposed for the data in Table 6. This plot indicates fairly good agreement except that 9 of the 12 data points are below the line of agreement.

Figure 2 shows the plot of the difference (HPLC−GC) vs. the mean of HPLC and GC for each subject. A visual inspection of Fig. 2 suggests that the within-subject repeatability is not associated with the size of the measurement, i.e., that (HPLC−GC) does not increase (or decrease) systematically as (HPLC+GC)/2 increases. The sample correlation between (HPLC−GC) and (HPLC+GC)/2 is $r = 0.113$ and the p-value for the test of H_0: $\rho = 0$ is 0.728. Therefore, the assumption of the independence between the difference and the average is not contradicted by the data. The "limits of agreement" are $\bar{d} - 2s_d = -11.9 - 2(34.2) = -80.3$ to $\bar{d} + 2s_d = -11.9 + 2(34.2) = 56.5$ and these are represented (along with $\bar{d}$) by dotted lines in Fig. 2. (Note that all of the differences fall within the limits $\bar{d} - 2s_d$ to $\bar{d} + 2s_d$.) If differences as large as 80.3 are not clinically relevant, then the two methods can be used interchangeably. Given the order of magnitude of the measurements in Table 6, it appears that a difference of 80 would be clinically important, so there is an indication of

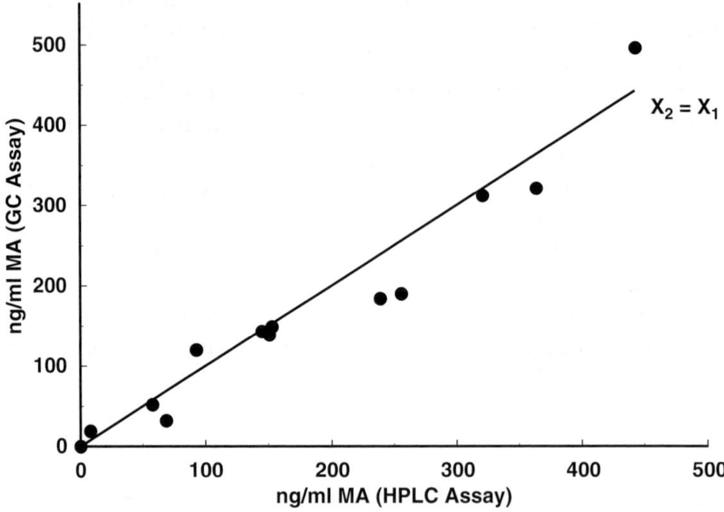

Fig. 1. Scatterplot of data on agreement between (HPLC)-based and (GC)-based assays for urinary muconic acid with the line of perfect agreement ($X_2 = X_1$) superimposed.

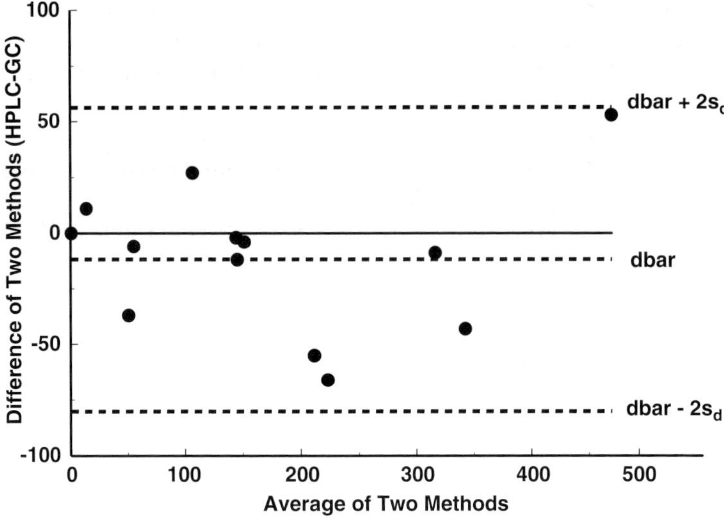

Fig. 2. Plot of difference vs. mean for data on agreement between (HPLC)-based and (GC)-based assays for urinary muconic acid.

inadequate agreement between the two methods. This was not obvious from the plot in Fig. 1.

2.3.2.3. Deming regression. Strike (1996) describes an approach for determining the type of disagreement that may be present when comparing two biomarkers.

These methods are most likely to be applicable when one of the methods (Method X) is a *reference* method, perhaps a biomarker that is already in routine use, and the other method (Method Y) is a *test* method, usually a new biomarker that is being evaluated. Any systematic difference (or *bias*) between the two biomarkers is relative in nature, since neither method can be thought of as representing the true exposure.

As in the Bland–Altman method described in Section 2.3.2.2, the first step is to construct a scatterplot of Y vs. X and superimpose the line $Y = X$. Any systematic discrepancy between the two biomarkers will be represented on this plot by a general shift in the location of the points away from the line $Y = X$. Strike assumes that systematic differences between the two biomarkers can be attributed to either *constant bias*, *proportional bias*, or both, and assumes the following models for each biomarker result:

$$X_i = \xi_i + \delta_i, \qquad 1 \le i \le n, \tag{8}$$

$$Y_i = \eta_i + \varepsilon_i, \qquad 1 \le i \le n,$$

where X_i is the observed value for biomarker X, ξ_i the true value of biomarker X, δ_i the random error for biomarker X, Y_i the observed value for biomarker Y, η_i the true value of biomarker Y, and ε_i the random error for biomarker Y.

Strike further assumes that the errors δ_i and ε_i are stochastically independent of each other and normally distributed with constant variance (σ_δ^2 and σ_ε^2, respectively) throughout the range of biomarker determinations in the study sample. [Strike points out that constant variance assumptions are usually unrealistic in practice and recommends a computationally intensive method for accounting for this lack of homogeneity. This method is incorporated into the MINISNAP software provided with Strike (1996).]

Strike assumes that any systematic discrepancy between Methods X and Y can be represented by

$$\eta_i = \beta_0 + \beta_1 \xi_i. \tag{9}$$

In this model, *constant bias* is represented by deviations of β_0 from 0 and *proportional bias* by deviations of β_1 from 1. [This is the same terminology used by Westgard and Hunt (1973).] If we now incorporate Eq. (9) into the equation for Y_i in Eq. (8), we have

$$Y_i = \beta_0 + \beta_1 X_i + (\varepsilon_i - \beta_1 \delta_i). \tag{10}$$

Model (2.10) is sometimes called a *functional errors-in-variables model* and assessing agreement between biomarkers X and Y requires the estimation of the parameters β_0 and β_1. Strike proposes a method that requires an estimate of the ratio of the error variances given by $\lambda = \sigma_\varepsilon^2/\sigma_\delta^2$. This method is generally referred to in the clinical laboratory literature as "Deming regression"; however, this is somewhat of a misnomer as Deming was concerned with generalizing the errors-in-variables model to non-linear relationships. Strike points out that the method he advocates for obtaining estimates of β_0 and β_1 is actually due to Kummel (1879).

The equations for estimating β_0 and β_1 are as follows:

$$\hat{\beta}_1 = \frac{(S_{yy} - \hat{\lambda}S_{xx}) + \sqrt{(S_{yy} - \hat{\lambda}S_{xx})^2 + 4\hat{\lambda}S_{xy}^2}}{2S_{xy}}, \tag{11}$$

$$\hat{\beta}_0 = \bar{Y} - \hat{\beta}_1\bar{X},$$

where

$$\hat{\lambda} = \frac{\hat{\sigma}_\varepsilon^2}{\hat{\sigma}_\delta^2},$$

$$S_{yy} = \sum_{i=1}^{n}(y_i - \bar{y})^2, \quad S_{xx} = \sum_{i=1}^{n}(x_i - \bar{x})^2, \quad S_{xy} = \sum_{i=1}^{n}(x_i - \bar{x})(y_i - \bar{y}).$$

The estimate $\hat{\lambda}$ can be obtained either from error variance estimates for each biomarker provided by the laboratory or by estimating each error variance using

$$\hat{\sigma}^2 = \frac{\sum_{i=1}^{n} d_i^2}{2n}$$

where d_i is the difference between the two determinations of the biomarker (replicates) for specimen i. (Note that the methodology proposed by Strike cannot be applied without an estimate of the ratio of error variances of the two biomarkers.)

To perform significance tests for β_0 and β_1, we need formulas for the standard errors (SEs) of $\hat{\beta}_0$ and $\hat{\beta}_1$. The approximations that Strike recommends for routine use are given by

$$\mathrm{SE}(\hat{\beta}_1) = \left\{\frac{\hat{\beta}_1^2((1 - r^2)/r^2)}{n - 2}\right\}^{1/2} \tag{12}$$

and

$$\mathrm{SE}(\hat{\beta}_0) = \left\{\frac{[\mathrm{SE}(\hat{\beta}_1)]^2 \sum_{i=i}^{n} x_i^2}{n}\right\}^{1/2},$$

where

$$r^2 = \left(\frac{S_{xy}}{\sqrt{S_{xx}S_{yy}}}\right)^2$$

is the usual "R^2" value for the regression of Y on X. Tests of $H_0 : \beta_1 = 1$ and $H_0 : \beta_0 = 0$ can be performed by referring $(\hat{\beta}_1 - 1)/\mathrm{SE}(\hat{\beta}_1)$ and $\hat{\beta}_0/\mathrm{SE}(\hat{\beta}_0)$, respectively, to the $t(n - 2)$ distribution.

As mentioned earlier, the approach described above is based on the assumption that the error variances σ_δ^2 and σ_ε^2 are constant throughout the range of biomarker determinations in the study sample. However, as Strike points out, this assumption is usually unrealistic in practice and recommends the "weighted Deming regression" methods of Linnet (1990, 1993) for accounting for this lack of homogeneity. These methods are incorporated into the MINISNAP software provided with Strike (1996); however, replicate measurements are required for each test specimen using both biomarkers in order to apply these methods.

As an example, consider the hypothetical data in Table 7. The scatterplot for these data in Fig. 3 indicates substantial lack of agreement between X and Y and

Table 7
Hypothetical data on the agreement between biomarkers A and B

Specimen Number	Biomarker A	Biomarker B
1	31	206
2	4	28
3	17	112
4	14	98
5	16	104
6	7	47
7	11	73
8	4	43
9	14	93
10	7	57
11	10	87

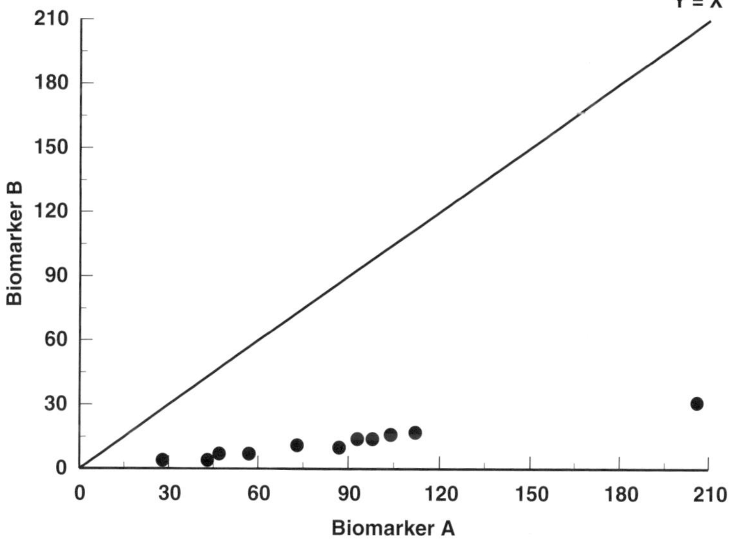

Fig. 3. Scatterplot of hypothetical data on agreement between biomarkers A and B with the line of perfect agreement ($Y = X$) superimposed.

this is borne out by Lin's coefficient, which indicates substantial disagreement ($r_c = 0.102$). (Note that $r = 0.989$, indicating near-perfect linear association. This illustrates one of the major deficiencies in using r as a measure of agreement.) We apply Strike's method to gain a better understanding of the lack of agreement between X and Y.

Applying Eqs (11) and (12), we obtain $\hat{\beta}_1 = 0.158$, $\text{SE}(\hat{\beta}_1) = 0.007$, $\hat{\beta}_0 = -1.342$, and $\text{SE}(\hat{\beta}_0) = 0.614$. For the test of $H_0 : \beta_1 = 1$, this yields

$$t_{\text{cal}} = \frac{\hat{\beta}_1 - 1}{\text{SE}(\hat{\beta}_1)} = \frac{0.158 - 1}{0.007} = -129.54,$$

and using a t-distribution with $n - 2 = 9$ degrees of freedom, we find $p < 0.0001$. Therefore, there is significant proportional bias (which in this case is negative since $\hat{\beta}_1 < 1.0$). For the test of $H_0 : \beta_0 = 0$, we have

$$t_{\text{cal}} = \frac{\hat{\beta}_0}{\text{SE}(\hat{\beta}_0)} = \frac{-1.342}{0.614} = -2.19,$$

and, again using a t-distribution with 9 degrees of freedom, we have $p = 0.056$. Thus, the constant bias is not statistically significant, but just misses the usual cutoff of 0.05.

3. Statistical methods for analyzing biomarker data

3.1. Testing distributional assumptions

It is well known that violating the distributional assumption(s) underlying a statistical procedure can have serious adverse effects on the performance of the procedure (Wilcox, 1987). Therefore, it is beneficial to attempt to verify such assumptions prior to beginning data analysis. However, in many analyses of biomarker data, the underlying distributional assumptions are typically ignored and/or no attempt is made to check the distributional assumptions before proceeding with the analyses. Some authors may state something to the effect that "due to the skewed nature of the data, nonparametric statistical methods were used," but usually no formal test of the distributional assumption was ever performed. For example, in their evaluation of hemoglobin adducts as biomarkers of exposure to tobacco smoke, Atawodi et al. (1998) state that "because the distribution of HPB-Hb adduct levels was not normal, we used the nonparametric Kruskal–Wallis test ..." (p. 819); however, they offer no justification for why they concluded that the adduct levels were not normally distributed.

3.1.1. Graphical methods for assessing normality

Several graphical methods for verifying the assumption of normality have been proposed (D'Agostino, 1986). One commonly used method is the *probability plot* (Gerson, 1975), of which the quantile–quantile (Q–Q) plot is a special case. Another graphical method that is not as widely used as the probability plot is the *normal density plot* (Jones and Daly, 1995; Hazelton, 2003), which is easier to interpret than a probability plot because it is based on a direct comparison of a certain plot of the sample data vs. the familiar bell-shaped curve of the normal distribution.

While graphical examination of data can be extremely valuable in assessing a distributional assumption, the interpretation of any plot or graph is inherently subjective. Therefore, it is not sufficient to base the assessment of a distributional assumption entirely on a graphical device. Bernstein et al. (1999) evaluated the use of a bile acid-induced apoptosis assay as a measure of colon cancer risk. They determined that their apoptotic index (AI) "had a Gaussian distribution, as assessed by a box plot, quantile–quantile plot, and histogram" (p. 2354). However, each of these methods is a graphical technique, and different data analysts could interpret the plots differently. One should always supplement the graphical examination of a distributional assumption with a formal statistical test, which may itself be based on the results of the graphical device that was used. For example, correlation coefficient tests based on probability plots have been shown to have good power for detecting departures from normality against a wide variety of non-normal distributions (Looney and Gulledge, 1985). Formal tests of the distributional assumption can also be based on a normal density plot (Jones and Daly, 1995; Hazelton, 2003).

3.1.2. The Shapiro–Wilk (S–W) test

Another formal test of the assumption of normality that we recommend for general use is the Shapiro–Wilk (S–W) test (Shapiro and Wilk, 1965). Several studies have demonstrated that the S–W test has good statistical power against a wide variety of non-normal distributions (e.g., Shapiro et al., 1968). Even though the S–W test is not based directly on a graphical method for assessing normality, it is a valuable adjunct to such methods. The S–W test has been used in several studies involving biomarker data (e.g., Buckley et al., 1995; Lagorio et al., 1998; MacRae et al., 2003), although at least one author incorrectly treated the S–W test as upper-tailed, rather than lower-tailed (Buckley et al., 1995).

To perform the S–W test for normality, assume that the sample is composed of n independent and identically distributed observations $(x_1, x_2, \ldots, x_n)$ from a normal distribution with unspecified mean and variance. If $x_{[1]}, x_{[2]}, \ldots, x_{[n]}$ represents the n observations arranged in ascending sequence, the test statistic is

$$W = \frac{\left[\sum_{i=1}^{n} a_i x_{[i]}\right]^2}{\sum_{i=1}^{n} (x_i - \overline{x})^2},$$

where the a_i's represent constants that are functions of n (see Royston, 1982). The null hypothesis of normality is rejected for small values of W. Although not normally distributed under the null hypothesis (even asymptotically), W can be transformed to approximate normality when $7 \leqslant n \leqslant 2{,}000$ (Royston, 1982, 1992). For $3 \leqslant n \leqslant 6$, the methods described by Wilk and Shapiro (1968) should be used to find the lower-tailed *p*-value. It is especially important to account for the presence of ties when applying the S–W test (Royston, 1989). The S–W test can be performed using StatXact or the UNIVARIATE procedure within SAS.

3.1.3. Remedial measures for violation of a distributional assumption

If it has been determined that a violation of the distributional assumption underlying a statistical procedure has occurred, and that this departure is important enough to adversely affect the results of the proposed statistical analyses, at least three approaches have been recommended: (a) attempt to find a transformation of the data that will result in a new random variable that does appear to follow the assumed underlying distribution (usually the normal), (b) attempt to find a statistical procedure that is more robust to the distributional assumption, or (c) use a distribution-free test that is not dependent on the assumption of an underlying statistical distribution. Robust methods are beyond the scope of this chapter and will not be treated here; for a general treatment of these techniques, see Huber (1996). Distribution-free (also called *non-parametric*) alternatives to normal-theory-based methods for measuring association and for comparing groups are described in Sections 3.2.3.2 and 3.3, respectively. Methods for identifying an appropriate transformation for biomarker data that appear to violate a distributional assumption are discussed in the following section.

3.1.4. Choosing a transformation

A transformation based on the logarithm (usually the "natural" logarithm, $\log_e$) is commonly used in the analysis of biomarker data (e.g., Atawodi et al., 1998; MacRae et al., 2003; Strachan et al., 1990). However, authors usually provide no justification for such a transformation other than that it is commonly used in analyzing the type of data collected in the study. At the very least, the log-transformed data should be tested for normality as described in Sections 3.1.1 and 3.1.2 above. If one concludes that the log-transformed data are not normally distributed, then there are many other possible transformations that one could try. Several families of possible transformations have been proposed, including the Box–Cox family (Box and Cox, 1964), the Tukey "ladder of powers" (Tukey, 1977, pp. 88–93), the Johnson S_u family (Johnson, 1949), and the Pearson family (Stuart and Ord, 1987, pp. 210–220). The Box–Cox approach is particularly attractive, in that there is a formal statistical test for determining if the chosen transformation is "statistically significant"; however, selecting the appropriate transformation can be computationally difficult (Atkinson, 1973). (A SAS module for selecting the appropriate Box–Cox transformation parameter is available from the first author.) The Tukey "ladder of powers" is also attractive in that it requires that one consider only a small number of possible transformations. Whatever method is used to select a transformation, the transformed data should be tested for normality before proceeding to the next stage of the analysis, as was done in MacRae et al. (2003).

Table 8
Association between dichotomized cotinine level and diagnosis of depression using the Diagnostic Interview Survey (DIS), female subjects only

	DIS Diagnosis		
Cotinine $\geqslant$15	Positive	Negative	Total
Yes	27	202	229
No	7	121	128
Total	34	323	357

Source: Adapted from Table 4 of Pérez-Stable et al. (1995) with permission from Elsevier.

3.2. Analyzing cross-classified categorical data

3.2.1. Comparing two independent groups in terms of a binomial proportion

It is often of interest in the analysis of biomarker data to compare two independent groups in terms of a binomial proportion. (The comparison of dependent proportions is treated in Section 2.2.1 of this chapter.) For example, Pérez-Stable et al. (1995) compared smokers and non-smokers in terms of the proportion diagnosed with depression using the Depression Interview Schedule (DIS) (Table 8). As is commonly done with data of this type, they performed the comparison using the χ^2 test. However, this test is known to have very poor statistical properties, especially if the number of subjects in either group is small (Mehrotra et al., 2003), and is not recommended for general use. A preferred method is the "exact" version of Fisher's exact test, as implemented in StatXact or SAS. This test is described below.

Suppose that we wish to perform an exact test of the null hypothesis H_0: $\pi_1 = \pi_2$. Following the argument in Mehta and Patel (2005), denote the common probability of success for the two populations by $\pi = \pi_1 = \pi_2$. Under the null hypothesis, the probability of observing the data in Table 8 is

$$f_0(x_{11}, x_{12}, x_{21}, x_{22}) = \binom{n_1}{x_{11}}\binom{n_2}{x_{21}}\pi^{x_{11}+x_{21}}(1-\pi)^{x_{12}+x_{22}}, \tag{13}$$

where x_{ij} denotes the count in cell (i,j) of the 2×2 table, and n_1 and n_2 denote the sample sizes in the two groups being compared. In order to calculate the exact p-value for any test of H_0, we will need to calculate the probability of obtaining a 2×2 table at least as extreme as the observed table given in Table 8. The probability of any such table will involve the parameter π, as in Eq. (13). The "conditional" approach to exact inference for 2×2 tables involves eliminating π from the probability calculations by conditioning on its sufficient statistic (Cox and Hinkley, 1974, Chapter 2). This is the approach implemented in many of the exact statistical procedures in StatXact, and one that is recommended here. After conditioning on the sufficient statistic for π, we find that the exact distribution of x_{11} (the test statistic for Fisher's exact test) is hypergeometric.

For the upper-tailed alternative H_a: $\pi_1 > \pi_2$, any 2×2 table with the same marginal row and column totals as the observed table that has a count in the (1,1) cell that is greater than or equal to x_{11} in the observed table will be favorable to H_a. The hypergeometric probability for each of these tables should then be accumulated when calculating the upper-tailed p-value. The reference set under the conditional approach is defined to be any 2×2 table with the same marginal row and column totals as the observed table.

In Table 8, the test statistic for Fisher's exact test is $x_{11} = 27$. Then, the exact upper-tailed p-value for the test of H_0 would be found by accumulating the hypergeometric probabilities for all possible values in the (1,1) position that are greater than 27, assuming that the row and column totals remain at the same values as in Table 8. This yields an exact upper-tailed p-value of 0.0355, and a two-tailed p-value of 0.0710.

Fisher's exact test as formulated here is known to be conservative (Agresti, 1996, pp. 41–44). That is, the hypergeometric distribution used to calculate the exact p-values is highly discrete, especially when n_1 or n_2 is small. This means that there will be only a small number of possible values that x_{11} can assume, leading to a small number of possible p-values, and hence a small number of possible significance levels, none of which may be close to 0.05. By convention, we choose the upper-tailed significance level that is closest to, but less than or equal to 0.025. For example, for the data in Table 8, examination of the exact conditional null distribution of x_{11} based on the hypergeometric distribution indicates that the upper-tailed significance level closest to, but less than, 0.025 is 0.013 (obtained using a critical value of $x_{11} = 28$).

To help diminish the effect of the conservativeness of Fisher's exact test, we follow the recommendation of Agresti (2002, p. 94) that one use the *mid-p-value*, which is equal to the appropriate exact p-value, minus half the exact point probability of the observed value of the test statistic. For the data in Table 8, this yields a one-tailed mid-p-value of $0.0355 - (1/2)(0.0222) = 0.0244$. The two-tailed mid-$p$-value is $2(0.0244) = 0.0488$.

3.2.2. Testing for trend in proportions

Tunstall-Pedoe et al. (1995) examined the association between passive smoking, as measured by level of serum cotinine, and the presence or absence of several adverse health outcomes (chronic cough, coronary heart disease, etc.). Serum cotinine level was classified into four ordinal categories: "non-detectable," and 0.01–1.05, 1.06–3.97, or 3.98–17.49 ng/ml. The authors calculated odds ratios for the comparison of each serum cotinine category vs. "non-detectable" in terms of the odds of each health outcome. However, an additional analysis that we recommend for data of this type is to perform a test for trend across the serum cotinine categories in terms of the prevalence of the outcomes. Such an analysis would be especially helpful in establishing dose–response relationships between passive smoking and the adverse outcomes. Tunstall-Pedoe et al. (1995) speak in terms of a "gradient" across exposure categories, but perform no statistical test to determine if their data support the existence of such a gradient.

Recommended procedures for testing for trend include the permutation test (Gibbons and Chakraborti, 2003, Chapter 8) and the Cochran–Armitage test (Cochran, 1954; Armitage, 1955).

To perform the Cochran–Armitage (C–A) test, let k denote the number of ordinal categories for the biomarker, and suppose that a score x_i has been assigned to the ith category ($i = 1, 2, \ldots, k$). Within the ith category, assume that r_i specimens out of a total of n_i have been detected as "positive" using the biomarker. Then the total sample size $n = \sum_{i=1}^{k} n_i$. Let $r = \sum_{i=1}^{k} r_i$ denote the total number of positive specimens in the sample of size n, and let

$$\bar{x} = \frac{\sum_{i=1}^{k} n_i x_i}{n}$$

denote the weighted average of the x-values. Then the test statistic for the C–A test for trend is given by

$$X^2_{\text{trend}} = \frac{\left(\sum_{i=1}^{k} r_i x_i - r\bar{x}\right)^2}{p(1-p)\left(\sum_{i=1}^{k} n_i x_i^2 - n\bar{x}^2\right)}, \tag{14}$$

where $p = r/n$ denotes the overall proportion of "positive" findings in the sample. To perform the asymptotic test for significant trend in proportions, the test statistic given in Eq. (14) is compared with a χ^2 distribution with 1 degree of freedom (upper-tailed test only). An exact test for trend based on the test statistic in Eq. (14) can be performed by using the same conditioning argument as was used for the exact version of Fisher's exact test in Section 3.2.1. The permutation test (Gibbons and Chakraborti, 2003, Chapter 8) can also be used to perform an exact test for trend in proportions across ordinal levels of a biomarker. Both the permutation test and the exact version of the C–A test are available in StatXact and the exact version of the C–A test is available in the FREQ procedure in SAS.

For the Tunstall-Pedoe et al. study described above, scores corresponding to the midpoint were assigned to each serum cotinine category (0.00, 0.53, 2.52, and 10.74 ng/ml) and then the C–A test was performed. The results indicate a highly significant increasing trend in the prevalence of "diagnosed coronary heart disease" as serum cotinine level increases ($p<0.001$), a finding that was not reported by the authors.

One difficulty with the C–A test is that it requires preassigned fixed scores. In some cases, there may be no reasonable way to select the scores. In addition, the C–A test is more powerful when the scores and the observed binomial proportions follow a similar observed trend (Neuhäuser and Hothorn, 1999). Alternative methods that can be used without specifying scores that are robust with respect to the dose–response shape have been proposed by Neuhäuser and Hothorn (1999). However, these methods are not currently available in any widely used statistical software package, so we are unable to recommend their general use at this time.

3.2.3. Testing for linear-by-linear association

Cook et al. (1993) examined the association between the number of smokers to whom children had been exposed and their salivary cotinine measured in ng/ml. The "number of smokers" was categorized as 0, 1, 2, and $\geqslant 3$, and salivary cotinine was categorized as "non-detectable," 0.1–0.2, 0.3–0.6, 0.7–1.7, 1.8–4.0, 4.1–14.7, and >14.7. The authors state that "salivary cotinine concentration was strongly related to the number of smokers to whom the child was usually exposed" (p. 16). However, they provide no numerical summary or statistical test to justify this assertion. One method that could be used to test for significant association between these two variables would be the linear-by-linear association test (Agresti et al., 1990). An alternative method would be to use Spearman's correlation to produce a single numerical summary of this association, and to perform a test of the null hypothesis that the population value of Spearman's correlation is different from zero.

3.2.3.1. Linear-by-linear association test. To perform the linear-by-linear association test, assume that the rows and columns of the $r \times c$ contingency table can be ordered according to some underlying variable. In the example from Cook et al. (1993) described above, there is a natural ordering in both the rows ("number of smokers") and columns (salivary cotinine level). Following the notation of Mehta and Patel (2005), let x_{ij} denote the count in the (i,j) position of the "ordered" contingency table and consider the test statistic

$$T(x) = \sum_{i=1}^{r} \sum_{j=1}^{c} u_i v_j x_{ij}, \tag{15}$$

where u_i, $i = 1, 2, \ldots, r$, are row scores, and v_j, $j = 1, 2, \ldots, c$, are column scores. Let m_i, $i = 1, 2, \ldots, r$, denote the row totals, and n_j, $j = 1, 2, \ldots, c$, denote the column totals. Under the null hypothesis of no association between the row and column variables, the test statistic given in Eq. (15) has mean

$$E[T] = \frac{\sum_{i=1}^{r} u_i m_i \sum_{j=1}^{c} v_j n_j}{n},$$

and variance

$$\mathrm{Var}[T] = \frac{\left[\sum_{i=1}^{r} u_i^2 m_i - \frac{\left(\sum_{i=1}^{r} u_i m_i\right)^2}{n}\right]\left[\sum_{j=1}^{c} v_j^2 n_j - \frac{\left(\sum_{j=1}^{c} v_j n_j\right)^2}{n}\right]}{n-1}$$

where

$$n = \sum_{j=1}^{c} n_j = \sum_{i=1}^{r} m_i$$

is the total sample size.

Since the test statistic given by

$$Z^* = \frac{T - E(T)}{\sqrt{\mathrm{Var}(T)}} \tag{16}$$

has an asymptotically standard normal distribution under the null hypothesis, one can compare the calculated value of Z^* in Eq. (16) with the standard normal tables to obtain an approximate p-value. Exact p-values can be obtained for the linear-by-linear test by considering the conditional permutation distribution of the test statistic T under the null hypothesis. Consistent with our earlier discussion of exact distributions, the reference set is defined to be the set of all $r \times c$ contingency tables with the same row and column totals as the observed table.

3.2.3.2. Spearman's correlation. There are many equivalent ways to define Spearman's correlation coefficient. (We denote the population value by ρ_s and the sample value by r_s.) One of the most useful definitions of r_s is the Pearson correlation coefficient calculated on the observations after both the x and y values have been ordered from smallest to largest and replaced by their ranks. Let u_1, $u_2, \ldots, u_n$ denote the ranks of the n observed values of X and let $v_1, v_2, \ldots, v_n$ denote the ranks of the n observed values of Y. Then Spearman's sample coefficient is defined by

$$r_s = \frac{S_{uv}}{\sqrt{S_u^2 S_v^2}}, \tag{17}$$

where S_{uv} is the sample covariance between the u's and v's, S_u^2 the sample variance of the u's, and S_v^2 the sample variance of the v's. If ties are present in the data, a modified version of Eq. (17) should be used (Gibbons and Chakraborti, 2003, pp. 429–431), although this will typically have little effect on the calculated value of r_s unless there are a large number of ties. Fisher's z transformation can be applied to Spearman's coefficient and then used to calculate approximate p-values for hypothesis tests involving ρ_s and to find approximate CIs for ρ_s. Fisher's z transformation applied to r_s is given by

$$z_s = \frac{1}{2}\ln\left(\frac{1 + r_s}{1 - r_s}\right),$$

which is approximately normally distributed with mean 0 and SE $\hat{\sigma}_s = 1.03/\sqrt{n - 3}$. The exact distribution of r_s can be derived using enumeration (Gibbons and Chakraborti, 2003, pp. 424–428). Both the approximate and exact inference results for ρ_s are available in StatXact. Hypothesis tests and CIs based on the Fisher's z transformation for Spearman's coefficient are available in SAS.

For the data presented in Table 1 of Cook et al. (1993), the linear-by-linear association test indicates a strongly significant association between the "number of smokers" and salivary cotinine ($Z^* = 31.67$, $p < 0.001$). Similar results were obtained for Spearman's correlation: $r_s = 0.72$, 95% CI 0.70–0.74, $p < 0.001$.

3.3. Comparison of mean levels of biomarkers across groups

It is widely assumed that the optimal methods for comparing the means of normally distributed variables across groups are the *t*-test in the case of two groups and the analysis of variance (ANOVA) in the case of three or more groups. The proper application of both the *t*-test and ANOVA, as they are usually formulated, is based on two assumptions: (a) that the data in all groups being compared are normally distributed, and (b) that the population variances in all groups being compared are equal (Sheskin, 1997). In this section, we discuss the importance of these assumptions, and provide recommendations for alternative procedures to use when these assumptions appear to be violated.

3.3.1. Importance of distributional assumptions

The performance of both the *t*-test and ANOVA is generally robust against violations of the normality assumption; however, the presence of certain types of departures from normality can seriously affect their performance (Algina et al., 1994). If the methods for testing the assumption of normality described in Sections 3.1.1 and 3.1.2 above indicate a significant departure from normality in any of the groups being compared, we recommend that one consider applying distribution-free alternatives to the *t*-test and the ANOVA *F*-test.

For example, the Mann–Whitney–Wilcoxon (M–W–W) test has been used in biomarker studies when comparing two groups in terms of a continuous variable that appears to be non-normally distributed (e.g., Granella et al., 1996; Qiao et al., 1997). Similarly, the Kruskal–Wallis (K–W) test has been used with biomarker data when comparing more than two groups (e.g., Amorim and Alvarez-Leite, 1997; Atawodi et al., 1998). To perform either the M–W–W or K–W tests, all of the observations are combined into one sample and ranked from smallest (1) to largest (n), where n is the combined sample size. Tied observations are assigned the midrank, i.e., the average rank of all observations having the same value. The test statistic for the M–W–W test is

$$T = \sum_{i=1}^{n_1} w_{i1},$$

where the w_{i1}'s represent the rank order of the observations in Group 1. The mean of T is

$$\mu_T = \frac{n_1(n+1)}{2},$$

and the standard deviation of T is

$$\sigma_T = \sqrt{\frac{n_1(n+1)n_2}{12}}$$

if there are no ties. If ties are present, then

$$\sigma_T = c\sqrt{\frac{n_1(n+1)n_2}{12}},$$

where

$$c = \sqrt{1 - \frac{\sum(t^3 - t)}{n(n^2 - 1)}}, \tag{18}$$

and t denotes the multiplicity of a tie and the sum is calculated over all sets of t ties.

The exact null distribution for the M–W–W test can be obtained using enumeration (or by network algorithms when enumeration is not feasible) and is available in StatXact and the NPAR1WAY procedure in SAS. Approximate p-values for the M–W–W test can be obtained by standardizing the observed value of T using μ_T and σ_T as defined above and then using the standard normal to calculate the appropriate area under the curve. This normal approximation has been found to be "reasonably accurate for equal group sizes as small as 6" (Gibbons and Chakraborti, 2003, p. 273).

To apply the K–W test (appropriate in situations in which $k \geqslant 3$ groups are being compared in terms of their biomarker determinations), let R_i denote the sum of the ranks of the observations in Group i, $i = 1, 2, \ldots, k$. Then the test statistic for the K–W test is

$$H = \frac{12}{n(n+1)} \sum_{i=1}^{k} \frac{1}{n_i} \left[R_i - \frac{n_i(n+1)}{2} \right]^2$$

if there are no ties, and $(1/c)H$, where c is given by Eq. (18), if ties are present. The exact distribution of H can be obtained using a permutation argument and is available in StatXact and the NPAR1WAY procedure in SAS. It can also be shown that H has an approximate $\chi^2(k-1)$ distribution under the null hypothesis.

One interesting feature of any distribution-free test based on ranks (of which the M–W–W and K–W tests are examples) is that applying a monotonic transformation (such as the logarithm) to the data does not affect the results of the analysis. Atawodi et al. (1998) were apparently unaware of this fact when they applied the K–W test to both the original and log-transformed data and obtained "virtually identical results" (p. 820).

It is recommended that exact p-values be used for all of the distribution-free methods mentioned in this section whenever possible; many commonly used statistical packages are able to produce only approximate p-values for distribution-free methods. This may explain the discrepancies found by Atawodi et al. (1998) when they compared the results of the K–W test for the original and log-transformed data.

A characteristic of both the M–W–W and K–W tests that is often overlooked is that these tests are most effective in detecting "shift alternatives"; i.e., the assumption is made that the populations being compared have identical shapes and the alternative hypothesis is that at least one of the populations is a "shifted" version of the others. If the "shift alternative" does not appear to be the appropriate alternative hypothesis, another method that can be used to test the null hypothesis that the parent populations are identical is the Kolmogorov–Smirnov test (Conover, 1999, pp. 428–438; Gibbons and Chakraborti, 2003, pp. 239–246). The exact version of the two-sample Kolmogorov–Smirnov test is available in both StatXact and the NPAR1WAY procedure in SAS and the exact version of the k-sample Kolmogorov–Smirnov test is available in the NPAR1WAY procedure.

3.3.2. The importance of homogeneity of variances in the comparison of means

3.3.2.1. Two-group comparisons in the presence of heterogeneity. The performance of the "usual" t-test (sometimes called the "equal variance t-test") depends very strongly on the underlying assumption of equal population variances (sometimes called *homogeneity*) between the groups (Moser et al., 1989). One approach would be to attempt to use the F-test for testing equality of population variances or another method to verify the homogeneity assumption before applying the equal variance t-test (Moser and Stevens, 1992). If the hypothesis of equal variances is not rejected, then one would apply the "usual" t-test. If the hypothesis of equal variances is rejected, then one would use an alternative approach that does not depend on the homogeneity assumption. One such alternative is the "unequal variance t-test" [sometimes referred to as the "Welch test" or "Satterthwaite approximation" (Moser and Stevens, 1992)], which is generally available in any statistical package that can perform the equal variance t-test. However, Moser and Stevens demonstrate that the preliminary F-test of equality of variances contributes nothing of value and that, in fact, the unequal variance t-test can be used any time the means of two groups are being compared since the test performs almost as well as the equal variance t-test when the population variances in the two groups are equal, and outperforms the equal variance t-test when the variances are unequal. Hence, we follow their advice and recommend that the unequal variance t-test be used routinely whenever the means of two groups are being compared and the data appear to be normally distributed in both the groups. If the data are not normally distributed in either group, a distribution-free alternative to the t-test such as the M–W–W test (Section 3.3.1) can be used instead.

The test statistic for the unequal variance t-test recommended here is given by

$$t^* = \frac{(\bar{x} - \bar{y})}{\sqrt{(s_x^2/n_1) + (s_y^2/n_2)}}, \tag{19}$$

where $\bar{x}$, s_x^2, and n_1 denote the mean, variance, and sample size, respectively, for the biomarker levels in Group 1, and $\bar{y}$, s_y^2, and n_2 the mean, variance, and sample size, respectively, for the biomarker levels in Group 2. To perform the test of the null hypothesis that the mean biomarker level is the same in the two groups, compare the observed value of t^* in Eq. (19) with a Student's t distribution with the following degrees of freedom:

$$\upsilon = \frac{\left((1/n_1) + (u/n_2)\right)^2}{\left(1/n_1^2(n_1 - 1)\right) + \left(u^2/n_2^2(n_2 - 1)\right)}$$

where $u = s_y^2/s_x^2$.

Salmi et al. (2002) evaluated the potential usefulness of soluble vascular adhesion protein-1 (sVAP-1) as a biomarker to monitor and predict the extent of ongoing artherosclerotic processes. The investigators compared two groups: diabetic study participants on insulin treatment only ($n = 7$) vs. diabetic study participants on other treatments ($n = 41$). They used the "usual" (equal-variance) t-test to compare the mean sVAP-1 levels of the two groups: mean $\pm$ S.D. 148 ± 114 vs. 113 ± 6; $t = 2.06$, $\text{df} = 46$, one-tailed $p = 0.023$, a statistically significant result. However, they ignored the fact that the variances in the two groups they were comparing were quite different (12,996 vs. 36, $F = 361$, $\text{df} = (6,40)$, $p < 0.001$). If the unequal variance t-test is used, as recommended by Moser and Stevens (1992), one obtains $t^* = 0.81$, $\upsilon = 6$, one-tailed $p = 0.224$, a non-significant result. Given the extremely strong evidence that the two population variances are unequal, the latter results provide a more valid comparison of the two study groups.

3.3.2.2. Multiple comparisons in the presence of heterogeneity. It is often of interest to compare three or more groups in terms of the mean level of a biomarker. For example, Bernstein et al. (1999) compared the mean levels of AI across three groups: (a) "normal" subjects; that is; those with no previous history of polyps or cancer; (b) patients with a history of colorectal cancer; and (c) patients with colorectal adenomas. They used the Tukey method to perform all possible pairwise comparisons among the three groups. The Tukey method is the technique of choice if the population variances of the three groups are equal (Dunnett, 1980a); however, if they are not equal, the methods known as Dunnett's C and Dunnett's T3 are preferable (Dunnett, 1980b). These two methods are very similar to the unequal variance t-test recommended in the previous section. The Tukey, Dunnett's C, and Dunnett's T3 procedures are all available in SPSS (SPSS Inc., Chicago, IL).

Let μ_i and σ_i^2 denote the population mean and population variance, respectively, in the ith group. Let $\bar{x}_i$ denote the sample mean and let s_i^2 denote the unbiased estimate of σ_i^2 based on υ_i degrees of freedom in the ith group. We wish to find a set of $100(1-\alpha)\%$ joint CI estimates for the $k(k-1)/2$ differences $\mu_i - \mu_j$, $1 \leqslant i < j \leqslant k$. Both Dunnett's C and T3 methods involve constructing joint CI estimates of the form

$$\bar{y}_i - \bar{y}_j \pm c_{ij,\alpha,k}\sqrt{\frac{s_i^2}{n_i} + \frac{s_j^2}{n_j}},$$

where $c_{ij,\alpha,k}$ is a "critical value" chosen so that the joint confidence coefficient is as close as possible to $1 - \alpha$.

For Dunnett's C procedure,

$$c_{ij,\alpha,k} = \frac{\mathrm{SR}_{\alpha,k,\upsilon^*_{ij}}}{\sqrt{2}},$$

where

$$\mathrm{SR}_{\alpha,k,\upsilon^*_{ij}} = \frac{\left(\mathrm{SR}_{\alpha,k,\upsilon_i} s_i^2/n_i\right) + \left(\mathrm{SR}_{\alpha,k,\upsilon_j} s_j^2/n_j\right)}{\left(s_i^2/n_i\right) + \left(s_j^2/n_j\right)}$$

and $\mathrm{SR}_{\alpha,k,\upsilon}$ denotes the upper α-percentage point of the distribution of the Studentized range of k normal variates with an estimate of the variance based on υ degrees of freedom.

For Dunnett's T3 procedure,

$$c_{ij,\alpha,k} = \mathrm{SMM}_{\alpha,k^*,\hat{\upsilon}_{ij}},$$

where $\mathrm{SMM}_{\alpha,k^*,\hat{\upsilon}_{ij}}$ denotes the upper α-percentage point of the Studentized maximum modulus distribution of $k^* = k(k-1)/2$ uncorrelated normal variates with degrees of freedom $\hat{\upsilon}_{ij}$ given by

$$\hat{\upsilon}_{ij} = \frac{\left((s_i^2/n_i) + (s_j^2/n_j)\right)^2}{\left(s_i^4/n_i^2(\upsilon_i)\right) + \left(s_j^4/n_j^2(\upsilon_j)\right)}.$$

Tables of the percentage points of the SMM distribution are available in Stoline and Ury (1979). As recommended by Dunnett (1980b), percentage points of the SMM distribution for fractional degrees of freedom can be obtained by quadratic interpolation on reciprocal degrees of freedom for percentage points in the published tables.

3.4. Use of correlation coefficients in analyzing biomarker data

It is often of interest in studies involving biomarkers to examine the association between two continuous variables, at least one of which is the numerical value of a particular biomarker. For example, Salmi et al. (2002) correlated observed levels of sVAP-1 with risk factors for coronary heart disease, measures of liver dysfunction, diabetic parameter levels, etc. If both variables are normally distributed, then the appropriate measure of association to use is the Pearson correlation coefficient r. However, if the data for either variable are non-normally distributed, then a non-parametric measure of association such as Spearman's r_s should be used instead (Siegel and Castellan, 1988, pp. 224–225). In the study by Buss et al. (2003), the authors correctly used Spearman correlation in their evaluation of 3-chlorotyrosine in tracheal aspirates from preterm infants as a biomarker for protein damage by myeloperoxidase; they stated that they used Spearman's r_s "because the data were not normally distributed" (p. 5). The calculation of r_s was described in Section 3.2.3.2.

In the following sections, we consider three challenges frequently encountered when correlation coefficients are used in the analysis of biomarker data: (a) proper methods of analysis and interpretation of the results, (b) sample size determination, and (c) comparison of related correlation coefficients.

3.4.1. Proper methods of analysis and interpretation of results

Salmi et al. (2002) determined the "significance" of their correlation coefficients by testing the null hypothesis $H_0 : \rho = 0$, where ρ denotes the population correlation coefficient. However, there are several problems with this approach, the primary one being that correlations of no practical significance may be declared to be "significant" simply because the p-value is less than 0.05 (Looney, 1996). We have found the classification scheme presented by Morton et al. (1996) to be useful in interpreting the magnitude of correlation coefficients in terms of their practical significance. They classify correlations between 0.0 and 0.2 as "negligible," between 0.2 and 0.5 as "weak," between 0.5 and 0.8 as "moderate," and between 0.8 and 1.0 as "strong." In their sample of 411 Finnish men, Salmi et al. (2002) found a "significant" correlation of 0.108 between sVAP-1 and carbohydrate-deficient transferrin, a measure of liver dysfunction. While this correlation is statistically significant ($p = 0.029$), it would be considered "negligible" according to the Morton et al. criteria mentioned above, raising doubt about the practical significance of the result.

In addition to testing $H_0 : \rho = 0$, one should also construct a CI for the population correlation in order to get a sense of the precision of the correlation estimate, as well as a reasonable range of possible values for the population correlation. In the example taken from Salmi et al. (2002) mentioned above, the 95% CI for ρ is (0.01–0.20). Thus, the entire CI falls within the "negligible" range according to the Morton et al. criteria, casting further doubt on the practical significance of the observed correlation.

As discussed in Looney (1996), another problem with declaring a correlation to be significant simply because $p < 0.05$ is that smaller correlations may be declared to be "significant" even when n is fairly small, resulting in CIs that are too wide to be of any practical usefulness. In the study by Salmi et al. (2002) mentioned above, the value of r for the correlation between sVAP-1 and ketone bodies in a sample of 38 observations taken from diabetic children and adolescents was 0.34 ($p = 0.037$), a statistically significant result. However, a 95% CI for ρ is (0.02–0.60), which indicates that the population correlation could be anywhere between "negligible" and "moderate," according to the Morton et al. criteria. A CI of such large width provides very little useful information about the magnitude of the population correlation.

3.4.2. Sample size issues in the analysis of correlation coefficients

One way to avoid the difficulties described in the previous section is simply to perform a sample size calculation prior to beginning the study. There is no justification of the sample sizes used in the study by Salmi et al. (2002), so one must assume that no such calculation was done. Looney (1996) describes several approaches that typically yield sample sizes that provide more useful information about the value of the population correlation coefficient and the practical significance of the results than if one simply bases the sample size calculation on achieving adequate power for the test that the population correlation is zero. These include basing the sample size calculation on (a) the desired width of the CI for the population correlation, or (b) tests of null hypotheses other than that the population correlation is zero. (For example, one might test the null hypothesis $H_0 : \rho \leq 0.2$; rejecting this null hypothesis would indicate that the population correlation is "non-negligible.")

To perform a sample size calculation for the test of $H_0 : \rho = \rho_0$, where $\rho_0 \neq 0$, we recommend using Fisher's z-transformation applied to r as a test statistic; in other words,

$$z(r) = \frac{1}{2} \ln\left(\frac{1+r}{1-r}\right).$$

The following formula could then be used to determine the minimum sample size n required for achieving power of $100(1-\beta)\%$ for detecting an alternative correlation value of $\rho_1 > \rho_0$ using a one-tailed test of H_0 at significance level α:

$$n = 3 + \left[\frac{(z_\alpha + z_\beta)}{z(\rho_1) - z(\rho_0)}\right]^2,$$

where z_γ denotes the upper γ-percentage point of the standard normal and $z(\rho)$ the Fisher z-transform of ρ. If one wished to base the sample size calculation on the desired width of a CI for ρ, then one could use the approximate method described in Looney (1996), or the more precise method recommended by Bonett and Wright (2000).

3.4.3. Comparison of related correlation coefficients

In some studies involving biomarker data, it has been of interest to compare "related" correlation coefficients; that is, the correlation of variable X with Y vs. the correlation of variable X with Z. For example, Salmi et al. (2002) found "significant" correlations of sVAP-1 with both glucose ($r = 0.57$, $p < 0.001$) and ketone bodies ($r = 0.34$, $p = 0.037$) in their sample of 38 observations taken from diabetic children and adolescents. They concluded that there was a "less-marked" correlation of sVAP-1 with ketone bodies than with glucose. However, they did not perform any statistical test to determine if, in fact, the corresponding population correlation coefficients were different from each other. Had they performed such a test, as described in Steiger (1980), they would have found no significant difference between the two correlations ($p = 0.093$). (SAS code for performing comparisons of related correlation coefficients is available from the first author.)

The null hypothesis for the test of dependent correlations can be stated as

$$H_0 : \rho_{uv} = \rho_{uw}, \tag{20}$$

where ρ_{uv} denotes the population correlation between the random variables U and V and ρ_{uw} the population correlation between the random variables U and W.

In the example taken from Salmi et al. described above, $U=$ sVAP-1, $V=$ ketone bodies, and $W=$ glucose. Let r_{uv} and r_{uw} denote the sample correlations between U and V and between U and W, respectively, and let $\bar{r}_{uv,uw}$ denote the mean of r_{uv} and r_{uw}. Denote by z_{uv} and z_{uw}, the Fisher's z-transforms of r_{uv} and r_{uw}, respectively. Then the test statistic recommended by Steiger (1980) for the null hypothesis in Eq. (20) is given by

$$Z^* = \frac{(z_{uv} - z_{uw})\sqrt{n-3}}{\sqrt{2(1 - \bar{s}_{uv,uw})}}, \tag{21}$$

where $\bar{s}_{uv,uw}$ is an estimate of the covariance between z_{uv} and z_{uw} given by

$$\bar{s}_{uv,uw} = \frac{\hat{\psi}_{uv,uw}}{(1 - \bar{r}^2_{uv,uw})^2}$$

where

$$\hat{\psi}_{uv,uw} = r_{vw}(1 - 2\bar{r}^2_{uv,uw}) - \frac{1}{2}(\bar{r}^2_{uv,uw})(1 - 2\bar{r}^2_{uv,uw} - r^2_{vw}).$$

The test of H_0 in Eq. (20) is performed by comparing the sample value of Z^* in Eq. (21) with the standard normal distribution. For example, using the results given in Salmi et al. (2002), $r_{uv} = 0.57$, $r_{uw} = 0.34$, $r_{vw} = 0.55$, $n = 38$, and $\bar{s}_{jk,jh} = 0.4659$, yielding $Z^* = 1.68$ and $p = 0.093$, as mentioned previously.

3.5. Dealing with non-detectable values in the analysis of biomarker data

In analyzing biomarker data, there may be samples for which the concentration of the biomarker is below the analytic limit of detection (LOD), i.e., left-censored at the LOD. These observations are commonly referred to as non-detects, or *ND's*. For example, Amorim and Alvarez-Leite (1997) examined the correlation between *o*-cresol and hippuric acid concentrations in urine samples of individuals exposed to toluene in shoe factories, painting sectors of metal industries, and printing shops. Out of 54 samples in their study, *o*-cresol concentrations were below its LOD (0.2 μg/ml) in 39. In 4 of these samples, the hippuric acid concentration was also below its LOD (0.1 mg/ml). In another study, Atawodi et al. (1998) compared 18 smokers with 52 "never smokers" in terms of their levels of hemoglobin adducts, which were being evaluated as biomarkers of exposure to tobacco smoke. In 7 of the 52 never smokers, adduct levels were below the LOD (9 fmol HPB/g Hb).

Unfortunately, methods that are commonly used in the biomarker literature for handling ND's are flawed. Perhaps the most commonly used method is to ignore the missing value(s) and analyze only those samples with complete data. This was the method used by Lagorio et al. (1998) in their examination of the correlations among the concentrations of *trans,trans* muconic acid (t,t-MA) obtained from the urine of 10 Estonian shale oil workers using three different preanalytical methods. Another commonly used method is to impute a value in place of the missing data and then apply the "usual" statistical analyses.

The values commonly imputed include the LOD (Amorim and Alvarez-Leite, 1997; Atawodi et al., 1998) and LOD/2 (Cook et al., 1993).

Other methods that have been proposed for handling ND's include the "non-parametric approach," in which one treats all ND's as if they were tied at the LOD. Thus, if one wished to correlate two biomarkers, at least one of which was undetectable in some samples, one would calculate Spearman's r_s using the ranks of the entire data set, where all ND's were assigned the smallest midrank. If one wished to compare mean levels of a biomarker that was subject to ND's across two groups, one would apply the M–W–W test after computing the ranks of the two combined samples in this way. This is the method used by Atawodi et al. (1998) in their evaluation of hemoglobin adducts as biomarkers of exposure to tobacco smoke.

Recent simulation results (Wang, 2006) suggest that none of the methods described above for correlating two biomarkers that are both subject to left-censoring are satisfactory, especially if the two biomarkers are strongly correlated ($\rho \geqslant 0.5$). Instead, we recommend the maximum likelihood (ML) approach developed by Lyles et al. (2001) for estimating the correlation coefficient. A similar approach developed by Taylor et al. (2001) can be adapted to group comparisons of means and is also likely to be preferred to applying a non-parametric test to the data after replacing the ND's by the LOD. Other more advanced methods, such as multiple imputation (Scheuren, 2005), could be applied if the appropriate missing data mechanism is present. However, these methods are beyond the scope of this chapter. In this section, we briefly describe the estimation method proposed by Lyles et al. (2001).

Let X and Y denote the two biomarkers to be correlated, and denote the two fixed detection limits as L_x and L_y. Assuming a bivariate normal distribution, Lyles et al. proposed that one estimates the population parameter vector $\boldsymbol{\theta} = [\mu_x, \mu_y, \sigma_x^2, \sigma_y^2, \rho]'$ using ML estimation applied to a random sample (x_i, y_i); $i = 1, \ldots, n$. In their derivation of the likelihood function, they noted that there are four types of observed pairs of (x,y) values: (1) pairs with both x and y observed, (2) pairs with x observed and $y < L_y$, (3) pairs with y observed and $x < L_x$, and (4) pairs with $x < L_x$ and $y < L_y$. Following the notation in Lyles et al. (2001), the contribution of each pair of type 1 is given by

$$t_{i1} = (2\pi\sigma_x\sigma_{y|x})^{-1} \exp\left\{-0.5\left[\frac{(y_i - \mu_{y|x_i})^2}{\sigma_{y|x}^2} + \frac{(x_i - \mu_x)^2}{\sigma_x^2}\right]\right\},$$

where $\mu_{y|x_i} = \mu_y + \rho(\sigma_y/\sigma_x)(x_i - \mu_x)$ and $\sigma_{y|x}^2 = \sigma_y^2(1 - \rho^2)$.

The contribution of each pair of type 2 is given by

$$t_{i2} = (2\pi\sigma_x^2)^{-1/2} \exp\left[-0.5\frac{(x_i - \mu_x)^2}{\sigma_x^2}\right] \times \Phi\left(\frac{L_y - \mu_{y|x_i}}{\sigma_{y|x}}\right),$$

where $\Phi(\cdot)$ denotes the standard normal distribution function. Similarly, the contribution of each pair of type 3 is given by

$$t_{i3} = (2\pi\sigma_y^2)^{-1/2} \exp\left[-0.5\frac{(y_i - \mu_y)^2}{\sigma_y^2}\right] \times \Phi\left(\frac{L_x - \mu_{x|y_i}}{\sigma_{x|y}}\right),$$

where $\mu_{x|y_i} = \mu_x + \rho(\sigma_x/\sigma_y)(y_i - \mu_y)$ and $\sigma_{x|y}^2 = \sigma_x^2(1 - \rho^2)$.

Finally, each pair of type 4 contributes

$$t_4 = \int_{-\infty}^{L_y} \Phi\left\{\frac{L_x - [\mu_x + (\rho\sigma_x(y - \mu_y)/\sigma_y)]}{\sigma_x\sqrt{1-\rho^2}}\right\} \times (2\pi\sigma_y^2)^{-1/2} \exp\left[-0.5\frac{(y - \mu_y)^2}{\sigma_y^2}\right] \mathrm{d}y.$$

Without loss of generality, suppose the data are ordered and indexed by i so that pairs of type 1 come first, followed by pairs of types 2, 3, and 4. Further, assume that there are n_j terms of type j ($j = 1, 2, 3, 4$) and define $n_{k\bullet} = \sum_{j=1}^{k} n_j$ for $k = 2, 3$. Then, the total likelihood can be written as

$$\mathrm{L}(\boldsymbol{\theta}|\mathbf{x},\mathbf{y}) = \left(\prod_{i=1}^{n_1} t_{i1}\right)\left(\prod_{i=n_1+1}^{n_{2\bullet}} t_{i2}\right)\left(\prod_{i=n_{2\bullet}+1}^{n_{3\bullet}} t_{i3}\right) t_4^{n_4},$$

where $\mathbf{x}$ is the vector of observed x-values and $\mathbf{y}$ the vector of observed y-values.

Once the ML estimates and the corresponding estimated SEs are obtained, one can construct an approximate $100(1-\alpha)\%$ Wald-type CI for ρ by using $\hat{\rho}_{\mathrm{ML}} \pm z_{\alpha/2}\widehat{\mathrm{SE}}(\hat{\rho}_{\mathrm{ML}})$. Lyles et al. also considered profile likelihood CIs since Wald-type CIs are known to be potentially suspect when the sample size is small and they found that they generally performed better than the Wald-type intervals. For the data given in the study by Amorim and Alvarez-Leite (1997), the method developed by Lyles et al. yields $\hat{\rho}_{\mathrm{ML}} = 0.79$ and an approximate 95% CI(ρ) of (0.67, 0.91). Analyzing only the 15 cases with complete data yields $r = 0.76$ with an approximate 95% CI(ρ) of (0.40, 0.92).

4. Concluding remarks

In this chapter, we have not attempted to provide a comprehensive treatment of statistical methods that could be used in analyzing biomarker data; certainly, this entire volume could have been devoted to this task. Nor is this chapter intended to be a primer on how to perform elementary statistical analyses of biomarker data. Basic statistical methods, when properly applied, will usually suffice for this purpose. [For a good treatment of basic statistical methods and their proper application to environmental exposure data (for which biomarkers are frequently used), see Griffith et al. (1993).] Rather, we have focused our discussion on what we feel are some important analytic issues that we have encountered in our examination of biomarker data, and on some statistical techniques that we have found to be useful in dealing with those issues. It is hoped that the recommendations provided here will prove to be useful to statisticians, biomarker researchers, and other workers who are faced with the often challenging task of analyzing biomarker data.

Because of space limitations, we were unable to say very much in this chapter about power and sample size calculations. Fortunately, both StatXact and the POWER procedure within SAS are capable of carrying out power and sample size calculations for many of the procedures discussed in this chapter. Goldsmith (2001) provides a good general discussion of power and sample size considerations and provides an extensive list of references.

References

Agresti, A. (1996). *An Introduction to Categorical Data Analysis.* Wiley, New York.

Agresti, A. (2002). *Categorical Data Analysis*, 2nd ed. Wiley, Hoboken, NJ.

Agresti, A., Mehta, C.R., Patel, N.R. (1990). Exact inference for contingency tables with ordered categories. *Journal of the American Statistical Association* **85**, 453–458.

Algina, J., Oshima, T.C., Lin, W. (1994). Type I error rates for Welch's test and James's second-order test under nonnormality and inequality of variance when there are two groups. *Journal of Educational and Behavioral Statistics* **19**, 275–291.

Altman, D.G., Bland, J.M. (1983). Measurement in medicine: The analysis of method comparison studies. *The Statistician* **32**, 307–317.

Amorim, L.C.A., Alvarez-Leite, E.M. (1997). Determination of *o*-cresol by gas chromatography and comparison with hippuric acid levels in urine samples of individuals exposed to toluene. *Journal of Toxicology and Environmental Health* **50**, 401–407.

Armitage, P. (1955). Test for linear trend in proportions and frequencies. *Biometrics* **11**, 375–386.

Atawodi, S.E., Lea, S., Nyberg, F., Mukeria, A., Constantinescu, V., Ahrens, W., Brueske-Hohlfeld, I., Fortes, C., Boffetta, P., Friesen, M.D. (1998). 4-Hydroxyl-1-(3-pyridyl)-1-butanone-hemoglobin adducts as biomarkers of exposure to tobacco smoke: Validation of a method to be used in multicenter studies. *Cancer Epidemiology Biomarkers & Prevention* **7**, 817–821.

Atkinson, A.C. (1973). Testing transformations to normality. *Journal of the Royal Statistical Society Series B* **35**, 473–479.

Bartczak, A., Kline, S.A., Yu, R., Weisel, C.P., Goldstein, B.D., Witz, G. (1994). Evaluation of assays for the identification and quantitation of muconic acid, a benzene metabolite in human urine. *Journal of Toxicology and Environmental Health* **42**, 245–258.

Bartko, J.J. (1991). Measurement and reliability: Statistical thinking considerations. *Schizophrenia Bulletin* **17**, 483–489.

Bartko, J.J. (1994). General methodology II. Measures of agreement: A single procedure. *Statistics in Medicine* **13**, 737–745.

Benowitz, L. (1999). Biomarkers of environmental tobacco smoke exposure. *Environmental Health Perspectives* **107**(Suppl 2), 349–355.

Bernstein, C., Bernstein, H., Garewal, H., Dinning, P., Jabi, R., Sampliner, R.E., McCluskey, M.K., Panda, M., Roe, D.J., L'Heureux, L.L., Payne, C. (1999). A bile acid-induced apoptosis assay for colon cancer risk and associated quality control studies. *Cancer Research* **59**, 2353–2357.

Bland, J.M., Altman, D.G. (1986). Statistical methods for assessing agreement between two methods of clinical measurement. *The Lancet* (February 8, 1986), 307–310.

Bland, J.M., Altman, D.G. (1990). A note on the use of the intraclass correlation coefficient in the evaluation of agreement between two methods of measurement. *Computers in Biology and Medicine* **20**, 337–340.

Bonett, D.G., Wright, T.A. (2000). Sample size requirements for estimating Pearson, Kendall, and Spearman correlations. *Psychometrica* **65**, 23–28.

Box, G.E.P., Cox, D.R. (1964). An analysis of transformations. *Journal of the Royal Statistical Society Series B* **26**, 211–252.

Buckley, T.J., Waldman, J.M., Dhara, R., Greenberg, A., Ouyang, Z., Lioy, P.J. (1995). An assessment of a urinary biomarker for total human environmental exposure to benzo[*a*]pyrene. *International Archives of Occupational and Environmental Health* **67**, 257–266.

Buss, I.H., Senthilmohan, R., Darlow, B.A., Mogridge, N., Kettle, A.J., Winterbourn, C.C. (2003). 3-Chlorotyrosine as a marker of protein damage by myeloperoxidase in tracheal aspirates from preterm infants: Association with adverse respiratory outcome. *Pediatric Research* **53**, 455–462.

Byrt, T., Bishop, J., Carlin, J.B. (1993). Bias, prevalence, and kappa. *Journal of Clinical Epidemiology* **46**, 423–429.

Cheng, N.F., Gansky, S.A. A SAS macro to compute Lin's concordance correlation with confidence intervals. UCSF CAN-DO website. Accessed December 29, 2006. http://www.ucsf.edu/cando/resources/software/linscon.doc

Cicchetti, D.V., Feinstein, A.R. (1990). High agreement but low kappa: II. Resolving the paradoxes. *Journal of Clinical Epidemiology* **43**, 551–558.

Cochran, W.G. (1954). Some methods for strengthening the common χ^2 tests. *Biometrics* **10**, 417–454.

Cohen, J. (1960). A coefficient of agreement for nominal scales. *Educational and Psychological Measurement* **20**, 37–46.

Conover, W.J. (1999). *Practical Nonparametric Statistics*, 3rd ed. Wiley, New York.

Cook, D.G., Whincup, P.H., Papacosta, O., Strachan, D.P., Jarvis, M.J., Bryant, A. (1993). Relation of passive smoking as assessed by salivary cotinine concentration and questionnaire to spirometric indices in children. *Thorax* **48**, 14–20.

Cox, D.R., Hinkley, D.V. (1974). *Theoretical Statistics*. Chapman & Hall, London.

D'Agostino, R.B. (1986). Graphical analysis. In: D'Agostino, R.B., Stephens, M.A. (Eds.), *Goodness-of-Fit Techniques*. Marcel Dekker, New York, pp. 7–62.

Dunnett, C.W. (1980a). Pairwise multiple comparisons in the homogeneous variance, unequal sample size case. *Journal of the American Statistical Association* **75**, 789–795.

Dunnett, C.W. (1980b). Pairwise multiple comparisons in the unequal variance case. *Journal of the American Statistical Association* **75**, 796–800.

Feinstein, A.R., Cicchetti, D.V. (1990). High agreement but low kappa: I. The problems of two paradoxes. *Journal of Clinical Epidemiology* **43**, 543–549.

Fleiss, J.L. (1971). Measuring nominal scale agreement among many raters. *Psychological Bulletin* **76**, 378–382.

Gerson, M. (1975). The techniques and uses of probability plots. *The Statistician* **24**, 235–257.

Gibbons, J.D., Chakraborti, S. (2003). *Nonparametric Statistical Inference*, 4th ed. Marcel Dekker, New York.

Goldsmith, L.J. (2001). Power and sample size considerations in molecular biology. In: Looney, S.W. (Ed.), *Methods in Molecular Biology, Vol. 184: Biostatistical Methods*. Humana Press, Totowa, NJ, pp. 111–130.

Graham, P., Bull, B. (1998). Approximate standard errors and confidence intervals for indices of positive and negative agreement. *Journal of Clinical Epidemiology* **51**, 763–771.

Granella, M., Priante, E., Nardini, B., Bono, R., Clonfero, E. (1996). Excretion of mutagens, nicotine and its metabolites in urine of cigarette smokers. *Mutagenesis* **11**, 207–211.

Griffith, J., Aldrich, T.E., Duncan, R.C. (1993). Epidemiologic research methods. In: Aldrich, T., Griffithh, J., Cooke, C. (Eds.), *Environmental Epidemiology and Risk Assessment*. Van Nostrand Reinhold, New York, pp. 27–60.

Hagan, J.L., Looney, S.W. (2004). Frequency of use of statistical techniques for assessing agreement between continuous measurements. *Proceedings of the American Statistical Association*. American Statistical Association, Alexandria, VA, pp. 344–350.

Hazelton, M.L. (2003). A graphical tool for assessing normality. *The American Statistician* **57**, 285–288.

Huber, P.J. (1996). *Robust Statistical Procedures*, 2nd ed. Society for Industrial and Applied Mathematics, Philadelphia.

Johnson, N.L. (1949). Systems of frequency curves generated by methods of translation. *Biometrika* **36**, 149–176.

Jones, M.C., Daly, F. (1995). Density probability plots. *Communications in Statistics – Simulation and Computation* **24**, 911–927.

Kraemer, H.C. (1980). Extension of the kappa coefficient. *Biometrics* **36**, 207–216.

Kummel, C.H. (1879). Reduction of observation equations which contain more than one observed quantity. *The Analyst* **6**, 97–105.

Lagorio, S., Crebelli, R., Ricciarello, R., Conti, L., Iavarone, I., Zona, A., Ghittori, S., Carere, A. (1998). Methodological issues in biomonitoring of low level exposure to benzene. *Occupational Medicine* **8**, 497–504.

Landis, J.R., Koch, G.G. (1977). The measurement of observer agreement for categorical data. *Biometrics* **33**, 159–174.

Last, J.M. (1995). *A Dictionary of Epidemiology*, 3rd ed. Oxford University Press, New York.

Lehmann, E.L. (1975). *Nonparametrics: Statistical Methods Based on Ranks*. Holden-Day, San Francisco, pp. 267–270.

Lin, L.I. (1989). A concordance correlation coefficient to evaluate reproducibility. *Biometrics* **45**, 255–268.

Lin, L.I. (2000). A note on the concordance correlation coefficient. *Biometrics* **56**, 324–325.

Linnet, K. (1990). Estimation of the linear relationship between the measurements of two methods with proportional errors. *Statistics in Medicine* **9**, 1463–1473.

Linnet, K. (1993). Evaluation of regression procedures for methods comparison studies. *Clinical Chemistry* **39**, 424–432.

Looney, S.W. (1996). Sample size determination for correlation coefficient inference: Practical problems and practical solutions. *Proceedings of the Statistical Computing Section, American Statistical Association*. American Statistical Association, Alexandria, VA, pp. 240–245.

Looney, S.W. (Ed.) (2001). Statistical methods for assessing biomarkers. *Methods in Molecular Biology, Vol. 184: Biostatistical Methods*. Humana Press, Totowa, NJ, pp. 81–109.

Looney, S.W., Gulledge, T.R. (1985). Use of the correlation coefficient with normal probability plots. *The American Statistician* **39**, 75–79.

Lyles, R.H., Williams, J.K., Chuachoowong, R. (2001). Correlating two viral load assays with known detection limits. *Biometrics* **57**, 1238–1244.

MacRae, A.R., Gardner, H.A., Allen, L.C., Tokmakejian, S., Lepage, N. (2003). Outcome validation of the Beckman Coulter access analyzer in a second-trimester Down syndrome serum screening application. *Clinical Chemistry* **49**, 69–76.

Mehrotra, D.V., Chan, I.S.F., Berger, R.L. (2003). A cautionary note on exact unconditional inference for a difference between two independent binomial proportions. *Biometrics* **59**, 441–450.

Mehta, C., Patel, N. (2005). *StatXact 7*. CYTEL Software Corporation, Cambridge, MA.

Morton, R.F., Hebel, J.R., McCarter, R.J. (1996). *A Study Guide to Epidemiology and Biostatistics*, 4th ed. Aspen Publishers, Gaithersburg, MD, pp. 92–97.

Moser, B.K., Stevens, G.R. (1992). Homogeneity of variance in the two-sample means test. *The American Statistician* **46**, 19–21.

Moser, B.K., Stevens, G.R., Watts, C.L. (1989). The two-sample *t* test versus Satterthwaite's approximate *F* test. *Communications in Statistics Part A-Theory and Methods* **18**, 3963–3975.

Neuhäuser, M., Hothorn, L.A. (1999). An exact Cochran–Armitage test for trend when dose–response shapes are a priori unknown. *Computational Statistics and Data Analysis* **30**, 403–412.

Pérez-Stable, E.J., Benowitz, N.L., Marín, G. (1995). Is serum cotinine a better measure of cigarette smoking than self-report. *Preventive Medicine* **24**, 171–179.

Qiao, Y-L., Tockman, M.S., Li, L., Erozan, Y.S., Yao, S., Barrett, M.J., Zhou, W., Giffen, C.A., Luo, X., Taylor, P.R. (1997). A case-cohort study of an early biomarker of lung cancer in a screening cohort of Yunnan tin miners in China. *Cancer Epidemiology, Biomarkers & Prevention* **6**, 893–900.

Royston, J.P. (1982). An extension of Shapiro and Wilk's W test for normality to large samples. *Applied Statistics – Journal of the Royal Statistical Society Series C* **31**, 115–124.
Royston, J.P. (1989). Correcting the Shapiro–Wilk *W* for ties. *Journal of Statistical Computation and Simulation* **31**, 237–249.
Royston, J.P. (1992). Approximating the Shapiro–Wilk's W test for non-normality. *Statistics and Computing* **2**, 117–119.
Salmi, M., Stolen, C., Jousilahti, P., Yegutkin, G.G., Tapanainen, P., Janatuinen, T., Knip, M., Jalkanen, S., Salomaa, V. (2002). Insulin-regulated increase of soluble vascular adhesion protein-1 in diabetes. *The American Journal of Pathology* **161**, 2255–2262.
Scheuren, F. (2005). Multiple imputation: How it began and continues. *The American Statistician* **59**, 315–319.
Shapiro, S.S., Wilk, M.B. (1965). An analysis of variance test for normality (complete samples). *Biometrika* **52**, 591–611.
Shapiro, S.S., Wilk, M.B., Chen, H.J. (1968). A comparative study of various tests for normality. *Journal of the American Statistical Association* **63**, 1343–1372.
Sheskin, D.J. (1997). *Handbook of Parametric and Nonparametric Statistical Procedures*. CRC Press, Boca Raton, FL.
Shoukri, M.M. (2004). *Measures of Interobserver Agreement*. Chapman & Hall/CRC, Boca Raton, FL.
Siegel, S., Castellan, N.J. (1988). *Nonparametric Statistics for the Behavioral Sciences*, 2nd ed. McGraw-Hill, New York.
Steiger, J.H. (1980). Tests for comparing elements of a correlation matrix. *Psychological Bulletin* **87**, 245–251.
Stoline, M.R., Ury, H.K. (1979). Tables of the studentized maximum modulus distribution and an application to multiple comparisons among means. *Technometrics* **21**, 87–93.
Strachan, D.P., Jarvis, M.J., Feyerabend, C. (1990). The relationship of salivary cotinine to respiratory symptoms, spirometry, and exercise-induced bronchospasm in seven-year-old children. *The American Review of Respiratory Disease* **142**, 147–151.
Strike, P.W. (1996). *Measurement in Laboratory Medicine: A Primer on Control and Interpretation*. Butterworth-Heinemann, Oxford, pp. 147–172.
Stuart, A., Ord, J.K. (1987). *Kendall's Advanced Theory of Statistics*. Oxford University Press, New York, pp. 210–220.
Suissa, S., Shuster, J. (1991). The 2×2 matched-pairs trial: Exact unconditional design and analysis. *Biometrics* **47**, 361–372.
Taylor, D.J., Kupper, L.L., Rappaport, S.M., Lyles, R.H. (2001). A mixture model for occupational exposure mean testing with a limit of detection. *Biometrics* **57**, 681–688.
Tockman, M.S., Gupta, P.K., Myers, J.D., Frost, J.K., Baylin, S.B., Gold, E.B., Chase, A.M., Wilkinson, P.H., Mulshine, J.L. (1988). Sensitive and specific monoclonal antibody recognition of human lung cancer antigen on preserved sputum cells: A new approach to early lung cancer detection. *Journal of Clinical Oncology* **6**, 1685–1693.
Tukey, J.W. (1977). *Exploratory Data Analysis*. Addison-Wesley, Reading, MA.
Tunstall-Pedoe, H., Brown, C.A., Woodward, M., Tavendale, R. (1995). Passive smoking by self-report and serum cotinine and the prevalence of respiratory and coronary heart disease in the Scottish heart health study. *Journal of Epidemiology and Community Health* **49**, 139–143.
Wang, H. (2006). Correlation analysis for left-censored biomarker data with known detection limits. Unpublished Masters thesis, Louisiana State University Health Sciences Center, Biostatistics Program, School of Public Health.
Westgard, J.O., Hunt, M.R. (1973). Use and interpretation of common statistical tests in method-comparison studies. *Clinical Chemistry* **19**, 49–57.
Wilcox, R.R. (1987). *New Statistical Procedures for the Social Sciences*. Lawrence Erlbaum Associates, Hillsdale, NJ.
Wilk, M.B., Shapiro, S.S. (1968). The joint assessment of normality of several independent samples. *Technometrics* **10**, 825–839.

Handbook of Statistics, Vol. 27
ISSN: 0169-7161

DOI: 10.1016/S0169-7161(07)27005-1

5

Linear and Non-Linear Regression Methods in Epidemiology and Biostatistics

Eric Vittinghoff, Charles E. McCulloch, David V. Glidden and Stephen C. Shiboski

Abstract

This chapter describes a family of statistical techniques called linear and non-linear regression that are commonly used in medical research. Regression is typically used to relate an outcome (or dependent variable or response) to one or more predictor variables (or independent variables or covariates). We examine several ways in which the standard linear model can be extended to accommodate non-linearity. These include non-linear transformation of predictors and outcomes within the standard linear model framework; generalized linear models, in which the mean of the outcome is modeled as a non-linear transformation of the standard linear function of regression parameters and predictors; and fully non-linear models, in which the mean of the outcome is modeled as a non-linear function of the regression parameters. We also briefly discuss several special topics, including causal models, models with measurement error in the predictors, and missing data problems.

1. Introduction

This chapter describes a family of statistical techniques called linear and non-linear regression that are commonly used in medical research. Regression is typically used to relate an outcome (or dependent variable or response) to one or more predictor variables (or independent variables or covariates). The goal might be prediction, testing for a relationship with a single predictor (perhaps while adjusting for other predictors), or in modeling the relationship between the outcome and all the predictors. We begin with an example.

1.1. Example: Medical services utilization

The most acutely ill patients treated by a hospital system use a highly disproportionate amount of resources – often in ways that can be prevented.

For example, persons without insurance may use the emergency room for non-emergency care. Sorenson et al. (2003) and Masson et al. (2004) described the utilization of medical resources in 190 patients enrolled in a randomized trial of a managed care intervention designed to improve access to healthcare. Measurements were taken at baseline, as well as at 6, 12, and 18 months after randomization. Outcomes included cost of care, number of emergency room visits, and death. Predictors included treatment group (managed care or not), gender, the Beck depression inventory (BDI), and whether the person was homeless. A primary focus was on the treatment effect, while adjusting for the effects of the other predictors. A secondary goal was to assess the impact of all the predictors on the outcomes.

1.2. Linear and non-linear regression methods

The choice of an appropriate regression model depends on both the type of outcome being modeled, which governs the random portion of the model, and how the parameters to be estimated enter the model, which governs whether it is a linear or non-linear model. In our example, cost is likely to be highly skewed right, while the logarithm of cost might be more approximately normally distributed. Death during the 18 months of follow-up is binary or could be analyzed as time to death. And number of emergency room visits is a count variable, for which we might consider a Poisson distribution appropriate. A further complication in our example is that we have repeated measurements over time on the same patient (e.g., number of emergency room visits during the preceding 6 months is collected at 6, 12, and 18 months), so that the data need to be treated as correlated.

Each of these different outcome types – continuous and skewed right, continuous and approximately normally distributed, binary, time-to-event, or count – would typically need a different style of regression analysis. Treating log(cost) at 6 months as approximately normally distributed might suggest using the usual linear regression model

$$\log \text{cost}_i = \beta_0 + \beta_1 x_{1i} + \beta_2 x_{2i} + \beta_3 x_{3i} + \beta_4 x_{4i} + \varepsilon_i, \tag{1}$$

where cost_i is the 6-month cost of medical care for patient i, x_{1i} is 1 if the patient was in the case management group and 0 otherwise, x_{2i} is 1 if the patient is female and 0 otherwise, x_{3i} is the patient's BDI at baseline, x_{4i} is 1 if the patient was homeless at baseline and 0 otherwise, and ε_i is an error term. The parameters to be estimated (the βs) enter Eq. (1) as a linear combination, hence the name *linear regression.*

Re-expressing Eq. (1) as a model for cost_i by exponentiating both sides of the equation gives

$$\begin{aligned}\text{cost}_i &= e^{\beta_0} e^{\beta_1 x_{1i}} e^{\beta_2 x_{2i}} e^{\beta_3 x_{3i}} e^{\beta_4 x_{4i}} e^{\varepsilon_i} \\ &= \gamma_0 \gamma_1^{x1i} \gamma_2^{x2i} \gamma_3^{x3i} \gamma_4^{x4i} \delta_i, \end{aligned} \tag{2}$$

where $\gamma_k = e^{\beta_k}$ and $\delta_i = e^{\varepsilon_i}$.

This is somewhat different, as we elaborate in Section 3.1, from the *non-linear regression* equation, below, which assumes (incorrectly) that cost_i is homoscedastic and normally distributed:

$$\text{cost}_i = \alpha_0 \alpha_1^{x_{1i}} \alpha_2^{x_{2i}} \alpha_3^{x_{3i}} \alpha_4^{x_{4i}} + \upsilon_i \quad \text{with} \quad \upsilon_i \sim \text{i.i.d.} \mathcal{N}(0, \sigma_\upsilon^2). \tag{3}$$

On the other hand, treating death during the 18-month follow-up period as a binary outcome would usually be handled with a *logistic regression* model, in which the probability of death is modeled in the form

$$P(D_i) = \frac{1}{1 + \exp(-[\beta_0 + \beta_1 x_{1i} + \beta_2 x_{2i} + \beta_3 x_{3i} + \beta_4 x_{4i}])}, \tag{4}$$

where D_i is 1 if the ith patient died and 0 otherwise, and these are not the same βs as in Eq. (1). Clearly the parameters to be estimated for this model (the βs) enter in a non-linear fashion. There is no error term in this model, because the randomness is captured by the Bernoulli distribution with the appropriate probability of death given by Eq. (4).

This is an example of a *generalized linear model* (GLM) because we can transform the mean response (which is just the probability for a binary variable like D_i) to get a model that *is* linear in the parameters:

$$\log \frac{P(D_i)}{1 - P(D_i)} = \beta_0 + \beta_1 x_{1i} + \beta_2 x_{2i} + \beta_3 x_{3i} + \beta_4 x_{4i}. \tag{5}$$

The left-hand side of Eq. (5) is the log of the ratio of the probability of death compared to the probability of survival, or the log of the *odds* of death. Therefore the logistic regression model is a linear model for the log odds and the parameters have interpretations in terms of the difference in log odds of the outcome associated with a one-unit change in the predictor (holding the other variables "constant").

The various regression models are clearly different but still share important features. The accommodation of multiple predictors and continuous or categorical predictors is similar. Techniques for adjustment by variables to control confounding and incorporate interactions, and methods for predictor selection are similar. Finally, all regression analyses are used to answer the same broad classes of practical questions involving multiple predictors.

1.3. Overview

This chapter provides a practical survey of linear and non-linear regression analysis in biomedical studies and to provide pointers to the other, more detailed chapters on special types of regression models elsewhere in this book. We start by introducing the idea of linear regression, in which the model for the mean of the outcome is a linear combination of the parameters, an example of which is Eq. (1), when the outcome is log(cost). In this context we describe inference, model checking, extensions to repeated measures data, and choice of predictors. Next, we show how building a linear model for transformations of the outcome, such as the model for log(cost), induces a non-linear model for the untransformed outcome, e.g., cost itself. Non-linear models are then developed, with identification of the important special case of generalized linear models, i.e., a model in which a transformation of the mean is a linear combination of the parameters. We also cover some models capable of handling censored data, as well as models where no transformation of the mean is linear in the parameters. Finally, we discuss recent developments such as the use of classification and regression trees (CART), generalized additive models (GAMs), and segmented and asymptotic regression, as well as computing for regression analyses.

2. Linear models

In the multiple linear regression model, the expected value of the outcome for observation i, given a set of predictors $\mathbf{x}_i' = (x_{1i}, x_{2i}, \ldots, x_{pi})$, is specified by a linear combination of the parameters $\beta_0, \beta_1, \ldots, \beta_p$:

$$E[Y_i|\mathbf{x_i}] = \beta_0 + \beta_1 x_{1i} + \beta_2 x_{2i} + \cdots + \beta_p x_{pi}. \tag{6}$$

In Eq. (6), the coefficient β_j gives the change in $E[Y_i|\mathbf{x}_i]$ for an increase of one unit in predictor x_{ji}, holding other factors in the model constant. The intercept β_0 gives the value of $E[Y|\mathbf{x}]$ if all the predictors were equal to zero. Considering all observations in the sample ($i = 1, \ldots, N$), we can write

$$E[\mathbf{Y}|\mathbf{X}] = \mathbf{X}\boldsymbol{\beta}, \tag{7}$$

where the outcomes are written as vector $\mathbf{Y}$ of order N; $\mathbf{X}$ is the *model matrix* of order N by $p+1$ with ith row $\mathbf{x}_i'$; and $\boldsymbol{\beta}$ is the vector of $p+1$ regression coefficients.

Random departures of the outcomes from their expectations may result from measurement error as well as unmeasured determinants of the outcome. Thus

$$\mathbf{Y} = \mathbf{X}\boldsymbol{\beta} + \boldsymbol{\varepsilon}, \tag{8}$$

where the vector of random errors $\boldsymbol{\varepsilon}$ has mean $\mathbf{0}$ and variance–covariance matrix $\mathbf{V}$. Note that given $\mathbf{X}$, $\mathbf{Y}$ also has variance–covariance matrix $\mathbf{V}$. In the basic form of the multiple linear regression model we usually assume that $\boldsymbol{\varepsilon} \sim \mathcal{N}(\mathbf{0}, \sigma^2\mathbf{I})$, where $\mathbf{I}$ is the identity matrix of order N; that is, the random errors are normally distributed with mean zero and constant variance σ^2, and are independent across observations.

In contrast to the outcome, no distributional assumptions are made about the predictors. However, we do formally assume that the predictors are measured without error. This is often not very realistic, and the effects of violations are the subject of ongoing statistical research. In Section 4.2, we briefly discuss the issue of measurement error.

2.1. Maximum likelihood (ML) under normality

Under the assumption that **Y** has a multivariate normal distribution – that is,

$$\mathbf{Y} \sim \mathcal{N}(\mathbf{X}\boldsymbol{\beta}, \sigma^2\mathbf{I}) \tag{9}$$

the likelihood function is

$$L = L(\boldsymbol{\beta}, \sigma^2) = \frac{\exp\left[-\frac{1}{2}(\mathbf{Y} - \mathbf{X}\boldsymbol{\beta})'(\mathbf{I}/\sigma^2)(\mathbf{Y} - \mathbf{X}\boldsymbol{\beta})\right]}{(2\pi\sigma^2)^{N/2}}. \tag{10}$$

Thus the log-likelihood is

$$l = \log\ L = -\frac{N}{2}\log(2\pi) - \frac{N}{2}\log\sigma^2 - \frac{1}{2}(\mathbf{Y} - \mathbf{X}\boldsymbol{\beta})'(\mathbf{Y} - X\boldsymbol{\beta})/\sigma^2 \tag{11}$$

Setting the vector of partial derivatives of the log-likelihood with respect to the elements of $\boldsymbol{\beta}$ equal to $\mathbf{0}$ gives the *score* equation for $\boldsymbol{\beta}$:

$$\frac{\partial l}{\partial \boldsymbol{\beta}} = \frac{\mathbf{X}'\mathbf{Y} - \mathbf{X}'\mathbf{X}\boldsymbol{\beta}}{\sigma^2} = \mathbf{0} \tag{12}$$

with solution

$$\hat{\boldsymbol{\beta}} = (\mathbf{X}'\mathbf{X})^{-1}\mathbf{X}'\mathbf{Y} \tag{13}$$

if $(\mathbf{X}'\mathbf{X})^{-1}$ exists. See McCulloch and Searle (2000) for a full development of important cases where **X** is not full rank and generalized inverses of $\mathbf{X}'\mathbf{X}$ must be used.

For σ^2 the score equation is

$$\frac{\partial l}{\partial \sigma^2} = \frac{(\mathbf{Y} - \mathbf{X}\boldsymbol{\beta})'(\mathbf{Y} - \mathbf{X}\boldsymbol{\beta})}{2\sigma^4} - \frac{N}{2\sigma^2} = 0 \tag{14}$$

with solution

$$\hat{\sigma}^2_{ml} = (\mathbf{Y} - \mathbf{X}\hat{\boldsymbol{\beta}})'(\mathbf{Y} - \mathbf{X}\hat{\boldsymbol{\beta}})/N \tag{15}$$

In practice the unbiased *restricted maximum likelihood* (REML) estimate (McCulloch and Searle, 2000) is more often used. In REML, $\boldsymbol{\beta}$ is removed from the likelihood by considering the likelihood of

$$\left[\mathbf{I} - \mathbf{X}(\mathbf{X}'\mathbf{X})^{-1}\mathbf{X}'\right]\mathbf{Y}, \tag{16}$$

in this simple case giving

$$\hat{\sigma}^2 = \frac{(\mathbf{Y} - \mathbf{X}\hat{\boldsymbol{\beta}})'(\mathbf{Y} - \mathbf{X}\hat{\boldsymbol{\beta}})}{N - (p+1)} \tag{17}$$

Finally, under regularity conditions, $\hat{\boldsymbol{\beta}}$ is a consistent estimator of $\boldsymbol{\beta}$, with asymptotic variance–covariance estimator $\hat{\sigma}^2(\mathbf{X}'\mathbf{X})^{-1}$ based on the Hessian of the log-likelihood – that is, the matrix of its second partial derivatives with respect to $\boldsymbol{\beta}$.

2.2. Ordinary least squares

Estimation of the regression parameters in the multiple linear regression model can also be understood in terms of *ordinary least squares* (OLS), meaning that $\hat{\boldsymbol{\beta}}$ is the value of $\boldsymbol{\beta}$ that minimizes the *residual sum of squares* under the proposed linear model:

$$\text{RSS} = (\mathbf{Y} - \mathbf{X}\boldsymbol{\beta})'(\mathbf{Y} - \mathbf{X}\boldsymbol{\beta}). \tag{18}$$

Setting the vector of partial derivatives of Eq. (18) with respect to $\boldsymbol{\beta}$ equal to $\mathbf{0}$ gives

$$\hat{\boldsymbol{\beta}} = (\mathbf{X}'\mathbf{X})^{-1}\mathbf{X}'\mathbf{Y}. \tag{19}$$

Thus the OLS criterion motivates the same estimator of $\boldsymbol{\beta}$, without making distributional assumptions, as does maximum likelihood in the case where $\mathbf{Y}$ is multivariate normal.

The variance of $\hat{\boldsymbol{\beta}}$ can be written as

$$\begin{aligned}\Sigma &= \text{var}[(\mathbf{X}'\mathbf{X})^{-1}\mathbf{X}'\mathbf{Y}] \\ &= (\mathbf{X}'\mathbf{X})^{-1}\mathbf{X}'\,\text{var}[\mathbf{Y}]\mathbf{X}(\mathbf{X}'\mathbf{X})^{-1} \\ &= (\mathbf{X}'\mathbf{X})^{-1}\mathbf{X}'\mathbf{V}\mathbf{X}(\mathbf{X}'\mathbf{X})^{-1}\end{aligned} \tag{20}$$

Clearly Σ simplifies to $\sigma^2(\mathbf{X}'\mathbf{X})^{-1}$ when $\mathbf{V} = \sigma^2\mathbf{I}$.

If $E[\mathbf{Y}|\mathbf{X}]$ is of the form $\mathbf{X}\boldsymbol{\beta}$ and $\mathbf{X}$ is full rank, $\hat{\boldsymbol{\beta}}$ is unbiased:

$$\begin{aligned}E[\hat{\boldsymbol{\beta}}] &= E[(\mathbf{X}'\mathbf{X})^{-1}\mathbf{X}'\mathbf{Y}] \\ &= (\mathbf{X}'\mathbf{X})^{-1}\mathbf{X}'E[\mathbf{Y}] \\ &= (\mathbf{X}'\mathbf{X})^{-1}\mathbf{X}'\mathbf{X}\boldsymbol{\beta} \\ &= \boldsymbol{\beta}\end{aligned} \tag{21}$$

Under the assumptions of independence and constant variance – that is, $\mathbf{V} = \sigma^2\mathbf{I}$ – the OLS estimates are minimally variable among linear unbiased estimators. They are also well-behaved in large samples when the normality assumptions concerning $\mathbf{Y}$ are not precisely met. A potentially important drawback of OLS is sensitivity to influential data points.

2.3. Tests and confidence intervals

At least in large samples, the estimates of the regression parameters have a multivariate normal distribution. This follows on theoretical grounds if the outcome $\mathbf{Y}$ is multivariate normal as in Eq. (9), regardless of sample size. Otherwise, the OLS estimators converge in distribution to multivariate normality as the sample size increases under fairly mild assumptions. If the outcome is short-tailed, then the tests and confidence intervals may be valid with as few as 30–50 observations. However, with long-tailed or skewed outcomes, samples of at least 100 may be required. Factors influencing the precision of the estimates are made clear by writing the variance of a particular $\hat{\beta}_j$ as:

$$\text{Var}(\hat{\beta}_j) = \frac{\sigma^2}{(N-1)s_{x_j}^2(1-r_j^2)}. \tag{22}$$

In Eq. (22), $s_{x_j}^2$ is the sample variance of x_j, and r_j is the multiple correlation of x_j with the other predictors; $1/(1-r_j^2)$ is known as the *variance inflation factor*. In brief, the parameter β_j is more precisely estimated when the residual variance σ^2 is small, the sample size N and sample variance of x_j are large, and x_j is minimally correlated with the other predictors in the model.

When **Y** is multivariate normal, the ratio of $\hat{\beta}_j - \beta_j$ to its standard error (defined as the square root of the estimate of Eq. (22), using Eq. (17) for σ^2) has a t-distribution with $N-(p+1)$ degrees of freedom. This reference distribution is used for Wald tests of H_0: $\beta_j = 0$, and to compute confidence intervals for β_j as

$$\hat{\beta}_j \pm t_{\alpha/2,N-(p+1)}\sqrt{\hat{\text{Var}}(\hat{\beta}_j)}, \tag{23}$$

where $t_{\alpha/2,N-(p+1)}$ is the $\alpha/2$ quantile of the reference t-distribution. By extension, the variance of a linear combination $c = \mathbf{a}'\hat{\boldsymbol{\beta}}$ of the parameter estimates is $\mathbf{a}'\Sigma\mathbf{a}$, providing analogous hypothesis tests and confidence intervals for c.

The F-test is used to test composite null hypotheses involving more than one parameter, including tests for heterogeneity in the mean of the outcome across levels of multilevel categorical predictors. Suppose the categorical predictor has $k > 2$ levels and is represented by $k-1$ indicator variables $x_{2i}, x_{3i}, \ldots, x_{ki}$, with $x_{ji} = 1$ if observation i is in category j ($j = 2, \ldots, k$) and 0 otherwise. The corresponding parameters are $\beta_2, \beta_3, \ldots, \beta_k$; x_{1i} and β_1 correspond to the reference level and are omitted. Then the F-statistic for the test of $H_0: \beta_2 = \beta_3 = \cdots = \beta_k = 0$ is

$$F = \frac{(\text{RSS}_r - \text{RSS}_f)/(k-1)}{\text{RSS}_f/(N-(p+1))} \tag{24}$$

where RSS_f is the residual sum of squares from the full model including the $k-1$ indicator variables $x_2, x_3, \ldots, x_k$ and RSS_r is from the reduced model excluding these covariates. The statistic is compared to the F-distribution with $k-1$ and $N-(p+1)$ degrees of freedom. Within the maximum likelihood framework, the F-statistic can be derived as a monotonic transformation of the likelihood-ratio statistic (McCulloch and Searle, 2000).

These exact methods for inference when **Y** is multivariate normal do not apply to non-linear models, nor to linear models used with unbalanced repeated measures data. For those cases, hypothesis testing with either maximum likelihood or restricted maximum likelihood utilizes the large sample theory of maximum likelihood estimators. Typical are Wald tests, in which the estimators divided by their standard errors are treated as approximately normal to form z-statistics. Likewise, approximate confidence intervals are based on normality by calculating the estimate ± 1.96 standard errors. Standard errors typically come from the Hessian of the log-likelihood. Kenward and Roger (1997) have suggested adjustments to improve the small sample performance of the Wald statistics in extensions of the linear model for repeated measures (see Section 2.5). Alternatively, likelihood-ratio tests and confidence regions based on the likelihood are also commonly used to form test statistics and confidence regions for $\boldsymbol{\beta}$. These are regarded as more reliable than the Wald procedures and should be used in circumstances where the two procedures give discrepant results (Cox and Hinkley, 1974).

2.4. Checking model assumptions and fit

In the multiple linear regression model (Eq. (8)), we start with assumptions that $E[\mathbf{Y}|\mathbf{X}]$ changes linearly with each continuous predictor and that the errors $\boldsymbol{\varepsilon}$ are independently multivariate normal with mean zero and constant variance. Violations of these assumptions have the potential to bias regression coefficient estimates and undermine the validity of confidence intervals and p-values, and thus may motivate the use of non-linear models. Residuals are central to detecting violations of these assumptions and also assessing their severity. Model assumptions rarely hold exactly, and small departures can be benign, especially in large datasets. Nonetheless, careful attention to model assumptions can prevent us from being seriously misled, and help us to decide when non-linear methods need to be used.

Linearity. In single predictor models, checks for departures from linearity could be carried out using a non-parametric smoother, such as LOWESS (Cleveland, 1981) of the outcome on the single predictor, approximating the regression line under the weaker assumption that it is smooth but not necessarily linear. Substantial and systematic deviations of the non-parametric estimate from the linear fit indicate departures from linearity. Smoothing the residuals rather than the outcome may give a more sensitive assessment, and extends this strategy to the multiple linear regression model, providing a check on linearity after the effects of covariates have been taken into account. In this context, we smooth the residuals against each continuous predictor (*residual* vs *predictor* plots) as well as the fitted values (*residual* vs *fitted* plots). Related diagnostic plots include *component plus residual* plots (Larsen and McCleary, 1972), in which the contribution of the predictor of interest to each fitted value is added back into the corresponding residual, which is then smoothed against the predictor. In all cases, a well-behaved smoother with skillfully chosen smoothness is important for detecting non-linearity.

Departures from linearity can often be corrected using transformations of the continuous predictors causing problems. For strictly positive predictors, log transformation is useful for modeling "diminishing returns," in which the mean of the outcome changes more and more slowly as the predictor increases. In polynomial models, we may add quadratic, cubic, and even higher-order terms in the predictor. For mild non-linearities, addition of a quadratic term in the predictor is often adequate. However, for highly non-linear response patterns, polynomial models may not provide adequate flexibility, or provide it only at the cost of poor performance in the extremes of the predictor range.

In contrast to polynomial models, *splines* provide more flexibility where the predictor values are concentrated and better performance at the extremes, by fitting local polynomial models under constraints that preserve continuity and smoothness, often making the results more plausible. Simplest are *linear splines*, which model the mean response to the predictor as continuous and piecewise linear, changing slope at *knots*, or cutpoints in the range of the predictor, but linear within the intervals between knots. In the simplest cases, the knots are placed by the analyst at sample quantiles or at inflections in diagnostic smooths; however, automatic, adaptive methods are also available. *Cubic splines* are local third-order polynomials, constrained to have continuous first and second derivatives at the knots; only the third derivative is allowed to jump. *Natural cubic splines* are constrained to be linear beyond the outermost knots, for better behavior in the tails. These spline models are implemented using a linear combination of *basis* functions defined for each value of the continuous predictor, and thus remain linear in the parameters. *Smoothing splines* can be understood as cubic splines with a knot at each unique value of the predictor, but incorporating a penalty in the log-likelihood to prevent overfitting (Hastie et al., 2001). This results in shrinkage of the parameter estimates corresponding to the basis functions of the spline toward zero. The penalty parameter determining the degree of smoothness is commonly chosen by cross-validation, discussed below.

Normality. Residuals are also central to the evaluation of normality and constant variance. *Quantile–quantile* plots provide the most direct assessment of normality of the residuals; also potentially useful are histograms and nonparametric density plots. Long tails and skewness are more problematic for linear models than short-tailed distributions, with reduced efficiency the most likely result. However, both types of violation become less important with increasing sample size. In addition to diagnostic plots, which can be difficult to interpret, particularly in small samples, numerous statistical tests for non-normality are available. A disadvantage of these tests is that they lack sensitivity in small samples, where violations are relatively important, and may in contrast "detect" trivial violations in large samples.

Departures from normality can sometimes be corrected by transforming the outcome. Log and fractional power (square and cube root) transformations are commonly used for right-skewed outcome variables. Rank transformation, resulting in a uniform distribution, can be used when both tails are too long, though this incurs some loss of information. When no normalizing transformation can be found, the generalized linear models discussed in more detail below are often used.

Constant variance. Reduced efficiency as well as mistaken inferences can result from serious violations of this assumption, in particular when the mean of the outcome is being compared across subgroups of unequal size with substantially different residual variance. The OLS estimates remain unbiased but naive standard errors can be seriously misleading. In contrast to violations of the normality assumption, the adverse effects of unequal variance are not mitigated by increasing sample size.

The constant variance assumption can be checked by assessing patterns in the spread of the residuals in the residual vs. predictor and residual vs. fitted plots also used to assess linearity; similarly, the variance of the residuals within levels of categorical predictors can be compared. As for normality, tests for heteroscedasticity are available (White, 1980), but have low power in small datasets and are thus not recommended.

One often-used approach to rectifying non-constant variance is transformation of the outcome. In many situations, the variance grows approximately in proportion to the mean. In that case, the log transformation is ideal in that it will remove heteroscedasticity. Often, other model assumptions hold on the transformed scale, although this is not guaranteed.

Alternatively, if the variance matrix of the errors is known, inference can proceed by weighted least squares, which will produce unbiased and efficient point estimates of $\hat{\boldsymbol{\beta}}$. However, the required variance matrix is usually unknown. For that case, a variety of asymptotic estimators, variants of the robust or "sandwich" variance estimator (Huber, 1967) explained in more detail below, are consistent in the presence of heteroscedasticity. In this case $\mathbf{V}$ in Eq. (20) is a diagonal matrix with element v_{ii} estimated by some function of $e_i = (Y_i - \mathbf{x}'_i\hat{\boldsymbol{\beta}})$, the residual for observation i. While the various estimators are asymptotically equivalent, their behavior in small sample sizes can vary considerably. In extensive simulations, Long and Ervin (2000) show that the basic robust HC0 estimator, with $\hat{v}_{ii} \equiv e_i^2$, performs poorly in samples as large as 250 observations. They find that the more conservative HC3 estimator developed by MacKinnon and White (1985) has the best properties and should be used when subject-matter knowledge or exploratory data analysis suggests heteroscedasticity. In the HC3 estimator, $\hat{v}_{ii} = (e_i/(1 - h_{ii}))^2$, where h_{ii} is the ith diagonal element of the *hat* or *projection* matrix $\mathbf{H} = \mathbf{X}(\mathbf{X}'\mathbf{X})^{-1}\mathbf{X}'$.

Influential points. We would mistrust regression results – which purport to summarize the information in the entire dataset – if they change substantively when one or a few observations are omitted from the analysis. This can happen when *high-leverage* observations with extreme values of one or more of the predictors, or an anomalous combination of predictor values, also have large residuals. Especially in small datasets, the OLS coefficient estimates may unduly reflect minimization of the contribution of these observations to RSS. In linear models it is easy to compute the exact changes in each of the regression coefficient estimates, called *DFBETAs*, when each of the N observations is omitted; in logistic regression and other GLMs easily computed approximations are available. Boxplots of these *DFBETA* statistics for each predictor can then be used to identify influential points. Statistics that summarize the influence of each observation on all coefficient estimates include *DFITS* (Welsch and Kuh, 1977), *Cook's distance* (Cook, 1977), and *Welsch distance* (Welsch, 1982). Identifying influential *sets* of observations that are influential in combination but not necessarily individually remains a difficult computational problem.

2.5. Repeated measures

It is not unusual to collect repeated measurements on the same individuals, at the same centers, or from the same doctors. For example, in the medical services utilization example, measurements were taken on the same person at baseline, 6, 12, and 18 months after randomization. Outcomes measured on the same person, center, or doctor (sometimes called a cluster) are almost certain to be correlated and this needs to be accommodated in the analysis. Another feature of such data is that predictors can be measured at the observation level (e.g., length of time post-randomization or whether the person was homeless a majority of the preceding 6 months) or at the cluster level (gender, treatment group).

Consider an elaboration of the introductory model to accommodate the repeated measures:

$$Y_{it} = \log\ \text{cost}_{it} = \beta_0 + \beta_1 x_{1i} + \beta_2 x_{2i} + \beta_3 x_{3it} + \beta_4 x_{4it} + \delta_{it}, \tag{25}$$

where cost_{it} is the cost of medical care during the previous 6 months for $t = 6$, 12, or 18, x_{1i} is 1 if the patient was in the case management group and 0 otherwise, x_{2i} is 1 if the patient is female and 0 otherwise, x_{3it} is the patient's BDI at time t, x_{4it} is 1 if the patient was homeless a majority of the past six months and 0 otherwise, and δ_{it} is an error term.

So far there is nothing in the model to incorporate the potential correlation among measurements within a subject. One method is to directly assume a correlation among the error terms:

$$\text{var}\begin{pmatrix} \delta_{i6} \\ \delta_{i12} \\ \delta_{i18} \end{pmatrix} = \Sigma_\delta = \begin{pmatrix} \sigma_{\delta,6,6} & \sigma_{\delta,6,12} & \sigma_{\delta,6,18} \\ \sigma_{\delta,12,6} & \sigma_{\delta,12,12} & \sigma_{\delta,12,18} \\ \sigma_{\delta,18,6} & \sigma_{\delta,18,6} & \sigma_{\delta,18,18} \end{pmatrix}. \tag{26}$$

Another common strategy is to induce a variance–covariance structure by hypothesizing the existence of random effects. Essentially we decompose the error term, δ_{it} into two pieces, a subject-specific term, b, and an observation-specific term, ε:

$$\delta_{it} = b_i + \varepsilon_{it}, \tag{27}$$

with $b_i \sim$ i.i.d. $\mathcal{N}(0, \sigma_b^2)$ independent of $\varepsilon_{it} \sim$ i.i.d. $\mathcal{N}(0, \sigma_\varepsilon^2)$. The b_i are called *random effects* since we have assigned them a distribution. In this case, (25) would be called a *mixed model*, since it would include random effects as well as the usual *fixed* effects $x_1, \ldots, x_4$.

From this model is it easy to calculate the covariance between two observations on the same subject: $\text{cov}(Y_{it}, Y_{is}) = \text{cov}(\delta_{it}, \delta_{is}) = \sigma_b^2$. Note that this result holds without needing the assumption of normality of b_i or ε_{it}. In a similar manner it is straightforward to calculate the variance of Y_{it} or Y_{is} as $\sigma_b^2 + \sigma_e^2$ and the correlation between them as $\sigma_b^2/(\sigma_b^2 + \sigma_e^2)$.

So Eq. (27) corresponds to a special case of Eq. (26) with

$$\Sigma_\delta = \mathbf{I}\sigma_\varepsilon^2 + \mathbf{J}\sigma_b^2 = \begin{pmatrix} \sigma_\varepsilon^2 + \sigma_b^2 & \sigma_b^2 & \sigma_b^2 \\ \sigma_b^2 & \sigma_\varepsilon^2 + \sigma_b^2 & \sigma_b^2 \\ \sigma_b^2 & \sigma_b^2 & \sigma_\varepsilon^2 + \sigma_b^2 \end{pmatrix}, \tag{28}$$

where $\mathbf{J}$ is a matrix of all ones.

2.5.1. Estimation

Whether we formulate the model as Eq. (26) or the special case of Eq. (27), how should we fit the model and conduct statistical inference? OLS does not accommodate the correlated data. If the variance–covariance matrix, $\mathbf{V}$, were known, then weighted least squares could be used, weighting by the inverse of the variance–covariance matrix. This would yield:

$$\hat{\boldsymbol{\beta}}_V = (\mathbf{X}'\mathbf{V}^{-1}\mathbf{X})^{-1}\mathbf{X}'\mathbf{V}^{-1}\mathbf{Y}. \tag{29}$$

Or with a full parametric specification (i.e., that the data are multivariate normal) a logical method is maximum likelihood or a variant mentioned earlier, restricted maximum likelihood.

Consider a general model for the situation with correlated data and a linear model for the mean:

$$\mathbf{Y} \sim \mathcal{N}(\mathbf{X}\boldsymbol{\beta}, \mathbf{V}). \tag{30}$$

For the medical utilization example, if each of the N subjects had exactly three observations that followed model (26), and if the data vector $\mathbf{Y}$ were ordered by subject, then $\mathbf{V} = \mathbf{I}_N \otimes \Sigma_\delta$, with $\otimes$ denoting a Kronecker product, i.e., $\mathbf{A}\otimes\mathbf{B}$ is a partitioned matrix with entries $a_{ij}\mathbf{B}$. In particular $\mathbf{V} = \mathbf{I}_N \otimes \Sigma_\delta$ implies that $\mathbf{V}$ is block diagonal with $\boldsymbol{\Sigma}_\delta$ on the diagonal.

It is easy to show that the OLS estimator is unbiased, even in the presence of correlated data: Eq. (21) remains valid in this case. It is also straightforward to show that its variance is given by Eq. (20); in this case, of course, $\mathbf{V}$ does not simplify to $\sigma^2\mathbf{I}$. Similar calculations show that the weighted least squares estimator, Eq. (29), which is optimal under normality, is also unbiased and has variance equal to $(\mathbf{X}'\mathbf{V}^{-1}\mathbf{X})^{-1}$. Interestingly the OLS estimator often retains nearly full efficiency compared to the weighted least squares estimator (Diggle et al., 2002).

In practical situations the variance–covariance matrix of the data is never known and must be estimated. Typically $\mathbf{V}$ is a function of parameters $\boldsymbol{\theta}$, and as long as the parameters $\boldsymbol{\theta}$ are not functionally related to $\boldsymbol{\beta}$, the ML equations for $\boldsymbol{\beta}$ take the form:

$$\hat{\boldsymbol{\beta}}_{\hat{V}} = (\mathbf{X}'\hat{\mathbf{V}}^{-1}\mathbf{X})^{-1}\mathbf{X}'\hat{\mathbf{V}}^{-1}\mathbf{Y}, \tag{31}$$

where $\hat{\mathbf{V}}$ is the ML estimator of $\mathbf{V}$, i.e., $\mathbf{V}$ with the ML estimator of $\boldsymbol{\theta}$ substituted for $\boldsymbol{\theta}$ (McCulloch and Searle, 2000).

The ML equations for $\boldsymbol{\theta}$ are considerably more complicated and depend on the specific parametric form of $\mathbf{V}$ so we will not elaborate here, but refer the reader to McCulloch and Searle (2000) or Searle et al. (1992). Often the REML log-likelihood based on Eq. (16), and introduced in Section 2.1, is maximized to find an estimate of $\boldsymbol{\theta}$, which is then used in Eq. (31). Again, see Searle et al. (1992) for details.

2.5.2. *Prediction*

One of the advantages of the random effects approach, Eq. (27), is the ability to generate predicted values for each of the random effects, b_i, which we do not get to observe directly. Mixed models are used, for example, in rating the performance of hospitals or doctors (Normand et al., 1997; Hofer et al., 1999). In such a situation the outcome is a performance measure for the hospital, e.g., average log cost, and the random effects would represent, after adjustment for the fixed factors in the model, how a particular hospital or doctor deviated from the average.

Predicted values from random effects models are so-called shrinkage estimators because they are typically closer to a common value than estimates based on raw or adjusted averages. The shrinkage factor depends on the random effects variance and the sample size per cluster. When there is little variation from cluster to cluster and/or when the sample sizes are small, the shrinkage is greatest, reflecting the facts that clusters with extreme outcome values are likely to be due to chance in those circumstances. On the other hand, with sufficient data per cluster or evidence that clusters are quite different, the predicted values exhibit little shrinkage and are closer to raw or adjusted averages. So with varying sample sizes per cluster, estimates based on smaller sample sizes will show more shrinkage. Shrinkage predictions can be shown theoretically (Searle et al., 1992) to give more accurate predictions than those derived from the raw data. This occurs, especially with small cluster sizes, because information from other clusters is used to improve the prediction; this is sometimes called "borrowing strength" from the other clusters.

2.5.3. *Robust and sandwich variance estimators*

The fact that the OLS estimator is unbiased and often fairly efficient suggests that it could be used in practice. The problem with using the usual OLS regression packages is that they get the standard errors and hence tests and confidence intervals wrong by assuming all the data are independent.

In the case of longitudinal data, where we have independent data on M different subjects, a direct estimator of the true variance of the OLS estimator, Eq. (20) can be formed. Let $\mathbf{Y}_i$ denote the n_i outcomes for the ith subject, so that the number of observations $N = \sum_{i=1}^{M} n_i$. Then the model for the ith subject, using a corresponding model matrix $\mathbf{X}_i$, is

$$\begin{aligned} \mathbf{Y}_i &= \mathbf{X}_i\boldsymbol{\beta} + \varepsilon_i \quad i = 1, \ldots, M \\ \text{var}[\varepsilon_i] &= \mathbf{V}_i. \end{aligned} \tag{32}$$

In this case the OLS estimator $\hat{\boldsymbol{\beta}} = (\mathbf{X}'\mathbf{X})^{-1}(\mathbf{X}'\mathbf{Y})$ can be written as

$$\left(\sum_i \mathbf{X}_i'\mathbf{X}_i\right)^{-1}\left(\sum_i \mathbf{X}_i'\mathbf{Y}_i\right) \tag{33}$$

with variance

$$\left(\sum_i \mathbf{X}_i'\mathbf{X}_i\right)^{-1}\left(\sum_i \mathbf{X}_i'\mathbf{V}_i\mathbf{X}_i\right)\left(\sum_i \mathbf{X}_i'\mathbf{X}_i\right)^{-1}. \tag{34}$$

A crude estimator of $\mathbf{V}_i$ can be formed as $\hat{\mathbf{V}}_i = (\mathbf{Y}_i - \mathbf{X}_i\hat{\boldsymbol{\beta}})(\mathbf{Y}_i - \mathbf{X}_i\hat{\boldsymbol{\beta}})'$ giving

$$\hat{\text{var}}[\hat{\boldsymbol{\beta}}] = \left(\sum_i \mathbf{X}_i'\mathbf{X}_i\right)^{-1}\left(\sum_i \mathbf{X}_i'\hat{\mathbf{V}}_i\mathbf{X}_i\right)\left(\sum_i \mathbf{X}_i'\mathbf{X}_i\right)^{-1} \tag{35}$$

Even though $\hat{\mathbf{V}}_i$ is a crude estimator, Eq. (35) is often a good estimator of the variance of $\hat{\boldsymbol{\beta}}$ due to the averaging over the M subjects and the "averaging" that takes place when pre- and post-multiplying by $\mathbf{X}_i$. This is called the "sandwich" estimator due to the sandwiching of the $\mathbf{X}'\mathbf{V}^{-1}\mathbf{X}$ piece between $(\mathbf{X}'\mathbf{X})^{-1}$ terms and is a robust estimator in the sense that it is asymptotically (as $M \to \infty$) valid without making assumptions about the variance–covariance structure. As such, it is quite useful for sensitivity checks against model assumptions. When M is not large, inferences based on the robust variance estimator may be liberal. This is consistent with the results cited in Section 2.4 for the HC0 estimator, to which Eq. (35) reduces when there is only one outcome per subject (see Kaucrmann and Carroll, 2001).

2.5.4. Repeated measures ANOVA

Correlated data analyses can sometimes be handled by repeated measures analysis of variance (ANOVA). When the data are balanced and appropriate for ANOVA, statistics with exact null hypothesis distributions (as opposed to asymptotic, likelihood based) are available for testing. However, the variance–covariance structure is typically estimated by the method of moments, which may be less efficient than maximum likelihood. For unbalanced data, tests are approximate, and, even though approximations have been developed (e.g., the Geisser–Greenhouse correction; Greenhouse and Geisser, 1959), may not achieve nominal significance levels. Also, in the specification of approximate F-statistics, it is not always straightforward to specify a denominator mean square (i.e., what is the "right" error term?).

Maximum likelihood estimation generates test statistics relatively automatically and gives better predictions of the random effects. Maximum likelihood methods also generalize naturally to non-normally distributed outcomes (see, e.g., McCulloch and Searle, 2000), unlike repeated measures ANOVA. See McCulloch (2005) for further discussion.

2.6. Model selection

Many more potential predictor variables are commonly measured than can reasonably be included in a multivariable regression model. In the introductory example, many factors in addition to gender, the BDI, and homelessness are likely to influence medical services utilization, including having health insurance and the range of health conditions driving the need for such services. The difficult problem of how to select predictors can be resolved to serve three distinct uses of regression. First, *prediction*: Can we identify which types of patients will use the most medical resources? Regression is a powerful and general tool for using multiple measured predictors to make useful predictions for future observations. Second, *isolating the effect of a single predictor*: What is the effect of the case management treatment on use of the emergency room, after adjusting for whether the patients in the two treatment groups (although randomized) differ with regard to gender, depression, or homeless status? Regression is a method to isolate the effect of one predictor (treatment) while adjusting for other differences. And third, *understanding multiple predictors*: Are the homeless at an increased risk of mortality and does the case management especially help the homeless? Regression is a method for understanding the joint and combined associations of all the predictors with the outcome.

2.6.1. Prediction

Here the primary issue is minimizing prediction error rather than causal interpretation of the predictors in the model. *Prediction error* (*PE*) measures how well the model is able to predict the outcome for a new, randomly selected observation that was not used in estimating the parameters of the prediction model. In this context, inclusive models that minimize confounding may not work as well as models with smaller numbers of predictors. This can be understood in terms of the *bias-variance trade-off*. Bias is often reduced when more variables are included, but as less important covariates are added, precision may suffer without commensurate decreases in bias. The larger models may be *overfitted* to the data, reflecting random error to such an extent that they are less able to predict new observations than models with fewer predictors that give slightly biased estimates but are less reflective of randomness in the current data.

Because R^2, the proportion of variance explained, increases with each additional covariate, even if it adds minimal information about the outcome, a model that maximizes R^2 is unlikely to minimize *PE*. Alternative measures include adjusted R^2, which works by penalizing R^2 for the number of predictors in the model. Thus when a variable is added, adjusted R^2 increases only if the increment in R^2 outweighs the added penalty. Mallow's C_p, the Akaike information criterion (AIC), and the Bayesian information criterion (BIC) are analogs which impose respectively stiffer penalties for each additional variable, and thus lead to selection of smaller models. Measures of concordance of the observed and predicted outcomes for the logistic and Cox models include the *c*-statistic and Somer's D (Harrell et al., 1996), as well as adaptations of the Brier score (Graf et al., 1999).

More direct estimates of *PE* are based on *cross-validation* (CV), a class of methods that work by using distinct sets of observations to estimate the model and to evaluate *PE*. The most straightforward example is the learning set/test set (LS/TS) approach, in which the parameter estimates are obtained from the learning set and then used to evaluate *PE* in the test set. In linear regression, computing *PE* is straightforward, using $\hat{\beta}$ from the learning set to compute the predicted value $\hat{y}$ and corresponding residual for each observation in the test set. The learning and test sets are sometimes obtained by splitting a single dataset, often with two-thirds of the observations randomly assigned to the learning set. However, using an independent sample as the test set may give more generalizable estimates of *PE*, since the test set is generally not sampled from exactly the same population as the learning set.

An alternative to LS/TS is leave-one-out or *jackknife* methods, in which all but one observation are used to estimate the model, and then *PE* is evaluated for the omitted observation; this is done in turn for each observation. In linear regression models, the resulting predicted residual sum of squares (PRESS) can be computed for the entire dataset with minimal extra computation. In logistic and Cox models, fast one-step approximations are available.

Midway between LS/TS and the jackknife is *h-fold cross-validation* (hCV). The dataset is divided into h mutually exclusive subsets and a measure of *PE* is evaluated in each subset, using parameter estimates obtained from the remaining observations. A global estimate of *PE* is then found by averaging over the h subset estimates. Typically values of h from 5 to 10 are used.

Bootstrap methods provide a potentially more efficient alternative to cross-validation for estimating prediction error (Efron, 1986; Harrell et al., 1996). Prediction models are developed using the methods employed with the original data but applied to bootstrap samples, and then evaluated using both the bootstrap and original data. The estimated prediction error of the rule both developed and evaluated using the original data is then corrected by the average difference between the two prediction error estimates for the bootstrap datasets.

Modern computing power makes it possible to use CV or the bootstrap not just to validate a prediction model using independent data but to guide iterative predictor selection procedures. Among them, Breiman (2001) describes modern methods that do not follow the paradigm motivated by the bias-variance trade-off that smaller models are better for prediction. The newer methods tend to keep all the predictors in play, while using various methods to avoid overfitting and control variance; cross-validation plays a central role throughout.

The so-called shrinkage procedures also play an important role in prediction, especially those made on the basis of small datasets. In this approach over-fitting is avoided and prediction improved by shrinking the estimated regression coefficients toward zero, rather than eliminating weak predictors from the model. Variants of shrinkage include the *non-negative garrote* (Breiman, 1995) and the *LASSO* method, short for *least absolute shrinkage and selection operator* (Tibshirani, 1997). An alternative to direct shrinkage implements *penalties* in the fitting procedure against coefficient estimates which violate some measure of smoothness. This achieves something like shrinkage of the estimates and thus better predictions; see Le Cessie and Van Houwelingen (1992) and Verweij and Van Houwelingen (1994) for applications to logistic and Cox regression. These methods derive from *ridge regression* (Hoerl and Kennard, 1970), a method for obtaining slightly biased but stabler estimates in linear models with highly correlated predictors.

Finally, Altman and Royston (2000) give an excellent discussion of validating prediction models from a broader perspective, focusing on the ways in which these models may or may not be useful in clinical and other practical applications.

2.6.2. Isolating the effect of a single predictor

In observational data, the main problem in evaluating a predictor of primary interest is to rule out non-causal explanations of an association between this predictor and the outcome as persuasively as possible – that is, *confounding* of the association by the true causal factors, or correlates of such factors. Confounders are associated with the predictor of interest and independently associated with the outcome, and thus may explain all or part of the unadjusted association of the primary predictor and the outcome. As a result, addition of the confounder to the model typically affects the estimate for the primary predictor; in most cases, the adjusted estimate is smaller. Potential confounders to be considered include factors identified in previous studies or hypothesized to matter on substantive grounds, as well as variables that behave like confounders by the statistical measures. Two classes of covariates would not be considered for inclusion in the model: covariates which are essentially alternative measures of either the outcome or the predictor of interest, and those hypothesized to *mediate* its effect – that is, to lie on a causal pathway between the predictor of interest and the outcome.

To rule out confounding more effectively, a liberal criterion of $p < 0.2$ for inclusion of covariates in the model makes sense (Maldonado and Greenland, 1993). A comparably effective alternative is to retain variables if removing them changes the coefficient for the predictor of interest by more than 10% or 15% (Greenland, 1989; Mickey and Greenland, 1989). These inclusive rules are particularly important in small datasets, where even important confounders may not meet the usual criterion for statistical significance. Among the common procedures that could be used to select covariates, backward selection (that is, starting with the full model and sequentially eliminating the least important remaining variable) has the advantage that *negatively confounded* variables are less likely to be omitted from the final model (Sun et al., 1999). Negatively confounded variables appear *more* important when they are included in the model together, in contrast to the more common case in which addition of a confounder to the model attenuates the estimate for the predictor of interest.

Randomized experiments including clinical trials represent a special case where the predictor of primary interest is the intervention; confounding is not usually an issue, but covariates are sometimes included in the model for other reasons. These include design variables in stratified experiments, including clinical center in multicenter randomized trials, necessary for obtaining valid standard errors, p-values, and confidence intervals. In linear models inclusion of important prognostic variables can also substantially reduce residual error and thus increase power; Hauck et al. (1998) emphasize, however, that the adjusted model should be pre-specified in the study protocol. Furthermore, adjustment in experiments with binary or failure time outcomes can avoid attenuation of treatment effect estimates in logistic (Neuhaus and Jewell, 1993; Neuhaus, 1998) and Cox models (Gail et al., 1984; Schmoor and Schumacher, 1997; Henderson and Oman, 1999). Hypothesis tests remain valid when there is no treatment effect (Gail et al., 1988), but power is lost in proportion to the importance of the omitted covariates (Lagakos and Schoenfeld, 1984; Begg and Lagakos, 1993). Note, however, that adjustment for *im*balanced covariates can potentially increase as well as decrease the treatment effect estimate, and can erode both precision and power. Finally, adjusted or de-attenuated treatment effect estimates are more nearly interpretable as *subject-specific* – in contrast to *population-averaged* (Hauck et al., 1998).

2.6.3. Understanding multiple predictors

This is the most difficult case, and one in which both causal interpretation and statistical inference are most problematic. When the focus is on isolating the effect of a single predictor, covariates are included in order to obtain a minimally confounded estimate. However, broadening the focus to multiple important predictors of an outcome can make selecting a single best model considerably more difficult. For example, inferences about most or all of the predictors retained in the model are now of primary interest, so overfitting and false-positive results are more of an issue, particularly for novel and seemingly implausible associations. Interaction – that is, the dependence of the effect of one predictor on the value of another – will usually be of interest, but systematically assessing the large number of possible interactions can easily lead to false-positive findings, some at least not easily rejected as implausible. It may also be difficult to choose between alternative models that each include one variable from a collinear pair or set. Mediation is also more difficult to handle, to the extent that both the overall effect of a predictor as well as its direct and indirect effects may be of interest. In this case, models which both exclude and include the mediator may be required to give a full picture. Especially in the earlier stages of research, modeling these complex relationships is difficult, prone to error, and likely to require considerable re-analysis in response to input from subject-matter experts.

2.6.4. Number of predictors

The rationale for inclusive predictor selection rules, whether we are isolating the effect of single predictor or trying to understand multiple predictors, is to obtain minimally confounded estimates. However, this can make regression coefficient estimates less precise, especially for highly correlated predictors. At the extreme, model performance can be severely degraded by the inclusion of too many predictors. Rules of thumb have been suggested for number of predictors that can be safely included as a function of sample size or number of events. A commonly used guideline prescribes ten observations for each predictor; with binary or survival outcomes the analogous guideline specifies ten events per predictor (Peduzzi et al., 1995, 1996; Concato et al., 1995). The rationale is to obtain adequately precise estimates, and in the case of the logistic and Cox models, to ensure that the models behave properly.

However, such guidelines are too simple. Their primary limitation is that the precision of coefficient estimates depends on other factors as well as the number of observations or events per predictor. In particular, the variance of a coefficient estimate in a linear model (Eq. (22)) depends on the residual variance of the outcome, which is generally reduced by the inclusion of important covariates. Precision also depends on the multiple correlation between a predictor of interest and other variables in the model, which figures in the denominator of Eq. (22). Thus addition of covariates that are at most weakly correlated with the primary predictor but explain substantial outcome variance can actually improve the precision of the estimate for the predictor of interest. In contrast, addition of just one collinear predictor can degrade its precision unacceptably. In addition, the allowable number of predictors depends on effect size, with larger effects being more robust to multiple adjustments than smaller ones.

In many contexts where these guidelines might be violated, power is low, in which case misleading inferences can usually be avoided if confidence intervals are used to interpret negative findings (Hoenig and Heisey, 2001). However, when statistically significant associations are found despite the inclusion of more predictors than this rule allows – with 5 or more events per variable – only a modest degree of extra caution appears to be warranted (Vittinghoff and McCulloch, 2007).

2.6.5. Model selection complicates inference

Underlying the confidence intervals and *p*-values which play a central role in interpreting regression results is the assumption that the predictors to be included in the model were specified a priori without reference to the data. In *confirmatory* analyses in well-developed areas of research, including phase-III clinical trials, prior determination of the model is feasible and important. In contrast, at earlier stages of research, data-driven predictor selection and checking are reasonable, even obligatory, and certainly widely used. However, some of the issues raised for inference include the following:

- The chance of at least one type-I error can greatly exceed the nominal level used to test each term.
- In small datasets precision and power are often poor, so important predictors may be omitted from the model, especially if a restrictive inclusion criterion is used.
- Parameter estimates can be biased away from the null, owing to selection of estimates that are large by chance (Steyerberg et al., 1999).
- Choices between predictors can be poorly motivated, especially between collinear variables, and are potentially sensitive to addition or deletion of a few observations. Altman and Andersen (1989) propose bootstrap methods for assessing this sensitivity.

Breiman (2001) is skeptical of modeling causal pathways using such procedures, and argues that computer-intensive methods validated strictly in terms of prediction error not only give better predictions but may also be more reliable guides to "variable importance" – another term for understanding multiple predictors, and with implications for assessing isolating the effect of a single predictor.

Finally, we note that these issues in predictor selection apply broadly, to non-linear as well as linear models.

3. Non-linear models

3.1. Introduction: A salary analysis

One of us recently completed an analysis of salary data for the compensation plan at our university to check for inequities in pay between males and females. Not surprising, the salary data is highly skewed right with a few extreme salaries (mostly MDs who generate large amounts of clinical income). The traditional method of handling such data is to consider a log transformation of the outcome, which made the data approximately normally distributed. Here is an overly simplistic version of the analysis to illustrate the basic points, adjusting only for faculty rank before looking for a gender effect. The model uses a reference group of assistant professor and is given by

$$\log(\text{salary}_i) = \beta_0 + \beta_1 x_{1i} + \beta_2 x_{2i} + \beta_3 x_{3i} + \varepsilon_i, \tag{36}$$

where salary_i is the monthly salary of the ith faculty member, and x_{1i}, x_{2i}, and x_{3i} are the indicator functions for the faculty member being an associate professor, being a full professor, and being male, respectively.

The gender effect, β_3, was estimated to be 0.185 with a 95% confidence interval of (0.116, 0.254). How do we interpret this result? It is unsatisfying to interpret log(dollars) so the inclination is to back transform both sides of Eq. (36) giving

$$\begin{aligned} \text{salary}_i &= \exp\{\beta_0 + \beta_1 x_{1i} + \beta_2 x_{2i} + \beta_3 x_{3i} + \varepsilon_i\} \\ &= e^{\beta_0} e^{\beta_1 x_{1i}} e^{\beta_2 x_{2i}} e^{\beta_3 x_{3i}} e^{\varepsilon_i} \\ &= \gamma_0 \gamma_1^{x_{1i}} \gamma_2^{x_{2i}} \gamma_3^{x_{3i}} \delta_i, \end{aligned} \tag{37}$$

here $\gamma_j = e^{\beta_j}$ and $\delta_i = e^{\varepsilon i}$. Ignoring the error term, δ, for the moment, and taking the ratio of the model equation, Eq. (37), for males and females of the same rank gives

$$\gamma_3 = \frac{\gamma_0 \gamma_1^{x_1} \gamma_2^{x_2} \gamma_3^1}{\gamma_0 \gamma_1^{x_1} \gamma_2^{x_2} \gamma_3^0} \tag{38}$$

In words, males make, on average, $e^{0.185} = 1.203$ or about 20% more with a confidence interval of (1.123, 1.289).

Being more careful, in Eq. (38), we have taken the ratio of values of $\exp\{E[\log(\text{salary})]\}$, which is not the same as $E[\text{salary}]$. However, if the log transformation makes the errors, ε_i, normally distributed (or, more generally symmetrically distributed) as it did in this example, then the mean and the median are the same. So we can also interpret the model as a model for median log(salary). Since

$$\exp\{\text{median}[\log(\text{salary})]\} = \exp\{\log(\text{median}[\text{salary}])\} = \text{median}[\text{salary}] \tag{39}$$

we can interpret γ_3 in terms of median salaries. In particular, males have a median salary that is, on average, about 20% higher than females.

This is a very reasonable interpretation and is, in many cases, preferred to a model for mean salary, which is sensitive to the few extreme salaries. Furthermore, the ratio interpretation (20% more for males) is a common way of thinking about salaries as opposed to an additive one (e.g., \$1,800 more per month) since, for example, raises are often decided on a percentage basis.

However, what about the medical center administrator in charge of making sure the compensation plan generates enough revenue to pay all the faculty? Clearly, she is concerned with *mean* salary since the total revenue has to exceed the mean salary times the number of faculty. What models are available if we require a model for mean salary?

The ratio form of the model, but for the mean salary, could be retained by fitting a model of the form

$$\text{salary}_i = \gamma_0^* \gamma_1^{*x_{1i}} \gamma_2^{*x_{2i}} \gamma_3^{*x_{3i}} + \varepsilon_i^*, \tag{40}$$

Non-linear least squares could be used and would give consistent estimates even though we would not feel comfortable assuming that the ε_i^* were homoscedastic and normally distributed. So confidence intervals or tests for γ_3 based on normality assumptions would be suspect but inferences could still be achieved, e.g., through bootstrapping. Fitting model (40) to the salary data gave $\hat{\gamma}_3^* = 1.165$ with a bootstrap confidence interval of (1.086, 1.244).

But it might be more satisfying to make mild, but reasonable assumptions about the form of the distribution, for example that the salaries had a gamma distribution with mean μ_i given by a multiplicative model and constant coefficient of variation:

$$\begin{aligned} &\text{salary}_i \sim \text{Gamma}(\mu_i) \\ &\log(\mu_i) = \beta_0^{**} + \beta_1^{**} x_{1i} + \beta_2^{**} x_{2i} + \beta_3^{**} x_{3i}. \end{aligned} \tag{41}$$

Fitting this model gives an estimate $\exp\{\hat{\beta}_3^{**}\} = 1.223$ with a model based confidence interval of (1.138, 1.314) and a bootstrap confidence interval of (1.142, 1.310).

Models (40) and (41) differ from (36) in that they model the mean salary rather than the median salary and by the fact that they are non-linear in the parameters. Model (41) differs from (40) in that it is a generalized linear model: a known transformation of the mean is linear in the parameters ($\log(\mu_i)$ is linear in the β_j^{**} whereas the log of the mean of model (40) is not linear in the γ_j^*). In the next section, we present a model for survival times which is analogous to model (41) but can also be written as a linear model with a log-transformed outcome and non-normal errors.

3.2. The accelerated failure time model

Consider examining the effect of the managed care intervention on survival among homeless patients. Survival times typically have a right-skewed distribution; hence we might use a model similar to the last model (41) proposed for faculty salaries:

$$\begin{aligned}&\text{survival}_i \sim \text{exponential}(\mu_i)\\&\log(\mu_i) = \beta_0 + \beta x_{1i} + \beta_2 x_{2i} + \beta_3 x_{3i}\end{aligned} \tag{42}$$

In Eq. (42), x_{1i} is the intervention indicator, x_{2i} is the BDI, and x_{3i} indicates if the subject is homeless. The exponential distribution is an important special case for survival data because the so-called hazard function is constant under this model (see Chapter 9 of this book on survival analysis).

However, an important difference between the salary and survival time outcome variables is that many subjects either drop out prior to or survive past the end of the study, so we only know that their actual survival times are greater than their observed follow-up time Y_i. In the salary example, this would amount to knowing only that some of the faculty were earning more than, say, \$500,000 per year. These survival times are said to be *right-censored.*

The *accelerated failure time* (AFT) model can be written in terms of the so-called survival function, $S_i(t) = P(\text{survival}_i > t)$. Under the AFT,

$$P(\text{survival}_i > t|\mathbf{x}_i) = S_i(t) = S_0\big(t \exp(\mathbf{x}_i'\boldsymbol{\beta})\big) \tag{43}$$

where $S_0(t) = P(\text{survival}_i > t|\mathbf{x}_i = 0)$ is the baseline survival function. The baseline survival function plays the role of the intercept β_0 in other regression models, and represents the survival function for a subject with all covariate values equal to 0; this can be made interpretable by centering covariate values. The effect of the covariates in the model is to multiply t by $\exp(\mathbf{x}_i'\boldsymbol{\beta})$, in some sense speeding up or slowing down time, depending on the sign of $\mathbf{x}_i'\boldsymbol{\beta}$. The interpretation is similar to the equivalence of 1 dog and 7 human years – for the dog, time is accelerated.

The AFT model can also be written as a linear model with log-transformed outcome:

$$\log(\text{survival}_i) = -\mathbf{x}_i'b + \varepsilon_i \tag{44}$$

where ε_i follows some distribution. In particular, if survival_i follows an exponential distribution, then ε_i follows the extreme-value distribution. When the distribution of ε (or, equivalently $S_0(\cdot)$) is parametrically specified, maximum likelihood estimation of $\boldsymbol{\beta}$ is straightforward. The likelihood of the possibly censored follow-up time Y_i has the form

$$f_i(Y_i)^{\Delta_i} S_i(Y_i)^{(1-\Delta_i)} \tag{45}$$

where $f_i(t) = -\partial S_i(t)/\partial t$ is the density function, and Δ_i is 0 if subject i is censored and 1 otherwise. Intuitively, the likelihood contribution for a censored observation is just $P(\text{survival}_i > t_i)$.

For example, under the exponential AFT model, with baseline survival function $S_0(t) = \exp(-\lambda t)$, the log-likelihood based on Eq. (45) is

$$\sum_{i=1}^{N} \Delta_i\{\log \lambda + \mathbf{x}_i'\boldsymbol{\beta} - \lambda Y_i \exp(\mathbf{x}_i'\boldsymbol{\beta})\} + (1 - \Delta_i)\{-\lambda Y_i \exp(\mathbf{x}_i'\boldsymbol{\beta})\}. \tag{46}$$

This simplifies to

$$\sum_{i=1}^{N} \Delta_i(\log \lambda + \mathbf{x}_i'\boldsymbol{\beta}) - \lambda Y_i \exp(\mathbf{x}_i'\boldsymbol{\beta}) \tag{47}$$

and is straightforward to maximize numerically.

In general, AFT models have proved useful in industrial applications and have been advocated for biomedical research (Wei, 1992). However, when the distribution of ε is unspecified, estimation becomes a complex problem. Considerable interest has centered on rank-based estimation in the semi-parametric case where ε follows an unspecified distribution. Estimation there has proven difficult due to non-monotone, non-differentiable estimation functions (Lin and Geyer, 1992). Recently, more computationally feasible approaches have been developed (Jin et al., 2003).

3.3. Generalized linear models

We return to the example of Section 1.1 on utilization of health resources. Recall that interest focused on an intervention to reduce health care costs, number of emergency room visits, and death. How should we model the outcome of number of emergency room visits as a function of the predictors: intervention group, gender, baseline depression score, and homeless status?

This outcome is a count variable and skewed to the right. Furthermore, in subsets of the data in which the mean value is higher (e.g., among homeless persons) the variability is higher. Both of these features make a linear regression model assuming normality and homoscedasticity of the outcome an unattractive strategy.

We might consider a transformation of the outcome to try to make it more approximately normally distributed and to achieve variance homogeneity. This strategy will not work in cases where a large percentage of observations are zero, as they were for this dataset. The most a transformation will do is move the large percentage of data exactly equal to zero to a different value. For example the square root transformation, a common transformation for count data, would leave the same large percentage of zeros at zero.

The typical linear regression model for the mean is also unattractive for this example. The mean number of emergency room visits for any particular configuration of the predictors must be positive, but a linear regression model will not be so constrained.

3.3.1. *Modeling a transformation of the mean*

A solution is to separately define the distribution of the data and then model some function of the mean instead of the mean itself. For simplicity we will consider just the first measurement (at 6 months) and accordingly define Y_i as the number of emergency room visits for patient i between the baseline and 6-month visits.

Since the data are counts, we might consider a Poisson distribution as a first step. With a small mean value, this may accurately model the large percentage of zeroes. A common and useful function of the mean to model is the logarithm, which we will justify later. That leads us to

$$\begin{aligned} &Y_i \sim \text{indep. Poisson}(E[Y_i]) \\ &\log E[Y_i] = \beta_0 + \beta_1 x_{1i} + \beta_2 x_{2i} + \beta_3 x_{3i} + \beta_4 x_{4i}. \end{aligned} \tag{48}$$

where x_{1i}, x_{2i}, and x_{3i} are the indicators for being in the case management group, female, and homeless, respectively, and x_{4i} is the patient's BDI at baseline.

Back transforming the mean in Eq. (48) gives the following non-linear regression equation relating the mean rate in 6 months to the predictors:

$$\begin{aligned} E[Y_i] &= \exp\{\beta_0 + \beta_1 x_{1i} + \beta_2 x_{2i} + \beta_3 x_{3i} + \beta_4 x_{4i}\} \\ &= \mathrm{e}^{\beta_0}\mathrm{e}^{\beta_1 x_{1i}}\mathrm{e}^{\beta_2 x_{2i}}\mathrm{e}^{\beta_3 x_{3i}}\mathrm{e}^{\beta_4 x_{4i}} \\ &= \gamma_0 \gamma_1^{x_{1i}} \gamma_2^{x_{2i}} \gamma_3^{x_{3i}} \gamma_4^{x_{4i}}, \end{aligned} \tag{49}$$

with $\gamma_k \equiv e^{\beta_k}$.

Although many of the data points are zero (and hence not acceptable to log transform) the mean value will not be exactly zero, allowing the use of the log function. Also, the exponential in Eq. (49) keeps the mean value positive, allowing flexible linear models for log $E[Y_i]$.

Model (49) is clearly a multiplicative model in the parameters and the coefficients have a ratio interpretation. As an example we calculate the ratio of the means, holding intervention group, gender, and homeless status as fixed and evaluating the BDI at the values $x^* + 1$ and x^*:

$$\begin{aligned} \frac{E[Y|x_4 = x^* + 1]}{E[Y|x_4 = x^*]} &= \frac{\exp\{\beta_0 + \beta_1 x_1 + \beta_2 x_2 + \beta_3 x_3 + \beta_4(x^* + 1)\}}{\exp\{\beta_0 + \beta_1 x_1 + \beta_2 x_2 + \beta_3 x_3 + \beta_4 x^*\}} \\ &= \exp\{\beta_4\} \\ &= \gamma_4. \end{aligned} \tag{50}$$

So γ_4 has the interpretation as the relative rate of emergency room visits (per 6 months) when BDI is increased by 1. The other coefficients are interpreted similarly, for example, γ_3 is the relative rate for homeless compared to non-homeless. So we see that modeling the log transformation of the mean, called using a log *link*, has two attractive features: it keeps the mean values positive and provides a relative rate interpretation.

It has a different, more subtle advantage. This is a model for the number of emergency room visits per half year. What if the subject is followed for only 2 months before dying? Let t_i be the amount of time that subject i is followed. Then we would like to build a model for the rate of emergency room visits per unit time, namely, $E[Y_i]/t_i$. When using the log link the model then can be rearranged to

$$\begin{aligned} \log\big(E[Y_i]/t_i\big) &= \beta_0 + \beta_1 x_{1i} + \beta_2 x_{2i} + \beta_3 x_{3i} + \beta_4 x_{4i}, \\ \log E[Y_i] &= \beta_0 + \beta_1 x_{1i} + \beta_2 x_{2i} + \beta_3 x_{3i} + \beta_4 x_{4i} + \log\ t_i. \end{aligned} \tag{51}$$

Notably, we can still model the mean of a Poisson variate (Y_i/t_i is not Poisson distributed since it can take non-integer values) as long as we include a term, $\log t_i$, on the right-hand side of the equation. This is not quite a predictor or covariate because it has no coefficient multiplying it and so it is called an *offset.* Statistical analysis programs that fit such models usually allow the specification of an offset so the program does not estimate an associated coefficient.

3.3.2. A log link binary data model

We now consider a similar model, but for binary data. Recall that in Section 1.1 we posited a logistic regression model for the binary outcome of death. This model had multiplicative interpretations in terms of odds so that exponentiating a coefficient gave the odds ratio of death associated with increasing the predictor by 1. But some analysts find odds ratios hard to interpret and instead prefer *relative risks*, namely the ratio of the risk of death under two different scenarios. We now investigate the consequences of using a log link for binary outcome data:

$$\begin{aligned} &Y_i = 1 \quad \text{if subject } i \text{ dies in the first 6 months and 0 otherwise} \\ &Y_i \sim \text{indep. Bernoulli}(\mathrm{E}[Y_i]) \\ &\log\ \mathrm{E}[Y_i] = \beta_0 + \beta_1 x_{1i} + \beta_2 x_{2i} + \beta_3 x_{3i} + \beta_4 x_{4i}. \end{aligned} \tag{52}$$

Using arguments the same as in Eq. (50) we see that $\gamma_3 = e^{\beta_3}$ gives the relative risk of death for homeless compared to non-homeless.

The log link is not as attractive in this scenario as it is for the Poisson model. While the log link keeps the model for the mean (which is the probability of the outcome for a binary data model) positive, as is required, it does not constrain the probabilities to be less than 1 (which the logistic model does). So Eq. (52) is mainly useful when the outcome is rare and probabilities near or above 1 will not be estimated in a reasonable range of the model; otherwise the model can be unstable to fit.

3.3.3. A general approach

Models like the one developed in this section are called *generalized linear models* because a model that is linear in the parameters is assumed to hold for a known function of the mean of the outcome. Besides the generality gained by using a different function of the mean, this approach has the advantage of separating the decision as to the distribution of the outcome and what sort of model to create for the mean. In particular, we illustrated two possible models for the Bernoulli distribution, using either a logit or log link.

The key to use of a generalized linear model program is the specification of the relationship of the variance to the mean. As examples, the Poisson distribution assumes the mean (μ) and variance (σ^2) are equal; the Bernoulli assumes $\sigma^2 = \mu(1 - \mu)$; and the Gamma assumes $\sigma \propto \mu$. Most programs use this information as input to an iteratively re-weighted least squares algorithm and base inferences on a quasi-likelihood (which does not require specification of a full probabilistic model). The variance-to-mean relationship may be implied by the distribution (as with a binary outcome), inferred from past experience (e.g., if lipid measures are known to have standard deviation proportional to the mean), or assessed using the data, for example by plotting subgroup standard deviations against their means.

Generalized linear models have been extended to accommodate correlated data using two main approaches. The first is by including random effects along with likelihood estimation (e.g., McCulloch and Searle, 2000). The second approach is the use of the robust variance estimate (as in Section 2.5.3) using so-called generalized estimating equations (Diggle et al., 2002).

3.4. Transformations of predictors resulting in non-linear models

In the generalized linear models just described, a function of $E[Y_i|\mathbf{x_i}]$ is specified by a linear combination of the regression parameters, and thus is similar to a linear model. And in a previous section we described spline models which, despite using elaborate transformations of continuous predictors, nonetheless retain this property. However, some methods of transforming predictors induce models which are intrinsically non-linear, in that no transformation of the mean of the outcome can be represented as a linear function of the regression parameters. These include *segmented regression models*, *GAMs*, *CART*, and other non-linear models.

Segmented regression models. With segmented regression models, we postulate that the mean of the outcome is a series of connected line segments (much like linear regression splines). However, in segmented regression the general form is specified, but with knots as well as slopes unknown. Segmented regression is thus useful in problems where inference on the placement of the knots is of interest. The technique has been used to examine if there were trends in cancer diagnosis over time and, if so, which were the years of the change points (Hankey et al., 1999). Such problems are not linear because the mean cannot be represented as a linear function of the knots.

Generalized additive models (GAMs). An interesting class of models, termed GAMs (Hastie and Tibshirani, 1990) relax the assumptions of the classic generalized linear model. These models take the form

$$g(E[y|\mathrm{x}]) = f_0 + f_1(x_1) + \cdots + f_p(x_p) \tag{53}$$

where $g(\cdot)$ is known but the $f_j(\cdot)$ are unspecified but smooth functions. These models make it possible to examine the response as a non-linear function of the predictors. The approach is useful for simultaneous non-parametric exploration of the effects of predictors on the outcome. A description of the effect of the jth covariate is given in the form of $\hat{f}_j$.

Classification and regression trees (CART) (Breiman et al., 1984) divide the predictor space into a series of mutually exclusive and exhaustive subsets. Given the subsets, the model can be written as linear in a series of indicator functions. The splits (or nodes) defined by CART are arrived at by recursive partitioning of the predictor space based on a splitting criterion which measures homogeneity within the nodes (e.g., the sum of the squared residuals). The approach is appealing because it seamlessly handles many different predictor types and missing values, automatically detects interactions and avoids distributional assumptions. *Pruning* of the tree based on cross-validation is commonly used to avoid over-fitting.

3.5. Other non-linear models

In many situations, scientific knowledge about a biological phenomenon of interest suggests an appropriate form for the regression relationship between outcome and predictors. Because many such models cannot be reduced to the linear additive form familiar from conventional regression, alternate techniques for estimation and inference are often required. An example is provided by analyses of left ventricular pressure data aimed at estimating clinically relevant features indicative of cardiac performance (Takeuchi et al., 1991). The basic data are in the form of pressure data obtained from cardiac catheterization, and are in the form of *loops* corresponding to individual heartbeats. A typical example is illustrated in Fig. 1. The points represent the observed data for a single beat, and the line gives the theoretical pressure curve. The latter cannot be observed directly because in a typical ventricular contraction, the heart valves release before maximum pressure is attained and observed pressure drops accordingly. The labeled quantity $P_{\max}$ represents the maximum pressure that the ventricular contraction can theoretically generate. The goal of the analysis is to fit a plausible model to the observed data (typically using multiple beats for a given individual), and use it to estimate $P_{\max}$. A model for pressure, $P(t)$, as a function of time, t, has been proposed by Takeuchi et al. (1991), which takes the following form:

$$P(t) = 1/2P_{\max}[1 - \cos(\omega t + C)] + \mathrm{EDP}. \tag{54}$$

Here, $P_{\max}$, ω, and C represent the amplitude, angular frequency, and phase shift angle of the theoretical pressure curve, respectively. EDP refers to end-diastolic ventricular pressure, which is defined as the distance from the lowest point of the curve to the horizontal axis in the figure. The angular frequency $\omega = 2\pi/T$, where T is the duration of the approximated pressure curve. The quantities ω and EDP are typically obtained from separate measurements, leaving C and $P_{\max}$ as the primary unknown parameters to be estimated from the observed pressure data.

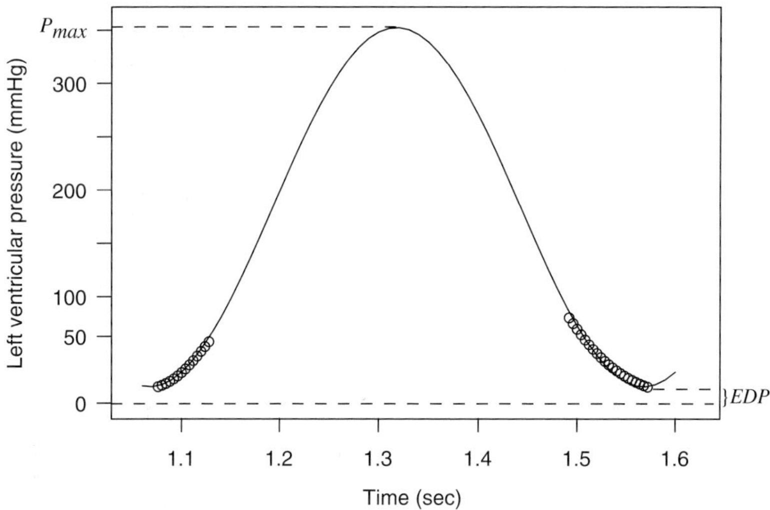

Fig. 1. Ventricular pressure data for a single heart beat.

The model (55) can be viewed as a special case of the following general non-linear regression model:

$$Y_i = f(\mathbf{x}_i; \boldsymbol{\theta}) + \varepsilon_i \quad i = 1, \ldots, N, \tag{55}$$

where f is a non-linear function of predictor variables $\mathbf{x}$, $\boldsymbol{\theta}$ is a vector of parameters, and the errors ε are typically assumed to be i.i.d. normally distributed. Estimation is typically performed via non-linear least squares, where the estimate $\hat{\boldsymbol{\theta}}$ is obtained as the minimizer of the following equation:

$$\hat{\boldsymbol{\theta}} = \operatorname{argmin} \sum_{i=1}^{N} (Y_{\mathrm{i}} - f(\mathbf{x}_i; \boldsymbol{\theta}))^2 \tag{56}$$

When the errors ε are normally distributed this yields the maximum likelihood estimate of $\boldsymbol{\theta}$. Even in situations where this is not the case, estimation is typically based on Eq. (56). For the data presented in Fig. 1, the estimates (approximate standard errors) for $P_{\max}$ and C were 337.2 (6.87) and −7.3 (0.007).

The *asymptotic regression* model, Eq. (57), provides another example of an inherently non-linear model:

$$Y_i = \beta_0 + \beta_2 e^{\beta_2 x_i} \tag{57}$$

For negative values of β_2, Y reaches the asymptote β_0 as x increases. This model is commonly applied in analyses of growth curves.

Additional examples arise in a number of applications where models of biological phenomena exist. For instance, studies of pharmacokinetic properties of drugs often focus on quantities such as the rate of drug metabolism as a function of applied dose. This relationship can frequently be described using simple differential equation models, the parameters of which are useful in summarizing characteristics of the drug. The *Michaelis–Menten* model is an example (Pinheiro and Bates, 2000). Other examples include models of carcinogenesis (Day, 1990) and of infectious disease spread (Becker, 1989). Techniques for estimation and inference for such models are reviewed in a number of books, including Seber and Wild (2003) and Bates and Watts (1988).

4. Special topics

4.1. Causal models

Regression models used to isolate the effect of a predictor or understand multiple predictors often have the implicit goal of assessing possible causal relationships with the outcome. The difficulties of achieving this goal are clearly recognized in epidemiology as in other fields relying on observational data: in particular the requirement that all confounders must have been measured and adequately adjusted for in the model. The superiority of experiments, including clinical trials, for determining causation stems from random assignment to treatment or experimental condition, more or less ensuring that all other determinants of the outcome are balanced across the treatment groups, and thus could not confound treatment assignment. In contrast, treatment actually received could be confounded; estimating the causal effect of treatment in trials with poor adherence poses problems similar to those posed by inherently observational data.

Propensity scores (Rosenbaum and Rubin, 1983) attempt to avoid potential difficulties in adequately adjusting for all confounders of a non-randomized treatment by adjusting instead for an estimate of the probability of receiving the treatment, given the full range of confounders (that is, the propensity score); related strategies are to stratify by or match on the scores (D'Agostino, 1998). Closely related *inverse probability of treatment weighted* (IPTW) models weight observations in inverse proportion to the estimated probability of the treatment actually received (Hernan et al., 2001; Robins et al., 2000). Propensity scores are most clearly an improvement over conventional regression adjustment when the outcome is binary and rare, limiting our ability to adjust adequately, but treatment is relatively common, so that the propensity score is relatively easy to model. However, this approach does not avoid the crucial requirement that all confounders are measured. Moreover, variability in the effect of treatment across levels of the propensity score, as well as gross dissimilarity between the treated and untreated subsamples, can invalidate the analysis (Kurth et al., 2005).

Instrumental variables are an alternative method for estimating causal effects from observational data (Greenland, 2000). An instrumental variable is associated with the treatment received, but uncorrelated with the outcome after controlling for treatment received. Because treatment assignment meets these criteria, instrumental variable arguments can be used to motivate a well-known estimator of the causal effect of treatment in trials with all-or-nothing adherence in which the observed treatment–control difference in the mean value of the outcome is inflated by the inverse of the proportion adherent. In observational settings, identification and validation of the instrumental variable is of course crucial. Chapter 2 by Rubin on causal effects provides a complete discussion of these issues.

4.2. Measurement error and misclassification

Data collected in many experimental and observational studies in epidemiology and medicine are based on measurements subject to error. Errors may occur in both the outcome and predictors of regression models, and may arise from a number of sources, including laboratory instruments and assays, medical devices and monitors, and from participant responses to survey questions. The presence of measurement error raises a legitimate concern that estimates from fitted regression models may be biased, and that associated inferences may be incorrect.

There is a wealth of published research on the impacts of measurement error in predictors in the context of linear models (Fuller, 1987). Most of this relies on the *classical error model*, in which the observed (and error prone) predictor W is related to the actual predictor X via the additive model

$$W = X + U, \tag{58}$$

in which U is a random variable with conditional (given X and other predictors measured without error) mean zero and variance σ_u^2. In the linear regression model (8) with a single predictor X, regression of the outcome Y on the error-contaminated W in Eq. (58) yields an attenuated estimate β^* of the true coefficient β, defined as $E[Y|X = x + 1] - E[Y|X = x]$. The degree of attenuation is described by the multiplicative factor

$$\frac{\sigma_\varepsilon^2}{\sigma_\varepsilon^2 + \sigma_u^2} < 1. \tag{59}$$

An additional impact of this type of measurement error is inflation of the residual variance of the outcome, resulting in reduced precision of estimates. In practice, the impact of measurement error in this context depends on a number of factors, including the nature of the assumed measurement error model, presence of additional predictors, and bias in W as an estimate of X.

In the case of non-linear models (e.g., generalized linear models with links other than the identity), the effects of measurement error are more complex than in the situation just described. Although these are usually manifested as attenuation in estimated coefficients and inflation of associated variances, the nature of the bias depends on the model, the type of parameter, and the assumed error model. The book by Carroll et al. (2006) provides broad coverage of this topic for non-linear models.

Measurement error can also occur in the outcome variable Y. In the case of linear models, this is generally handled via modifications of the conditional error distribution. Approaches for non-linear models are discussed in Carroll et al. (2006) and illustrated in Magder and Hughes (1997).

4.3. Missing data

For the medical services utilization example, consider a regression model for the effect of depression on the cost of care. It is possible that some subjects may have missing values for cost and/or depression, as measured by the BDI. The possible causes for these missing values could be missed visits or declining to fill out a sensitive item on a questionnaire. When the fact that the data are missing is related to the outcomes of interest, loss of efficiency or serious distortion of study results can occur. Therefore it is useful to classify the mechanism of missing data to understand these relationships and to inform analytic approaches. An exhaustive treatment is given by Little and Rubin (1986).

Denote the complete data as $\mathbf{Y}_{\text{full}}$. In the example, this would be the values of depression and cost of care on all subjects. The available values of cost and depression are denoted by $\mathbf{Y}_{\text{obs}}$ while the missing values are denoted as $\mathbf{Y}_{\text{miss}}$. The variable $\mathbf{R}_i$ indicates the pattern of missing data for subject i; in particular, $\mathbf{R}_i = (0,0)$ if both cost and BDI are available, (1, 0) if only cost is missing; (0, 1) if only BDI is missing; and (1, 1) if both are missing. Let $g(\mathbf{R};\gamma)$ denote the distribution of $\mathbf{R}$.

Missing data fall into three broad classes. Data are said to be *missing completely at random* (MCAR) if the distribution of $\mathbf{R}$ depends on neither $\mathbf{Y}_{\text{miss}}$ nor $\mathbf{Y}_{\text{obs}}$: that is, $g(\mathbf{R}|\mathbf{Y}_{\text{miss}}, Y_{\text{obs}}; \gamma) = g(\mathbf{R};\gamma)$. If the data are *missing at random* (MAR) the distribution of $\mathbf{R}$ does not depend on $\mathbf{Y}_{\text{miss}}$ after conditioning on $\mathbf{Y}_{\text{obs}}$. Formally, this implies that $g(\mathbf{R}|\mathbf{Y}_{\text{miss}}, \mathbf{Y}_{\text{obs}}; \gamma) = g(\mathbf{R}|\mathbf{Y}_{\text{obs}}; \gamma)$. Both of these are *ignorable* missing data mechanisms, in the sense, explained in more detail below, that we can consistently estimate the regression parameters of interest without loss of efficiency while ignoring $g(\mathbf{R}|\mathbf{Y}_{\text{obs}}; \gamma)$. Otherwise, the data are said to have a non-ignorable missing data mechanism, or to be missing not at random (MNAR).

It can be shown that if data are MCAR, then naive approaches which just delete observations with missing values (so-called complete case analyses) will yield unbiased estimates. However, this can be quite inefficient if the number of omitted observations is large. Further, the MCAR assumption is not credible in many practical situations. Fortunately, it can be shown that for data which are MAR, likelihood-based methods will yield correct inferences. This is because the likelihood

$$f(\mathbf{Y}_{\text{obs}}; \boldsymbol{\theta}) = \int f(\mathbf{Y}_{\text{obs}}, \mathbf{Y}_{\text{miss}}, \boldsymbol{\theta}) \mathrm{d}\mathbf{Y}_{\text{miss}} \tag{60}$$

is proportional to the full data log-likelihood

$$f(\mathbf{R}, \mathbf{Y}_{\text{obs}}; \boldsymbol{\theta}) = \int f(\mathbf{Y}_{\text{obs}}, \mathbf{Y}_{\text{miss}}, \boldsymbol{\theta}) g(\mathbf{R}|\mathbf{Y}, \mathbf{Y}_{\text{obs}}, \mathbf{Y}_{\text{miss}}; \gamma) \mathrm{d}\mathbf{Y}_{\text{miss}} \tag{61}$$

which under the MAR mechanism is then

$$\int f(\mathbf{Y}_{\text{obs}}, \mathbf{Y}_{\text{miss}}; \boldsymbol{\theta}) g(\mathbf{R}|\mathbf{Y}_{\text{obs}}; \gamma) \mathrm{d}\mathbf{Y}_{\text{miss}} \tag{62}$$

which simplifies to the observed data likelihood

$$f(\mathbf{Y}_{\text{obs}}, \boldsymbol{\theta}) g(\mathbf{R}|\mathbf{Y}_{\text{obs}}; \gamma) \tag{63}$$

Provided there are no common elements in the parameter vectors $\boldsymbol{\theta}$ and γ, we can safely maximize Eq. (60) while ignoring $g(\mathbf{R}|\mathbf{Y}_{\text{obs}}; \gamma)$. Many statistical approaches are likelihood-based and thus can easily handle MAR data without modeling the missing data mechanism.

In some cases, it is difficult to calculate or maximize the likelihood for the observed data; however, it would be easy to calculate the likelihood estimates for the complete data. In such cases, the EM algorithm (Dempster et al., 1977) is a useful approach to ML estimation. The EM algorithm alternates between an E (expectation) step and an M (maximization) step. In the E-step, we calculate the expected values of the sufficient statistics (i.e., the data or data summaries) of the complete data log-likelihood, conditional on the observed data and current parameter estimates. Then in the M-step the parameters of the complete data log-likelihood are maximized, using the expected values from the E-step. The algorithm is iterated to convergence and produces parameter estimates which can be shown to maximize the observed data log-likelihood.

To see how the EM algorithm might work, consider the exponential AFT model for censored survival times presented in Section 3.2. When the survival times are censored, the observed data consist of ($\mathbf{Y}$, $\boldsymbol{\Delta}$, $\mathbf{X}$), where $Y_i = T_i$, the actual survival time, only for uncensored subjects (i.e. $\Delta_i = 1$), and $\mathbf{X}$ is the familiar matrix of predictors. In contrast, the full data are just ($\mathbf{T}$, $\mathbf{X}$). The log-likelihood for the full data is

$$\sum_{i=1}^{n} \log \lambda + \mathbf{x}_i'\boldsymbol{\beta} - \lambda T_i \exp(\mathbf{x}_i'\boldsymbol{\beta}) \tag{64}$$

The more complicated log-likelihood for the observed data, Eq. (46), could be maximized by repeated maximization of Eq. (64) using the EM algorithm. In the pth iteration of the E-step, we calculate $\widetilde{\mathbf{T}}^{(p)}$, the expected value of $\mathbf{T}$, given the observed data and the current parameter estimates $(\hat{\lambda}^{(p)}, \hat{\boldsymbol{\beta}}^{(p)})$. Under the exponential AFT,

$$\begin{aligned} \widetilde{T}_i^{(p)} &= E\left(T_i | Y_i, \Delta_i, \mathbf{x}_i; \hat{\lambda}^{(p)}, \hat{\boldsymbol{\beta}}^{(p)}\right) \\ &= \begin{cases} Y_i & \Delta_i = 1 \\ Y_i + \exp\left(-\mathbf{x}_i'\hat{\boldsymbol{\beta}}^{(p)}\right)/\hat{\lambda}^{(p)} & \Delta_i = 0 \end{cases} \end{aligned} \tag{65}$$

In the pth iteration of the M-step, updated parameter estimates $(\hat{\lambda}^{(p+1)}, \hat{\boldsymbol{\beta}}^{(p+1)})$ are obtained by maximizing Eq. (64) over the parameters, using $\widetilde{\mathbf{T}}^{(p)}$ in place of $\mathbf{T}$. The two-step algorithm is iterated to convergence, yielding estimates $(\hat{\lambda}_{em}, \hat{\boldsymbol{\beta}}_{em})$ that maximize Eq. (46).

An alternative approach is to augment the data by *multiple imputation* (Rubin, 1987; Schafer, 1999). In this method, we sample the missing values from $f\{\mathbf{Y}_{\text{full}}|\mathbf{Y}_{\text{obs}}\}$, resulting in several "completed" datasets, each of which is analyzed using complete-data methods. Summary parameter estimates are found by averaging over the estimates from each of the imputations; in addition, the averaged standard errors are inflated by a function of the between-imputation variability in the parameter estimates, to reflect that fact that some of the data are imputed, not observed, and thus only known approximately. This approach can be used in settings where the E-step is difficult to calculate analytically, as well as in MNAR problems where the missingness mechanism can be specified.

Many techniques discussed in this chapter (e.g., generalized estimating equations) are not likelihood based. Robins et al. (1994) proposed an approach in which an explicit model for the missingness is postulated. Weights inversely proportional to the estimated probability that each subject is observed are then incorporated explicitly in the analysis. This approach is adapted from classic methods for survey sampling developed by Horvitz and Thompson (1952). By incorporating the inverse weights, non-likelihood based methods such as GEE are valid for MAR data.

Analysis of MNAR data requires detailed specification of the missing data mechanism. Two alternative approaches stem from different decompositions of the full-data likelihood. The decomposition Eq. (61) represents a so-called selection model (Little, 1995), because the missingness or selection mechanism is specified by $g(\mathbf{R}|\mathbf{Y}_{\text{obs}},\mathbf{Y}_{\text{miss}};\gamma)$; results are known to be sensitive to this specification (Kenward, 1998). Under the alternative *pattern mixture model*, the complete data likelihood is decomposed as

$$f(\mathbf{R},\mathbf{Y}_{\text{obs}};\boldsymbol{\theta}) = \int f^*(\mathbf{Y}_{\text{obs}},\mathbf{Y}_{\text{miss}}|\mathbf{R};\boldsymbol{\theta}^*)g^*(\mathbf{R};\gamma^*)\mathrm{d}\mathbf{Y}_{\text{miss}} \qquad (66)$$

(Little, 1993). In this case summary parameter estimates are weighted averages over the various missing data patterns. The two strategies are closely related but pattern mixture models typically are more computationally feasible (Schafer and Graham, 2002).

As an example of the pattern mixture model, consider a randomized placebo-controlled trial of clopidogrel, an antiplatelet agent, administered in the first 24 hours following a mild stroke. One objective of the trial is to assess the effect of clopidogrel on cognitive function, as measured by the Digit Symbols Substitution Test (DSST). The DSST will be administered at enrollment, 1 month, and 3 months. Denote the DSST values for subject i by $\mathbf{Y}_i' = (Y_{0i}, Y_{1i}, Y_{2i})$. Pattern mixture models specify the distribution of $\mathbf{Y}$ conditional on the pattern of missing data. Nearly all subjects will have a baseline DSST, so missing data will involve missing values of Y_1 and Y_2. We again denote patterns of missing data by $\mathbf{R}_i$, the vector of missing data indicators, with values (0, 1, 0), (0, 0, 1), or (0, 1, 1), when the second, third, or both follow-up DSST values are missing, respectively. We index those three patterns of missing data as $M = 1, 2, 3$, respectively; subjects with complete data (i.e., $R = (0, 0, 0)$) are indexed as pattern $M = 0$.

Then the pattern mixture model is the product of a multinomial model for M and a model for $f(\mathbf{Y}|\mathbf{M})$. One possibility might be to estimate $\mu = E(\mathbf{Y})$ and $\boldsymbol{\Sigma} = \text{cov}(\mathbf{Y})$, the mean and variance of $\mathbf{Y}$, the first of which can be expressed as

$$\mu = \sum_{m=0}^{3} \mu^{(m)} P(M = m). \tag{67}$$

where $\boldsymbol{\mu}^{(m)} = E(Y|M = m)$. The pattern mixture approach obtains MLEs of $\boldsymbol{\mu}$ through likelihood-based estimates of the parameters of the mixture model (68).

The MLEs of $P(M = m)$ are just the observed frequencies of the missing data patterns. However, the parameters $\boldsymbol{\mu}^{(m)}$ are under-identified by this model. For instance, there are no data on Y_2 in the subsample with $M = 2$, so $\mu_2^{(2)} = E(\mathrm{Y}_2|\mathrm{M} = 2)$ cannot be estimated. To estimate all parameters, *identifying restrictions* must be imposed. For example, we might assume that the trend over time is the same for $M = 2$ as for $M = 1$. Other potential restrictions encompass the familiar MCAR and MAR assumptions; if the data are MCAR, the parameterization is simplified because $\boldsymbol{\mu}^{(m)}$ and $\boldsymbol{\Sigma}^{(m)}$ are identical for all patterns. It is also possible to specify pattern mixture models which allow for more general ignorable and non-ignorable missingness mechanisms (Little, 1993). An important advantage of these models, especially compared with selection models, is the fact that the identifying restrictions are explicitly specified. Furthermore, the likelihoods for these models are straightforward to maximize as compared to those for selection models.

The weighting approach described earlier can also be applied to MNAR data; see Bang and Robins (2005) for a review. This approach is related to selection models, but handles missingness using a weighted analysis. As before, data points are weighted in inverse proportion to the estimated probability of being observed. Approaches such as these are discussed more fully in Chapter 2 of this volume, which deals with causal inference.

4.4. Computing

Regression problems have been one of the major driving forces in many of the recent advances in numerical computing. Books by Gentle (2005), Monahan (2001), and Thisted (1988) cover many of these, and provide details on computational techniques used in many of the methods covered here.

The continued expansion in the number of software tools to perform statistical analyses coupled with increases in the processing speed and capacity of modern computer hardware has made what were once considered insurmountable tasks practical even for many desktop machines. Major commercial statistical software packages with extensive facilities for many of the regression methods described here include SAS (SAS Institute Inc., 2005), Stata (StataCorp LP., 2005), SPSS (SPSS Inc., 2006), and S-PLUS (Insightful Corporation, 2006). The R statistical programming language (R Development Core Team, 2005) is public domain software most similar to S-PLUS. Despite substantial overlap in regression-oriented features, these packages are quite different in terms of programming

Table 1
Regression features of several major statistical software packages

Regression Technique	SAS	Stata	SPSS	S-PLUS	R
Linear	X	X	X	X	X
Generalized linear	X	X	X	X	X
Non-linear	X	X	X	X	X
Mixed effects linear	X	X	X	X	X
Mixed effects non-linear	X	X	–	X	X
Non-parametric	X	X	–	X	X

style and user interface. SAS, SPSS, and Stata have generally more developed and "user friendly" interfaces, while S-PLUS and R are more akin to interpreted programming languages that provide many "canned" procedures, but also allow great flexibility in user-defined functions (including support for linking with external routines written in compiled languages such as C and FORTRAN).

Table 1 summarizes capabilities for many of the methods covered here. Although all offer similar features for standard regression methods and generalized linear models, the depth of coverage of more specialized techniques varies considerably. In the area of mixed-effects regression, the *MIXED* and *NLMIXED* procedures in SAS are more fully featured than competitors. Stata is distinguished by the implementation of generalized estimating equation and robust variance methods as an option with most of the included regression commands. In addition, methods for bootstrap, jackknife, and permutation testing are implemented in a very accessible way. Because of their extensibility and the availability of a large range of procedures written by researchers, S-PLUS and R tend to have more functionality in the areas of non-parametric regression, smoothing methods, alternative variable selection procedures, and approaches for dealing with missing data and measurement error.

In addition to the major packages covered here, there are a number of specialized software offerings that target particular regression methods or related numerical computations. These include CART (Steinberg and Colla, 1995) software for classification and regression tree methods and the LogXact (Mehta and Patel, 1996) program for exact logistic regression. Additional packages that focus more generally on numerical computation, but that also provide more limited regression capabilities (and also support user-defined regression functions) include Matlab (MathWorks, 2006), Mathematica (Wolfram Research Inc., 2005), and Maple (Maplesoft, 2003).

References

Altman, D.G., Andersen, P.K. (1989). Bootstrap investigation of the stability of the Cox regression model. *Statistics in Medicine* **8**, 771–783.

Altman, D.G., Royston, P. (2000). What do we mean by validating a prognostic model? *Statistics in Medicine* **19**, (453–473.

Bang, H., Robins, J.M. (2005). Doubly robust estimation in missing data and causal inference models. *Biometrics* **61**, 962–973.

Bates, D., Watts, D. (1988). *Nonlinear Regression Analysis and its Applications*. Wiley, Chichester, New York.

Becker, N. (1989). *Analysis of Infectious Disease Data*. Chapman & Hall/CRC, London.

Begg, M.D., Lagakos, S. (1993). Loss in efficiency caused by omitted covariates and misspecifying exposure in logistic regression models. *Journal of the American Statistical Association* **88**(421), 166–170.

Breiman, L. (1995). Better model selection using the nonnegative garrote. *Technometrics* **37**, 373–384.

Breiman, L. (2001). Statistical modeling: The two cultures. *Statistical Science* **16**(3), 199–231.

Breiman, L., Friedman, J.H., Olshen, R.A., and Stone, C.J. (1984). *Classification and Regression Trees*. Statistics/Probability Series. Wadsworth Publishing Company, Belmont, CA.

Carroll, R., Rupprt, D., Stefanski, L., Crainiceanu, C. (2006). *Measurement Error in Nonlinear Models: A Modern Perspective*, 2nd ed. Chapman & Hall/CRC, London.

Cleveland, W.S. (1981). Lowess: A program for smoothing scatterplots by robust locally weighted regression. *The American Statistician* **35**, 45–54.

Concato, J., Peduzzi, P., Holfold, T.R. (1995). Importance of events per independent variable in proportional hazards analysis. I. background, goals, and general strategy. *Journal of Clinical Epidemiology* **48**, 1495–1501.

Cook, R.D. (1977). Detection of influential observations in linear regression. *Technometrics* **19**, 15–18.

Cox, D.R., Hinkley, D.V. (1974). *Theoretical Statistics*. Chapman & Hall, London, New York.

D'Agostino, R.B. (1998). Propensity score methods for bias reduction in the comparison of a treatment to a non-randomized control group. *Statistics in Medicine* **17**, 2265–2281.

Day, N. (1990). The Armitage-Doll multistage model of carcinogenesis. *Statistics in Medicine* **83**, 677–689.

Dempster, A.P., Laird, N., Rubin, D. (1977). Maximum-likelihood from incomplete data via the em algorithm. *Journal of the Royal Statistical Society, Series B* **39**(1–38).

Diggle, P., Heagerty, P., Liang, K.-Y., Zeger, S.L. (2002). *Analysis of Longitudinal Data*, 2nd ed. Oxford University Press, Oxford.

Efron, B. (1986). Estimating the error rate of a prediction rule: Improvement on cross-validation. *Journal of the American Statistical Association* **81**, 316–331.

Fuller, W. (1987). *Measurement Error Models*, 2nd ed. Wiley, New York.

Gail, M.H., Tan, W.Y., Piantodosi, S. (1988). Tests for no treatment effect in randomized clinical trials. *Biometrika* **75**, 57–64.

Gail, M.H., Wieand, S., Piantodosi, S. (1984). Biased estimates of treatment effect in randomized experiments with nonlinear regressions and omitted covariates. *Biometrika* **71**, 431–444.

Gentle, J. (2005). *Elements of Computational Statistics*, 1st ed. Springer, New York.

Graf, E., Schmoor, C., Sauerbrei, W., Schumacher, M. (1999). Assessment and comparison of prognostic classification schemes for survival data. *Statistics in Medicine* **18**, 2529–2545.

Greenhouse, S.W., Geisser, S. (1959). On methods in the analysis of profile data. *Psychometrika* **32**, 95–112.

Greenland, S. (1989). Modeling and variable selection in epidemiologic analysis. *American Journal of Public Health* **79**(3), 340–349.

Greenland, S. (2000). An introduction to instrumental variables for epidemiologists. *International Journal of Epidemiology* **29**, 722–729.

Hankey, B.F., Feuer, E.J., Clegg, L.X., Hayes, R.B., Legler, J.M., Prorok, P.C., Ries, L.A., Merrill, R.M., Kaplan, R.S. (1999). Cancer surveillance series: Interpreting trends in prostate Cancer. Part I: Evidence of the effects of screening in recent prostate cancer incidence, mortality, and survival rates. *Journal of the National Cancer Institute* **91**, 1017–1024.

Harrell, F.E., Lee, K.L., Mark, D.B. (1996). Multivariable prognostic models: Issues in developing models, evaluating assumptions and adequacy, and measuring and reducing errors. *Statistics in Medicine* **15**, 361–387.

Hastie, T., Tibshirani, R. (1990). *Generalized Additive Models*. Chapman & Hall, New York.

Hastie, T., Tibshirani, R., Friedman, J.H. (2001). *The Elements of Statistical Learning: Data Mining, Inference, and Prediction*. Springer, New York.

Hauck, W.W., Anderson, S., Marcus, S.M. (1998). Should we adjust for covariates in nonlinear regression analyses of randomized trials? *Controlled Clinical Trials* **19**, 249–256.

Henderson, R., Oman, P. (1999). Effect of frailty on marginal regression estimates in survival analysis. *Journal of the Royal Statistical Society, Series B, Methodological* **61**, 367–379.

Hernan, M.A., Brumback, B., Robins, J.M. (2001). Marginal structural models to estimate the joint causal effect of nonrandomized treatments. *Journal of the American Statistical Association* **96**, 440–448.

Hoenig, J.M., Heisey, D.M. (2001). The abuse of power: The pervasive fallacy of power calculations for data analysis. *The American Statistician* **55**(1), 19–24.

Hoerl, A.E., Kennard, R.W. (1970). Ridge regression: Biased estimates for nonorthogonal problems. *Technometrics* **12**, 55–67.

Hofer, T., Hayward, R., Greenfield, S., Wagner, E., Kaplan, S., Manning, W. (1999). The unreliability of individual physician "report cards" for assessing the costs and quality of care of a chronic disease. *Journal of the American Medical Association* **281**, 2098–2105.

Horvitz, D.G., Thompson, D.J. (1952). A generalization of sampling without replacement from a finite universe. *Journal of the American Statistical Association* **47**, 663–685.

Huber, P.J. (1967). The behaviour of maximum likelihood estimates under nonstandard conditions. In: Le Cam, L., Neyman, J. (Eds.), *The Fifth Berkeley Symposium in Mathematical Statistics and Probability*. University of California Press, Berkeley.

Insightful Corporation. (2006). *S-PLUS version 7.0 for Windows*. Seattle, Washington.

Jin, Z., Lin, D.Y., Wei, L.J., Ying, Z. (2003). Rank-based inference for the accelerated failure time model. *Biometrika* **90**, 341–353.

Kauermann, G., Carroll, R.J. (2001). A note on the efficiency of sandwich covariance matrix estimation. *Journal of the American Statistical Association* **96**(456), 1387–1396.

Kenward, M.G. (1998). Selection models for repeated measurements with non-random dropout: An illustration of sensitivity. *Statistics in Medicine* **17**, 2723–2732.

Kenward, M.G., Roger, J.H. (1997). Small sample inference for fixed effects from restricted maximum likelihood. *Biometrics* **53**, 983–997.

Kurth, T., Walker, A.M., Glynn, R.J., Chan, K.A., Gaziano, J.M., Berger, K., Robins, J.M. (2005). Results of multivariable logistic regression, propensity matching, propensity adjustment, and propensity-based weighting under conditions of nonuniform effect. *American Journal of Epidemiology* **163**, 262–270.

Lagakos, S.W., Schoenfeld, D.A. (1984). Properties of proportional-hazards score tests under misspecified regression models. *Biometrics* **40**, 1037–1048.

Larsen, W.A., McCleary, S.J. (1972). The use of partial residual plots in regression analysis. *Technometrics* **14**, 781–790.

Le Cessie, S., Van Houwelingen, J.C. (1992). Ridge estimators in logistic regression. *Applied Statistics* **41**, 191–201.

Lin, D.Y., Geyer, C.J. (1992). Computational methods for semiparametric linear regression with censored data. *Journal of Computational and Graphical Statistics* **1**, 77–90.

Little, R.J.A. (1993). Pattern-mixture models for multivariate incomplete data. *Journal of the American Statistical Association* **88**, 125–134.

Little, R.J.A. (1995). Modeling the drop-out mechanism in longitudinal studies. *Journal of the American Statistical Association* **90**, 1112–1121.

Little, R.J.A., Rubin, D.B. (1986). *Statistical Analysis with Missing Data*. Wiley, New York.

Long, J.S., Ervin, L.H. (2000). Using heteroscedasticity consistent standard errors in the linear regression model. *The American Statistician* **54**, 217–224.

MacKinnon, J.G., White, H. (1985). Some heteroskedasticity consistent covariance matrix estimators with improved finite sample properties. *Journal of Econometrics* **29**, 53–57.

Magder, L., Hughes, J. (1997). Logistic regression when the outcome is measured with uncertainty. *American Journal of Epidemiology* **146**, 195–203.

Maldonado, G., Greenland, S. (1993). Simulation study of confounder-selection strategies. *American Journal of Epidemiology* **138**, 923–936.

Maplesoft. (2003). *Maple 9 Getting Started Guide.* Waterloo, ON, Canada.

Masson, C., Sorensen, J., Phibbs, C., Okin, R. (2004). Predictors of medical service utilization among individuals with co-occurring HIV infection and substance abuse disorders. *AIDS Care* **16**(6), 744–755.

MathWorks. (2006). *MATLAB version 7.2.* Natick, MA.

McCulloch, C.E. (2005). Repeated measures ANOVA, R.I.P.? *Chance* **18**, 29–33.

McCulloch, C.E., Searle, S.R. (2000). *Generalized, Linear, and Mixed Models.* Wiley, Chichester, New York.

Mehta, C., Patel, N. (1996). *LogXact for Windows.* Cytel Software Corporation, Cambridge, MA.

Mickey, R.M., Greenland, S. (1989). The impact of confounder selection on effect estimation. *American Journal of Epidemiology* **129**(1), 125–137.

Monahan, J. (2001). *Numerical Methods of Statistics*, 1st ed. Cambridge University Press, Cambridge.

Neuhaus, J. (1998). Estimation efficiency with omitted covariates in generalized linear models. *Journal of the American Statistical Association* **93**, 1124–1129.

Neuhaus, J., Jewell, N.P. (1993). A geometric approach to assess bias due to omitted covariates in generalized linear models. *Biometrika* **80**, 807–815.

Normand, S.-L.T., Glickman, M.E., Gatsonis, C.A. (1997). Statistical methods for profiling providers of medical care: Issues and applications. *Journal of the American Statistical Association* **92**, 803–814.

Peduzzi, P., Concato, J., Feinstein, A.R. (1995). Importance of events per independent variable in proportional hazards regression analysis. II. Accuracy and precision of regression estimates. *Journal of Clinical Epidemiology* **48**, 1503–1510.

Peduzzi, P., Concato, J., Kemper, E., Holford, T.R., Feinstein, A.R. (1996). A simulation study of the number of events per variable in logistic regression analysis. *Journal of Clinical Epidemiology* **49**, 1373–1379.

Pinheiro, J., Bates, D. (2000). *Mixed-effects models in S and S-PLUS.* Springer, New York.

R Development Core Team. 2005. *R: A Language and Environment for Statistical Computing.* R Foundation for Statistical Computing, Vienna, Austria. ISBN 3-900051-07-0.

Robins, J.M., Hernan, M.A., Brumback, B. (2000). Marginal structural models and causal inference in epidemiology. *Epidemiology* **11**, 550–560.

Robins, J.M., Rotnitzky, A., Zhao, L.P. (1994). Estimation of regression coefficients when some regressors are not always observed. *Journal of the American Statistical Association* **89**, 846–866.

Rosenbaum, P.R., Rubin, D.B. (1983). The central role of the propensity score in observational studies for causal effects. *Biometrika* **70**, 41–55.

Rubin, D.B. (1987). *Multiple Imputation for Nonresponse in Surveys.* Wiley, Chichester, New York.

SAS Institute Inc. (2005). *SAS/STAT Software, Version 9.* Cary, NC.

Schafer, J.L. (1999). Multiple imputation: A primer. *Statistical Methods in Medical Research* **8**, 3–15.

Schafer, J.L., Graham, J.W. (2002). Missing data: Our view of the state of the art. *Psychological Methods* **7**, 147–177.

Schmoor, C., Schumacher, M. (1997). Effects of covariate omission and categorization when analysing randomized trials with the Cox model. *Statistics in Medicine* **16**, 225–237.

Searle, S.R., Casella, G., McCulloch, C.E. (1992). *Variance Components.* Wiley, Chichester, New York.

Seber, G., Wild, C. (2003). *Nonlinear Regression*, 2nd ed. Wiley, Chichester, New York.

Sorensen, J., Dilley, J., London, J., Okin, R., Delucchi, K., Phibbs, C. (2003). Case management for substance abusers with HIV/AIDS: A randomized clinical trial. *The American Journal of Drug And Alcohol Abuse* **29**, 133–150.

SPSS Inc. (2006). *SPSS for Windows, Rel. 14.0.* Chicago, IL.

StataCorp LP. (2005). *Stata Statistical Software: Release 9.* College Station, TX.

Steinberg, D., Colla, P. (1995). *CART: Tree-Structured Nonparametric Data Analysis.* Salford Systems, San Diego, CA.

Steyerberg, E.W., Eijkemans, M.J.C., Habbema, J.D.F. (1999). Stepwise selection in small datasets: a simulation study of bias in logistic regression analysis. *Journal of Clinical Epidemiology* **52**, 935–942.

Sun, G.W., Shook, T.L., Kay, G.L. (1999). Inappropriate use of bivariable analysis to screen risk factors for use in multivariable analysis. *Journal of Clinical Epidemiology* **49**, 907–916.

Takeuchi, M., Igarashi, Y., Tomimoto, S., Odake, M., Hayashi, T., Tsukamoto, T., Hata, K., Takaoka, H., Fukuzaki, H. (1991). Single-beat estimation of the slope of end-systolic pressure-volume relation in the human left ventricle. *Circulation* **83**, 202–212.

Thisted, R. (1988). *Elements of Statistical Computing: Numerical Computation*, 1st ed. Chapman & Hall, New York.

Tibshirani, R. (1997). The LASSO method for variable selection in the Cox model. *Statistics in Medicine* **16**, 385–395.

Verweij, P.J.M., Van Houwelingen, H.C. (1994). Penalized likelihood in Cox regression. *Statistics in Medicine* **13**, 2427–2436.

Vittinghoff, E., McCulloch, C.E. (2007). Relaxing the rule of ten events per variable in logistic and Cox regression. *American Journal of Epidemiology* **165**(6), 710–718.

Wei, L.J. (1992). The accelerated failure time model: A useful alternative to the Cox regression model in survival analysis. *Statistics in Medicine* **11**, 1871–1879.

Welsch, R.E. (1982). Influence functions and regression diagnostics. In: Launer, R.L., Siegel, A.F. (Eds.), *Modern Data Analysis*. Academic Press, New York, pp. 149–169.

Welsch, R.E., Kuh, E. (1977). Linear Regression Diagnostics. Technical report 923-77, Sloan School of Management, Massachusetts Insititute of Technology, Cambridge, MA.

White, H. (1980). A heteroskedastic-consistent covariance matrix estimator and a direct test of heteroskedasticity. *Econometrica* **48**, 817–838.

Wolfram Research Inc. (2005). *Mathematica Version 5.2*. Champaign, IL.

Handbook of Statistics, Vol. 27
ISSN: 0169-7161

DOI: 10.1016/S0169-7161(07)27006-3

6

Logistic Regression

Edward L. Spitznagel Jr.

Abstract

This chapter provides an introduction to logistic regression, which is a powerful modeling tool paralleling ordinary least squares (OLS) regression. The difference between the two is that logistic regression models categorical rather than numeric outcomes. First, the case of a binary or dichotomous outcome will be considered. Then the cases of unordered and ordered outcomes with more than two categories will be covered. In all three cases, the method of maximum likelihood replaces the method of least squares as the criterion by which the models are fitted to the data. Additional topics include the method of exact logistic regression for the case in which the maximum likelihood method does not converge, probit regression, and the use of logistic regression for analysis of case–control data.

1. Introduction

Logistic regression is a modeling tool in which the dependent variable is categorical. In most applications, the dependent variable is binary. However, it can have three or more categories, which can be ordered or unordered. Except for the nature of the dependent variable, logistic regression closely resembles ordinary least squares (OLS) regression.

A comparison with OLS regression can lead to a better understanding of logistic regression. In both types of regression, the fitted models consist of intercept and slope coefficients. In OLS regression, the fitting criterion is the principle of least squares. In least squares, the intercept and slope coefficients are chosen to minimize the sum of squared deviations of the dependent variable's values from the values given by the regression equation. In logistic regression, the fitting criterion is the principle of maximum likelihood. In maximum likelihood, the intercept and slope coefficients are chosen to maximize the probability of obtaining the observed data. For OLS regression, the principles of maximum likelihood and least squares coincide if the assumptions of normality, equal variance, and independence are satisfied. Therefore, the use of maximum likelihood for logistic regression can be regarded as a natural extension of the fitting method used in OLS regression.

In OLS regression, the model coefficients can be estimated by solving a system of linear equations, called the *normal* equations. In logistic regression, there is no counterpart to the normal equations. Model coefficients are estimated by searching iteratively for the values that maximize the likelihood. Modern software usually finds the maximum in less than a half dozen iterative steps.

In OLS regression, hypotheses about coefficients are tested by using sums of squared deviations to compute test statistics known as F ratios. In logistic regression, hypotheses about coefficients are tested by using likelihoods to compute test statistics known as likelihood ratio χ^2.

In both OLS and logistic regression, every coefficient estimate has an associated standard error. In the case of OLS regression, these standard errors can be used to perform Student's t-tests on the coefficients and to compute t-based confidence intervals. In logistic regression, these standard errors can be used to perform approximate Z (or χ^2) tests on the coefficients and to compute approximate Z-based confidence intervals.

2. Estimation of a simple logistic regression model

The example below illustrates how these ideas are used in logistic regression. Consider an experiment in which disease-vector mosquitoes are exposed to 9 different levels of insecticide, 50 mosquitoes per dose level, with the results shown in Table 1.

In Fig. 1, the vertical axis shows the number killed at each dose level, from 1 at the lowest level to 50 at the highest level. Owing to the curvature at the low and high levels of insecticide, a straight line produced by a linear function will not give an adequate fit to this data. In fact, a straight line would imply that for very low doses of insecticide, the number of kills would be less than 0, and for very high doses of insecticide, the number of kills would be larger than the number of mosquitoes exposed to the dose.

The natural bounds on the probability of kill, 0 and 1, constrain the model so that no linear function can adequately describe the probability. However, we can solve this problem by replacing probability with a function that has no lower or upper bounds. First, if we replace probability with odds ($=p/(1-p)$), we open up the range on the upper end to $+\infty$. The lower end remains at 0, and

Table 1
Relationship between insecticide dose and number of mosquitoes killed

Dosage	1	2	3	4	5	6	7	8	9
Mosquitoes	50	50	50	50	50	50	50	50	50
Killed	1	2	4	17	26	39	42	48	50

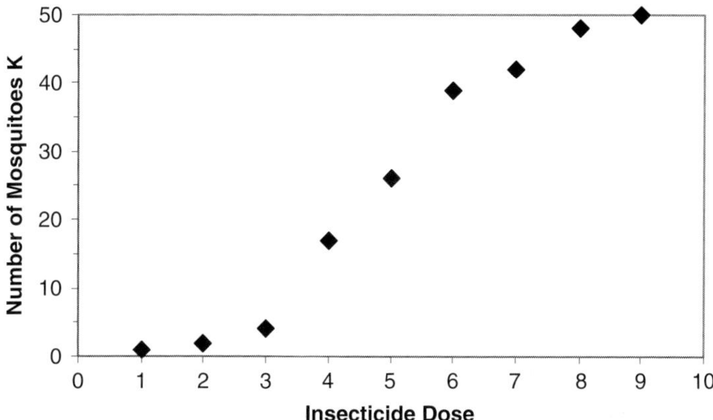

Fig. 1. Graph of proportion killed as a function of insecticide dose.

probability = 1/2 corresponds to odds of 1. To open up the range on the lower end and symmetrize it at the same time, we can take the natural logarithm of odds, known as the *logit* function, $\ln(p/(1-p))$. When p ranges from 0 to 1, the logit function ranges from $-\infty$ to $+\infty$, in symmetric fashion. The logit of 1/2 is equal to 0. The logits of complementary probabilities, such as 1/3 and 2/3, have the same size but opposite signs: $\pm\ln(2) = \pm 0.693$.

Using the SAS LOGISTIC procedure (SAS Institute Inc., 2004), we obtain the following output estimating the logit as a linear function of dose:

Parameter	df	Estimate	Standard Error	χ^2	$Pr > \chi^2$
Intercept	1	−5.0870	0.4708	116.7367	<0.0001
Dose	1	1.0343	0.0909	129.3662	<0.0001

The estimated log-odds of death is

$$\text{logit} = -5.0870 + 1.0343 \times \text{dose}.$$

From this formula we can estimate the probability of mosquito death for any dose level, including but not limited to the actual doses in the experiment. Suppose, for example, that we would like to know the probability (= expected fraction) of insect kill with 6.5 units of insecticide. The estimated logit is $-5.0870 + 1.0343 \times 6.5 = 1.636$. To convert into probability, we reverse the two steps that took us from probability to the logit. First, we exponentiate base-e to convert to odds: $\exp(1.636) = 5.135$. Second, we convert odds to probability by the formula $p = \text{odds}/(\text{odds}+1)$: $5.135/6.135 = 0.8346$. Thus, with a 6.5 unit dose, we expect 83.46% of insects to be killed. Figure 2 demonstrates the close agreement between actual numbers killed and the computed probabilities multiplied by 50.

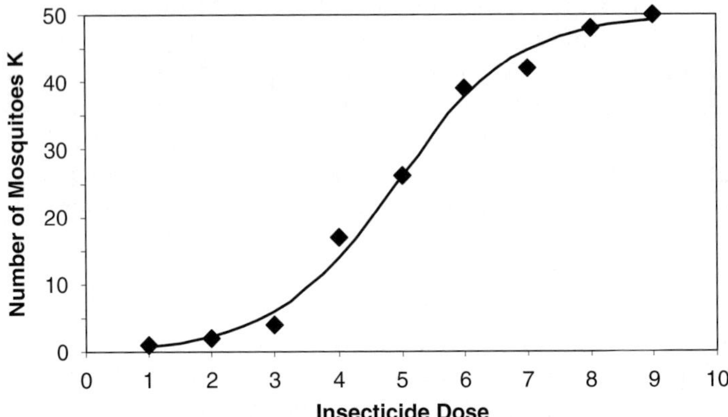

Fig. 2. Logistic regression curve fitted to insecticide lethality data.

The coefficient of dose, 1.0343, estimates the increase in log-odds per unit of dose. The exponential of this number, $\exp(1.0343) = 2.813$, estimates the multiplicative increase in odds of insect death per unit of dose. This value is called the *odds ratio*. It is the most commonly used number in logistic regression results, usually reported along with approximate 95% confidence limits. These limits can be obtained by adding and subtracting 1.96 standard errors from the slope estimate, then exponentiating: $\exp(1.0343 \pm 1.96 \times 0.0909) = (2.354, 3.362)$. Most statistics packages will compute both odds ratios and confidence limits, either automatically or as options.

If we divide the coefficient 1.0343 by its standard error, 0.0909, we obtain the value of an asymptotically standard normal test statistic $Z = 1.0343/0.0909 = 11.38$ for testing the null hypothesis that the true value of the slope is equal to 0. Some statistics packages report the square of this statistic, $11.38^2 = 129.4$ in the table above, which has an asymptotic χ^2 distribution with 1 df, and is called a *Wald* χ^2. The *p*-value will be the same, whichever statistic is used.

As we discussed earlier, estimation of a logistic regression model is achieved through the principle of maximum likelihood, which can be thought of as a generalization of the least squares principle of linear regression. In maximum likelihood estimation, we search over all values of intercept and slope until we reach the point where the likelihood of obtaining the observed data is largest. This occurs when the intercept is -5.0870 and the slope is 1.0343. This maximized likelihood is very small, 3.188×10^{-67}. Such small values are typical in maximum likelihood calculations. Accordingly, in lieu of the likelihood itself, most statistical software reports the natural logarithm of the likelihood, which in our case is $\ln(3.188 \times 10^{-67}) = -153.114$.

Besides being the means of estimating the logistic regression coefficients, the likelihood also furnishes us a means of testing hypotheses about the model. If we wish to test the null hypothesis of no relationship between dose and insect mortality, we re-fit the model with the slope coefficient constrained equal to 0.

Doing so produces an intercept estimate of 0.0356 and the smaller log-likelihood of −311.845. To compare the two models, we multiply the difference in log-likelihoods by 2, $2 \times (-153.114 - (-311.845)) = 2 \times 158.731 = 317.462$. If the null hypothesis being tested is true, we would have an asymptotic χ^2 distribution with degrees of freedom equal to the number of coefficient constraints, which in this case equals 1. This is known as a *likelihood ratio* χ^2, as it is equal to twice the log of the ratio of the two likelihoods, unconstrained to constrained.

Taking advantage of the analogy with OLS, the likelihood ratio χ^2 value of 317.462 is the counterpart of the *F*-ratio obtained by computing sums of squares with and without constraints, whereas the earlier values of $Z = 11.38$ and the Wald χ^2 $Z^2 = 129.4$, are the counterparts of Student's *t* and its square, computed by comparing a coefficient estimate with its standard error. In the case of OLS, the two different computations give identical and exact results. In the case of maximum likelihood, the two different computations give different, and asymptotic, rather than exact results. Ordinarily, we would expect the two different χ^2 to be approximately equal. The primary reason for the large difference between them is the strength of the dose–mortality relationship. Should it ever happen that the likelihood ratio and Wald χ^2 lead to opposite conclusions in a hypothesis test, the likelihood ratio χ^2 is usually preferred.

3. Two measures of model fit

In our example, both χ^2 test statistics provide strong evidence of the relationship between dose and mortality, but they do not provide an estimate of how strong the relationship is. The reason is that test statistics in general depend on sample size (if the null hypothesis of no relationship is false). In OLS regression, the coefficient of determination, R^2, is the most commonly used measure of the strength of relationship. For maximum likelihood estimation, Cox and Snell (1989) proposed an analog of R^2 computed from the likelihood ratio χ^2:

$$\text{Cox}-\text{Snell } R^2 = 1 - \exp(-\chi^2/n) = 1 - \exp(-317.462/450) = 0.5061.$$

Nagelkerke (1991) pointed out that, in the case of discrete models such as logistic regression, the maximum value possible with this definition will be less than 1. He proposed that the Cox–Snell R^2 be divided by its maximum possible value, to produce a closer analog of the R^2 of least-squares regression. In our example, the Nagelkerke $R^2 = 0.6749$. Both Cox–Snell and Nagelkerke R^2 values are readily available in most statistics packages.

Logistic regression also has a direct and natural measure of relationship strength called the coefficient of concordance *C*. It stems from the purpose of logistic regression, to estimate probabilities of an outcome from one or more independent variables. The coefficient of concordance measures the fraction of pairs with different outcomes in which the predicted probabilities are consistent with the outcomes. For a pair of mosquitoes, one dead and the other alive, if the calculated probability of death for the dead mosquito is greater than the

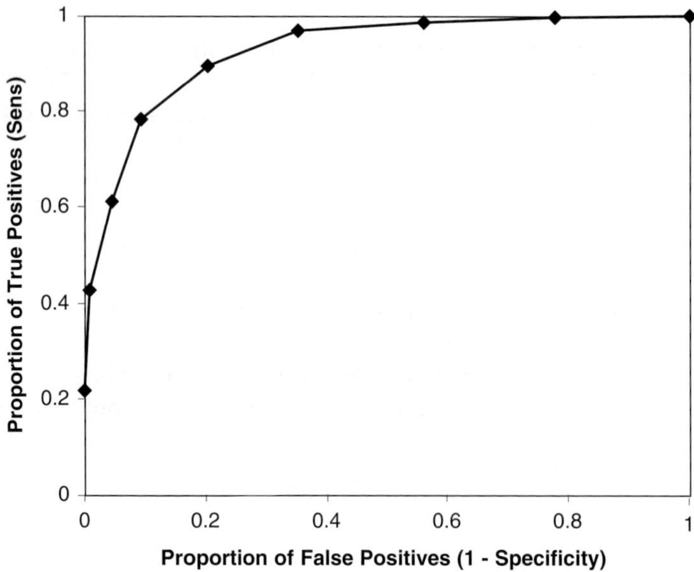

Fig. 3. Interpretation of logistic regression in terms of a receiver-operating characteristic curve.

calculated probability of death for the live one, those probabilities would be consistent with the outcomes in that pair.

In our example, of 450 mosquitoes, 221 survived and 229 died. We thus have $221 \times 229 = 50{,}609$ pairs with different outcomes. The great majority of these pairs, 45,717, were concordant, with the dead mosquito having the higher probability of death. A much smaller number, 2,517, were discordant, with the live mosquito having the higher probability of death. There were also 2,375 ties, in which the dead and live mosquitoes had exactly the same probability of death. The ties are counted as half concordant and half discordant, and so the coefficient of concordance is $C = (45{,}717 + 2{,}375/2)/50{,}609 = 0.927$.

Like R^2, the coefficient of concordance has range 0–1, but, unlike R^2, its expected value under the null hypothesis of no relationship is 0.5 rather than 0. When logistic regression is used in medical diagnosis, a graph called the receiver operating characteristic (ROC) curve is used to portray the effectiveness of the regression model. This graph, in Fig. 3, shows the tradeoff in the proportion of true positives (sensitivity) versus the proportion of false positives ($= 1-$specificity). The area beneath this curve is equal to C. A value of C close to 1 means the diagnosis can have simultaneously high sensitivity and high specificity. Further information regarding the use of ROC curves can be found in Chapter 5 of Hosmer and Lemeshow (2000) and in McNeil et al. (1975).

4. Multiple logistic regression

As with OLS regression, logistic regression is frequently used with multiple independent variables. Suppose in our example we had treated 25 male

Table 2
Differential lethality of insecticide for males and females

Dosage	1	2	3	4	5	6	7	8	9
Males killed	1	1	3	11	16	21	22	25	25
Females killed	0	1	1	6	10	18	20	23	25

and 25 female mosquitoes at each dose level, with the results shown in Table 2.

Within each group, there is a dose–response relation between insecticide and mosquito deaths, with more deaths among the males than among the females at almost every dosage level. Using the SAS LOGISTIC procedure, we obtain the following output estimating the logit as a linear function of dose and sex:

Testing Global Null Hypothesis (Beta = 0)

Test	χ^2	df	$\Pr>\chi^2$
Likelihood ratio	326.8997	2	<0.0001

Parameter	df	Estimate	Standard Error	χ^2	$Pr>\chi^2$
Intercept	1	−5.7186	0.5465	109.4883	<0.0001
Dose	1	1.0698	0.0950	126.8817	<0.0001
Male	1	0.9132	0.3044	9.0004	0.0027

The sex of the insect was coded as 0 = female, 1 = male. Hence, the choice of variable name "male." In terms of the probabilities estimated from the model, it does not matter whether the sex variable is coded 1 for being male or 1 for being female. The coefficients will change so that the logits and the probabilities come out the same. Also, the χ^2 values will come out the same, except for that of the intercept term. (Testing the intercept coefficient being equal to 0 is not particularly meaningful, in any event.)

Since the coefficient for male is positive, males are more susceptible to the insecticide than females are throughout the dose range. For example, at a dose of five units, the logit of a male mosquito dying is $-5.7816+1.0698 \times 5+0.9132 = 0.4806$. This corresponds to an odds of 1.6170 and a probability of 0.6179. At a dose of five units, the logit of a female dying is $-5.7816+1.0698 \times 5 = -0.4326$. This corresponds to odds of 0.6488 and probability of 0.3935. Figure 4 shows the estimated probabilities of death for males and females over the entire dose range. Across the entire range of dosing, the ratio of male odds to female odds is $\exp(0.9132) = 2.492$. (Verifying at dose = 5 units, we have explicitly $1.6179/0.6488 = 2.494$.)

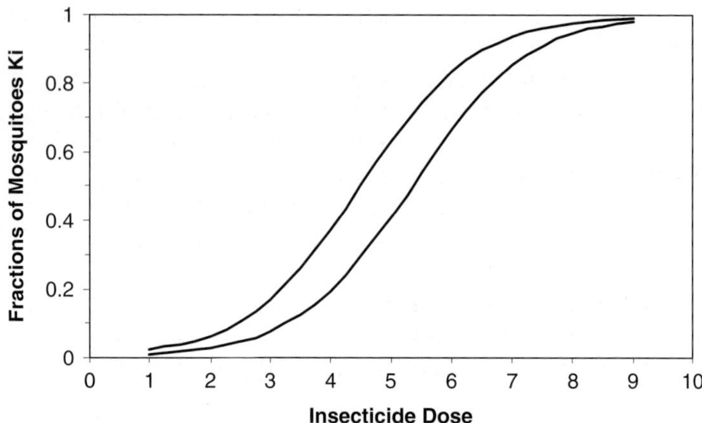

Fig. 4. Logistic regression curves fitted to males and females separately, with curve for males above that for females.

5. Testing for interaction

The fitted model above is an additive, or non-interactive, model. It assumes that if we graph the logit versus dose separately for males and females, we get parallel lines. To test the possibility that the two lines are not parallel, we can include an interaction term obtained by multiplying dose by male, and rerunning the regression with that term included:

Testing Global Null Hypothesis (Beta = 0)

Test	χ^2	df	$Pr > \chi^2$
Likelihood ratio	326.9221	3	<0.0001

Parameter	df	Estimate	Standard Error	χ^2	$Pr > \chi^2$
Intercept	1	−5.6444	0.7322	59.4229	<0.0001
Dose	1	1.0559	0.1321	63.9266	<0.0001
Male	1	0.7735	0.9816	0.6209	0.4307
Interaction	1	0.0284	0.1900	0.0224	0.8812

By two different but related criteria, there is no evidence for the existence of an interaction. First, we have the Wald χ^2 value 0.0224 (and P-value = 0.8812) for testing the hypothesis that the interaction is equal to 0. Second, we can "partition" the likelihood ratio χ^2 in the same fashion as calculating partial sums of squares in OLS regression: $326.9221 - 326.8995 = 0.0226$. This difference has degrees of freedom $3 - 2 = 1$. The conclusion again is that there is no evidence for an interaction.

In the above model, the coefficient and standard error for the variable male have changed dramatically from what they were in the earlier additive model, leading to a non-significant χ^2 value for the sex effect. This is typical in testing for interactions using simple product terms, which are usually highly correlated with one or both variables they are generated from. Since we have concluded that we should return to the additive model, there is no problem for us. Had the interaction been statistically significant, meaning we need to use the more complex model, we could redefine our variables by shifting them to have means of zero, which reduces the correlation between them and their product, the interaction. This yields a model whose coefficients are simpler to interpret.

6. Testing goodness of fit: Two measures for lack of fit

In OLS regression, there are two aspects to assessing the fit of a model. The first is the fraction of variation explained by the model, denoted by R^2. Section 3 above described the logistic regression counterpart of R^2, as well as the coefficient of concordance (which is not a counterpart to anything in OLS regression). The larger these measures, the better the fit. However, even a very large value is not a guarantee that a modification of the existing model may not produce even a better fit.

The second aspect of assessing model fit speaks to the possibility that the existing model might not be the best available. The goodness of fit of an OLS regression model can be based on examination of residuals. By plotting residuals against expected values, deviations from the assumptions of independence and identical distribution (IID) can easily be detected. In logistic regression, the goodness of fit can be assessed in two ways, the first based on contingency tables, the second based on a cumulative plot of the number of positives versus the sum of predicted probabilities.

The approach based on contingency tables is called the Hosmer–Lemeshow test (Hosmer and Lemeshow, 1980). The data are first sorted by predicted probabilities and then divided into 10 (or possibly fewer) groups of approximately equal size. Within each group, the numbers of dead and alive ("observed frequencies") are compared with the sums of the probabilities of dead and alive ("expected frequencies"). The usual χ^2 test for goodness of fit is then calculated. Its degrees of freedom are equal to the number of groups minus two. Using the logistic regression of insects killed on dose and sex, the observed and expected frequencies are given in Table 3.

The value of χ^2 is 4.3001 with $9-2=7$ degrees of freedom and p-value $= 0.7446$. Therefore, there is no evidence that the model can be improved using the existing two independent variables, dose and sex. Note that the software generated nine rather than ten groups. This is due to the tabular nature of the data, which resulted in large numbers of ties. Normally there will be 10 groups, with $10 - 2 = 8$ degrees of freedom.

Table 3
Details of the Hosmer–Lemeshow test for goodness of fit

Group	1	2	3	4	5	6	7	8	9
Observed dead	1	2	4	17	26	39	42	48	50
Observed alive	49	48	46	33	24	11	8	2	0
Expected dead	0.82	2.30	6.09	14.08	26.03	37.55	44.76	48.05	49.31
Expected alive	49.18	47.70	43.91	35.92	23.97	12.45	5.24	1.95	0.69

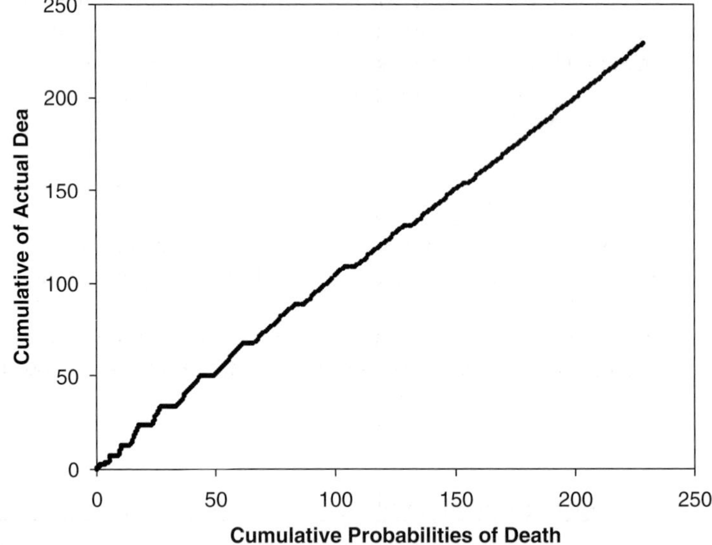

Fig. 5. Graphic assessment of goodness of fit.

An alternative to the Hosmer–Lemeshow test is a graphical procedure that plots the cumulative number of positives versus the sum of predicted probabilities. The diagonal straight line plot in Fig. 5 indicates that no improvement in the model is possible using existing variables. This diagnostic plot is in the same spirit as residual plots in OLS regression and therefore may be preferred by those who are accustomed to reading residual plots. Using cumulatives smooth the plot, making it easier to read.

7. Exact logistic regression

On occasion, the method of maximum likelihood may fail to converge, or it may yield coefficient estimates that are totally unrealistic. This is usually the result of some combination of independent variables being associated with only one category of response. The simplest example occurs in a 2×2 table containing a cell with a frequency of 0, as in Table 4.

Table 4
Example of quasi-complete separation

Survival	Dead	Alive
Treatment A	4	16
Treatment B	0	20

If we code Dead as 0 and Alive as 1, and code Treatments A and B as 0 and 1 respectively, we can attempt to fit a logistic regression model to predict survival status from treatment. The odds ratio from this table is $(20/0)/(16/4) = \infty$. Since the slope coefficient in logistic regression is the log of the odds ratio, the corresponding logistic regression model should be non-estimable, and the software will warn us of this.

Model Convergence Status
Quasi-complete separation of data points detected
Warning: The maximum likelihood estimate may not exist

Warning	The LOGISTIC procedure continues in spite of the above warning. Results shown are based on the last maximum likelihood iteration. Validity of the model fit is questionable

Testing Global Null Hypothesis (Beta = 0)

Test	χ^2	df	$Pr > \chi^2$
Likelihood ratio	5.9905	1	0.0144

Analysis of Maximum Likelihood Estimates

Parameter	df	Estimate	Standard Error	χ^2	$Pr > \chi^2$
Intercept	1	1.3863	0.5590	6.1498	0.0131
X	1	11.9790	178.5	0.0045	0.9465

Warning: The validity of the model fit is questionable

There are in fact three distinct warnings. The term "quasi-complete separation" in the first warning refers to the fact that in our sample, all subjects who received Treatment B are alive. That is, the lower left frequency in the table, representing deaths among subjects receiving Treatment B, is 0. (If the upper right cell also were 0, we would have the even more extreme case of "complete separation.")

In categorical data, there are two distinct kinds of zero frequencies. One is called a structural zero. Structural zeros are zero frequencies that by logic cannot possibly be non-zero. For example, if we were to crosstabulate gender by common surgical procedures, the cell for male hysterectomies would of necessity be 0, as would the cell for female prostatectomies. (These cells are logically zero because males do not have uteruses, and females do not have prostates.)

The other type of zero is a sampling zero, which we could argue is the kind of zero frequency that occurred in our example. While Treatment B has an impressive success rate, 20 alive out of 20 trials, we have no doubt that in further trials, some deaths must surely occur. Therefore, we are convinced that the true odds ratio cannot be infinite, and we would like to use the information from our data to estimate it.

A similar situation can happen with estimating a binomial success probability. Suppose, for example, that out of 20 independent trials there are 20 successes and no failures. The maximum likelihood estimate would be 1, and the estimate of its standard error would be 0. The conventional confidence interval (of any degree of confidence) is the totally uninformative interval $1 \pm 0 = (1,1)$. An alternative approach to calculating a confidence interval in this case is to base it on the value(s) p_L and p_U of the success probability, obtained from the binomial distribution, that form the boundary between accepting and rejecting the null hypotheses $H_0 : p = p_L$ and $H_0 : p = p_U$. The lower 95% confidence limit for the success probability is $p_L = 0.8315$, and the upper confidence limit p_U is taken to be equal to 1 (since no value, no matter how close to 1, can lead to rejection of H_0). Technically, this makes the interval have 97.5% confidence, but in all cases where the sample proportion is *close* to 1, both limits will exist and yield 95% confidence. For example, if out of 20 trials there are 19 successes and one failure, we would find $p_L = 0.7513$, and $p_U = 0.9987$. This confidence interval is more satisfying than the standard-error based interval, as the latter has upper limit 1.0455, which is substantially larger than 1. Thus, exact methods are appropriate not just for the case of zero frequencies, but whenever sample sizes and frequencies are too small for asymptotic methods to work.

Exact logistic regression is based on similar logic: Although the odds ratio from the sample may involve a division by zero and therefore be "infinite," the observed data are consistent with a range of odds ratios extending to infinity. This is a generalization of the well-known Fisher exact test, which we consider first. Under the fixed marginals of 20, 20, 36, and 4, the probability of obtaining the table we have observed is the hypergeometric, (20! 20! 36! 4!)/(40! 4! 16! 0! 20!) = 0.0530. The null hypothesis for the Fisher exact test corresponds to a population odds ratio of 1. Calculating an exact lower 95% (or technically 97.5%) confidence limit for the population odds ratio entails finding a value for the odds ratio for which a calculation similar to the above hypergeometric probability (but incorporating an arbitrary odds ratio) becomes equal to 0.025. The upper confidence limit is equal to infinity, analogous to the case where 20 successes out of 20 trials has upper confidence limit for proportion $p_U = 1$.

The results obtained from adding an exact option to our logistic regression are as follows:

Exact Parameter Estimates

Parameter	Estimate	95% Confidence Limits		*p*-value
Intercept	1.3863	0.2549	2.7999	0.0118
X	1.8027*	−0.3480	Infinity	0.1060

Exact Odds Ratios

Parameter	Estimate	95% Confidence Limits		*p*-value
Intercept	4.000	1.290	16.442	0.0118
X	6.066*	0.706	Infinity	0.1060

* Indicates a median unbiased estimate.

The 95% (actually 97.5%) confidence interval for the true odds ratio is reported as (0.706, ∞). The number 0.706 was obtained by searching for the odds ratio that made the probability of the crosstable equal to 0.025. The "median unbiased estimate" of 6.066 was obtained by searching for the value of the odds ratio that made the probability of the crosstable equal to 0.5. The *p*-value reported is the same as the *p*-value from the two-sided "Fisher Exact Test," which is the test customarily used when expected frequencies are too small to justify using a χ^2 test. Thus, although our point estimate of the odds ratio, 6.066, is much larger than 1, both the lower confidence limit for the odds ratio and the hypothesis test indicate that we cannot reject the null hypothesis that the odds ratio is equal to 1.

The point estimate of the log-odds ratio β is reported as 1.8027, and the confidence interval for β is reported as $(-0.3480, \infty)$. These values are the logarithms of the estimate and confidence limits for the odds ratio.

The intercept estimates are based on the odds of success for Treatment A, $16/4 = 4$, and the corresponding confidence intervals are exact intervals based on the binomial distribution. Thus, our estimated logistic regression model is:

$$\text{log-odds of survival} = 1.3863 + 1.8027 \times (0 \text{ for Treatment A}, 1 \text{ for Treatment B}).$$

Exact logistic regression is valuable even beyond the extreme case of quasi-complete separation. For small sample sizes and/or rare events, maximum likelihood methods may not exhibit the asymptotic behavior guaranteed by theory. Suppose, for example, we have the 2×2 crosstabulation seen in Table 5,

Table 5
Example of small cell frequencies

Survival	Dead	Alive
Treatment A	3	17
Treatment B	1	19

in which two cells have low frequencies, particularly one cell containing a single observation.

The marginal frequencies are the same as before, but now there is no cell containing 0. Two cells have very small expected frequencies, each equal to 2. These are too small for the method of maximum likelihood to give good estimates, and too small to justify using a χ^2 test. Below is the result of the exact logistic regression, and, for comparison purposes, below it is the result of the maximum likelihood logistic regression.

Exact Logistic Regression:

Exact Parameter Estimates

Parameter	Estimate	95% Confidence Limits		p-value
Intercept	1.7346	0.4941	3.4072	0.0026
X	1.1814	−1.4453	5.2209	0.6050

Exact Odds Ratios

Parameter	Estimate	95% Confidence Limits		p-value
Intercept	5.667	1.639	30.181	0.0026
X	3.259	0.236	185.105	0.6050

Maximum Likelihood Logistic Regression:

Testing Global Null Hypothesis (Beta = 0)

Test	χ^2	df	$\Pr > \chi^2$
Likelihood ratio	1.1577	1	0.2820

Parameter	df	Estimate	Standard Error	Wald χ^2	$Pr > \chi^2$
Intercept	1	1.7346	0.6262	7.6725	0.0056
X	1	1.2097	1.2020	1.0130	0.3142

Odds Ratio Estimates

Effect	Point Estimate	95% Wald Confidence Limits	
X	3.353	0.318	35.358

The two estimates of the odds ratio, 3.259 and 3.353, are very similar. However, the two confidence intervals are very different, with the length of the exact interval being much larger. Consistent with the differing lengths of the confidence intervals, the *p*-values for testing the null hypothesis that the odds ratio is equal to 1 are quite different, 0.6050 from the exact logistic regression, and 0.2820 (LR χ^2) and 0.3142 (Wald χ^2) from the maximum likelihood logistic regression. As with the earlier exact logistic regression, the *p*-value 0.6050 is the same as the *p*-value from the Fisher exact test.

8. Ordinal logistic regression

Although the dependent variable is usually binary, logistic regression has the capability to handle dependent variables with more than two categories. If the categories have a natural ordering, such as levels "none," "mild," "moderate," and "severe," the natural first step in building a model is to see if an *ordinal* logistic regression model fits the data. In an ordinal logistic regression model, there is one set of slope coefficients but multiple intercepts. The number of intercepts is always one less than the number of categories. In conjunction with the slopes, the intercepts determine the probabilities of an observation being in the various categorical levels.

As an example, we will use a measure of drinking constructed in the 2001 College Alcohol Study, (Wechsler, 2001), called DRINKCAT. This variable has four levels: 0 = Abstainer or no drinking within the last year, 1 = Drinking within the last year but no binge drinking in the previous two weeks, 2 = Binge drinking once or twice within the last two weeks, 3 = Binge drinking more than twice within the last two weeks.

We will use three binary variables as independent variables: A2 = male gender, A5 = sorority/fraternity membership, B8 = living in "alcohol-free" housing. There is an interaction between A2 and A5, which we will omit in order to make the example simpler. For further simplicity, we will also omit effects due to weighting and to clustering by institution.

Following is the result of fitting an ordinal logistic regression model to this data:

Response Profile

Ordered Value	DRINKCAT	Total Frequency
1	3.00	2365
2	2.00	2258
3	1.00	4009
4	0.00	2039

Probabilities modeled are cumulated over the lower ordered values

Score Test for the Proportional Odds Assumption

χ^2	df	$Pr > \chi^2$
80.4140	6	<0.0001

Testing Global Null Hypothesis (Beta = 0)

Test	χ^2	df	$Pr > \chi^2$
Likelihood ratio	336.6806	3	<0.0001

Analysis of maximum likelihood estimates

Parameter	df	Estimate	Standard Error	Wald χ^2	$Pr > \chi^2$
Intercept 3.00	1	−1.3848	0.0292	2250.9331	<0.0001
Intercept 2.00	1	−0.3718	0.0257	209.2745	<0.0001
Intercept 1.00	1	1.3749	0.0294	2185.4249	<0.0001
A2	1	0.1365	0.0366	13.9106	0.0002
A5	1	0.8936	0.0540	274.3205	<0.0001
B8	1	−0.3886	0.0486	64.0554	<0.0001

Odds Ratio Estimates

Effect	Point Estimate	95% Wald Confidence Limits	
A2	1.146	1.067	1.231
A5	2.444	2.199	2.716
B8	0.678	0.616	0.746

The first test labeled, "Score Test for the Proportional Odds Assumption," is a check on the validity of the ordinal logistic model. This test is statistically significant, which means that there is a better-fitting model, namely, the multinomial logistic regression model discussed below. We will, however, study the additional output from this ordinal logistic model in order to compare results with those from the more appropriate multinomial logistic.

The likelihood ratio χ^2 for testing the overall model is 336.6806 with 3 degrees of freedom and p-value less than 0.0001. This tells us that the overall model fits better than we would expect by chance alone. We can then proceed to the assessment of the three variables A2 (male gender), A5 (Greek membership), and B8 (alcohol-free housing). All three are statistically significant, with A2 and A5 being risk factors and B8 being protective.

Because there is only one set of slope coefficients (rather than 3) for A2, A5, and B8, it is necessary to compute all probabilities using this single set of slope coefficients combined with the three different intercept estimates. The three intercept estimates yield the estimated log odds, odds and probabilities that: DRINKCAT = 3 (from the first intercept, −1.3848), DRINKCAT ≥ 2 (from the second intercept, −0.3718), and DRINKCAT ≥ 1 (from the third intercept, 1.3749). Once these estimated probabilities have been determined, the probabilities that DRINKCAT is equal to 0, 1, or 2 can be obtained by subtractions.

Suppose we have a subject who is at highest risk of heavy drinking. That would be a male who is a member of a Greek organization and who does not live in alcohol-free housing. For that person, we have:

$$\text{log-odds}(\text{DRINKCAT} = 3) = -1.3848 + 0.1365 \times 1 + 0.8936 \times 1 - 0.3886 \times 0 = -0.3547$$

$$\text{log-odds}(\text{DRINKCAT} \geq 2) = -0.3718 + 0.1365 \times 1 + 0.8936 \times 1 - 0.3886 \times 0 = 0.6583$$

$$\text{log-odds}(\text{DRINKCAT} \geq 1) = 1.3749 + 0.1365 \times 1 + 0.8936 \times 1 - 0.3886 \times 0 = 2.4050$$

$$\text{odds}(\text{DRINKCAT} = 3) = \exp(-0.3547) = 0.7014;\quad P(\text{DRINKCAT} = 3) = 0.7014/1.7014 = 0.4122$$

$$\text{odds}(\text{DRINKCAT} \geq 2) = \exp(0.6583) = 1.9315;\quad P(\text{DRINKCAT} \geq 2) = 1.9315/2.9315 = 0.6589$$

$$\text{odds}(\text{DRINKCAT} \geq 1) = \exp(2.4050) = 11.0784;\quad P(\text{DRINKCAT} \geq 1) = 11.0784/12.0784 = 0.9172.$$

Finally we obtain the individual probabilities by subtractions:

$$P(\text{DRINKCAT} = 0) = 1 - 0.9172 = 0.0828$$

$$P(\text{DRINKCAT} = 1) = 0.9172 - 0.6589 = 0.2583$$

$$P(\text{DRINKCAT} = 2) = 0.6589 - 0.4122 = 0.2467$$

$$P(\text{DRINKCAT} = 3) = 0.4122$$

By contrast, the four probabilities for a person with the lowest risk of heavy drinking – a female who is not a sorority member and lives in alcohol-free housing – are:

$$P(\text{DRINKCAT} = 0) = 0.2716$$

$$P(DRINKCAT = 1) = 0.4098$$

$$P(DRINKCAT = 2) = 0.1734$$

$$P(DRINKCAT = 3) = 0.1451$$

9. Multinomial logistic regression

If the categories of the dependent variable do not have a natural ordering, the single set of slopes of ordinal logistic regression must be replaced with multiple sets of slopes, producing what is called a multinomial logistic regression model. The number of slopes for each independent variable will always be one less than the number of categories of the dependent variable, matching the number of intercepts. In effect, a multinomial logistic regression model looks like a set of binary logistic regressions. The advantages of fitting one multinomial model over fitting several binary models are that there is one likelihood ratio χ^2 for the fit of the entire model, and there is opportunity to test hypotheses about equality of slopes.

Even if the categories of the dependent variable are ordered, a multinomial model may be necessary to provide a better fit to the data than the ordinal logistic regression may afford. One way to investigate this possibility is to fit both ordered logistic and multinomial logistic models and calculate the difference in the likelihood ratio χ^2. Another way is to look for a test of the "proportional odds assumption" in the ordinal logistic regression. If the χ^2 statistic from that test is significant, there is evidence that one set of slopes is insufficient, and the correct model is multinomial rather than ordinal.

In the ordinal logistic regression above, we remarked that the test for the proportional odds assumption had quite a large χ^2. Its value was 80.4140 with 6 degrees of freedom and p-value less than 0.0001. This is evidence that we will obtain a better-fitting model by using multinomial logistic regression, even though the categories of DRINKCAT are naturally ordered.

Following is the result of running a multinomial logistic regression on the Harvard College Drinking Study data:

Response Profile

Ordered Value	DRINKCAT	Total Frequency
1	0.00	2039
2	1.00	4009
3	2.00	2258
4	3.00	2365

Logits modeled use DRINKCAT = 0.00 as the reference category

Testing Global Null Hypothesis (Beta = 0)

Test	χ^2	df	$Pr>\chi^2$
Likelihood	Ratio	415.5538	9<0.0001

Type 3 Analysis of Effects

Effect	df	Wald χ^2	$Pr>\chi^2$
A2	3	68.8958	<0.0001
A5	3	266.3693	<0.0001
B8	3	87.2105	<0.0001

Analysis of Maximum Likelihood Estimates

Parameter	DRINKCAT	df	Estimate	Standard Error	Wald χ^2	$Pr>\chi^2$
Intercept	1.00	1	0.8503	0.0373	519.4807	<0.0001
Intercept	2.00	1	0.0800	0.0430	3.4632	0.0627
Intercept	3.00	1	0.0731	0.0430	2.8970	0.0887
A2	1.00	1	−0.3120	0.0572	29.7276	<0.0001
A2	2.00	1	0.0514	0.0632	0.6597	0.4167
A2	3.00	1	0.0609	0.0629	0.9353	0.3335
A5	1.00	1	0.3462	0.1049	10.8943	0.0010
A5	2.00	1	0.9812	0.1064	85.0242	<0.0001
A5	3.00	1	1.3407	0.1027	170.4737	<0.0001
B8	1.00	1	−0.5220	0.0702	55.2565	<0.0001
B8	2.00	1	−0.5646	0.0811	48.5013	<0.0001
B8	3.00	1	−0.6699	0.0819	66.9267	<0.0001

Odds Ratio Estimates

Effect	DRINKCAT	Point Estimate	95% Wald Confidence Limits	
A2	1.00	0.732	0.654	0.819
A2	2.00	1.053	0.930	1.192
A2	3.00	1.063	0.939	1.202
A5	1.00	1.414	1.151	1.736
A5	2.00	2.668	2.165	3.286
A5	3.00	3.822	3.125	4.674
B8	1.00	0.593	0.517	0.681
B8	2.00	0.569	0.485	0.666
B8	3.00	0.512	0.436	0.601

The likelihood ratio χ^2 for this model is 415.5583 with 9 degrees of freedom. We can compare this value with the χ^2 value of 336.6806 with 3 degrees of freedom for the ordinal logistic regression model. Their difference, 415.5583–336.6806 = 78.8732 has degrees of freedom 9 − 3 = 6, in close agreement with the χ^2 80.4140 with 6 df that tested the proportional odds assumption in the ordinal logistic regression. Thus, from two different perspectives, we are led to the conclusion that multinomial logistic regression is more appropriate for our data.

Interpreting the model coefficients is best done by thinking of the multinomial model as a collection of three binomial models. Each binomial model estimates probabilities of the DRINKCAT values 1, 2, and 3 relative to value 0. For example, consider the three log-odds ratio coefficients −0.5220, −0.5646, and −0.6699 for the variable B8, living in alcohol-free housing. These correspond to odds ratios of 0.593, 0.569, and 0.512, meaning that for those living in alcohol-free housing the odds of being in any of the positive drinking categories (DRINKCAT = 1, 2, or 3) are about 40–50% less than being in the non-drinking category. The big drop in risk, of about 40%, occurs between DRINKCAT = 0 and DRINKCAT = 1, with small further drops in risk of being in DRINKCAT = 2 and DRINKCAT = 3. A formal test of the hypothesis that the three slopes are equal is not statistically significant, leading us to conclude that alcohol-free housing has "threshold" protective effect of reducing the risk of all three levels of drinking by the same amount.

By contrast, the three log-odds coefficients for the variable A5 show a large monotone increasing pattern, from 0.3462 to 0.9812, and finally to 1.3407, meaning that fraternity or sorority membership shows a pattern of increasing risks of the more severe drinking behaviors. A formal test of the null hypothesis that the three slopes are equal to each other rejects the null hypothesis. Based on the final odds ratio of exp(1.3407) = 3.822, members of Greek organizations have almost four times the risk of extreme binge drinking than do non-members.

Finally, the coefficients for the variable A2 show that males have reduced odds of moderate drinking, and somewhat greater odds of each level of binge drinking. A formal test of the null hypothesis that the three slopes are equal rejects the null hypothesis.

10. Probit regression

Earlier we introduced the logit function as a means of "opening up" the probability range of [0,1] to $(-\infty, +\infty)$. This can also be done by using the inverse standard normal function. Although the logit and the inverse normal (sometimes called *normit* or *probit*) have very different behavior in the extreme tails, in actual practice, they yield nearly the same predicted probabilities. If we use the inverse standard normal function in place of the logit for our insecticide data, the result is:

Testing global null hypothesis (Beta = 0)

Test	χ^2	df	$Pr>\chi^2$
Likelihood ratio	327.4488	2	<0.0001

Parameter	df	Estimate	Standard Error	χ^2	$Pr > \chi^2$
Intercept	1	−3.2286	0.2759	136.9310	<0.0001
Dose	1	0.6037	0.0471	164.6159	<0.0001
Male	1	0.5126	0.1686	9.2450	0.0024

The likelihood ratio χ^2 is very close to that from the additive logit model, 326.8997, but the estimated model coefficients are very different. This difference is due to the fact that the standard normal density function has standard deviation equal to 1, whereas the logit density function has standard deviation equal to $\pi/\sqrt{3} = 1.8138$. Despite the differences in model coefficients, probabilities estimated from the two models come out nearly the same.

For example, in the logit model, we found that at a dose of five units, the logit of a male mosquito dying is $-5.7816 + 1.0698 \times 5 + 0.9132 = 0.4806$. This corresponded to a probability of 0.6179. From our current model, at a dose of five units, the Z-score, or probit, of a mosquito dying is $-3.2286 + 0.6037 \times 5 + 0.5126 = 0.3025$. This corresponds to a probability of 0.6189, almost identical with 0.6179.

The Hosmer–Lemeshow goodness of fit test yields a value of χ^2 is 4.1243 with 7 degrees of freedom and p-value = 0.7654. Not only is the test non-significant, the χ^2 value itself is virtually identical with the Hosmer–Lemeshow χ^2 4.3001 that we calculated from the logistic regression model.

Given that in most cases there is little difference between the probability estimates from logit and probit models; most users of logistic regression prefer the logit model as simpler to understand. Its coefficients can be directly interpreted in terms of odds ratios, and the odds ratios can be multiplied to estimate overall risk.

Most statistical software provides a third link function option called the complementary log–log function (or "Gompertz" function). This also opens up the probability range of [0,1] to $(-\infty, +\infty)$, but it does so in a non-symmetric fashion. It is useful for special purposes but should not be considered a natural alternative to logit and probit models. In particular, it does not fit our example data as well as the logit and probit models do.

11. Logistic regression in case–control studies

Risk factors for rare disorders are frequently determined through case–control studies. For example, there is considerable literature on the interrelationship of asbestos exposure, smoking, and lung cancer. Since the prevalence of lung cancer is relatively low, most studies have compared lung cancer patients with comparable cancer-free control subjects. Many of these studies have involved shipyard workers because of asbestos exposure in shipbuilding. Smoking was fairly common among these blue-collar employees, so smoking was investigated along with asbestos exposure as another risk factor.

Table 6
Case–control data showing the relationship of asbestos exposure and smoking with lung cancer

Exposure(s)	A^-S^-	A^+S^-	A^-S^+	A^+S^+
Cases	50	11	313	84
Controls	203	35	270	45

Since odds ratios are marginal-independent, they do not change if a factor is over or under represented. Thus, we can use "caseness" as a response variable in logistic regression without introducing bias in our estimates of the logistic regression slope coefficients. The only coefficient that is biased is the intercept term, and we ordinarily are not interested in estimating it anyway.

Table 6 contains data from Blot et al. (1978), as reproduced in Lee (2001).

A full logistic regression model would attempt to predict lung cancer (caseness) from asbestos exposure, smoking, and the interaction between asbestos and smoking. In this full model, the interaction term is not statistically significant, and the final model is the additive model estimated in the following output:

Testing global null hypothesis (BETA = 0)

Test	χ^2	df	$Pr > \chi^2$
Likelihood ratio	118.2789	2	<0.0001

Analysis of maximum likelihood estimates

Parameter	df	Estimate	Standard Error	Wald χ^2	$Pr > \chi^2$
Intercept	1	−1.4335	0.1476	94.3817	<0.0001
Smoke	1	1.5902	0.1626	95.6905	<0.0001
Asbestos	1	0.4239	0.1769	5.7437	0.0165

Odds ratio estimates

Effect	Point Estimate	95% Wald Confidence Limits	
Smoke	4.904	3.566	6.745
Asbestos	1.528	1.080	2.161

We conclude that smoking is by far the more potent risk factor, increasing risk of lung cancer, in the sense of odds, almost five-fold. Asbestos exposure is also a statistically significant risk factor, but it increases risk by 53%. Furthermore, the number 1.528 is a point estimate of the odds ratio, but the 95% confidence interval for the true asbestos-exposure odds ratio ranges from a low of 1.08 to a high of 2.16.

Case–control studies are normally performed for disorders that are rare in the general population. For rare disorders, the odds ratio is a good approximation (a slight overestimate, always) to relative risk. Therefore, in these settings, it is very common to treat the odds ratio as being a surrogate for relative risk. For example, suppose a disease has a base prevalence of exactly 1%, and a certain risk factor changes its prevalence to 2%. By definition, the relative risk is exactly equal to 2. The odds ratio is $(0.02/0.98)/(0.01/0.99) = 2.02$ and therefore serves as an excellent approximation to relative risk.

More complex case–control designs involve matching individual cases with controls, either on a one-to-one basis or even a one-to-many basis. Logistic regression can also be used to analyze these more complicated designs. Chapters 6 and 7 of Hosmer and Lemeshow (2000) contain a wealth of information regarding the use of logistic regression in case–control studies.

References

Blot, W.J., Harrington, J.M., Toledo, A., Hoover, R., Heath, C.W., Fraumeni, J.F. (1978). Lung cancer after employment in shipyards during World War II. *The New England Journal of Medicine* **299**, 620–624.

Cox, D.R., Snell, E.J. (1989). *The Analysis of Binary Data*, 2nd ed. Chapman & Hall, London.

Hosmer, D.W., Lemeshow, S. (1980). A goodness-of-fit test for the multiple logistic regression model. *Communications in Statistics* **A10**, 1043–1069.

Hosmer, D.W., Lemeshow, S. (2000). *Applied Logistic Regression*, 2nd ed. Wiley, New York.

Lee, P.N. (2001). Relation between exposure to asbestos and smoking jointly and the risk of breast cancer. *Occupational and Environmental Medicine* **58**, 145–153.

McNeil, B.J., Keller, E., Adelstein, S.J. (1975). Primer on certain elements of medical decision making. *The New England Journal of Medicine* **293**, 211–215.

Nagelkerke, N.J.D. (1991). A note on a general definition of the coefficient of determination. *Biometrika* **78**, 691–692.

SAS Institute Inc. (2004). *SAS/STAT® 9.1 User's Guide*. SAS Institute, Cary, NC.

Wechsler, H. (2001). *Harvard School of Public Health College Alcohol Study*. ICPSR, Ann Arbor.

Handbook of Statistics, Vol. 27
ISSN: 0169-7161

DOI: 10.1016/S0169-7161(07)27007-5

7

Count Response Regression Models

Joseph M. Hilbe and William H. Greene

Abstract

Count response regression models refer to regression models having a count as the response; e.g., hospital length of stay, number of bacterial pneumonia cases per zip code in Arizona from 2000 to 2005. Poisson regression is the basic model of this class. Having an assumption of the equality of the distributional mean and variance, Poisson models are inappropriate for many count-modeling situations. Overdispersion occurs when the variance exceeds the nominal mean. The negative binomial (NB2) is commonly employed to model overdispersed Poisson data, but NB models can themselves be overdispersed. A wide variety of alternative count models have been designed to accommodate overdispersion in both Poisson and NB models; e.g., zero-inflated, zero-truncated, hurdle, and sample selection models. Data can also be censored and truncated; specialized count models have been designed for these situations as well. In addition, the wide range of Poisson and NB panel and mixed models has been developed. In the chapter we provide an overview of the above varieties of count response models, and discuss available software that can be used for their estimation.

1. Introduction

Modeling counts of events can be found in all areas of statistics, econometrics, and throughout the social and physical sciences. Some familiar applications include:

- the incidence of diseases in specific populations,
- numbers of patents applied for,
- numbers of regime changes in political units,
- numbers of financial 'incidents' such as defaults or bankruptcies,
- numbers of doctor visits,
- numbers of incidents of drug or alcohol abuse, and so on.

The literatures in all these fields and many more are replete with applications of models for counts. The signature feature of all of these is that familiar linear regression techniques that would relate the measured outcomes to appropriate covariates – smoking and disease or research and development to patents for examples – would not be applicable because the response variable is discrete, not continuous. Nonetheless, a related counterpart to the familiar regression model is a natural departure point. The Poisson regression model has been used throughout the research landscape to model counts in applications such as these. The Poisson model is a nonlinear, albeit straightforward and popular modeling tool. It is ubiquitous enough that estimation routines are built into all well-known contemporary computer programs. This chapter will survey models and methods for analyzing counts, beginning with this basic tool.

The Poisson model provides the platform for modeling count data. Practical issues in 'real' data have compelled researchers to extend the model in several directions. The most fundamental extension involves augmenting the model to allow a more realistic treatment of variation of the responses variable. The Poisson model, at its heart, describes the mean of the response. A consequence of the specification is that it implies a wholly unsatisfactory model for the variance of the response variable. Models such as the NB model are designed to accommodate a more complete description of the distribution of observed outcomes. Observed data often present other forms of 'nonPoissonness.' An important example is the 'excess zeros' case. Survey data often contain more zero responses (or more of some other responses) than would be predicted by a Poisson or a NB model. For example, the incidence of hypertension in school age children, or credit card default, are relatively rare events. The count response is amenable to modeling in this framework; however, an unmodified Poisson model will underpredict the zero outcome. In another interesting application, Poisson-like models are often used to model family size; however, family size data in Western societies will often display excess twos in the number of children, where, once again, by 'excess' we mean in excess of what would typically be predicted by a Poisson model. Finally, other data and situation-driven applications will call for more than one equation in the count model. For example, in modeling health care system utilization, researchers often profitably employ 'two part models' in which one part describes a decision to use the health care system and a second equation describes the intensity of system utilization given the decision to use the system at all.

This chapter will survey these count models. The analysis will proceed as follows: Section 2 details the fundamental results for the Poisson regression model. Section 3 discusses the most familiar extension of models for counts, the NB model. Section 4 considers the types of broad model extensions suggested above including the important extensions to longitudinal (panel) data. Section 5 presents several additional more specialized model extensions. Section 5 describes some of the available software tools for estimation. Rather than collecting an extended example in one place at the end of the survey, we will develop some applications as part of the ongoing presentations. Our analyses are done with LIMDEP statistical software. Section 5 describes this and a few other packages in some more detail. Section 6 concludes.

2. The Poisson regression model

The Poisson model derives from a description of how often events occur per unit of time. Consider, for example, a service window at a bank, or an observer watching a population for the outbreak of diseases. The 'interarrival time' is the amount of time that elapses between events, for example, the duration between arrivals of customers at the teller window or the amount of time that passes between 'arrivals' of cases of a particular disease. If the interarrival time is such that the probability that a new incident will occur in the next instant of time is independent of how much time has passed since the last one, then the process is said to be 'memoryless.' The exponential distribution is used to describe such processes. Now, consider not the interarrival time, but the number of arrivals that occur in a fixed length interval of time. Under the assumptions already made, if the length of time is short, then the 'Poisson' distribution will be an appropriate distribution to use to model the number of arrivals that occur during a fixed time interval.[1]

More formally, suppose the process is such that the expected interarrival time does not vary over time. Say θ is this value. Then, the number of arrivals that can be expected to arrive per unit of time is $\lambda = 1/\theta$. The distribution of the number of arrivals, Y, in a fixed interval is the Poisson distribution

$$f(Y) = Prob[Y = y] = \frac{\exp(-\lambda)\lambda^y}{y!}, \quad y = 0, 1, \ldots; \quad \lambda > 0. \tag{1}$$

The Poisson model describes the number of arrivals per single unit of time. Suppose that the observer observes T consecutive intervals. Then, the expected number of arrivals would naturally be λT. Assuming the process is not changing from one interval to the next, the appropriate distribution to model a window of length T, rather than 1, would be

$$f(Y) = Prob[Y = y] = \frac{\exp(-\lambda T)(\lambda T)^y}{y!}, \quad y = 0, 1, \ldots; \quad \lambda > 0. \tag{2}$$

One can imagine a sampling process such that successive observers watched the population or process for different amounts of time. The appropriate model for the number of observed events in such a sample would necessarily have to account for the different lengths of time. A sample of observations would be $(y_1,T_1), \ldots (y_N,T_N)$. The joint observations would consist of an observed count variable and an observed 'exposure' variable. (For reasons that are far from obvious, such a variable is often called an 'offset' variable – see, e.g., the documentation for *Stata* or *SAS*.) An analogous process would follow if the

[1] Another way to develop the Poisson model from first principles is to consider a Bernoulli sampling process in which the success probability, π, becomes small while the number of trials, T, becomes large such that πT is constant. The limiting process of this binomial sampling scheme is the Poisson model. By treating the 'draws' as specific short intervals of time, we can view this as an alternative view of the exponential model suggested earlier.

observation were designed so that each observation was based on a count of occurrences in a group of size T_i, where T_i is allowed to differ from one observation to another. Larger groups would tend to produce larger counts, not because the process had changed, but because of the increased 'exposure' to the same process.

The Poisson random variable has mean

$$E[Y] = \lambda T \tag{3}$$

and variance

$$\text{Var}[Y] = \lambda T. \tag{4}$$

These are derived for the case $T = 1$ in any basic statistics book. For convenience at this point, we will focus on that case as well. Where necessary, we will reinstate the exposure as part of the model for a particular sampling process. Note, in particular, that the variance equals the mean, a fact that will become important in the next section of this survey.

To extend this model to a regression context, consider once again the health application. For any group observed at random in a population in a given time interval, suppose the Poisson model, is appropriate. To consider a concrete example, suppose we observe new cancer cases per unit of time or per group. The overall average number of cases observed per unit of time may be well described with a fixed mean, λ. However, for the assumed case, three significant comorbidity factors, age, weight, and smoking, stand out as possible explanatory variables. For researchers observing different populations in different places, one might surmise that the parameter, λ, which is the mean number of new cases per unit of time, would vary substantively with these covariates. This brings us to the point of 'model' building, and, in particular, since we have surmised that the mean of the distribution is a function of the covariates, regression modeling.

Precisely, how the covariates in the model should enter the mean is an important question. Suppose we denote average age, average weight, and percent who smoke in the different observed groups suggested by the example, for convenience, as (x_1,x_2,x_3), it would be tempting to write the mean of the random variable as

$$\lambda = \beta_0 + \beta_1 x_1 + \beta_2 x_2 + \beta_3 x_3. \tag{5}$$

However, a crucial feature of the model emerges immediately. Note in (1), and for obvious reasons, $\lambda > 0$. This is the mean of a nonnegative random variable. It would not be possible to insure that the function in (5) is positive for all values of the parameters and any data. The constraint is more important yet in view of (4). The commonly accepted solution, and the conventional approach in modeling count data, is to use

$$\lambda = \exp(\boldsymbol{\beta}'\mathbf{x}), \tag{6}$$

where the vector notation is used for convenience, and $\boldsymbol{\beta}$ and $\mathbf{x}$ are assumed to include a constant term.[2]

To summarize, then, the Poisson regression model that is typically used to model count data is

$$f(Y|\mathbf{x}) = Prob[Y = y] = \frac{\exp(-\lambda T)(\lambda T)^y}{y!}, \quad y = 0, 1, \ldots;$$
$$\lambda = \exp(\boldsymbol{\beta}'\mathbf{x}) > 0. \tag{7}$$

This is a nonlinear regression which has conditional mean function

$$E[Y|\mathbf{x}] = \lambda = \exp(\boldsymbol{\beta}'\mathbf{x}) \tag{8}$$

and heteroskedastic conditional variance

$$\mathrm{Var}[Y|\mathbf{x}] = \lambda. \tag{9}$$

2.1. Estimation of the Poisson model

The parameters of the nonlinear Poisson regression model, $\boldsymbol{\beta}$, can, in principle, be estimated by nonlinear least squares by minimizing the conventional sum of squares. With a sample of N observations, $(y_1,\mathbf{x}_1), \ldots, (y_N,\mathbf{x}_N)$, we would minimize

$$\mathrm{SS}(\boldsymbol{\beta}) = \sum_{i=1}^{N}[y_i - \exp(\boldsymbol{\beta}'\mathbf{x}_i + \log\ T_i)]^2. \tag{10}$$

However, maximum likelihood estimation is the method of most common choice for this model. The log-likelihood function for a sample of N observations may be characterized as

$$\log\ L(\boldsymbol{\beta}) \sum_{i=1}^{N} y_i(\boldsymbol{\beta}'\mathbf{x}_i + \log\ T_i) - \exp(\boldsymbol{\beta}'\mathbf{x}_i + \log\ T_i) - \log(y_i!). \tag{11}$$

Note how the exposure variable enters the model, as if it were a covariate having a coefficient of one. As such, accommodating data sets that are heterogeneous in this respect does not require any substantial modification of the model or the estimator. For convenience in what follows, we will assume that each observation is made in an interval of one period (or one observation unit; $T_i = 1$; $\ln T_i = 0$). As noted earlier, this is a particularly straightforward model to estimate, and it is available as a built-in option in all modern software.

[2] This implies that the model is a 'log-linear' model in the development of McCullagh and Nelder (1983) – indeed, in the history of log-linear modeling, the Poisson model might reasonably be regarded as *the* log-linear model. The Poisson model plays a central role in the development of the theory. As we will not be exploring this aspect of the model in any depth in this review, we note this feature of the model at this point only in passing.

The conditional mean function for the Poisson model is nonlinear

$$E[y|\mathbf{x}] = \exp(\boldsymbol{\beta}'\mathbf{x}). \tag{12}$$

For inference purposes, e.g., testing for the significance of average weight in the incidence of disease, the coefficients, β, provide the appropriate metric. For analysis of the behavior of the response variable, however, one typically examines the partial effects

$$\boldsymbol{\delta}(\mathbf{x}) = \frac{\partial E[y|\mathbf{x}]}{\partial \mathbf{x}} = \exp(\boldsymbol{\beta}'\mathbf{x}) \times \boldsymbol{\beta}. \tag{13}$$

As in any regression model, this measure is a function of the data point at which it is evaluated. For analysis of the Poisson model, researchers typically use one of the two approaches: The marginal effects, computed at the mean, or the center of the data are

$$\boldsymbol{\delta}(\bar{\mathbf{x}}) = \frac{\partial E[y|\bar{\mathbf{x}}]}{\partial \bar{\mathbf{x}}} = \exp(\boldsymbol{\beta}'\bar{\mathbf{x}}) \times \boldsymbol{\beta}, \tag{14}$$

where $\bar{\mathbf{x}} = (1/N)\Sigma_{i=1}^{N}\mathbf{x}_i$ is the sample mean of the data. An alternative, commonly used measure is the set of average partial effects,

$$\bar{\boldsymbol{\delta}}(\mathbf{X}) = \frac{1}{N}\sum_{i=1}^{N}\frac{\partial E[y|\mathbf{x}_i]}{\partial \mathbf{x}_i} = \frac{1}{N}\sum_{i-1}^{N}\exp(\boldsymbol{\beta}'\mathbf{x}_i) \times \boldsymbol{\beta}. \tag{15}$$

Although the two measures will generally not differ by very much in a practical setting, the two measures will not converge to the same value as the sample size increases. The estimator in (15) will converge to that (13) plus a term that depends on the higher order moments of the distribution of the covariates.

We note two aspects of the computation of partial effects that are occasionally overlooked in applications. Most applications of count models involve individual level data. The typical model will involve dummy variables, for example, sex, race, education, marital status, working status, and so on. One cannot differentiate with respect to a binary variable. The proper computation for the partial effect of a binary variable, say z_i is

$$\Delta(z_i) = E[y|\mathbf{x}, z = 1] - E[y|\mathbf{x}, z = 0].$$

In practical terms, the computation of these finite differences will usually produce results similar to those that use derivatives – the finite difference is a crude derivative. Nonetheless, the finite difference presents the more accurate picture of the desired result. Second, models often include nonlinear functions of the independent variables. In our applications below, for example, we have a tezrm $\beta_1\text{AGE} + \beta_2\text{AGE}^2$. In this instance, neither coefficient, nor the associates marginal effect, is useful by itself for measuring the impact of education. The appropriate computation would be

$$\delta(\text{AGE}) = \exp(\boldsymbol{\beta}'\mathbf{x}_i)[\beta_1 + 2\beta_2\text{AGE}].$$

2.2. Statistical inference

For basic inference about coefficients in the model, the standard trinity of likelihood-based tests, likelihood ratio, Wald and Lagrange multiplier (LM), are easily computed.[3] For testing a hypothesis, linear or nonlinear, of the form

$$H_0 : \mathbf{c}(\boldsymbol{\beta}) = \mathbf{0}, \tag{16}$$

the likelihood-ratio statistic is the obvious choice. This requires estimation of β subject to the restrictions of the null hypothesis, for example, subject to the exclusions of a null hypothesis that states that certain variables should have zero coefficients – that is, that they should not appear in the model. Then, the likelihood-ratio statistic is

$$\chi^2[J] = 2(\log\ L - \log\ L_0), \tag{17}$$

where $\log L$ is the log-likelihood computed using the unrestricted estimator, $\log L_0$ the counterpart based on the restricted estimator and the degrees of freedom, J, the number of restrictions (an example appears below).

Each predictor, including the constant, can have a calculated Wald statistic, defined as $[\beta_j/\mathrm{SE}(\beta_j)]^2$, which is distributed as χ^2. $[\beta_j/\mathrm{SE}(\beta_j)]$ defines both the t or z statistic, respectively distributed as t or normal. For computation of Wald statistics, one needs an estimate of the asymptotic covariance matrix of the coefficients. The Hessian of the log-likelihood is

$$\frac{\partial^2 \log L}{\partial \boldsymbol{\beta} \partial \boldsymbol{\beta}'} = -\sum_{i=1}^{N} \lambda_i \mathbf{x}_i \mathbf{x}_i', \tag{18}$$

where $\lambda_i = \exp(\boldsymbol{\beta}'\mathbf{x}_i)$. Since this does not involve the random variable, y_i, (18) also gives the expected Hessian. The estimated asymptotic covariance matrix for the maximum likelihood, based on the Hessian, is

$$\mathbf{V}_{\mathrm{H}} = \mathrm{Est.Asy.Var}[\hat{\boldsymbol{\beta}}_{\mathrm{MLE}}] = \left[\sum_{i=1}^{N} \hat{\lambda}_i \mathbf{x}_i \mathbf{x}_i'\right]^{-1}, \tag{19}$$

where $\hat{\lambda}_i = \exp(\hat{\boldsymbol{\beta}}'\mathbf{x}_i)$. Although in practice, one normally uses the variance matrices discussed in Section 2.4, a commonly used alternative estimator based on the first derivatives is the BHHH, or outer products estimator,

$$\mathbf{V}_{\mathrm{OPG}} = \mathrm{Est.Asy.Var}[\hat{\boldsymbol{\beta}}_{\mathrm{MLE}}] = \left[\sum_{i=1}^{N} (y_i - \hat{\lambda}_i)^2 \mathbf{x}_i \mathbf{x}_i'\right]^{-1}. \tag{20}$$

Researchers often compute asymptotic standard errors for their estimates of the marginal effects. This is a moderately complicated exercise in some cases. The

[3] The presentation here is fairly terse. For more detailed derivations of these results, the reader may refer many of the sources that develop this model in detail, including Hilbe (2007), Winkelmann (2003), or Greene (2003, Chapter 21).

most straightforward case is based on (14). To use the delta method to estimate the asymptotic covariance matrix for $\hat{\boldsymbol{\delta}}(\bar{\mathbf{x}})$, we would require the Jacobian,

$$\hat{\mathbf{G}} = \frac{\partial \hat{\boldsymbol{\delta}}(\bar{\mathbf{x}})}{\partial \hat{\boldsymbol{\beta}}} = \hat{\lambda}(\bar{\mathbf{x}})(I + \hat{\boldsymbol{\beta}}\bar{\mathbf{x}}'). \tag{21}$$

Then, the desired asymptotic covariance matrix is computed using

$$\text{Est.Asy.Var}[\hat{\boldsymbol{\delta}}(\bar{\mathbf{x}})] = \hat{\mathbf{G}}\mathbf{V}\hat{G}'. \tag{22}$$

The analogous computation can be done for the average partial effect in (15). To do this, note that in the sample mean computed there, all N terms are based on the same estimator of β. As such, the computation of an asymptotic analogous to (22) must have N^2 terms. The result will be

$$\text{Est.Asy.Var}[\hat{\bar{\boldsymbol{\delta}}}(\mathbf{X})] = \frac{1}{N^2}\sum_{i=1}^{N}\sum_{j=1}^{N}\hat{\mathbf{G}}_i\mathbf{V}\hat{\mathbf{G}}_j'. \tag{23}$$

An alternative method of computing an asymptotic covariance matrix for such a function of the estimated parameters suggested by Krinsky and Robb (1986) is to sample from the estimated asymptotic variance distribution of and compute $\hat{\boldsymbol{\beta}}$ the empirical variance of the observations on $\hat{\boldsymbol{\delta}}(\bar{\mathbf{x}})$. This method does not appear to be widely employed in this setting.

To compute a LM statistic, also referred to as a score test, we note that the bracketed matrix (uninverted) in either (18) or (19) is an estimator of the asymptotic covariance matrix of the score vector

$$\mathbf{g}(\boldsymbol{\beta}) = \frac{\partial \log L}{\partial \boldsymbol{\beta}} = \sum_{i=1}^{N} e_i\mathbf{x}_i, \tag{24}$$

where e_i is the generalized (as well as the simple) residual, $e_i = y_i - \exp(\boldsymbol{\beta}'\mathbf{x}_i)$. The LM statistics for tests of restrictions are computed using the χ^2 statistic

$$\text{LM} = \mathbf{g}(\hat{\boldsymbol{\beta}}_0)'[\mathbf{V}_0]^{-1}\mathbf{g}(\hat{\boldsymbol{\beta}}_0), \tag{25}$$

where $\hat{\boldsymbol{\beta}}_0$ is the estimator of $\boldsymbol{\beta}$ with the restrictions imposed, and $\mathbf{V}_0$ is either of the matrices in (18) or (19) evaluated at $\hat{\boldsymbol{\beta}}_0$ (not $\boldsymbol{\beta}$). In view of (24), the LM statistic based on (19) has an interesting form

$$\begin{aligned}\text{LM} &= \left(\sum_{i=1}^{N} e_i\mathbf{x}_i\right)'\left(\sum_{i=1}^{N} e_i^2\mathbf{x}_i\mathbf{x}_i'\right)\left(\sum_{i=1}^{N} e_i\mathbf{x}_i\right)\\ &= \mathbf{i}'\mathbf{X}^*(\mathbf{X}^{*\prime}\mathbf{X}^*)^{-1}\mathbf{X}^{*\prime}\mathbf{i},\end{aligned} \tag{26}$$

where $\mathbf{i}$ is a column of ones and $\mathbf{X}^*$ a matrix of derivatives; each row is one of the terms in the summation in (24). This is the NR^2 in a linear regression of a column of ones on the first derivatives, $\mathbf{g}_i = e_i\mathbf{x}_i$.

2.3. Fit and prediction in the Poisson model

Like any nonlinear model, the Poisson regression specification does not imply an obvious counterpart to R^2 for measuring the goodness of fit of the model to the data. One measure that has become very popular is the

$$\text{Pseudo} - R^2 = \frac{1 - \log L_0}{\log L}, \tag{27}$$

where $\log L_0$ is the log-likelihood for a model that contains only a constant and $\log L$ the log-likelihood for the model as a whole. Note that for this measure to 'work,' the latter must actually contain a constant term. As happens in the linear model as well, if the regression does not contain a constant, then fit measures, such as these, can be negative or larger than one, depending on how they are computed. By construction, the pseudo$-R^2$ is between zero and one, and increases toward one as variables are added to a model. Beyond that, it is difficult to extend the analogy to the R^2 in a linear model, since the maximum likelihood estimation (MLE) in the Poisson model is not computed so as to maximize the fit of the model to the data, nor does it correspond to a proportion of variation explained. Nonetheless, it is current practice to report this statistic with one's other results.

Two other statistics related to the lack of fit of the model are often computed. The deviance measure is

$$G^2 = 2\sum_{i=1}^{N} y_i \log\left(\frac{y_i}{\hat{\lambda}_i}\right) \tag{28}$$

(where it is understood that $0 \times \log 0 = 0$). The Pearson goodness-of-fit statistic is

$$C^2 = \sum_{i=1}^{N} \frac{(y_i - \hat{\lambda}_i)^2}{\hat{\lambda}_i}. \tag{29}$$

The second of these resembles the familiar fit measure in discrete response analysis

$$C_*^2 = \sum_{i=1}^{N} \frac{(\text{Observed}_i - \text{Expected}_i)^2}{\text{Expected}_i}. \tag{30}$$

Both of these statistics have limiting χ^2 distributions. They can be translated to aggregate fit measures by dividing each by the counterpart measure that uses the simple mean as the prediction. Thus,

$$R^2_{\text{Deviance}} = 1 - \frac{\sum_{i=1}^{N} y_i \log(y_i/\hat{\lambda}_i)}{\sum_{i=1}^{N} y_i \log(y_i/\bar{y})} \tag{31}$$

and

$$R^2_{\text{Pearson}} = 1 - \frac{\sum_{i=1}^{N} (y_i - \hat{\lambda}_i)^2/\hat{\lambda}_i}{\sum_{i=1}^{N} (y_i - \bar{y})^2/\bar{y}}. \tag{32}$$

We note, although there is no obvious counterpart to R^2 in the linear model, with regard to 'explained variation,' one can compute the correlation between the actual and fitted values in the Poisson model easily enough by using the conditional mean function as the prediction. The statistic would be

$$r_{y,\hat{\lambda}} = \frac{\sum_{i=1}^{N}(y_i - \bar{y})(\hat{\lambda}_i - \bar{y})}{\sqrt{\sum_{i=1}^{N}(y_i - \bar{y})^2 \sum_{i=1}^{N}(\hat{\lambda}_i - \bar{y})^2}} \tag{33}$$

(where we have made use of the first-order condition, $\bar{\hat{\lambda}} = \bar{y}$).

The Wald, likelihood ratio and LM tests developed in Section 2.2 are used to analyze the specification of the conditional mean function by testing restrictions on the parameters. Nonnested (and nested) models are often compared on the basis of the 'information criteria' statistics, which are, in the realm of maximum likelihood estimation, rough counterparts to adjusted R^2s. A frequently used statistic is the Akaike information criterion (AIC),

$$\mathrm{AIC} = \frac{-2\log L + 2K}{N}, \tag{34}$$

where K is the full number of parameters in the model (see Hardin and Hilbe, 2007; McCullagh and Nelder, 1989).

2.4. *Specification testing and robust covariance matrix estimation*

A crucial part of the specification of the Poisson model, the assumption that the conditional mean and variance are equal (to λ_i), cannot be tested in this fashion. Nonetheless, this is generally viewed as the fundamental shortcoming of the model, and is always subjected to close scrutiny. There are several ways of addressing the question of over- (or under-) dispersion. Section 3 considers a direct approach of specifying a more general model. Alternatively, one can begin the analysis by examining the estimated Poisson model itself to ascertain whether it satisfies the assumption. In the same manner that the squares of OLS regression residuals can be examined for evidence of heteroskedasticity, the squared residuals in the Poisson model can provide evidence of overdispersion. Cameron and Trivedi (1990) suggested a pair of statistics to examine this relationship. In the linear regression of $z_i = [(y_i - \hat{\lambda}_i)^2 - y_i]/\hat{\lambda}\sqrt{2}$ on $w_i = g(\hat{\lambda}_i)/\hat{\lambda}_i\sqrt{2}$, if the equidispersion assumption of the model is correct, then the coefficient on w_i should be close to zero, regardless of the choice of $g(.)$. The authors suggest two candidates for $g(\hat{\lambda}_i)$, $\hat{\lambda}_i$, and $\hat{\lambda}_i^2$. A simple t-test of the restriction that the coefficient is zero is equivalent to a test of the equidispersion hypothesis. (The literature contains many other suggested tests, most based on this idea. See Hilbe (2007) or Winkelmann (2003) for discussion of some others.)

Another concern about the estimator of the model parameters is their robustness to failures of the assumption of the model. Specifically, if the specification of the Poisson model is incorrect, what useful information can be retained from the

MLE? For a certain failure of the assumptions, namely the equidispersion restriction, the Poisson maximum likelihood estimator remains consistent. However, the estimated asymptotic covariance matrix based on (18) or (19) may miss-estimate the appropriate matrix. An estimator based on both (18) and (19) – now colorfully called the 'sandwich estimator' – solves the problem. The robust covariance matrix based on this result is

$$\text{Est.Asy.Var}[\hat{\boldsymbol{\beta}}_{\text{MLE}}] = \left[\sum_{i=1}^{N} \hat{\lambda}_i \mathbf{x}_i \mathbf{x}_i'\right]^{-1} \left[\sum_{i=1}^{N} (y_i - \hat{\lambda}_i)^2 \mathbf{x}_i \mathbf{x}_i'\right] \left[\sum_{i=1}^{N} \hat{\lambda}_i \mathbf{x}_i \mathbf{x}_i'\right]^{-1}. \tag{35}$$

We emphasize, this is not a cureall for all possible model misspecification, and if we do use (35), then the likelihood-ratio and LM tests in Section 2.2 are no longer valid. Some, such as endogeneity of the covariates, missing variables, and many others, render the MLE inconsistent. In these cases, 'robust' covariance matrix is a moot point.

A related issue that gets considerable attention in the current literature is the so-called 'cluster effects.' Suppose observations in the sample of N are grouped in sets of N_i in some fashion such that observations within a group are correlated with each other. Once again, we have to assume that in spite of this, the (now, pseudo-) MLE remains consistent. ['pseudo-' is used since the cluster nature of the data violates the ***iid*** assumption of likelihood theory.] It will follow once again that the estimated asymptotic covariance matrix is inaccurate. A commonly used alternative to (18) or (19) is related to (32). In the clustering case, the center matrix in (35) is replaced with

$$\mathbf{C} = \left[\sum_{r=1}^{G} \sum_{i=1}^{N_g} (\mathbf{g}_{ir} - \bar{\mathbf{g}}_r)(\mathbf{g}_{ir} - \bar{\mathbf{g}}_r)'\right] \tag{36}$$

where there are G groups or clusters, the number of observations in cluster 'r' is N_r, $\mathbf{g}_{ir} = e_{ir}\mathbf{x}_{ir}$, and $\bar{\mathbf{g}}_r = (1/N_r)\sum_{i=1}^{N_r} \mathbf{g}_{ir}$.

2.5. An application

To illustrate this model (and several extensions), we will employ the data used in the study by Ripahn et al. (2003). The raw data are published on the *Journal of Applied Econometrics* data archive website, http://qed.econ.queensu.ca/jae/ [4] The .zip file contains the single data file **rwm.data**.[5] The data file contains raw data on variables (original names) (Table 1).

---

[4] The URL for the data file is http://qed.econ.queensu.ca/jae/2003-v18.4/riphahn-wambach-million/ This URL provides links to a text file which describes the data, http://qed.econ.queensu.ca/jae/2003-v18.4/riphahn-wambach-million/readme.rwm.txt and the raw data, themselves, which are in text form, zipped in the file http://qed.econ.queensu.ca/jae/2003-v18.4/riphahn-wambach-million/rwm-data.zip.

[5] Data handling and aspects of software usage are discussed in Section 5.

Table 1
Data used in applications

id	person – identification number
female	female = 1; male = 0
year	calendar year of the observation
age	age in years
hsat	health satisfaction, coded 0 (low) – 10 (high)
handdum	handicapped = 1; otherwise = 0
handper	degree of handicap in percent (0–100)
hhninc	household nominal monthly net income in German marks/1000
hhkids	children under age 16 in the household = 1; otherwise = 0
educ	years of schooling
married	married = 1; otherwise = 0
haupts	highest schooling degree is high school; degree = 1; else = 0
reals	highest schooling degree is college degree = 1; else = 0
fachhs	highest schooling degree is technical degree = 1; else = 0
abitur	highest schooling degree is trade school = 1; otherwise = 0
univ	highest schooling degree is university degree = 1; otherwise = 0
working	employed = 1; otherwise = 0
bluec	blue collar employee = 1; otherwise = 0
whitec	white collar employee = 1; otherwise = 0
self	self employed = 1; otherwise = 0
beamt	civil servant = 1; otherwise = 0
docvis	number of doctor visits in last three months
hospvis	number of hospital visits in last calendar year
public	insured in public health insurance = 1; otherwise = 0
addon	insured by add-on insurance = 1; otherwise = 0

The data file contains 27,326 observations. They are an unbalanced panel, with group sizes ranging from 1 to 7 with frequencies T: $1 = 1525$, $2 = 2158$, $3 = 825$, $4 = 926$, $5 = 1051$, $6 = 1000$, and $7 = 987$. Additional variables created in the data set included year dummy variables, sex = female + 1, and age^2/1000. For the purpose of this illustration, we are interested in the count variable DOCVIS, which is the number of doctor visits in the last three months. A histogram of this variable appears in Fig. 1.

The model in Table 2 is based on the authors' specification in the paper. The estimator of the asymptotic covariance matrix is based on the second derivatives, as in (18). The likelihood-ratio test of the hypothesis that all of the coefficients are zero is computed using the log-likelihood for the full model, −89,431.01, and the log-likelihood for the model that contains only the constant term, −108,662.1. The χ^2 statistic of 38,462.26 is far larger than the 95% critical value for the χ^2 distribution with 16 degrees of freedom, 26.29. There are two alternative methods of testing this hypothesis. The Wald statistic will be computed using

$$W = (\hat{\boldsymbol{\beta}}_0 - \mathbf{0})[\text{Est.Asy. Var}(\hat{\boldsymbol{\beta}}_0 - \mathbf{0})]^{-1}(\hat{\boldsymbol{\beta}}_0 - 0), \tag{37}$$

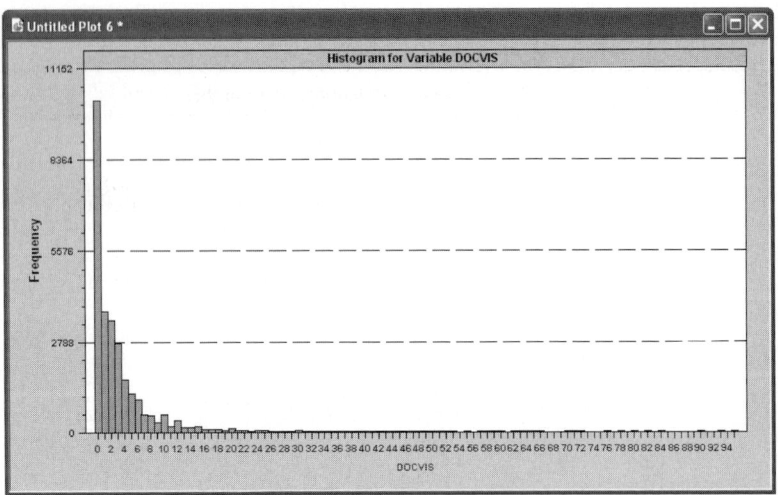

Fig. 1. Histogram of doctor visits.

where $\hat{\boldsymbol{\beta}}_0$ is all coefficients save the intercept (the latter 16 of them) and Est.Asy.Var$(\hat{\boldsymbol{\beta}}_0 - \mathbf{0})$ is the 16×16 part of the estimated covariance matrix that omits the constant term. The result is 41,853.37, again with 16 degrees of freedom. As before, this is far larger than the critical value, so the hypothesis is rejected. Finally, the LM statistic is computed according to (18) and (23), giving a value of 44,346.59. As is typical, the three statistics are reasonably close to one another.

The coefficient estimates are shown at the left of the table. Standard tests of the hypothesis that each is zero are shown in the third column of results. Most of the individual significance tests decisively reject the hypothesis that the coefficients are zero, so the conclusions drawn above about the coefficient vector as a whole are not surprising. The partial effects reported at the right of the table are average partial effects, as defined in (15), with standard errors computed using (22). As these are a straightforward multiple of the original coefficient vector, conclusions drawn about the impacts of the variables on the response variable follow those based on the estimate of $\boldsymbol{\beta}$. The multiple, 3.1835 is, in fact, the sample mean of the response variable. (This is straightforward to verify. The necessary condition for maximization of $\log L$ in (24) implies that $\Sigma_i e_i = \Sigma_i(y_i - \lambda_i) = 0$ at the MLE. The claimed result follows immediately. Note that this does not occur if the model does not contain a constant term – the same result that occurs in a linear regression setting.) As noted earlier, since AGE enters this model nonlinearly, neither the coefficients nor the partial effects for AGE or AGESQ give the right measure for the impact of AGE. The partial effects evaluated at the means would be

$$\delta(\bar{\mathbf{x}}, \overline{\mathrm{AGE}}) = (\beta_3 + 2\beta_4\overline{\mathrm{AGE}}/1000) \times \exp(\boldsymbol{\beta}'\bar{\mathbf{x}}), \tag{37a}$$

which we compute at the mean of age of 43.5256898. The resulting estimate is 0.012924. In order to compute a standard error for this estimator, we would use the delta method. The required derivatives are $(g_1, g_2, \ldots, g_{17})$, where all 17 components

Table 2
Estimated Poisson regression model

	Coeff.	Std. Err.	b/Std. Err.	Robust SE	Cluster SE	Partial Effect	SE Partial[a]
Constant	2.48612758	.06626647	37.517	.17631321	.21816313	0.	0.
FEMALE	.28187106	.00774175	36.409	.02448327	.03106782	.89734351	.03529496**
AGE	−.01835519	.00277022	−6.626	.00804534	.00983497	−.05843420	.01121654**
AGESQ	.26778487	.03096216	8.649	.09134073	.11183550	.85249979	.12576669**
HSAT	−.21345503	.00141482	−150.871	.00449869	.00497983	−.67953940	.01375581**
HANDDUM	.09041129	.00963870	9.380	.02960213	.02873540	.28782659	.03917770**
HANDPER	.00300153	.00017626	17.029	.00057489	.00073815	.00955544	.00073483**
MARRIED	.03873812	.00881265	4.396	.02752875	.03325271	.12332377	.03558146**
EDUC	−.00342252	.00187631	−1.824	.00489031	.00639244	−.01089568	.00756284
HHNINC	−.16498398	.02291240	−7.201	.06072932	.07060708	−.52523061	.09283605**
HHKIDS	−.09762798	.00862042	−11.325	.02555567	.03154185	−.31080111	.03519498**
SELF	−.23243199	.01806908	−12.864	.05225385	.06470690	−.73995303	.07402117**
BEAMT	.03640374	.01921475	1.895	.04994140	.06426340	.11589220	.07745533
BLUEC	−.01916882	.01006783	−1.904	.02922716	.03577130	−.06102440	.04058392
WORKING	.00041819	.00941149	.044	.02808178	.03266767	.00133132	.03792298
PUBLIC	.14122076	.01565581	9.020	.03926803	.04593042	.44957981	.06360250**
ADDON	.02584454	.02544319	1.016	.05875837	.06596606	.08227672	.10253177

[a] ** indicates the ratio of estimate to standard error as larger than 2.0.

Diagnostic Statistics for Poisson Regression	
Number of observations	27,326
Log-likelihood function	−89,431.01
Restricted log-likelihood	−10,8662.1
χ^2	38,462.26
Akaike information criterion	6.54673
McFadden pseudo R^2	.176981
χ^2 based on Pearson residuals	184,919.711
R^2 based on Pearson residuals	.3345
G^2 based on deviance	25,823.429
R^2 based on deviance	.2341
Overdispersion test: $g = \lambda_i$	22.899
Overdispersion test: $g = \lambda_i^2$	23.487

equal $\delta(\bar{\mathbf{x}}, \overline{\text{AGE}})$ times the corresponding element of $\bar{\mathbf{x}}$ save for the third and fourth (corresponding to the coefficients on AGE and $\text{AGE}^2/1000$, which are

$$g_3 = \partial\delta(\bar{\mathbf{x}}, \overline{\text{AGE}})/\partial\beta_3 = \lambda(\bar{\mathbf{x}}, \overline{\text{AGE}}) + \delta(\bar{\mathbf{x}}, \overline{\text{AGE}}) \times \overline{\text{AGE}} \tag{37b}$$

$$g_4 = \partial\delta(\bar{\mathbf{x}}, \overline{\text{AGE}})\partial\beta_4 = \lambda(\bar{\mathbf{x}}, \overline{\text{AGE}}) + 2\overline{\text{AGE}}/1000 + \delta(\bar{\mathbf{x}}, \overline{\text{AGE}}) \times \overline{\text{AGE}}^2/1000. \tag{37c}$$

The estimated standard error is 0.001114. (There is a large amount of variation across computer packages in the ease with which this kind of secondary computation can be done using the results of estimation.)

These data are a panel, so, in fact, the motivation for the cluster robust covariance matrix in (32) or (33) would apply here. These alternative estimates of the standard errors of the Poisson regression coefficients are given in Table 2. As is clearly evident, these are substantially larger than the 'pooled' counterparts. While not a formal test, these results are strongly suggestive that the Poisson model as examined so far should be extended to accommodate these data.

The two Cameron and Trivedi tests of overdispersion also strongly suggest that the equidispersion assumption of the Poisson model is inconsistent with the data. We will pursue this now, in the next section. Together, these results are convincing that the specification of the Poisson model is inadequate for these data. There are two directions to be considered. The overdispersion tests suggest that a model that relaxes this restriction, such as the NB model discussed below, should be considered. The large increase in the standard errors implied by the cluster corrected estimator would motivate this researcher to examine a formal panel data specification, such as those detailed in Section 4.

3. Heterogeneity and overdispersion

The test results in the preceding example that suggest overdispersion in the Poisson model are typical – indeed it is rare not to find evidence of over- (or under-) dispersion in count data. The equidispersion assumption of the model is a fairly serious shortcoming. One way to approach the issue directly is to allow the Poisson mean to accommodate unmeasured heterogeneity in the regression function. The extended model appears

$$E[y|\mathbf{x},\varepsilon] = \exp(\boldsymbol{\beta}'\mathbf{x} + \varepsilon), \qquad \mathrm{Cov}[\mathbf{x},\varepsilon] = \mathbf{0}, \tag{38}$$

where the unmeasured ε plays the role of a regression disturbance. More to the point here, it plays the role of the unmeasured heterogeneity in the Poisson model. How the model evolves from here depends crucially on what is assumed about the distribution of ε. In the linear model, a normal distribution is typically assumed. That is possible here as well (see ESI, 2007), however, most contemporary applications use the log-gamma density to produce an empirically manageable formulation. With the log-gamma assumption, as we show below, the familiar NB model emerges for the unconditional (on the unobserved ε) distribution of the observed variable, y. The NB model has become the standard device for accommodating overdispersion in count data since its implementation into commercial software beginning with *LIMDEP* (1987), *Stata* Corp. (1993), and *SAS* (1998).

3.1. The negative binomial model

The Poisson model with log-gamma heterogeneity may be written

$$\begin{aligned} f(y_i|\mathbf{x}_i,u_i) &= Prob[Y = y_i|\mathbf{x}_i,u_i] \\ &= \frac{\exp(-\lambda_i u_i)(\lambda_i u_i)^{y_i}}{y_i!}, \qquad y = 0,1,\ldots. \end{aligned} \tag{39}$$

The log-gamma assumption for ε implies that $u_i = \exp(\varepsilon_i)$ has a gamma distribution. The resulting distribution is a Poisson-gamma mixture model. The gamma noise, which is mixed with the Poisson distribution, is constrained to have a mean of one. The conditional mean of y_i in (38), given the gamma heterogeneity, is therefore given as $\lambda_i u_i$ rather than the standard Poisson mean, λ_i. (We can thus see that this will preserve the Poisson mean, λ_i, but induce additional variation, which was the purpose.) In order to estimate the model parameters (and use the model), it must be written in terms of the observable variables (so that we can construct the likelihood function). The unconditional distribution of y_i is obtained by integrating u_i out of the density. Thus,

$$\begin{aligned} f(y_i|\mathbf{x}_i) &= \int_n f(y_i|\mathbf{x}_i, u_i) g(u_i)\,\mathrm{d}u_i \\ &= \int_u \frac{\exp(-\lambda_i u_i)(\lambda_i u_i)^{y_i}}{y_i!} g(u_i)\,\mathrm{d}u_i, \qquad y_i = 0, 1, \ldots. \end{aligned} \tag{40}$$

The gamma density is a two-parameter distribution; $g(u) = [\theta^\gamma/\Gamma(\gamma)]\exp(\text{-}\theta u)\, u^{\gamma-1}$. The mean is γ/θ, so to impose the restriction that the mean is equal to one, we set $\gamma = \theta$. With this assumption, we find the unconditional distribution as

$$f(y_i|\mathbf{x}_i) = \int_0^\infty \frac{\exp(-\lambda_i u_i)(\lambda_i u_i)^{y_i}}{\Gamma(y_i+1)} \frac{\theta^\theta}{\Gamma(\theta)} \exp(-\theta u_i) u_i^{\theta-1}\,\mathrm{d}u_i, \quad y_i =, 0, 1, \ldots. \tag{41}$$

The variance of the gamma distribution is $\gamma/\theta^2 = 1/\theta$, so the smaller is θ, the larger is the amount of overdispersion in the distribution. (Note we have used the identity $y_i! = \Gamma(y_i + 1)$.) Using properties of the gamma integral and a bit of manipulation, we can write this as.

$$f(y_i|\mathbf{x}_i) = \frac{\Gamma(y_i+\theta)}{\Gamma(y_i+1)\Gamma(\theta)} \left(\frac{\theta}{\lambda_i+\theta}\right)^\theta \left(\frac{\lambda_i}{\lambda_i+\theta}\right)^{y_i}, \qquad y_i = 0, 1, \ldots. \tag{42}$$

By dividing all terms by θ, we obtain another convenient form,

$$f(y_i|\mathbf{x}_i) = \frac{\Gamma(y_i+\theta)}{\Gamma(y_i+1)\Gamma(\theta)} \left(\frac{1}{1+(\lambda_i/\theta)}\right)^\theta \left(1 - \frac{1}{1+(\lambda_i/\theta)}\right)^{y_i}, \quad y = 0, 1, \ldots. \tag{43}$$

By defining the dispersion parameter $\alpha = 1/\theta$ so that there will be a direct relationship between the model mean and α, we can obtain another convenient form of the density,

$$f(y_i|\mathbf{x}_i) = \frac{\Gamma(y_i+1/\alpha)}{\Gamma(y_i+1)\Gamma(1/\alpha)} \left(\frac{1}{1+\alpha\lambda_i}\right)^{1/\alpha} \left(\frac{\alpha\lambda_i}{1+\alpha\lambda_i}\right)^{y_i}, \qquad y = 0, 1, \ldots. \tag{44}$$

One of the important features of the NB model is that the conditional mean function is the same as in the Poisson model,

$$E[y_i|x_i] = \lambda_i. \tag{45}$$

The implication is that the partial effects are computed the same way.

3.2. Estimation of the negative binomial model

Direct estimation of the NB model parameters ($\boldsymbol{\beta}$,α) can be done easily with a few modern software packages including *LIMDEP*, *Stata*, and *SAS*. The likelihood equations for the algorithm are revealing

$$\frac{\partial \log L}{\partial \boldsymbol{\beta}} = \sum_{i=1}^{N} \left(\frac{(y_i - \lambda_i)}{1 + \alpha\lambda_i} \right) \mathbf{x}_i = \mathbf{0}. \tag{46}$$

We can see immediately, as might be expected, that these are not the same as for the Poisson model, so the estimates will differ. On the other hand, note that as α approaches zero, the condition approaches that for the Poisson model – a point that will become important below. The other necessary condition for estimation is the derivative with respect to α,

$$\frac{\partial \log L}{\partial \alpha} = \sum_{i=1}^{N} \left\{ \frac{1}{\alpha^2} \left[\log(1 + \alpha\lambda_i) - \log\left(\frac{\Gamma(y_i + 1/\alpha)}{\Gamma(1/\alpha)} \right) \right] - \left(\frac{y_i - \lambda_i}{\alpha(1 + \alpha\lambda_i)} \right) \right\}. \tag{47}$$

Second derivatives or outer products of the first derivatives can be used to estimate the asymptotic covariance matrix of the estimated parameters. An example appears below.

3.3. Robust estimation of count models

The conditional mean in the mixture model is $E[y_i|\mathbf{x}_i,u_i] = \lambda_i u_i$. By a simple application of the law of iterated expectations, we find $E[y_i|\mathbf{x}_i] = \mathrm{E}_u[\lambda_i u_i|u_i] = \lambda_i E[u_i] = \lambda_i$. (Since the terms are independent, the mean is just the product of the means.) The fact that the conditional mean function in the NB model is the same as in the Poisson model has an important and intriguing implication. It follows from the result that the Poisson MLE is a generalized mixed models (GMM) estimator for the NB model. In particular, the conditional mean result for the NB model implies that the score function for the Poisson model,

$$\mathbf{g} = \sum\nolimits_i (y_i - \lambda_i)\mathbf{x}_i \tag{48}$$

has mean zero even in the presence of the the overdispersion. The useful result for current purposes is that as a consequence, the Poisson MLE of $\boldsymbol{\beta}$ is consistent even in the presence of the overdispersion. (The result is akin to the consistency of ordinary least squares in the presence of heteroskedastic errors in the linear model for panel data.) The Poisson MLE is robust to this kind of model misspecification. The asymptotic covariance matrix for the Poisson model is not appropriate, however. This is one of those rare instances in which the increasingly popular 'robust' covariance matrix (see (35)) is actually robust to something specific that we can identify. The upshot of this is that one can estimate the parameters, an appropriate asymptotic covariance matrix, and appropriate partial effects for the slope parameters of the NB model just by fitting the Poisson model and using (32).

Why then would one want to go the extra distance and effort to fit the NB model? One answer is that the NB estimator will be more efficient. Less obvious is that we do not have a test with demonstrable power against the equidispersion hypothesis in the Poisson model. With the NB model, we can begin to construct a test statistic, though as shown below, new problems do arise.

3.4. Application and generalizations

Table 3 presents both Poisson and negative binomial estimates of the count model for doctor visits. As anticipated, the estimates do differ noticeably. On the other hand, we are using quite a large sample, and both sets of estimates are consistent. The large differences might make one suspect that something else is amiss with the model; perhaps a different specification is called for, and neither estimator is consistent. Unfortunately, this cannot be discerned internally based on just these estimates, and a more detailed analysis would be needed. In fact, the differences persist in the partial effects – in some cases, these are quite large as well. We might add here that there is an efficacy gain from the NB2 model since the standard errors are roughly 25% less than the heteroskedasticity-robust standard errors for the Poisson.

Testing for the specification of the NB model against that of the Poisson model has a long and wide history in the relevant literature (see Anscombe, 1949; Blom, 1954). Unfortunately, none of the tests suggested, save for the Cameron and Trivedi tests used earlier, are appropriate in this setting. These tests include the LM tests against the negative binomial for overdispersed data, and against the Katz system for underdispersed data. Hilbe (2007) discusses a generalized Poisson which can also be used for underdispersed data. Regardless, the problem is that the relevant parameter, α, is on the edge of the parameter space, not in its interior. The test is directly analogous to a test for a zero variance. In practical terms, the LM test cannot be computed because the covariance matrix of the derivatives is singular at $\alpha = 0$. The Wald and likelihood-ratio tests can be computed, but again, there is the issue of the appropriate distribution for the test statistic. It is not $\chi^2(1)$. For better or worse, practitioners routinely compute these statistics in spite of the ambiguity.[6] It is certainly obvious that the hypothesis $\alpha = 0$ would be rejected by either of these tests.

Table 3 also presents robust standard errors for the NB model. For the pooled data case, these differ only slightly from the uncorrected standard errors. This is to be expected, since the NB model already accounts for the specification failure (heterogeneity) that would be accommodated by the robust standard errors. This does call into question why one would compute a robust covariance matrix for the NB model. Any remaining violation of the model assumptions is likely to produce inconsistent parameter estimates, for which robust standard errors provide dubious virtue.

[6] Stata reports one half the standard $\chi^2[1]$ statistic. While this surely is not the appropriate test statistic, one might surmise that it is a conservative result. If the hypothesis that $\alpha = 0$ is rejected by this test, it seems extremely that it would not be rejected by the appropriate χ^2 test, whatever that is.

Table 3
Poisson and negative binomial models

	Poisson			Negative Binomial Model (NB-2)			Robust Standard Errors	
	Coeff.	Std. Err.	Part. Eff.	Coeff.	Std. Err.	Part. Eff.	Robust SE	Cluster SE
Constant	2.48612758	.06626647	0.	2.93815327	.14544040	0.	.14550426	.17427529
FEMALE	.28187106	.00774175	.89734351	.35108438	.01643537	1.14442153	.01680855	.02128039
AGE	−.01835519	.00277022	−.05843420	−.03604169	.00610034	−.11748426	.00616981	.00737181
AGESQ	.26778487	.03096216	.85249979	.46466762	.07006707	1.51466615	.07108961	.08528665
HSAT	−.21345503	.00141482	−.67953940	−.22320535	.00339028	−.72757725	.00344216	.00387560
HANDDUM	.09041129	.00963870	.28782659	.03863554	.02154854	.12593935	.02155752	.02070723
HANDPER	.00300153	.00017626	.00955544	−.00598082	.00050291	.01949555	.00050309	.00064984
MARRIED	.03873812	.00881265	.12332377	.05048344	.01856803	.16455967	.01857855	.02249464
EDUC	−.00342252	.00187631	−.01089568	−.01126970	.00390703	−.03673558	.00393156	.00495663
HHNINC	−.16498398	.02291240	−.52523061	−.01356497	.00472261	−.04421742	.00489946	.00556370
HHKIDS	−.09762798	.00862042	−.31080111	−.09439713	.01724797	−.30770411	.01781272	.02144006
SELF	−.23243199	.01806908	−.73995303	−.24001686	.03042783	−.78237732	.03128019	.03727414
BEAMT	.03640374	.01921475	.11589220	.04321571	.03494549	.14086922	.03531910	.04368996
BLUEC	−.01916882	.01006783	−.06102440	−.00355440	.02073448	−.01158621	.02083167	.02530838
WORKING	.00041819	.00941149	.00133132	.02487987	.02060004	.08110034	.02086701	.02435497
PUBLIC	.14122076	.01565581	.44957981	.11074510	.03041037	.36099319	.03066638	.03558399
ADDON	.02584454	.02544319	.08227672	.03713781	.06968404	.12105726	.07002987	.07939311
α	0.	0.	0.	1.46273783	.01654079	0.	.04080414	.04893952
$\log L$		−89,431.01			−57,982.79			

NB Model Form	α	P	$\log L$
Negbin – 0	0.0000	0.0000	−89,431.01
	(.00000)	(0.0000)	
Negbin – 1	4.8372	1.0000	−57,861.96
	(.05306)	(.00000)	
Negbin – 2	1.4627	2.0000	−57,982.79
	(.01654)	(.00000)	
Negbin – P	2.6380	1.4627	−57,652.60
	(.05891)	(.01663)	

The literature, mostly associating the result with Cameron and Trivedi's (1986) early work, defines two familiar forms of the NB model. Where

$$\lambda_i = \exp(\boldsymbol{\beta}'\mathbf{x}_i), \tag{49}$$

the *Negbin 2* or NB-2 form of the probability is the one we have examined thus far

$$\text{Prob}(Y = y_i|\mathbf{x}_i) = \frac{\Gamma(\theta + y_i)}{\Gamma(\theta)\Gamma(y_i + 1)} u_i^{\theta}(1 - u_i)^{y_i}, \tag{50}$$

where $u_i = \theta/(\theta + \lambda_i)$ and $\theta = 1/\alpha$. This is the default form of the model in most (if not all) of the received statistics packages that provide an estimator for this model. The signature feature of the model is the relationship between the mean and the variance of the model,

$$\text{Var}[y_i|\mathbf{x}_i] = \lambda_i[1 + \alpha\lambda_i^{P-1}]. \tag{51}$$

Thus, when $\alpha = 0$, we revert to the Poisson model. The model considered thus far has $P = 2$, hence the name NB-2. The *Negbin 1* form of the model results if θ in the preceding is replaced with $\theta_i = \theta\lambda_i$. Then, u_i becomes $u = \theta/(1 + \theta)$, and the density becomes

$$\text{Prob}(Y = y_i|\mathbf{x}_i) = \frac{\Gamma(\theta\lambda_i + y_i)}{\Gamma(\theta\lambda_i)\Gamma(y_i + 1)} w^{\theta\lambda_i}(1 - w)^{y_i}, \tag{52}$$

where $w = \theta/(\theta + 1)$. In this instance, $P = 1$, and the model is one of a more pure form of overdispersion,

$$\text{Var}[y_i|\mathbf{x}_i] = \lambda_i[1 + \alpha]. \tag{53}$$

Note that this is not a simple reparameterization of the model – it is a NB model of a different form. The general Negbin P or NB-P model is obtained by allowing P in (51) to be a free parameter. This can be accomplished by replacing θ in (50) with $\theta\lambda^{2-P}$. For convenience, let $Q = 2 - P$. Then, the density is

$$\text{Prob}(Y = y_i|\mathbf{x}_i) = \frac{\Gamma(\theta\lambda_i^Q + y_i)}{\Gamma(\theta\lambda_i^Q)\Gamma(y_i + 1)} \left(\frac{\theta\lambda_i^Q}{\theta\lambda_i^Q + \lambda_i}\right)^{\theta\lambda_i^Q} \left(\frac{\lambda}{\theta\lambda_i^Q + \lambda_i}\right)^{y_i}. \tag{54}$$

(As of this writing, this model is only available in *LIMDEP*.) The table following the parameter estimates shows this specification analysis for our application. Though the NB-1 and NB-2 specifications cannot be tested against each other, both are restricted cases of the NB-P model. The likelihood-ratio test is valid in this instance, and it decisively rejects both models (see Hilbe, 1993; Hilbe, 1994; Lawless, 1987; Long and Freese, 2006).

4. Important extensions of the models for counts

The accommodation of overdispersion, perhaps induced by latent unobserved heterogeneity, is arguably the most important extension of the Poisson model for the applied researcher. But, other practicalities of 'real' data have motivated analysts to consider many other varieties of the count models. We will consider four broad areas here that are often encountered in received data: censoring and truncation, zero inflation, two part models, and panel data applications. In this section, we will turn to a sample of more exotic formulations that are part of the (very large) ongoing frontier research.

4.1. Censoring and truncation

Censoring and truncation are generally features of data sets that are modified as part of the sampling process. Data are censored when values in certain ranges of the distribution of outcomes are collapsed into one (or fewer) values. For example, we can see in Fig. 1 for the doctor visits data that the distribution of outcomes has an extremely long (perhaps implausibly so) right tail. Perhaps if one were skeptical of the data gathering process, or even if just to restrict the influence of outliers, they might recode all values above a certain value, say 15 in those data, down to some upper limit (such as 8). Values in a data set may be censored at either or both tails, or even in ranges within the distribution (see, e.g., Greene's (2003, pp. 774–780) analysis of Fair's (1978) data on extramarital affairs). The most common applications of censoring in counts will, however, involve recoding the upper tail of the distribution, as suggested in our example.

Truncation, in contrast, involves not masking a part of the distribution of outcomes, but discarding it. Our health care data suggest two possibilities. The number of zeros in our data is extremely large, perhaps larger than a Poisson model could hope to predict. One (perhaps not very advisable, but we are speaking theoretically here) modeling strategy might be simply to discard those zeros, as not representative. The distribution that describes the remaining data is truncated – by construction, only values greater than zero will be observed. In fact, in many quite reasonable applications, this is how data are gathered. In environmental and recreation applications, researchers are often interested in numbers of visits to sites. Data are gathered on site, so, again, by construction, it is not possible to observe a zero. The model, however, constructed, applies only to value 1,2, ... One might, as well truncate a distribution at its upper tail. Thus, in our data set, again referring to the histogram in Fig. 1, rather than censor the values larger than 15, we might just discard them. The resulting distribution then applies to the values 0,1, ..., 15, which is a truncated distribution.

Estimation of count models for censored or truncated distributions requires a straightforward extension of the base model. We illustrate for the Poisson case, but by a simple change of the function, the results can be extended to negative binomial or, in fact, any other specification.

The applicable distribution for the random variable that is censored is formed by using the laws of probability to produce a density that sums to one. For example, suppose the data are censored at an upper value, U. Thus, any actual value that is U or larger is recorded as U. The probability distribution for this set of outcomes is

$$
\begin{aligned}
f(Y|\mathbf{x}_i) = Prob[Y = y|\mathbf{x}_i] &= \frac{\exp(-\lambda_i)\lambda_i^y}{y!}, \quad && y = 0, 1, \ldots, U - 1, \\
Prob[Y = U|\mathbf{x}_i] &= \sum_{u=U}^{\infty} \frac{\exp(-\lambda_i)\lambda_i^u}{u!}, && \lambda_i = \exp(\boldsymbol{\beta}'\mathbf{x}_i) > 0.
\end{aligned} \tag{55}
$$

The log-likelihood is formulated by using these probabilities for the observed outcomes. Note that the upper tail involves an infinite number of terms. This is transformed to a finite sum by noting that

$$
\mathrm{Prob}[Y = U|\mathbf{x}_i] = 1 - \mathrm{Prob}[Y < U|x_i]. \tag{56}
$$

(For a detailed development of this result, see Econometric Software, Inc., 2007, Chapter 25). There are three important implications of this specification:

- Estimation of the model ignoring the censoring produces an inconsistent estimator of β. The result is precisely analogous to ignoring censoring in the linear regression model (see Greene, 2003, Chapter 22)
- Under this specification, the mean of Y is no longer λ_i. It is easy to see based on how the model is constructed that the mean must be less than λ_i. Intuitively, large values are being converted into small ones, so this must shrink the mean. (The opposite would be true if the censoring were in the lower tail.)
- Because the conditional mean is affected by the censoring, the partial effects are also. A full development of the appropriate partial effects is fairly complicated (see, again, Econometric Software, Inc. (ESI), 2007). The end result is that the censoring dampens the partial effects as well.

The analysis here parallels the development of the censored regression (Tobit) model for continuous data. See Terza (1985) for extensive details. (An alternative representation of censoring in count models in terms of discrete survival models can be found in Hilbe (2007).)

The truncation case is handled similarly. In this case, the probability distribution must be scaled so that the terms sum to one over the specified outcomes. Suppose, for example, that the distribution is truncated at lower value L. This means that only values $L+1$, $L+2, \ldots$ appear in an observed sample. The appropriate probability model would be

$$
\begin{aligned}
f(Y|\mathbf{x}_i) = Prob[Y = y|\mathbf{x}_i] &= \frac{\left[\exp(-\lambda_i)\lambda_i^y\right]/y!}{Prob[Y > L]}, \qquad y = L + 1, L + 2, \ldots, \\
\lambda_i &= \exp(\boldsymbol{\beta}'\mathbf{x}_i) > 0.
\end{aligned} \tag{57}
$$

Once again, we use complementary probabilities to turn infinite sums into finite ones. For example, consider the common case of truncation at zero. The applicable distribution for the observed counts will be

$$\begin{aligned} f(Y|\mathbf{x}_i) = \text{Prob}[Y = y|\mathbf{x}_i] &= \frac{[\exp(-\lambda_i)\lambda_i^y]/y!}{\text{Prob}[Y > 0]} \\ &= \frac{[\exp(-\lambda_i)\lambda_i^y]/y!}{1 - \text{Prob}[Y = 0]} \\ &= \frac{[\exp(-\lambda_i)\lambda_i^y]/y!}{1 - \exp(-\lambda_i)}, \qquad Y = 1, 2, \ldots. \end{aligned} \tag{58}$$

As in the censoring case, truncation affects both the conditional mean and the partial effects. (A detailed analysis appears in ESI, 2007.) Note, finally, these (and the cases below) are among those noted earlier in which computing a 'robust' covariance matrix does not solve the problem of nonrobustness. The basic MLE that ignores the censoring or truncation is inconsistent, so it is not helpful to compute a robust covariance matrix.

To demonstrate these effects, we continue the earlier application of the Poisson model. Table 4 shows the impact of censoring at 8 in the distribution. This masks about 10% of the observations, which is fairly mild censoring. The first set of results in the table at the left is based on the original uncensored data. The center set of results is based on the censored data, but ignore the censoring. Thus, the comparison to the first set shows the impact of ignoring the censoring. There is no clear generality to be drawn in the table, because it is clear that some of the changes in the coefficients are quite large, while others are quite small. The partial effects, however, tell a somewhat different story. These change quite substantially. Note, for example, that the estimated partial effect of income (HHNINC) falls by 80% while that of children (HHKIDS) falls by half. The third set of results in Table 4 is based on the corrected likelihood function. In principle, these should replicate the first set. We see, however, that for these data, the full MLEs for the censored data model actually more closely resemble those for the estimator that ignored the censoring. One might expect this when the censoring is only a small part of the distribution. The impact of the censoring is likely to be more severe when a larger proportion of the observations are censored.

Table 5 repeats the calculations for the truncation at zero case. The zeros are 37% of the sample (about 10,200), so we would expect a more noticeable impact. Indeed, the effect of ignoring the truncation is quite substantial. Comparing the left to the center set of estimates in Table 5, we see that some coefficients change sign, while others change considerably. The third should replicate the first. However, truncating 37% of the distribution quite substantively changes the distribution, and the replication is not particularly good. One might suspect, as we explore below, that the data process that is producing the zeros actually differs from that underlying the rest of the distribution.

Hilbe (2007) developed a survival parameterization of the censored Poisson and NB models. Rather than having cut points below or above which censored observations fall, and observation in the data may be censored. Characterized after traditional survival models such as the Cox proportional hazards model and

Table 4
The effect of censoring on the Poisson model

	Poisson Based on Uncensored Data			Poisson Model Ignoring Censoring			Censored Data (at 8) Poisson Model		
	Coeff.	Std. Err.	Part. Eff.	Coeff.	Std. Err.	Part. Eff.	Coeff.	Std. Err.	Part. Eff.
Constant	2.48612758	.06626647	0.	2.14986800	.07524413	0.	2.25968677	.07596690	0.
FEMALE	.28187106	.00774175	.89734351	.27709347	.00894003	.66233310	.29202937	.00904040	.66106102
AGE	−.01835519	.00277022	−.05843420	−.03211408	.00318455	−.07676189	−.03403051	.00322451	−.07703417
AGESQ	.26778487	.03096216	.85249979	.42280492	.03578592	1.01062538	.44605854	.03627228	1.00973377
HSAT	−.21345503	.00141482	−.67953940	−.15716683	.00166910	−.37567393	−.16927552	.00171922	−.38318561
HANDDUM	.09041129	.00963870	.28782659	.03913318	.01132602	.09353955	.04291882	.01147955	.09715448
HANDPER	.00300153	.00017626	.00955544	.00308629	.00021489	.00737711	.00353402	.00022065	.00799989
MARRIED	.03873812	.00881265	.12332377	.05122800	.01024523	.12244965	.05587384	.01038134	.12648049
EDUC	−.00342252	.00187631	−.01089568	−.00021599	.00211001	−.00051628	.00072296	.00212106	.00163656
HHNINC	−.16498398	.02291240	−.52523061	−.02645213	.02544113	−.06322820	−.03024873	.02566863	−.06847344
HHKIDS	−.09762798	.00862042	−.31080111	−.06493632	.00985764	−.15521648	−.06795371	.00994926	−.15382544
SELF	−.23243199	.01806908	−.73995303	−.24973460	.02038677	−.59693753	−.25682829	.02045212	−.58137705
BEAMT	.03640374	.01921475	.11589220	−.00855232	.02140198	−.02044250	−.00464199	.02148378	−.01050797
BLUEC	−.01916882	.01006783	−.06102440	−.03340251	.01151415	−.07984161	−.03558453	.01159109	−.08055198
WORKING	.00041819	.00941149	.00133132	.03061167	.01080953	.07317070	.02669552	.01090431	.06043012
PUBLIC	.14122076	.01565581	.44957981	.06153310	.01722210	.14708182	.06893203	.01729248	.15604004
ADDON	.02584454	.02544319	.08227672	.08361017	.02824989	.19985236	.08126672	.02852185	.18396185

Table 5
The effect of truncation on the Poisson model

	Poisson Based on Original Data			Poisson Model Ignoring Truncation			Truncated (at 0) Poisson Model		
	Coeff.	Std. Err.	Part. Eff.	Coeff.	Std. Err.	Part. Eff.	Coeff.	Std. Err.	Part. Eff.
Constant	2.48612758	.06626647	0.	2.25206660	.06654230	0.	2.24409704	.06888683	0.
FEMALE	.28187106	.00774175	.89734351	.12026803	.00772833	.60860197	.12711629	.00795253	.54174405
AGE	−.01835519	.00277022	−.05843420	.00595941	.00278220	.03015687	.00668132	.00286642	.02847444
AGESQ	.26778487	.03096216	.85249979	−.04163927	.03115181	−.21071054	−.04695040	.03201880	−.20009316
HSAT	−.21345503	.00141482	−.67953940	−.14637618	.00144060	−.74071918	−.15271640	.00148358	−.65084657
HANDDUM	.09041129	.00963870	.28782659	.10255607	.00969572	.51897271	.10904012	.00990456	.46470706
HANDPER	.00300153	.00017626	.00955544	.00153298	.00017760	.00775747	.00145161	.00017977	.00618647
MARRIED	.03873812	.00881265	.12332377	−.01292896	.00882816	−.06542545	−.01233626	.00906142	−.05257467
EDUC	−.00342252	.00187631	−.01089568	−.00555201	.00189701	−.02809531	−.00598173	.00197010	−.02549295
HHNINC	−.16498398	.02291240	−.52523061	−.20206192	.02308216	−1.0225102	−.21657724	.02408796	−.92300865
HHKIDS	−.09762798	.00862042	−.31080111	−.05706609	.00865236	−.28877613	−.06100208	.00893594	−.25997858
SELF	−.23243199	.01806908	−.73995303	−.08128493	.01803489	−.41133269	−.08960050	.01886738	−.38185930
BEAMT	.03640374	.01921475	.11589220	.06077767	.01916495	.30755811	.06449740	.01999381	.27487497
BLUEC	−.01916882	.01006783	−.06102440	.00182451	.01002870	.00923271	.00230018	.01034645	.00980291
WORKING	.00041819	.00941149	.00133132	−.02881502	.00936256	−.14581498	−.02827975	.00963105	−.12052261
PUBLIC	.14122076	.01565581	.44957981	.11278164	.01557239	.57071800	.12294551	.01629795	.52396906
ADDON	.02584454	.02544319	.08227672	−.09224023	.02542136	−.46677065	−.09827798	.02645306	−.41884099

Note: Where Q is the regime probability and $P(0)$ the Poisson, negative binomial, or other probability.

parametric survival models such as exponential, Weibull, gamma, log-logistic, and so forth, the censored Poisson and censored NB response is parameterized in terms of a discrete count. For example, a typical count response in health care analysis is hospital length of stay data. The response we have been using for our examples, number of patient visits to the hospital, is also appropriate for modeling censored count models. If various counts are lost to a length of stay study after reaching a certain time in the hospital, these counts may be considered as right censored. In modeling LOS data, it is important to take into account the days that were counted for particular patients, even though records are lost thereafter.

Survival parameterized censored count models will differ from what has been termed (Hilbe, 2007) the econometric parameterization as earlier discussed in that the values of censored responses are not recast to the cut level. This method changes the values of censored data. Table 6 shows the results of survival censored Poisson and NB models using the same data as in Tables 4 and 5. Note the much better fit using the censored negative binomial. The AIC and BIC statistics have significantly lower values than the Poisson. Derivation of the respective likelihoods as well as a discussion of both methods can be found in Hilbe (2007). Supporting software is at http://ideas.repec.org/s/boc/bocode.html or at http://econpapers.repec.org/software/bocbocode/.

4.2. Zero inflation

The pattern in Fig. 1 might suggest that there are more zeros in the data on DOCVIS than would be predicted by a Poisson model. Behind the data, one might, in turn, surmise that the data contain two kinds of respondents, those who would never visit a doctor save for extreme circumstances, and those who regularly (or even more often) visit the doctor. This produces a kind of 'mixture' process generating the data. The data contain two kinds of zeros: a certain zero from individuals who never visit the physician and an occasional zero from individuals who for whatever reason, did not visit the doctor that period, but might in some other. (The pioneering study of this kind of process is Lambert's (1992) analysis of process control in manufacturing – the sampling mechanism concerned the number of defective items produced by a process that was either under control (y always zero) or not under control (y sometimes zero).)

The probability distribution that describes the outcome variable in a zero-inflated Poisson (ZIP) or zero-inflated negative binomial (ZINB) model is built up from first principles: The probability of observing a zero is equal to the probability that the individual is in the always zero group plus the probability that the individual is not in that group times the probability that the count process produces a zero anyway. This would be

$$\mathrm{Prob}[y = 0] = Q + [1 - Q] \times P(0), \tag{59}$$

where Q is the regime probability and $P(0)$ the Poisson, negative binomial, or other probability for the zero outcome in the count process. The probability of a

Table 6
Survival parameterization of censored Poisson and negative binomial

Docvis Censored at Value of 8				Number of obs = 27,326		
Censored Poisson Regression				Wald $\chi^2(16) = 41{,}967.07$		
Log-likelihood = −87,520.01				Prob > $\chi^2 = 0.0000$		
docvis	Coeff.	Std. Err.	z	$P>\|z\|$	[95% CI]	
female	.2962892	.0078474	37.76	0.000	.2809086	.3116699
age	−.0201931	.0028097	−7.19	0.000	−.0257001	−.0146861
agesq	.2893301	.0314347	9.20	0.000	.2277191	.350941
hsat	−.2245135	.0014598	−153.80	0.000	−.2273746	−.2216523
handdum	.0935722	.0097864	9.56	0.000	.0743912	.1127532
handper	.0034529	.000181	19.08	0.000	.0030981	.0038076
married	.0464825	.0089499	5.19	0.000	.0289411	.0640239
educ	−.0022596	.0018888	−1.20	0.232	−.0059617	.0014425
hhninc	−.0163339	.0023175	−7.05	0.000	−.0208761	−.0117917
hhkids	−.1008135	.008725	−11.55	0.000	−.1179143	−.0837128
self	−.240174	.0181211	−13.25	0.000	−.2756908	−.2046572
beamt	.0402636	.0192906	2.09	0.037	.0024547	.0780725
bluec	−.0210752	.0101502	−2.08	0.038	−.0409693	−.0011812
working	−.0064606	.0095068	−0.68	0.497	−.0250937	.0121725
public	.1480981	.0157224	9.42	0.000	.1172827	.1789134
addon	.0189115	.0256716	0.74	0.461	−.0314039	.0692269
_cons	2.578406	.0670071	38.48	0.000	2.447075	2.709738
AIC statistic = 6.407 6				BIC statistic = −103,937.		
LM value = 17,2762.665				LM $\chi^2(1) = 0.000$		
Score test OD = 428,288.802				Score $\chi(1) = 0.000$		

Censored Negative Binomial Regression

Log-likelihood = −55,066.082

Number of obs = 27,326
Wald $\chi^2(16)$ = 3472.65
Prob > χ^2 = 0.0000

docvis	Coeff.	Std. Err.	z	$P>\|z\|$	[95% CI]	
xb						
female	.2918081	.0244625	11.93	0.000	.2438626	.3397537
age	.0037857	.0089505	0.42	0.672	−.0137569	.0213284
agesq	−.0294051	.1015427	−0.29	0.772	−.2284252	.169615
hsat	−.252314	.0052074	−48.45	0.000	−.2625204	−.2421077
handdum	.0752106	.032167	2.34	0.019	.0121645	.1382567
handper	.0065435	.0007127	9.18	0.000	.0051466	.0079404
married	.0236717	.0276851	0.86	0.393	−.0305901	.0779335
educ	−.0375634	.0058873	−6.38	0.000	−.0491023	−.0260244
hhninc	−.0628296	.0066091	−9.51	0.000	−.0757832	−.049876
hhkids	−.2249677	.0260514	−8.64	0.000	−.2760276	−.1739078
self	−.0766637	.0518638	−1.48	0.139	−.1783148	.0249875
beamt	.2819248	.0579536	4.86	0.000	.1683378	.3955118
bluec	.1135119	.0302827	3.75	0.000	.0541589	.1728649
working	−.1079542	.0284011	−3.80	0.000	−.1636193	−.052289
public	.3378024	.0452985	7.46	0.000	.249019	.4265858
addon	−.2807842	.0797627	−3.52	0.000	−.4371163	−.1244522
_cons	4.62027	.2161169	21.38	0.000	4.196689	5.043851
lnalpha						
_cons	1.574162	.0117548	133.92	0.000	1.551123	1.597201
alpha	4.826693	.0567366	4.716763	4.939186		

AIC statistic = 4.032

BIC statistic = −168,835.3

nonzero observation is, then

$$\text{Prob}[y = j > 0] = [1 - Q] \times P(j). \tag{60}$$

It remains to specify Q, then we can construct the log-likelihood function. Various candidates have been suggested (see ESI, 2007, Chapter 25); the most common is the logistic binary choice model,

$$\begin{aligned} Q_i &= \text{Prob}[\text{Regime } 0] \\ &= \frac{\exp(\boldsymbol{\gamma}'\mathbf{z}_i)}{1 + \exp(\boldsymbol{\gamma}'\mathbf{z}_i)}, \end{aligned} \tag{61}$$

where $\mathbf{z}_i$ is a set of covariates – possibly the same as $\mathbf{x}_i$ that is believed to influence the probability of the regime choice and $\boldsymbol{\gamma}$ is a set of parameters to be estimated with $\boldsymbol{\beta}$.

The log-likelihood for this model based on the Poisson probabilities is

$$\begin{aligned} \log L = &\sum_{y_i=0} \log\left[\frac{\exp(\boldsymbol{\gamma}'\mathbf{z}_i)}{1 + \exp(\boldsymbol{\gamma}'\mathbf{z}_i)} + \frac{\exp(-\lambda_i)}{1 + \exp(\boldsymbol{\gamma}'\mathbf{z}_i)}\right] \\ &+ \sum_{y_i>0} \log\left[\frac{\exp(-\lambda_i)\lambda_i^{y_i}}{[1 + \exp(\boldsymbol{\gamma}'\mathbf{z}_i)]y_i!}\right]. \end{aligned} \tag{62}$$

This formulation implies several new complications. First, its greater complexity is apparent. This log-likelihood function is much more difficult to maximize than that for the Poisson model. Second, the conditional mean function in this model is now

$$E[y|\mathbf{x}, \mathbf{z}] = Q_i\lambda_i = \frac{\exp(\boldsymbol{\gamma}'\mathbf{z}_i)\exp(\boldsymbol{\beta}'\mathbf{x}_i)}{1 + \exp(\boldsymbol{\gamma}'\mathbf{z}_i)}, \tag{63}$$

which is much more involved than before, and involves both the original covariates and the variables in the regime model. Partial effects are correspondingly more involved;

$$\frac{\partial E[y|\mathbf{x}, \mathbf{z}]}{\partial\begin{pmatrix}\mathbf{x}\\ \mathbf{z}\end{pmatrix}} = \lambda_i Q_i \begin{pmatrix}\boldsymbol{\beta}\\ Q_i(1 - Q_i)\boldsymbol{\gamma}\end{pmatrix}. \tag{64}$$

If there is any overlap between $\mathbf{x}$ and $\mathbf{z}$, the partial effect of that variable is the sum of the two effects shown.

The zero inflation model produces a substantial change in the specification of the model. As such, one would want to test the specification if possible. There is no counterpart to the LM test that would allow one to test the model without actually estimating it. Moreover, the basic model is not a simple restricted version of the ZIP (ZINB) model. Restricting γ to equal zero in the model above, for example produces $Q = 1/2$, not $Q = 0$, which is what one would hope for. Common practice is to use the Vuong (1989) test for these nonnested models. The statistic is computed as follows, based on the log-likelihood functions for the two models. Let

$\log L_{i0}$ be an individual contribution (observation) in the log-likelihood for the basic Poisson model, and let $\log L_{i1}$ denote an individual contribution to the log-likelihood function for the zero inflation model. Let $m_i = (\log L_{i1} - \log L_{i0})$. The statistic is

$$Z = \frac{\sqrt{N}\bar{m}}{s_m} \tag{65}$$

where $\bar{m} = (1/N)\Sigma_i m_i$ and $s_m = (1/N)\Sigma_i(m_i - \bar{m})^2$. In large samples, the statistic converges to standard normal. Under the assumption of the base model, Z will be large and negative, while under the assumption of the zero inflation model, Z will be large and positive. Thus, large positive values (greater than 2.0) reject the Poisson model in favor of the zero inflation model.

To illustrate the ZIP model, we extend the Poisson model estimated earlier with a regime splitting equation

$$Q_i = \Lambda(\gamma_1 + \gamma_2\text{FEMALE} + \gamma_3\text{HHNINC} + \gamma_4\text{EDUC} + \gamma_5\text{ADDON}), \tag{66}$$

where $\Lambda(t)$ is the logistic probability shown in (60). The estimated model is shown in Table 7.

The log-likelihood for the ZIP model is −77,073.779 compared to −89,431.005 for the Poisson model, which implies a difference of well over 12,000. On this basis, we would reject the Poisson model. However, as noted earlier, since the models are not nested, this is not a valid test. The Vuong statistic is +39.08, which does decisively reject the Poisson model. One can see some quite large changes in the results, particularly in the marginal effects. These are different models. On the specific point of the specification, the estimation results (using LIMDEP) indicate that the data contain 10,135 zero observations. The Poisson model predicts 2013.6 zeros. This is computed by multiplying the average predicted probability of a zero across all observations times the sample size. The zero inflation model predicts 9581.9 zeros, which is, as might be expected, much closer to the sample proportion.

4.3. Two part models

Two models that are related to the zero inflation model, hurdle models and sample selection models play important roles in the contemporary literature. A hurdle model (Mullahy, 1986) specifies the observed outcome as the result of two decisions, a participation equation and a usage equation. This is a natural variant of the ZIP model considered above, but its main difference is that the regime split is not latent. The participation equation determines whether the count will be zero or positive. The usage equation applies to the positive count outcomes. Thus, the formal model determining the observed outcomes is

$$\begin{aligned}
&\text{Prob}(y = 0) = R_i,\\
&\text{Prob}(y > 0) = 1 - R_i,\\
&\text{Prob}[y = j | y > 0][1 - R_i]P_i(j)/[1 - P_i(0)].
\end{aligned} \tag{67}$$

Table 7
Estimated zero-inflated Poisson model

	Base Poisson Model			Poisson Count Model		Zero Regime Equation		Partial Effect
	Coeff.	Std. Err.	Part. Eff.	Coeff.	Std. Err.	Coeff.	Std. Err.	
Constant	2.48612758	.06626647	0.	2.27389204	.02824420	−.86356818	.07269384	0.
FEMALE	.28187106	.00774175	.89734351	.14264681	.00289141	−.58033790	.02817964	.97216018
AGE	−.01835519	.00277022	−.05843420	.00194385	.00110859			.0056986
AGESQ	.26778487	.03096216	.85249979	.01169342	.01220742			.03428056
HSAT	−.21345503	.00141482	−.67953940	−.15791310	.00053102			−.46293957
HANDDUM	.09041129	.00963870	.28782659	.10648551	.00358290			.31217396
HANDPER	.00300153	.00017626	.00955544	.00158480	.597360D−04			.00464603
MARRIED	.03873812	.00881265	.12332377	−.00596092	.00334023			−.01747509
EDUC	−.00342252	.00187631	−.01089568	−.00335247	.00084300	.04090428	.00614014	−.04887430
HHNINC	−.16498398	.02291240	−.52523061	−.17752186	.01001860	.04894552	.08141084	−.56714692
HHKIDS	−.09762798	.00862042	−.31080111	−.05709710	.00342170			−.16738641
SELF	−.23243199	.01806908	−.73995303	−.12653617	.00764267			−.37095465
BEAMT	.03640374	.01921475	.11589220	.06028953	.00831117			.17674537
BLUEC	−.01916882	.01006783	−.06102440	.00195719	.00396727			.00573772
WORKING	.00041819	.00941149	.00133132	−.01322419	.00359116			−.03876818
PUBLIC	.14122076	.01565581	.44957981	.12484058	.00712261			.36598386
ADDON	.02584454	.02544319	.08227672	−.09812657	.01187915	−.51567053	.11710229	.20457682

The participation equation is a binary choice model, like the logit model used in the previous section. The count equation is precisely the truncated at zero model detailed in Section 4.1. This model uses components that have already appeared. The log-likelihood function separates the probabilities into two simple parts:

$$\log L = \sum_{y=0} \log R_i + \sum_{y>0} \log[1 - R_i] - \log[1 - P_i(0)] + \log P_i(j). \tag{68}$$

The four terms of the log-likelihood partition into two log-likelihoods,

$$\log L = \sum_{d=0} \log R_i + \sum_{d=1} \log[1 - R_i] + \sum_{d=1} \log P_i(j) - \log[1 - P_i(0)], \tag{69}$$

where the binary variable d_i equals zero if y_i equals zero and one if y_i is greater than zero. Notice that the two equations can be estimated separately: a binary choice model for d_i and a truncated at zero Poisson (or negative binomial) model for the positive values of y_i.

We shall illustrate this model with the same specification as the ZIP model. The hurdle equation determines whether the individual will make any visits to the doctor. Then, the usage equation is, as before, a count model for the number of visits. This model differs from the ZIP model in that the main equation applies only to the positive counts of doctor visits. Not surprisingly, the model results are quite similar. The hurdle model and the zero inflation model are quite similar both in the formulation and in how the models are interpreted (Table 8).

Models for sample selection differ considerably from the frameworks we have considered so far. Loosely, while the two part models considered so far concern the utilization decision, the sample selection models can be viewed as a two part model in which the first involves a decision whether or not to be in the observed sample. A second crucial aspect of the model is that the effects of the first step are taken to operate on the unmeasured aspects of the usage equation, not directly in the specified equations.

To put this in a context, suppose we hypothesize that in our health care data, individuals who have insurance make their utilization decisions differently from those who do not, in ways that are not completely accounted for in the observed covariates. An appropriate model might appear as follows:

$$\text{Insurance decision } (0/1) = F(\boldsymbol{\alpha}'\mathbf{w}_i + u_i), \tag{70}$$

where $\mathbf{w}_i$ is the set of measured covariates and u_i is the unmeasured element of the individual's decision to have insurance. Then, the usage equation holds that

$$\text{Doctor visits (count)} = G(\boldsymbol{\beta}'\mathbf{x}_i + \varepsilon_i), \tag{71}$$

where ε_i accounts for those elements of the usage decision that are not directly measured by the analyst. The second equation is motivated by the same

Table 8
Estimated hurdle Poisson model

	Base Poisson Model			Poisson Count Model		Participation Equation		Partial Effect
	Coeff.	Std. Err.	Part. Eff.	Coeff.	Std. Err.	Coeff.	Std. Err.	
Constant	2.48612758	.06626647	0.	2.24409689	.02803268	.80374458	.06710834	0.
FEMALE	.28187106	.00774175	.89734351	.12711631	.00274746	.59195506	.02599107	.95763200
AGE	−.01835519	.00277022	−.05843420	.00668133	.00108985			.01821318
AGESQ	.26778487	.03096216	.85249979	−.04695053	.01195589			−.12798632
HSAT	−.21345503	.00141482	−.67953940	−.15271640	.00052262			−.41630224
HANDDUM	.09041129	.00963870	.28782659	.10904010	.00345227			.29724142
HANDPER	.00300153	.00017626	.00955544	.00145161	.586338D−04			.00395706
MARRIED	.03873812	.00881265	.12332377	−.01233627	.00316579			−.03362846
EDUC	−.00342252	.00187631	−.01089568	−.00598172	.00081933	−.04518713	.00566753	−.06295579
HHNINC	−.16498398	.02291240	−.52523061	−.21657725	.00981680	−.11523583	.07381806	−.70935153
HHKIDS	−.09762798	.00862042	−.31080111	−.06100214	.00326811			−.16629077
SELF	−.23243199	.01806908	−.73995303	−.08960050	.00698770			−.24424941
BEAMT	.03640374	.01921475	.11589220	.06449742	.00833036			.17581884
BLUEC	−.01916882	.01006783	−.06102440	.00230015	.00387887			.00627017
WORKING	.00041819	.00941149	.00133132	−.02827977	.00354930			−.07709015
PUBLIC	.14122076	.01565581	.44957981	.12294552	.00715542			.33514735
ADDON	.02584454	.02544319	.08227672	−.09827801	.01187417	.43208724	.10043663	.17816867

considerations that underlie the overdispersion models, such as the NB model. There can be unmeasured, latent elements in the usage equation that influence the outcome, but are not observable by the analyst. In our earlier application, this induced overdispersion, which was easily accommodated by extending the Poisson model to the NB framework. The effect is more pernicious here. If our estimation sample for the count variable contained only those individuals who have insurance, and if the unmeasured effects in the two equations are correlated, then the sampling mechanism becomes nonrandom. In effect, under these assumptions, the variables $\mathbf{w}_i$ will be acting in the background to influence the usage variable, and will distort our estimates of $\boldsymbol{\beta}$ in that equation.[7]

It is a bit ambiguous how the unmeasured aspects of the usage decision should enter the model for the count outcome. Note there is no 'disturbance' in (7)–(9). On the other hand, the presence of the latent heterogeneity in the overdispersion models in Section 3 provides a suitable approach. The following two part model for a count variable embodies these ideas:

$$z_i^* = \boldsymbol{\alpha}'\mathbf{w}_i + u_i,$$
$$z_i = 1 \text{ if } z_i^* > 0,\ 0 \text{ otherwise (a standard binary choice model)} \tag{72}$$

$$\text{Prob}[y_i = j | z_i = 1, \mathbf{x}_i, \varepsilon_i] = P(\boldsymbol{\beta}'\mathbf{x}_i + \sigma\varepsilon_i) \text{ (Poisson count model)}, \tag{73}$$

where the data for the count model are only observed when $z_i = 1$, e.g., only for the insured individuals in the larger sample. The first equation is the participation equation. The second is the usage equation. The model is made operational by formal distributional assumptions for the unobserved components; (u_i, ε_i) are assumed to be distributed as joint standard normal with correlation ρ. It is the nonzero ρ that ultimately induces the complication of the selection effect.

Estimation of this model is considerably more involved than those considered so far. The presence of the unobserved variable makes familiar maximum likelihood methods infeasible. The model can be estimated by maximum simulated likelihood. (Development of the method is beyond the scope of our presentation here. Readers may refer to Greene (1994, 2003 or 2006) or ESI (2007) for details.) To illustrate the selection model, we have estimated a restricted version of the count model used earlier for doctor visits; the participation equation for whether or not the individual has PUBLIC health insurance is based on

$$\mathbf{w} = (\text{Constant, AGE, HHNINC, HHKIDS, EDUC}). \tag{74}$$

The usage equation includes

$$\mathbf{x} = (\text{Constant, AGE, FEMALE, HHNINC, HHKIDS, WORKING, BLUEC, SELF, BEAMT}). \tag{75}$$

[7] In Greene (1994), this method is used to model counts of derogatory reports in credit files for a sample of individuals who have, in an earlier screening, applied for a specific credit card. The second step of the analysis is applied only to those individuals whose credit card application was approved.

The estimates are given in Table 9. The leftmost estimates are obtained by the Poisson regression model ignoring the selection issue. The point of comparison is the second set of results for the Poisson model. (These are computed jointly with the probit equation at the far right of the table.) It can be seen that the effect of the selection correction is quite substantial; the apparently significant income effect in the first equation disappears; the effect of kids in the household becomes considerably greater; the positive and significant effect of BLUEC becomes negative and significant; and the insignificant BEAMT coefficient changes sign and becomes significant in the modified equation. Apparently, the latent effect of the insurance decision is quite important in these data. The estimate of ρ is $-.3928$, with a standard error of .0282. Based on a simple t-test, we would decisively reject the hypothesis of no correlation, which reinforces our impression that the selection effect in these data is indeed substantial. The fairly large negative estimate suggests that the latent effects that act to increase the likelihood that the individual will have insurance act in turn to reduce the number of doctor visits. A theory based on moral hazard effects of insurance would have predicted a positive coefficient, instead.

4.4. Panel data

The health care data we have been using are a panel. Data sets such as this one are becoming increasingly common in applications of count models. The main virtues of panel data are that they allow a richer specification of the model that we have been using so far, and they allow, under suitable assumptions, the researcher to learn more about the latent sources of heterogeneity that are not captured by the measured covariates already in the model. We shall examine the two most familiar approaches here, fixed effects and random effects. A wider variety of panel models is presented in Stata and ESI (2007). As suggested by the application, we assume that the sample contains N individuals, indexed by $i = 1, \ldots, N$. The number of observations available for each individual is denoted T_i; this may vary across individuals, as it does in our data set. [Note that T_i is used here differently than in Section 2.1.]

In general terms, the availability of panel data allows the analyst to incorporate individual heterogeneity in the model. For the fixed effects case, this takes the form of an individual-specific intercept term.

$$\log \lambda_{it} = \alpha_i + \boldsymbol{\beta}'\mathbf{x}_{it}(+\varepsilon_{it} \text{ for the negative binomial model}). \tag{76}$$

where α_i can be interpreted as the coefficient on a binary variable, d_i, which indicates membership in the ith group. A major difference between this and the linear regression model is that this model cannot be fit by least squares using deviations from group means – the transformation of the data to group mean form in this context brings no benefits at all. Two approaches are used instead. One possibility is to use a conditional maximum likelihood approach – the model conditioned on the sum of the observations is free of the fixed effects and has a closed form that is a function of $\boldsymbol{\beta}$ alone. This is provided for both Poisson and negative binomial (see Hausman et al., 1984). A second approach is direct, brute force estimation of the full model including the fixed effects. The *unconditional* estimator is obtained by a

Table 9
Estimated sample selection model

	Poisson Model; Subsample		Poisson Model; Maximum Likelihood		Probit Insurance Equation		Reestimated Probit Insurance Equation	
	Coeff.	Std. Err.	Coeff.	Std. Err.	Coeff.	Std. Err.	Coeff.	Std. Err.
Constant	.62950929	.02172139	−.25578895	.03277438	3.62691256	.07326231	3.60039973	.07232337
AGE	.01649406	.00035426	.01861389	.00052927	.00079753	.00104823	.00074654	.00108170
FEMALE	.23541478	.00783352	.33195368	.01057008				
HHNINC	−.35832703	.02330320	.01529087	.03513743	−.98823990	.05500769	−.98247429	.04954413
HHKIDS	−.16894816	.00843149	−.21559300	.01213431	−.07928466	.02276865	−.07028879	.02238365
WORKING	−.19400071	.00918292	−.22010784	.01272314				
BLUEC	.02209633	.00974552	−.03595214	.01371389				
SELF	−.26437394	.01978391	−.36281283	.02770759				
BEAMT	.03168950	.02771184	−.12155827	.04288937				
EDUC					−.17148226	.00403598	−.16970876	.00402272
σ	0.	0.					1.31093146	.00494213
ρ	0.	0.					−.39283049	.02820212
$\log L$	−94,322.56		−62,584.14		−8320.77794			
N	24,203		27,326		27,326			

direct maximization of the full log-likelihood function and estimating all parameters including the group-specific constants. A result that is quite rare in this setting is that for the Poisson model (and few others), the conditional and unconditional estimators are numerically identical. The choice of approach can be based on what feature is available in the computer package one is using. The matter is more complicated in the NB case. The conditional estimator derived in HHG is not the same as the brute force estimator. Moreover, the underlying specifications are different. In HHGs specification, the fixed effect (dummy variable) coefficients appear directly in the distribution of the latent heterogeneity variable, not in the regression function as shown above. Overall, the fixed effects, negative binomial (FENB) appears relatively infrequently in the count data literature. Where it does occur, current practice appears to favor the HHG approach.

We note before turning to random effects models two important aspects of fitting FE models. First, as in the linear regression case, variables in the equation that do not differ across time become collinear with the individual-specific dummy variables. Thus, FE models cannot be fit with time invariant variables. (There is one surprising exception to this. The HHG FENB models can be fit with a full set of individual dummy variable and an overall constant – a result which collides with familiar wisdom. The result occurs because of the aforementioned peculiarity of the specification of the latent heterogeneity.) The second aspect of this model is relatively lightly documented phenomenon known as the incidental parameters problem (see Greene, 1995). The full unconditional maximum likelihood estimator of models that contain fixed effects is usually inconsistent – the estimator is consistent in T (or T_i), but T is usually taken to be fixed and small. The Poisson model is an exception to this rule, however. It is consistent even in the presence of the fixed effects. (One could deduce this from the discussion already. The brute force estimator would normally suffer from the incidental parameter problem. But, since it is numerically identical to the conditional estimator, which does not, the brute force estimator must be consistent as well.)

The random effects model is

$$\log \lambda_{it} = \boldsymbol{\beta}'\mathbf{x}_{it} + u_i. \tag{77}$$

Once again, the approach used for the linear model, in this case, two-step generalized least squares, is not usable. The approach is to integrate out the random effect and estimate by maximum likelihood the parameters of the resulting distribution (which, it turns out, is the NB model when the kernel is Poisson and the effect is log-gamma). The bulk of the received literature on random effects is based on the Poisson model, though HHG and modern software (e.g., LIMDEP and Stata) do provide estimators for NB models with random effects.

The random effects model for the count data framework is

$$\log \lambda_{it} = \boldsymbol{\beta}'\mathbf{x}_{it} + u_i, \quad i = 1, \ldots, N, \quad t = 1, \ldots, T_i, \tag{78}$$

where u_i is a random effect for the ith group such that $\exp(u_i)$ has a gamma distribution with parameters (θ,θ). Thus, $E[\exp(u_i)$ has mean 1 and variance $1/\theta = \alpha$. This is the framework, which gave rise to the NB model earlier, so that, with minor modifications, this is the estimating framework for the Poisson model with random effects.

For the NB model, Hausman et al. proposed the following approach: We begin with the Poisson model with the random effects specification shown above. The random term, u_i is distributed as gamma with parameters (θ_i,θ_i), which produces the NB model with a parameter that varies across groups. Then, it is assumed that $\theta_i/(1+\theta_i)$ is distributed as beta (a_n,b_n), which layers the random group effect onto the NB model. The random effect is added to the NB model by assuming that the overdispersion parameter is randomly distributed across groups. The two random effects models discussed above may be modified to use the normal distribution for the random effect instead of the gamma, with $u_i \sim N[0,\sigma^2]$. For the Poisson model, this is an alternative to the log-gamma model which gives rise to the negative binomial.

Table 10 displays estimates for fixed and random effects versions of the Poisson model, with the original model based on the pooled data. Both effects models lead to large changes in the coefficients and the partial effects. As usually occurs, the FE model brings the larger impact. In most cases, the fit of the model will improve dramatically – this occurs in linear models as well. The pooled model is a restriction on either of the panel models. Note that the log-likelihood function has risen from −89,431 in the pooled case to −45,480 for the FE model. The χ^2 statistic for testing for the presence of the fixed effects is about 87,900 with 7292 degrees of freedom. The 95% critical value is about 7500, so there is little question about rejecting the null hypothesis of the pooled model. The same result applies to the random effects model. The fixed effects and random effects are not nested, so one cannot use a likelihood-ratio test to test for which model is preferred. However, the Poisson model is an unusual nonlinear model in that the FE estimator is consistent – there is no incidental parameters problem. As such, in the same fashion as in the linear model, one can use a Hausman (1978) (see also Greene, 2003, Chapter 13) test to test for fixed vs. random effects. The appropriate statistic is

$$H = (\hat{\boldsymbol{\beta}}_{\text{FE}} - \hat{\boldsymbol{\beta}}_{\text{RE}})'[\text{Est.Var}(\hat{\boldsymbol{\beta}}_{\text{FE}}) - \text{Est.Var}(\hat{\boldsymbol{\beta}}_{\text{RE}})]^{-1}(\hat{\boldsymbol{\beta}}_{\text{FE}} - \hat{\boldsymbol{\beta}}_{\text{RE}}). \tag{79}$$

(Note the constant term is removed from the random effects results.) Applying this computation to the models in Table 10 produces a χ^2 statistic of 114.1628. The critical value from the table, with 16 degrees of freedom is 26.296, so the hypothesis of the random effects model is rejected in favor of the FE model.

Texts providing a thorough discussion of fixed and random effects models and generalized estimating equations (GEE) with an emphasis in health analysis include Zeger et al. (1988), Hardin and Hilbe (2003), Twist (2003), and Hilbe (2007). Texts discussing multilevel count models include Skrondal and Rabe-Hesketh (2005). Hilbe (2007) is the only source discussing multilevel NB models.

5. Software

Count response regression models include Poisson and NB regression, and all of the enhancements to each that are aimed to accommodate some violation in the

Table 10
Poisson models with fixed and random effects

	Pooled Poisson Model with No Effects			Fixed Effects Poisson Model			Random Effects Poisson Model		
	Coeff.	Std. Err.	Part. Eff.	Coeff.	Std. Err.	Part. Eff.	Coeff.	Std. Err.	Part. Eff.
Constant	2.48612758	.06626647	0.				2.24392235	.07371198	
FEMALE	.28187106	.00774175	.89734351	.51658559	.11586172	1.64456306	.30603129	.02119303	.97425823
AGE	−.01835519	.00277022	−.05843420	−.00645204	.00660632	−.02054024	−.02242192	.00240763	−.07138075
AGESQ	.26778487	.03096216	.85249979	.31095952	.06972973	.98994735	.39324433	.02574887	1.25190310
HSAT	−.21345503	.00141482	−.67953940	−.14713933	.00222146	−.46842172	−.16059023	.00074867	−.51124299
HANDDUM	.09041129	.00963870	.28782659	.05697301	.01101687	.18137500	.04903557	.00442617	.15610595
HANDPER	.00300153	.00017626	.00955544	−.00123990	.00034541	−.00394724	.00058881	.00011537	.00187449
MARRIED	.03873812	.00881265	.12332377	−.02568156	.02186501	−.08175789	−.02623233	.00773198	−.08351126
EDUC	−.00342252	.00187631	−.01089568	−.03829432	.01670290	−.12191093	−.01343872	.00427488	−.04278251
HHNINC	−.16498398	.02291240	−.52523061	−.12296257	.04266832	−.39145439	−.07074651	.01754451	−.22522326
HHKIDS	−.09762798	.00862042	−.31080111	.00275859	.01602765	.00878203	−.02970393	.00580292	−.09456319
SELF	−.23243199	.01806908	−.73995303	−.11580970	.03538353	−.36868304	−.16546368	.01330546	−.52675775
BEAMT	.03640374	.01921475	.11589220	−.07260535	.05533064	−.23114092	−.01814889	.02270099	−.05777745
BLUEC	−.01916882	.01006783	−.06102440	−.01636891	.01947144	−.05211084	−.01456716	.00775266	−.04637491
WORKING	.00041819	.00941149	.00133132	−.05009017	.01635782	−.15946331	−.04212169	.00711048	−.13409546
PUBLIC	.14122076	.01565581	.44957981	.09352915	.03072334	.29775238	.10688932	.01320990	.34028480
ADDON	.02584454	.02544319	.08227672	−.07453049	.03631482	−.23726967	−.05483927	.01859563	−.17458217
α							.87573201	.01570144	
$\log L$		−89,431.01			−45,480.27			−68,720.91	

distributional assumptions of the respective models. The most commonly used extended Poisson and NB models include zero-truncated, zero-inflated, and panel data models. Hurdle, sample selection, and censored models are used less frequently, and thus find less support in commercial software. The heterogeneous NB regression is a commonly used extension that has no Poisson counterpart. Other count model extensions that have been crafted have found support in *LIMDEP*, which has far more count response models available to its users than other commercial software.

LIMDEP and Stata are the only commercial statistical packages that provide their respective users with the ability to model Poisson, negative binomial, as well as their extensions. *LIMDEP* offers all of the enhanced models mentioned in this chapter, while Stata offers most of the models, including both base models, NB-1, zero-truncated and zero-inflated Poisson and negative binomial, a full suite of count panel data models, mixed models, and heterogeneous negative binomial. Stata users have written hurdle, censored, sample selection, and Poisson mixed model procedures. Both software packages provide excellent free technical support, have exceptional reference manual support with numerous interpreted examples, and have frequent incremental upgrades.

Unfortunately, other commercial programs provide limited support for count response models. *SAS* has Poisson and negative binomial as families within its *SAS/STAT GENMOD* procedure, *SAS*'s generalized linear models (GLM) and GEE facility. *SAS* also supports Poisson panel data models. *SPSS* provides no support for count response regression models, but is expected to release a GLM program in its next release, thereby providing the capability for Poisson regression. *GENSTAT* supports Poisson and NB regression, together with a variety of Poisson panel and mixed models.

R is a higher language statistical software environment that can be freely downloaded from the web. It enjoys worldwide developmental and technical support from members of academia as well as from statisticians at major research institutions or agencies. R statistical procedures are authored by users; thus its statistical capabilities depend entirely on the statistical procedures written and filed in user-supported R libraries. Although R has a rather complete suite of statistical procedures, it is at present rather weak in its support of count response models. R has software support for Poisson and NB regression, but not for any of the extensions we have discussed. A basic NB-2 model in R is provided as part of the *MASS* software package, based on the work of Venables and Ripley (2002). We expect, though, that this paucity of count response model offerings is only temporary and that most if not all of the extensions mentioned in this chapter will be available to users in the near future.

Other commercial statistical software either fails to support count response models, or provides only the basic models, and perhaps a GEE or fixed/random effects Poisson panel data module.

When evaluating software for its ability to model counts, care must be taken to check if the model offered has associated goodness-of-fit statistics and if it allows the user to generate appropriate residuals for model evaluation. Several of the software packages referenced in the previous paragraph may offer Poisson or NB regression, yet fail to provide appropriate fit statistics in their output. A model without fit analysis is statistically useless, and fosters poor statistical practice.

A caveat should be given regarding NB regression capability from within the framework of GLM. Since GLMs are one-parameter models, and the negative binomial has two parameters to estimate, the heterogeneity parameter, α, must be entered into the GLM algorithm as a constant. If the software also has a full maximum likelihood NB procedure, one may use it to obtain an estimate of α, and then insert it into the GLM negative binomial algorithm as the heterogeneity parameter constant. The value of adopting this two-stage procedure is that GLM procedures typically have a variety of goodness-of-fit output and residual analysis support associated with the procedure. Model evaluation may be enhanced. On the other hand, software such as *LIMDEP* provides extensive fit and residual support for all of its count regression models, thereby making the two-stage modeling task unnecessary. We advise the user of statistical software to be aware of the capability, as well as the limitations, of any software being used for modeling purposes.

With the increased speed of computer chips and the availability of cheap RAMs has made available the ability of statistical software to estimate highly complex models based on permutations. Cytel Corp has recently offered users of its *LogXact* program, the ability to model Poisson regression based on exact statistics. That is, the procedure calculates parameter estimate standard errors, and hence confidence intervals, based on exact calculations, not on traditional asymptotics. This is a particularly valuable tool when modeling small or ill-defined data sets. Software such as *SAS*, *SPSS*, *Stata*, and *StatXact* have exact statistical capabilities for tables, but only *LogXact* and *Stata* (version 10) provide exact statistical support for logistic and Poisson models. Cytel intends to extend *LogXact* to provide exact NB regression, but as of this writing the research has not yet been done to develop the requisite algorithms.

We have provided an overview of the count response regression capabilities currently available in commercial statistical software. *LIMDEP* and *Stata* stand far above other packages in the number of count models available, but also in their quality; i.e., providing a full range of goodness-of-fit statistics and residuals. As the years pass, other software vendors will likely expand their offerings to include most of the count models discussed in this chapter. As we mentioned before though, before using statistical software to model count responses, be certain to evaluate its fit analysis capability as well as its range of offerings.

6. Summary and conclusions

We have surveyed the most commonly used models related to the regression of count response data. The foundation for this class of models is Poisson regression. Though it has provided the fundamental underpinning for modeling counts, the equidispersion assumption of the Poisson model is a severe limitation. This shortcoming is generally overcome by the NB model, which can be construed as the unconditional result of conditioning the Poisson regression on unobservable heterogeneity, or simply as a more general model for counts that is not limited by the Poisson assumption on the variance of the response variable. We also considered the most common extensions of these two basic count models: zero inflation models, sample selection, two part (hurdle) models, and the most familiar panel data applications. The applications presented above focused on the Poisson model, though all of them have been extended to the NB model as well. The basic models are available in most commercial software packages, such as Stata, LIMDEP, GENSTAT, and SAS. The more involved extensions tend to be in more limited availability, with the most complex count response models only supported in LIMDEP and Stata.

The literature, both applied and theoretical, on this subject is vast. We have omitted many of the useful extensions and theoretical frontiers on modeling counts. (See, e.g., Winkelmann (2003), which documents these models in over 300 pages, Hilbe (2007), which provides detailed examples, most related to health data, for each major count response model, particularly all of the varieties of NB regression, or Cameron and Trivedi (1998), which has been a standard text on count response models, but emphasizes economic application.) Recent developments include many models for panel data, mixed models, latent class models, and a variety of other approaches. Models for counts have provided a proving ground for development of an array of new techniques as well, such as random parameters models and Bayesian estimation methods.

References

Anscombe, F.J. (1949). The statistical analysis of insect counts based on the negative binomial distribution. *Biometrics* **5**, 165–173.

Blom, G. (1954). Transformations of the binomial, negative binomial, Poisson, and χ^2 distributions. *Biometrika* **41**, 302–316.

Cameron, A., Trivedi, P. (1986). Econometric models based on count data: Comparisons and applications of some estimators and tests. *Journal of Applied Econometrics* **1**, 29–54.

Cameron, A., Trivedi, P. (1990). Regression based tests for overdispersion in the Poisson model. *Journal of Econometrics* **46**, 347–364.

Cameron, C., Trivedi, P. (1998). *Regression Analysis of Count Data*. Cambridge University Press, New York.

Econometric Software, Inc (1987). *LIMDEP*, version 4, Plainview, NY.

Econometric Software, Inc (2007). *LIMDEP and NLOGIT*. Plainview, New York.

Fair, R. (1978). A theory of extramarital affairs. *Journal of Political Economy* **86**, 45–61.

Greene, W. (1994). Accounting for excess zeros and sample selection in Poisson and negative binomial regression models. Working Paper No. EC-94-10, Department of Economics, Stern School of Business, New York University.

Greene, W. (1995). Sample selection in the Poisson regression model. Working Paper No. EC-95-6, Department of Economics, Stern School of Business, New York University.

Greene, W. (2003). *Econometric Analysis*, 5th ed. Prentice-Hall, Englewood Cliffs.

Greene, W. (2006). A general approach to incorporating selectivity in a model. Working Paper No. EC-06-10, Stern School of Business, Department of Economics.

Hardin, J., Hilbe, J. (2003). *Generalized Estimating Equations*. Chapman & Hall/CRC, London, UK.

Hardin, J., Hilbe, J. (2007). *Generalized Linear Models and Extensions*, 2nd ed. Stata Press, College Station, TX.

Hausman, J. (1978). Specification tests in econometrics. *Econometrica* **46**, 1251–1271.

Hausman, J., Hall, B., Griliches, Z. (1984). Economic models for count data with an application to the patents–R&D relationship. *Econometrica* **52**, 909–938.
Hilbe, J. (1994). Negative binomial regression., *Stata Technical Bulletin* **STB-18**, sg16.5.
Hilbe, J. (2007). *Negative binomial regression.* Cambridge University Press, Cambridge, UK.
Hilbe, J.M. (1993). Log negative binomial regression as a generalized linear model. Technical Report COS 93/94-5-26, Department of Sociology, Arizona State University.
Hilbe, J.M. (1994). Generalized linear models. *The American Statistician* **48**(3), 255–265.
Krinsky, I., Robb, A.L. (1986). On approximating the statistical properties of elasticities. *Review of Economics and Statistics* **68**, 715–719.
Lambert, D. (1992). Zero-inflated Poisson regression, with an application to defects in manufacturing. *Technometrics* **34**(1), 1–14.
Lawless, J.F. (1987). Negative binomial and mixed Poisson regression. *The Canadian Journal of Statistics* **15**(3), 209–225.
Long, J.S., Freese, J. (2006). *Regression Models for Categorical Dependent Variables using Stata*, 2nd ed. Stata Press, College Station, TX.
McCullagh, P., Nelder, J. (1983). *Generalized Linear Models.* Chapman & Hall, New York.
McCullagh, P., Nelder, J.A. (1989). *Generalized Linear Models*, 2nd ed. Chapman & Hall, New York.
Mullahy, J. (1986). Specification and testing of some modified count data models. *Journal of Econometrics* **33**, 341–365.
Rabe-Hesketh, S., Skrondal, A. (2005). *Multilevel and Longitudinal Modeling Using Stata.* Stata Press, College Station, TX.
Ripahn, R., Wambach, A., Million, A. (2003). Incentive effects in the demand for health care: A bivariate panel count data estimation. *Journal of Applied Econometrics* **18**(4), 387–405.
SAS Institute (1998). *SAS.* SAS Institute, Cary, NC.
Skrondal, A., Rabe-Hesketh, S. (2004). *Generalized Latent Variable Modeling.* Chapman & Hall/CRC, Boca Raton, FL.
Stata Corp., (1993, 2006). *Stata.* Stata Corp., College Station, TX.
Terza, J. (1985). A Tobit type estimator for the censored Poisson regression model. *Economics Letters* **18**, 361–365.
Twist, J. (2003). *Applied Longitudinal Data Analysis for Epidemiology.* Cambridge University Press, Cambridge, UK.
Vuong, Q. (1989). Likelihood ratio tests for model selection and non-nested hypotheses. *Econometrica* **57**, 307–334.
Venables, W., Ripley, B. (2002). *Modern Applied Statistics with S*, 4th ed. Springer, New York.
Winkelmann, R. (2003). *Econometric Analysis of Count Data*, 4th ed. Springer, Heidelberg, Germany.
Zeger, S.L., Liang, K-Y., Albert, P.S. (1988). Models for longitudinal data: A generalized equation approach. *Biometrics* **44**, 1049–1060.

Handbook of Statistics, Vol. 27
ISSN: 0169-7161

DOI: 10.1016/S0169-7161(07)27008-7

8

Mixed Models

Matthew J. Gurka and Lloyd J. Edwards

Abstract

This paper provides a general overview of the mixed model, a powerful tool for analyzing correlated data. Numerous books and other sources exist that cover the mixed model comprehensively. However, we aimed to provide a relatively concise introduction to the mixed model and describe the primary motivations behind its use. Recent developments of various aspects of this topic are discussed, including estimation and inference, model selection, diagnostics, missing data, and power and sample size. We focus on describing the mixed model as it is used for modeling normal outcome data linearly, but we also discuss its use in other situations, such as with discrete outcome data. We point out various software packages with the capability of fitting mixed models, and most importantly, we highlight many important articles and books for those who wish to pursue this topic further.

1. Introduction

1.1. The importance of mixed models

Why mixed models? Simply put, mixed models allow one to effectively model data that are not independent. Of course, such a statement is quite general, and the actual use of mixed models varies widely across fields of study. Data suited for analysis via mixed models usually have some multilevel or hierarchical organization (hence mixed models are often times referred to as multilevel or hierarchical models). This usually means that this kind of data can be organized into different levels, or clusters. Observations made within a cluster are usually assumed to be dependent, whereas clusters themselves are assumed to be independent of one another.

One may wonder what kind of data lend themselves to such a cluster arrangement. The most convenient and common example of this sort of hierarchical organization is longitudinal data, in which observations are collected over time on a subject. Obviously characteristics unique to that subject or individual dictate that multiple observations collected over time on that individual will be correlated. Because of this, mixed models have become one common method for analyzing many types of longitudinal data, particularly from medical research.

But, mixed model analysis is by no means limited to longitudinal studies. Mixed models are often used in settings in which data are collected on families, schools, or hospitals. In using the individuals that comprise those groups, it is recommended that one take into account the natural correlation of those individuals from the same family, school, or hospital, depending on the motivation of the analysis. Mixed models can accommodate data from such studies easily and in a straightforward fashion that is easy to interpret.

Our aim for this chapter was to generally introduce the mixed model for the reader who is not an expert on such an analysis tool. In doing so, we describe the main aspects of the model, such as estimation and inference. We also discuss areas of research within the mixed model that are ongoing, such as model selection and power analysis. Our main goal was to provide a fairly comprehensive and current reference to textbooks, journal articles, and other sources of information that give details on more specific topics related to the mixed model for the reader who wishes to learn more about this popular method of analyzing data.

1.2. "Mixed" models

In introducing mixed models, one should discuss what makes a model "mixed." A model is "mixed" because it contains different types of effects to be estimated: namely, "fixed" effects and "random" effects. What sets apart a mixed model from a typical univariate or multivariate model is the addition of the random effects. While introducing the concept of linear mixed models, it is most straightforward to discuss with reference to linear models. However, mixed models can be applied to nonlinear models as well, and this concept will be introduced later.

In the case of the univariate linear model, the following form is typically observed:

$$\boldsymbol{y} = \boldsymbol{X\beta} + \varepsilon. \tag{1}$$

Here, we are fitting a model to data from N sampling units (subjects), considered to be independent of one another. In model (1), $\boldsymbol{y}$ is the $(N \times 1)$ vector of responses from the N subjects, $\boldsymbol{X}$ the $(N \times p)$ design matrix of known variables, $\boldsymbol{\beta}$ a $(p \times 1)$ vector of fixed, unknown parameters, and ε the $(N \times 1)$ vector whose rows represent unobservable random variables that capture the subject-specific deviation from the expected value. So, each row of $\boldsymbol{y}$, $\boldsymbol{X}$, and ε correspond to a subject. Typically, the rows of ε are assumed to be normally distributed with mean 0 and common variance σ^2; i.e., $\varepsilon \sim \mathcal{N}(0, \sigma^2 \mathcal{I})$.

Now, the linear mixed model, in the common form developed by Laird and Ware (1982) for longitudinal data analysis, is as follows:

$$\boldsymbol{y}_i = \boldsymbol{X}_i\boldsymbol{\beta} + \boldsymbol{Z}_i\boldsymbol{b}_i + e_i. \tag{2}$$

Here, $i \in \{1, \ldots, m\}$, where m is the number of independent sampling units (subjects), $\boldsymbol{y}_i$ an $n_i \times 1$ vector of observations on the ith subject; $\boldsymbol{X}_i$ an $n_i \times p$

known, constant design matrix for the ith subject with rank p; $\boldsymbol{\beta}$ a $p \times 1$ vector of unknown, constant population parameters; $\boldsymbol{Z}_i$ an $n_i \times q$ known, constant design matrix for the ith subject with rank q corresponding to $\boldsymbol{b}_i$, a $q \times 1$ vector of unknown, random individual-specific parameters (the "random effects"); and $\boldsymbol{e}_i$ an $n_i \times 1$ vector of random "within-subject," or "pure," error terms.

Additionally, let $\varepsilon_I = \boldsymbol{Z}_i\boldsymbol{b}_i + \boldsymbol{e}_i$ be the "total" error term of model (2). The following distributional assumptions are usually held: $\boldsymbol{b}_i$ is normally distributed with mean vector 0 and covariance matrix $\boldsymbol{D}$ and $\boldsymbol{b}_i$ independent of $\boldsymbol{b}_j$, $i \neq j$. Also, $\boldsymbol{e}_i$ is distributed normally with mean vector 0 and covariance matrix $\boldsymbol{R}_i$, independent of $\boldsymbol{b}_i$. The covariance matrices $\boldsymbol{D}$ and $\boldsymbol{R}_i$ are typically assumed to be characterized by unique parameters contained in the $k \times 1$ vector θ. Often, a "conditionally independent" model is assumed; i.e., $\boldsymbol{R}_i = \sigma^2 \boldsymbol{I}_{n_i}$. The total variance for the response vector in (2) is $\mathrm{var}(\mathbf{y}_i) = \mathrm{var}(\varepsilon_i) = \Sigma_i(\theta) = \boldsymbol{Z}_i\boldsymbol{D}(\theta)\boldsymbol{Z}_i' + \boldsymbol{R}_i(\theta)$. It is common to write $\Sigma_i = \Sigma_i(\theta)$, $\boldsymbol{D} = \boldsymbol{D}\,(\theta)$, and $\boldsymbol{R}_i = \boldsymbol{R}_i(\theta)$ so that $\Sigma_i = \boldsymbol{Z}_i\boldsymbol{D}\boldsymbol{Z}_i' + \boldsymbol{R}_i$.

As alluded to in Section 1.1, the utility of the mixed model is primarily in its applicability to non-independent data. So, the standard univariate linear model (1) is valid when one observation each is collected on numerous "subjects" that are independent of one another.

A subject here can be a person, a family, a hospital, or so on. When multiple observations are collected on each person/family/hospital, independence of observations, at least taken from the same subject, can no longer be assumed. The mixed model (2), then, with its additional source of variation represented by the random effects ($\boldsymbol{b}_i$) can accommodate such data.

1.3. An example

The mixed model is especially useful when fitting longitudinal data. It allows an analyst to not only make inferences about the population, but it also accommodates estimation and inference about subject-specific level deviation from the population estimates of typical interest. An especially useful property for the mixed model, particularly in longitudinal data analysis, is the fact that it can accommodate missing data. Missing data, usually in the form of withdrawals or drop outs, are a common characteristic of most studies collecting information on individuals over time. To be discussed later, depending on the nature of the missingness, mixed models can allow for missing data.

To exemplify the use of the mixed model in a repeated measures setting, we introduce an application to obesity research. In the United States, the prevalence of obesity has reached epidemic levels (Flegal et al., 2002). Additionally, obesity is a major risk factor for type 2 diabetes (Mokdad et al., 2001). Lifestyle treatment with modest weight loss has been shown to prevent type 2 diabetes (Knowler et al., 2002), and can thus be seen as a crucial element for diabetes control in obese individuals.

Improving Control with Activity and Nutrition (ICAN) was a randomized control trial designed to assess the efficacy of a modestly priced, registered dietician (RD)-led case management (CM) approach to lifestyle change in patients with type 2 diabetes (Wolf et al., 2004). The primary goal of the study was to compare the intervention to usual medical care with respect to weight loss for obese patients with type 2 diabetes. Weight in kilograms and waist circumference (cm) were recorded on 124 individuals at the beginning of the study, and then at 4, 6, 8, and 12 months following baseline. A significant overall difference was found in weight loss over the period of the trial favoring lifestyle CM over usual care (UC).

The primary focus of the study and the subsequent analysis of the data were in differences between the two groups, the lifestyle CM group and the UC group, with respect to weight loss over time. To do this, one would estimate and make inferences about the "fixed effects" portion of the model. One could with such a model fit a linear trend over time for each group and then compare groups, or one could examine polynomial effects over time.

It would also prove interesting to study the variation observed in the data as well. Namely, we could examine whether the variability in weight loss over time was different between the two groups. Such an examination would allow investigators to make decisions on the overall effectiveness of the CM intervention in facilitating consistent weight loss. The mixed model allows for separate models of the variation for the two intervention groups, and one could then make conclusions based on the resulting estimates. Similarly, examination of outliers in both groups using random effect estimates (i.e., subject-specific deviations from the average trend over time for the group) could also be useful in helping to identify underlying individual factors that may influence the response to such an intervention.

In order to achieve such goals, a linear mixed model was fitted to the data. Previous experience with the data coupled with careful model fitting strategies resulted in the following model of interest:

$$\begin{aligned} y_{ij} = {} & \beta_1(\text{BASELINE WEIGHT})_i + \beta_2(\text{BASELINE AGE})_i + \beta_3(\text{UC}_i) \\ & + \beta_4(\text{CM}_i) + (\beta_5\text{UC}_i + \beta_6\text{CM}_i)t_{ij} + b_{1i}(\text{UC}_i) + b_{2i}(\text{CM}_i) + e_{ij}. \end{aligned} \quad (3)$$

Here, y_{ij} is the change from baseline weight (kg) observed for individual i at month t_{ij} ($t_{ij} = 4,6,8,12$). CM_i and UC_i are indicator variables for those subjects in the CM and UC groups, respectively. The among-unit variation was modeled separately for each group; i.e., $\text{var}(b_{1i}) = \sigma^2_{b,\text{UC}}$ for those individuals in the UC group and $\text{var}(b_{2i}) = \sigma^2_{b,\text{CM}}$ for those individuals in the CM group. This variation, stemming from the random intercept included in the model (b_{1i} and b_{2i}, depending on the group assignment for subject i), represents the variation of the deviations of each subject's estimated intercept from the population intercepts (β_3 and β_4). In this instance, we assumed a constant within-unit variation between the two groups. Thus, $\text{var}(e_{ij}) = \sigma^2_e$.

In the majority of applications, as is the case here, primary interest lies in inference about the fixed effects; namely, we wish to know if there is a difference between the two groups with respect to weight loss over time. So, we wish to make inferences about the intercept and time parameters for the two groups. With this particular mixed model, we assume a linear change in weight loss over time for both groups, on average. But, the mixed model allows for individual deviations from these population estimates. Here, we only allow for deviation from the intercept; each individual has a random intercept estimate that will represent that person's deviation from the estimate of the average initial weight loss (intercept) for that particular group. However, one could add a number of random effects to account for multiple sources of variation that one believes can be modeled in such a fashion. In this particular case, we could have included a random slope term that represented the subject's deviation from the population slope estimate. As we will discuss later, there are methods to assess the necessity for including such random effects. In doing so, we decided that a random intercept term was only required, but we allowed for the random intercept's variation to differ between the two groups.

Figure 1 displays model-predicted weight loss at the mean values of age and weight (50 years old and 105 kg, respectively) for both groups, as well as a random sampling of individual profiles. These individual observations over time allow for estimation of average changes over time per group as well as estimation of variation from those average changes. The figure displays that in the UC group, there is no discernable pattern of weight change over the span of the study, as to be expected since this group of subjects did not receive any intervention more than what is considered "usual care." However, the subjects in the CM

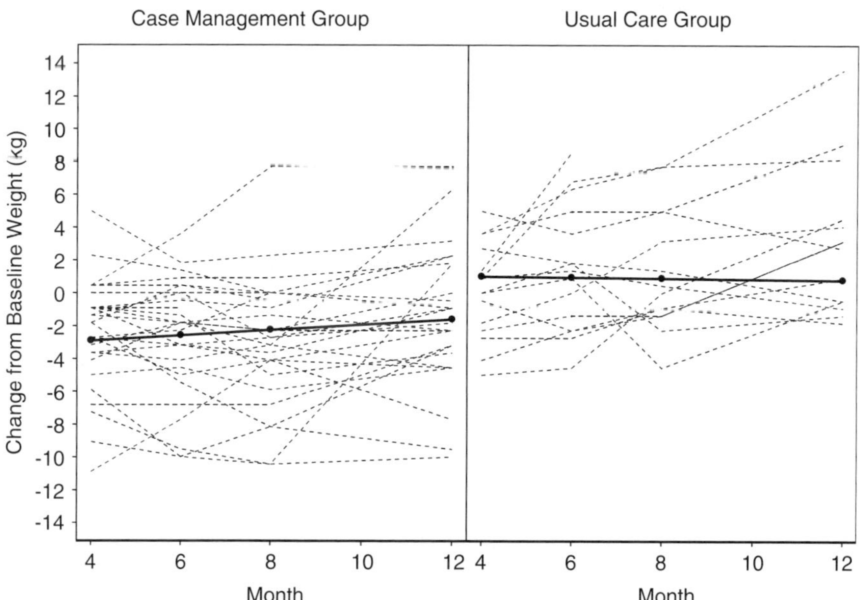

Fig. 1. Random sample of individual profiles of weight change from ICAN study along with estimated average weight loss (based on mixed model (3), using the mean values of age and weight (50 years old and 105 kg, respectively)).

Dashed lines represent observed weights for each individual over the span of the study. Solid lines represent the model-estimated weight change from baseline for each group. The individual profiles seen here represent only a random sampling of the entire set of subjects used to estimate the parameters of model (3).

Table 1
ICAN mixed model (3) parameter estimates

Effect	Parameter	Estimate	Standard Error
Baseline weight	β_1	−0.008	0.013
Baseline age	β_2	−0.084	0.042
Intercepts			
UC group	β_3	6.121	3.042
CM group	β_4	1.458	3.054
Month effect			
UC group	β_5	−0.025	0.069
CM group	β_6	0.164	0.076
Var(b_{1i})	σ_b^2,UC	8.626	2.035
Var(b_{2i})	σ_b^2,CM	10.404	2.477
Var(e_{ij})	σ_e^2	10.573	0.798

group on average lost more weight than those in the UC group. The figure of the individual profiles is extremely helpful in determining the appropriate model of the data. As one can see, there is considerable variation of the measurements for both groups over time, both among subjects as well as within-subjects.

Table 1 includes the estimates of the parameters in model (3). After using inference techniques described later, we can conclude from this model that there is a significantly greater initial amount of weight loss at four months in the CM group, compared to the UC group. However, there is no significant difference in the two population slopes, signifying that the two groups do not differ in weight loss/gain over time after the initial weight change at four months. In fact, the subjects in the CM group actually gained weight throughout the rest of the study on average, while the patients in the UC group remained relatively stable in terms of weight change throughout the year. Thus, we can conclude based on the fixed effect estimates that the intervention to be tested is effective at initial weight loss on average, but that those who received this intervention could not maintain this weight loss over the span of the study. Additionally, we observe that the subjects in the CM group experienced greater variation in their initial weight loss than those in the UC group. We could then look at actual random intercept estimates (not displayed) to determine those subjects who experienced the most weight loss.

1.4. Marginal versus hierarchical

To begin, it is worth writing the linear mixed model (2) again:

$$\boldsymbol{y}_i = \boldsymbol{X}_i\boldsymbol{\beta} + \boldsymbol{Z}_i\boldsymbol{b}_i + \boldsymbol{e}_i.$$

The motivation behind the analysis or scientific question of interest will drive the interpretation of the estimates resulting from fitting model (2) to the data. As alluded to in the discussion of the ICAN example, most often analysts are interested in estimation and inference about the fixed effects parameters, β, and possibly the "variance components," the variance parameters of θ. In this setting, model (2) with $\varepsilon_i = \boldsymbol{Z}_i\boldsymbol{b}_i + \boldsymbol{e}_i$, i.e., $\boldsymbol{y}_i = \boldsymbol{X}_i\boldsymbol{\beta} + \varepsilon_i$, is often referred to as the marginal model (Verbeke and Molenberghs, 2000), or the population-averaged model (Zeger et al., 1988). Here, the following distributional assumptions are all that are needed in making the conclusions necessary from the analysis of the data:

$$y_i \sim \mathcal{N}\left(\boldsymbol{X}_i\boldsymbol{\beta}, \Sigma_i = \boldsymbol{Z}_i\boldsymbol{D}\boldsymbol{Z}_i' + \boldsymbol{R}_i\right). \tag{4}$$

Use of the marginal model does not imply that random effects are unnecessary for such an analysis. On the contrary, proper modeling of the random effects provides for a typically intuitive way of modeling variation of complex data that allows for accurate estimation and inference on the parameters of interest, $\boldsymbol{\beta}$, and sometimes $\boldsymbol{\theta}$. Although not explicitly defined or needed in this case, random effects make it convenient in modeling the variation of multilevel data.

But, many times it is also important for one to focus on the random effects themselves. In this case, we should view (2) as a "hierarchical" model (Verbeke and Molenberghs, 2000), or a "subject-specific" model (Vonesh and Chinchilli, 1997). Rather than explicitly ignore the random effects in the model, $\boldsymbol{b}_i$, we now define the distributional assumptions of the model conditional on $\boldsymbol{b}_i$:

$$\begin{aligned} \mathbf{y}_i|\boldsymbol{b}_i &\sim \mathcal{N}(\boldsymbol{X}_i\boldsymbol{\beta} + \boldsymbol{Z}_i\boldsymbol{b}_i,\ \boldsymbol{R}_i); \\ \boldsymbol{b}_i &\sim \mathcal{N}(0, \boldsymbol{D}). \end{aligned} \tag{5}$$

Notice that here, $y_i \sim \mathcal{N}(\boldsymbol{X}_i\boldsymbol{\beta},\ \Sigma_i)$, which is the same distributional assumption of the marginal model. However, the marginal model and the hierarchical model are not equivalent, at least in terms of interpretation and utility of the models. When we discuss the potential for using the mixed model, specifically the random effects portion of it, to focus on individual-specific deviation from the mean profiles (fixed effects), it is in the context of the hierarchical perspective. The hierarchical model then accommodates analyses to identify outlying individuals and to make predictions on the individual level.

Naturally, one may place certain restrictions on the structure and the number of parameters of both covariance matrices, $\boldsymbol{D}$ and $\boldsymbol{R}_i$. The structure of $\boldsymbol{D}$ is often dictated by the number of random effects included in the model. For example, in the context of longitudinal data, if one included only a random intercept, then one only needs to estimate the variance of this random intercept term. However, if one also includes a random slope as well, then one must decide whether or not to allow the two random effects to covary. Most software can accommodate many different specified parametric models of both covariance matrices of the mixed model. For more detailed information, see Verbeke and Molenberghs (2000).

2. Estimation for the linear mixed model

Seminal papers by Harville (1976, 1977) developed the linear mixed model as is written in (2), and Laird and Ware (1982) discussed its use for longitudinal data. Harville (1976) extended the Gauss–Markov theorem to cover the random effects, $\boldsymbol{b}_i$, in estimating linear combinations of $\boldsymbol{\beta}$ and $\boldsymbol{b}_i$. The prediction of $\boldsymbol{b}_i$ is also derived in an empirical Bayesian setting. Harville (1977) provided a review of the maximum likelihood (ML) approach to estimation in the linear mixed model. For model (2), the maximum log-likelihood is written as

$$l_{ML}(\boldsymbol{\theta}) = -\frac{N}{2}\log(2\pi) - \frac{1}{2}\sum_{i=1}^{m}\log|\Sigma_i| - \frac{1}{2}\sum_{i=1}^{m}(\boldsymbol{y}_i - \boldsymbol{X}_i\boldsymbol{\beta})'\Sigma_i^{-1}(\boldsymbol{y}_i - \boldsymbol{X}_i\boldsymbol{\beta}). \quad (6)$$

Maximization of $l_{ML}(\boldsymbol{\theta})$ produces ML estimators (MLEs) of the unknown parameters $\boldsymbol{\beta}$ and $\boldsymbol{\theta}$. When $\boldsymbol{\theta}$ is known, the MLE of $\boldsymbol{\beta}$ is given by

$$\hat{\boldsymbol{\beta}} = \left(\sum_{i=1}^{m}\boldsymbol{X}_i'\Sigma_i^{-1}\boldsymbol{X}_i\right)^{-1}\sum_{i=1}^{m}\boldsymbol{X}_i'\Sigma_i^{-1}\boldsymbol{y}_i. \quad (7)$$

Kackar and Harville (1984) stated that the best linear unbiased estimators of the fixed and random effects are available when the true value of the variance parameter, $\boldsymbol{\theta}$, is known. In the usual case when $\boldsymbol{\theta}$ is unknown, Σ_i is simply replaced with its estimate, $\hat{\Sigma}_i$. Kackar and Harville (1984) concluded that if $\boldsymbol{\theta}$ needs to be estimated, the mean squared error of the estimates of $\boldsymbol{\beta}$ and $\boldsymbol{b}_i$ becomes larger. They also provided an approximation of this decrease in precision.

Harville (1974) also introduced the use of the restricted, or residual, maximum likelihood (REML) developed by Patterson and Thompson (1971) in estimating the covariance parameters of the linear mixed model. ML estimations of $\boldsymbol{\theta}$ are biased downward since the loss of degrees of freedom resulting from the estimation of the fixed effects is not taken into account. REML estimation acknowledges this loss of degrees of freedom and hence leads to less biased estimates. The REML estimator of $\boldsymbol{\theta}$ is calculated by maximizing the likelihood function of a set of error contrasts of $\boldsymbol{y}_i$, $\boldsymbol{u}'\boldsymbol{y}_i$, chosen so that $E(\boldsymbol{u}'\boldsymbol{y}_i) = 0$. The resulting function, not dependent on $\boldsymbol{\beta}$, is based on a transformation of the original observations that lead to a new set of $N-p$ observations. Harville (1974) showed that the restricted log-likelihood function can be written in the following form based on the original observations:

$$l_{REML}(\boldsymbol{\theta}) = -\frac{N-p}{2}\log(2\pi) + \frac{1}{2}\log\left|\sum_{i=1}^{m}\boldsymbol{X}_i'\boldsymbol{X}_i\right| - \frac{1}{2}\sum_{i=1}^{m}\log|\Sigma_i| - \frac{1}{2}\log\left|\sum_{i=1}^{m}\boldsymbol{X}_i'\Sigma_i^{-1}\boldsymbol{X}_i\right| - \frac{1}{2}\sum_{i=1}^{m}(\boldsymbol{y}_i - \boldsymbol{X}_i\hat{\boldsymbol{\beta}})'\Sigma_i^{-1}(\boldsymbol{y}_i - \boldsymbol{X}_i\hat{\boldsymbol{\beta}}), \quad (8)$$

where $\hat{\boldsymbol{\beta}}$ is of the form given above (7).

Laird and Ware (1982) introduced the linear mixed model in a general setting as it applies to longitudinal data, discussing how the model can be reduced to both growth curve models and repeated measures models. This two-stage random effects model is touted as being superior to ordinary multivariate models in its fitting of longitudinal data since it can handle unbalanced situations that typically arise when one gathers serial measurements on individuals. A unified approach to fitting the linear mixed model is the primary theme, comparing estimation of the model parameters using ML as well as empirical Bayes methods.

Harville (1977) noted that estimating the parameters of the linear mixed model via ML methods has computational disadvantages by requiring the solution of a nonlinear problem, an issue that is not as detrimental today with advances in computer technology that have dramatically increased the speed of estimation algorithms. Laird and Ware (1982) discussed the use of the Expectation-Maximization (EM) algorithm for estimation in the linear mixed model for longitudinal data. The EM algorithm was originally introduced by Dempster et al. (1977) as an iterative algorithm that can be used for computing ML estimates in the presence of incomplete data. Laird et al. (1987) attempted to improve the speed of convergence of the EM algorithm, noting the rate of convergence is dependent on the data and the specified forms of the covariance matrices, $\boldsymbol{D}$ and $\boldsymbol{R}_i$.

Lindstrom and Bates (1988) proposed an efficient version of the Newton–Raphson (NR) algorithm for estimating the parameters in the linear mixed model via both ML and REML. They also developed computationally stable forms of both the NR and EM algorithms and compared the two in terms of speed and performance. While the NR algorithm is concluded to require fewer iterations to achieve convergence, it is not guaranteed to converge, whereas the EM algorithm will always converge to a local maximum of the likelihood. The faster convergence time of the NR algorithm has made it the preferred estimation method of choice for most mixed model fitting procedures.

3. Inference for the mixed model

3.1. Inference for the fixed effects

As stated previously, it is extremely common to be primarily interested in making conclusions regarding the fixed effects of the model. Not surprisingly, then, inference tools for the fixed effect parameters in the mixed model have received most of the attention methodologically. Likelihood ratio tests (LRTs) can compare two nested mixed models (Palta and Qu, 1995; Vonesh and Chinchilli, 1997; Verbeke and Molenberghs, 2000) with ML estimation and are assumed to exhibit a χ^2 distribution.

McCarroll and Helms (1987) evaluated a "conventional" LRT with a linear covariance structure via simulation studies. They showed that the LRT inflates Type I error rates. In addition, the LRT gave observed power values that were usually higher than the hypothesized values. McCarroll and Helms (1987) recommended using tests other than the LRT.

Use of the LRT based on the REML log-likelihood function is not valid when interest lies in the comparison of models with different sets of fixed effects. Welham and Thompson (1997) proposed adjusted LRTs for the fixed effects using REML, while Zucker et al. (2000) developed what they termed "refined likelihood ratio tests" in order to improve small sample inference. The adjusted tests of Welham and Thompson (1997) are reasonably well approximated by χ^2 variables. Zucker et al. (2000) found that an adjusted LRT based on the Cox–Reid adjusted likelihood produced Type I error rates lower than nominal. Consequently, a Bartlett correction greatly improved the Type I error rates of the adjusted LRT. Though the techniques appear promising, new and extensive analytic work seems required for each specific class of model.

Approximate Wald and F-statistics allow testing hypotheses regarding $\boldsymbol{\beta}$. However, Wald tests can underestimate the true variability in the estimated fixed effects because they do not take into account the variability incurred by estimating $\boldsymbol{\theta}$ (Dempster et al., 1981). The approximate F-test is more commonly used. The null hypothesis H_0: $\boldsymbol{C\beta} = 0$, with $\boldsymbol{C}$ a $a \times p$ contrast matrix, can be tested with

$$T_F = a^{-1}(\boldsymbol{C}\hat{\boldsymbol{\beta}})' \left[\boldsymbol{C} \left(\sum_{i=1}^{m} \boldsymbol{X}_i' \hat{\Sigma}_i^{-1} \boldsymbol{X}_i \right)^{-1} \boldsymbol{C}' \right]^{-1} (\boldsymbol{C}\hat{\boldsymbol{\beta}}). \tag{9}$$

Under the null hypothesis, it is assumed that T_F has an approximate F-distribution with a numerator degrees of freedom, and v denominator degrees of freedom, denoted $F(a,v)$. The denominator degrees of freedom, v, have to be estimated from the data. Determining the denominator degrees of freedom has been a source of research and debate for many years, with no clear consensus. However, in the analysis of longitudinal data, Verbeke and Molenberghs (2000, Section 6.2.2, p. 54) noted that "... different subjects contribute independent information, which results in numbers of degrees of freedom which are typically large enough, whatever estimation method is used, to lead to very similar p-values." Unfortunately, the approximate F-statistic is known to result in inflated Type I errors and poor power approximations in small samples, even for complete and balanced data (McCarroll and Helms, 1987; Catellier and Muller, 2000). Finally, Vonesh (2004) concluded that the denominator degrees of freedom of the F-test in the linear mixed model should be the number of independent sampling units minus "something" and we simply do not know what that "something" is.

Kenward and Roger (1997) presented a scaled Wald statistic with an approximate F-distribution for testing fixed effects with REML estimation that performs well, even in small samples. The Wald statistic uses an adjusted estimator of the covariance matrix to reduce the small sample bias. A drawback occurs when the variance components are constrained to be nonnegative and estimates fall on a boundary. In such cases the Taylor series expansions underlying the approximations may not be accurate. In addition, the procedure can fail to behave well with a nonlinear covariance structure. The technique has been implemented in popular mixed model fitting procedures such as SAS PROC MIXED (SAS Institute, 2003b). However, even this inference technique is not ideal, as documented performance of the Kenward–Roger F-statistic for some small sample cases has revealed inflated Type I error rates with various covariance model selection techniques (Gomez et al., 2005).

3.2. Inference for the random effects

When one is interested in the random effects themselves in the mixed model, then one needs to make inferences from the hierarchical model perspective. It is most convenient to estimate the random effects using Bayesian techniques, resulting in the following form of the estimates of $\boldsymbol{b}_i$, assuming $\boldsymbol{\theta}$ is known:

$$\hat{\boldsymbol{b}}_i = \boldsymbol{D}\boldsymbol{Z}_i'\Sigma_i^{-1}(\boldsymbol{y}_i - \boldsymbol{X}_i\boldsymbol{\beta}). \tag{10}$$

The variance of $\hat{\boldsymbol{b}}_i$ is then approximated by

$$v(\hat{\boldsymbol{b}}_i) = \boldsymbol{D}\boldsymbol{Z}_i'\left\{\Sigma_i^{-1} - \Sigma_i^{-1}\boldsymbol{X}_i\left(\sum_{i=1}^{m}\boldsymbol{X}_i'\Sigma_i^{-1}\boldsymbol{X}_i\right)^{-1}\boldsymbol{X}_i'\Sigma_i^{-1}\right\}\boldsymbol{Z}_i\boldsymbol{D}. \tag{11}$$

As noted by Laird and Ware (1982), (11) underestimates the variability in $\hat{\boldsymbol{b}}_i - \boldsymbol{b}_i$ because it ignores the variation of $\boldsymbol{b}_i$. Consequently, inference about $\boldsymbol{b}_i$ is typically based on

$$v(\hat{\boldsymbol{b}}_i - \boldsymbol{b}_i) = \boldsymbol{D} - v(\hat{\boldsymbol{b}}_i). \tag{12}$$

As with inference for the fixed effects, we typically do not know $\boldsymbol{\theta}$ beforehand. And, in this particular setting, we most often do not know $\boldsymbol{\beta}$. So, we usually replace $\boldsymbol{\theta}$ and $\boldsymbol{\beta}$ with their ML or REML estimates in the above equations. In this case, $\hat{\boldsymbol{b}}_i$ in (10) is known as the "empirical Bayes" estimate of $\boldsymbol{b}_i$. Again, as is the case when making inference about the fixed effects, when we use $\hat{\boldsymbol{\theta}}$ in place of $\boldsymbol{\theta}$, we then underestimate the variability of $\hat{\boldsymbol{b}}_i$. In this setting too, then, it is recommended that inference on the random effects be based on approximate F-tests with specific procedures for the estimation of the denominator degrees of freedom (Verbeke and Molenberghs, 2000).

3.3. Inference for the covariance parameters

Even though focus typically lies on the fixed effects, it is important to effectively model the variation of the data via the variance parameters in such a model. Making valid conclusions about the variability of the data are important information in itself, but it also leads to proper inference about the fixed effects as well. As discussed in Verbeke and Molenberghs (2000), likelihood theory allows for the distribution of both the ML and REML estimators of $\boldsymbol{\theta}$, $\hat{\boldsymbol{\theta}}$, to be approximated by a normal distribution with mean vector $\boldsymbol{\theta}$ and covariance matrix equaling the inverse of the Fisher information matrix. Thus, techniques such as LRTs and Wald tests can be used to make inferences about $\boldsymbol{\theta}$. Of course, there are restrictions to the possible values of the parameters contained in $\boldsymbol{\theta}$, most commonly that variance components be strictly positive. To demonstrate, in the example model (3), we assume $\text{var}(b_{1i}) = \sigma^2_{b,\text{UC}} > 0$. Of course, in practice, when one fits the data using a mixed model procedure in a software package, if a value of a variance parameter is close to the boundary space (e.g., the variance is close to 0), this indicates that the source of variation may not need to be modeled. In the case when a negative value of the variance component parameter is not allowed, Verbeke and Molenberghs (2003) discuss the use of one-sided tests, in particular the score test.

In the context of a generalized nonlinear mixed model (to be discussed), Vonesh and Chinchilli (1997, Section 8.3.2) proposed a pseudo-likelihood ratio test (PLRT) used by Vonesh et al. (1996) to assess goodness-of-fit of the modeled covariance structure. The idea was to compare the robust "sandwich" estimator of the fixed effects covariance matrix to the usual estimated covariance matrix. The fixed effects covariance matrix is $\Omega = v(\hat{\boldsymbol{\beta}})$. The usual estimate and the robust "sandwich" estimator of the fixed effects covariance matrix for (2) are given by

$$\hat{\Omega} = \left(\sum_{i=1}^{m} \boldsymbol{X}_i' \hat{\Sigma}_i^{-1} \boldsymbol{X}_i \right)^{-1} \tag{13}$$

and

$$\hat{\Omega}_R = \hat{\Omega} \left[\sum_{i=1}^{m} \boldsymbol{X}_i' \hat{\Sigma}_i^{-1} (\boldsymbol{y}_i - \boldsymbol{X}_i \hat{\boldsymbol{\beta}})(\boldsymbol{y}_i - \boldsymbol{X}_i \hat{\boldsymbol{\beta}})' \hat{\Sigma}_i^{-1} \boldsymbol{X}_i \right] \hat{\Omega}. \tag{14}$$

By comparing the closeness of the estimators using a PLRT, one can evaluate the goodness-of-fit of the modeled covariance matrix Σ_i. Assuming that $m\hat{\Omega}_R$ has an approximate Wishart distribution, the PLRT is approximately distributed as a chi-square with $p(p+1)/2$ degrees of freedom. One advantage of the technique is that it does not require repeated fittings of models. The authors suggested that the PLRT should not be used when the outcomes exhibit a non-normal distribution. More work needs to be done to assess the performance of the PLRT for the mixed model in general. For more details of the technique, the reader is directed to Vonesh and Chinchilli (1997, Section 8.3.2).

4. Selecting the best mixed model

Discussion of estimation and inference on the parameters of the linear mixed model naturally falls under the discussion of model selection. Often, we usually perform hypothesis tests on model parameters to decide whether or not their inclusion in the model is necessary. Inference tools discussed previously are useful in linear mixed models when the parameters of note are nested. However, in the context of mixed models, it is common to want to compare models that are not nested, particularly when trying to determine the best model of the covariance.

4.1. Information criteria

Information theoretic criteria have played a prominent role in mixed model selection due to their relative validity in comparing non-nested models. Most practitioners use the Akaike Information Criterion (AIC, Akaike, 1974) and the Bayesian Information Criterion (BIC, Schwarz, 1978). Many variations have

Table 2
General formulas for commonly used information criteria in mixed model selection

Criteria	Larger-is-Better Formula	Smaller-is-Better Formula
AIC	$l-s$	$-2l+2s$
AICC	$l-s(N^*/N^*-s-1)$	$-2l+2s(N^*/N^*-s-1)$
CAIC	$l-s(\log N^*+1)/2$	$-2l+s(\log N^*+1)$
BIC	$l-s(\log N^*)/2$	$-2l+s(\log N^*)$

Note: Here, l is either $l_{REML}(\boldsymbol{\theta})$ or $l_{ML}(\boldsymbol{\theta})$, s refers to the number of parameters of the model, and N^* a function of the number of observations.

been introduced, including the corrected AIC, or AICC (Hurvich and Tsai, 1989), and the consistent AIC, or CAIC (Bozdogan, 1987). In their original forms, a larger value of the criteria for a given model indicates a better fit of the data. However, it is common to see them presented in a "smaller-is-better" form when they are calculated directly from the $-2 \times$ log-likelihood. Table 2 displays the formulas for the AIC, AICC, CAIC, and BIC from both angles, based on formulas familiar to readers of Vonesh and Chinchilli (1997).

Here, l is either $l_{REML}(\boldsymbol{\theta})$ or $l_{ML}(\boldsymbol{\theta})$, s refers to the number of parameters of the model, and N^* is a function of the number of observations. When using ML estimation, most often $s = p+k$, the total number of parameters in the model. The proper formulas and application of these formulas under REML is still debated; see Gurka (2006) for a summary of the various viewpoints and forms specific to REML model selection. The general consensus (Vonesh and Chinchilli, 1997) is that under ML, $N^* = N$, the total number of observations, and under REML, $N^* = N-p$, given that the restricted likelihood is based on $N-p$ observations. However, this recommendation has not been consistently employed and needs further investigation (see Gurka, 2006 for more discussion). Shi and Tsai (2002) noted that Akaike (1974) used the likelihood function as a basis for obtaining the AIC, but just like the variance estimates of a linear mixed model when using the unrestricted likelihood, the estimator used in the criterion is biased. They then proposed a "residual information criterion" (RIC) that uses REML, applying it to the classical regression setting. Extension of the RIC for use with the linear mixed model is an area of future research.

When discussing model selection criteria, one should introduce the large-sample notions of efficiency and consistency. Efficient criteria target the best model of finite dimension when the "true model" (which is unknown) is of infinite dimension. In contrast, consistent criteria choose the correct model with probability approaching 1 when a true model of finite dimension is assumed to exist. Selection criteria usually fall into one of the two categories; for instance, the AIC and AICC are efficient criteria, while the BIC and CAIC are considered to be consistent criteria. Debate has ensued as to which characteristic is preferred, as opinions are largely driven by the field of application in which one is interested in applying model selection techniques. For further discussion, see Burnham and Anderson (2002) or Shi and Tsai (2002).

In Hjort and Claeskens (2003) and Claeskens and Hjort (2003), the authors discuss model selection, inference after model selection, and both frequentist and Bayesian model averaging. Claeskens and Hjort (2003) noted that traditional information criteria aim to select a single model with overall good properties, but do not provide insight into the actual use of the selected model. Claeskens and Hjort (2003) proposed to focus on the parameter of interest to form the basis of their model selection criterion, and introduce a selection criteria for this purpose denoted as the focused information criterion (FIC). Discussions that follow the article describe limitations of the frequentist model averaging estimator and the FIC (Shen and Dougherty, 2003).

Jiang and Rao (2003) developed consistent procedures for selecting the fixed and random effects in a linear mixed model. Jiang and Rao (2003) focused on two types of linear mixed model selection problems: (a) selection of the fixed effects while assuming the random effects have already been correctly chosen and (b) selection of both the fixed effects and random effects. Their selection criteria are similar to the generalized information criterion (GIC), with the main idea centering on the appropriate selection of a penalty parameter to adjust squared residuals. Owing to the inability to provide an optimal way of choosing the best penalty parameter for a finite set of data, the methods require further investigation before recommending its widespread use.

It is very common to see values for information criteria in standard output of many mixed model fitting procedures, such as SAS PROC MIXED. The applicability of information criteria for mixed model selection is apparent. However, as one can observe by the above summary of this area of research, much more work needs to be performed to consolidate the utility of information criteria to mixed model selection. Thus, we must caution the analyst in using the values of computed information criteria from standard procedures without a through investigation of the research to date in this area.

4.2. Prediction

The introduction of cross-validation methods (Stone, 1974; Geisser, 1975) led to ensuing research in model selection focused on the predictive ability of models (Geisser and Eddy, 1979; Stone, 1977; Shao, 1993). The predictive approach generally involves two steps. For a given number of independent sampling units, m, the data are split into two parts, with $m = m_c + m_v$. Sample size m_c is used for model construction and sample size m_v is used for model validation.

For modeling repeated measures data with correlated errors, Liu et al. (1999) generalized a cross-validation model selection method, the Predicted Residual Sum of Squares (*PRESS*). Allen (1971) originally suggested *PRESS* as a model selection criterion in the univariate linear model. *PRESS* is a weighted sum of squared residuals in which the weights are related to the variance of the predicted values. Though Liu et al. (1999) presented various definitions of *PRESS*, only *PRESS* for the fixed effects was developed since it could be applied to unbalanced designs and the distribution of the statistic yielded useful results. As a result, the *PRESS* statistic should not be used for selecting random effects in the linear mixed model. No conclusive evidence exists of its performance against other model selection criteria. As with the LRT and information criteria, *PRESS* requires repeated fittings of mixed models and hence does not allow model adequacy to be assessed using only the chosen model of interest.

Vonesh et al. (1996) proposed a weighted concordance correlation coefficient as a measure of goodness-of-fit for repeated measurements. The concordance correlation coefficient for the linear and nonlinear mixed effects model (Vonesh and Chinchilli, 1997), denoted by r_c, is a function of the observed outcomes, $\boldsymbol{y}_i$, and the model-predicted outcomes, $\hat{y}_i$. The r_c is a modification of Lin's (1989) proposed concordance correlation coefficient to assess the level of agreement between two bivariate measurements. In general, $-1 \leq r_c \leq 1$, with $r_c = 1$ being a perfect fit and $r_c \leq 0$ being significant lack of fit. Unlike the LRT, information criteria, or PRESS, r_c does not require repeated fittings of mixed models to evaluate adequacy of fit. However, r_c can be used to differentiate between different hypothesized models by choosing the model with the largest r_c. It does not appear that r_c has been widely implemented in the literature for linear mixed models, and its performance has not been assessed via any large-scale simulation studies.

Vonesh and Chinchilli (1997) also presented a modification of the usual R^2-statistic from the univariate linear model that is interpreted as the explained residual variation, or proportional decrease in residual variation. Unlike r_c, the R^2-statistic requires specification of a hypothesized model and a null model (one that is simple but consistent with the application). As with the r_c, the lack of evidence describing the performance of R^2 strongly discourages its use in selecting a linear mixed model. Vonesh and Chinchilli (1997) noted that r_c may be preferred since it equals a concordance correlation between observed and predicted values.

Xu (2003) and Gelman and Pardoe (2005) investigated measures to estimate the proportion of explained variation under the linear mixed model. Xu (2003) considered three types of measures and generalized the familiar R^2-statistic from the univariate linear model to the linear mixed model for nested models. In order to measure explained variation, the method by Xu (2003) relies upon defining a "null" model such as a model with only a fixed effect and random effect intercept. Gelman and Pardoe (2005) presented a Bayesian method of defining R^2 for each level of a multilevel (hierarchical) linear model, which includes the linear mixed model. The method is based on comparing variances in a single-fitted model rather than comparing to a null model. Xu's (2003) simulation results demonstrated that the R^2 measure gives good estimates with reasonably large cluster sizes, but overestimates the proportion of variation in $\boldsymbol{y}$ explained by the covariates if the cluster sizes are too small. Gelman and Pardoe (2005) performed no simulations to assess the performance of their R^2 measure. More investigation must be done.

Weiss et al. (1997) presented a Bayesian approach to model selection for random effect models. In a data analysis example, Weiss et al. (1997) found conflicting results, showing that the selected model was dependent on the chosen priors and hyperparameter settings. In comparing their technique to the LRT,

AIC, and BIC, the results were again mixed. There exists a lack of evidence that the Bayesian approach performs well in model selection for linear mixed models, since no in-depth simulation study or other additional comparative procedures have been conducted.

In the univariate linear model, Mallows' C_p criterion (Mallows, 1973) requires a pool of candidate models which are each separately nested within a single full model. It compares the mean square error (*MSE*) of each candidate model to the MSE of the full model, which then allows comparing one candidate to another. However, the MSE for the linear mixed model is not well defined since there are two independent sources of variation, one due to deviations about the population profile and one due to deviations about subject-specific profiles. Recently, Cantoni et al. (2005) suggested a generalized version of Mallows' C_p, denoted GC_p, for marginal longitudinal models. GC_p provides an estimate of a measure of adequacy of a model for prediction. Though the technique was developed for models fitted using generalized estimating equations (GEE), there is potential for considering the method in linear mixed model analysis.

The small sample characteristics of model selection methods based on predictive approaches require further investigation. Furthermore, in some cases the approach cannot be used. For example, in many small sample applications it is unacceptable to split the sample for determining model construction and model validation.

4.3. Graphical techniques

Graphical techniques have long been a component of model selection in both univariate and multivariate settings. Plotting the estimated response function or residuals against predicted values provides statisticians with visual aids that help in model selection. Similarly, graphical techniques can help select a linear mixed model. Plotting the estimated response function from the fixed effects and comparing it to a mean curve constructed using averages at selected time points provides one useful aid. For longitudinal data, plotting the collection of estimated individual response functions against the observed data can greatly help model selection.

For simple examples and some small sample applications, graphical techniques can work well, even though they are subjective aids. More complex scenarios make using graphical techniques either very challenging or render graphical techniques almost useless. In addition, due to the subjective nature of graphical procedures, perhaps the techniques can never be considered as a primary means of model selection. Grady and Helms (1995), Diggle et al. (2002) and Verbeke and Molenberghs (2000) gave expanded discussions of the use of graphical techniques.

5. Diagnostics for the mixed model

As is the case with ordinary linear regression, the linear mixed model has distributional assumptions that may or may not be valid when used with applied data. Unlike univariate linear regression, however, diagnostics to assess these assumptions, and consequent alternatives when violations of the assumptions are suspected have not been developed fully for the linear mixed model, primarily due to the relative youth of the analysis tool. An area that has received some attention is the assumed normality of the random effects, $\boldsymbol{b}_i$. Lange and Ryan (1989) described a method for assessing the distribution assumption of the random effects that uses standardized empirical Bayes estimates of $\boldsymbol{b}_i$. The assumed linearity of the covariance matrices of the observations, along with assuming $\boldsymbol{R}_i = \sigma^2 \boldsymbol{I}_{n_i}$, allows these standardized estimates to be independent across individuals. They then used classical goodness-of-fit procedures, in particular a weighted normal plot, to assess the normality of the random effects. Butler and Louis (1992) demonstrated that the normality assumption of the random effects has little effect on the estimates of the fixed effects; they did not investigate the effect on the estimates of the random effects themselves. Verbeke and Lesaffre (1996) investigated the impact of assuming a Gaussian distribution for the random effects on their estimates in the linear mixed model. They showed that if the distribution of the random effects is a finite mixture of normal distributions, then the estimates of $\boldsymbol{b}_i$ may be poor if normality is assumed. Consequently, they argued it is beneficial to assume a mixture of normal distributions and compare the fitted model to the model fit when assuming a Gaussian distribution.

Verbeke and Lesaffre (1997) showed that the ML estimates for the fixed effects as well as the variance parameters, $\boldsymbol{\theta}$, obtained when assuming normality of the random effects, are consistent and asymptotically normally distributed, even when the random effects distribution is not normal. But, they claimed that a sandwich-type correction to the inverse of the Fisher information matrix is needed in order to obtain the correct asymptotic covariance matrix. They showed through simulations that the obtained corrected standard errors are better than the uncorrected ones in moderate to large samples, especially for the parameters in $\boldsymbol{D}$. Very little work has been done on the performance of the linear mixed model in small sample settings when normality of the random effects is assumed but not achieved.

Little attention has been given to the distribution assumption of the pure errors, $\boldsymbol{e}_i$, in the linear mixed model. Often it is assumed that mixed models exhibit conditional independence, i.e., $\boldsymbol{R}_i = \sigma^2 \boldsymbol{I}_{n_i}$, as in some cases it is arguable that the correlation exhibited between observations within an individual can be accounted for fully by the random effects covariance structure. In certain instances this assumption is included simply for computational convenience. Chi and Reinsel (1989) developed a score test of the assumption of conditional independence compared to a model that assumes auto-correlation in the within-individual errors. They argued that assuming an auto-correlation structure for $\boldsymbol{R}_i$ can actually reduce the number of required random effects needed in the final model. One could note that not only does one assume independence when it is given that $\boldsymbol{R}_i = \sigma^2 \boldsymbol{I}_{n_i}$, but also that there is a constant within-unit error variance. Ahn (2000) proposed a score test for assessing this homoskedasticity of the within-unit errors.

Transformations have also been utilized in mixed model settings. Lipsitz et al. (2000) analyzed real longitudinal data by applying a Box–Cox transformation on the response of a marginal (population-averaged) model. Since the model did not explicitly contain random effects, the authors assumed the transformation achieved normality of the overall error term only. Gurka et al. (2006) discussed details that follow when extending the Box–Cox transformation to the linear mixed model. They showed that the success of a transformation may be judged solely in terms of how closely the total error, ε_i, follows a Gaussian distribution. Hence, the approach avoids the complexity of separately evaluating pure errors and random effects when one's primary interest lies in the marginal model. Oberg and Davidian (2000) extended the method for estimating transformations to nonlinear mixed effects models for repeated measurement data, employing the transform-both-sides model proposed by Carroll and Ruppert (1984).

6. Outliers

Of course, mixed models are sensitive to outlying observations. However, the multilevel structure of the mixed model allows for different definitions of outliers. When viewed as a marginal model, $\boldsymbol{y}_i - \boldsymbol{X}_i\hat{\boldsymbol{\beta}}$ is one form of a residual that measures deviation from the overall population mean. Likewise, $\boldsymbol{y}_i - \boldsymbol{X}_i\hat{\boldsymbol{\beta}} - \boldsymbol{Z}_i\hat{\boldsymbol{b}}_i$ measures the amount of difference from the observed value to a subject's predicted regression. As defined earlier, the random effect estimate itself, $\hat{\boldsymbol{b}}_i$, is also an estimate of deviation; in the longitudinal setting, it is a measure of the subject-specific deviation. As one can imagine, then, due to the many definitions of residuals in the mixed model, diagnostic techniques regularly used for the univariate linear model (leverage, Cook's distance, etc.) do not extend to the mixed model in a straightforward fashion. For a more detailed discussion of influence for the linear mixed model, the reader is directed to Chapter 11 in Verbeke and Molenberghs (2000).

As is the case in the univariate linear model, some researchers have examined robust estimation and inference procedures that will not be greatly affected by such influential observations for mixed models. But, since mixed models are a relatively modern statistical technique, the literature on robust estimation for the linear mixed model is sparse. Fellner (1986) proposed a method for limiting the influence of outliers with respect to the random components in a simple variance components model. A robust modification of restricted ML estimation, Fellner's method uses influence functions attributed to Huber (1981) without explicitly using the likelihood function. Richardson and Welsh (1995) introduced the definitions of robust ML and robust restricted ML in the context of mixed models that are also based on bounding the influence. They applied the methods to data and performed simulation studies to show the advantages of these robust procedures.

7. Missing data

As introduced previously, one common characteristic of study data, particularly longitudinal data, is missing data. This is especially the case in biomedical studies of human beings over time, as it is impossible to ensure 100% compliance with the study protocol. Subjects drop out of studies for many reasons, or may simply miss a visit and continue the study.

The mixed model can accommodate missing data, thus making it an ideal tool to analyze longitudinal data. Unlike other multivariate models, such as the general linear multivariate model (Muller and Stewart, 2006), complete data are not required when fitting a mixed model as long as the missing data are of a certain type. However, the validity of the parameter estimates of the mixed model depends on the nature of the missingness.

Standard classifications of missing data exist. For a more comprehensive look at missing data, see Little and Rubin (1987). The "best" type of missing data is data that are missing completely at random (MCAR). Simply put, with MCAR the fact that the data are missing has nothing to do with any of the effects (e.g., the treatment to be studied) or outcomes of interest. Data in which MCAR is present will not lead to biased estimates of the parameters of the mixed model. The next classification of missingness, one that is also not "bad" from a validity standpoint for the mixed model, is missing at random (MAR). For MAR, the missingness depends on previous values of the outcome, but the missingness is still independent of the model covariates of interest. Handling MAR data is not as simple as MCAR, as careful strategies must be taken in order for valid conclusions to be made from the fitted mixed model.

The type of missingness that results in biased estimates of the parameters of the mixed model is generally referred to as non-ignorable missingness. Generally speaking, missingness that is non-ignorable results when the pattern of missingness is directly related to the covariates of interest. There is no way to accommodate this type of missingness while fitting standard mixed models.

It would be most helpful to give examples of each type of missingness in the context of the ICAN study, where we are comparing two intervention groups with respect to weight loss over time. If a few patients in each intervention group dropped out of the study because they moved out of the area, this most likely would be classified as MCAR. However, since the study participants were obese type 2 diabetes patients, it is quite possible that some of the subjects were so overweight and unhealthy that they could not continue to make their regularly scheduled visits. This pattern of missingness is not directly related to the intervention group in which they belong, but rather the outcome (their weight), and hence most likely this would be classified most likely as MAR. Finally, if many of the patients in the CM group, the intervention that was more intensive, dropped out due to the intensity of this intervention, this type of missingness would be non-ignorable.

To summarize, mixed models are extremely powerful in analyzing longitudinal data in particular due to its ability to accommodate missing data. However, the analyst must be careful in determining which pattern of missingness is present in the data they wish to model. Analytical tools exist to model the incompleteness, thus providing insight into the nature of the missingness. Additionally, imputation methods exist to "fill in the holes," so to speak. As alluded to earlier, missing data are an expansive area of research in itself, and the reader is referred to other articles and texts that deal exclusively with missing data issues. For an excellent overview of missing data in the context of linear mixed models for longitudinal data, see Verbeke and Molenberghs (2002). Also, Diggle et al. (2002) discuss missing data in the longitudinal data setting.

8. Power and sample size

The research on power analysis for mixed models is sparse. Exact power calculations are not available for the mixed model simply because the exact distributions of the tests used in the mixed model are not known. That being said, all hope is not lost in calculating power based on tests of the mixed model. To our knowledge, research on power analysis for the linear mixed model has been limited to calculations based on tests of the fixed effects of the model. As previously discussed, the test of the form (9) follows an approximate F-distribution under the null hypothesis. Simulation results in Helms (1992) support the notion that (9) follows an approximate non-central F-distribution under the alternative hypothesis. We must point out again the uncertainty regarding the denominator degrees of freedom of (9). We have no reason to believe that this uncertainty does not carry over to its use when considering the power of the test. For additional discussion regarding power and the mixed model in this setting, see Stroup (1999) and Littell et al. (2006, Chapter 12).

Power analyses in general require many assumptions. For simple analyses such as a t-test or a univariate linear model, one must have an estimate of the variability of the data, and some idea of what is considered a meaningful effect size before determining the appropriate sample size for a given power. As one can imagine, in settings where the mixed model is ideal (e.g., longitudinal studies), the amount of parameters to make assumptions is relatively large, and the required assumptions become more complicated. For instance, one must make assumptions about the structure of the correlation of the data, and then determine reasonable values to base the power analysis. Such a task is neither simple nor straightforward. Unfortunately, little has been done in terms of laying out sound strategies to perform power calculations for complicated settings such as repeated measures studies.

Calculating sample size for the linear mixed model is directly related to computing power analysis. As noted before, since little has been done to obtain sound strategies for power analysis, the same is then true for computing sample size. Sample size requirements for the linear mixed model, depending on the motivation behind the analysis, can be quite large. However, it is not clear what is sufficiently large with regard to sample size in order to make valid inferences about the model parameters. The primary application of mixed models, the analysis of clustered or longitudinal data, makes this question even more challenging. Should one focus on obtaining more subjects or clusters, or should one try to gather more measurements per subject, or individuals within a cluster? We mentioned earlier that it is generally recognized that for valid inference about the fixed effects, one should perhaps target a larger number of independent sampling units (Vonesh, 2004). However, this has not been proven definitively beyond simulation studies. One useful discussion regarding sample size calculations for repeated measures designs can be found in Overall and Doyle (1994).

9. Generalized linear mixed models

The linear mixed model discussed thus far is primarily used to analyze outcome data that are continuous in nature. One can see from the formulation of the model (2) that the linear mixed model assumes that the outcome is normally distributed. As mentioned previously, researchers have studied the utility of the linear mixed model when the continuous outcome does not follow a Gaussian distribution.

Often times, however, one is interested in modeling non-continuous outcome data, such as binary data or count data. The generalized linear model is appropriate for modeling such data. The generalized linear model encompasses many commonly used models, such as logistic regression, Poisson regression, and in fact linear regression. For an introduction to the generalized linear model, see McCullagh and Nelder (1989).

In the same way the linear mixed model builds on the capabilities of the linear model by allowing for clustered or longitudinal data, the generalized linear mixed model accommodates clustered or longitudinal data that are not continuous. Similar to the linear mixed model, the generalized linear mixed model can be viewed from a marginal or a hierarchical standpoint. Remember that in the hierarchical case of the linear mixed model,

$$E(\boldsymbol{y}_i|\boldsymbol{b}_i) = \boldsymbol{X}_i\boldsymbol{\beta} + \boldsymbol{Z}_i\boldsymbol{b}_i.$$

Now, for the generalized linear mixed model (McCulloch and Searle, 2001), again assuming $\boldsymbol{b}_i \sim \mathcal{N}(0, \boldsymbol{D})$,

$$E(\boldsymbol{y}_i|\boldsymbol{b}_i) = f(\boldsymbol{X}_i\boldsymbol{\beta} + \boldsymbol{Z}_i\boldsymbol{b}_i), \tag{15}$$

where f is a function of the fixed and random effects of the model. The inverse of this function, say g, is typically called the "link" function. So, $g\{E(\boldsymbol{y}_i|\boldsymbol{b}_i)\} = \boldsymbol{X}_i\boldsymbol{\beta} + \boldsymbol{Z}_i\boldsymbol{b}_i$. There are many common link functions, each usually corresponding to an assumed distribution of $\boldsymbol{y}_i|\boldsymbol{b}_i$. The simplest function is $g\{E(\boldsymbol{y}_i|\boldsymbol{b}_i)\} = E(\boldsymbol{y}_i|\boldsymbol{b}_i)$, the identity link, where $\boldsymbol{y}_i|\boldsymbol{b}_i$ is assumed to be normally distributed. This simple case is the linear mixed model, a specific case of the generalized linear mixed model. For logistic regression, the link function is called the logit link, $g(x) = \log\{x/(1-x)\}$, where x is assumed to follow a binary distribution. Logistic regression is popular in many epidemiological and other biomedical studies where the outcome has two options, e.g., disease or no disease, and interest lies in estimating the odds of developing the disease. For Poisson regression, the link function is the log link, $g(x) = \log(x)$, where x is assumed to follow a Poisson distribution. Poisson regression is often used to model count or rate data.

There are many other link functions and corresponding distributions used in the case of generalized linear models, including generalized linear mixed models.

Again, the addition of the random effect term in this setting allows for clustered or repeated data. For instance, one may be interested in estimating the odds of developing a disease, but has data on multiple individuals from the same families. In this case, it may be unreasonable to assume that these individuals are independent of one another with respect to the risk of developing the disease. Here, then, the generalized linear mixed model allows the analyst to accommodate this dependence.

The above formulation applies to the hierarchical view of the mixed model, but the marginal view is applicable in this setting as well. In this case, we simply assume $E(\boldsymbol{y}_i) = f(\boldsymbol{X}_i b)$. If one is simply interested in population estimates (averages), then alternatives to the generalized linear mixed model exist, such as GEE. See Diggle et al. (2002) for a discussion of GEE. Thus, most often when generalized linear mixed models are used, the hierarchical standpoint is of interest; here the random effects included in the model are of importance and not just a nuisance.

Although at first glance the generalized linear mixed model, when using a link/distribution other than the identity/normal, does not seem to be much more complicated with respect to estimation and inference, the methodology involved for this model is actually quite a bit more complex. When using a link function other than the identity link, it is more difficult to express the likelihood of $\boldsymbol{y}_i$, which now involves an integral with respect to $\boldsymbol{b}_i$. The difficulty with expressing the likelihood, coupled with the lack of closed-form solutions, makes estimation much more computationally intensive. Sophisticated numerical techniques are necessary, and the body of literature in this area is relatively expansive. More in-depth introductions and discussions of generalized linear mixed models, along with estimation and inference about its parameters, can be found in many books (McCulloch and Searle, 2001; Diggle et al., 2002; Agresti, 2002; Demidenko, 2004; Molenberghs and Verbeke, 2005).

10. Nonlinear mixed models

Another version of the mixed model is the nonlinear mixed model. The nonlinear mixed model actually follows the same general form (15) as the generalized linear mixed model. However, the function f for a nonlinear mixed model is typically more complicated than the standard functions used for the generalized linear mixed model. It is common to see applications in which the data are best fitted by models that are nonlinear in the parameters of interest. As mentioned, generalized linear mixed models are one form of nonlinear mixed models. More complicated forms of nonlinear models are often used in pharmacokinetics and biological and agricultural growth models. In most of these cases, there is a known or suspected form, based on past experiences or theoretical knowledge, for how the parameters enter the model in a nonlinear fashion.

As an example of the applicability of the nonlinear mixed model in pharmacokinetic settings, Pinheiro and Bates (1995) fit what is referred to as a first-order compartment model to data on serum concentrations of the drug theophylline from 12 subjects observed over a 25-h period. The nonlinear mixed model in this case has the following form:

$$y_{it} = \left\{ \frac{Dk_{e_i} \cdot k_{a_i}}{Cl_i(k_{a_i} - k_{e_i})} \right\} \cdot \left\{ e^{(-k_{e_i} t)} - e^{(-k_{a_i} t)} \right\} + e_{it}. \tag{16}$$

Here, y_{it} is the observed serum concentration of the ith subject at time t, D the dose of theophylline, k_{e_i} the elimination rate constant, k_{a_i} the absorption rate constant, and Cl_i the clearance for subject i. Also, e_{it} represents the error term that is assumed to be normally distributed. The "mixed" model stems from the following assumed forms of k_{e_i}, k_{a_i}, and Cl_i:

$$\begin{aligned} Cl_i &= e^{(\beta_1 + b_{i1})}, \\ k_{e_i} &= e^{(\beta_2 + b_{i2})}, \\ k_{a_i} &= e^{(\beta_3 + b_{i3})}. \end{aligned} \tag{17}$$

Similar to the preceding treatment of linear mixed models, here β_1, β_2, and β_3 are fixed effect parameters representing population averages, and b_{i1}, b_{i2}, and b_{i3} are random effect parameters. As one can see, both the fixed effects and random effects of model (16) enter the model in a nonlinear fashion. Additionally, it is easy to imagine that estimating and inferring on the parameters of such a model is quite difficult from a computational perspective. Discussion of estimation and inference for the nonlinear mixed model is beyond the scope of this presentation on mixed models. However, the interested reader is referred to numerous texts that deal with the subject, including Davidian and Giltinan (1995), Vonesh and Chinchilli (1997) and Demidenko (2004). For demonstration of the analysis of data from this example, see Example 51.1 of the SAS online documentation (SAS OnlineDoc 9.1, SAS Institute Inc., 2003a, 2003b).

11. Mixed models for survival data

Random effects can also be included in models of time-to-event data as well. These types of models are often referred to as survival models, as one popular "event" of interest is death. The mixed model approach in estimating time to a certain event has two main uses, depending on the nature of the event to be modeled. When the event can only occur once, such as death, inclusion of random effects can be helpful when correlation among subjects may exist. For instance, subjects from the same hospital, nursing home, or even community may not be independent of one another, and this dependence might need to be taken into account depending on the motivation of the analysis. Mixed time-to-event models may also be useful when the event occurs repeatedly on the same individuals, and thus we have repeated durations that should be modeled accordingly.

For a detailed discussion of what is often referred to as "multilevel" survival data models, see Goldstein (2003, Chapter 10).

12. Software

As alluded to often in this discussion, many computational techniques for fitting mixed models exist. We wish not to create an exhaustive list, but rather highlight some of the more popular tools.

Tools for fitting linear mixed models are the most readily available. PROC MIXED in SAS (2003b), lme in S-PLUS (MathSoft, 2002) and R (R Development Core Team, 2006), and xtmixed in STATA (StataCorp, 2005) are just a few of the linear mixed model fitting procedures. Additionally, SPSS (2006) has the ability to fit linear mixed models to data. Most of these procedures have similar capabilities, with many distinctions between them too detailed to list here. Rest assured that developers of most of these statistical software packages are kept abreast of the current mixed model research, and these procedures are continuously being updated and improved.

Tools exist for the analysis of generalized and nonlinear mixed models as well, although one must be warned that due to the complicated nature of these modeling scenarios, such procedures should not be used without substantial knowledge of both the modeling process as well as the procedure itself. PROC GLIMMIX and PROC NLMIXED are now available in SAS (2003) to fit generalized linear mixed models and nonlinear mixed models, respectively. S-PLUS (MathSoft, 2002) and R (R Development Core Team, 2006) have the nlme function for nonlinear mixed models. For an overview of fitting mixed models using S and S-PLUS, see Pinheiro and Bates (2000). Again, we simply wanted to cite some of the available options without trying to show favor to one particular software package. There are almost assuredly other options available in other software packages.

13. Conclusions

The powerful set of statistical analysis tools that collectively fit into the category "mixed models" is indeed quite large, and the capabilities of these tools continue to grow. It is impossible to write a comprehensive exposition of the topic of mixed models in a book, let alone a chapter of a book. We simply wished to introduce the mixed model in general, providing details regarding its applicability and utility. At the same time, we attempted to introduce some of the more recent areas of research that have been performed on the mixed model. More importantly, we aimed to provide references for areas of mixed model research for the reader interested in more details.

The theory behind the mixed model has existed for decades; however, advances in computing have made the mixed model a popular analytical tool only in the past 10–15 years. Consequently, the availability of this powerful method of analysis has led to more sophisticated study designs which in turn has allowed for answers to hypotheses previously too complicated to be addressed using standard statistical techniques. For example, more and more studies involve repeated measurements taken on subjects, as tools such as the mixed model can provide valid analyses of such data. For someone familiar with univariate linear models in a simple sense, mixed models are fairly intuitive and thus have great appeal to data analysts working with researchers without an extensive background in statistics.

The primary focus of this chapter is on the most straightforward form of the mixed model, the linear mixed model for continuous outcome data. We also introduce more general and complicated forms of the linear mixed model, the generalized, and the nonlinear mixed models. Owing to the computational intensity necessary for these more advanced types of mixed models, their use has become more commonplace only recently. The relatively recent expanded use of mixed models makes it necessary to continue methodological research on aspects of these models. For example, much more study is required on power analysis for the mixed model, and inference, particularly for small samples, needs to be further refined. Model selection and diagnostic tools also should be addressed in more detail. However, the practical utility of the mixed model in a variety of applications coupled with its complexity makes the mixed model a very exciting statistical analysis tool for future study.

References

Agresti, A. (2002). *Categorical Data Analysis*, 2nd ed. Wiley InterScience, New Jersey.

Ahn, C.H. (2000) Score tests for detecting non-constant variances in linear mixed models. *ASA Proceedings of the Biopharmaceutical Section* **0**, 33–38.

Akaike, H. (1974). A new look at the statistical model identification. *IEEE Transaction on Automatic Control* **AC-19**, 716–723.

Allen, D. M. (1971). The Prediction Sum of Squares as a Criterion for Selecting Predictor Variables, Technical Report 23, Department of Statistics, University of Kentucky.

Bozdogan, H. (1987). Model selection and Akaike's information criterion: The general theory and its analytical extensions. *Psychometrika* **52**, 345–370.

Burnham, K.P., Anderson, D.R. (2002). *Model selection and multimodel inference: A practical information-theoretic approach*. Springer, New York.

Butler, S.M., Louis, T.A. (1992). Random effects models with non-parametric priors. *Statistics in Medicine* **11**, 1981–2000.

Cantoni, E., Mills Flemming, J., Ronchetti, E. (2005). Variable selection for marginal longitudinal generalized linear models. *Biometrics* **61**, 507–514.

Carroll, R.J., Ruppert, D. (1984). Power transformations when fitting theoretical models to data. *Journal of the American Statistical Association* **79**, 321–328.

Catellier, D.J., Muller, K.E. (2000). Tests for Gaussian repeated measures with missing data in small samples. *Statistics in Medicine* **19**, 1101–1114.

Chi, E.M., Reinsel, G.C. (1989). Models for longitudinal data with random effects and AR(1) errors. *Journal of the American Statistical Association* **84**, 452–459.

Claeskens, G., Hjort, N.L. (2003). The focused information criterion. *Journal of the American Statistical Association* **98**, 900–916.

Davidian, M., Giltinan, D.M. (1995). *Nonlinear Models for Repeated Measures Data*. Chapman & Hall, London.

Demidenko, E. (2004). *Mixed Models: Theory and Application.* Wiley, New York.
Dempster, A.P., Laird, N.M., Rubin, R.B. (1977). Maximum likelihood with incomplete data via the E–M algorithm. *Journal of the Royal Statistical Society, Series B* **39**, 1–38.
Dempster, A.P., Rubin, R.B., Tsutakawa, R.K. (1981). Estimation in covariance components models. *Journal of the American Statistical Association* **76**, 341–353.
Diggle, P.J., Heagerty, P., Liang, K.Y., Zeger, S.L. (2002). *Analysis of Longitudinal Data.* Oxford University Press, Oxford.
Fellner, W.H. (1986). Robust estimation of variance components. *Technometrics* **28**, 51–60.
Flegal, K.M., Carroll, M.D., Ogden, C.L., Johnson, C.L. (2002). Prevalence and trends in obesity among US adults, 1999–2000. *Journal of the American Medical Association* **288**(14), 1723–1727.
Geisser, S. (1975). The predictive sample reuse method with applications. *Journal of the American Statistical Association* **70**, 320–328.
Geisser, S., Eddy, W.F. (1979). A predictive approach to model selection. *Journal of the American Statistical Association* **74**, 153–160.
Gelman, A., Pardoe, I. (2005). Bayesian measures of explained variance and pooling in multilevel (hierarchical) models. *Technometrics* **48**, 241–251.
Goldstein, H. (2003). *Multilevel Statistical Models*, 3rd ed. Arnold, London.
Gomez, E.V., Schaalje, G.B., Fellingham, G.W. (2005). Performance of the Kenward–Roger method when the covariance structure is selected using AIC and BIC. *Communications in Statistics-Simulation and Computation* **34**, 377–392.
Grady, J.J., Helms, R.W. (1995). Model selection techniques for the covariance matrix for incomplete longitudinal data. *Statistics in Medicine* **14**, 1397–1416.
Gurka, M.J. (2006). Selecting the best linear mixed model under REML. *The American Statistician* **60**, 19–26.
Gurka, M.J., Edwards, L.J., Muller, K.E., Kupper, L.L. (2006). Extending the Box–Cox transformation to the linear mixed model. *Journal of the Royal Statistical Society, Series A* **169**, 273–288.
Harville, D.A. (1974). Bayesian inference for variance components using only error contrasts. *Biometrika* **61**, 383–385.
Harville, D.A. (1976). Extension of the Gauss–Markov theorem to include the estimation of random effects. *Annals of Statistics* **4**, 384–395.
Harville, D.A. (1977). Maximum likelihood approaches to variance component estimation and to related problems. *Journal of the American Statistical Association* **72**, 320–338.
Helms, R.W. (1992). Intentionally incomplete longitudinal designs: I. Methodology and comparison of some full span designs. *Statistics in Medicine* **11**, 1889–1913.
Hjort, N.L., Claeskens, G. (2003). Frequentist model average estimator. *Journal of the American Statistical Association* **98**, 879–899.
Huber, P.J. (1981). *Robust Statistics.* John Wiley, New York.
Hurvich, C.M., Tsai, C.L. (1989). Regression and time series model selection in small samples. *Biometrika* **76**, 297–307.
Jiang, J., Rao, J.S. (2003). Consistent procedures for mixed linear model selection. *The Indian Journal of Statistics* **65**, 23–42.
Kackar, R.N., Harville, D.A. (1984). Approximations for standard errors of estimators of fixed and random effect in mixed linear models. *Journal of the American Statistical Association* **79**, 853–862.
Kenward, M.G., Roger, J.H. (1997). Small sample inference for fixed effects from restricted maximum likelihood. *Biometrics* **53**, 983–997.
Knowler, W.C., Barrett-Connor, E., Fowler, S.E., Hamman, R.F., Lachin, J.M., Walker, E.A., Nathan, D.M. (Diabetes Prevention Program Research Group) (2002). Reduction in the incidence of type 2 diabetes with lifestyle intervention or metformin. *New England Journal of Medicine* **346**(6), 393–403.
Laird, N.M., Ware, J.H. (1982). Random-effects models for longitudinal data. *Biometrics* **38**, 963–974.
Laird, N.M., Lange, N., Stram, D. (1987). Maximum likelihood computations with repeated measures: Application of the EM algorithm. *Journal of the American Statistical Association* **82**, 97–105.
Lange, N., Ryan, L. (1989). Assessing normality in random effects models. *Annals of Statistics* **17**, 624–642.

Lin, L.I. (1989). A concordance correlation coefficient to evaluate reproducibility. *Biometrics* **45**, 255–268.
Lindstrom, M.J., Bates, D.M. (1988). Newton-Raphson and EM algorithms for linear mixed-effects models for repeated-measures data. *Journal of the American Statistical Association* **83**, 1014–1022.
Lipsitz, S.R., Ibrahim, J., Molenberghs, G. (2000). Using a Box-Cox transformation in the analysis of longitudinal data with incomplete responses. *Applied Statistics* **49**, 287–296.
Littell, R., Milliken, G., Stroup, W., Wolfinger, R., Schabenberger, O. (2006). *SAS for Mixed Models*, 2nd ed. SAS Institute Inc., Cary, NC, Chapter 12.
Little, R.J.A., Rubin, D.B. (1987). *Statistical Analysis with Missing Data*. John Wiley and Sons, New York.
Liu, H., Weiss, R.E., Jennrich, R.I., Wenger, N.S. (1999). PRESS model selection in repeated measures data. *Computational Statistics and Data Analysis* **30**, 169–184.
Mallows, C.L. (1973). Some comments on C_p. *Technometrics* **15**, 661–675.
MathSoft, Inc. (2002). *S-Plus (Release 6)*. MathSoft Inc., Seattle.
McCarroll, K.A., Helms, R.W. (1987). An evaluation of some approximate *F* statistics and their small sample distributions for the mixed model with linear covariance structure. *The Institute of Statistics Mimeo Series*. Department of Biostatistics, University of North Carolina, Chapel Hill, NC.
McCullagh, P., Nelder, J.A. (1989). *Generalized Linear Models*, 2nd ed. Chapman & Hall, New York.
McCulloch, C.E., Searle, S.R. (2001). *Generalized, Linear and Mixed Models*. Wiley, New York.
Mokdad, A.H., Bowman, B.A., Ford, E.S., Vinicor, F., Marks, J.S., Koplan, J.P. (2001). The continuing epidemics of obesity and diabetes in the United States. *Journal of the American Medical Association* **286**(10), 1195–1200.
Molenberghs, G., Verbeke, G. (2005). *Models for Discrete Longitudinal Data*. Springer, New York.
Muller, K.E., Stewart, P.W. (2006). *Linear Model Theory: Univariate, Multivariate, and Mixed Models*. Wiley, New York.
Oberg, A., Davidian, M. (2000). Estimating data transformations in nonlinear mixed effects models. *Biometrics* **56**, 65–72.
Overall, J.E., Doyle, S.R. (1994). Estimating sample sizes for repeated measurement designs. *Controlled Clinical Trials* **15**, 100–123.
Palta, M., Qu, R.P. (1995). Testing lack of fit in mixed effect models for longitudinal data. In: Tiit, E.-M., Kollo, T., Niemi, H. (Eds.), *New Trends in Probability and Statistics Volume 3: Multivariate Statistics and Matrices in Statistics (Proceedings of the 5th Tartu Conference)*. VSP International Science Publishers, Zeist, The Netherlands, pp. 93–106.
Patterson, H.D., Thompson, R. (1971). Recovery of inter-block information when block sizes are equal. *Biometrika* **58**, 545–554.
Pinheiro, J.C., Bates, D.M. (1995). Approximations to the log-likelihood function in the nonlinear mixed-effects model. *Journal of Computational and Graphical Statistics* **4**, 12–35.
Pinheiro, J.C., Bates, D.M. (2000). *Mixed Effects Models in S and S-Plus*. Springer, New York.
R Development Core Team (2006). *R: A Language and Environment for Statistical Computing*. R Foundation for Statistical Computing, Vienna.
Richardson, A.M., Welsh, A.H. (1995). Robust restricted maximum likelihood in mixed linear models. *Biometrics* **51**, 1429–1439.
SAS Institute Inc (2003a). *SAS OnlineDoc® 9.1*. SAS Institute Inc., Cary, NC.
SAS Institute Inc (2003b). *SAS/Stat User's Guide, Version 9.1*. SAS Institute Inc, Cary, NC.
Schwarz, G. (1978). Estimating the dimension of a model. *Annuals of Statistics* **6**, 461–464.
Shao, J. (1993). Linear model selection by cross-validation. *Journal of the American Statistical Association* **88**, 486–494.
Shi, P., Tsai, C.L. (2002). Regression model selectiona residual likelihood approach. *Journal of the Royal Statistical Society B* **64**(2), 237–252.
Shen, X., Dougherty, D.P. (2003). Discussion: Inference and interpretability considerations in frequentist model averaging and selection. *Journal of the American Statistical Association* **98**, 917–919.
SPSS for Windows (2006). *Rel. 14.0.1*. SPSS Inc., Chicago.
StataCorp (2005). *Stata Statistical Software: Release 9*. StataCorp LP., College Station, TX.

Stone, M. (1974). Cross-validatory choice and assessment of statistical predictions (with discussion). *Journal of the Royal Statistical Society, Series B* **36**, 111–147.

Stone, M. (1977). An asymptotic equivalence of choice of model by cross-validation and Akaike's criterion. *Journal of the Royal Statistical Society, Series B* **39**, 44–47.

Stroup, W.W. (1999). *Mixed model procedures to assess power, precision, and sample size in the design of experiments.* American Statistical Association, Alexandria, VA, (pp. 15–24).

Verbeke, G., Lesaffre, E. (1996). A linear mixed-effects model with heterogeneity in the random-effects population. *Journal of the American Statistical Association* **91**, 217–221.

Verbeke, G., Lesaffre, E. (1997). The effect of misspecifying the random-effects distribution in linear mixed models for longitudinal data. *Computational Statistics and Data Analysis* **23**, 541–556.

Verbeke, G., Molenberghs, G. (2000). *Linear Mixed Models for Longitudinal Data.* Springer, New York.

Verbeke, G., Molenberghs, G. (2003). The use of score tests for inference on variance components. *Biometrics* **59**, 254–262.

Vonesh, E.F. (2004). Hypothesis testing in mixed-effects models. Presented in Session 12: Estimation and Inference in Mixed-Effects Models. 2004 International Biometric Society Eastern North American Region Meetings, Pittsburgh, PA.

Vonesh, E.F., Chinchilli, V.M. (1997). *Linear and Nonlinear Models for the Analysis of Repeated Measurements.* Marcel Dekker, New York.

Vonesh, E.F., Chinchilli, V.M., Pu, K. (1996). Goodness-of-fit in generalized nonlinear mixed-effects models. *Biometrics* **52**, 572–587.

Weiss, R.E., Wang, Y., Ibrahim, J.G. (1997). Predictive model selection for repeated measures random effects models using Bayes factors. *Biometrics* **53**, 592–602.

Welham, S.J., Thompson, R. (1997). A likelihood ratio test for fixed model terms using residual maximum likelihood. *Journal of the Royal Statistical Society, Series B* **59**, 701–714.

Wolf, A.M., Conaway, M.R., Crowther, J.Q., Hazen, K.Y., Nadler, J.L., Oneida, B., Bovbjerg, V.E. (2004). Translating lifestyle intervention to practice in obese patients with type 2 diabetes: Improving control with activity and nutrition (ICAN) study. *Diabetes Care* **27**(7), 1570–1576.

Xu, R. (2003). Measuring explained variation in linear mixed effects models. *Statistics in Medicine* **22**, 3527–3541.

Zeger, S.L., Liang., K-Y., Albert, P.S. (1988). Models for longitudinal data: A generalized estimating equation approach. *Biometrics* **44**(4), 1049–1060.

Zucker, D.M., Lieberman, O., Manor, O. (2000). Improved small sample inference in the mixed linear model. *Journal of the Royal Statistical Society, Series B* **62**, 827–838.

Handbook of Statistics, Vol. 27
ISSN: 0169-7161

DOI: 10.1016/S0169-7161(07)27009-9

9

Survival Analysis

John P. Klein and Mei-Jie Zhang

Abstract

This paper presents an overview of statistical techniques for time-to-event data. We consider both the case where a single event such as death is of interest and the case of competing risks where a subject is at risk for a multiplicity of causes of failure. We consider univariate methods to summarize the survival experience, techniques to compare the outcomes of two or more treatments and a variety of models and methods to study the effects of covariates on outcome. We illustrate the methods on several data sets.

1. Introduction

Problems in survival analysis arise in many areas of epidemiology and medicine. The problems involve, for example, the time to death following diagnosis of a disease, the time to a complete recovery following a treatment, the time to treatment failure or simply the time to death. Analysis of this type of data is often complicated by censoring and/or truncation.

Censoring occurs when only partial information is available on each subject. Most common is right censoring where all that is known for some subjects is that the event of interest has yet to occur. If we let T be the potential time to event if there was no censoring and X the observed on study time, then for some cases all we know is that $T>X$. Special types of right censoring are *type I progressive censoring* where the on study time is fixed when the subject enters the study or *random censoring*, where each subject has a potential random censoring time, C, and we observe $X=\min(T,C)$ and $\delta=1$ if $X=T$ (a death) or 0 if $T>X=C$ (censored). Other censoring includes interval censoring where all that is known is that the event occurred in some interval and left censoring where all that is known is that the event occurred prior to some time.

Truncation, as opposed to censoring, arises when some intermediate event must occur for the subject to come under observation. Most common is left truncation where an event, V, must occur prior to the event time for the event to be observed. Subjects for whom the event V has not occurred prior to T are not observable. Left truncation is also called delayed entry or time-dependent stratification. An example of left truncation is the time to death after relapse in patients treated for disease. If time is measured from diagnosis only those patients who relapse are at risk for death and relapse is the truncating event. Left-truncated data requires special analysis.

Another type of data found in medicine is competing risks data. Here a subject is at risk of failure from J distinct causes. One observes for each subject an on study time, X, and an indicator, ε, which tells us which event was the cause of failure. Examples of competing risks are causes of death or relapse and death in remission in cancer studies. Since there is no way given data on X and ε alone to distinguish between independent and dependent competing risks, the marginal distribution of the time to failure from each cause is most often not estimated (see Basu and Klein, 1982). In the competing risks framework one typically summarizes the survival experience by J cumulative incidence functions defined as the chance a subject fails from a given cause in the presence of all other causes prior to time t (cf. Gooley et al., 1999; Pepe and Mori, 1993).

2. Univariate analysis

In this section, we examine univariate techniques for summarizing time to event data and competing risks data. We will discuss these methods in some detail for right-censored data and indicate extensions to other censoring or truncation schemes. For right-censored data we assume that the censoring mechanism is non-informative for the event of interest. The non-informative assumption means that the only information obtained from a censored observation is that the event time is larger than the censoring time and is in most cases satisfied by independence of T and C. This assumption is needed to ensure many of the properties of the estimators we shall discuss. For a sample of size n from a right-censored sample we observe (X_i, δ_i), $i = 1, \ldots, n$. Let $0 < t_1 < t_2 < \cdots < t_D$ be the observed event times. At an event time, t_i, let d_i be the observed number of events and Y_i be the number alive just prior to t_i.

For a survival time T, two functions are typically used to summarize a subject's survival experience. The first is the survival function, $S(t) = P[T > t]$, the chance a subject is alive at time t. The second is the hazard rate, $\lambda(t)$, which is the rate at which subjects are dying. The hazard rate is defined as

$$\lambda(t) = \lim_{\Delta t \to 0} \frac{P[t \leq T < t + \Delta t | T \geq t]}{\Delta t}. \tag{1}$$

For a continuous lifetime with a density $f(t)$ the two functions are related by

$$\lambda(t) = f(t)/S(t) = -d \ln[S(t)]/dt \tag{2}$$

The quantity $\lambda(t)dt$ is the approximate probability that an individual of age t will experience the event in the next instant. A related quantity is the cumulative hazard rate, $\Lambda(t) = \int_0^t \lambda(u)du$.

The survival function is estimated by the Kaplan–Meier (1958) estimator, which is also know as the product-limit estimator (PLE), and is defined by

$$\hat{S}(t) = \begin{cases} 1 & \text{if } t \leq t_1 \\ \prod_{t_i \leq t}\left[1 - \frac{d_i}{Y_i}\right] & \text{if } t_1 \leq t \end{cases}. \tag{3}$$

The variance of the PLE is estimated by Greenwood's (1926) formula given by

$$\hat{V}[\hat{S}(t)] = \hat{S}(t)^2 \sum_{t_i \leq t} \frac{d_i}{Y_i(Y_i - d_i)}. \tag{4}$$

This estimator is available in any package that allows for censored survival data.

The Kaplan–Meier estimator can be derived in a number of ways. It arises naturally from the theory of counting processes (see Aalen, 1978 or Andersen et al., 1993), by a self-consistency argument (see Efron, 1967) and via a redistribute to the right algorithm (see Efron, 1967). Under some regularity conditions it can be shown that the estimator is a non-parametric maximum likelihood estimator and that the estimator converges weakly to a Gaussian process. Small sample properties are studied, for example, in Guerts (1987) and Klein (1991).

While the logarithm of the PLE provides an estimator of the cumulative hazard rate, $\Lambda()$, a better estimator is the Nelson (1972)–Aalen (1978) estimator defined by

$$\tilde{\Lambda}(t) = \begin{cases} 0 & \text{if } t \leq t_1 \\ \sum\limits_{t_i \leq t} \frac{d_i}{Y_i} & \text{if } t_1 \leq t \end{cases}, \tag{5}$$

which has a variance estimated by

$$\hat{V}[\tilde{\Lambda}(t)] = \sum_{t_i \leq t} \frac{d_i}{Y_i^2}. \tag{6}$$

The estimator $\tilde{S}(t) = \exp[-\tilde{\Lambda}(t)]$ provides an alternative estimator of $S(t)$.

To illustrate these methods we consider a set of patients with cancers of the mouth (Sickle-Santanello et al., 1988). The outcome is the time from diagnosis to death in weeks. In this study, 52 patients had an aneuploid (abnormal) and 28 patients a diploid (normal) DNA profile for their tumor based on flow cytometry. There were 31 deaths in the aneuploid group and 22 in the diploid group. The data can be found on the website http://www.biostat.mcw.edu/homepgs/klein/tongue.html. Figure 1 shows both the product-limit and Nelson–Aalen estimates of survival for the two groups. Note that the PLE gives slightly lower estimates of survival.

Using either the PLE or the Nelson–Aalen estimators one can construct pointwise confidence intervals for the survival function or confidence bands for the entire curve. Borgan and Liestøl (1990) show that better coverage probabilities are obtained for the pointwise intervals if a variance-stabilizing transformation is made. Three forms are suggested for a $(1-\alpha)100\%$ confidence

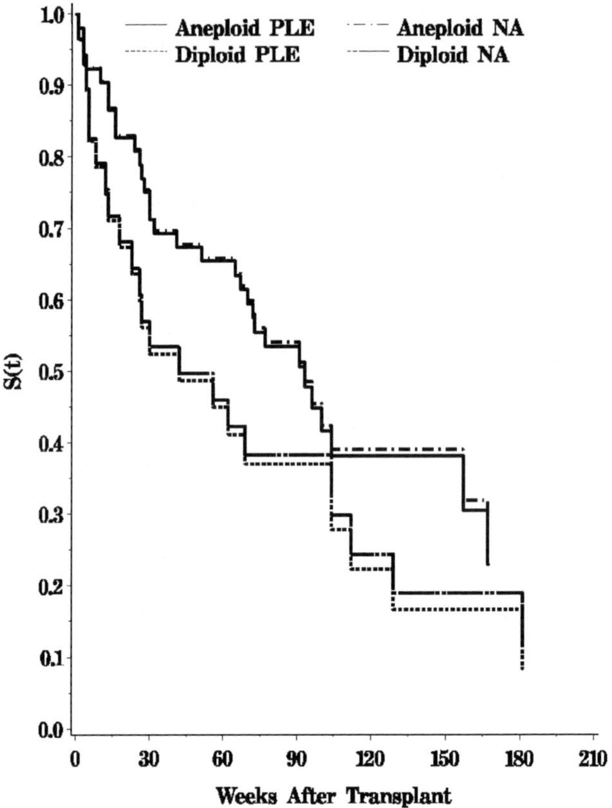

Fig. 1. Estimates of survival for patients with cancer of the mouth.

interval for $S(t_0)$:

$$\text{Naive}: \quad \left[\hat{S}(t_0) - Z_{\alpha/2}\sigma_s(t_0)\hat{S}(t_0), \hat{S}(t_0) + Z_{\alpha/2}\sigma_s(t_0)\hat{S}(t_0)\right]; \tag{7}$$

$$\text{Log-log transformed}: \quad \left[\hat{S}(t_0)^{1/\theta}, \hat{S}(t_0)^{\theta}\right], \quad \text{where } \theta = \exp\left\{\frac{Z_{\alpha/2}\sigma_s(t_0)}{\ln\left[\hat{S}(t_0)\right]}\right\} \tag{8}$$

and

$$\begin{array}{c} \text{Arc sine-square root}: \\ \sin^2\left\{\max\left[0, \arcsin\left(\hat{S}(t_0)^{1/2}\right) - 0.5Z_{\alpha/2}\sigma_s(t_0)\left[\frac{\hat{S}(t_0)}{1-\hat{S}(t_0)}\right]^{1/2}\right]\right\} \\ \leq S(t_0) \leq \\ \sin^2\left\{\max\left[0, \text{arsin}\left(\hat{S}(t_0)^{1/2}\right) + 0.5Z_{\alpha/2}\sigma_S(t_0)\left[\frac{\hat{S}(t_0)}{1-\hat{S}(t_0)}\right]^{1/2}\right]\right\} \end{array}. \tag{9}$$

Here $Z_{\alpha/2}$ is the upper $\alpha/2$th percentile of the standard normal distribution and $\sigma_s(t) = \hat{V}(\hat{S}(t))^{1/2}/\hat{S}(t)$. Both the arc sine-square root interval and the log–log transformed interval give about the correct coverage probabilities for samples as small as 25, while the naïve interval requires much larger sample sizes. These confidence intervals are available in SAS, STATA, SPlus and R.

Two formulations are used to construct confidence bands for the survival function. The first, suggested by Nair (1984) provides confidence bands parallel to the pointwise confidence intervals discussed above. The confidence band over the range T_L–T_U is constructed by replacing $Z_{\alpha/2}$ by $c_\alpha(a_L,a_U)$ in (7)–(9), where $a_M = n\sigma_s^2(T_M)/[1 + n\sigma_s^2(T_M)]$, $M = L$, U and $c_\alpha(a_L,a_U)$ is the αth fractile of the random variable $U = \sup\{|W^0(x)[x(1-x)]^{-1/2}|,\ a_L \leq x \leq a_U\}$, where $W^0()$ is a standard Brownian bridge.

The second interval is due to Hall and Wellner (1980). These intervals are constructed by replacing $Z_{\alpha/2}\sigma_s(t_0)$ by $k_\alpha(a_L, a_U)[1 + n\sigma_s^2(t)]/n^{1/2}$. Here $k_\alpha(a_L, a_U)$ is the upper αth fractile of a Brownian bridge over the range $a_L \leq x \leq a_U$ (see Chung, 1986).

Both confidence bands are available in SAS. Confidence coefficients for both approaches are tabulated in Klein and Moeschberger (2003). Borgan and Liestøl (1990) show that the naïve form of Nair's band requires a large sample size of at least 200 to ensure proper coverage probabilities. For the other forms of the bands, the coverage probability is correct for samples with as few as 20 events.

Figure 2 depicts the two confidence bands and a set of pointwise confidence intervals based on the arc sine-square root transformation for the aneuploid mouth cancer group. These were construct using Version 9 of SAS Proc Lifetest. Here we see clearly that the pointwise confidence interval, if taken as a confidence band, is too narrow and should not be used. The two confidence bands are quite close with the Hall–Wellner band being wider in either tail.

The PLE can also be used to obtain estimators of the mean survival times. For survival data the mean time to event is the area under the survival curve. With censored data the area under the estimated survival function provides an estimator of the mean survival time. When the largest on study time is censored then the PLE does not drop to zero and the area under the curve is not well defined. One approach is to complete the tail by some type of parametric curve (see Moeschberger and Klein, 1985). More often the inference is made to a restricted mean defined as the area under the survival function up to some time. This approach is taken in SAS, SPlus and R for example. With this approach one needs to be careful in that the default maximum time may change depending on what package is used to compute the mean. For example, SAS uses the largest death as a cut-off point, while STATA and SPlus use the largest on study time. The restricted mean up to time τ is then defined by

$$\hat{\mu}_\tau = \int_0^\tau \hat{S}(u)du, \tag{10}$$

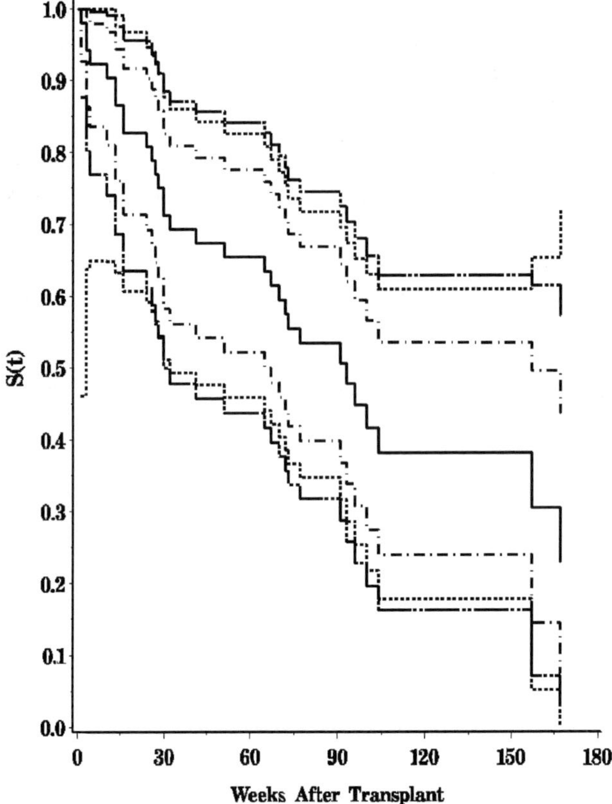

Fig. 2. Confidence intervals and bands for Aneuploid data. Kaplan-Meier estimate (—), 95% pointwise confidence interval (—•—•), 95% Nair's confidence band (—••—••), 95% Hall-Wellner confidence band (- - - -).

which has an estimated variance of

$$\hat{V}[\hat{\mu}_\tau] = \sum_{i=1}^{D} \left[\int_{t_i}^{\tau} \hat{S}(u)du \right]^2 \frac{d_i}{Y_i(Y_i - d_i)}. \tag{11}$$

For large samples $\hat{\mu}_\tau$ has an approximate normal distribution so that confidence intervals can be constructed by standard methods.

For the cancer of the mouth data the mean time to death from diagnosis restricted to the largest on study time in each group is 146.5 weeks (SE 28.1 weeks) in the aneuploid group and 86.8 weeks (SE 24.6 weeks) in the diploid group.

Estimators of survival can be found for other censoring schemes. For right-censored data with left truncation a simple modification of Y_i to be the number alive and entered into the study just prior to t_i is all that is needed to construct the PLE. Here the PLE estimates the conditional probability of death given a subject that has experienced the truncating event. There can be some problems for small t where the number at risk is small and Lai and Ying (1991) provide a possible modification to the PLE.

For interval censoring and/or mixes of right and left censoring an estimator can be constructed by using a self-consistency argument (see Turnbull, 1976, 1974). These estimators are available in SPlus and R. A more complete discussion and an example can be found in Chapter 5 of Klein and Moeschberger (2003).

For competing risks data we observe for each person the on study time T_i, the censoring indicator δ_i, and for those subjects observed to fail ($\delta_i = 1$) the cause of failure ε_i. To construct the estimators, let $t_1 < t_2 < \cdots < t_D$ be the distinct event times. We wish to summarize the survival experience for a particular cause of failure. At time t_i, let r_i be the number of subjects with an occurrence of the event of interest; q_i the number with an occurrence of any other competing risk and Y_i the number at risk just prior to time t_i. Subjects who are censored are counted in Y_i but not in r_i and q_i. If we assume that cause 1 is the cause of interest, the population cumulative incidence function (CIF) is given by

$$\mathrm{CI}_1(t) = P[X \le t, \varepsilon = 1]. \tag{12}$$

This can be estimated by

$$\hat{\mathrm{CI}}_1(t) = \begin{cases} 0 & \text{if } t \le t_1 \\ \sum_{t_i \le t} \hat{S}(t_i -)\dfrac{r_i}{Y_i} & \text{if } t_1 \le t \cdot \end{cases} \tag{13}$$

The variance of this estimator can be estimated by

$$\hat{V}[\mathrm{CI}_1(t)] = \sum_{t_i \le t} \hat{S}(t_i -)^2 \left\{ [\hat{\mathrm{CI}}_1(t) - \hat{\mathrm{CI}}_1(t_i)]^2 \frac{r_i + q_i}{Y_i^2} + [1 - 2(\hat{\mathrm{CI}}_1(t) - \hat{\mathrm{CI}}_1(t_i))] \frac{r_i}{Y_i} \right\}. \tag{14}$$

Here $\hat{S}()$ is the PLE obtained ignoring the cause (i.e. based on T and δ).

The CIF estimate can be obtained in a number of ways. The first derivation relies on the representation of the CIF in terms of the so-called crude hazard functions. Consider two competing risks and a time to event X. We define the crude hazard rate for cause j as the rate of occurrence of cause j among subjects at risk for either cause of failure. That is

$$\lambda_j(t) = \lim_{\Delta t \to 0} \frac{P[t \le X < t + \Delta t, \varepsilon = j | X \ge t]}{\Delta t}. \tag{15}$$

The CIF for cause j is related to the crude hazard rates of both risks by

$$\mathrm{CI}_j(t) = \int_0^t \lambda_j(u) \exp\left\{ - \int_0^u [\lambda_1(v) + \lambda_2(v)] dv \right\} du. \tag{16}$$

The crude hazard rates for causes 1 and 2 can be estimated at time t_i by r_i/Y_i and q_i/Y_i, respectively. Plugging these values into (16) and replacing the exponential integral with a product integral yield the estimator (13).

An alternative derivation of the estimated CIF is by the use of the method of inverse probability of censoring weighting (IPCW). This general technique, first proposed by Robins and Rotnizky (1992), is increasingly being used to develop estimators for censored data. Basically, this approach starts with a complete sample estimator of the quantity of interest. Censoring is adjusted for by reweighing the events to account for censoring. In the competing risk problem note that if we had a sample with no censoring then the cumulative incidence function for cause 1 is simply the fraction of the sample who fail from cause 1 prior to time t. That is

$$\hat{\mathrm{CI}}_1(t) = \frac{\sum_{i=1}^{n} I[T_i \le t, \varepsilon_i = 1]}{n}. \tag{17}$$

For right-censored data the IPCW technique estimator is given by

$$\hat{\mathrm{CI}}_1(t) = \left(\frac{1}{n}\right) \sum_{i=1}^{n} \frac{\delta_i I[X_i \le t, \varepsilon_i = 1]}{\hat{G}(X_i)}, \tag{18}$$

where $\hat{G}(t)$ is the Kaplan–Meier estimator of the censoring distribution. This estimator can be shown to be equivalent to the usual estimator of the cumulative incidence (13) (see Gooley et al., 1999).

To illustrate competing risk analysis we consider a data set of leukemia patients reported in Szydlo et al. (1997). The data set consists of 1225 HLA-identical sibling patients, 383 HLA-matched unrelated and 108 HLA-mismatched unrelated bone marrow transplant patients. The study has two competing risks: treatment-related death defined as death in complete remission, $n = 557/1716$ cases and relapse defined as recurrence of the primary disease, $n = 311/1716$ cases. We will focus on the HLA-matched sibling and unrelated samples. Figures 3a and 3b show the estimated cumulative incidence functions for relapse (3a) and death in remission (3b). Here we see clearly that the sibling donor cohort has slightly more relapse than the unrelated donor cohort but this is offset by much higher death in remission probabilities in the unrelated donor group.

3. Hypothesis testing

In this section, we shall investigate techniques for comparing two or more treatments. We will look at methods for right-censored survival data and for competing risks data.

We will discuss statistics used to test the equality of survival distributions between K-samples (treatment groups). The available data used to compare the K groups is from independent right-censored and possibly left-truncated samples. We shall focus on independent right-censored data in this article. The methods

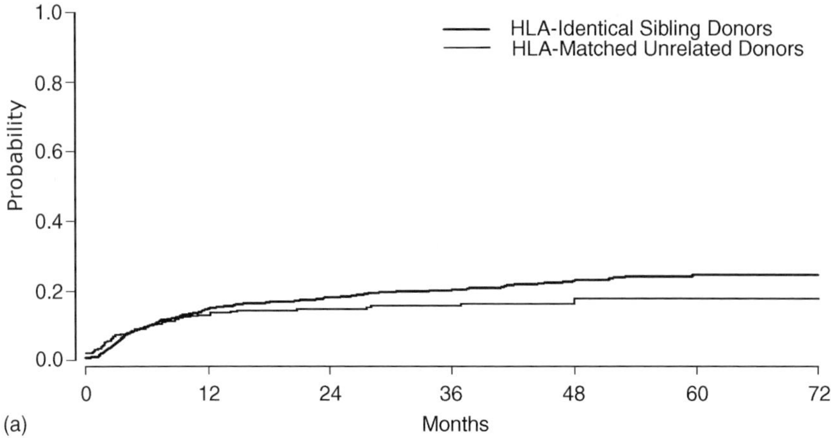

Fig. 3a. Cumulative incidence function for relapse.

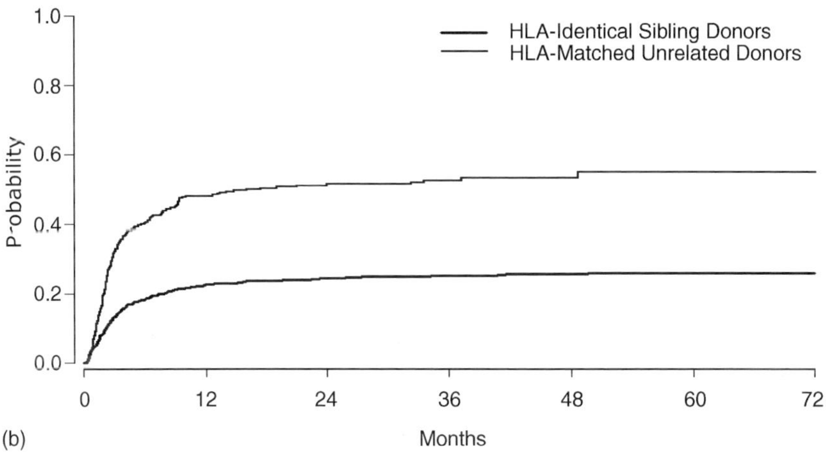

Fig. 3b. Cumulative incidence function for death in remission.

and results discussed here can be easily generalized to left-truncated data by adjusting the risk sets (Andersen et al., 1993).

The weighted log-rank test is the most commonly used testing procedure for analyzing time-to-event data. It is based on comparing differences in the hazard rates between groups. The hypothesis of interest is

$$\begin{aligned} &H_0 : \lambda_1(t) = \cdots = \lambda_K(t), \qquad \text{for all } t \le \tau, \text{ versus} \\ &H_A : \text{at least one of } \lambda_k(t) \text{ is different for some } t \le \tau, \end{aligned} \tag{19}$$

where $\lambda_k(.)$ is the hazard function of kth sample and τ the largest on study time. Let $t_1 < t_2 < \cdots < t_D$ be the distinct failure times in the pooled sample. At each failure time t_i, let $d_{i,k}$ be the observed number of events and $Y_{i,k}$ be the number alive just prior to t_i in the kth sample. The weighted log-rank test statistic is

$$Z_k = \sum_{i=1}^{D} w_k(t_i)\left\{\frac{d_{i,k}}{Y_{i,k}} - \frac{d_i}{Y_i}\right\}, \qquad k = 1, \ldots, K, \tag{20}$$

where $d_i = \sum_{k=1}^{K} d_{i,k}$, $Y_i = \sum_{k=1}^{K} Y_{i,k}$ and $w_k(t_i)$ is a predicable non-negative weight function. Commonly we take $w_k(t_i) = Y_{i,k}w(t_i)$, where $w()$ is a common weight function for all groups. Hence,

$$Z_k = \sum_{i=1}^{D} w(t_i)\left\{d_{i,k} - Y_{i,k}\left(\frac{d_i}{Y_i}\right)\right\}, \qquad k = 1, \ldots, K. \tag{21}$$

Aalen (1978) and Gill (1980) studied large sample properties of the weighted log-rank tests. Under independent censoring and the null hypothesis, the variance of Z_k and the covariance of Z_k, Z_l can be consistently estimated by

$$\hat{\sigma}_{kk} = \sum_{i=1}^{D} w(t_i)^2 \frac{Y_{i,k}}{Y_i}\left(1 - \frac{Y_{i,k}}{Y_i}\right)\left(\frac{Y_i - d_i}{Y_i - 1}\right)d_i, \qquad k = 1, \ldots, K$$

$$\hat{\sigma}_{kl} = -\sum_{i=1}^{D} w(t_i)^2 \frac{Y_{i,k}}{Y_i}\frac{Y_{i,l}}{Y_i}\left(\frac{Y_i - d_i}{Y_i - 1}\right)d_i, \qquad k \neq l. \tag{22}$$

Note that $(Y_i - d_i)/(Y_i - 1)$ is a correction for ties, and is equal to 1 when no two events occurred at the same time. Since $\sum_{k=1}^{K} Z_k = 0$, the log-rank test statistic can be constructed by selecting any $K-1$ of the Z_k's. The estimated variance–covariance matrix is the $(K-1) \times (K-1)$ matrix, $\hat{\Sigma}$, with the corresponding elements of $\hat{\sigma}_{kl}$. Under the null hypothesis, the test statistic

$$\chi^2 = (Z_1, \ldots, Z_{K-1})\hat{\Sigma}^{-1}(Z_1, \ldots, Z_{K-1})^T \tag{23}$$

has asymptotically a χ^2 distribution with $K-1$ degrees of freedom.

Several weight functions have been proposed and studied in the literature. The most common weight is $w(t) = 1$ for all t, which yields a standard log-rank test and is available in most statistical packages. Gehan (1965) generalized Mann–Whitney Wilcoxon's test with $w(t_i) = Y_i$. Tarone and Ware (1977) proposed a weight function of $w(t_i) = Y_i^{1/2}$. Peto and Peto (1972), Andersen et al. (1982), Kalbfleisch and Prentice (1980) and others proposed alternative weights that are based on the estimated survival function from the pooled sample. These weights are not affected by censoring patterns, which is a problem when using Gehan's weight. Fleming and Harrington (1981) proposed a class of weighted log-rank test that allows the weight to be very general and flexible. That is

$$w_{p,q}(t_i) = [\hat{S}(t_i-)]^p[1 - \hat{S}(t_i-)]^q, \quad p \geq 0, \ q \geq 0, \tag{24}$$

where $\hat{S}(t_i-) = \hat{S}(t_{i-1})$ is the Kaplan–Meier estimator in the pooled sample just prior to t_i. When $p = 0$ and $q = 0$, we have a standard log-rank test. When $p>0$ and $q = 0$, the test gives most weight to detecting an early difference in hazards,

Table 1
Two sample weighted log-rank tests comparing aneuploid and diploid tumors

Version	$w(t_i)$	χ^2	p-value
Log-rank	1	2.790	0.0949
Gehan	Y_i	3.305	0.0691
Tarone-ware	$Y_i^{1/2}$	3.118	0.0774
Fleming–Harrington ($P = 1$, $q = 0$)	$\hat{S}(t_i-)$	3.296	0.0694
Fleming–Harrington ($P = 0$, $q = 1$)	$1 - \hat{S}(t_i-)$	0.992	0.3192
Fleming–Harrington ($P = 1$, $q = 1$)	$\hat{S}(t_i-)\left[1 - \hat{S}(t_i-)\right]$	1.390	0.2374

while when $p = 0$ and $q > 0$ the test gives most weight to detecting late differences. Klein and Moeschberger (2003) gave a detailed review of the effects of all the commonly used weights. Log-rank tests are available in most commonly used statistical packages. The availability of weights is different across statistical packages (see Klein and Zhang, 2005).

To illustrate the weighted log-rank tests, we considered comparing the hazard rates for the aneuploid and diploid tumors of the mouth described in the previous section. Table 1 summarizes the results. The p-values of the tests range from 0.0601 to 0.3194. The tests with smaller p-values are those that give more weight to early differences between the tumor groups.

Log-rank test statistics are based on estimating weighted differences in hazard functions and are most sensitive when the hazard functions do not cross. Pepe and Fleming (1989) proposed a class of statistics that are sensitive if the survival functions of the two groups are stochastically ordered in the range of the data. Pepe and Fleming's test is based on the weighted difference of Kaplan–Meier estimates

$$\mathrm{WKM} = \sqrt{\frac{n_1 n_2}{n}} \int_0^{\tau} w(t)\left[\hat{S}_1(t) - \hat{S}_2(t)\right] dt, \tag{25}$$

where $n = n_1 + n_2$. Here $w(t)$ is a non-negative weight function with the property that $w(t) = 0$ if $\hat{G}_k(t) = 0$, for $k = 1, 2$, where $\hat{G}_k(.)$ is the Kaplan–Meier estimator of the censoring distribution for sample k. The WKM test statistics generalize the location test statistics. For uncensored data with a weight equal to 1 the WKM estimates the difference in mean survival time. The variance of WKM can be estimated from the unpooled samples or from the pooled sample. We only report the pooled variance estimator here since it has superior performance over the unpooled estimator (Pepe and Fleming, 1989)

$$\hat{\sigma}^2 = -\int_0^{\tau} \frac{\left[\int_0^{\tau} w(u)\hat{S}(u)du\right]^2}{\hat{S}(t)\hat{S}(t-)} \frac{n_1\hat{G}_1(t-) + n_2\hat{G}_2(t-)}{n\hat{G}_1(t-)\hat{G}_2(t-)} d\hat{S}(t), \tag{26}$$

where $\hat{S}(t-)$ is the pooled Kaplan–Meier estimator. Pepe and Fleming (1989) suggest that the weights to be a function of $\hat{G}_k$ to satisfy a stability constraint.

One suggestion is

$$w_c(t) = \frac{n\hat{G}_1(t-)\hat{G}_2(t-)}{n_1\hat{G}_1(t-) + n_2\hat{G}_2(t-)}. \tag{27}$$

For large sample sizes under the null hypothesis the statistic $\chi^2 = \mathrm{WKM}^2/\hat{\sigma}^2$ has a limiting χ^2 distribution with 1 degree of freedom.

We used the weighted Kaplan–Meier test and compare the aneuploid and diploid tumor groups for the cancer of the mouth data set discussed above. For this test we have a χ^2 statistic of 3.27 and a p-value of 0.0706.

For competing risks data tests can be based either on the crude hazard rates or the cumulative incidence functions. To compare crude hazard rates the weighted log-rank tests discussed above can be applied by treating failures from causes other than the cause of interest as censored observations. These tests are easy to apply and are available in most statistical packages tests. These tests, however, do not reflect differences in cumulative incidence functions since the product integral of the crude hazard rate is not equal to the cumulative incidence function. The CIF is a function of the crude hazards from all competing risks, so differences in crude hazard rates of a particular cause do not translate into differences in CIF.

Several tests have been suggested that directly compare CIF in the competing risks framework. The first is due to Gray (1988). Let $\mathrm{CI}_k(t)$, $k = 1, \ldots, K$ be the CIF for the cause of interest ($\varepsilon = 1$ for simplicity) for treatment k. The hypothesis of interest is

$$\begin{aligned} &\mathrm{H}_0: \ \mathrm{CI}_1(t) = \cdots = \mathrm{CI}_K(t), \quad \text{for all } \ t \leq \tau. \\ &\mathrm{H}_\mathrm{A}: \ \text{at least one of the } \mathrm{CI}_k^{'s}(\mathrm{t}) \text{ is different for some } t. \end{aligned} \tag{28}$$

Gray proposed a test based on the sub-distribution hazard function of $\mathrm{CI}_k(t)$ defined by

$$\lambda_k^*(t) = \frac{-d\log\{1 - \mathrm{CI}_k(t)\}}{dt} \tag{29}$$

and showed that an improper random variable X_{ik}^*, $i = 1, \ldots, n_k$, has a hazard rate of $\lambda_k^*(t)$, where $X_{ik}^* = T_{ik}$, if $\varepsilon_{ik} = 1$ and $X_{ik}^* = \infty$, if $\varepsilon_{ik} \neq 1$. The cumulative sub-distribution hazard $\Lambda_k^*(t) = \int_0^t \lambda_k^*(u)du$ is estimated by

$$\hat{\Lambda}_k^*(t) = \int_0^t \left[\left\{1 - \widehat{\mathrm{CI}}_k(u-)\right\} Y_k(u)\right]^{-1} \hat{S}_k(u-)dN_k(u), \tag{30}$$

where $N_k(u) = \sum_{i=1}^{n_k} I(X_{ik} \leq u, \varepsilon_{ik} = 1, \delta_{ik} = 1)$, $Y_k(u) = \sum_{i=1}^{n_k} Y_{ik}(u)$ and $\hat{S}_k(.)$ is the Kaplan–Meier estimator for all causes obtained by ignoring the cause of failure. Gray's test is given by

$$Z_k = \int_0^\tau w_k(u)\left\{d\hat{\Lambda}_k^*(u) - d\hat{\Lambda}_0^*(u)\right\}, \tag{31}$$

where $w_k(.)$ is a weight function and $\hat{\Lambda}_0^*(.)$ is estimated from the pooled sample. Gray suggests that the weight function be of the form $w_k(t) = L(t)R_k(t)$, where

$$R_k(t) = \frac{Y_k(t)\left[1 - \widehat{\mathrm{CI}}_k(t-)\right]}{\hat{S}_k(t-)}. \tag{32}$$

When $L(t) = 1$, Gray's test corresponds to an analogue of the log-rank test on the sub-distribution hazard.

Standard counting process techniques can be used to find the variance–covariance matrix (see Klein and Bajorunaite, 2004). That is

$$\begin{aligned} V(Z_k) = &\int_0^\tau \left[\frac{R\bullet(u) - R_k(u)}{R\bullet(u)}\right]^2 Y_k(u)\frac{d\hat{\mathrm{CI}}_1^0(u)}{\hat{S}_k(u-)} \\ &+ \int_0^\tau \left[\frac{R_k(u)}{R\bullet(u)}\right]^2 \sum_{i\neq k} Y_i(u)\frac{d\hat{\mathrm{CI}}_1^0(u)}{\hat{S}_i(u-)} \end{aligned} \tag{33}$$

and

$$\begin{aligned} \mathrm{Cov}(Z_h, Z_k) = &\int_0^\tau \left[-\frac{R_k(u)(R\bullet(u) - R_h(u))}{R\bullet(u)^2}\right] Y_h(u)\frac{d\hat{\mathrm{CI}}_1^0(u)}{\hat{S}_h(u-)} \\ &+ \int_0^\tau \left[-\frac{R_h(u)(R\bullet(u) - R_k(u))}{R\bullet(u)^2}\right] Y_k(u)\frac{d\hat{\mathrm{CI}}_1^0(u)}{\hat{S}_k(u-)}. \\ &+ \sum_{j\neq h,k}\int_0^\tau \left[\frac{R_k(u)R_h(u)}{R\bullet(u)^2}\right] Y_j(u)\frac{d\hat{\mathrm{CI}}_1^0(u)}{\hat{S}_j(u-)} \end{aligned} \tag{34}$$

Here $R\bullet(t)$ is the value of $R_i(t)$ summed over all K treatments and $\hat{\mathrm{CI}}_1^0(u)$ is the pooled sample estimate of the cumulative incidence function of the event of interest. The test statistic is

$$\chi^2 = (Z_1, \ldots, Z_{K-1})\Sigma^-(Z_1, \ldots, Z_{K-1})^t, \tag{35}$$

where Σ^- is the inverse of the correct part of the covariance matrix. The statistics has a large sample χ^2 distribution under the null hypothesis. Estimates of cumulative incidence function and the K-sample Gray's test are available in cmprsk R-library created by Robert Gray (see http://www.cran.r-project.org/doc/packages/cmprsk.pdf).

The second test is based on an analogue of the weighted Kaplan–Meier test discussed above. This test is originally due to Pepe (1991) and is based on the difference between cumulative incidence function in the two sample problem. The test statistic is given by

$$Z = \sqrt{\frac{n_1 n_2}{n}} \int_0^\tau \hat{w}(t)\left[\widehat{\mathrm{CI}}_{11}(t) - \widehat{\mathrm{CI}}_{12}(t)\right]dt, \tag{36}$$

where $\hat{w}(.)$ is a weight function. Here for the kth treatment we let CI_{1k} be the CIF of the cause of interest and CI_{2k} the CIF for all other causes. We let $\hat{\mathrm{CI}}_1^0$ be the estimate of the CIF of the cause of interest in the pooled sample, $\hat{S}_k$ the Kaplan–Meier estimator ignoring cause of failure in the kth sample and $Y_k(t)$ the number at risk at time t in the kth sample. Pepe (1991) suggested a method of moments type estimator of the variance of Z. Here we use an improved estimator presented in Bajorunaite and Klein (2007) based on a counting process formulation given (with $w() = 1$) by

$$\sigma_Z^2 = \left(\frac{n_1 n_2}{n_1 + n_2}\right) \sum_{k=1}^{2} \left[\begin{array}{l} \int_0^\tau \left\{(\tau - s)\frac{1-\hat{\mathrm{CI}}_{2k}(u)}{Y_k(s)} - \frac{1}{Y_k(s)}\int_s^\tau \hat{\mathrm{CI}}_{1k}(u)du\right\}^2 \frac{Y_k(s)}{\hat{S}_k(s)} d\hat{\mathrm{CI}}_1^0(s) + \\ \int_0^\tau \left\{(\tau - s)\frac{\hat{\mathrm{CI}}_1^0(u)}{Y_k(s)} - \frac{1}{Y_k(s)}\int_s^\tau \hat{\mathrm{CI}}_{1k}(u)du\right\}^2 \frac{Y_k(s)}{\hat{S}_k(s)} d\hat{\mathrm{CI}}_{2k}(s) \end{array} \right]. \tag{37}$$

The test statistics Z/σ_Z has an approximate standard normal distribution under the null hypothesis.

A third test is a Kolmogorov–Smirnov type test suggested by Lin (1997). The test statistic is

$$Z = \sup_{t \in [0,\tau]} \left| w(t)\left\{\widehat{\mathrm{CI}}_{11}(t) - \widehat{\mathrm{CI}}_{12}(t)\right\}\right|. \tag{38}$$

Lin shows that for large samples $\Delta_k(t) = \sqrt{n_k}\left[\hat{\mathrm{CI}}_{1k}(t) - \mathrm{CI}_{1k}\right]$ has the same limiting distribution as

$$\begin{aligned} \Delta_k(t) \approx \sqrt{n_k}\Bigg[& \int_0^\tau \frac{1 - \mathrm{CI}_{2k}(u)}{Y_k(u)} dM_{1k}(u) + \int_0^\tau \frac{1 - \mathrm{CI}_{1k}(u)}{Y_k(u)} dM_{1k}(u) \\ & -\mathrm{CI}_{1k}(t)\int_0^\tau \frac{dM_{1k}(u) + dM_{2k}(u)}{Y_k(u)}\Bigg] \end{aligned} \tag{39}$$

Here the $M_{jk}(t)$ are independent martingale. A Monte Carlo method is used to find the p-values. We replace the $M_{jk}(t)$'s by $\sum_{l=1}^{n_k} \zeta_{jk}^l N_{jk}^l(t)$, $j = 1,2$, $k = 1,2$, where the ζ_{jk}^l are independent standard normal random variables. Here $N_{jk}^l(t) = I[X_{lk} \le t, \varepsilon_{lk} = j, \delta_{lk} = 1]$. To generate the distribution of $\Delta_k(t)$, we repeatedly generate a large number, L, of realizations by repeatedly generating ζ's from the normal distribution with all other quantities fixed at their sample values. We obtain replicates of Δ_k using (39) which provides us with replicates of Z given by

$$\hat{Z}_l = \sup_{t \in [0,\tau]} \left| \frac{\Delta_{1l}(t)}{\sqrt{n_1}} - \frac{\Delta_{2l}(t)}{\sqrt{n_2}} \right|, \qquad l = 1, \ldots, L. \tag{40}$$

These are then compared to the observed value of Z to provide a Monte Carlo p-value.

We apply these competing risks tests to the comparison of relapse and treatment related mortality between the HLA-identical sibling and HLA-matched

Table 2
Test of hypothesis in BMT example

Test	Relapse	Treatment-Related Mortality
	p-value	p-value
Log-rank test	0.4702	<0.0001
Gray's test	0.1188	<0.0001
Pepe's test	0.0533	<0.0001
Kolmogorov test	0.0212	<0.0001

unrelated donor groups in the data set presented at the end of Section 2. Table 2 presents the results.

The log-rank test compares the crude hazard rates and in this example suggests no differences in the relapse hazard rates. The other four tests compare directly the cumulative incidence function and in most cases this is a primary interest. Gray's test, which compares the sub-distributional hazards, has the most power to detect proportional sub-distributional hazards and has little power to detect crossing sub-distributional hazards (or cumulative incidence curves), as we have here for relapse. The other two tests are more omnibus tests and have better power to detect crossing cumulative incidence functions. In this example, the cumulative incidence functions cross (see Fig. 3a) and these two tests indicate a significant difference in the relapse incidences.

4. Regression models

In this section, we review a number of models that are used to study the effects of covariates on outcome. Our data consists of $(X_i,\delta_i,\mathbf{Z}_i(t))$, for $i=1,\ldots,n$ where $\mathbf{Z}_i(t)=(Z_{i1}(t),\ldots,Z_{ip}(t))$ is a p-vector of explanatory covariates. These covariates may be fixed at time zero (e.g. gender, race, initial disease stage, etc.) or they may vary with time (most recent blood pressure, indicator of some intermediate event). For time-dependent covariates the value needs to be known for everyone at risk just prior to every event time.

In most biological applications a semi-parametric model is used to model the effect of the covariates on outcome. In these models a parametric form is assumed for the covariate effect but the distribution of the baseline survival rate is not specified. In the sequel we will focus on these methods.

The most common regression model is the Cox (1972) or proportional hazards model. For this model we assume that the covariates act in a multiplicative fashion on the hazard rate. That is we assume that

$$\lambda(t|\mathbf{Z}(t))=\lambda_0(t)\exp\{\boldsymbol{\beta}\mathbf{Z}(t)\}, \tag{41}$$

where $\lambda_0(t)$ is a baseline hazard rate and $\boldsymbol{\beta}$ a p-vector of parameter estimators. Note that for this model the relative risk for a subject with a covariate vector $\mathbf{Z}_1$

as compared to a subject with covariate vector $\mathbf{Z}_2$ is a constant given by

$$\frac{\lambda_0(t)\exp\{\boldsymbol{\beta}\mathbf{Z}_1\}}{\lambda_0(t)\exp\{\boldsymbol{\beta}\mathbf{Z}_2\}} = \exp\{\boldsymbol{\beta}[\mathbf{Z}_1 - \mathbf{Z}_2]\}. \tag{42}$$

For a binary covariate coded as (0,1), $\exp\{\boldsymbol{\beta}\}$ is the relative risk for a subject with the characteristic ($\mathbf{Z} = 1$) as compared to a subject with the baseline level of the characteristic ($\mathbf{Z} = 0$), all other covariates held the same. For continuous covariates, $\exp\{\boldsymbol{\beta}\}$ is the relative risk for a one unit change in the covariate. Because of the relationship between the hazard rate and the survival function, for fixed covariates, the relationship between $\mathbf{Z}$ and the survival function is

$$S(t|\mathbf{Z}) = S_0(t)^{\exp\{\boldsymbol{\beta}\mathbf{Z}\}}, \tag{43}$$

where $S_0(t) = \exp\{-\int_0^t \lambda_0(u)du\}$ is the baseline survival function.

The parameters of the proportional hazards model are estimated using a partial likelihood approach. We assume for simplicity that there are no tied event times and we have only fixed time covariates. As before let $t_1 < t_2 < \cdots < t_D$ be the ordered event times and $\mathbf{Z}_{(j)}$ the corresponding covariate associated with the subject who failed at t_j. Let $R(t_j)$ be the set of individuals at risk just prior to time t_j. The log partial likelihood is

$$\mathrm{LL}(\boldsymbol{\beta}) = \sum_{j=1}^{D} \boldsymbol{\beta}\mathbf{Z}_{(j)} - \sum_{j=1}^{D} \ln\left[\sum_{l\in R(t_j)} \exp(\boldsymbol{\beta}\mathbf{Z}_l)\right]. \tag{44}$$

When there are ties in the event times then modifications to (44) are given by Efron (1977), Breslow (1974) and Cox (1972) (see Klein and Moeschberger, 2003 for details).

The partial maximum likelihood estimators (pmle) of $\boldsymbol{\beta}, \hat{\boldsymbol{\beta}}$, are found by maximizing (44) or equivalently solving the score equations $\mathbf{U}(\boldsymbol{\beta}) = \partial\mathrm{LL}(\boldsymbol{\beta})/\partial\boldsymbol{\beta} = \mathbf{0}$. For large samples $\hat{\boldsymbol{\beta}}$ has an approximate multivariate normal distribution with a mean $\boldsymbol{\beta}$ and a variance estimated consistently by the inverse of the information matrix $\mathbf{I}(\hat{\boldsymbol{\beta}})$, where

$$\mathbf{I}(\boldsymbol{\beta}) = -\partial^2\mathrm{LL}(\boldsymbol{\beta})/\partial\boldsymbol{\beta}^2 = \partial\mathbf{U}(\boldsymbol{\beta})/\partial\boldsymbol{\beta}.$$

Global tests of the hypothesis H_0: $\boldsymbol{\beta} = \boldsymbol{\beta}_0$ can be made in three ways. The first test is a likelihood-ratio test with

$$\chi^2_{\mathrm{LR}} = 2[\mathrm{LL}(\hat{\boldsymbol{\beta}}) - \mathrm{LL}(\boldsymbol{\beta}_0)]. \tag{45}$$

The second is the Wald test with

$$\chi^2_W = (\hat{\boldsymbol{\beta}} - \boldsymbol{\beta}_0)^t\mathbf{I}(\hat{\boldsymbol{\beta}})(\hat{\boldsymbol{\beta}} - \boldsymbol{\beta}_0) \tag{46}$$

and the third is the score or Rao test with

$$\chi^2_{\mathrm{SC}} = \mathbf{U}(\boldsymbol{\beta}_0)^t\mathbf{I}^{-1}(\boldsymbol{\beta}_0)\mathbf{U}(\boldsymbol{\beta}_0). \tag{47}$$

Under the null hypothesis all three statistics have an approximate χ^2 distribution with p degrees of freedom.

Local tests of subsets of covariates can also be constructed in three forms. Let $\boldsymbol{\beta} = (\boldsymbol{\beta}_1, \boldsymbol{\beta}_2)$, where $\boldsymbol{\beta}_1$ is a q-vector of the $\boldsymbol{\beta}$'s of interest and $\boldsymbol{\beta}_2$ the vector of the remaining $\boldsymbol{\beta}$'s of interest. We wish to test H_0: $\boldsymbol{\beta}_1 = \boldsymbol{\beta}_{10}$. We partition the pmle into $\hat{\boldsymbol{\beta}} = (\hat{\boldsymbol{\beta}}_1, \hat{\boldsymbol{\beta}}_2)$ and the information matrix $\mathbf{I}$ as

$$\mathbf{I} = \begin{pmatrix} \mathbf{I}_{11} & \mathbf{I}_{12} \\ \mathbf{I}_{21} & \mathbf{I}_{22} \end{pmatrix}. \tag{48}$$

For the likelihood-ratio test we compute the pmle of $\boldsymbol{\beta}$ with the first q components fixed at $\boldsymbol{\beta}_{10}, \hat{\boldsymbol{\beta}}_2(\boldsymbol{\beta}_{10})$. The test statistic is

$$\chi^2_{\mathrm{LR}} = 2\left[\mathrm{LL}(\hat{\boldsymbol{\beta}}) - \mathrm{LL}(\boldsymbol{\beta}_{10}, \hat{\boldsymbol{\beta}}_2(\boldsymbol{\beta}_{10})\right]. \tag{49}$$

The Wald test is

$$\chi^2_W = (\hat{\boldsymbol{\beta}}_1 - \boldsymbol{\beta}_{10})^t \left[\mathbf{I}^{11}(\hat{\boldsymbol{\beta}})\right]^{-1} (\hat{\boldsymbol{\beta}}_1 - \boldsymbol{\beta}_{10}), \tag{50}$$

where $\mathbf{I}^{11}(\hat{\boldsymbol{\beta}})$ is the upper $q \times q$ submatrix of $\mathbf{I}^{-1}(\hat{\boldsymbol{\beta}})$.The score test is given by

$$\chi^2_{\mathrm{SC}} = \mathbf{U}[\boldsymbol{\beta}_{10}, \hat{\boldsymbol{\beta}}_2(\boldsymbol{\beta}_{10})]^t \mathbf{I}^{11}[\boldsymbol{\beta}_{10}, \hat{\boldsymbol{\beta}}_2(\boldsymbol{\beta}_{10})] \mathbf{U}[\boldsymbol{\beta}_{10}, \hat{\boldsymbol{\beta}}_2(\boldsymbol{\beta}_{10})]. \tag{51}$$

All three test statistics have a large sample χ^2 distribution with q degrees of freedom under the null hypothesis.

To illustrate the regression methods we consider a sample of 154 patients described in Ichida et al. (1993). The goal of the study was to evaluate a change in protocol in disinfectant practices for severe burn cases from a routine bathing care (initial 10% povidone–iodine cleaning followed by regular cleansing with Dial soap) to body cleansing with 4% chlohexidine gluconate. Of interest was a comparison of the distribution of the time to staphylococcus infection. Patients were censored by death or on leaving the hospital. The covariates to be considered are indicator variables for the type of treatment ($Z_1 = 1$ if body cleansing, 0 if routine care), gender ($Z_2 = 1$ if female, 0 if male), race ($Z_3 = 1$ if white, 0 otherwise), percent of total surface area burned (Z_4) and a time-dependent indicator of whether the burn had been excised or not ($Z_5(t) = 1$ if burned excised by time t, 0 otherwise). Note the value of $Z_5(t)$ is initially 0 and changes to 1 on the day the burn was excised.

A proportional hazards model with only the main effect, Z_1, finds an estimate of -0.56 (SE $= 0.29$). The likelihood ratio χ^2 is $\chi^2_{\mathrm{LR}} = 3.64$ ($p = 0.0541$), the Wald χ^2 $\chi^2_W = 3.64$ (0.0563) and the score χ^2 is $\chi^2_{\mathrm{SC}} = 3.74$ (0.0532). Note that when there are no ties in the event times the score χ^2 is equal to the usual log-rank χ^2. Here the estimated relative risk is $0.57 = \exp\{-0.56\}$ so patients are approximately half as likely to develop an infection on the new bath solution as compared to the old method. A 95% confidence interval can be found by exponentiation of the interval for β. The interval is $\exp\{-0.056 \pm 1.96\ 0.563\} = [0.32, 1.02]$.

Before additional analysis on the fixed covariates is performed it is useful to check the assumption of proportional hazards. One approach is to create an artificial time-dependent covariate, $Z_{PH}(t)$ for each fixed time covariate, Z. We let $Z_{PH}(t) = Z\phi(t)$, where $\phi(\cdot)$ is a known function. Typically, as suggested by Cox (1972), we use $\phi(t) = \ln(t)$ although we could use other functions such as $\phi(t) = t$ or $\phi(t) = I[t<t_0]$. Interested readers are directed to Therneau and Grambsch (2000) for a somewhat technical discussion of what type of departure from proportionality each choice of ϕ has the most power to detect. A local test of the hypothesis that the regression coefficient for $Z_{PH}(t)$ is equal to zero is a check of proportional hazards. When the proportional hazards assumption is suspect then one can model Z by a set of time-dependent covariates such as $Z_1(t) = ZI[t<t_0]$ and $Z_2(t) = ZI[t \geq t_0]$, where t_0 is usually found by maximizing the log partial likelihood (see Klein and Moeschberger, 2003). For the bathing solution data we have the following p-values of the Wald tests for proportional hazards suggesting there is no problem with this assumption (Table 3).

Table 4 gives the results of fitting the proportional hazards model to all five covariates. In this table we see that the main effect of method of care is not significant, that white patients are significantly more likely to have an infection (8.5 times more likely), that once patients have their wound excised they are less like to develop infections and that gender and percent surface area burned are not associated with the time to infection. Note that for Z_4 the relative risk of $\exp\{0.003\}$ is the increase risk per a change of 1% of body surface area burned. A more interpretable number may be $\exp\{10 \times 0.003\} = 1.03$, which is the increase in risk of infection per an increase of 10% in body surface area.

Table 3
Tests of proportional hazards

Effect	p-value
Z_1: Method of care	0.6323
Z_2: Gender	0.1900
Z_3: Race	0.2752
Z_4: Percent burned	0.3451

Table 4
Proportional hazards analysis of full model

Effect	β	SE	exp $\{\beta\}$	χ^2	p-value
Z_1: Method of care	−0.499	0.300	0.61	2.77	0.096
Z_2: Gender	−0.537	0.392	0.58	1.87	0.171
Z_3: Race	2.142	1.013	8.51	4.46	0.034
Z_4: Percent burned	0.003	0.007	1.00	0.23	0.632
$Z_5(t)$: Excision indicator	−0.898	0.485	0.41	3.43	0.064

Table 5
Proportional hazards analysis of final model

Effect	β	SE	exp $\{\beta\}$	χ^2	p-value
Z_1: Method of care	−0.483	0.300	0.62	2.65	0.103
Z_3: Race	2.180	1.012	8.90	4.67	0.031
$Z_5(t)$: Excision indicator	−0.998	0.483	0.37	4.26	0.039

Keeping the main effect of method of care and eliminating the non-significant factors in Table 4 using forward model selection we obtain the final model given in Table 5.

The proportional hazards model is perhaps one of the most studied models in the statistical literature. The reader is referred to the text books by Therneau and Grambsch (2000) or Klein and Moeschberger (2003) for details and discussions on regression diagnostics for this model. Software to fit the Cox model is available in most every package that deals with censored data.

Cox regression models can be developed for other censoring and truncation schemes. For left-truncated data all of the above results carry through. These models are available in SAS, for example. For interval-censored data special techniques have been developed for proportional hazards regression. These are detailed, for example, in Finkelstein (1986), Goggins and Finkelstein (2000) and in the book by Sun (2006).

A second set of models for survival data are the additive hazards models. These model the excess risk due to a factor rather than the relative risk. The model was originally proposed by Aalen (1989, 1993) with time-varying risk coefficients and modified to have fixed risk coefficients by Lin and Ying (1994, 1997). For this model we have

$$\lambda(t|\mathbf{Z}_i(t)) = \alpha_0(t) + \boldsymbol{\alpha}(t)\mathbf{Z}_i(t). \tag{52}$$

Here $\alpha_0()$ is a baseline rate and $\boldsymbol{\alpha}()$ is a p-vector of regression functions.

To estimate the regression parameters in the Aalen model (52) a least squares approach is used. For simplicity we will consider the case where all the covariates are fixed at time t. Let $Y_i(t)$ be the indicator that the ith subject is at risk at time t, and let $N_i(t) = 1$ if $X_i \leq t$ and $d_i = 1$. Let $\mathbf{N}(t) = [N_1(t), \ldots, N_n(t)]^t$, and let $\mathbf{X}(t)$ be the $n \times (p+1)$ matrix with ith row given by $[Y_i(t), \; Y_i(t)Z_{1i}, \ldots, Y_i(t)Z_{pi}]$, $i = 1, \ldots, n$. We shall estimate the cumulative regression function

$$\mathbf{A}(t) = \left\{ A_j(t) = \int_0^t \alpha_j(u)du \right\}, \qquad j = 0, 1, \ldots, p \tag{53}$$

by

$$\hat{\mathbf{A}}(t) = \int_0^t \mathbf{X}^-(u)d\mathbf{N}(u), \tag{54}$$

where $\mathbf{X}^{-}(t)$ is a generalized inverse of $\mathbf{X}$. While any generalized inverse maybe used in most applications, the inverse $\mathbf{X}^{-}(t) = [\mathbf{X}^{t}(t)\mathbf{X}(t)]^{-1}\mathbf{X}^{t}(t)$. Huffer and McKeague (1991) examined the use of other generalized inverses. The estimator is defined over the range of the data $[0,\tau]$, where $[\mathbf{X}^{t}(t)\ \mathbf{X}(t)]$ is non-singular. The variance–covariance matrix of $\hat{\mathbf{A}}$ is given by

$$\widehat{\mathrm{var}}(\hat{\mathbf{A}}(t)) = \sum_{T_i \le t} \left[\mathbf{X}^{t}(T_i)\mathbf{X}(T_i)\right]^{-1}\mathbf{X}^{t}(T_i)\mathbf{I}^{D}(T_i)\mathbf{X}(T_i)\left[\left[\mathbf{X}^{t}(T_i)\mathbf{X}(T_i)\right]^{-1}\right]^{t}, \tag{55}$$

where $\mathbf{I}^{D}(t)$ is a diagonal matrix with diagonal elements equal to 1 if subject i dies at time t. For large samples the estimates of $\mathbf{A}$ are approximately normal with a variance given by (55).

Figure 4 shows the estimated cumulative regression estimates for the time to infection data based on the four fixed covariates. Included in the figures is the point estimate of $A_i(t)$ and 95% pointwise confidence intervals constructed as $\hat{A}_i(t) \pm 1.96\widehat{\mathrm{var}}(\hat{A}_i(t))^{1/2}$. The slope of these estimates provides an estimator of $\alpha()$. Smother estimates of $\alpha()$ can be obtained by smoothing these crude estimates (see Klein and Moeschberger, 2003). From these graphs it appears that there is little effect of the method of care, gender or percent body surface since the curves and confidence intervals are close to the zero line. For race it appears there is a strong positive effect, at least in the first three weeks with an approximate estimate of $\alpha(t)$ of about $0.6/20 = 0.03$, after which the estimate of $\alpha()$ is close to zero.

Tests for the global hypothesis H_0: $\alpha_j(t) = 0$, $j = 1, \ldots, p$ or local hypotheses like H_{0j}: $\alpha_j(t) = 0$ can be constructed based on a weighted statistic as suggested first by Aalen (1993). Let $\mathbf{W}(t)$ be the $p \times p$ diagonal weight matrix with diagonal elements $(W_1(t), \ldots, W_p(t))$. The test statistic is a quadratic form in $\mathbf{U} = (U_1, \ldots, U_p)$ where

$$U_j(t) = \int_0^{\tau} W_j(u)d\hat{A}(u). \tag{56}$$

The covariance matrix is

$$\mathbf{V} = \sum_{T_i} \mathbf{W}(T_i)\left\{\left[\mathbf{X}^{t}(T_i)\mathbf{X}(T_i)\right]^{-1}\mathbf{X}^{t}(T_i)\mathbf{I}^{D}(T_i)\mathbf{X}(T_i)\left[\mathbf{X}^{t}(T_i)\mathbf{X}(T_i)\right]^{-1}\right\}^{t}\mathbf{W}(T_i) \tag{57}$$

and the test statistic is given by $X^2 = \mathbf{U}^{t}\mathbf{V}^{-1}\mathbf{U}$. Under the null hypothesis for large samples the statistic has a χ^2 distribution with p degrees of freedom. For the weight function Aalen (1993) proposed the diagonal elements of $[\mathbf{X}^{t}(t)\mathbf{X}(t)]^{-1}$, however Bhattacharyya and Klein (2005) show that in the one-way layout this may lead to test statistics that depend on which group is chosen as the baseline group. They show that weights which are multiples of the identity matrix do not have this problem. Such weights include $W_j(t) = 1$ for all t, $W_j(t) = Y(t)$, the total number at risk at time t and $W_j(t) = Y(t)^{1/2}$. Gandy et al. (2007) suggest a refinement of the additive model to eliminate this problem as well based on redefining the covariate vector.

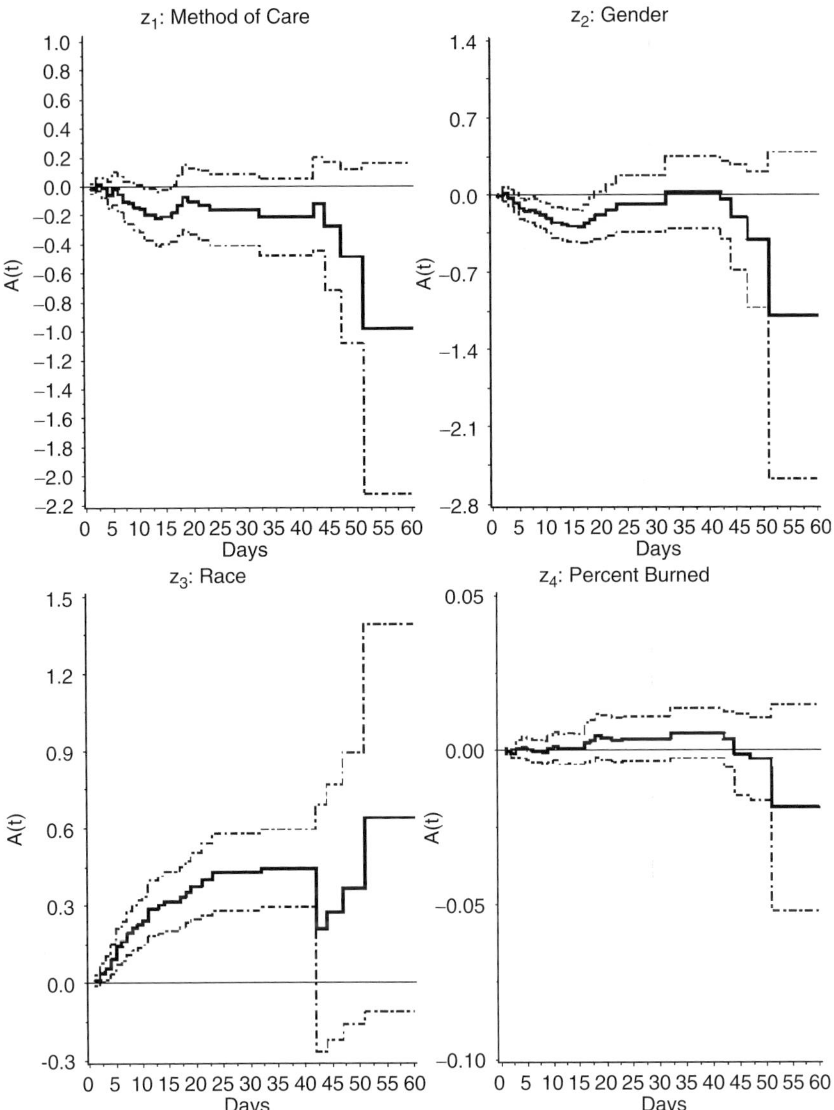

Fig. 4. Aalen's additive regression function estimates.

Table 6 gives the test statistics and p-values for the Aalen model using several weight functions. Note that there is rough agreement between these tests suggesting that gender is marginally significant, percent of area burned is not significant, race is strongly associated with outcome and the main effect of method of care is associated with infection.

The above computations were based on a SAS macro that can be found at http://www.biostat.mcw.edu/software/SoftMenu.html. An SPlus/R package is

Table 6
Tests for a regression effect in the Aalen model

Effect	Weight		
	$[\mathbf{X}^t(t)\mathbf{X}(t)]^{-1}$	$Y(t)$	$Y(t)^{1/2}$
Global test	$\chi^2 = 24{\cdot}7$ $p<0.0001$	$\chi^2 = 29{\cdot}62$ $p = <0.0001$	$\chi^2 = 12{\cdot}12$ $p = 0.0165$
Z_1: Method of care	$\chi^2 = 3{\cdot}95$ $p = 0.0468$	$\chi^2 = 4{\cdot}07$ $p = 0.0437$	$\chi^2 = 4{\cdot}15$ $p = 0.0416$
Z_2: Gender	$\chi^2 = 3{\cdot}44$ $p = 0.0634$	$\chi^2 = 4{\cdot}55$ $p = 0.0329$	$\chi^2 = 3{\cdot}00$ $p = 0.0831$
Z_3: Race	$\chi^2 = 21{\cdot}19$ $p<0.0001$	$\chi^2 = 25{\cdot}92$ $p = <0.0001$	$\chi^2 = 10{\cdot}12$ $p = 0.0015$
Z_4: Percent burned	$\chi^2 = 0{\cdot}18$ $p = 0.6681$	$\chi^2 = 0{\cdot}06$ $p = 0.8143$	$\chi^2 = 0{\cdot}29$ $p = 0.58$

available at http://www.med.uio.no/imb/stat/addreg/. A package timereg 0.1 for R available at http://www.med.uio.no/imb/stat/addreg/ includes routines to fit the additive model.

The second additive hazards model is the model of Lin and Ying (1994). In this model the effect of the covariates on the hazard rate is given by

$$\lambda(t|\mathbf{Z}) = \gamma_0(t) + \boldsymbol{\gamma}\mathbf{Z}(t). \tag{58}$$

Here γ_0 is an arbitrary baseline hazard function. Estimators of the model parameters are found by maximizing a pseudo partial score equation based on replacing the hazard rate in the Cox model by the model (58) in the score equations. The estimates are given by

$$\hat{\boldsymbol{\gamma}} = \mathbf{A}^{-1}\mathbf{B}^t, \tag{59}$$

where the p-vector $\mathbf{B}$ is given by

$$\mathbf{B}^t = \sum_{i=1}^{n} \delta_i\left[\mathbf{Z}_i - \bar{\mathbf{Z}}(X_i)\right]. \tag{60}$$

$\mathbf{A}$ is the $p \times p$ matrix

$$\mathbf{A} = \sum_{i=1}^{n}\sum_{j=1}^{i}(X_j - X_{j-1})[\mathbf{Z}_i - \bar{\mathbf{Z}}(X_j)]^t[\mathbf{Z}_i - \bar{\mathbf{Z}}(X_j)]. \tag{61}$$

Here we assume that the X_i's are ordered with $0 = X_0 < X_1 < \cdots < X_n$ and that

$$\bar{\mathbf{Z}}(t) = \frac{\sum_{i=1}^{n} \mathbf{Z}_i Y_i(t)}{\sum_{i=1}^{n} Y_i(t)}. \tag{62}$$

The variance of $\hat{\gamma}$ can be estimated consistently by

$$\widehat{\text{var}}(\hat{\gamma}) = \mathbf{A}^{-1}\mathbf{C}\mathbf{A}^{-1}, \tag{63}$$

where

$$\mathbf{C} = \sum_{i=1}^{n} \delta_i [\mathbf{Z}_i - \bar{\mathbf{Z}}(X_i)]^t [\mathbf{Z}_i - \bar{\mathbf{Z}}(X_i)]. \tag{64}$$

For large samples the estimators have a normal distribution with mean γ and a variance estimated by (63). Tests of hypothesis about model parameters can be based on the large sample normal distribution.

Applying the Lin–Ying model to the wound care problem gives the results in Table 7. Here we see that only the percent surface area burned is not associated with the time to infection. For the main effect of method of care the rate of occurrence of infection is reduced by 0.0091 by using the new cleaning method. These results are in agreement with the Aalen model using the weight function $Y(t)$ in testing.

Additive hazards models have been studied for other censoring and truncation schemes. In particular, for interval-censored data the paper by Sun et al. (2004) provides results for both additive models. A good survey of these results can be found in Sun (2006).

The Cox proportional hazard model and Aalen's additive hazards models are the two most commonly used semi-parametric regression models. The models complement each other and provide different interpretations of the effects of the covariates on the hazard rate. One advantage of the additive models is that it allows the covariates to have a time-varying effects that is easy to estimate. Scheike and Zhang (2002) proposed an additive–multiplicative intensity model that includes the Cox regression model as well as the additive Aalen model. We partition the covariates into two disjoint vectors, $\mathbf{Z}_1 = (1, Z_{11}, \ldots, Z_{1p})$ and $\mathbf{Z}_2 = (Z_{21}, \ldots, Z_{2q})$. We define the hazard function by

$$\lambda(t|\mathbf{Z}_1, \mathbf{Z}_2) = (\mathbf{Z}_1^t \boldsymbol{\alpha}(t)) \exp\{\mathbf{Z}_2^t \boldsymbol{\beta}\}. \tag{65}$$

For this model one first estimates $\boldsymbol{\beta}$ by solving the estimating equation

$$\mathbf{U}(\boldsymbol{\beta}) = \int_0^\tau \{\mathbf{Z}_2^t - \mathbf{Z}_2^t \mathbf{Y}(\boldsymbol{\beta}, t)\mathbf{Y}^-(\boldsymbol{\beta}, t)\} d\mathbf{N}(t) = 0, \tag{66}$$

Table 7
Estimates of regression effects in the Lin–Ying model

Effect	$\hat{\gamma}$	SE	$Z = \hat{\gamma}/\text{SE}$	p-value
Z_1: Method of care	−0.0091	0.0044	−2.30	0.0424
Z_2: Gender	−0.0082	0.0041	−1.99	0.0462
Z_3: Race	0.0134	0.0029	4.59	<0.0001
Z_4: Percent burned	0.0007	0.0001	0.55	0.5830

where $\mathbf{Y}(\boldsymbol{\beta}, t) = \left[Y_1(t)\mathbf{Z}_{11}\exp\{\mathbf{Z}_{21}^t\boldsymbol{\beta}\}, \ldots, Y_n(t)\mathbf{Z}_{1n}\exp\{\mathbf{Z}_{2n}^t\boldsymbol{\beta}\}\right]^t$. The estimate of $\mathbf{A}(t) = \int_0^t \boldsymbol{\alpha}(u)\,du$ is given by

$$\hat{\mathbf{A}}(t) = \int_0^t \mathbf{Y}^-(\hat{\boldsymbol{\beta}}, u)d\mathbf{N}(u). \tag{67}$$

Here $\mathbf{Y}^-(\boldsymbol{\beta}, s) = [\mathbf{Y}(\boldsymbol{\beta}, s)^t\mathbf{W}(s)\mathbf{Y}(\boldsymbol{\beta}, s)]^{-1}\mathbf{Y}(\boldsymbol{\beta}, s)^t\mathbf{W}(s)$, where $\mathbf{W}()$ is a diagonal weight matrix with elements $W_i(t) = Y_i(t)\exp\{-\mathbf{Z}_{2i}\boldsymbol{\beta}\}$. The variance of $\hat{\boldsymbol{\beta}}$ can be estimated by

$$\mathrm{Var}(\hat{\boldsymbol{\beta}}) = \mathbf{I}^{-1}(\hat{\boldsymbol{\beta}})\mathrm{var}[\mathbf{U}(\hat{\boldsymbol{\beta}})]\mathbf{I}^{-1}(\hat{\boldsymbol{\beta}}), \tag{68}$$

where

$$\mathbf{I}(\boldsymbol{\beta}) = -\partial\mathbf{U}(\boldsymbol{\beta})/\partial\boldsymbol{\beta},$$

$$\mathrm{var}[\mathbf{U}(\hat{\boldsymbol{\beta}})] = \int_0^\tau \left[\mathbf{Z}_2^t - \mathbf{S}^{(1)}(\hat{\boldsymbol{\beta}}, t)\mathbf{Y}^-(\hat{\boldsymbol{\beta}}, t)\right]\mathrm{diag}(d\mathbf{N}(t))\left[\mathbf{Z}_2^t - \mathbf{S}^{(1)}(\hat{\boldsymbol{\beta}}, t)\mathbf{Y}^-(\hat{\boldsymbol{\beta}}, t)\right]^t$$

and

$$\mathbf{S}^{(1)}(\hat{\boldsymbol{\beta}}, t) = \sum_{i=1}^n Y_i(t)\mathbf{Z}_{2i}\exp\{\mathbf{Z}_{2i}\boldsymbol{\beta}\}\mathbf{Z}_{1i}.$$

When $\mathbf{Z}_1$ is a vector of discrete-valued covariates the mixed additive–multiplicative model leads to stratified Cox model, which is available in most statistical package. The general mixed model can be fit using the cox.aalen-function in R created by Scheike (Martinussen and Scheike, 2006).

To illustrate this model, we consider the burn data with the covariates method of care, gender and race as having a multiplicative effect ($\mathbf{Z}_2$) and the covariate percent of surface area burned as having an additive effect (Z_1). The p-value testing for an effect of percent of area burned has a p-value of 0.95 in this model as compared to a p-value of 0.57 in a standard Cox model. As shown in Table 8, the estimates of the multiplicative effects are quite similar in the two models. This is not surprising since a test of the appropriateness of modeling the percentage of surface area burned as a time-varying effect discussed in Scheike and Zhang (2002) was not significant ($p = 0.63$).

Table 8
Illustration of the mixed model

Effect	Standard Cox Model			Mixed Model		
	Estimate	SE	p-value	Estimate	SE	p-value
Method of care	−0.61	0.30	0.0377	−0.60	0.30	0.0420
Gender	−0.64	0.39	0.1050	−0.62	0.39	0.1103
Race	2.11	1.00	0.0351	2.11	1.03	0.0370
Percent burned	0.004	0.007	0.5686	—	—	0.9500

An alternative to both the multiplicative and additive hazards models is the proportional odds model. This model, first suggested by Pettitt (1984) and Bennett (1983) allows for the effects of the covariates to diminish over time. The model assumes that

$$\frac{1 - S(t|\mathbf{Z})}{S(t|\mathbf{Z})} = \frac{1 - S_0(t)}{S_0(t)} \exp\{\boldsymbol{\beta}\mathbf{Z}\}. \tag{69}$$

Here $S_0(t)$ is a baseline survival function.

The proportional odds model can be viewed as a special model of the semi-parametric transformation models

$$\phi(T) = -\boldsymbol{\beta}\mathbf{Z} + E, \tag{70}$$

where ϕ is an unspecified monotone transformation function, and E a random variable with a known distribution independent of $\mathbf{Z}$. When $\phi(t) = \log(t)$ and E has a standard logistic distribution with probability density function $f(x) = \exp(x)/[1 + \exp(x)]^2$, this leads to a parametric proportional odds model.

Various authors have considered and studied the proportional odds models and general transformation models. The key references for semi-parametric inference in the transformation models are Pettitt (1984), Bennett (1983), Cheng et al. (1995), Rossini and Tsiatis (1996), Murphy et al. (1997), Fine et al. (1998), Yang and Prentice (1999), Bagdonavicius and Nikulin (1999) and Chen et al. (2002). To fit a semi-parametric proportional odds model with right-censored survival data, Cheng et al. (1995), Fine et al. (1998) and others suggested using a general approach based on IPCW techniques. Murphy et al. (1997) presented a profile likelihood approach, recently Bagdonavicius and Nikulin (1999) and Chen et al. (2002) considered an estimating equations approach based on a modified partial likelihood method. Martinussen and Scheike (2006) gave a detailed overview of semi-parametric analysis of transformation models with censored data.

Let $\Phi(t) = \exp(\phi(\mathrm{t}))$ be a strictly increasing positive function such that $\Phi(0) = 0$ and $\Phi(t) \rightarrow \infty$ as $t \rightarrow \infty$. For a transformation model, the hazard function of T given $\mathbf{Z}$ can be written as

$$\lambda(t|\mathbf{Z}) = \lambda_0(\exp[\boldsymbol{\beta}\mathbf{Z}])\exp[\boldsymbol{\beta}\mathbf{Z}]\Phi(t)\mathrm{d}\Phi(t), \tag{71}$$

where $\lambda_0(t)$ is the hazard associated with $\exp(E)$. In the case of a semi-parametric proportional odds model note that

$$\log\left\{\frac{1 - S(t|\mathbf{Z})}{S(t|\mathbf{Z})}\right\} = \log[\Phi(t)] + \boldsymbol{\beta}\mathbf{Z}, \tag{72}$$

where $\Phi(t) = 1 - S_0(t)/[1 - S_0(t)]$ and $S_0(t)$ is an unspecified survival function. The survival and hazard functions are

$$S(t|\mathbf{Z}) = \frac{1}{1 + \Phi(t)\exp(\boldsymbol{\beta}\mathbf{Z})} \quad \text{and} \quad \lambda(t|\mathbf{Z}) = \frac{d\Phi(t)}{\exp\{-\boldsymbol{\beta}\mathbf{Z}\} + \Phi(t)}. \tag{73}$$

The relative risk for two individual with covariates $\mathbf{Z}_2$ versus $\mathbf{Z}_1$ is

$$\mathrm{RR}(t) = \frac{\lambda(t|\mathbf{Z}_2)}{\lambda(t|\mathbf{Z}_1)} = \frac{\exp\{-\boldsymbol{\beta}\mathbf{Z}_2\} + \Phi(t)}{\exp\{-\boldsymbol{\beta}\mathbf{Z}_1\} + \Phi(t)}. \tag{74}$$

Thus, $\exp((\mathbf{Z}_2 - \mathbf{Z}_1)\boldsymbol{\beta})$ is the initial relative risk and the relative risk tends to 1 for very large time. This is an appealing property that the covariate effect diminishes over time.

We introduce an estimating equation approach for the general transformation models. Let

$$S^{(0)}(t, \boldsymbol{\beta}, \Phi) = \sum_{i=1}^{n} Y_i(t) \exp\{\boldsymbol{\beta}\mathbf{Z}_i\} \frac{d\Phi(t-)}{1 + \Phi(t-)\exp\{\boldsymbol{\beta}\mathbf{Z}_i\}}. \tag{75}$$

For known $\boldsymbol{\beta}$ we can estimate $\Phi()$ by a Breslow-type estimator

$$\tilde{\Phi}(t, \beta) = \int_0^t \frac{dN\bullet(u)}{S^{(0)}(u, \boldsymbol{\beta}, \tilde{\Phi})}. \tag{76}$$

Here the estimation is solved by moving recursively through time starting with $\tilde{\Phi}(t) = 0$ for times smaller than the first death. With an estimate of Φ in hand we estimate $\boldsymbol{\beta}$ using a score equation approach by maximizing

$$\mathbf{U}(\boldsymbol{\beta}) = \sum_{i=1}^{n} \int_0^{\tau} \left\{ \frac{\mathbf{Z}_i \exp\{-\boldsymbol{\beta}\mathbf{Z}_i\} - (\partial\tilde{\Phi}(t-, \boldsymbol{\beta})/\partial\boldsymbol{\beta})}{\exp\{-\boldsymbol{\beta}\mathbf{Z}_i\} - \tilde{\Phi}(t-, \boldsymbol{\beta}\}} - \frac{S^{(1)}(t, \boldsymbol{\beta}, \tilde{\Phi})}{S^{(0)}(t, \boldsymbol{\beta}, \tilde{\Phi})} \right\}, \tag{77}$$

where

$$S^{(1)}(t, \boldsymbol{\beta}, \tilde{\Phi}) = \frac{\partial S^{(0)}(t, \boldsymbol{\beta}, \tilde{\Phi})}{\partial\boldsymbol{\beta}}.$$

Estimation proceeds by iterating between (76) and (77). The asymptotic variance of $\boldsymbol{\beta}$ is estimated by a sandwich estimator (see Bagdonavicius and Nikulin, 1999; Martinussen and Scheike, 2006)

$$\widehat{\mathrm{Var}}(\boldsymbol{\beta}) = I^{-1}(\boldsymbol{\beta}) \hat{\sum} I^{-1}(\boldsymbol{\beta}), \tag{78}$$

where

$$\mathbf{I}(\boldsymbol{\beta}) = -\frac{\partial\mathbf{U}(\boldsymbol{\beta})}{\partial\boldsymbol{\beta}} \tag{79}$$

and

$$\hat{\sum} = \sum_{i=1}^{n} \int_0^{\tau} \left[\frac{\mathbf{Z}_i \exp\{-\boldsymbol{\beta}\mathbf{Z}_i\} - (\partial\tilde{\Phi}(t-, \boldsymbol{\beta})/\partial\boldsymbol{\beta})}{\exp\{-\boldsymbol{\beta}\mathbf{Z}_i\} - \tilde{\Phi}(t-, \boldsymbol{\beta})} - \tilde{q}(t, \boldsymbol{\beta}) \right]^{\otimes 2} dN_i(t), \tag{80}$$

where

$$\hat{q}(t,\boldsymbol{\beta}) = \frac{S^{(1)}(t,\boldsymbol{\beta},\tilde{\Phi})}{S^{(0)}(t,\boldsymbol{\beta},\tilde{\Phi})} - \left[\kappa(t,\boldsymbol{\beta})S_0(t,\boldsymbol{\beta},\tilde{\Phi})\right]^{-1}\int_0^{\tau} L(s,\boldsymbol{\beta})\kappa(s,\boldsymbol{\beta})d\tilde{\Phi}(s,\boldsymbol{\beta}),$$

$$\kappa(t,\boldsymbol{\beta}) = \exp\left\{-\int_0^t \frac{S_0^*(u,\boldsymbol{\beta})}{S^{(0)}(u,\boldsymbol{\beta},\tilde{G})} d\tilde{\Phi}(u-,\boldsymbol{\beta})\right\},$$

$$L(t,\boldsymbol{\beta}) = \frac{S^{(1)}(t,\boldsymbol{\beta},\tilde{\Phi})S_0^*(t,\boldsymbol{\beta}) - S^{(0)}(t,\boldsymbol{\beta},\tilde{\Phi})S_1^*(t,\boldsymbol{\beta})}{S^{(0)}(t,\boldsymbol{\beta},\tilde{\Phi})}, \tag{81}$$

and

$$S_j^*(t,\boldsymbol{\beta}) = \sum_{i=1}^{n} Y_i(t)\left[\frac{\mathbf{Z}_i\exp\{-\boldsymbol{\beta}\mathbf{Z}_i\} - (\partial\tilde{\Phi}(t-,\boldsymbol{\beta})/\partial\boldsymbol{\beta})}{\exp\{-\boldsymbol{\beta}\mathbf{Z}_i\} - \tilde{\Phi}(t-,\boldsymbol{\beta}\}}\right]^j$$
$$\exp\{2\boldsymbol{\beta}\mathbf{Z}\}\left\{\frac{\partial[1/(1+\tilde{\Phi}(t-)\exp\{\boldsymbol{\beta}\mathbf{Z}_i\})]}{\partial\boldsymbol{\beta}}\right\},$$

for $j = 0{,}1$; $\boldsymbol{\beta} = \hat{\boldsymbol{\beta}}$.

Parametric proportional odds model can be fit by a maximum likelihood method and are available in most statistical packages, such as SAS, SPlus and STATA (Klein and Zhang, 2005). Scheike's timereg package (Martinussen and Scheike, 2006) can be used to fit a semi-parametric proportional odds model with prop.odds function.

To illustrate this model we consider the burn data with four covariates. First, we fit a parametric proportional odds model using the SAS Proc Lifereg procedure and specify Dist = logistic as an option in the model statement. Next we fit a semi-parametric proportional odds model using timereg prop.odds function. Table 9 gives the results. Here we see again a strong effect of race and marginal effects of treatment and gender. Here $\exp\{-0.70\} = 0.50$ is the odds ratio in favor of survival for patients given the new treatment. That is, patients given the standard treatment have an odds 2 as large of having an infection than patients given standard treatment.

A quite general approach to censored data regression has recently been suggested by Andersen et al. (2003). This general technique can be applied to

Table 9
Illustration of the proportional odds model

Effect	Parametric Proportional Odds			Semi-Parametric Proportional Odds		
	Estimate	SE	p-value	Estimate	SE	p-value
Method of care	−0.67	0.35	0.0531	−0.70	0.37	0.0573
Gender	−0.86	0.44	0.0516	−0.85	0.44	0.0496
Race	2.39	1.02	0.0159	2.39	1.02	0.0191
Percent burned	0.003	0.008	0.6957	−0.005	0.009	0.5880

censored survival data and as discussed in the next section to competing risks data. The general formulation is as follows. Let $(T_i,\ i = 1, \ldots, n)$ be the independent and identically distributed random variables. Each T_i could be a scalar random variable, a vector $\mathbf{T}_i = (T_{ij},\ j = 1, \ldots, p)$ or a process $T_i = (\mathbb{X}_i(t), t \geq 0)$. We are interested in a regression model for θ the expectation of some function f of T_i. That is

$$\theta = E[f(T_i)], \tag{82}$$

which may also be multivariate or a function of time. We suppose that we have made available an (approximately) unbiased estimator, $\hat{\theta}$, for θ. Examples are T_i is continuous and f is the identity function which yields $\theta = E[T_i]$, the mean; T_i Bernoulli and $f(T_i) = I[T_i = 1]$ so $\theta = p = P[T_i = 1]$; and $T_1, \ldots,\ T_n$ are non-negative lifetimes and $f(T_i) = I[T_i > t]$ so $\theta = S(t) = P[T_i > t]$.

Suppose that in addition to T_i we have covariates $\mathbf{Z}_i$ that are an independent and identically distributed sample from a distribution Ω. Then

$$\theta = E[f(T_i)] = E[E[f(T_i|\mathbf{Z}]] = \int E[f(T_i)|\mathbf{Z}_i]d\Omega(\mathbf{Z}_i)$$

and $\hat{\theta}$ is an unbiased estimator for this marginal expectation. If we take Ω to be the empirical distribution function and we let

$$\theta_i = E[f(T_i|\mathbf{Z}_i], \tag{83}$$

then $\theta = \sum_i \theta_i/n$. This means that $E[\hat{\theta}] = \sum_i \theta_i/n$ and the "leave-one-out" statistics $\hat{\theta}_{-i}$ based on the sample of size $n-1$ with T_i removed from the sample is unbiased for $\sum_{l \neq i} \theta_l/(n-1)$. This implies that the so-called pseudo-observation, $\hat{\theta}_i$, defined by

$$\hat{\theta}_i = n\hat{\theta} - (n-1)\hat{\theta}_{-i} = \hat{\theta} + (n-1)(\hat{\theta} - \hat{\theta}_{-i}), \tag{84}$$

is an unbiased estimate for $\theta_i = E[f(T_i)|\mathbf{Z}_i]$.

We exploit the relationship (83) using a generalized linear model with a link function $\phi()$. That is

$$\phi(\theta_i) = \boldsymbol{\beta}^t \mathbf{Z}_i \tag{85}$$

with an inverse link function (mean function)

$$\mu_i = \phi^{-1}(\boldsymbol{\beta}^t \mathbf{Z}_i). \tag{86}$$

Here we are incorporating an intercept term by a column of 1's in $\mathbf{Z}_i$. We estimate model parameters using the theory of generalized estimating equation (GEE) methods (cf. Liang and Zeger, 1986; Zeger and Liang, 1986). The estimating equations to be solved are

$$\mathbf{U}(\boldsymbol{\beta}) = \sum_{i=1}^{n} \left[\frac{\partial \mu_i}{\partial \boldsymbol{\beta}}\right]^t \mathbf{V}_i = \sum_{i=1}^{n} \mathbf{U}_i(\boldsymbol{\beta}) = \mathbf{0}, \tag{87}$$

where $\mathbf{V}_i$ is a working covariance matrix for $\hat{\theta}_i$. In most applications $\mathbf{V}_i$ is the identity matrix. The estimator of $\boldsymbol{\beta}$ is found by solving (87). The covariance of the $\hat{\boldsymbol{\beta}}$ is found using a "sandwich estimator" defined by

$$\hat{\sum} = \mathbf{I}(\boldsymbol{\beta})^{-1}\widehat{\text{var}}(\mathbf{U}(\boldsymbol{\beta}))\mathbf{I}(\boldsymbol{\beta})^{-1} \tag{88}$$

where

$$\mathbf{I}(\boldsymbol{\beta}) = \sum_{i=1}^{n} \left[\frac{\partial \mu_i}{\partial \boldsymbol{\beta}}\right]^t \mathbf{V}_i^{-1} \left[\frac{\partial \mu_i}{\partial \boldsymbol{\beta}}\right] \tag{89}$$

and

$$\widehat{\text{var}}(\mathbf{U}(\boldsymbol{\beta})) = \sum_{i=1}^{n} \mathbf{U}_i(\hat{\boldsymbol{\beta}})^t \mathbf{U}(\hat{\boldsymbol{\beta}}). \tag{90}$$

This technique can be applied in a number of situations. One can use the approach to model the relationship between covariates and survival at a single point of time or at a grid of time points by using pseudo-observations based on the Kaplan–Meier estimator (3). One can develop additional regression models for the cumulative hazard rate by using pseudo-values based on the Nelson–Aalen estimator (5). In Andersen et al. (2003) and Andersen and Klein (2007) the technique is used to model multistate probabilities. In the next section, we will show how the approach can be used to model competing risk probabilities.

Here we shall look at modeling the effect of covariates on the mean time to an event or on the mean log-survival function in the infection data set (see Andersen et al., 2004). The models discussed earlier in this section induce regression models for the mean of the (log) survival time, but these models are highly non-linear and hard to interpret. We shall look at modeling the restricted mean defined by

$$\mu(\tau) = E[\min(T, \tau)] = \int_0^{\tau} S(u)du, \tag{91}$$

since when the last observation is censored the mean is not well defined. In our example we shall take $\tau = 60$ which is slightly larger than the largest death at day 51 but smaller than the largest on study time. We shall examine two models:

$$\mu(\tau|\mathbf{Z}) = \beta_0 + \boldsymbol{\beta}^t\mathbf{Z}$$

and

$$E[\ln(\min(T, \tau))|\mathbf{Z}] = \beta_0 + \boldsymbol{\beta}^t\mathbf{Z}.$$

The model for $E[\ln(T)]$ is the so-called accelerated failure model which is usually analyzed by assuming a parametric model for the residuals. Semi-parametric approaches to the accelerated failure time model can be found in Buckley and James (1979), Ritov (1990) and Leurgans (1987), but these approaches have a number of numerical difficulties. Here we construct pseudo-observation for $E[T]$ using the Kaplan–Meier estimator (3) in Eq. (84). For $E[\ln(T)]$ we compute

Table 10
Regression models for $E[T]$ and $E[\ln T]$

Effect	Models for $E[T]$			Models for $E[\ln(T)]$		
	β	SE	p-value	β	SE	p-value
Intercept	49.98	5.63		3.775	0.176	
Z_1: Method of care	9.22	4.01	0.0365	0.332	0.173	0.0544
Z_2: Gender	7.25	5.39	0.1789	0.355	0.185	0.0545
Z_3: Race	−15.90	5.57	0.0044	−0.708	0.150	<0.0001
Z_4: Percent burned	−0.06		0.5830	−0.002	0.005	0.7467

pseudo-observations from

$$\ln[t_1] + \int_{\ln[t_1]}^{\ln[\min(t_D,\tau)]} \hat{S}(u)du + (\tau - t_D)^+ \hat{S}(t_D), \tag{92}$$

where $t_1 < \cdots < t_D$ are the ordered event times. Once the pseudo-observations are computed we fit the GEE estimates using $V = 1$ in (87–90). Any package which computes GEE can be used in the second step. Note that the pseudo-observations are computed only once since they do not involve the **Z**'s.

Table 10 shows the results for both the $E[T]$ and $E[\ln T]$ models using the identity link. Here we see that patients with the new method of care have on average 9.22 more days free of infection than those given the old bath solution.

SAS macros to compute pseudo-values for the restricted mean and the survival function are available on our website at www.biostat.mcw/Software.html. Also available on our website are R functions to compute the pseudo-values for these parameters.

5. Regression models for competing risks

For competing risk data we often wish to model the effect of covariates for a specific cause of failure. For competing risks data we can model the cause-specific hazard rate for a given cause, we can model the cumulative incidence function indirectly by modeling each of the J crude hazard rates and combining them using (16), or we can model directly the effects of covariates on the cumulative incidence function. In this section, we will briefly discuss a few techniques to fit these models and provide some comments on the merits of these approaches. We assume, for simplicity, that the first competing risk is of interest and that all other risks can be combined into a second competing risk.

The first approach is to model the cause-specific hazard function (15). Here we can use any of the models and techniques discussed in the previous section with the modification that events from causes other than the cause of interest are treated as censored observations. No new software is needed for these models.

One needs, however, to interpret the results in terms of the cause-specific hazard rate only since the cumulative incidence function for the cause of interest is not a simple function of the cause-specific hazard rate for the cause of interest, but rather a function of all the J competing risks.

A second approach is to model the cumulative incidence function for the cause of interest by modeling the cause-specific hazards for all J risks and combining these using an Aalen–Johansen (1978) estimator. That is

$$\hat{\mathrm{C}}\mathrm{I}(t|\mathbf{Z}) = \int_0^t \exp\left\{ -\sum_{j=1}^{2} \hat{\Lambda}_j(u - |\mathbf{Z})\right\} d\hat{\Lambda}_1(u|\mathbf{Z}). \tag{93}$$

Cheng et al. (1998) proposed modeling $\mathrm{CI}(t|\mathbf{Z})$ using a proportional hazards regression model for all causes. In Shen and Cheng (1999), the additive model for the cause-specific hazards was considered. Scheike and Zhang (2003) proposed using the mixed additive–multiplicative model for the hazards. Andersen et al. (1993) derived a variance estimator for a general multistate model, which can be applied to estimate the standard error of $\hat{\mathrm{C}}\mathrm{I}(t|\mathbf{Z})$. With this approach the relationship between the covariates and the CIF is highly non-linear and quite difficult to interpret.

The third approach is to model the CIF directly. Here we discuss three methods to perform estimation for this approach.

The first is due to Fine and Gray (1999) and is based on modeling the sub-distribution hazard (29) defined in the discussion of Gray's test in Section 3. A proportional sub-distribution hazard model is given by

$$\lambda^*(t|\mathbf{Z}) = \lambda_0^*(t)\exp\{\boldsymbol{\beta}\mathbf{Z}\}, \tag{94}$$

where $\lambda_0^*(t)$ is an unknown baseline hazard function. Since

$$\mathrm{CI}(t|\mathbf{Z}) = \exp\left\{ -\int_0^t \lambda^*(u|\mathbf{Z})du \right\} = \left[\exp\left\{ -\int_0^t \lambda_0^*(u)du \right\}\right]^{\exp(\boldsymbol{\beta}\mathbf{Z})} \tag{95}$$

we can interpret the covariate effect on the CIF directly.

With complete data and no censoring, Fine and Gray (1999) proposed a modified partial likelihood method. A modified risk set at the time of failure for the ith individual is defined by $R_i = \{l\colon (X_l \geq X_i) \cup (X_l \leq X_i, \varepsilon_l \neq 1\}$. That is R_i is the set of all individuals yet to fail at time X_i or who failed from cause 2 prior to X_i. If we set $X_i = \infty$ if the ith individual failed from a cause other than that of interest, standard partial likelihood methods can be applied. This makes estimation available in all statistical packages.

For a censored sample, the counting process $N_i(t) = I[T_i \leq t, \varepsilon_i = 1]$ and the modified risk indicator $Y_i(t) = 1 - N_i(t-)$ are not always observable for censored individuals. Let C_i be the potential censoring time for the ith subject and define $r_i(t) = I[C_i \geq T_i \wedge t]$. Then $r_i(t)N_i(t)$ and $r_i(t)Y_i(t)$ are computable for all time points. Fine and Gray proposed estimating the regression parameter $\boldsymbol{\beta}$ by solving a modified score equation

$$\mathbf{U}(\boldsymbol{\beta}) = \sum_{i=1}^{n} \int_0^{\tau} \left\{ \mathbf{Z}_i - \frac{\sum_{l=1}^{n} w_l(s) Y_l(s) \mathbf{Z}_l \exp\{\boldsymbol{\beta}\mathbf{Z}_l\}}{\sum_{l=1}^{n} w_l(s) Y_l(s) \exp\{\boldsymbol{\beta}\mathbf{Z}_l\}} \right\} w_i(s) dN_i(s), \tag{96}$$

where $w_i(t) = r_i(t)\hat{G}(t)/\hat{G}(T_i \wedge t)$ and $\hat{G}(t)$ the Kaplan–Meier estimator of the survival function of the censoring distribution. The cumulative baseline sub-distribution hazard can be estimated by a Breslow-type estimator

$$\Lambda_0^*(t) = \sum_{i=1}^{n} \int_0^{t} \frac{w_i(u) dN_i(u)}{\sum_{l=1}^{n} w_l(s) Y_l(s) \exp\{\boldsymbol{\beta}\mathbf{Z}_l\}}. \tag{97}$$

Fine and Gray (1999) derived consistent variance estimators, which consider the variation caused by using an estimated censoring survival function. The estimator is given by the sandwich estimator

$$\widehat{\text{var}}(\hat{\boldsymbol{\beta}}) = \left[\mathbf{I}(\hat{\boldsymbol{\beta}})\right]^{-1} \hat{\Sigma} \left[\mathbf{I}(\hat{\boldsymbol{\beta}})\right]^{-1}. \tag{98}$$

Here we have

$$\mathbf{I}(\boldsymbol{\beta}) = -\partial \mathbf{U}(\boldsymbol{\beta})/\partial \boldsymbol{\beta}$$

and

$$\hat{\sum} = \sum_{i=1}^{n} (\hat{\boldsymbol{\eta}}_i + \hat{\boldsymbol{\psi}}_i)^t (\hat{\boldsymbol{\eta}}_i + \hat{\boldsymbol{\psi}}_i),$$

where

$$\hat{\boldsymbol{\eta}}_i = \int_0^{\tau} \left[\mathbf{Z}_i - \frac{S^{(1)}(\hat{\boldsymbol{\beta}}, t)}{S^{(0)}(\hat{\boldsymbol{\beta}}, t)} \right] w_i(t) d\hat{M}_i(t),$$

$$\hat{\boldsymbol{\psi}}_i = \int_0^{\tau} \frac{\left[-\sum_{l=1}^{n} \int_0^{\tau} \left[\mathbf{Z}_l - (S^{(1)}(\hat{\boldsymbol{\beta}}, t)/S^{(0)}(\hat{\boldsymbol{\beta}}, t)) \right] I(X_i < u \le t) w_l(t) d\hat{M}_l(t) \right]}{\sum_{l=1}^{n} I[X_l \ge u]} d\hat{M}_i^C(u)$$

$$S^{(0)}(\boldsymbol{\beta}, t) = \sum_{i=1}^{n} w_i(t) Y_i(t) \exp\{\boldsymbol{\beta}\mathbf{Z}_i\}, S^{(1)}(\boldsymbol{\beta}, t) = \sum_{i=1}^{n} w_i(t) \mathbf{Z}_i Y_i(t) \exp\{\boldsymbol{\beta}\mathbf{Z}_i\},$$

$$\hat{M}_i(t) = N_i(t) - \int_0^{t} Y_i(u) d\hat{\Lambda}_0^*(u)$$

and

$$\hat{M}_i^C(t) = N_i^c(t) - \int_0^t I[X_i \geq u]\left[\frac{\sum_{l=1}^{n} dN_l^c(u)}{\sum_{l=1}^{n} I[X_l \geq u]}\right] \quad \text{with } N_i^c(t) = I[X_i \leq t, \delta_i = 0].$$

Estimates of regression parameters in this model are available in the crr function of the cmprsk R-library created by Robert Gray. Sun et al. (2006) considered an alternative mixed sub-distribution hazard model of the form

$$\lambda_0^*(t|\mathbf{Z}_1, \mathbf{Z}_2) = \boldsymbol{\alpha}(t)\mathbf{Z}_1 + \lambda_0^*(t)\exp(\boldsymbol{\beta}\mathbf{Z}_2), \tag{99}$$

where $\boldsymbol{\alpha}(t)$ is an unknown q-vector of time-varying components representing the effects of covariates $\mathbf{Z}_1$ and $\boldsymbol{\beta}$ a p-vector of unknown regression parameters for the effects of covariates $\mathbf{Z}_2$.

A second approach to modeling the CIF is the pseudo-value approach discussed in Section 4. For competing risk data this approach is discussed in Klein and Andersen (2005) and Klein (2006). For competing risks data we consider a grid of time points, $\tau_1, \ldots, \tau_M$. At each grid time point we estimate the CIF using (13) based on the complete data set, $\hat{\mathrm{CI}}(\tau_h)$ and based on the sample of size $n-1$ obtained by deleting the ith observation, $\hat{\mathrm{CI}}^{(i)}(\tau_h)$, respectively. The pseudo-value for the ith subject at time τ_h is defined as $\hat{\theta}_{ih} = n\hat{\mathrm{CI}}(\tau_h) - (n-1)\hat{\mathrm{CI}}^{(i)}(\tau_h)$. Let $\theta_{ih} = \mathrm{CI}(\tau_h|\mathbf{Z}_i)$ be the outcome of interest. We model θ_{ih} by

$$\phi(\theta_{ih}) = \alpha_h + \boldsymbol{\gamma}\mathbf{Z}_i, \tag{100}$$

where ϕ is a known link function. Common link functions such as logit link with $\phi(\theta) = \log(\theta/(1-\theta))$ and the complementary log–log link with $\phi(\theta) = \log[-\log(1-\theta)]$ can be applied here. Note that the complimentary log–log link gives models equivalent to the proportional hazards models on the sub-distribution hazard. The logit link gives a proportional odds model for the CIF. Estimates of the $\boldsymbol{\alpha}$'s and $\boldsymbol{\gamma}$'s are obtained using the pseudo-score Eq. (87). The sandwich variance estimate (87)–(90) is used to estimate the standard error. To numerically apply this approach, Klein and Andersen (2005) suggested computing the pseudo-values at a preset grid time points first, and then using Proc GENMOD procedure in SAS for models with independent or empirical working covariance model. A SAS macro and an R function to compute the pseudo-values for the cumulative incidence function are also available on our website.

The third approach to direct regression modeling of the cumulative incidence function is based on the IPCW approach discussed at the end of Section 2. We will illustrate using a generalized additive model

$$\phi(\mathrm{CI}(t|\mathbf{Z})) = \mathbf{A}(t)\mathbf{Z}, \tag{101}$$

where ϕ is a known link function, $\mathbf{A}(t)$ a $p+1$ dimensional vector of regression effects and $\mathbf{Z}=(1, Z_1, \ldots, Z_p)$ has the first element equal to 1 to allow for a baseline cumulative incidence. The $\log(\phi(x)=\ln(1-x))$, logit $(\phi(x)=\ln(x/(1-x))$ or the complimentary log–log function $(\phi(x)=\ln(-\ln(1-\mathrm{x}))$ are commonly used link functions. The log-link function gives a model like Aalen's additive model (52) in the non-competing risk framework.

Scheike and Zhang (2006) proposed estimating $\mathbf{A}()$ by solving a pseudo-score equation at each distinct event time, $t_1<t_2<\cdots<t_D$. That is one solves $\mathrm{U}(t_i, \boldsymbol{\beta})=0$

$$\mathbf{U}(t_i, \boldsymbol{\beta})=\sum_{l=1}^{n} \frac{\partial\phi^{-1}(\mathbf{A}(t_i)\mathbf{Z}_l)}{\partial\mathbf{A}(t_i)}\left\{\frac{I[X_l \leq t_i, \varepsilon_l=1]I[\mathrm{C}_l \geq X_l \wedge t_i]}{\hat{G}(X_l \wedge t_i)}-\partial\phi^{-1}(\mathbf{A}(t_i)\mathbf{Z}_l)\right\}, \tag{102}$$

where $\hat{G}$ is an estimate of the survival function of the censoring times. To estimate the variance define

$$\mathbf{I}(t, \mathbf{A}(t))=\sum_{i=1}^{n}\left[\frac{\partial\phi^{-1}(\mathbf{A}(t)\mathbf{Z}_i)}{\partial\mathbf{A}(t)}\right]\left[\frac{\partial\phi^{-1}(\mathbf{A}(t)\mathbf{Z}_i)}{\partial\mathbf{A}(t)}\right]^t, \tag{103}$$

then we can estimate the variance of $\hat{\mathbf{A}}(t)$ by

$$\hat{\Sigma}(t)=\sum_{i=1}^{n} \hat{\mathbf{W}}_i^A(t)\hat{\mathbf{W}}_i^A(t)^t, \tag{104}$$

Table 11
Regression models for relapse

	Crude Hazard Cox Model			Fine and Gray			Andersen and Klein		
	β	SE	p	β	SE	p	β	SE	p
Donor type									
Matched unrelated	0.011	0.153	0.94	−0.32	0.16	<0.01	−0.037	0.16	0.02
Mismatched unrelated	−0.944	0.364	0.01	−1.37	0.38	<0.01	−1.61	0.45	<0.01
Disease									
AML	−0.0271	0.145	0.06	−0.17	0.15	0.24	−0.17	0.15	0.27
CML	−0.721	0.157	<0.001	−0.75	0.16	<0.01	−0.66	0.17	<0.01
Stage of disease									
Intermediate	0.640	0.153	<0.001	0.51	0.15	<0.01	0.54	0.16	<0.01
Advanced	1.8487	0.150	<0.001	1.51	0.15	<0.01	1.55	0.15	<0.01
Karnofsky									
>90	−0.118	0.142	0.41	0.17	0.15	0.26	0.28	0.16	0.07

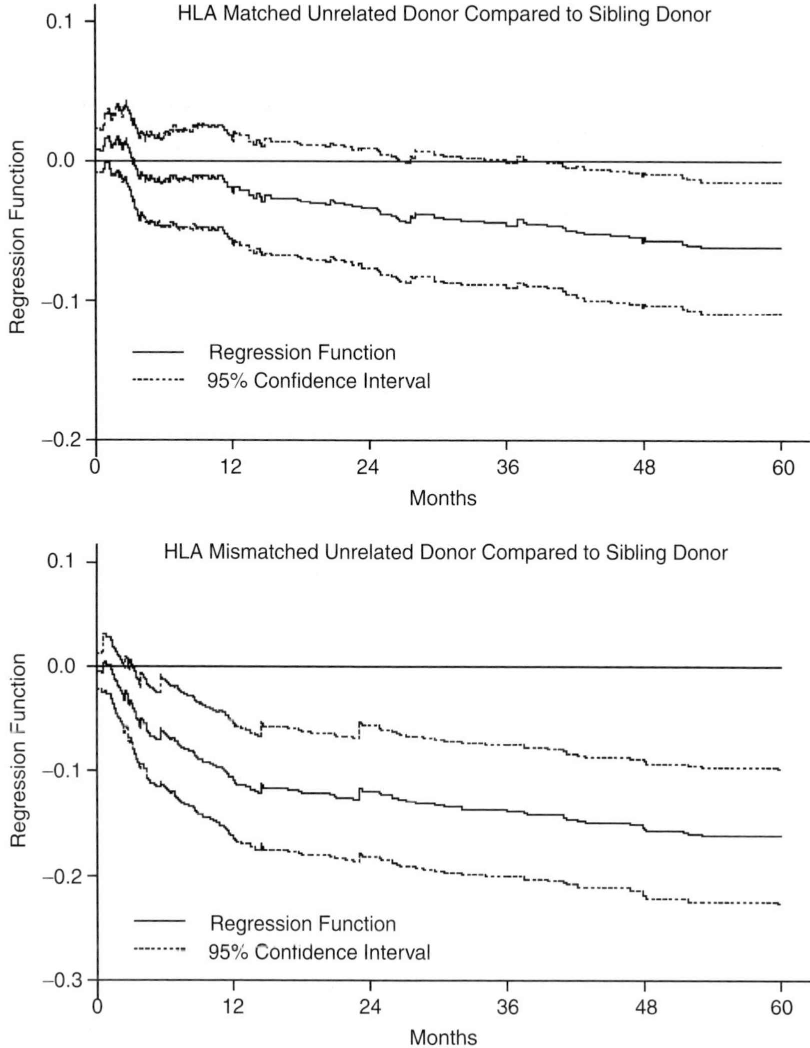

Fig. 5a. Regression function estimates for treatment related mortality CIF using log link function.

where

$$\mathbf{W}_i^A(t) = \{\mathbf{I}(t, \mathbf{A}(t))\}^{-1}\{\xi_i(t) + \psi_i(t)\},$$

$$\xi_i(t) = \frac{\partial \phi^{-1}(\mathbf{A}(t)\mathbf{Z}_i)}{\partial \mathbf{A}(t)} \left\{ \frac{I[X_i \leq t, \varepsilon_i = 1]I[C_i \geq X_i \wedge t]}{\hat{G}(X_i \wedge t)} - \partial \phi^{-1}(\mathbf{A}(t)\mathbf{Z}_i) \right\}$$

and

$$\psi_i(t) = \int_0^t \left\{ \sum_{l=1}^n \frac{\partial \phi^{-1}(\mathbf{A}(t)\mathbf{Z}_l) I[X_l \leq t, \varepsilon_l = 1] I[\mathrm{C}_l \geq X_l \wedge t]}{\partial \mathbf{A}(t) \qquad \hat{G}(X_l \wedge t)} I(u \leq X_l \leq t) \right\} \frac{d\hat{M}_i^C(u)}{\sum_{l=1}^n I[X_l \geq u]}.$$

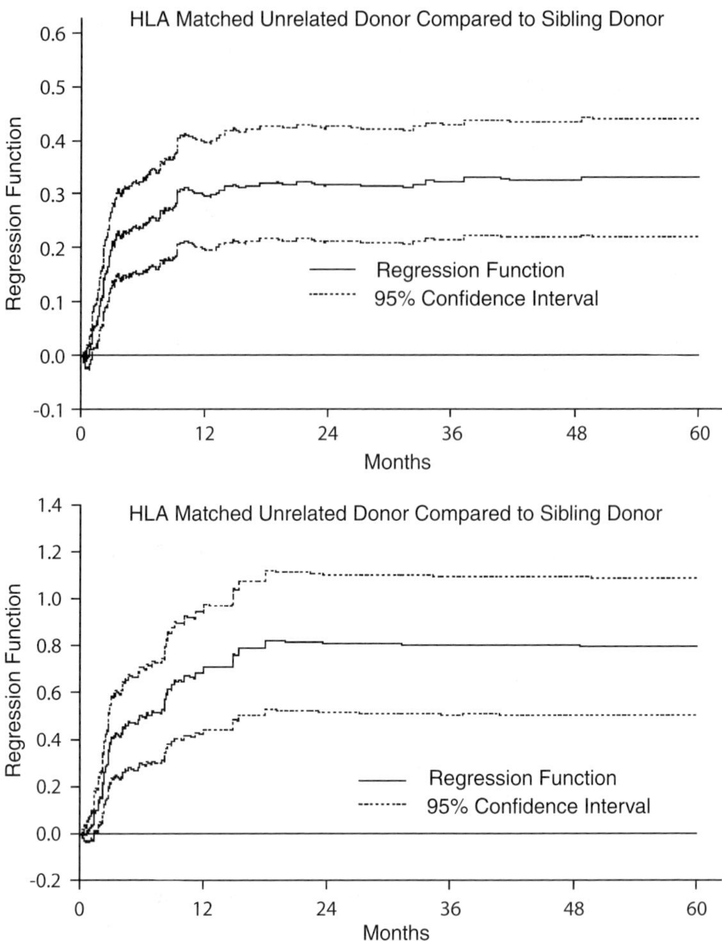

Fig. 5b. Regression function estimates for relapse using log link function.

One drawback of this approach is that one needs to estimate the censoring distribution for each individual. This is done by using a Kaplan–Meier estimator.

We illustrate these methods using the bone marrow transplant data set. Recall that the data set consists of 1715 patients with 1225, 383 and 108 patients receiving HLA-identical sibling, HLA-matched unrelated and HLA-mismatched unrelated transplant, respectively. The initial Karnofsky score was greater than or equal to 90 in 1382 cases. The study had 537 patients with acute lymphoblastic leukemia (ALL), 340 with acute myelogenous leukemia (AML) and 838 with chronic myelogenous leukemia (CML). Patients were transplanted in an early (1026), intermediate (410) or advanced (279) disease state.

The study has two competing risks, treatment-related death (death in complete remission, $n = 557/1716$ cases) and relapse (recurrence of the primary disease, $n = 311/1716$ cases). For illustration purpose, we only report the results of donor effect on relapse based on: (1) fitting a Cox proportional hazard model to the crude relapse rate; (2) fitting a Fine and Gray proportional sub-distributional hazards regression and (3) the Klein and Andersen's pseudo-value approach using a complementary log–log model with the identity working covariance matrix on $1-\mathrm{CI}(t)$, which is equivalent to Fine and Gray's model. For the pseudo-value model, 10 equally spaced points on the event scale were used. The results are in Table 11. In Fig. 5a and 5b, we present the estimated regression function and 95% pointwise confidence intervals for $\mathbf{A}(t)$ based on fitting model (101) using the link $\phi(x) = -\log(1-x)$. Here we show only the curves for donor type. Note that the Cox model based on the crude hazard rate suggests no difference between the HLA-matched sibling and the matched unrelated groups. The other methods suggest that the matched unrelated group has a lower relapse cumulative incidence perhaps due to more of a graft-versus-leukemia effect.

Acknowledgements

This research was partially supported by a grant (R01 CA54706-12) from the National Cancer Institute.

References

Aalen, O.O. (1978). Nonparametric inference for a family of counting processes. *The Annals of Statistics* **6**, 701–726.

Aalen, O.O. (1989). A linear regression model for the analysis of life times. *Statistics in Medicine* **8**, 907–925.

Aalen, O.O. (1993). Further results on the non-parametric linear regression model in survival analysis. *Statistics in Medicine* **12**, 1569–1588.

Aalen, O.O., Johansen, S. (1978). An empirical transition matrix for nonhomogeneous Markov chains based on censored observations. *Scandinavian Journal of Statistics* **5**, 141–150.

Andersen, P.K., Borgan, Ø., Gill, R.D., Keiding, N.Linear non-parametric tests for comparison of counting processes, with application to censored survival data (with discussion). *International Statistical Review* **50**, 219–258, Amendment: 1984, 52, 225.

Andersen, P.K., Borgan, Ø., Gill, R.D., Keiding, N. (1993). *Statistical Models Based on Counting Processes*. Springer, New York.

Andersen, P.K., Hansen, M.A., Klein, J.P. (2004). Regression analysis of restricted mean survival time based on pseudo-observations. *Lifetime Data Analysis* **10**, 335–350.

Andersen, P.K., Klein, J.P. (2007). Regression analysis for multistate models based on a pseudo-value approach, with applications to bone marrow transplantation studies. *Scandinavian Journal of Statistics* **34**, 3–16.

Andersen, P.K., Klein, J.P., Rosthøl, S. (2003). Generalized linear models for correlated pseudo-observations with applications to multi-state models. *Biometrika* **90**, 15–27.

Bagdonavičius, V.B., Nikulin, M.S. (1999). Generalized proportional hazards model based on modified partial likelihood. *Lifetime Data Analysis* **5**, 329–350.

Bajorunaite, R., Klein, J.P. (2007). Two sample tests of the equality of two cumulative incidence functions. *Computational Statistics and Data Analysis* **51**, 4209–4281.

Basu, A.P., Klein, J.P. (1982). Some recent results in competing risk theory. In: Crowley, J., Johnson, R. (Eds.), *Survival Analysis*. IMS, NY, pp. 216–229.

Bennett, S. (1983). Analysis of survival data by the proportional odds model. *Statistics in Medicine* **2**, 273–277.

Bhattacharyya, M., Klein, J.P. (2005). A note on testing in Aalen's additive hazards regression model. *Statistics in Medicine* **24**, 2235–2240.

Borgan, Ø., Liestøl, K. (1990). A note on confidence intervals and bands for the survival curve based on transformations. *Scandinavian Journal of Statistics* **17**, 35–41.

Breslow, N.E. (1974). Covariance analysis of censored survival data. *Biometrics* **30**, 89–99.

Buckley, J., James, I. (1979). Linear regression with censored data. *Biometrika* **66**, 429–436.

Chen, K., Jin, Z., Ying, Z. (2002). Semiparametric analysis of transformation models with censored data. *Biometrika* **89**, 659–668.

Cheng, S.C., Fine, J.P., Wei, L.J. (1998). Prediction of cumulative incidence function under the proportional hazards model. *Biometrics* **54**, 219–228.

Cheng, S.C., Wei, L.J., Ying, Z. (1995). Analysis of transformation models with censored data. *Biometrika* **92**, 835–845.

Chung, C.F. (1986). Formulae for probabilities associated with Wiener and Brownian bridge processes. Technical Report 79, Laboratory for Research in Statistics and Probability, Carleton University, Ottawa, Canada.

Cox, D.R. (1972). Regression models and life-tables (with discussion). *Journal of the Royal Statistical Society B* **34**, 187–220.

Efron, B. (1967). The two sample problem with censored data. In: Le Cam, L.M., Neyman, J. (Eds.), *Proceedings of the Fifth Berkeley Symposium on Mathematical Statistics and Probability*. vol. 4. Prentice-Hall, New York, pp. 831–853.

Efron, B. (1977). The efficiency of Cox's likelihood function for censored data. *Journal of the American Statistical Association* **72**, 557–565.

Fine, J., Ying, Z., Wei, L.J. (1998). On the linear transformation model with censored data. *Journal of American Statistical Association* **85**, 980–986.

Fine, J.P., Gray, J.P. (1999). A proportional hazards model for the sub distribution of a competing risks. *Journal of the American Statistical Association* **94**, 496–509.

Finkelstein, D.M. (1986). A proportional hazards model for interval-censored failure time data. *Biometrics* **42**, 845–854.

Fleming, T.R., Harrington, D.P. (1981). A class of hypothesis tests for one and two samples of censored survival data. *Communications in Statistics* **10**, 763–794.

Gandy, A., Therneau, T., Aalen, O. (2007). Global tests in the additive hazards regression model. *Statistics in Medicine* (in press).

Gehan, E.A. (1965). A generalized Wilcoxon test for comparing arbitrarily singly censored samples. *Biometrika* **52**, 203–223.

Gill, R.D. (1980). *Censoring and Stochastic Integrals*. Mathematisch Centrum, Mathematical Centre Tracts, Amsterdam, p. 124.

Goggins, W.B., Finkelstein, D.M. (2000). A proportional hazards model for multivariate interval-censored failure time data. *Biometrics* **56**, 940–943.

Gooley, T.A., Leisenring, W., Crowley, J., Storer, B. (1999). Estimation of failure probabilities in the presence of competing risks: New representations of old estimators. *Statistics in Medicine* **18**, 695–706.

Gray, R.J. (1988). A class of K-sample tests for comparing the cumulative incidence of a competing risk. *The Annals of Statistics* **16**, 1140–1154.

Greenwood, M. (1926). The natural duration of cancer. In: *Reports on Public Health and Medical Subjects*, vol. 33. His Majesty's Stationery Office, London, pp. 1–26.

Guerts, J.H.L. (1987). On the small sample performance of Efron's and Gill's version of the product limit estimator under proportional hazards. *Biometrics* **43**, 683–692.

Hall, W.J., Wellner, J.A. (1980). Confidence bands for a survival curve from censored data. *Biometrika* **67**, 133–143.

Huffer, F.W., McKeague, I.W. (1991). Weighted least squares estimation for Aalen's additive risk model. *Journal of the American Statistical Association* **86**, 114–129.

Ichida, J.M., Wassell, J.T., Keller, M.D., Ayers, L.W. (1993). Evaluation of protocol change in burn-care management using the Cox proportional hazards model with time-dependent covariates. *Statistics in Medicine* **12**, 301–310.

Kalbfleisch, J.D., Prentice, R.L. (1980). *The Statistical Analysis of Failure Time Data.* Wiley, New York.

Kaplan, E.L., Meier, P. (1958). Non-parametric estimation from incomplete observations. *Journal of the American Statistical Association* **53**, 457–481.

Klein, J.P. (1991). Small sample moments of some estimators of the variance of the Kaplan–Meier and Nelson–Aalen estimators. *Scandinavian Journal of Statistics* **18**, 333–340.

Klein, J.P. (2006). Modeling competing risks in cancer studies. *Statistics in Medicine* **25**, 1015–1034.

Klein, J.P., Andersen, P.K. (2005). Regression modelling of competing risks data based on pseudo-values of the cumulative incidence function. *Biometrics* **61**, 223–229.

Klein, J.P., Bajorunaite, R. (2004). Chapter 23 inference for competing risks. In: Balakrishnam, N., Rao, C.R. (Eds.), *Handbook of Statistics. Vol. 23, Advances in Survival Analysis.* Elsevier Science, NY, pp. 291–312.

Klein, J.P., Moeschberger, M.L. (2003). *Survival Analysis: Statistical Methods for Censored and Truncated data*, 2nd ed. Springer, New York.

Klein, J.P., Zhang, M.J. (2005). Survival analysis, software. In: Armitage, P., Colton, T. (Eds.), *Encyclopedia of Biostatistics*, 2nd ed., vol. 8. Wiley, New York, pp. 5377–5382.

Lai, T.L., Ying, Z. (1991). Estimating a distribution function with truncated and censored data. *The Annals of Statistics* **19**, 417–442.

Leurgans, S. (1987). Linear models, random censoring and synthetic data. *Biometrika* **74**, 301–309.

Liang, K.Y., Zeger, S.L. (1986). Longitudinal data analysis using generalized linear models. *Biometrika* **73**, 13–22.

Lin, D.Y. (1997). Non-parametric inference for cumulative incidence functions in competing risks studies. *Statistics in Medicine* **16**, 901–910.

Lin, D.Y., Ying, Z. (1994). Semiparametric analysis of the additive risk model. *Biometrika* **81**, 61–71.

Lin, D.Y., Ying, Z. (1997). Additive regression models for survival data. In: Lin, D.Y., Fleming, T.R. (Eds.), *Proceedings of the First Seattle Symposium in Biostatistics: Survival Analysis* Springer, New York, pp. 185–198.

Martinussen, T., Scheike, T.H. (2006). *Dynamic Regression Models for Survival Data.* Springer, New York.

Moeschberger, M.L., Klein, J.P. (1985). A comparison of several methods of estimating the survival function when there is extreme right censoring. *Biometrics* **41**, 253–259.

Murphy, S., Rossini, A., Van der Vaart, A. (1997). Maximum likelihood estimation in the proportional odds model. *Journal of American Statistical Association* **92**, 968–976.

Nair, V.N. (1984). Confidence bands for survival functions with censored data: A comparative study. *Technometrics* **14**, 265–275.

Nelson, W. (1972). Theory and applications of hazard plotting for censored failure data. *Technometrics* **14**, 945–965.

Pepe, M.S. (1991). Inference for events with dependent risks in multiple endpoint. *Journal of the American Statistical Association* **86**, 770–778.

Pepe, M.S., Fleming, T.R. (1989). Weighted Kaplan–Meier statistics: A class of distance tests for censored survival data. *Biometrics* **45**, 497–507.

Pepe, M.S., Mori, M.K. (1993). Marginal or conditional probability curves in summarizing competing risks failure time data? *Statistics in Medicine* **12**, 737–751.

Peto, R., Peto, J. (1972). Asymptotically efficient rank invariant test procedures (with discussion). *Journal of the Royal Statistical Society A* **135**, 185–206.

Pettitt, A.N. (1984). Proportional odds models for survival data and estimates using ranks. *Applied Statistics* **33**, 169–175.

Ritov, Y. (1990). Estimation in a linear regression model with censored data. *The Annals of Statistics* **18**, 303–328.

Robins, J., Rotnizky, A. (1992). Recovery of information and adjustment for dependent censoring using surrogate markers. In: Jewell, N., Dietz, K., Farewell, V. (Eds.), *AIDS Epidemiology – Methodological Issues*. Birkhauser, Boston, MA, pp. 298–331.

Rossini, A.J., Tsiatis, A.A. (1996). A semiparametric proportional odds regression model for the analysis of current status data. *Journal of the American Statistical Association* **91**, 713–721.

Scheike, T.H., Zhang, M.J. (2002). An additive multiplicative Cox–Aalen regression model. *Scandinavian Journal of Statistics* **29**, 75–88.
Scheike, T.H., Zhang, M.J. (2003). Extensions and applications of the Cox–Aalen survival model. *Biometrics* **59**, 1036–1045.
Scheike, T., Zhang, M.J. (2007). Directly modelling the regression effects in multistate models. *Scandinavian Journal of Statistics* **34**, 17–32.
Shen, Y., Cheng, S.C. (1999). Confidence bands for cumulative incidence curves under the additive risk model. *Biometrics* **55**, 1093–1100.
Sickle-Santanello, B.J., Farrar, W.B., Keyhani-Rofagha, S., Klein, J.P., Pearl, D., Laufman, H., Dobson, J., O'Toole, R.V. (1988). A reproducible system of flow cytometric DNA. Analysis of paraffin embedded solid tumors: Technical improvements and statistical analysis. *Cytometry* **9**, 594–599.
Sun, J.G. (2006). *The Statistical Analysis of Interval-Censored Failure Time Data*. Springer, New York.
Sun, L.Q., Kim, Y.J., Sun, J.G. (2004). Regression analysis of doubly censored failure time data using the additive hazards model. *Biometrics* **60**, 637–643.
Sun, L.Q., Liu, J.X., Sun, J.G., Zhang, MJ. (2006). Modeling the sub distribution of a competing risk. *Statistica Sinica* **16**(4).
Szydlo, R., Goldman, J.M., Klein, J.P., Gale, R.P., Ash, R.C., Bach, F.H., Bradley, B.A., Casper, J.T., Flomenberg, N., Gajewski, J.L., Gluchman, E., Henslee-Downey, P.J., Hows, J.M., Jacobsen, N., Kolb, H.-J., Lowenberg, B., Masaoka, T., Rowlings, P.A., Sondel, P.M., Van Bekkum, D.w., Van Rood, J.J., Vowels, M.R., Zhang, M.J., Horowitz, M.M. (1997). Results of allogeneic bone marrow transplants for leukemia using donors other than HLA-identical siblings. *Journal of Clinical Oncology* **15**, 1767–1777.
Tarone, R.E., Ware, J.H. (1977). On distribution-free tests for equality for survival distributions. *Biometrika* **64**, 156–160.
Therneau, T.M., Grambsch, P.M. (2000). *Modeling Survival Data: Extending the Cox Model*. Springer, New York.
Turnbull, B.W. (1974). Nonparametric estimation of a survivorship function with doubly censored data. *Journal of the American Statistical Association* **69**, 169–173.
Turnbull, B.W. (1976). The empirical distribution function with arbitrarily grouped, censored and truncated data. *Journal of the Royal Statistical Society B* **38**, 290–295.
Yang, S., Prentice, R.L. (1999). Semiparametric inference in the proportional odds regression model. *Journal of the American Statistical Association* **94**, 125–136.
Zeger, S.L., Liang, K.Y. (1986). Longitudinal data analysis for discrete and continuous outcomes. *Biometrics* **42**, 121–130.

Handbook of Statistics, Vol. 27
ISSN: 0169-7161

DOI: 10.1016/S0169-7161(07)27010-5

10

A Review of Statistical Analyses for Competing Risks

Melvin L. Moeschberger, Kevin P. Tordoff and Nidhi Kochar

Abstract

This paper reviews the statistical analyses of competing risks data. There is an extensive history of this topic; however, the literature is often confusing partially because it evolved over time. The available data for competing risks is in the form of time until event occurrence where T is the time from some suitable starting point until some cause of failure for each individual who fails, and δ_i *is an indicator variable equal to 1 if failure is due to the* ith *cause, 0 otherwise. In the latent failure time approach, one assumes that there are* k *potential failure times,* $X_1, X_2, \ldots, X_k$, *associated with each risk.* T *is then the min* $(X_1, X_2, \ldots, X_k)$ *and* δ_i *is an indicator variable equal to 1 if failure is due to the* ith *cause, 0 otherwise. References for the latent failure time model prior to the 1970s may be found in David and Moeschberger (1978), and more recently in Klein and Moeschberger (2003).*

The direction of the statistical analyses of competing risks studies changed dramatically after the identifiability problem for marginal distributions of the latent failure time model was pointed out by Tsiatis (1975), Prentice et al. (1978), and many others. At that time, interest centered on estimating identifiable competing risk probabilities. Most of the references cited in this paper deal with the more recent attempts to analyze competing risks data.

> I simply wish that, in a matter which so closely concerns the well being of the human race, no decision shall be made without all the knowledge which a little analysis and calculation can provide.
>
> Daniel Bernoulli (1766)

1. Introduction

In the competing risk problem, an individual or an experimental unit (referred to in this discussion as the subject) is observed until a particular event occurs in the presence of several events. Such events may preclude the occurrence of the main event of interest. A variety of disciplines may encounter problems involving competing risks. These include cancer research, reliability of physical equipment, economics, insurance assessments, and outcomes of preventive behaviors, among many other areas. Assessing the importance of these risks over a period of time has long been a concern of biostatisticians, demographers, vital statisticians, and actuaries.

The problem of assessing the effect of what the mortality pattern of a population would be if smallpox could be eradicated dates back to Daniel Bernoulli (1700–1782), one of the great scientists of the 18th century. Just a few years before Jenner inoculated an eight-year-old boy named James Phipps with cowpox; Bernoulli wrote a mathematical analysis of the problem and also encouraged the universal inoculation against smallpox. His analysis was first presented at the Royal Academy of Sciences in Paris during 1760 and later published in Bernoulli (1766).

As noted earlier, the subject under consideration is often exposed to several risks, but the eventual failure of the subject is attributed to only one of the risks, usually called the *cause of failure*. The available data for competing risks is in the form of time until event occurrence where T is the time from some suitable starting point until some cause of failure for each individual who fails, and δ_i is an indicator variable equal to 1 if failure is due to the ith cause, 0 otherwise. In the latent failure time approach, one assumes that there are k potential failure times, $X_1, X_2, \ldots, X_k$, associated with each risk. T is then the min $(X_1, X_2, \ldots, X_k)$ and δ_i is an indicator variable equal to 1 if failure is due to the ith cause, 0 otherwise. References for the latent failure time model prior to the 1970s may be found in David and Moeschberger (1978) and more recently in Klein and Moeschberger (2003).

The direction of the statistical analyses of competing risks studies changed dramatically after the identifiability problem for marginal distributions of the latent failure time model was pointed out by Tsiatis (1975), Prentice et al. (1978), and many others. At that time, interest centered on estimating identifiable competing risk probabilities. Such probabilities are represented by the crude (or cause-specific) hazard rate for cause i in the latent failure time model by

$$h_i(t) = \lim_{\Delta t \to 0} \frac{\Pr[t \leq X_i < t + \Delta t | T \geq t]}{\Delta t} \tag{1}$$

which is the conditional rate of occurrence for the ith cause of failure in the presence of all possible causes of failure, or by the cumulative incidence function

$$C_i(t) = \Pr[T \leq t, \delta_i = 1] = \int_0^t h_i(u) \exp\left\{ -\int_0^u \sum_{i=1}^k h_i(v) \mathrm{d}v \right\} \mathrm{d}u \tag{2}$$

Estimating the cumulative incidence function is of primary interest in most clinical studies. The Kaplan–Meier method can be used to obtain a nonparametric estimate of the cumulative incidence when the data consists of subjects who experience an event and the censoring mechanism is assumed to be noninformative (a special case of which is if the time at which a subject experiences an event is assumed to be independent of a mechanism that would cause the patient to be censored).

Gooley et al. (1999) discuss the appropriateness of the cumulative incidence function in survival analysis as opposed to routinely using the Kaplan–Meier estimator. They present a representation of both the cumulative incidence and Kaplan–Meier functions utilizing the concept of censored observations being "redistributed to the right." They claim that these interpretations "allow a more intuitive understanding of each estimate and therefore an appreciation of why the Kaplan–Meier method is inappropriate for estimation purposes in the presence of competing risks, while the cumulative incidence estimate is appropriate."

Model-based approaches such as the Cox proportional hazards model (Cox, 1972), or a refinement of this model, are also often used for the analysis of competing risks data. These models are particularly attractive in situations where one observes additional covariates which may be related to the event of interest.

Another alternative approach is to assume an additive hazard model presented by Aalen (1989), McKeague (1988), and more recently explored by Klein (2006). The latter author argues that additive models for either the hazard rates or the cumulative incidence functions are more natural and that these models properly partition the effect of a covariate on treatment failure into its component parts. The use and interpretation of such models are explored in detail in a study of the efficacy of two preparative regimes for hematopoietic stem cell transplantation.

Sun et al. (2004) also present an additive hazards model for competing risks analyses of the case-cohort design. This design may be applicable when the proportional hazards model does not provide a good fit for the observed survival data. Methods are presented for estimating regression parameters and cumulative baseline hazard functions, as well as cumulative incidence functions. The proposed estimators are shown to be consistent and asymptotically normal using the martingale central limit theory. The simulation studies conducted suggest that the proposed methods perform well.

Gichangi and Vach (2007) present a guided tour to the analysis of competing risk data. They point out that "there is still a great deal of uncertainty in the medical research and biostatistical community about how to approach this type of data."

In their opinion, there are three main reasons for this uncertainty

(1) The analysis of competing risks data does often not allow one to answer all research questions of interest, as we are unable to analyze associations or relationships among different risks. This general research methodological problem is often confused with a lack of adequate statistical methodology.
(2) Some standard methods of survival analysis like the log-rank test and the Cox model can be used in analyzing competing risks while other standard methods, especially the Kaplan–Meier estimator, have limited use. This is very confusing from a pedagogical point of view.
(3) Most papers on competing risks are written on a rather formal mathematical level. This is a natural consequence of the fact that the basic problem in analyzing competing risks is the proper definition of the quantities of interest.

However, the formal mathematical level makes many papers difficult to understand for many researchers.

This paper is certainly worth a close reading since the authors seem to have an appreciation for the difficulty and practical understanding of the issues inherent in sorting out this very real problem.

2. Approaches to the statistical analysis of competing risks

Refinements and extensions of the cumulative incidence approach have been considered by various authors. We present a brief discussion of these methods.

Several authors have discussed the topic of competing risks and the estimation of the cumulative incidence of an event. The theoretical concepts underlying the estimation of the cumulative incidence of an event using a variety of models is reviewed by Gail (1975) and Benichou and Gail (1990). Prentice et al. (1978) have discussed the likelihood inference approach to examine the effect of prognostic factors on the event of interest in the presence of competing risk events. A variety of probability models for summarizing competing risk data are described by Pepe and Mori (1993). A method to estimate the cumulative incidence of a specific event based on an extension of Cox proportional hazards regression model has been developed by Tai et al. (2001). Their findings suggest that the estimates obtained using the Kaplan–Meier approach are numerically larger than those accounting for competing risk events.

An alternative approach that accounts for informative censoring is given in the paper by Satagopan et al. (2004). They discuss cumulative incidence estimation in the presence of competing risk events. This approach is based on work done by Kalbfleisch and Prentice (2002) and Marubini and Valsecchi (1995). They outline a two-step process in which the first step involves calculating the Kaplan–Meier estimate of the overall survival from any event (where both the event of interest and the competing risk event are considered 'events'), while the second step involves calculating the conditional probabilities of experiencing the event of interest. The cumulative incidences are then estimated using these probabilities.

Often we are interested in comparing the risk of failure from a particular cause over two or more groups. The cumulative incidences in the various groups can be calculated by a variety of methods. If we are calculating incidences based on the Kaplan–Meier approach when the risks are noninformative, then the log-rank test is appropriate. However, when calculating incidences in the presence of competing risks, a modified test based on Gray's (1988) paper may be used. Both these methods are nonparametric and not based on any specific model.

Another approach that has been developed by Fine and Gray (1999) is a modification of the Cox proportional hazards model. This model directly assesses the effect of covariates on the cumulative incidence function, or subdistribution function, of a particular type of failure in the presence of competing risks. The basic model assumes that the subdistribution with covariates is a constant shift on the complementary log(−log) scale from some baseline subdistribution function.

Fine (2001) proposes a semi-parametric transformation model for the crude failure probabilities of a competing risk, conditional on covariates. This model is developed as an extension of the standard approach to survival data with independent right censoring. The procedures are useful for subgroup analyses of cumulative incidence functions which may be complex under a cause-specific hazards formulation. Estimation of the regression coefficients is achieved using a rank-based least squares criterion. The new estimating equations are computationally simpler than the partial likelihood procedure in Fine and Gray (1999), and simulations show that the procedure works well with practical sample sizes.

Pepe (1991) presents an alternative approach to estimating the cumulative incidence functions in a competing risk situation. The author develops inferential procedures for functions which are not simply survival, cumulative incidence, or cumulative hazard functions, but that can be expressed as simple functions of several of them. This paper's strong contribution is that it develops the asymptotic distribution theory for estimators of these constituent functions when there is a dependence structure among the multiple time-to-event endpoints.

Heckman and Honore (1989) show under certain regularity conditions, that for both proportional hazards and accelerated failure time models, if there is an explanatory variable whose support is the real line then the joint distribution of the competing risk times may be identifiable under certain conditions.

Abbring and van den Berg (2003) prove identification of dependent competing risks models in which each risk has a mixed proportional hazard specification with regressors, and the risks are dependent by way of the unobserved heterogeneity, or frailty, components. The authors also show that the conditions for identification given by Heckman and Honore, discussed above, can be relaxed.

Lunn and McNeil (1995) present two methods for the joint estimation of parameters in survival analysis models with competing risks. They demonstrate that it is possible to analyze survival data with competing risks using existing programs for fitting Cox's proportional hazards regression model with censored data. Two vectors of regression coefficients may be defined depending on the type of failure. The first procedure discussed runs a Cox regression stratified by the type of the failure. The second procedure uses unstratified Cox regression assuming that the hazard functions associated with the two types of failure have a constant ratio, which is an assumption that is often too stringent.

Jewell et al. (2003) provide an analysis with current status data (an extreme form of censoring which arises where the only information on studied individuals is their current survival status at a single monitoring time) in the context of competing risks. They look at simple parametric models and compare the results to nonparametric estimation. In addition to simulation results, the authors establish asymptotic efficiency of smooth functionals of the subdistribution functions.

Gilbert et al. (2004) provide tests for comparing mark-specific hazards and cumulative incidence functions. The authors develop nonparametric tests for the problem of determining whether there is a relationship between a hazard rate function or a cumulative incidence function, and a mark variable which is only observed at uncensored failure times. They consider the case where the mark variable is continuous.

There are several software packages available that estimate the cumulative incidence functions for an event of interest. Some of these include R (The R Foundation for Statistical Computing; http://www.r-project.org/), S-plus (Insightful Corporation; http://www.insightful.com), Stata (StataCorp LP; http://www.stata.com), and SAS (SAS Institute Inc.; http://www.sas.com). A popular software technique that has experienced widespread usage has been made available in R by Gray (1988, 2004; http://biowww.dfci.harvard.edu/~gray/). This software, along with others, will be implemented for the example discussed in the following section.

Several authors have suggested extensions of the above software. Rosthoj et al. (2004) suggest SAS macros for estimation of the cumulative incidence functions based on a Cox regression model for competing risks survival data. They describe how to estimate the parameters in this model when some of the covariates may, or may not, have exactly the same effect on several causes of failure. In their paper, two SAS macros are presented. The first macro named 'CumInc' is for estimation of the cumulative incidences, and a second macro named 'CumIncV' is for estimation of the cumulative incidences as well as the variances of those estimated cumulative incidences.

Klein and Andersen (2005) argue that the estimates from regression models for competing risks outcomes based on proportional hazards models for the crude hazard rates do not agree with impressions drawn from plots of cumulative incidence functions for each level of a risk factor. They present a technique which models the cumulative incidence function directly by using pseudovalues from a jackknife statistic constructed from the cumulative incidence curve. They then study the properties of this estimator and apply the technique to a study dealing with the effect of alternative donors on relapse for leukemia patients that were given a bone marrow transplant.

Two interesting papers by Andersen et al. (2002, 2003) show how the competing risks model may be viewed as a special case of a multi-state model. The properties of this model are reviewed and contrasted to the so-called latent failure time approach. The relation between the competing risks model and right-censoring is discussed, and a regression analysis of the cumulative incidence function is also reviewed.

Freidlin and Korn (2005) have pointed out that in certain circumstances when testing for treatment effects in the presence of competing risks, the popular cumulative incidence based approach may be problematic. However it would seem that more investigation is required to ascertain when, and under what circumstances, the cumulative incidence approach possesses the bias that is spoken of in this research study.

Steele et al. (2004) propose a general discrete time model for multilevel event history data. This model is developed for the analysis of longitudinal repeated episodes within individuals where there are multiple states and multiple types of events (competing risks) which may vary across states. The different transitions are modeled jointly to allow for correlation across transitions in unobserved individual risk factors. This model is then applied to the analysis of contraceptive use dynamics in Indonesia where transitions from two states, contraceptive use and nonuse, are of interest.

Escarela and Carriere (2003) propose fitting a fully parametric model for competing risks with an assumed copula. Using the assumed copula, the authors show how the dependence structure between the cause-specific survival times can be modeled. Features include: identifiability of the problem, accessible understanding of the dependence structure, and flexibility in choosing marginal survival functions. The model is constructed in such a way that it allows us to adjust for concomitant variables and a dependence parameter to assess the effect that these have on each marginal survival model and on the relationships between the causes of death.

The following two papers deal with sample sizes for competing risks. First, Pintilie (2002) presents a method to calculate the sample size for testing the effect of a covariate on an outcome in the presence of competing risks. Secondly, Latouche et al. (2004) present approximate sample size formulas for the proportional hazards modeling of competing risk subdistributions, considering either independent or correlated covariates. The validity of these approximate formulas is investigated through numerical simulations.

3. Example

To illustrate some of the methods previously described, we considered the mouse carcinogenicity data set published by Hoel (1972). The data were obtained from a laboratory experiment on two groups of RFM strain male mice which had received a radiation dose of 300 r at an age of 5–6 weeks. The mice were randomly assigned to either a conventional laboratory environment or a germ-free environment, and the number of days until death was recorded for each mouse. Two major causes of death were considered, namely thymic lymphoma and reticulum cell sarcoma, while all other causes of death were combined into a single group. Thus, the data consisted of three variables: number of days until death, cause of death, and type of environment.

A total of $n = 181$ mice were randomly assigned to either a conventional laboratory environment or a germ-free environment. Of the 99 mice that were randomly assigned to the conventional laboratory environment, 22 died as a result of thymic lymphoma while 38 died as a result of reticulum cell sarcoma. The remaining 39 mice assigned to the conventional laboratory environment experienced deaths attributed to other causes. Of the 82 mice that were randomly assigned to the germ-free environment, 29 died as a result of thymic lymphoma while 15 died as a result of reticulum cell sarcoma. The remaining 38 mice assigned to the germ-free environment experienced deaths attributed to other causes.

We begin by analyzing the data using nonparametric methods that are implemented in widely available software packages such as R 2.1.0 and Stata/SE 9.2. We will then consider other nonparametric methods of analyses described in the literature and compare their results to those given by the software

Table 1
Gray's test statistics and p-values for comparing the environment groups

Tests:	Stat	pv	df
1	2.895483	0.0888281369	1
2	13.885342	0.0001943080	1
3	6.640314	0.0099696340	1

Notes: Test 1 corresponds to death due to thymic lymphoma.
Test 2 corresponds to death due to reticulum cell sarcoma.
Test 3 corresponds to death due to other causes.

packages. Lastly, we will analyze the data using two semi-parametric methods also described in recent literature, and again compare their results to those previously obtained.

We first analyzed the data using the method described in Gray (1988). Gray's method can be performed using the 'cmprsk' package found in the R 2.1.0 statistical software package. Specifically, the 'cuminc' function provides statistical tests, estimates of the cumulative incidences, and variance estimates for the different environment groups. The 'plot.cuminc' function was then used to plot the cumulative incidence functions for the three failure types within each of the two environment groups. The output from the 'cuminc' function is given in Tables 1–3 while the plots are displayed in Figs. 1–3. Although so many significant digits would not typically be recorded in the Tables, we have included the actual R output strictly for the benefit of the reader. From the p-values given in Table 1, we see that there are significant differences between the environment groups in terms of death due to reticulum cell sarcoma and death due to other causes. By examining Figs. 2 and 3, we see that in both cases, the germ-free environment appears to improve survival time over the conventional environment. However, there is not enough evidence to suggest any significant differences between the environment groups in terms of death due to thymic lymphoma. In fact, Fig. 1 appears to suggest that the conventional environment may even be preferred when considering death due to thymic lymphoma.

Again using the Hoel data, we were able to estimate the cumulative incidence functions in the presence of competing risks by downloading the 'st0059' package available in the Stata/SE 9.2 software program. Specifically, the 'stcompet' function provides estimates of the cumulative incidence functions and their standard errors, as well as upper and lower confidence bounds for the cumulative incidences based on a log(-log) transformation. The resulting estimated cumulative incidence functions are displayed in Figs. 4–6. Note that these plots are in agreement with those produced using Gray's method. The lone difference being the convention with which the two software packages determine the largest time on study to be used in the extension of the plots. Whereas Gray's method in R 2.1.0 extends the plots out until the largest time on study within each treatment group regardless of cause, Stata/SE 9.2 uses the largest *cause-specific* time on study within each of the treatment groups.

Table 2
Gray's cumulative incidence estimates

		200	400	600	800	1000
1	1	0.05050505	0.18181818	0.22222222	NA	NA
2	1	0.06097561	0.23170732	0.31707317	0.3536585	0.3536585
1	2	0.00000000	0.03030303	0.15151515	NA	NA
2	2	0.00000000	0.00000000	0.02439024	0.1585366	0.1829268
1	3	0.06060606	0.17171717	0.30303030	NA	NA
2	3	0.01219512	0.04878049	0.07317073	0.2682927	0.4390244

Notes: In Table 2, the first column indicates that the estimates are for the two environment groups (1 corresponds to conventional and 2 corresponds to germ-free). The second column indicates that the estimates are for the three causes of death (1 corresponds to thymic lymphoma, 2 corresponds to reticulum cell sarcoma, and 3 corresponds to other causes). Also for Table 2, the first row of each table indicates the time points for which the respective estimates are given.

Table 3
Gray's estimated variances of the cumulative incidence estimates

		200	400	600	800	1000
1	1	0.0004897504	0.0015219666	0.0017700850	NA	NA
2	1	0.0007072238	0.0022024528	0.0026829906	0.002840750	0.002840750
1	2	0.0000000000	0.0003012409	0.0013277692	NA	NA
2	2	0.0000000000	0.0000000000	0.0002957942	0.001674860	0.001933082
1	3	0.0005811311	0.0014549986	0.0021697718	NA	NA
2	3	0.0001487210	0.0005743169	0.0008405426	0.002460062	0.003147561

Notes: In Table 3, the first column indicates that the estimates are for the two environment groups (1 corresponds to conventional and 2 corresponds to germ-free). The second column indicates that the estimates are for the three causes of death (1 corresponds to thymic lymphoma, 2 corresponds to reticulum cell sarcoma, and 3 corresponds to other causes). Also for Table 3, the first row of each table indicates the time points for which the respective estimates are given.

We then analyzed the same data set using the cumulative incidence estimator described in Klein and Moeschberger (2003). This method produced the same estimates as those obtained using Gray's method. The resulting cumulative incidence plots due to Klein and Moeschberger are given in Figs. 7–9. Klein and Moeschberger also provide a SAS macro for computing cumulative incidence on their web-site (http://www.biostat.mcw.edu/homepgs/klein/book.html), however this macro is written for the special case of only one competing risk. Therefore as an example, we considered only the deaths due to thymic lymphoma or reticulum cell sarcoma and again performed the analysis using Gray's method as well as the SAS macro provided by Klein and Moeschberger. Again, the estimates were identical. The cumulative incidence plots obtained from Gray's method when considering only thymic lymphoma and reticulum cell sarcoma are given in Figs. 10 and 11, while those obtained from Klein and Moeschberger's SAS macro are displayed in Figs. 12 and 13.

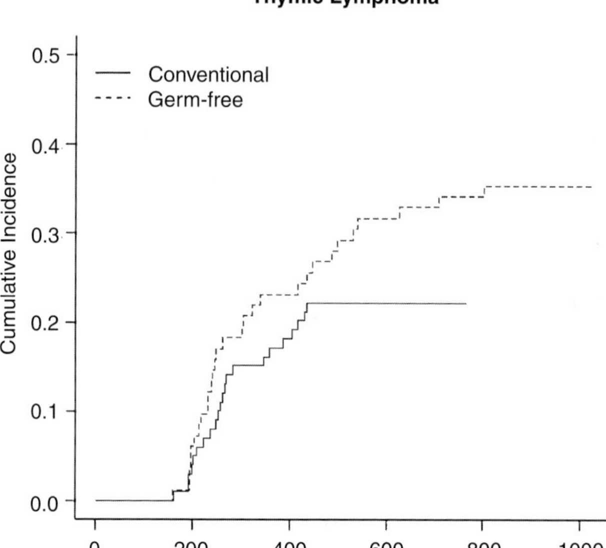

Fig. 1. Cumulative incidence estimates for the thymic lymphoma failure type (Gray).

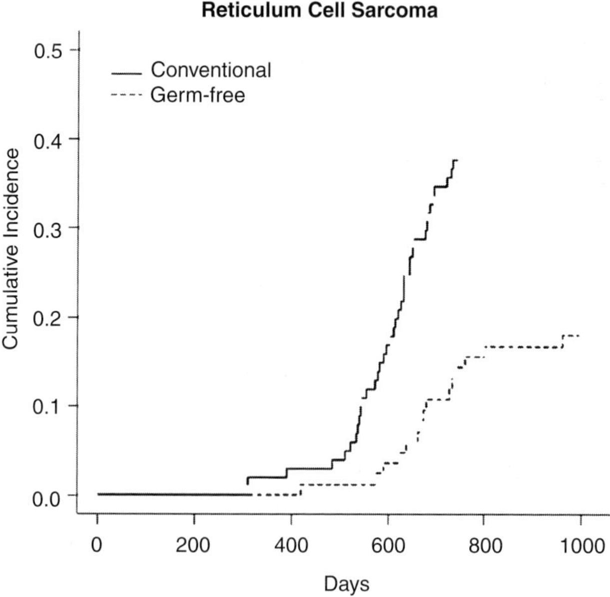

Fig. 2. Cumulative incidence estimates for the reticulum cell sarcoma failure type (Gray).

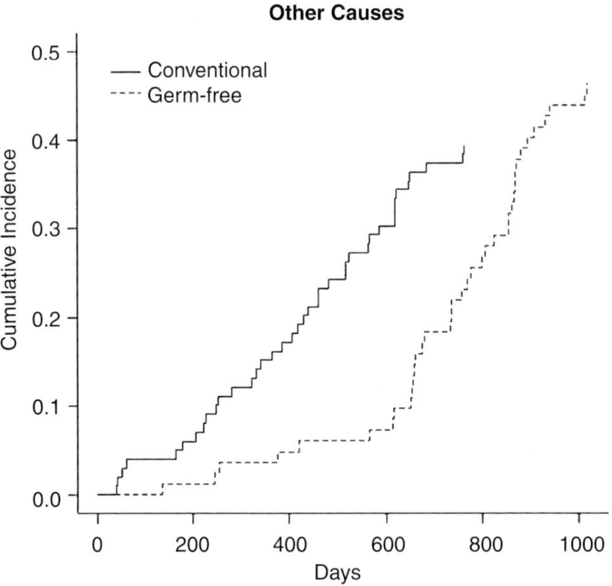

Fig. 3. Cumulative incidence estimates for the other causes failure type (Gray).

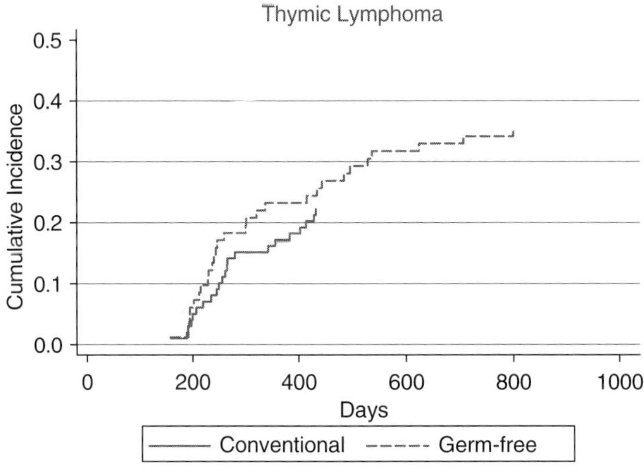

Fig. 4. Cumulative incidence estimates for the thymic lymphoma failure type (Stata/SE 9.2).

Once again using the complete data set given in Hoel (1972), we applied the 'crr' function in R 2.1.0 to fit the proportional subdistribution hazards regression model described in Fine and Gray (1999). The output from the 'crr' function is given in Tables 4–6 while the estimated cumulative incidence plots are displayed in Figs. 14–16. From the p-values given in Tables 4 and 5, we see that there are marginal differences between the environment groups in terms of death due to

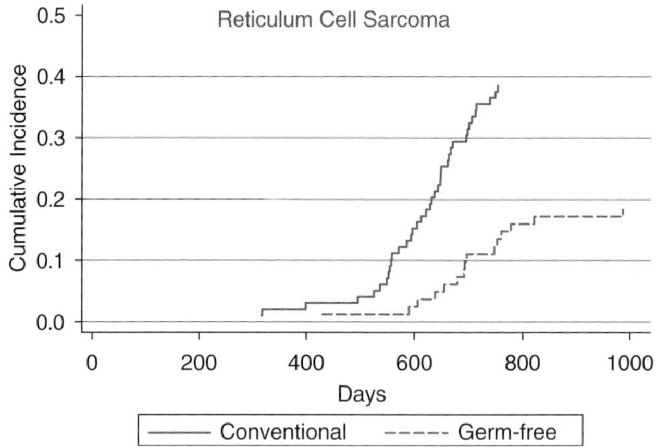

Fig. 5. Cumulative incidence estimates for the reticulum cell sarcoma failure type (Stata/SE 9.2).

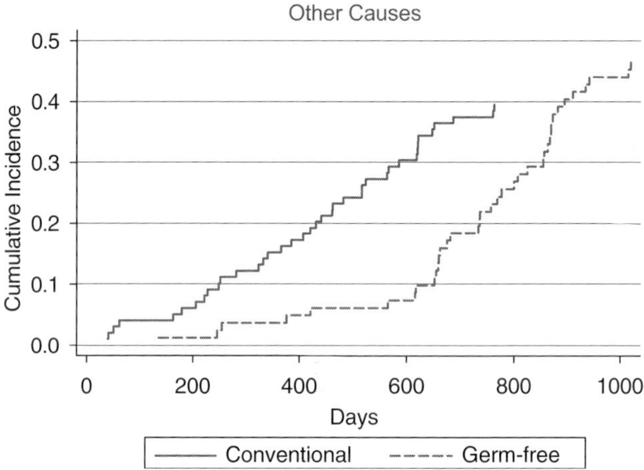

Fig. 6. Cumulative incidence estimates for the other causes failure type (Stata/SE 9.2).

thymic lymphoma and significant differences for death due to reticulum cell sarcoma. By examining Fig. 14, we see that in the case of thymic lymphoma, the conventional environment appears to improve survival time over the germ-free environment. However, Fig. 15 suggests that the germ-free environment is preferred in the case of reticulum cell sarcoma. The p-value and plot associated with other causes are also displayed in Table 6 and Fig. 16, respectively. Their examination does not suggest any significant differences between the environment groups in terms of death due to other causes. Note that for thymic lymphoma and reticulum cell sarcoma, the cumulative incidence estimates and conclusions based on this semi-parametric method due to Fine and Gray are quite similar, though not identical, to those drawn from the nonparametric method developed by Gray (1988). On the other hand, for deaths due to other causes, Gray's nonparametric

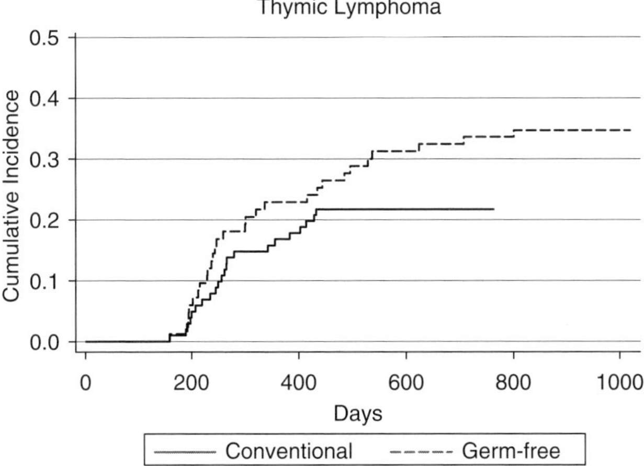

Fig. 7. Cumulative incidence estimates for the thymic lymphoma failure type (Klein and Moeschberger).

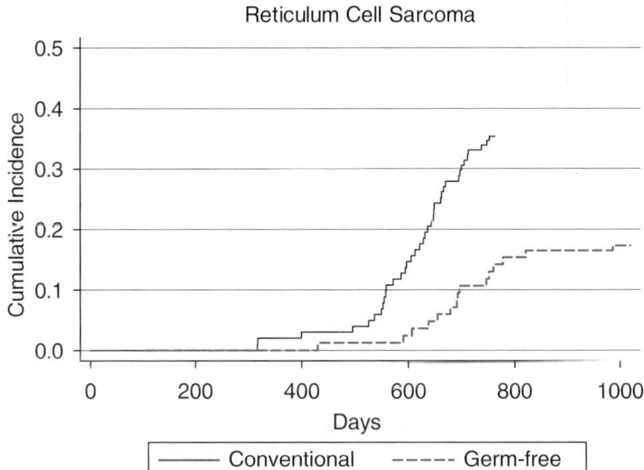

Fig. 8. Cumulative incidence estimates for the reticulum cell sarcoma failure type (Klein and Moeschberger).

method suggested a significant effect due to environment while the semi-parametric method due to Fine and Gray does not. Also note that the plots produced using Fine and Gray's method are extended out until the largest cause-specific time on study regardless of treatment group.

We again estimated the cumulative incidence functions for each cause of failure using a method proposed by Rosthoj et al. (2004). In their paper, the authors provide two SAS macros which can be used for estimating the cumulative incidence functions based on a Cox regression model for competing risks survival data. The 'CumInc' macro was used in SAS to obtain the cumulative incidence estimates for each cause of death within both the conventional and germ-free

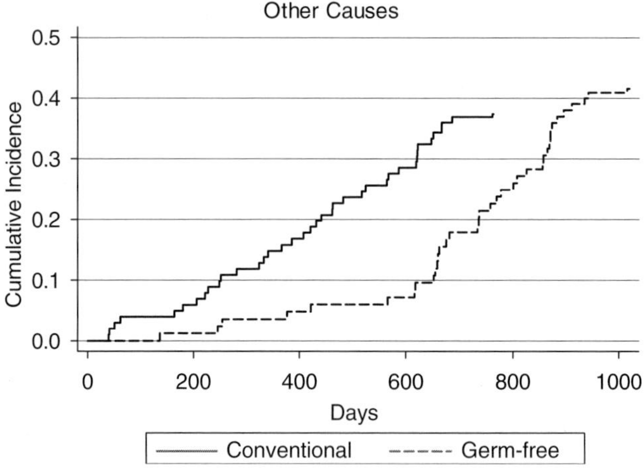

Fig. 9. Cumulative incidence estimates for the other causes failure type (Klein and Moeschberger).

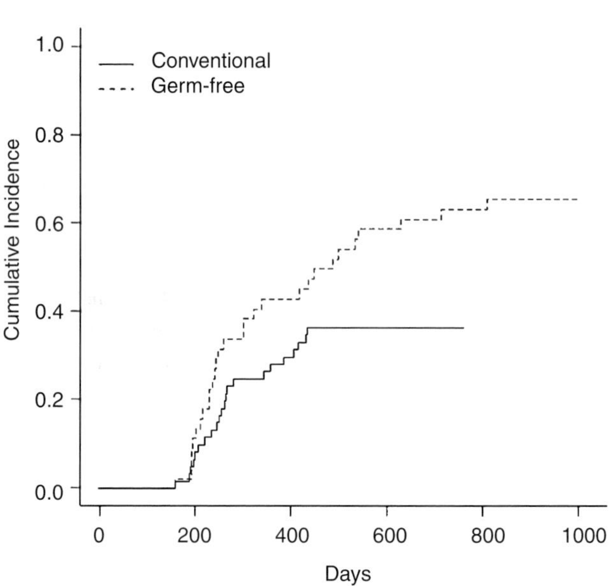

Fig. 10. Cumulative incidence estimates for the thymic lymphoma failure type when other causes are excluded (Gray).

environments. The resulting plots are very similar to those produced using Gray's (1988) method and are displayed in Figs. 17–19. Fig. 17 suggests that for death due to thymic lymphoma, the conventional environment may improve survival time over the germ-free environment. However, Figs. 18 and 19 suggest that when considering death due to reticulum cell sarcoma or other causes, the germ-free

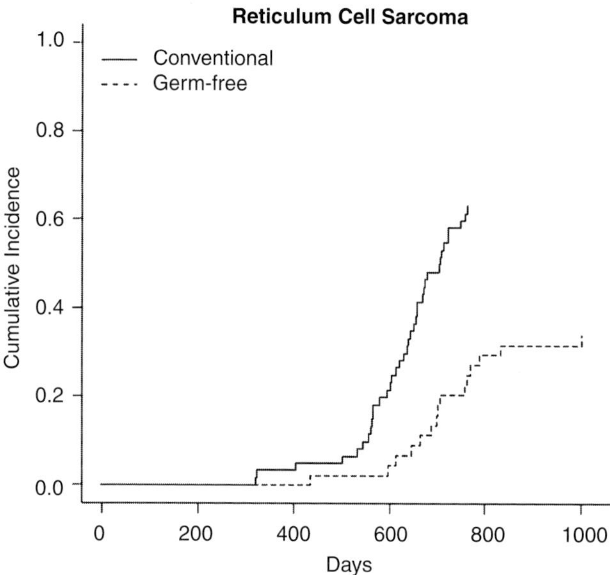

Fig. 11. Cumulative incidence estimates for the reticulum cell sarcoma failure type when other causes are excluded (Gray).

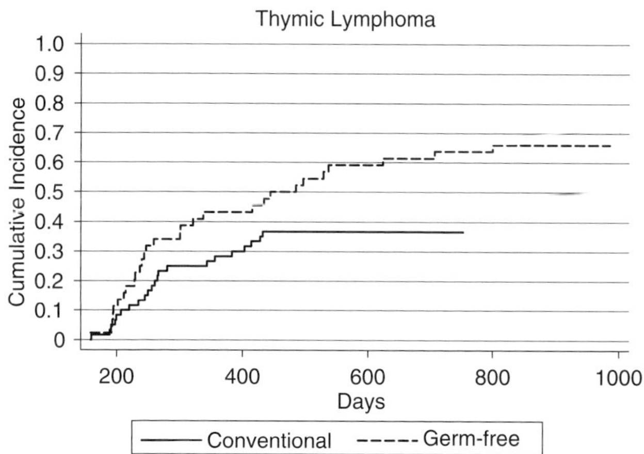

Fig. 12. Cumulative incidence estimates for the thymic lymphoma failure type when other causes are excluded (Klein and Moeschberger SAS macro).

environment may actually be preferred. One noticeable difference between the plots produced using the techniques described by Rosthoj and Gray's method is the crossing of the cumulative incidence functions for other causes in Fig. 19. This is explained by the convention employed by Rosthoj, which extends the

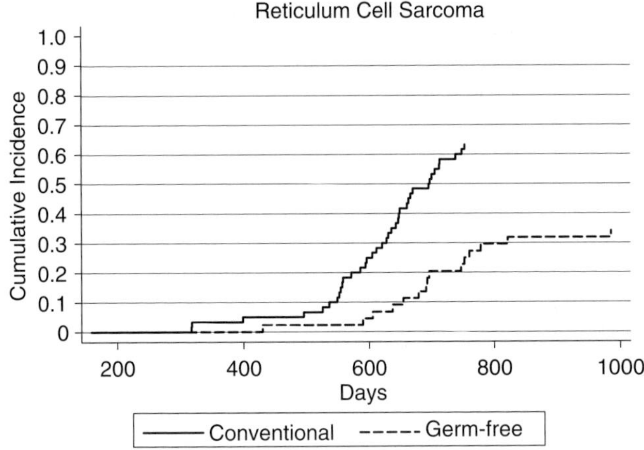

Fig. 13. Cumulative incidence estimates for the reticulum cell sarcoma failure type when other causes are excluded (Klein and Moeschberger SAS macro).

Table 4
Fine and Gray's estimated regression coefficients, standard errors, and p-values for comparing the environment groups with respect to thymic lymphoma

Coefficients:
[1] 0.5192
Standard errors:
[1] 0.282
Two-sided p-values:
[1] 0.066

Table 5
Fine and Gray's estimated regression coefficients, standard errors, and p-values for comparing the environment groups with respect to reticulum cell sarcoma

Coefficients:
[1] −0.9336
Standard errors:
[1] 0.2966
Two-sided p-values:
[1] 0.0016

Table 6
Fine and Gray's estimated regression coefficients, standard errors, and p-values for comparing the environment groups with respect to other causes

Coefficients:
[1] 0.004542
Standard errors:
[1] 0.227
Two-sided p-values:
[1] 0.98

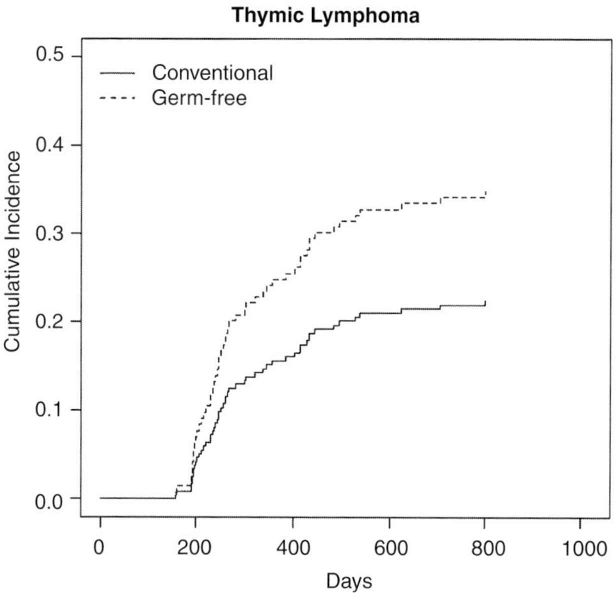

Fig. 14. Cumulative incidence estimates for the thymic lymphoma failure type (Fine and Gray).

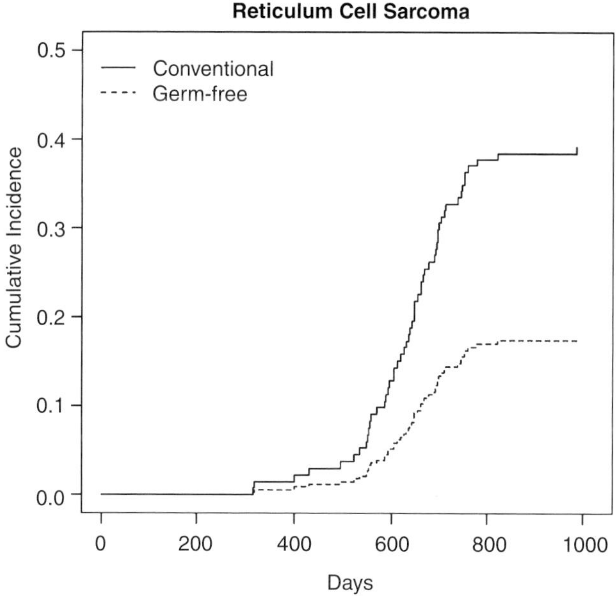

Fig. 15. Cumulative incidence estimates for the reticulum cell sarcoma failure type (Fine and Gray).

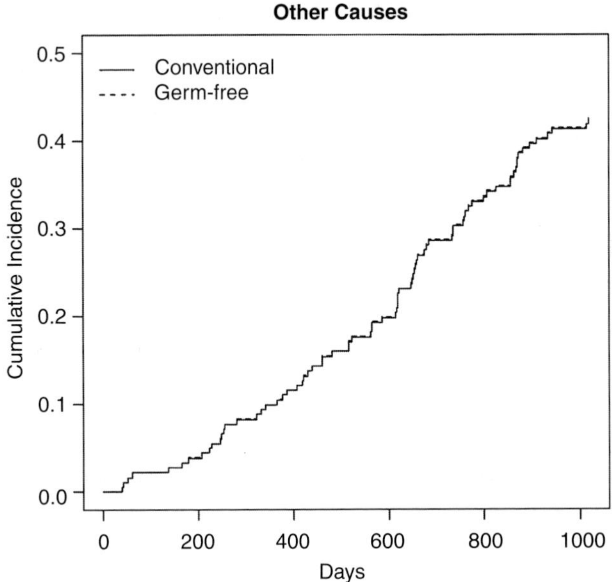

Fig. 16. Cumulative incidence estimates for the other causes failure type (Fine and Gray).

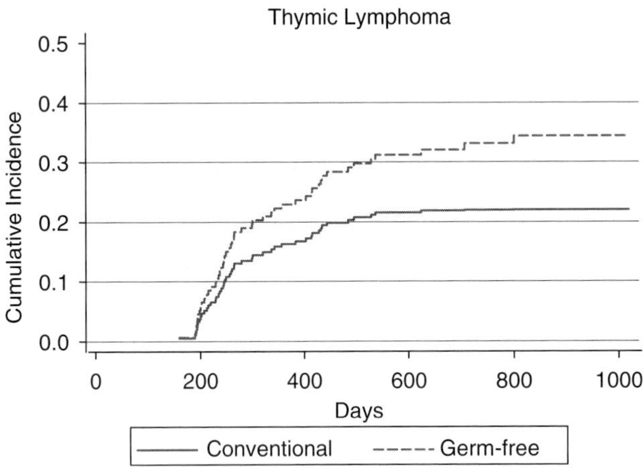

Fig. 17. Cumulative incidence estimates for the thymic lymphoma failure type (Rosthoj).

cumulative incidence functions out until the largest time on study regardless of the specific cause or treatment group.

As a final note, we point out that the cumulative incidence plots published in Hoel (1972) may be reproduced by considering separate data sets for each specific cause of death (thymic lymphoma, reticulum cell sarcoma, and other causes) and

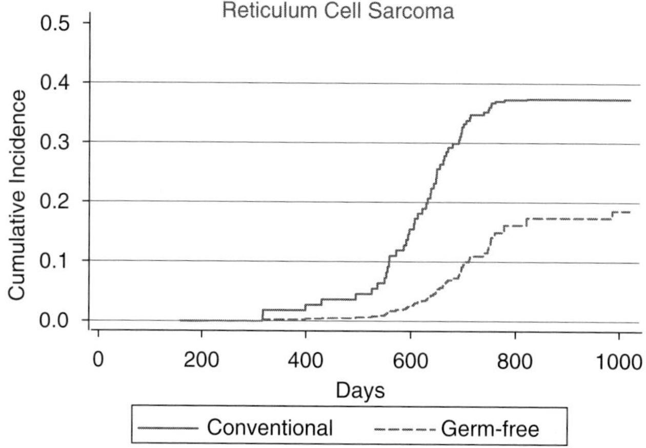

Fig. 18. Cumulative incidence estimates for the reticulum cell sarcoma failure type (Rosthoj).

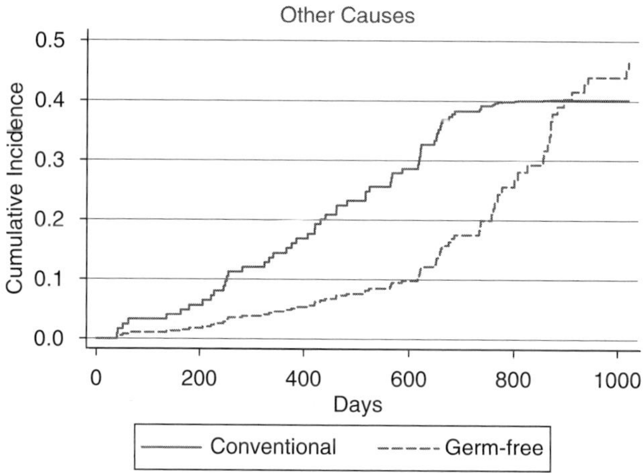

Fig. 19. Cumulative Incidence estimates for the other causes failure type (Rosthoj).

performing Gray's method. This technique, however, fails to estimate the cumulative incidence functions in a simultaneous fashion.

4. Conclusion

At this time, it is our recommendation that the technique described in Gray (1988) be the preferred method for estimating cumulative incidence curves in the presence of competing risks. Although several of the methods described above produced similar results, the recommendation to use Gray's method is based primarily on the fact that it is nonparametric in nature. Therefore no assumption of proportional hazards is required. We believe that the bias alluded to by other authors would require further investigation before any alternate recommendations could be made. For that reason, we are currently preparing a simulation study to determine if, and when, such biases occur.

References

Aalen, O.O. (1989). A linear regression model for analysis of lifetimes. *Statistics in Medicine* **8**, 907–925.

Abbring, J.H., van den Berg, G.J. (2003). The identifiability of the mixed proportional hazards competing risks model. *Journal of Royal Statistical Society Series B* **65**, 701–710.

Andersen, P.K., Abildstrom, S.Z., Rosthoj, S. (2002). Competing risks as a multi-state model. *Statistical Methods in Medical Research* **11**, 203–215.

Anderson, P.K., Klein, J.P., Rosthoj, S. (2003). Generalized linear models for correlated pseudo-observations, with applications to multi-state models. *Biometrics* **90**, 15–27.

Benichou, J., Gail, M.H. (1990). Estimates of absolute cause-specific risk in cohort studies. *Biometrics* **46**, 813–826.

Bernoulli, D. (1766) Essai d'une nouvelle analyse de la mortalité causée par la petite vérole. *Mém. Math. Phy. Acad. Roy. Sci. Paris,* 1–45. (English translation entitled 'An attempt at a new analysis of the mortality caused by smallpox and of the advantages of inoculation to prevent it' in: Bradley, L. (1971) Smallpox Inoculation: An Eighteenth Century Mathematical Controversy.)

Cox, D.R. (1972). Regression models and life tables (with discussion). *Journal of Royal Statistical Society Series B* **34**, 187–220.

David, H.A., Moeschberger, M.L. (1978). *The theory of competing risks*. Charles Griffin, London.

Escarela, G., Carriere, J.F. (2003). Fitting competing risks with an assumed copula. *Statistical Methods in Medical Research* **12**, 333–349.

Fine, J.P. (2001). Regression modeling of competing crude failure probabilities. *Biostatistics* **2**, 85–97.

Fine, J.P., Gray, R.J. (1999). A proportional hazards model for the sub-distribution of a competing risk. *Journal of the American Statistical Association* **94**, 496–509.

Freidlin, B., Korn, E. (2005). Testing treatment effects in the presence of competing risks. *Statistics in Medicine* **24**, 1703–1712.

Gail, M. (1975). A review and critique of some models used in competing risk analysis. *Biometrics* **31**, 209–222.

Gichangi, A., Vach, W. (2007) The analysis of competing risks data: A guided tour. Under Review.

Gilbert, P.B., Mckeague, I.W., Sun, Y. (2004). Test for comparing mark-specific hazards and cumulative incidence functions. *Lifetime Data Analysis* **10**, 5–28.

Gooley, T.A., Leisenring, W., Crowley, J., Storer, B.E. (1999). Estimation of failure probabilities in the presence of competing risks: New representations of old estimators. *Statistics in Medicine* **18**, 695–706.

Gray, B. (2004) The cmprsk Package.

Gray, R.J. (1988). A class of k-sample tests for comparing the cumulative incidence of a competing risk. *Annals of Statistics* **16**, 1141–1154.

Heckman, J.J., Honore, B.E. (1989). The identifiability of the competing risks model. *Biometrika* **76**, 325–330.

Hoel, D.G. (1972). A representation of mortality data by competing risks. *Biometrics* **28**, 475–488.

Insightful Corporation. 1700 Westlake Ave. N., Suite 500. Seattle, WA 98109. http://www.insightful.com.

Jewell, N.P., van der Laan, M., Henneman, T. (2003). Nonparametric estimation from current status data with competing risks. *Biometrika* **90**, 183–197.

Kalbfleisch, J.D., Prentice, R.L. (2002). *The statistical analysis of failure time data*, 2nd ed. Wiley, New York.

Klein, J.P. (2006). Modeling competing risks in cancer studies. *Statistics in Medicine* **25**, 1015–1034, Wiley.

Klein, J., Andersen, P.K. (2005). Regression modeling of competing risks data based on pseudo values of the cumulative incidence function. *Biometrics* **61**, 223–229.

Klein, J.P., Moeschberger, M.L. (2003). *Survival analysis: Statistical methods for censored and truncated data*, 2nd ed. Springer, New York.

Latouche, A., Porcher, R., Chevret, S. (2004). Sample size formula for proportional hazards modeling of competing risks. *Statistics in Medicine* **23**, 3263–3274.

Lunn, M., McNeil, D. (1995). Applying cox regression to competing risks. *Biometrics* **51**, 524–532.

Marubini, E., Valsecchi, M.G. (1995). *Analyzing survival data from clinical trials and observational studies.* Wiley, New York.

McKeague, I.W. (1988). Asymptotic theory for weighted least-squares estimators in Aalen's additive risk model. *Contemporary Mathematics* **80**, 139–152.

Pepe, M.S. (1991). Inference for events with dependent risks in multiple endpoint studies. *Journal of the American Statistical Association* **86**, 770–778.

Pepe, M.S., Mori, M. (1993). Kaplan Meier, marginal or conditional probability curves in summarizing competing risks failure time data? *Statistics in Medicine* **12**, 737–751.

Pintilie, M. (2002). Dealing with competing risks: Testing covariates and calculating sample size. *Statistics in Medicine* **21**, 3317–3324.

Prentice, R.L., Kalbfleisch, J.D., Peterson, A.V., Flournoy, N., Farewell, V.T., Breslow, N.E. (1978). The analysis of failure times in the presence of competing risks. *Biometrics* **34**, 541–554.

Rosthoj, S., Andersen, P.K., Abildstrom, S.Z. (2004). SAS macros for estimation of the cumulative incidence functions based on a Cox regression model for competing risks survival data. *Computer Methods and Programs in Biomedicine* **74**, 69–75.

SAS Institute Inc. 100 SAS Campus Drive. Cary, NC 27513. http://www.sas.com.

Satagopan, J.M., Ben-Porat, L., Berwick, M., Robson, M., Kutler, D., Auerbach, A.D. (2004). A note on competing risks in survival data analysis. *British Journal of Cancer* **91**, 1229–1235.

StataCorp LP. 4905 Lakeway Drive. College Station, TX 77845. http://www.stata.com.

Steele, F., Goldstein, H., Brown, W. (2004). A general multilevel multistate competing risks model for event history data, with an application to a study of contraceptive use dynamics. *Statistical Modeling* **4**, 145–159.

Sun, J., Sun, L., Flournoy, N. (2004). Additive hazards model for competing risks analysis of the case-cohort design. *Communication in Statistics* **33**, 351–366.

Tai, B.-C., Machin, D., White, I., Gebski, V. (2001). Competing risks analysis of patients with osteosarcoma: A comparison of four different approaches. *Statistics in Medicine* **20**, 661–684.

The R Foundation for Statistical Computing. Technische Universitat Wien. 1040 Vienna, Austria. http://www.r-project.org/.

Tsiatis, A.A. (1975). Aspect of the problem of competing risks. *Proceedings of the National Academy of Sciences* **72**, 20–22.

Handbook of Statistics, Vol. 27
ISSN: 0169-7161

DOI: 10.1016/S0169-7161(07)27011-7

11

Cluster Analysis

William D. Shannon

Abstract

This chapter introduces cluster analysis algorithms for finding subgroups of objects (e.g., patients, genes) in data such that objects within a subgroup are more similar to each other than to objects in other subgroups. The workhorse of cluster analysis are the proximity measures that are used to indicate how similar or dissimilar objects are to each other. Formulae for calculating proximities (distances or similarities) are presented along with issues related to scaling and normalizing variables. Three classes of clustering are presented next – hierarchical clustering, partitioning, and ordination or scaling. Finally, some recent examples from a broad range of epidemiology and medicine are very briefly described.

1. Introduction

In medicine and epidemiology, the concept of patient subgroups is well established and used in practice. In cancer tumor staging the goal is to determine treatment strategy and prognosis based on the patient subgroup. The National Heart, Lung and Blood Institute at the NIH classifies (during the writing of this chapter) blood pressure levels as normal (<120/80), pre-hypertension (120/80–139/89), Stage 1 hypertension (140/90–159/99), and Stage 2 hypertension (>159/99). In spatial epidemiology, disease clusters are found for planning healthcare delivery or for identifying causes of the disease.

To understand and motivate this work, it is valuable to have a basic overview of some modern statistical clustering algorithms. These tools can be applied to biomedical data to identify patients within subgroups who are likely to have similar natural history of their disease, similar treatment responses, and similar prognoses. This chapter addresses the problem of cluster analysis or unsupervised learning where the goal is to find subgroups or clusters within data when group membership is not known *a priori*. These might be clusters of patients, genes, disease groups, species, or any other set of objects that we wish to put into homogeneous subsets. The assumption of any cluster analysis is that the objects within a cluster are in some sense more similar to each other than to objects in other subgroups.

In contrast to cluster analysis is the classification or supervised learning problem. In classification the object's subgroup membership is known from the data, such as cases versus controls in an epidemiological study or responder versus non-responder in a clinical trial. The goal of the classification model is to use covariates or features of the objects with known class membership to develop a mathematical model to predict class membership in future objects where their true classification is not known. There are a large number of statistical and computational approaches for classification ranging from classical statistical linear discriminant analysis (Fisher, 1936) to modern machine-learning approaches such as support vector machines (Cristianini and Shawe-Taylor, 2000) and artificial neural networks (Bishop, 1996). Classification models as described here are distinct from cluster analysis and will not be discussed further in this chapter. However, cluster analysis or unsupervised learning is often referred to as classification, leading to confusion, though the context of the problem should make it clear which is being considered – if the data contains a variable with a class membership label then the classification is referring to that described in this paragraph. When no class membership variable is present in the data, then cluster analysis is being referred to. The remainder of this paper will focus on cluster analysis.

The concept of cluster analysis is most easily understood through a visual representation. In fact, cluster analysis should be thought of as an exploratory data analysis tool for data reduction where multivariate data are being displayed to uncover patterns (Tukey, 1977). In Fig. 1, we show visual clustering of 2-dimensional data (x, y) with four distinct clusters labeled A, B, C, and D. It is clear that the objects within each cluster are more similar to each other in terms of their X, Y values then they are to objects in the other clusters. Each of these three methods are discussed in more detail later in this chapter.

In multivariate data with more than 2 or 3 variables, the ability to identify clusters through direct visualization is impossible requiring a cluster analysis program. There are three major classes of cluster analysis – hierarchical, partitioning, and ordination or scaling – displayed in Fig. 1. *Hierarchical cluster analysis* clusters objects by proximity, in this case a distance measure, and displays them in a tree or dendrogram (e.g., Everitt et al., 2001; Gordon, 1999). Objects labeled at the tips of the tree are connected to each other by the branches of the dendrogram. Objects connected early or at a lower height are more similar as is seen with the four subgroups A–D. Objects connected at a higher level are further apart such as the objects between the four subgroups. *Cluster analysis by partitioning* produces boundaries between clusters so that points on one side of a boundary belong to one cluster while points on the other side of the boundary belong to the other cluster (Hartigan, 1975; Hartigan and Wong, 1979). In this example the boundaries are precise, though boundaries can be fuzzy or defined by probability vectors. *Cluster analysis by ordination or scaling* uses a projection of the data from many dimensions onto a few dimensions that can be displayed visually (Cox and Cox, 2001). In this example we projected the 2 dimensional X, Y data onto the X-axis, though in practice ordination often projects multi-dimensional data onto linear combinations of the dimensions or new arbitrary dimensions.

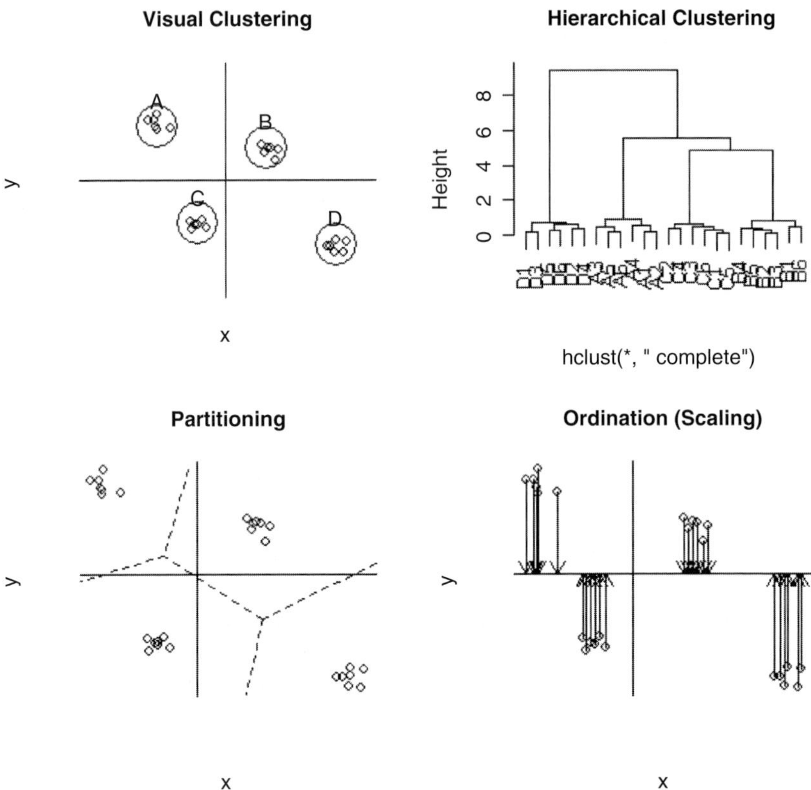

Fig. 1. Display of the three classes of cluster analysis discussed in this chapter.

For a broad overview of the multivariate statistics used in cluster analysis, the reader is referred toTimm (2002). For a broad overview of both unsupervised and supervised learning methods from both the statistics and machine-learning literature, the reader is referred to Hastie et al. (2001). For a broad overview of the application of these methods to biological data the reader is referred to Legendre and Legendre (1998). Each of these references covers hierarchical and other clustering methods in more mathematical detail than presented here and show their application to data for illustration.

2. Proximity measures

2.1. Some common distance measures

Fundamental to cluster analysis is the concept of proximity of two objects to each other measured in terms of a numerical value indicating the distance or similarity between the pair. For example, let two objects x and y be represented by points in the Euclidean n-dimensional space $x = (x_1, x_2, \ldots, x_n)$ and $y = (y_1, y_2, \ldots, y_n)$. The

Table 1
Three commonly used distance measures on continuous variables

Distance	Formula	Common Name
1 – norm	$\sum_{i=1}^{n} \lvert x_i - y_i \rvert$	Manhattan distance
2 – norm	$\left(\sum_{i=1}^{n} \lvert x_i - y_i \rvert^2\right)^{1/2}$	Euclidean distance
Infinity norm	$\lim_{p\to\infty} \left(\sum_{i=1}^{n} \lvert x_i - y_i \rvert^p\right)^{1/p} = \max(\lvert x_1 - y_1 \rvert, \lvert x_2 - y_2 \rvert, \ldots, \lvert x_n - y_n \rvert)$	Chebyshev distance

commonly used Minkowski distance of order p, or p-norm, distance are defined in Table 1 where $p \geq 1$.

Each of the example Minkowski distances (e.g., Manhattan, Euclidean, Chebyshev) has an intuitive sense of proximity. The Manhattan distance is how many blocks one would travel walking through downtown Manhattan, if blocks were laid out as a grid (i.e., go three blocks east and turn north for two blocks). The Euclidean distance is our normal sense of distance as measured by a ruler. The Chebyshev distance represents the distance along the largest dimension. These are illustrated for a distance between points X and Y, denoted by $d(x, y)$, in Fig. 2.

Distances can also be calculated using categorical variables (Table 2). Let our objects $x = (x_1, x_2, \ldots, x_n)$ and $y = (y_1, y_2, \ldots, y_n)$ be points on an n-dimensional space where each dimension is represented by a categorical variable. If we let $w_j = 1$ if neither x_j and y_j are missing, and $w_j = 0$ otherwise, then we can calculate 'matching' distances between objects X and Y. In the simplest example think of the objects vectors $x = (x_1, x_2, \ldots, x_n)$ and $y = (y_1, y_2, \ldots, y_n)$ as strings of 0's and 1's so that

$$\delta^i_{xy} = \begin{cases} 0 & \text{if} \quad x_i = y_i = 0 \text{ or } x_i = y_i = 1 \\ 1 & \text{if} \quad x_i = 0, y_i = 1 \text{ or } x_i = 1, y_i = 0 \end{cases}.$$

The Hamming and matching distances for this is the number of non-matching variables between x_j and y_j either weighted by the number of non-missing cases (matching metric) or not weighted (Hamming distance). Numerous other categorical distance measures are available and often based on contingency table counts (e.g., Jaccard distance).

In many applied problems there is a mixture of continuous and categorical variables. Distances can still be calculated between pairs of objects in this case using the Gower distance metric, which combines distances obtained using a

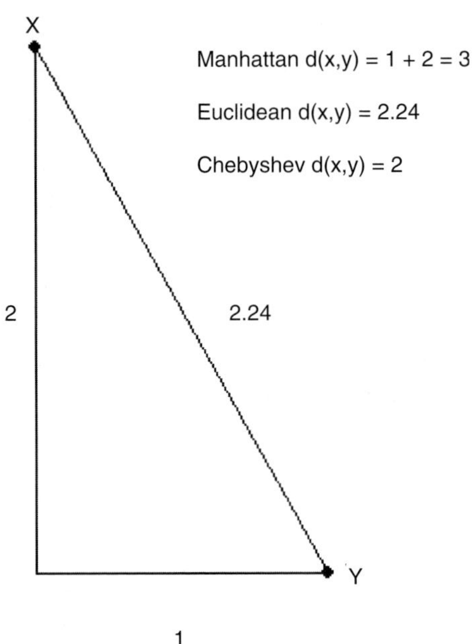

Fig. 2. Geometric display of three common distance measures.

Table 2
Two commonly used distance measures on categorical variables

Distance	Formula
Hamming	$\sum_{i=1}^{n} w_i\delta^i_{xy},\ \delta^i_{xy} = \begin{cases} 0 & \text{if } x_i = y_i \\ 1 & \text{if } x_i \neq y_i \end{cases}$
Matching	$\dfrac{\sum_{i=1}^{n} w_i\delta^i_{xy}}{\sum_{i=1}^{n} w_i},\ \delta^i_{xy} = \begin{cases} 0 & \text{if } x_i = y_i \\ 1 & \text{if } x_i \neq y_i \end{cases}$

standard p-norm metric on the continuous variables (e.g., Euclidean), and distances obtained using a matching-type distance measure on the categorical variables (e.g., Hamming).

2.2. *Definition of distance measures*

The above list of distance measures (also called metrics) was not meant to be comprehensive in any sense, but rather an introduction to the commonly used distances and the idea of distance measured on categorical and mixed data types.

Table 3
Criterion for distance measures

Rule	Definition
$d(x,y) \geq 0$	The distances between two objects X and Y is positive, and equal to 0 only when the two objects are the same, i.e., $X = Y$
$d(x,y) = d(y,x)$	The distance between two objects is symmetric where going from X to Y is the same distance as going from Y to X
$d(x,y) \leq d(x,z) + d(y,z)$	The distance between two objects X and Y will always be less than or equal to the distances between X and Z and between Y and Z (triangle inequality)

Implicit in each of the distance measures, however, is the necessity to meet certain formal criteria which are presented here.

Let objects $x = (x_1, x_2, \ldots, x_n)$, $y = (y_1, y_2, \ldots, y_n)$, and $z = (z_1, z_2, \ldots, z_n)$ be points on an n-dimensional space. Denote the distance between any pair of them by $d(a, b)$. Then $d(a, b)$ is a distance measure if each of the criterion in Table 3 are true.

A fourth criterion $d(x,y) \leq \max\{d(x,z), d(y,z)\}$, known as the strong triangle or ultrametric inequality, makes the space ultrametric. This states that every triangle in the ultrametric space connecting any three objects is isosceles (i.e., at least two of the sides have equal length, $d(x,y) = d(y,z)$ or $d(x,z) = d(y,z)$ or $d(x,y) = d(z,x)$). Ultrametric spaces have nice mathematical properties that make them amenable to certain types of problems (e.g., phylogenetic tree construction in evolution), but are not routinely used in medicine and epidemiology, though could be a valuable addition to biostatistical data analysis. An example of an ultrametric cluster analysis in medicine would be that all patients within a disease subgroup are equally distant from all patients in a different disease subgroup. This may have the potential to refine disease prognosis into more homogeneous subgroups but as far as we know it has not been formally explored.

2.3. Scaling

Although clustering methods can be applied to the raw data, it is often more useful to precede the analysis by standardizing the data. Standardization in statistics is a commonly used tool to transform data into a format needed for meaningful statistical analysis (Steele and Torrie, 1980). For example, *variance stabilization* is needed to fit a regression model to data where the variance for some values of the outcome Y may be large, say for those values of Y corresponding to large values of the predictor variable X, while the variance of Y is small for those values corresponding to small values of X (i.e., heteroscedasticity). Another use of standardization is to *normalize* the data so that a simple statistical test (e.g., t-test) can be used.

Scaling or transformation of data for cluster analysis has a different purpose than those used to meet assumptions of statistical tests as described in the previous paragraph. Cluster analysis depends on a distance measure that is most likely sensitive to differences in the absolute values of the data (scale). Consider a hypothetical situation where multiple lab tests have been measured on a patient where each test has a continuous value. Suppose further that the values for all but one test are normally distributed with mean 100 and variance 1, and the values for the remaining test is normally distributed with mean 100 and variance 10. Using the raw data the distance becomes dependent nearly exclusively on this one test with high variance as illustrated in Fig. 3, where each patient's lab values are shown connected by the line. On visual inspection, we see that the distances between patients on the first 5 lab tests will be small compared to the distances between patients for the lab test 6. If distances were calculated only on lab tests 1–5, the average Euclidean distance would be 3.24 while including lab test 6 the average Euclidean distance is 10.64 resulting in the cluster analysis being driven primarily by this last lab test.

To avoid this complication the analyst can weight the variables in the distance calculation (all distance measures described above have a corresponding variable weighting formulation that can be found in any standard cluster analysis reference, e.g., Everitt et al., 2001) or find an appropriate data transformation to have the variables scaled equivalently. In the case where the variables are all normally distributed, as in this example, a z-score transformation would be appropriate.

A second scaling issue is easily shown in time series data, though applies to any type of data. Suppose a lab test measured on a continuous scale is done at multiple times in patients. The goal of this study might be to find clusters of

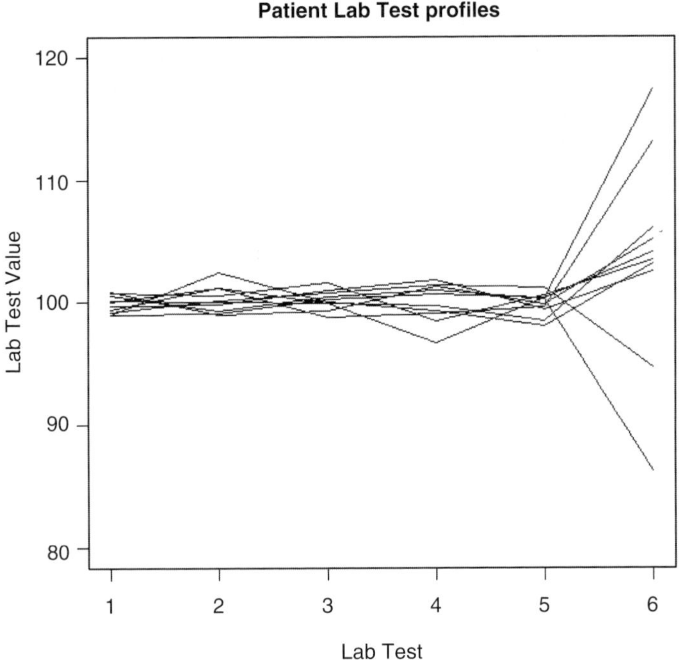

Fig. 3. The effect of high variability in different variables between subject distances.

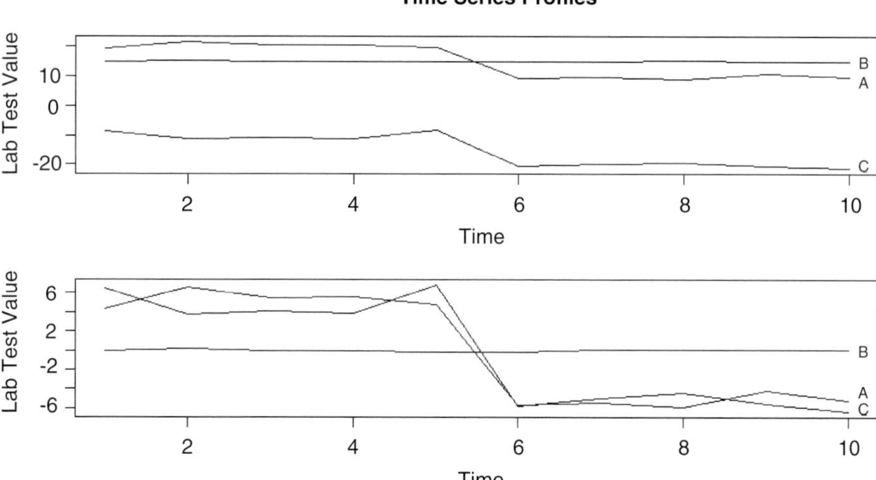

Fig. 4. The effect of standardization on outcome profiles.

patients with the same absolute values of the lab tests or to find patients with the same time series pattern of the lab tests. In Fig. 4 we display three patients, two of whom (A and C) show a decrease in their lab values at the sixth time point, and one (B) who shows no change. In the top graph showing the raw values patients A and B are more similar. In the bottom graph where we have shifted the profiles to be centered at 0 we see that patients A and C are more similar. The result is that clustering on the un-shifted data will find clusters of patients with similar raw lab values, while clustering on the shifted lab values will find clusters of patients with similar changes in pattern over time.

This section introduced the concept of scaling and shifting variables in cluster analysis. The important point to remember is that the cluster analysis results will be drastically affected by the choice of scale of the data. In the first example distances are dominated by the variance in a single variable and in the second example distances are dominated by the value locations. No single rule for transforming the data exists but it is important for the analyst to think through these issues and understand that the choices made will impact significantly the results obtained. By stating clearly before the analysis what the goal is (e.g., find patients with similar lab values or find patients with similar changes in patterns) the appropriate transformations can likely be found.

2.4. Proximity measures

Implicit in any cluster analysis is the concept of proximity, whether defined in terms of distance or similarity. Several cluster analysis methods, such as hierarchical clustering and some ordination methods, require in addition to a way to calculate proximities between objects, the calculation of a proximity (say distance) matrix giving pairwise distances between all pairs of objects. The clustering algorithm uses this matrix as the input to find the clusters.

If O_i, $i = 1, \ldots, N$ denote the objects to be clustered (e.g., patients), X_j, $j = 1, \ldots, P$ denote the variables measured on the objects, and $x_{i,j}$ denote the value of variable X_j in object O_i, then the Euclidean distance, say, between two objects i,i' is $d_{i,i'} = \sqrt{(x_{i,1} - x_{i',1})^2 + (x_{i,2} - x_{i',2})^2 + \cdots + (x_{i,P} - x_{i',P})^2}$. By repeating this calculation for all pairs, the $N \times P$ raw data table is transformed into the object pairwise distances matrix D:

$$
\begin{array}{c}
\text{Object} \\
1 \\ 2 \\ 3 \\ 4 \\ 5 \\ \vdots \\ N
\end{array}
\quad
\begin{array}{c}
\begin{array}{cccc} X_1 & X_2 & \cdots & X_P \end{array} \\
\begin{bmatrix}
x_{1,1} & x_{1,2} & \cdots & x_{1,P} \\
x_{2,1} & x_{2,2} & \cdots & x_{2,P} \\
x_{3,1} & x_{3,2} & \cdots & x_{3,P} \\
x_{4,1} & x_{4,2} & \cdots & x_{4,P} \\
x_{5,1} & x_{5,2} & \cdots & x_{5,P} \\
\vdots & \vdots & \ddots & \vdots \\
x_{N,1} & x_{N,2} & \cdots & x_{N,P}
\end{bmatrix}
\end{array}
\Rightarrow D =
\begin{bmatrix}
0 & d_{1,2} & d_{1,3} & d_{1,4} & d_{1,5} & \cdots & d_{1,N} \\
 & 0 & d_{2,3} & d_{2,4} & d_{2,5} & \cdots & d_{2,N} \\
 & & 0 & d_{3,4} & d_{3,5} & \cdots & d_{3,N} \\
 & & & 0 & d_{4,5} & \cdots & d_{4,N} \\
 & & & & 0 & \cdots & d_{5,N} \\
 & & & & & \ddots & \vdots \\
 & & & & & & 0
\end{bmatrix},
$$

where $d_{1,2}$ is the distance between objects 1 and 2, $d_{1,3}$ the distance between objects 1 and 3, etc. Only the upper triangle of the distance matrix is shown because of symmetry where $d_{1,2} = d_{2,1}$, $d_{1,3} = d_{3,1}$, etc. The diagonal for a distance matrix is 0 since the distance from an object to itself is 0. A similarity matrix often scales similarities to lie between 0 and 1 making the diagonal elements all 1.

A proximity matrix measured on N objects will have $n(n-1)/2$ entries in the upper triangle. The size of the distance matrix becomes a problem when many objects are to be clustered. The increase in the number of distances limits hierarchical clustering and some ordination methods to a small number of objects. To illustrate, for $N = 10$ there are $10*9/2 = 45$ pairwise distances, for $N = 100$ there are 4,950 pairwise distances, for $N = 1{,}000$ there are 499,500 pairwise distances, and for $N = 10{,}000$ there are 49,995,000 pairwise distances. When the number of pairwise proximities becomes too large to calculate and process efficiently partitioning methods that do not require pairwise distance matrices (e.g., k-means clustering) should be used for the cluster analysis. What this size is will depend on the computer resources available to the data analyst.

3. Hierarchical clustering

3.1. Overview

One of the major cluster analysis tools used is hierarchical clustering (Everitt and Rabe-Hesketh, 1997) where objects are either joined sequentially into clusters (agglomerative algorithms) or split from each other into subgroups (divisive clustering). In most applications agglomerative clustering is predominant and will be the focus of this section. Agglomerative clustering begins with each object separate and finds the two objects that are nearest to each other. These two objects are joined (agglomerated) to form a cluster, which is now treated as a new object. The distances between the new object and the other objects are calculated and the process repeated by joining the two nearest objects. This algorithm repeats until every object is joined. Several examples of hierarchical clustering algorithms are presented in Table 4.

An example of hierarchical clustering would be to identify prognosis subgroups where development of additional symptoms results in different diagnoses. In this case the presence of severe symptoms could be viewed hierarchically as being a subset of patients with less severe symptoms.

We illustrate this iterative process in Fig. 5 using a centroid cluster analysis algorithm (this and other cluster algorithms will be defined below). In the first step objects A and B which are nearest each other are joined (as indicated by the line) and a new object at the midpoint on this line is used to represent this cluster. In the second step objects D and E are joined. In the third step the new cluster AB is joined to object C. In the fourth and last step the cluster ABC is joined with cluster DE.

For this 2-dimensional problem it is easy to visualize the clustering in a scatter plot. For higher dimensional data (as well as 1 and 2 dimensional like Fig. 5), the dendrogram is able to represent the clustering process. In Fig. 6 the average cluster analysis performed on the objects A–E in Fig. 5 is shown. Here, we see the same pattern in the iterative process where cluster AB is formed first at the lowest height, followed by DE, then ABC, and finally ABCDE. The advantage of the dendrogram over the scatter plot representation is that the dendrogram includes a measure of distance at which objects are merged on the vertical axis.

In each step of the clustering as objects are merged the proximity matrix is modified to reflect the new number of objects and the new measures of proximity. In the first step we merged A and B whose distance was the smallest at 0.44.

$$\begin{bmatrix} & A & B & C & D & E \\ A & 0 & 0.44 & 1.12 & 3.33 & 3.49 \\ B & & 0 & 1.43 & 3.47 & 3.50 \\ C & & & 0 & 2.33 & 2.73 \\ D & & & & 0 & 1.06 \\ E & & & & & 0 \end{bmatrix}$$

The AB cluster was formed and the distance matrix updated to show the distance between AB and the other objects. From this the objects D and E are merged whose distance is smallest at 1.06.

$$\begin{bmatrix} & AB & C & D & E \\ AB & 0 & 1.26 & 3.39 & 3.49 \\ C & & 0 & 2.33 & 2.72 \\ D & & & 0 & 1.06 \\ E & & & & 0 \end{bmatrix}$$

Table 4
Five commonly used hierarchical clustering algorithms

Algorithm	Formula	Description
Average linkage	$D_{KL} = \frac{1}{N_K N_L} \sum_{i \in C_k} \sum_{j \in C_L} d(x_i, x_j)$	The distance between two clusters is the average of all the pairwise distances of all the members of one cluster with all the members of the other cluster. These tend to be small clusters with equal variance
Centroid method	$D_{KL} = \lVert \bar{x}_K - \bar{x}_L \rVert^2$	The distance between two clusters is the distance between the clusters centroids or mean vectors and are resistant to outliers
Complete linkage	$D_{KL} = \max_{i \in C_K} \max_{j \in C_L} d(x_i, x_j)$	The distance between two clusters equals the maximum distance between all the members of one cluster with all the members of the other cluster. These tend to be clusters with equal diameters across the space of the objects but are subject to distortion by outliers
Single linkage	$D_{KL} = \min_{i \in C_K} \min_{j \in C_L} d(x_i, x_j)$	The distance between two clusters equals the minimum distance between all the members of one cluster with all the members of the other cluster. These tend to be 'stringy' elongated clusters and have difficulty finding small compact clusters
Ward's minimum-variance method	$D_{KL} = \frac{\lVert \bar{x}_K - \bar{x}_L \rVert^2}{(1/N_K) + (1/N_L)}$	This method combines clusters with similar variances to produce homogeneous clusters. It assumes that the variables are distributed as multivariate normal and clusters tend to have similar size and distinct separation

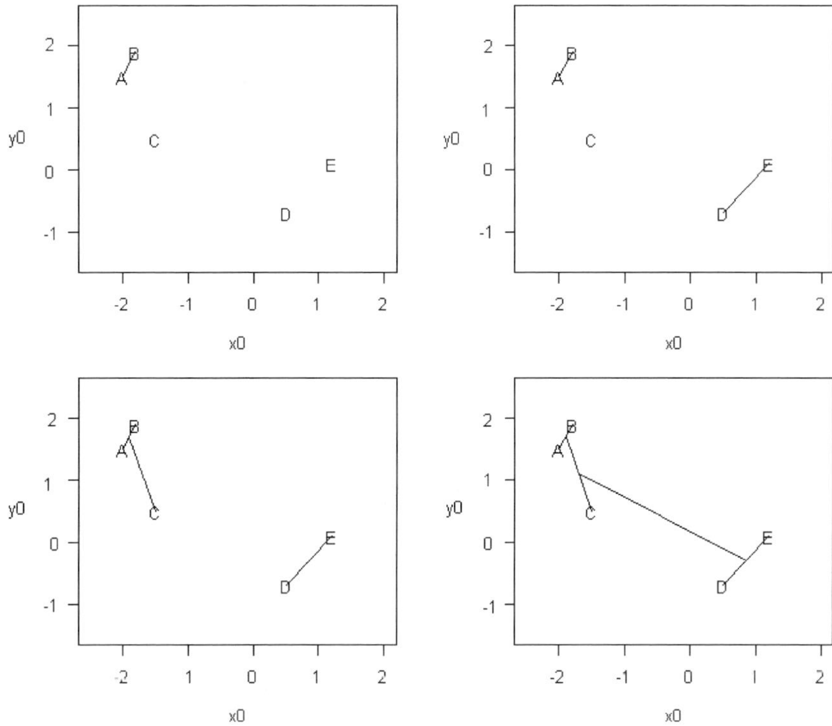

Fig. 5. Example of clustering order of five objects.

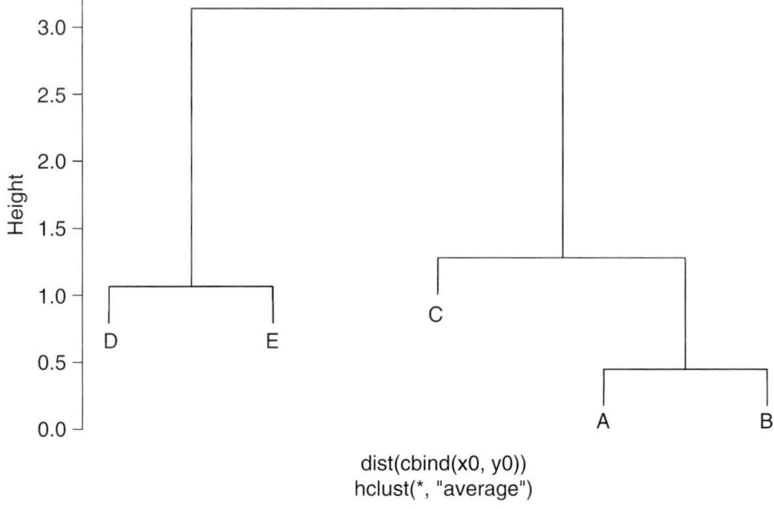

Fig. 6. Dendrogram representation of the clustering of the five objects in Fig. 5.

In the next step objects AB and C are merged with smallest distance 1.26.

$$\begin{bmatrix} & AB & C & DE \\ AB & 0 & 1.26 & 3.40 \\ C & & 0 & 2.48 \\ DE & & & 0 \end{bmatrix}$$

In the final step clusters ABC and DE were merged completing the algorithm.

$$\begin{bmatrix} & ABC & DE \\ ABC & 0 & 2.90 \\ DE & & 0 \end{bmatrix} \Rightarrow \begin{bmatrix} & ABCDE \\ ABCDE & 0 \end{bmatrix}$$

Once a dendrogram is fit to the data the decision as to where to cut it to produce distinct clusters is made. In Fig. 7, we fit a dendrogram to the data from Fig. 1 that were visually clustered into four distinct subgroups labeled A, B, C, and D. Within each cluster were six objects labeled A1–A6, B1–B6, etc. The horizontal dashed lines in Fig. 7 show how the dendrogram can be cut to produce from 1 to 4 clusters. In addition, we could decide anywhere between not cutting the dendrogram and have all the objects merged into a single cluster to cutting at the right height to keep each object in its own cluster. Criteria for deciding how to cut dendrograms will be discussed below.

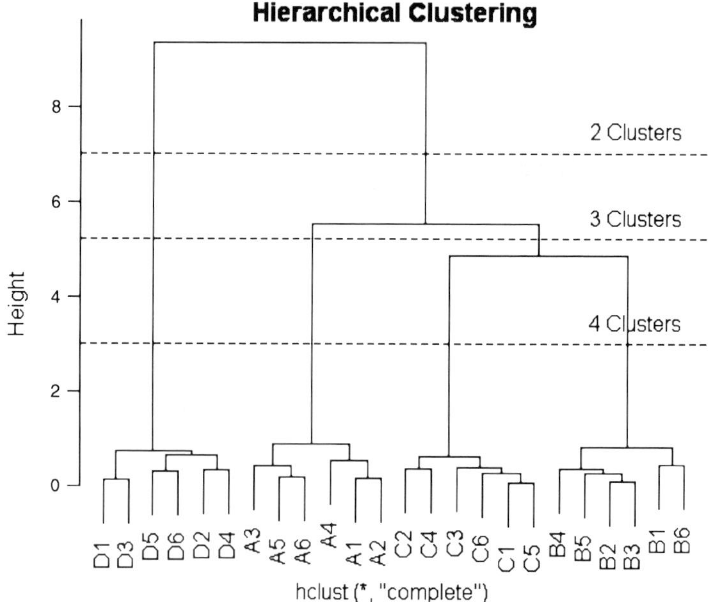

Fig. 7. How hierarchical clustering is split into different cluster numbers (stopping rule).

4. Partitioning

Hierarchical clustering algorithms proceed by sequentially merging objects or clusters into larger clusters based on some distance criterion. These algorithms however tend to be computationally intensive and begin breaking down for larger datasets (the size depending on the computer resources available). In addition, these algorithms tend to be less dependent on data distributions, with the exception of a few such as Ward's method, and so do not take advantage of probability models. In this section, we will introduce two types of partitioning clustering – *k*-means and model-based clustering – that can be used for very large datasets or when a probability model is assumed.

Partitioning attempts to split the space directly into regions where objects falling in the same region belong to the same cluster. The boundaries defining these regions can be defined differently and may be hard thresholds or based on probability of membership. In Fig. 8, data are generated from one of four bivariate normal distributions. Two decision boundaries are over-laid on the data. The solid straight lines represent the type of boundary obtained from a *k*-means clustering where objects are clustered according to the side of these lines they fall on. The dashed contour lines represent probability distributions and are the type of decision boundaries obtained from a model-based clustering. Each object has a probability of belonging to each of the four groups and is assigned to that group for which it has the highest probability of belonging to.

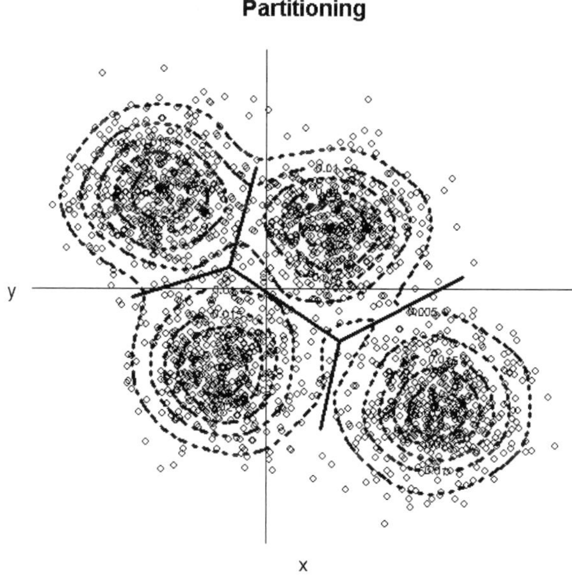

Fig. 8. Display of both a *k*-means partition (solid line boundary) and model-based clustering (dashed lines indicating density estimates).

4.1. k-Means clustering

The k-means algorithm directly partitions the space into k non-overlapping regions where k is specified by the analyst. This algorithm is useful for very large datasets where a hierarchical relationship is not being sought. This might include problems of clustering patients by disease category where the development of one category is not dependent on passing through a different category. In contrast hierarchical clustering assumes that lower branches or clusters on the dendrogram possess the same symptoms as clusters above it on the dendrogram.

The k-means algorithm is simple to implement. Assume each object is represented by a vector $x = (x_1, x_2, \ldots, x_n)$ and the analyst wants to divide them into k clusters. The algorithm starts with either k random or user-specified vectors from the space to represent the starting cluster centers which we denote by $\bar{x}_k$ for the kth cluster, $k = 1, \ldots, K$. The distance from each object to each of these initial centers, $d(x_i, \bar{x}_k)$, is calculated with each object being assigned to the center that it is closest to. If we define a cluster of objects as $C_{k,}$ a subset of all objects $\{1,2, \ldots, N\}$, then the k-means algorithm assigns individual objects x_i to the nearest cluster mean, i.e., $(C_K : \min_{k=1, \ldots, K} d(x_i, \bar{x}_k)$. All objects assigned to the same center form a distinct cluster. The algorithm recalculates the cluster centers $\bar{x}_k$ by averaging the individual vectors $x = (x_1, x_2, \ldots, x_n) \in C_k$. The algorithm repeats by calculating the distance of each object to the new cluster centers, reassigns each object to its new nearest cluster center, and iterates this process until none of the objects change clusters.

In Fig. 9 we see three iterations of the k-means algorithm in the first column for $k = 4$. We initialized this algorithm with four centers located at $(-1, 1)$, $(1, 1)$, $(1, -1)$, and $(-1, -1)$ defining the four clusters by the quadrants (i.e., all objects in the upper right quadrant belong to the $(1, 1)$ cluster). After the first iteration the clusters centers (dark dots) have moved part of the way towards the 'true' cluster centers located at $(-2.5, 2.5)$, $(1.5, 1.5)$, $(-1, -2)$, and $(4, -3)$. Overlaying this plot is the decision boundary which assigns objects to one of the four cluster centers. In the second iteration the cluster centers have converged on the true centers and the decision boundary finalized.

Any appropriate distance measure can be used in k-means clustering. However, there is often an assumption of multivariate normality in the data and the algorithm is implemented using the Mahalanobis distance measure. Let $x = (x_1, x_2, \ldots, x_n)$ be the object and $\bar{x}_k$ be the cluster means as above, and let $\hat{\Sigma}_k^{-1}$ be the inverse of the estimated covariance matrix for the kth cluster. Then the Mahalanobis distance, used routinely in multivariate normal distribution theory, is defined as $D_{ik}^2 = (x_i - \bar{x}_k)^T \Sigma_k^{-1} (x_i - \bar{x}_k)$.

4.2. Model-based clustering

If we assume the data from cluster k was generated by a probability model $f_k(x{:}\theta)$ with parameters θ, model-based clustering allows a maximum likelihood estimation approach to determine cluster membership. For our objects $x = (x_1, x_2, \ldots, x_n)$, we can define a vector of cluster assignments by $\gamma = (\gamma_1, \gamma_2, \ldots, \gamma_n)^T$ where $\gamma_I = k$ if object x_i belongs to cluster k. The parameters θ and cluster

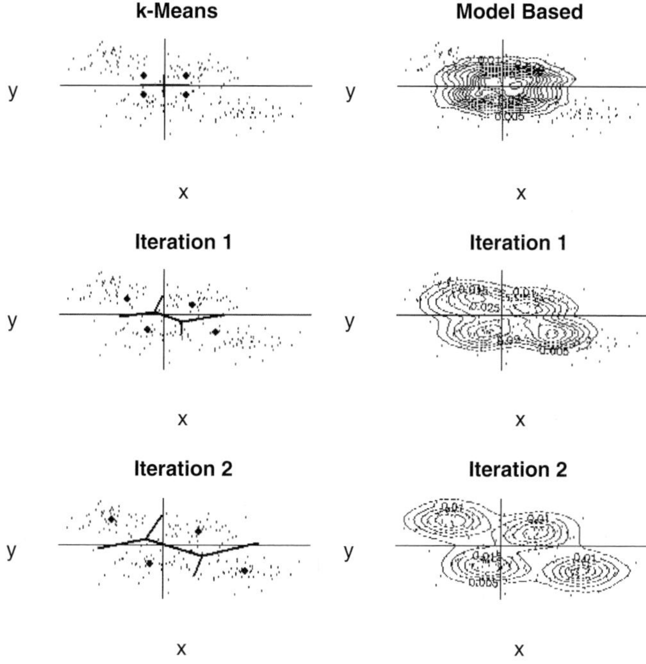

Fig. 9. Iterative process of k-means and model-based partitioning.

membership vector γ can be estimated by maximizing the likelihood

$$L(x;\theta,\gamma) = \prod_{k=1}^{K} f_{\gamma_k}(x;\theta),$$

where f_{γ_k} is the distribution for the objects in cluster k.

If we assume the distributions for each of the K clusters is multivariate normal then the likelihood function is

$$L(x;\mu_1,\ldots,\mu_K,\Sigma_1,\ldots,\Sigma_k,\gamma) = \prod_{k=1}^{K}\prod_{i\in C_k}(2\pi)^{-p/2}|\Sigma_k|^{-1/2} \times \exp\left\{-\frac{1}{2}(x_i-\mu_k)^T\Sigma_k^{-1}(x_i-\mu_k)\right\},$$

where C_k is the subset of objects in cluster k. This imposes significant structure assumptions on the data. However, accurate algorithms exist (e.g., EM) for maximum likelihood estimation of the parameters, including the class membership vector γ. In most applications the user will specify the covariance structure desired which defines other criteria to be optimized.

Whichever criterion is optimized the model-based search is an iterative process like the k-means algorithm. The left column of plots (Fig. 9) shows how the iterations for the same data used in the k-means example might appear in the model-based clustering. In this example the three iterations of k-mean cluster centers were used as $\hat{\bar{x}}_1, \ldots, \hat{\bar{x}}_K$ and we assumed that $\Sigma = \begin{bmatrix} 1 & 0 \\ 0 & 1 \end{bmatrix}$. In the first plot the probability densities appear as one and as we move to the second and third iteration we see a clear separation the probability masses into four distinct clusters.

An excellent general reference for model based clustering is McLachlan and Peel (2000).

5. Ordination (scaling)

Ordination or scaling methods project data from many dimensions to one, two, or a few dimensions while maintaining relevant distances between objects. Two objects that are far apart (close together) in the high dimensional space will be far apart (close together) in the lower dimensional space. In this lower dimensional space visual clustering can be done. Perhaps the best-known ordination method in multivariate statistics is principal components analysis (PCA) where variables are linearly transformed into new coordinates where hopefully the first two or three contain the majority of the information present in all the variables.

5.1. Multi-dimensional scaling

Multi-dimensional scaling (MDS) takes a proximity matrix measured on a set of objects and displays the object in a low dimensional space such that the relationships of the proximities in this low dimensional space matches the relationships of the distances in the original proximity matrix. A classical example of MDS is the visualization of cities determined by the flying distances between them. In the distance matrix we show the distances between 10 US cities, where Atlanta is 587 miles to Chicago, 1,212 miles to Denver, etc (Table 5).

This distance matrix defines a set of pairwise relationships for this set of cities but offers no clue as to their location in the US – their latitude and longitude. However, MDS can display these cities in a 2-dimensional projection to see if the physical locations can be estimated. In Fig. 10, we show the result of this projection and observe that in fact this does approximately reproduce their locations relative to each other.

MDS models are fit by finding a data matrix in fewer dimensions, say 2 dimensions, that produces a proximity matrix similar to that obtained, whether generated from an existing data matrix or given directly such as is found in many psychological experiments where a subject is asked to state the similarity of objects. Let $d_{i,\ j}$ be the distance between objects i and j obtained either by calculating distances between the object vectors $x = (x_1, x_2, \ldots, x_n)$ or obtained directly through a judgment experiment. MDS searches for a data representation for each object, say $y = (y_1, y_2)$, so that the distances between the objects are similar to the $d_{i,j}$'s, and so the objects can be displayed in a 2-dimensional scatter plot. If we let $d_{i,j}$ be the original distances (or proximities) we are working with,

Table 5
Flying mileage between 10 American cities

	Atlanta	Chicago	Denver	Houston	Los Angeles	Miami	New York	San Francisco	Seattle	Washington, DC
Atlanta	0	587	1212	701	1936	604	748	2139	2182	543
Chicago		0	920	940	1745	1188	713	1858	1737	597
Denver			0	879	831	1726	1631	949	1021	1494
Houston				0	1374	968	1420	1645	1891	1220
Los Angeles					0	2339	2451	347	959	2300
Miami						0	1092	2594	2734	923
New York							0	2571	2408	205
San Francisco								0	678	2442
Seattle									0	2329
Washington, DC										0

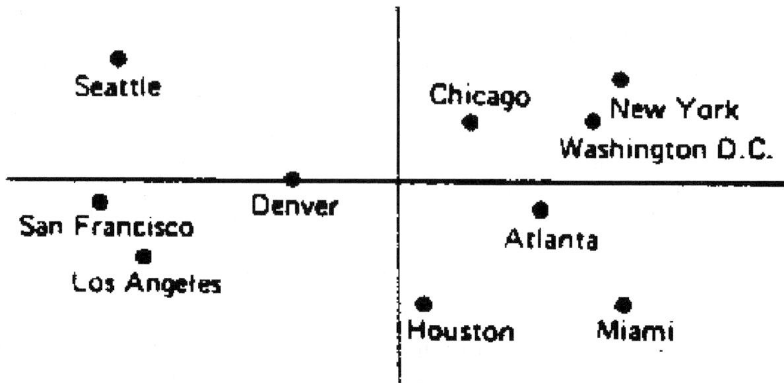

Fig. 10. Example of multi-dimensional scaling assigning relative positions of the US cities.

and $d_{i,j}(y)$ be the distances calculated on our new data points $y = (y_1, y_2)$, classical MDS attempts to find the data vectors $y = (y_1, y_2)$ such that the following is minimized:

$$E_M = \sum_{i \neq j} \left[d_{i,j} - d_{i,j}(y)\right]^2.$$

This represents the square-error cost associated with the projection. Note that the scale and orientation of the $y = (y_1, y_2)$ are arbitrary and the map of the US cities in the above example may just have easily been flipped from top to bottom and left to right. The goal of the MDS is not to obtain the exact values of the possibly unknown data vectors $x = (x_1, x_2, \ldots, x_n)$, but rather to obtain their pairwise spatial relationships.

Other criterion for MDS exists that addresses specific data requirements. For example, Kruskal showed that if the data are ordinal the projected distances $d_{i,j}(y)$ should only match the observed distances $d_{i,j}$ on a rank ordering. By imposing a monotonically increasing function on the observed distances, denoted by $f(d_{i,j})$, that preserves the rank order of them, then the criterion for the non-metric MDS is

$$E_N = \frac{1}{\sum_{i \neq j} \left[d_{i,j}(y)\right]} \sum_{i \neq j} \left[f(d_{i,j}) - d_{i,j}(y)\right]^2.$$

Another commonly used MDS-like algorithm is known as Sammon's mapping or normalization where the normalization allows small distances to be preserved and not overwhelmed by minimizing squared-error costs associated with large distances. Sammon mapping minimizes:

$$E_S = \sum_{i \neq j} \frac{\left[d_{i,j} - d_{i,j}(y)\right]^2}{d_{i,j}}.$$

Table 6
Caithness, Scotland, cross-classified by eye and hair color

		Hair Color				
		Fair	Red	Medium	Dark	Black
Eye Color	Blue	326	38	241	110	3
	Light	688	116	584	188	4
	Medium	343	84	909	412	26
	Dark	98	48	403	681	85

Finding the points $y = (y_1, y_2)$ requires a search. If the original data $x = (x_1, x_2, \ldots, x_n)$ are available, the search might begin with the first two principal components. If it is not available the starting points $y = (y_1, y_2)$ may be randomly generated. The search proceeds by iteration where the new set of points $y = (y_1, y_2)$ are generated by the previous set using one of several search algorithms until the change in the goodness-of-fit criterion falls below a user defined threshold.

5.2. Correspondence analysis

Another important ordination procedure for categorical data, analogous to PCA and MDS, is correspondence analysis (CA). Table 6 shows a cross-classification of people in Caithness, Scotland, cross-classified by eye and hair color (Fisher, 1940). This region of the UK is particularly interesting as there is a mixture of people of Nordic, Celtic, and Anglo-Saxon origin. In this table we find 326 people with blue eyes and fair hair, 38 with blue eyes and red hair, etc.

Ignoring the computational details we find the projection of this variables produces the scatter plot in Fig. 11. From this display we find that people with blue or light eye color tend to have fair hair, people with dark eyes tend to have black eye color, etc. The distances between these variables on this 2-dimensional projection gives a relative strength of the relationships. For example, blue eyes and fair hair are strongly related but blue eyes and dark hair are weakly related. Medium eye and hair color are strongly related and moderately related to the other colors as indicated by their appearance somewhat near the middle of the scatter plot.

Like MDS this projection places the points on arbitrary scales. Also, in this example two categorical variables are used for illustration but multiple variables can be projected onto a lower dimensional space.

6. How many clusters?

The author of this chapter believes that cluster analysis is an exploratory data analysis tool only and that methods to date to impose formal statistical inference to determine the correct number of clusters have not been fully developed and framed in such a way that they can be generally applied. This includes work by the author that attempts to use a graph-valued probability model to decide the

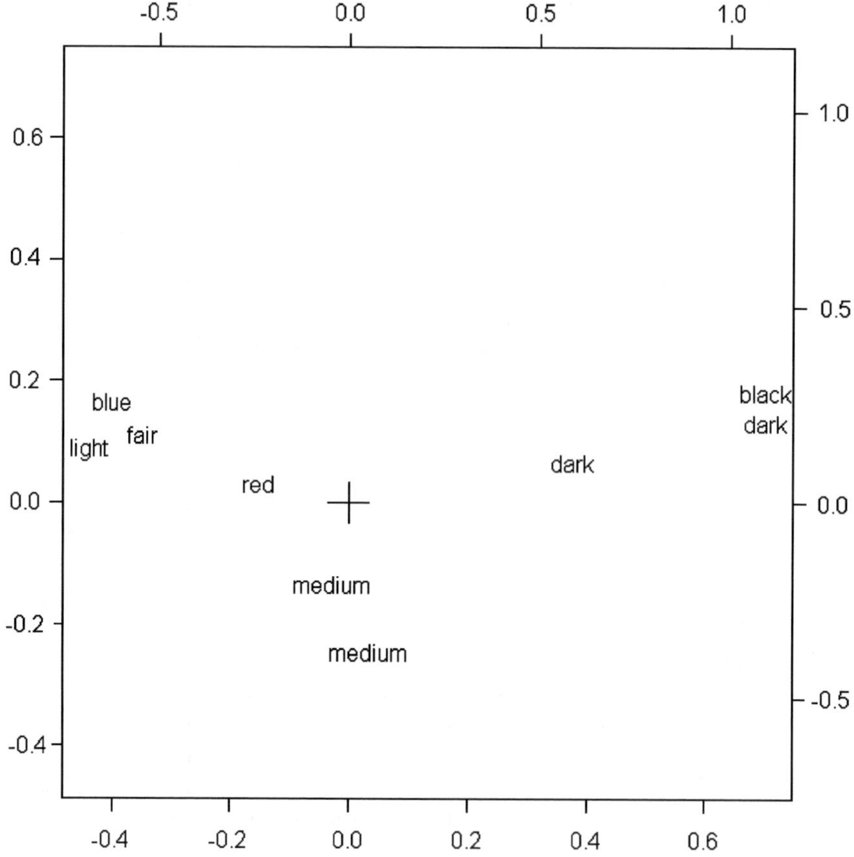

Fig. 11. Correspondence analysis display relating hair and skin color.

number of clusters by maximum likelihood (Shannon and Banks, 1999). However, many people make use of heuristic strategies for deciding the number of clusters that will be discussed in this section.

6.1. Stopping rule

In hierarchical clustering the 'stopping rule' indicates where to split the tree. The dendrogram in Fig. 7 could be cut to form 1, 2, 3, or 4 clusters (indicated by the dashed horizontal lines). (In fact it could produce more clusters by cutting lower on the vertical axis.) Several methods have been suggested for deciding among these choices and are defined and tested in the work by Milligan (1981). These generally are a modification of squared error or variance terms. Using definitions given before in this chapter, three stopping rule criteria for deciding how many clusters in the data are defined for each cut of the dendrogram:

$$R^2 = 1 - \frac{\left(\sum_K \sum_{i \in C_k} \|x_i - \bar{x}_k\|^2\right)}{\|x_i - \bar{x}\|^2},$$

$$pseudo - F = \frac{\left(\left(\|x_i - \bar{x}\|^2 - \sum_K \sum_{i \in C_k} \|x_i - \bar{x}_k\|^2\right) \Big/ K - 2\right)}{\left(\sum_K \sum_{i \in C_k} \|x_i - \bar{x}_k\|^2 \Big/ (n - K)\right)},$$

and,

$$pseudo - t^2 = \frac{\left(\sum_{i \in C_k \cup C_L} \left\|x_i - \bar{x}_{C_k \cup C_L}\right\|^2 - \sum_{i \in C_k} \left\|x_i - \bar{x}_{C_k}\right\|^2 - \sum_{i \in C_L} \left\|x_i - \bar{x}_{C_L}\right\|^2\right)}{\left(\sum_{i \in C_k} \left\|x_i - \bar{x}_{C_k}\right\|^2 + \sum_{i \in C_L} \left\|x_i - \bar{x}_{C_L}\right\|^2\right) \Big/ (n_K + n_L - 2)}.$$

These might be useful heuristics and the number of clusters which maximize these might be a reasonable number to use in the analysis. However, these are not distributed according to any known distribution (e.g., F, t) and it is important not to assign probabilities with these. See Milligan and Cooper (1985) and Cooper and Milligan (1988) for a detailed examination of these statistics and others regarding their performance in estimating the number of clusters.

6.2. Bayesian information criterion

When model-based clustering is used more formal likelihood criteria are available. The Schwartz Information Criterion (also called the Bayesian Information Criterion) is one of those which is often used. Recall that if we are modeling K multivariate normal clusters then the likelihood function is

$$L(x; \mu_1, \ldots, \mu_K, \Sigma_1, \ldots, \Sigma_k, \gamma) = \prod_{k=1}^{K} \prod_{i \in C_k} (2\pi)^{-p/2} |\Sigma_k|^{-1/2} \times \exp\left\{-\frac{1}{2}(x_i - \mu_k)^T \Sigma_k^{-1} (x_i - \mu_k)\right\}$$

Let $\log(L)$ denote the log-likelihood, $m = 2k + 1$ be the sum of number of estimated parameters, and n be the number of objects. Then the Schwartz Information Criterion is

$$-2\log(L) + m\log(n).$$

We select K clusters that maximizes this criterion.

7. Applications in medicine

A search of the NIH PUBMED publication database using the MESH term 'cluster analysis' resulted in 14,405 citations covering a wide range of areas of medicine. Here we provide a brief snapshot to some of them for reference.

Bierma-Zeinstra et al. (2001) used cluster analysis to analyze data on 224 consecutive patients being seen for hip pain. Ward's method for cluster analysis using medical history and physical exam results uncovered 10 distinct subgroups of patient. Subsequent examination of variables derived from X-rays and sonograms of their hip and knee regions showed significant correlation with these clusters. The medical history and physical exam results can then be used to classify patients into likely diagnostic group without waiting for expensive imaging data.

Lei et al. (2006) used hierarchical and k-means clustering to determine what size of lumbar disc replacement prosthesis appliances can be used in patients. Analyzing radiological data on 67 patients they were able to identify seven distinct device sizes that are widely used. If validated this will reduce the number of disc replacement sizes that need to be manufactured and stocked resulting in a possible improvement in healthcare delivery services.

Kaldjian et al. (2006) identified a list of factors that facilitate and impede voluntary physician disclosure of medical errors for patient safety, patient care, and medical education. Using a literature search they identified 316 articles reporting physician errors and extracted 91 factors from them and an additional 27 factors from a focus group thought to be related to error reporting. Several hierarchical clustering algorithms were used, but what is unique about this paper (versus the others reported here) was the distance measure used. In this study, 20 physicians grouped the factors into from 5 to 10 groups based on factor similarity, in essence a 'conceptual' proximity. The results of this research identified responsibility to the patient, to themselves, to the profession, and to the community as factors that facilitated error reporting. Attitude, helplessness, anxiety and fear, and uncertainty were identified as factors impeding error reporting.

Other applications include medication adherence (Russell et al., 2006), prediction of post-traumatic stress disorder (Jackson et al., 2006), microarry data analysis (Shannon et al., 2002; Shannon et al., 2003), and clarification of the obsessive compulsive disorders spectrum (Lochner et al., 2005). This small sample is presented to show the range of applications and introduce the reader to additional literature in the medical field to see how cluster analysis is applied.

8. Conclusion

This chapter has provided a brief overview of cluster analysis focusing on hierarchical, partitioning, and ordination methods. An overview of distance measures and the construction of pairwise distance matrices was presented since these are fundamental tools within the field of cluster analysis. Also, a very brief exposure to stopping rules for determining how many clusters and applications in medicine was presented to allow the reader entry into the literature for these areas. Anyone new to cluster analysis and planning on using these tools will be able to find many introductory textbooks to the field, and most statistical software packages have clustering algorithm procedures in them. Those readers wanting to become more involved with cluster analysis are encouraged to visit the *Classification Society of North America's* web page at http://www.classification-society.org/csna/csna.html.

References

Bierma-Zeinstra, S., Bohnen, A., Bernsen, R., Ridderikhoff, J., Verhaar, J., Prins, A. (2001). Hip problems in older adults: Classification by cluster analysis. *Journal of Clinical Epidemiology* **54**, 1139–1145.

Bishop, C. (1996). *Neural Networks for Pattern Recognition*. Oxford University Press, Oxford.

Cooper, M.C., Milligan, G.W. (1988). The effect of error on determining the number of clusters. *Proceedings of the International Workshop on Data Analysis, Decision Support and Expert Knowledge Representation in Marketing and Related Areas of Research*. pp. 319–328.

Cox, M.F., Cox, M.A.A. (2001). *Multidimensional Scaling*. Chapman & Hall, New York City.

Cristianini, N., Shawe-Taylor, J. (2000). *An Introduction to Support Vector Machines and Other Kernel-based Learning Methods*. Cambridge University Press, Cambridge, England.

Everitt, B., Rabe-Hesketh, S. (1997). *The Analysis of Proximity Data*. Wiley, New York City.

Everitt, B., Landau, S., Leese, M. (2001). *Cluster Analysis*, 4th ed. Edward Arnold Publishers Ltd, London.

Fisher, R. (1936). The use of multiple measurements in taxonomic problems. *Annals of Eugenics* **7**, 179–188.

Fisher, R.A. (1940). The precision of discriminant functions. *Annals of Eugenics (London)* **10**, 422–429.

Gordon, A.D. (1999). *Classification*, 2nd ed. Chapman & Hall/CRC Press, London.

Hartigan, J.A. (1975). *Clustering Algorithms*. Wiley, New York.

Hartigan, J., Wong, M. (1979). A *k*-means clustering algorithm. *Applied Statistics* **28**, 100–108.

Hastie, T., Tibshirani, R., Friedman, J. (2001). *The Elements of Statistical Learning*. Springer, New York City.

Jackson, C., Allen, G., Essock, S., Foster, M., Lanzara, C., Felton, C., Donahue, S. (2006). Clusters of event reactions among recipients of project liberty mental health counseling. *Psychiatric Services* **57**(9).

Kaldjian, L., Jones, E., Rosenthal, G., Tripp-Reimer, T., Hillis, S. (2006). An empirically derived taxonomy of factors affecting physicians' willingness to disclose medical errors. *Journal of General Internal Medicine: Official Journal of the Society for Research and Education in Primary Care Internal Medicine* **21**, 942–948.

Legendre, P., Legendre, L. (1998). *Numerical Ecology*. Elsevier, New York City.

Lei, D., Holder, R., Smith, F., Wardlaw, D., Hukins, D. (2006). Cluster analysis as a method for determining size ranges for spinal implants: Disc lumbar replacement prosthesis dimensions from magnetic resonance images. *Spine* **31**(25), 2979–2983.

Lochner, C., Hemmings, S., Kinnear, C., Niehaus, D., Nel, D., Corfield, V., Moolman-Smook, J., Seedat, S., Stein, D. (2005). Cluster analysis of obsessive compulsive spectrum disorders in patients with obsessive-compulsive disorder: Clinical and genetic correlates. *Comprehensive Psychiatry* **46**, 14–19.

McLachlan, G., Peel, D. (2000). *Finite Mixture Models*. Wiley and Sons, New York City.

Milligan, G. (1981). A monte carlo study of thirty internal criterion measures for cluster analysis. *Psychometrica* **46**(2), 187–199.

Milligan, G.W., Cooper, M.C. (1985). An examination of procedures for determining the number of clusters in a data set. *Psychometrika* **50**, 159–179.

Russell, C., Conn, V., Ashbaugh, C., Madsen, R., Hayes, K., Ross, G. (2006). Medication adherence patterns in adult renal transplant recipients. *Research in Nursing and Health* **29**, 521–532.

Shannon, W., Banks, D. (1999). Combining classification trees using maximum likelihood estimation. *Statistics in Medicine* **18**(6), 727–740.

Shannon, W., Culverhouse, R., Duncan, J. (2003). Analyzing microarray data using cluster analysis. *Pharmacogenomics* **4**(1), 41–51.

Shannon, W., Watson, M., Perry, A., Rich, K. (2002). Mantel statistics to correlate gene expression levels from microarrays with clinical covariates. *Genetic Epidemiology* **23**(1), 87–96.

Steele and Torrie (1980). *Principles and Procedures of Statistics: A Biometrical Approach*. McGraw-Hill, New York City.

Timm, N. (2002). *Applied Multivariate Analysis*. Springer, New York City.

Tukey, J.W. (1977). *Exploratory Data Analysis*. Addison-Wesley, Bosten, MA.

Handbook of Statistics, Vol. 27
ISSN: 0169-7161

DOI: 10.1016/S0169-7161(07)27012-9

12

Factor Analysis and Related Methods

Carol M. Woods and Michael C. Edwards

Abstract

This chapter introduces exploratory and confirmatory factor analysis (EFA and CFA) with brief mention of the closely related procedures principle components analysis and multidimensional item response theory. For EFA, emphasis is on rotation, the principle factors criterion, and methods for selecting the number of factors. CFA topics include identification, estimation of model parameters, and evaluation of model fit. EFA and CFA are introduced for continuous variables, and then extensions are described for non-normal continuous variables, and categorical variables. Study characteristics that influence sample size (for EFA or CFA) are discussed, and example analyses are provided which illustrate the use of three popular software programs.

1. Introduction

Factor analysis (FA) refers to a set of latent variable models and methods for fitting them to data. Factors are latent variables: Unobservable constructs presumed to underlie manifest variables (MVs). The objective of FA is to identify the number and nature of the factors that produce covariances or correlations among MVs. The variance of each MV is partitioned into *common variance* which is shared with other MVs, and *unique variance*, which is both random error and systematic variance unshared with other MVs (called *specific variance*). Because specific variance and random error are not modeled separately in FA, unique variance is often considered "error" variance. *Common factors* represent common variance and *unique factors* represent unique variance.

The FA model is:

$$\sum\nolimits_{xx} = \Lambda\Phi\Lambda^{\mathrm{T}} + \mathbf{D}_{\psi}, \tag{1}$$

where $\mathbf{\Sigma}_{xx}$ is the $p \times p$ covariance matrix among MVs $x_1, x_2, \ldots, x_p$, $\mathbf{\Lambda}$ is a $p \times m$ matrix of regression coefficients called *factor loadings* that relate each factor to each MV, $\mathbf{\Phi}$ is an $m \times m$ matrix of correlations among m factors, and $\mathbf{D}_{\psi}$ is a $p \times p$

diagonal matrix of unique variances (one for each MV). The model could be fitted to a matrix of correlations instead of covariances; this standardizes the factor loadings and elements of $\mathbf{D}_\psi$. Standardized unique variances are referred to as *uniquenesses*. The sum of squared standardized factor loadings, incorporating the correlations among factors (i.e., $\mathbf{\Lambda\Phi\Lambda}^{\mathrm{T}}$) gives the *communalities* for the MVs. The communality for an MV is the proportion of total variance it shares with other MVs, or its reliability. Notice that the communality and the uniqueness sum to 1.

Classic FA is applicable to continuous MVs and is analogous to multivariate linear regression, except that the predictors are unobservable. Assumptions comparable to those made in linear regression are made in FA: Common and unique factors are presumed uncorrelated, unique factors are presumed uncorrelated with one another, and MVs are assumed to be linearly related to the (linear combination of) factors. Additional assumptions are needed to identify the model because latent variables have no inherent scale. The scale of the common factors is often identified by fixing the mean and variance to 0 and 1, respectively. The mean of the unique factors is also usually fixed to 0, but the variance is estimated. The variance of a unique factor is usually interpreted as the error variance of the MV.

FA can be exploratory or confirmatory depending on the degree to which investigators have prior hypotheses about the number and nature of the underlying constructs. Although some of the methods used in exploratory and confirmatory factor analysis (EFA and CFA) are distinct, the boundary between them is often blurred. Rather than imagining them as completely separate techniques, it is useful to think of EFA and CFA as opposite ends of the same continuum.

In EFA, a preliminary sense of the latent structure is obtained, often without significance testing. Additional research is needed to make definitive claims about the number and nature of the common factors. In CFA, a hypothesized model is tested, and sometimes compared to other hypothesized models. CFA is a special case of a structural equation model (SEM); thus many principles of SEM also apply to CFA. CFA models are evaluated using significance tests and other indices of fit. Though replication and cross-validation is important for both types of FA, results from CFA are more definitive because prior hypotheses are tested.

2. Exploratory factor analysis (EFA)

EFA is performed when investigators are unable or unwilling to specify the number and nature of the common factors. A key task is to select the number of common factors (m) that best accounts for the covariance among MVs. Several models with differing m are fitted to the same data and both statistical information and substantive interpretability are used to select a model. The goal is to identify the number of major common factors such that the solution is not only parsimonious, but also plausible and well matched to the data. Typically, all pm elements of $\mathbf{\Lambda}$ are estimated rather than constrained to a particular value. Unique variances and correlations among factors are also estimated.

Once the parameters of a model with a particular m are estimated, the solution is rotated to improve substantive interpretability. Rotated, not un-rotated, factor loadings aid in the selection of m. The term *factor rotation* was coined during an era when FA was carried out by hand. FA models were represented graphically in m-dimensional space with an axis for each factor and a point for each MV. Axes were literally rotated to a subjective, *simple structure* solution. Thurstone (1947) specified formal criteria for simple structure, but essentially, each factor should be represented by a distinct subset of MVs with large factor loadings, subsets of MVs defining different factors should overlap minimally, and each MV should be influenced by only a subset of common factors.

In contemporary FA, rotation is objective and automated by computer software. The matrix of rotated loadings is produced by multiplying $\mathbf{\Lambda}$ by an $m \times p$ *transformation matrix*, $\mathbf{T}$. The elements of $\mathbf{T}$ are chosen to either maximize a *simplicity* function or minimize a *complexity* function. These functions mathematically specify simple structure, or its opposite (complexity) in the pattern of loadings.

The EFA model is *rotationally indeterminate*, meaning that if a single $\mathbf{\Lambda}$ can be found that satisfies the model for a particular $\mathbf{\Sigma}_{xx}$, then infinitely many other $\mathbf{\Lambda}$s exist that satisfy the model equally well. Procedures used to estimate EFA model parameters (discussed in a subsequent section) impose criteria to obtain unique values; however, an infinite number of alternative $\mathbf{\Lambda}$s could replace the initial solution.

Numerous rotation methods have been developed (see Browne, 2001). One major distinction among them is whether factors are permitted to correlate. *Orthogonal* rotations force factors to be uncorrelated whereas *oblique* rotations permit nonzero correlations among factors. Orthogonal rotations are primarily of didactic or historical interest; they are easier and were developed first. It is usually best to use an oblique rotation because factors are typically correlated to some degree, and correlation estimates will be 0 if they are not. A few of the most popular oblique rotation procedures are described next.

2.1. Rotation

The two-stage *oblique Promax rotation* procedure (Hendrikson and White, 1964) is frequently used and widely implemented in software. Orthogonal rotation is carried out first, followed by a procedure that permits correlations among factors. The first stage consists of rotating loadings to an orthogonal criterion called "Varimax" (Kaiser, 1958). The transformation matrix for *orthogonal Varimax rotation* maximizes the sum of the variances of the squared factor loadings on each factor. The simplicity criterion is:

$$V = \sum_{k=1}^{m} \frac{1}{p} \sum_{j=1}^{p} (\lambda_{jk}^2 - \bar{\lambda}_{.k}^2)^2, \quad \text{where } \bar{\lambda}_{.k}^2 = \frac{1}{p} \sum_{k=1}^{m} \lambda_{jk}^2 \tag{2}$$

and λ_{jk} is an element of $\mathbf{\Lambda}$ for the jth MV and the kth factor. Greater variability in the magnitude of the squared loadings indicates better simple structure.

The second stage of the Promax procedure is to raise Varimax-rotated loadings to a power (often the 4th), restore the signs, and estimate new loadings that are as close as possible to the powered loadings. Least squares estimation is used to minimize the sum of squared differences between the Varimax-rotated loadings and the powered (target) loadings, t_{jk}, which is the complexity function:

$$P = \sum_{k=1}^{m} \sum_{j=1}^{p} (\lambda_{jk}^2 - t_{jk})^2. \tag{3}$$

Because variables with larger communalities have more influence on the rotated solution than variables with smaller communalities, each row of $\mathbf{\Lambda}$ is standardized before rotation and returned to the original scale after rotation. Loadings for each MV are divided by the square root of the communality (called a *Kaiser weight*) before rotation, and then multiplied by the Kaiser weight after rotation. This process of *row standardization* was originally introduced for orthogonal Varimax rotation, but is now commonly used with most rotations, both orthogonal and oblique.

Other popular oblique rotations are members of a family described by Crawford and Ferguson (1970). The general complexity function is:

$$\mathrm{CF} = (1-\kappa) \sum_{j=1}^{p} \sum_{k=1}^{m} \sum_{\substack{\ell=1 \\ k \neq \ell}}^{m} \lambda_{jk}^2 \lambda_{j\ell}^2 + \kappa \sum_{k=1}^{m} \sum_{j=1}^{p} \sum_{\substack{h=1 \\ j \neq h}}^{p} \lambda_{jk}^2 \lambda_{hk}^2 , \tag{4}$$

where κ weights MV complexity (first term) and factor complexity (second term), and $0 \leq \kappa \leq 1$. MV complexity is minimized when there is a single nonzero loading in each row of $\mathbf{\Lambda}$; factor complexity is minimized when there is a single nonzero loading in each column of $\mathbf{\Lambda}$.

Researchers select κ and specify whether the rotation is orthogonal or oblique. When $\kappa = 1/p$, and orthogonal rotation is specified, the Crawford–Ferguson (CF) criterion is the same as the orthogonal Varimax criterion. Oblique Varimax rotation is also possible. When $\kappa = 0$, complexity in the MVs, but not the factors, is minimized. Oblique rotation renders the CF criterion equivalent to the oblique quartimax criterion (also called "quartimin" or "direct quartimin"), introduced by Jennrich and Sampson (1966).

Some FA experts prefer oblique quartimax rotation (e.g., Browne, 2001), but the best approach may depend on the particular data set and the goals of the FA. It is sometimes useful to use two or three different rotation criteria and then select the most substantively interpretable solution.

We turn now to methods for estimating the parameters of EFA models. The two most common methods are iterative principle factors and maximum likelihood (ML) estimation. Typically, correlations rather than covariances are analyzed because factor loadings are easier to interpret when standardized. Also, note that the columns of $\mathbf{\Lambda}$ (i.e., the factors) are always uncorrelated following initial estimation. In EFA, correlations among factors are introduced only by oblique rotation.

2.2. Principle factors

Because the EFA model is rotationally indeterminate, an additional criterion is imposed when the parameters are estimated so that initial factor loadings are unique. By the *criterion of principle factors*, each common factor should account for the maximum possible amount of variance in the MVs. Only one $\mathbf{\Lambda}$ satisfies the principle factors criterion. A principle factors solution uses eigenvalues and eigenvectors to estimate $\mathbf{\Lambda}$. If $\mathbf{S}$ is a symmetric matrix and $\mathbf{Su} = \ell\mathbf{u}$, then ℓ is an eigenvalue of $\mathbf{S}$ and $\mathbf{u}$ is an eigenvector of $\mathbf{S}$.

In EFA, eigenvalues and eigenvectors of the *reduced correlation matrix*, $\mathbf{R}_{xx}$, are used to compute $\mathbf{\Lambda}$. $\mathbf{R}_{xx}$ has communalities for each MV on the diagonal (rather than 1's). For a given m, $\mathbf{\Lambda}$ is constructed from the m largest eigenvalues and the corresponding eigenvectors: $\mathbf{\Lambda} = \mathbf{UD}_\ell^{1/2}$. $\mathbf{U}$ is a $p \times m$ orthogonal matrix with columns equal to eigenvectors, and $\mathbf{D}_\ell^{1/2}$ is an $m \times m$ diagonal matrix with nonzero elements equal to square roots of eigenvalues. An eigenvalue is equal to the sum of squared loadings down each column of $\mathbf{\Lambda}$, interpreted as the proportion of variance accounted for by each factor.

A complication inherent in the procedure just described is that communalities are needed prior to the computation of factor loadings. These so-called prior communalities must be estimated. Guttman (1940) showed that the squared multiple correlation (R^2) from the regression of an MV on the $p-1$ other MVs is a lower bound for the communality. Though somewhat conservative, R^2s from these regressions are usually used as estimates of prior communalities.

A newer way to estimate prior communalities is the *partitioning method* (Cudeck, 1991), which may be used only if $p \geq 2m+1$. For each MV, the remaining $p-1$ MVs are divided into two mutually exclusive subsets of m variables (because the method is contingent upon m, it must be repeated for every different m under consideration). The jth MV for which a communality is sought is subset 1, and the other mutually exclusive sets of MVs are subsets 2 and 3. The communality for the jth MV is given by $\boldsymbol{\rho}_{13}\mathbf{P}_{23}^{-1}\boldsymbol{\rho}_{21}$, where $\boldsymbol{\rho}_{13}$ is the vector of correlations between subsets 1 and 3, $\boldsymbol{\rho}_{21}$ is the vector of correlations between subsets 1 and 2, and $\mathbf{P}_{23}^{-1}$ is the (inverse of) the $m \times m$ matrix of correlations between subsets 2 and 3.

The set of procedures described thus far is referred to as *principle factors conditional on prior communalities* (or simply, conditional principle factors). However, a closely related method, *iterative principle factors*, can provide better answers. Iterative principle factors minimizes the sum of squared residuals, which are discrepancies between sample correlations (or covariances) and a particular solution for the FA model:

$$\mathrm{RSS} = \sum_{i=1}^{p}\sum_{j=1}^{p}[\mathbf{R}_{xx} - (\mathbf{\Lambda\Phi\Lambda}^{\mathrm{T}})]_{ij}^2, \tag{5}$$

where RSS is the residual sums of squares, $\mathbf{\Phi}$ is diagonal (prior to rotation), and $\mathbf{D}_\psi$ is not shown because it has been subtracted from the full correlation matrix to create $\mathbf{R}_{xx}$. A key feature of the iterative approach is that communalities placed on the diagonal of $\mathbf{R}_{xx}$ are estimated simultaneously with the factor loadings.

The iterative approach begins as conditional principle factors. Then the initial estimate of $\mathbf{\Lambda}$ is used to estimate new communalities as the sum of squared loadings across each row. These are placed on the diagonal of $\mathbf{R}_{xx}$, eigenvalues and eigenvectors are obtained as before, and $\mathbf{\Lambda}$ is re-estimated. This process continues until the communalities change minimally from one iteration to the next (i.e., converge).

2.3. *Normal theory maximum likelihood (ML) estimation*

One advantage of principle factors methods is that no distributional assumption about the MVs is needed. However, the disadvantage is that no standard errors (SEs), significance tests, or confidence intervals (CIs) are available. If MVs can be assumed to jointly follow a multivariate normal distribution, EFA parameters can be estimated as in conditional principle factors, with the additional requirement that they maximize a multivariate normal likelihood function. Normal theory ML estimation is the same as iterative principle factors except that loadings are chosen to maximize the likelihood function rather than to minimize RSS. The joint likelihood is

$$L = \prod_{i=1}^{N} \frac{|\mathbf{\Sigma}_{xx}|^{.5}}{(2\pi)^{.5p}} \exp\left(-\frac{1}{2}(\mathbf{x}_i - \boldsymbol{\mu})^{\mathrm{T}} \Sigma_{xx}^{-1} (\mathbf{x}_i - \boldsymbol{\mu}) \right), \tag{6}$$

where N is the total number of observations, $\mathbf{x}_i$ the vector of MV scores for observation i, and $\boldsymbol{\mu}$ is the vector of MV means.

When ML is used, a likelihood ratio (LR) test statistic and numerous descriptive indices may be used to evaluate global model fit. Two versions of the LR statistic are used. The classic LR statistic is $(N-1)(-2)[\log(L)]$, and Bartlett's (1950) corrected version is $(N - ((2p + 11)/6) - (2m/3)) - (2)[\log(L)]$. L is (Eq. (6)) evaluated at the maximum. With sufficient N, the LR statistic is approximately χ^2-distributed with degrees of freedom:

$$df = \frac{1}{2}p(p + 1) - \left\{ p + pm - \frac{1}{2}m(m - 1) \right\} = \frac{(p - m)^2 - (p + m)}{2} \tag{7}$$

Bartlett's correction may increase the degree to which the LR statistic is χ^2-distributed. The LR statistic may be used to test the null hypothesis (H_0) that the FA model with m factors holds. Rejection of H_o indicates that $\mathbf{\Sigma}_{xx}$ has no particular structure or that more factors are needed. Thus, failing to reject H_0 is desirable. However, this test of perfect fit is sensitive to N. Virtually any parsimonious model is rejected if N is large enough, and substantial misfit is missed if N is small.

Numerous descriptive indices of model fit have been developed that should be consulted along with, or instead of, the χ^2-test. These indices are usually studied or discussed in the context of CFA rather than EFA; thus it is more natural to review them when describing CFA. However, the indices are also useful for EFA, and are the primary method by which the number of factors is decided upon when ML is used. ML also provides SEs for the factor loadings and inter-factor correlations (following oblique rotation), which aids in the often subjective process of assigning MVs to factors in EFA.

2.4. *Tools for choosing m*

Three statistical tools used to choose m (which may be used with either principle factors or ML) are residuals, a scree plot, and parallel analysis. Smaller residuals indicate better model fit. A summary statistic, such as the root mean square residual or the maximum absolute residual, can be compared for models with different m. Examination of residuals for each correlation or covariance may help to identify specific areas of model misfit. The best model typically has many small residuals and no particularly large ones. Many software programs standardize residuals, which aid in the interpretation of their magnitude. Typically, a standardized residual greater than about 2 is considered large.

Another tool, the *scree plot* (Cattell, 1966), is a graph of the eigenvalues of $\mathbf{R}_{xx}$. Figure 1 shows an example for 9 MVs. The vernacular definition of "scree" is an accumulation of loose stones or rocky debris lying on a slope or at the base of a hill or cliff. In a scree plot, it is desirable to find a sharp reduction in the size of the eigenvalues (like a cliff), with the rest of the smaller eigenvalues constituting rubble. When the eigenvalues drop dramatically in size, an additional factor would add relatively little to the information already extracted. Because scree plots can be subjective and arbitrary to interpret, their primary utility is in providing two or three reasonable values of m to consider. The plot in Fig. 1 suggests that a useful model for these data may have 3 or 4 factors.

Parallel analysis (Horn, 1965) helps to make the interpretation of scree plots more objective. The eigenvalues of $\mathbf{R}_{xx}$ are plotted with eigenvalues of the reduced correlation matrix for simulated variables with population correlations of 0 (i.e., no common factors). An example is displayed in Fig. 2. The number of

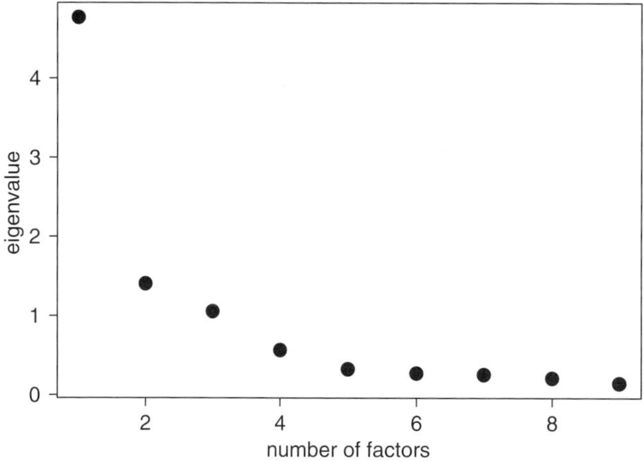

Fig. 1. Example scree plot.

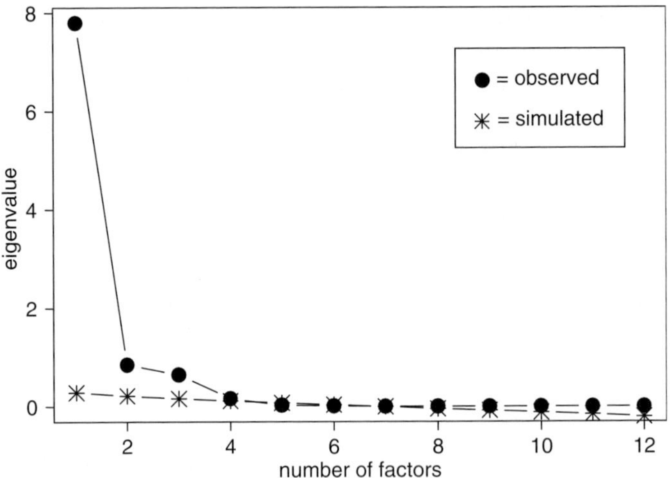

Fig. 2. Example of parallel analysis.

eigenvalues above the point where the two lines intersect (3 for the example in Fig. 2) is the suggested *m*. The rationale for parallel analysis is that useful factors account for more variance than could be expected by chance. Recall that an eigenvalue is the proportion of variance explained by each factor. Only factors with eigenvalues greater than those from uncorrelated data are useful.

We are not aware of a commercial computer program that implements parallel analysis, but any software that will simulate data from a normal distribution and compute eigenvalues may be used. To carry out parallel analysis, generate *N* observations from a normal distribution for *p* variables (*N* and *p* for the simulated data match those for the observed data). Then compute the reduced correlation matrix among simulated MVs and its eigenvalues, repeat this process approximately 100 times, and average the eigenvalues for each simulated MV. It is these mean eigenvalues that are plotted against the eigenvalues of $\mathbf{R}_{xx}$. Syntax for parallel analysis using SPSS (SPSS Incorporated, 2006), or SAS software (SAS Institute, 2006) was published by O'Connor (2000).

Additional tools are available to help select *m* when ML is used. Global indices of model fit may be compared among models with differing *m*. Increasing *m* improves model fit to some degree, but the goal is to identify *m* such that one fewer factor results in substantially poorer fit and one additional factor has little impact on the fit. Additionally, nested models can be statistically compared using a χ^2-difference test. The difference between the LR statistics for a model with *k* factors and a model with $k-1$ factors is approximately χ^2-distributed with degrees of freedom (*df*) equal to the difference between the *df* for the two models. A significant difference suggests that fit is better for the model with *k* factors. Otherwise, the more parsimonious model is preferred. The final model selected should fit in an absolute, as well as relative, sense.

We conclude this section with a warning about an approach commonly employed to select *m*, which is theoretically unjustifiable and likely to be misleading.

The eigenvalue-greater-than-one rule (also called the Kaiser criterion or the Kaiser–Guttman rule) leads researchers to select m equal to the number of eigenvalues of $\mathbf{R}_{xx}$ that exceed 1. The number of eigenvalues greater than 1 is a lower bound for the number of *components* to extract in *principle components analysis* (discussed next), but it should never be used as the sole criterion to select m for EFA.

3. Principle components analysis (PCA)

PCA is a data reduction method sometimes confused with EFA. Conditional principle factors EFA is mathematically similar to PCA. For both, parameters interpreted as standardized regression coefficients are calculated from eigenvectors and eigenvalues of a correlation matrix. However, EFA analyzes the *reduced* correlation matrix, with prior communalities on the diagonal, whereas PCA analyzes the *full* correlation matrix, with 1's on the diagonal. Because a communality is the proportion of MV variance that is reliable, PCA treats MVs as error-free. Thus, what may seem like a small technical difference between PCA and EFA has important implications for interpretation.

The purpose of EFA and PCA differs, as does interpretation of the results. EFA seeks to explain covariation among MVs and is useful for understanding underlying structure in the data. Total MV variance is separated into common and unique elements, and common factors are constructs thought to give rise to MVs. In contrast, PCA is useful for reducing a large number of variables into a smaller set. Instead of separating common and unique variance, total MV variance is reorganized into linear combinations called *components*. A component is a linear combination of MVs, not a latent variable. Component loadings are standardized regression coefficients indicating the strength of relation between each MV and each component. However, a component has no particular interpretation beyond "linear combination of" MVs. When the goal of an analysis is to understand underlying dimensions implied by correlations (or covariances) among MVs, and interpret the dimensions as constructs, FA is applicable and PCA is not.

4. Confirmatory factor analysis (CFA)

CFA is used to test a hypothesized model. Investigators specify the number of factors, and typically constrain many factor loadings to 0. Thus, fewer loadings are estimated in CFA than in EFA because not all factors are hypothesized to underlie all MVs. MVs with nonzero loadings on a factor are *indicators* of the factor. Researchers decide when fitting the model to data which parameters are *free* (i.e., to be estimated) and which are *fixed* (i.e., constrained to some value).

Because more restrictions are placed on the parameters than in EFA, CFA models are not rotationally indeterminate. Thus, eigenvalues and eigenvectors are not used in CFA, and correlations among factors are not introduced by rotation. Instead, researchers specify whether correlations among factors are free or fixed. Typically, unique variances are estimated as in EFA and correlations among them can be estimated if relationships are hypothesized. An important consideration in CFA that influences how many parameters can be freed is model identification.

4.1. Identification

A CFA model is *identified* if parameter estimates are unique, otherwise the model is *unidentified* (also called *under-identified*) and the results are not trustworthy. At a minimum, there must be more known quantities (e.g., non-redundant elements of $\boldsymbol{\Sigma}_{xx}$) than unknown quantities (i.e., parameters to estimate). This is a necessary but not sufficient condition for model identification. Bollen (1989) describes conditions that are sufficient but not necessary for identification that are useful for models matching these criteria. Models with $m > 1$ are identified if there are 3 or more indicators per factor, each indicator has a nonzero loading on only 1 factor, and unique variances are uncorrelated. Only 2 indicators per factor are acceptable if either all the factors are correlated (i.e., $\boldsymbol{\Phi}$ has no zeros), or each row of $\boldsymbol{\Phi}$ has at least one nonzero off-diagonal element.

Many possible models can be specified and identified which do not match Bollen's (1989) criteria above. Identification can be proven by matrix algebra, but this is tedious, error-prone, and unrealistic for some users. Most software programs detect some types of under-identification and warn users that re-specification may be needed. If identification is uncertain, Jöreskog and Sörbom (1986) suggest fitting the model to data, computing the model-implied covariance matrix, and then re-fitting the model treating the model-implied covariances as if they were observed. If parameter estimates from the two fittings differ, the model is not identified.

In addition to model identification, the scales of all latent variables must be identified in CFA. Typically, unique factors are handled as in EFA: Means are fixed to 0 and variances are free. The scales of common factors also may be identified as in EFA, by fixing the means and variances to 0 and 1, respectively. Alternatively, a common factor can be assigned the scale of one MV to which it is highly related by fixing that MV's loading to 1. This permits estimation of the common-factor variance which is sometimes of interest. Model fit is unaffected by the procedure used to identify the scales of the factors.

4.2. Estimation

A CFA model is usually fitted to data with ML under the assumption that MVs are continuous and multivariate normal. The likelihood is:

$$L_{\text{CFA}} = \log\left|\hat{\boldsymbol{\Sigma}}_{xx}\right| + \text{tr}(\boldsymbol{\Sigma}_{xx}\hat{\boldsymbol{\Sigma}}_{xx}^{-1}) - \log|\boldsymbol{\Sigma}_{xx}| - p, \tag{8}$$

where $\boldsymbol{\Sigma}_{xx}$ is the observed covariance matrix, $\hat{\boldsymbol{\Sigma}}_{xx}$ the model-implied covariance matrix, and "tr" refers to the trace (i.e., sum of diagonal elements). Thus, SEs for factor loadings and inter-factor correlations are available, as is an LR statistic for evaluating model fit that is χ^2-distributed in large samples. The LR statistic is $(N-1)L_{\text{CFA}}$ (where L_{CFA} is (Eq. (8)) evaluated at the maximum) with *df* equal to the number of nonredundant elements in $\mathbf{\Sigma}_{xx}$ less than the number of free parameters, t:

$$df = \frac{1}{2}p(p+1) - t \tag{9}$$

CFA models should be fitted to covariance, not correlation, matrices, unless one's software is known to handle correlation matrices correctly (Cudeck, 1989). The statistical theory that justifies CFA does not apply to correlation matrices without modification. Because the procedures are more complicated for correlation versus covariance matrices, many computer programs do not handle correlation matrices appropriately and will provide incorrect SEs (and possibly an incorrect LR statistic). The RAMONA program (Browne et al., 1994) and PROC CALIS in SAS (SAS Institute, 2006) handle correlation matrices appropriately, but with most software programs, it is best to fit a CFA model to a covariance matrix to ensure a proper analysis.

4.3. Evaluation of model fit

After a CFA model has been specified, identification has been addressed, and parameters have been estimated, a fundamental concern is how well the model fits the data. First, there should be no improper parameter estimates. If a correlation is outside the range −1 to 1, or a variance is negative (called a *Heywood case*), the solution should not be interpreted and causes of the problem should be explored. Improper estimates can occur when the population parameter is near the boundary, when outliers or influential observations are present in the data, when the model is poorly specified, or because of sampling variability.

If all parameter estimates are within permissible ranges, global model fit is evaluated. As in EFA, the χ^2-test of absolute fit is sensitive to sample size and could provide misleading results. However, the difference between LR statistics for two nested models provides a useful χ^2-difference test (for large samples) with *df* equal to the difference in *df*s for the two models. A significant difference supports the larger model; otherwise, the more parsimonious model is preferred.

Absolute fit is evaluated using descriptive indices. Available options are abundant and sometimes contradict one another. However, Hu and Bentler (1998, 1999) extensively studied many indices and provide guidance for selecting and interpreting a manageable subset. They recommend reporting one residuals-based measure such as the standardized root mean square residual (SRMR; Bentler, 1995; Jöreskog and Sörbom, 1981), and one or more of the following: (a) the root mean square error of approximation (RMSEA; Browne and Cudeck, 1993; Steiger, 1990; Steiger and Lind, 1980), (b) the Tucker–Lewis (1973) incremental fit index (TLI; also known as the non-normed fit index due to Bentler and Bonett, 1980), (c) Bollen's (1988) non-normed index (Δ_2), and (d) Bentler's (1990) comparative fit index (CFI).

The SRMR summarizes the differences between the observed and model-implied covariance matrices:

$$\text{SRMR} = \sqrt{\frac{2}{p(p+1)}\left\{\sum_{i=1}^{p}\sum_{j=1}^{i}\left[\frac{(\sigma_{ij}-\hat{\sigma}_{ij})}{\sigma_{ii}\sigma_{jj}}\right]^2\right\}}, \tag{10}$$

where σ_{ij} is an element of $\boldsymbol{\Sigma}_{xx}$ and $\hat{\sigma}_{ij}$ is an element of $\hat{\Sigma}_{xx}$. Values closer to 0 indicate better fit; Hu and Bentler (1999) suggested that fit is good if SRMR $\leq$ about .09.

The RMSEA indicates the degree of discrepancy between the model and the data per degree of freedom:

$$\text{RMSEA} = \sqrt{\frac{-2L_{\text{CFA}} - \frac{df}{N-1}}{df}}, \tag{11}$$

where L_{CFA} is (Eq. (8)) evaluated at the maximum. Values closer to 0 indicate better fit.

Roughly, model fit is quantified as close (RMSEA $<$ .05), reasonably good (.05 $<$ RMSEA $<$ .08), mediocre (.08 $<$ RMSEA $<$ .10), or unacceptable (RMSEA $>$ .10) (Browne and Cudeck, 1993). Hu and Bentler (1999) suggested that RMSEA $\leq$ about .06 indicates good fit. The RMSEA is unique because under certain assumptions, its sampling distribution is known; thus, CIs can be computed (Browne and Cudeck, 1993; Curran et al., 2003).

The TLI, CFI, and Δ_2 are the incremental fit indices that measure the proportionate improvement in fit by comparing our model to a more restricted, hypothetical baseline model. Usually the baseline model has independent MVs, thus 0 factors. The TLI and Δ_2 indicate where our model lies on a continuum between a hypothetical worst (baseline) model and a hypothetical perfect model, for which the LR statistic equals its *df* (thus, the ratio is 1):

$$\text{TLI} = \frac{\frac{\chi_b^2}{df_b} - \frac{\chi_m^2}{df_m}}{\frac{\chi_b^2}{df_b} - 1}, \tag{12}$$

and

$$\Delta_2 = \frac{\chi_b^2 - \chi_m^2}{\chi_b^2 - df_m}. \tag{13}$$

Subscripts "*b*" and "*m*" refer to the baseline model and the fitted model with *m* factors.

The CFI shows how much less misfit there is in our model than in the worst-fitting (baseline) model:

$$\text{CFI} = \frac{(\chi_b^2 - df_b) - (\chi_m^2 - df_m)}{\chi_b^2 - df_b}. \tag{14}$$

If our model fits perfectly, $\chi^2_m = df_m$ and CFI = 1. The worst possible fit for our model is $\chi^2_m = \chi^2_b$ with $df_m = df_b$; thus, CFI = 0. The TLI and Δ_2 are also typically between 0 and 1 with larger values indicating better fit, but values outside that range are possible. Hu and Bentler (1999) suggested that values of TLI, CFI, or Δ_2 equal to at least .95 indicate good fit.

It is possible for a model that fits well globally to fit poorly in a specific region; thus additional elements of model fit should be evaluated. Parameter estimates should make sense for the substantive problem, and most factor loadings should be statistically significant. It is useful to screen for extreme residuals, because specific misfit may not be reflected in the SRMR summary statistic. Models that are well matched to the data have moderate to large R^2s for each MV and reliable factors that explain substantial variance in the MVs.

The R^2 is the proportion of total variance in an MV that is accounted for by the common factors (i.e., the communality). Larger values are generally preferred. Fornell and Larcker (1981) recommend interpreting a reliability coefficient, ρ_η, for each factor:

$$\rho_\eta = \frac{\left(\sum_{j=1}^{p} \lambda_j\right)^2}{\left(\sum_{j=1}^{p} \lambda_j\right)^2 + \sum_{j=1}^{p} \sigma^2_{jj}}, \tag{15}$$

where σ^2_{jj} is the (estimated) unique variance for the jth MV. A rule of thumb is that .7 or larger is good reliability (Hatcher, 1994). Fornell and Larcker (1981) suggest an additional coefficient, $\rho_{\mathrm{vc}(\eta)}$, as a measure of the average variance explained by each factor in relation to the amount of variance due to measurement error:

$$\rho_{vc(\eta)} = \frac{\sum_{j=1}^{p} \lambda_j^2}{\sum_{j=1}^{p} \lambda_j^2 + \sum_{j=1}^{p} \sigma^2_{jj}}. \tag{16}$$

If $\rho_{\mathrm{vc}(\eta)}$ is less than .50, the variance due to measurement error is larger than the variance measured by the factor; thus, the validity of both the factor and its indicators is questionable (Fornell and Larcker, 1981, p. 46).

5. FA with non-normal continuous variables

In practice, MVs are often not approximately multivariate normal. This should be evaluated before methods described in the previous sections are applied. If ML estimation is used to fit an FA model to non-normal (continuous) data, the LR statistic and SEs are likely to be incorrect (Curran et al., 1996; Yuan et al., 2005; West et al., 1995). Thus, significance tests, CIs, and indices of model fit are potentially misleading. Coefficients and tests of multivariate skewness and kurtosis (e.g., Mardia, 1970) are available in many computer programs and should be used routinely. Outliers can cause non-normality, so screening for outliers also should be common practice.

If non-normality is detected in CFA, one alternative is a weighted least squares estimator called asymptotically distribution free (ADF) (Browne, 1982, 1984). Parameter estimates minimize the sum of squared deviations between $\mathbf{\Sigma}_{xx}$ and $\hat{\Sigma}_{xx}$, weighted by approximate covariances among elements of $\mathbf{\Sigma}_{xx}$. However, with large p, it becomes impractical to invert the $p \times p$ weight matrix, and it appears that large sample sizes (e.g., 1,000–5,000) are needed for the ADF method to perform well (Curran et al., 1996; West et al., 1995).

A more generally applicable alternative is to use ML with a correction to the LR statistic and SEs. The Satorra–Bentler correction (Satorra and Bentler, 1988; Satorra, 1990) has performed well with moderate sample sizes such as 200–500 (Chou et al., 1991; Curran et al., 1996; Hu et al., 1992; Satorra and Bentler, 1988). It is implemented in the EQS (Bentler, 1989) and Mplus (Muthén and Muthén, 2006) programs for CFA. ML with the Satorra–Bentler correction can also be used for EFA and is implemented in Mplus. If SEs and an LR statistic are not needed, conditional or iterative principle factors could be used for EFA because multivariate normality is not required.

6. FA with categorical variables

Both EFA and CFA are commonly used to assess the dimensionality of questionnaires and surveys. Typically, such items have binary or ordinal response scales; thus, classic FA is not appropriate for several reasons. For one, linear association is not meaningful because absolute distances between categories are unknown. Thus, the classic model of linear association among MVs, and between each MV and the factor(s), is inapplicable. Also, Pearson correlations are attenuated for categorical data, which can lead to underestimates of factor loadings if classic FA is applied. Strictly speaking, discrete variables cannot follow the continuous multivariate normal distribution. Serious biases can result when standard ML is used for FA with Pearson correlations computed from categorical data (DiStefano, 2002; West et al., 1995). An alternative to classic FA is needed for categorical data.

One solution is to posit that a continuous but unobserved distribution underlies the observed categories. In other words, in addition to an observed categorical MV, x, there is an unobserved continuous variable, x^*. It is assumed that the categorization occurs such that:

$$x_1 = \begin{cases} 1, & \text{if } x_1^* \leq \tau_1 \\ 2, & \text{if } \tau_1 < x_1^* \leq \tau_2 \\ \cdots & \cdots \\ c-1, & \text{if } \tau_{c-2} < x_1^* \leq \tau_{c-1} \\ c, & \text{if } \tau_{c-1} < x_1^* \end{cases} \tag{17}$$

where τ_j is the threshold separating category j from $j+1$ and $j = 1, 2, \ldots, c$. While a linear relationship between x and the latent construct(s) is untenable, linearity is reasonable for x^*.

If it can be assumed for a given research context that the observed categorical data arose through a categorization of unobserved continuous data, and that every pair of unobserved variables is bivariate normal, then the correlations among the underlying, continuous variables can be estimated by *polychoric correlations* (called *tetrachoric correlations* when both variables are binary). Typically, a polychoric correlation is computed in two stages (Olsson, 1979). First, τs are estimated for each MV based on the proportions of people responding in each category (and the normality assumption). Second, the correlation between each pair of underlying variables is estimated by ML. The likelihood is a function of the τs and the bivariate frequencies. The classic FA model is then fitted to the matrix of polychoric correlations. However, an alternate estimator is also needed.

Unweighted least squares requires no distributional assumptions about the MVs and produces consistent estimates of the factor loadings. However, SEs, significance tests, and most fit indices are not available; thus, it is only useful for EFA. Weighted least squares (WLS) is a popular alternative that may be used for EFA or CFA. When the asymptotic covariance matrix (i.e., the covariances among all the elements in the covariance matrix among MVs) is used as the weight matrix, WLS can provide accurate estimates of the SEs and the LR statistic. Unfortunately, inversion of the weight matrix (required for WLS) becomes increasingly difficult as the number of MVs increases, and very large sample sizes are needed for accurate estimation (West et al., 1995).

A compromise solution, called diagonally weighted least squares (DWLS; Jöreskog and Sörbom, 2001), uses only the diagonal elements of the asymptotic covariance matrix; thus, the weight matrix is much easier to invert. This results in a loss of statistical efficiency, but corrective procedures (e.g., the Satorra–Bentler correction) can be used to obtain accurate estimates of the SEs and the LR statistic. DWLS with these corrections is sometimes called *robust DWLS*. Recent simulations suggested that robust DWLS performs well, and better than WLS based on a full weight matrix (Flora and Curran, 2004). Robust DWLS is implemented in the LISREL (Jöreskog and Sörbom, 2005) and Mplus (Muthén and Muthén, 2006) programs.

Another way to evaluate the latent dimensionality of categorical MVs is with models and methods in the domain of item response theory (IRT; Embretson and Reise, 2000; Thissen and Wainer, 2001). Unlike FA, IRT models were originally developed for categorical data. As in FA, IRT models are based on the premise that latent variables give rise to observed data, and parameters provide information about relationships between MVs and factor(s). The exploratory–confirmatory continuum described for FA also applies in IRT. In certain circumstances, FA parameters may be converted by simple algebra to IRT parameters (McLeod, Swygert, and Thissen, 2001; Takane and de Leeuw, 1987). Multidimensional IRT (MIRT) methods (i.e., those involving more than one common factor) are sometimes referred to as full information item factor analysis (Bock et al., 1988; Muraki and Carlson, 1995) in acknowledgment of the similarities between classic FA and IRT. "Full information" reflects the fact that IRT models are fitted to the raw data directly rather than to summary statistics such as polychoric correlations. An ML-based estimation scheme described by Bock and Aitkin (1981) is typically used to fit the models.

MIRT is not as widely used as categorical FA, probably because software development has lagged behind that for FA. At the time of this writing, the commercially available TESTFACT program (v.4; Bock et al., 2002) performs exploratory MIRT and fits one very specific type of hierarchical confirmatory model known as the bi-factor model (Holzinger and Swineford, 1937; Gibbons and Hedeker, 1992). However, the only models implemented are for binary MVs. The ltm package (Rizopoulos, 2006) for *R* offers slightly more flexibility in the factor structure, but is limited to dichotomous variables and a maximum of two latent factors. The POLYFACT program (Muraki, 1993) performs exploratory MIRT for ordinal MVs, but this program has not been as widely distributed. Software for general kinds of confirmatory MIRT models is not readily available.

MIRT methods are appealing because the model is fitted to the data directly, thus polychoric correlations need not be calculated. However, the disadvantage is that m-dimensional numerical integration is required ($m =$ number of factors); thus, solutions are more difficult to obtain as m increases. Nevertheless, Markov chain Monte Carlo estimation methods may hold promise for use with MIRT models (Edwards, 2006), and we anticipate advancements in software for MIRT in future years.

7. Sample size in FA

For classic FA (without assumption violations), how many observations are needed for accurate estimation? Historically, minimum *N*s have been suggested such as 100 (Gorsuch, 1983; Kline, 1979), 200 (Guilford, 1954), 250 (Cattell, 1978), or 300 (Comrey and Lee, 1992), or minimum ratios of N to p such as 3 (Cattell, 1978), or 5 (Gorsuch, 1983; Kline, 1979). More recently, MacCallum, Widaman, Zhang, and Hong (1999) astutely pointed out that such rules of thumb are meaningless because the optimal N depends on characteristics of the study. These authors showed that under certain conditions 60 observations can be adequate, whereas in other situations, more than 400 observations are needed. Results apply to both EFA and CFA.

The theoretical arguments presented by MacCallum et al., 1999 (see also MacCallum and Tucker, 1991) are based on the fact that nonzero correlations between common and unique factors, and among unique factors, are a major source of error in the estimation of factor loadings. The correlations tend to be farther from zero with smaller N. However, small uniquenesses (e.g., $\leq .3$), and highly *overdetermined* factors, having four or more indicators with large loadings, can offset the limitations of small samples. Uniquenesses act as weights on the matrices of correlations between unique and common factors and among unique factors. The less these correlations are weighted, the less impact they have on the FA results. Further, with the number of MVs held constant, increasing the number of indicators per factor reduces m, which reduces the number of correlations among common and unique factors and among unique factors, giving them less overall influence on results.

MacCallum et al. (1999) found that when uniquenesses were small (.2, .3, or .4), accurate recovery of $\mathbf{\Lambda}$ could be achieved with around 60 observations with highly overdetermined factors, and 100 observations with weakly determined factors having 2 or 3 indicators. When uniquenesses were large (.6, .7, or .8), 400 observations were inadequate for recovery of $\mathbf{\Lambda}$ unless the factors had 6 or 7 strong indicators each, in which case $N \geq 200$ was required. When uniquenesses varied over MVs (.2, .3, …, .8), $N = 60$ provided pretty good recovery of $\mathbf{\Lambda}$ for factors with 6 or 7 strong indicators, but $N \geq 200$ was needed with weakly determined factors. These results were observed both with (MacCallum et al., 2001) and without (MacCallum et al., 1999) mis-specification of the model in the population.

The sample size question is perhaps even more crucial when analyzing categorical MVs. As mentioned above, WLS requires many observations (perhaps several thousand) for stable parameter estimates (Potthast, 1993), primarily because of the potentially massive number of parameters in the weight matrix. Robust DWLS has performed well with smaller samples. For example, Flora and Curran (2004) found that a sample size of 200 was adequate for relatively simple CFA models (e.g., 10 or 20 MVs and 1 or 2 factors), MVs with 2 or 5 categories, and communalities of .49.

With either WLS or robust DWLS, adequate sample size is needed for estimation of polychoric correlations because sparseness in the 2-way contingency tables used in their computation can cause serious instability in the correlation estimate. Sparseness is especially problematic for two dichotomous MVs, because a tetrachoric correlation is inestimable when there is a zero cell in the 2×2 contingency table. In addition, no easily implemented method exists to deal with missingness, and the common practice of listwise deletion can further exacerbate the problem. Robust DWLS is a relatively new procedure and additional research on the sample-size question is warranted.

8. Examples of EFA and CFA

In this section we present three example FAs. Many software packages are capable of estimating some (or all) of the FA models discussed in this chapter. We selected CEFA (Browne et al., 2004) because it is one of the most flexible EFA programs, and we chose LISREL (Jöreskog and Sörbom, 2005), and Mplus (Muthén and Muthén, 2006) to illustrate CFA because they are very popular, easy to use, and have many features. Other popular software programs that perform EFA and CFA include SAS (SAS Institute, 2006), Splus (Insightful Corporation, 2005), and R (R Development Core Team, 2005); all SEM programs carry out CFA. Our examples use only a fraction of currently available options in the selected programs and the software is always expanding and improving. Nevertheless, these examples should provide a valuable introduction to persons unfamiliar with the software or with FA.

8.1. EFA with continuous variables using CEFA

The first example is an EFA carried out using CEFA.[1] Continuous multivariate normal data were simulated using Mplus from a model with three correlated factors and 18 MVs ($N = 400$). For each factor, six different MVs had nonzero loadings, and all other MVs had zero loadings. The population factor loadings and communalities are given in Table 1. Population correlations among factors i and j (ρ_{ij}) were: $\rho_{12} = .3$, $\rho_{13} = .5$, and $\rho_{23} = .4$. The total sample of 400 was divided in half to provide one sample for EFA and another for a follow-up CFA (described in the next section).

For EFA, we analyzed a Pearson correlation matrix using ML (presuming multivariate normality). A scree plot of the eigenvalues, given in Fig. 3, suggests that no more than four factors should be extracted. Table 2 compares the fit of models with between one and four factors. The maximum absolute residual is in a correlation metric; thus, values of .33 and .29 are very large. The information in Table 2 indicates that fit is very poor for the one- and two-factor models. However, the three-factor model fits well, and is not significantly improved upon by the addition of a fourth factor. A χ^2-difference test comparing the three- and four-factor (nested) models is nonsignificant ($\chi^2(15) = 21.99$, $p = .108$). With real data, the substantive interpretability of the rotated factor loadings with different numbers of factors is as important as the fit and should be considered as part of model selection.

Estimated factor loadings, their SEs, and communalities for the three-factor model are given in Table 1. The loadings have been rotated using the oblique quartimax criterion. The estimated parameters match up well with the values used to generate the data. The estimated correlations among factors and their SEs were: $r_{12} = .37$ (.06), $r_{13} = .47$ (.07), and $r_{23} = .44$ (.07). These are also close to the population values.

CEFA is unusual among EFA programs because it provides SEs (and CIs) for the parameters which can be useful for assigning MVs to factors. Often, factor assignment is done using an arbitrary criterion such as "MVs with a loading of .30 or larger load on the factor". Arbitrary criteria are still needed when SEs are available, but sampling variability can be incorporated into the process. In Table 1, the MVs we assigned to each factor are highlighted in bold. In this case, loadings are either small or large so factor assignment is fairly straightforward.

8.2. CFA with continuous variables using LISREL

Once a structure has been determined from an EFA, it is useful to cross-validate it with CFA using a new sample. Splitting the initial sample in half is often a practical way to cross-validate EFA results. In this section, the other half of the simulated data described in the previous section is analyzed with CFA using LISREL.

Performing CFA in LISREL is a two-stage process. In the first stage, a covariance matrix is estimated from the raw data using the PRELIS program, which is distributed with LISREL. The PRELIS syntax we used is given in Appendix A.

[1] The CEFA software and user's manual may be downloaded for free from http://faculty.psy.ohio state.edu/browne/software.php.

Table 1
Factor loadings and communalities for the EFA example

MV	Population Values				Sample Estimates ($N = 200$)			
	λ_{j1}	λ_{j2}	λ_{j3}	h_j^2	$\hat{\lambda}_{j1}(SE)$	$\hat{\lambda}_{j2}(SE)$	$\hat{\lambda}_{j3}(SE)$	$\hat{h}_j^2$
1	.6	0	0	.36	**.61** (.06)	−.02 (.07)	.07 (.07)	.41
2	.6	0	0	.36	**.63** (.06)	−.03 (.07)	.04 (.07)	.40
3	.6	0	0	.36	**.48** (.07)	−.12 (.08)	.23 (.08)	.33
4	.7	0	0	.49	**.71** (.06)	.05 (.06)	−.02 (.06)	.52
5	.7	0	0	.49	**.64** (.06)	.07 (.07)	−.05 (.07)	.42
6	.7	0	0	.49	**.71** (.06)	.04 (.06)	−.03 (.06)	.51
7	0	.7	0	.49	−.05 (.05)	**.70** (.06)	.05 (.06)	.50
8	0	.7	0	.49	−.08 (.04)	**.81** (.05)	−.01 (.05)	.60
9	0	.7	0	.49	.07 (.05)	**.65** (.07)	.10 (.06)	.53
10	0	.8	0	.64	.04 (.04)	**.81** (.05)	−.04 (.05)	.65
11	0	.8	0	.64	.05 (.04)	**.80** (.05)	−.03 (.05)	.65
12	0	.8	0	.64	.04 (.04)	**.76** (.05)	−.06 (.05)	.65
13	0	0	.6	.36	−.11 (.06)	.08 (.06)	**.72** (.06)	.50
14	0	0	.6	.36	−.02 (.06)	−.05 (.06)	**.67** (.07)	.41
15	0	0	.6	.36	.06 (.07)	.22 (.08)	**.42** (.08)	.34
16	0	0	.8	.64	.03 (.06)	.10 (.06)	**.65** (.06)	.50
17	0	0	.8	.64	.01 (.05)	.01 (.05)	**.80** (.05)	.66
18	0	0	.8	.64	.11 (.05)	−.06 (.05)	**.75** (.06)	.61

Note: MV, measured variable; λ_{jk}, true factor loading for MV j on factor k; $\boldsymbol{h_j^2}$, true communality for MV j; $\hat{\boldsymbol{\lambda}}_{\boldsymbol{jk}}(\boldsymbol{SE})$, estimated factor loading for MV j on factor k, with its standard error; $\hat{\boldsymbol{h}}_{\boldsymbol{j}}^{\boldsymbol{2}}$, estimated communality for MV j. The estimated loadings have been rotated using the oblique quartimax criterion.

The first two lines are the title, followed by a data format line (DA) that specifies the number of indicators (NI), the number of observations (NO), and where the data are stored (FI). The last line tells PRELIS to output (OU) a sample covariance matrix (CM) from the data described in the preceding line. The output file will be created in the same folder as the syntax file.

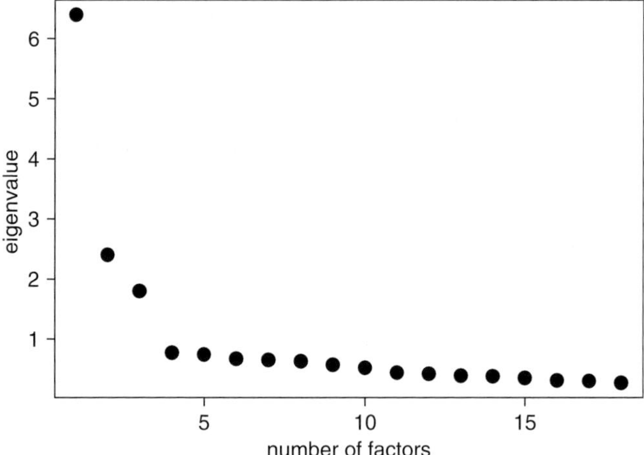

Fig. 3. Scree plot for EFA example.

Table 2
Comparisons among EFA models with differing numbers of factors

m	$\chi^2(df)$	Max. Residual	RMSEA (90% CI)
1	645.64 (135)	.33	.14 (.13, .15)
2	300.69 (118)	.29	.09 (.08, .10)
3	105.58 (102)	.08	.01 (.00, .04)
4	83.59 (87)	.09	.00 (.00, .04)

Note: *m*, number of factors; Max. Residual, maximum absolute correlation residual (range: 0–1); RMSEA (90% CI), root mean square error of approximation, with 90% confidence interval.

The second stage is to estimate the CFA model in LISREL. The syntax we used is given in Appendix A. The first line provides a title (TI) for the output file. The second line describes the data (DA) being used in terms of number of indicators (NI), number of observations (NO), number of groups (NG), and the kind of matrix (MA) that is to be analyzed. The third line specifies the file that contains the matrix to be analyzed. The next line contains a model statement (MO) that describes the CFA generally. In addition to indicating the number of MVs to be modeled (NX) and the number of factors (NK), this line indicates how the factor loading matrix (LX), error covariance matrix (TD), and the inter-factor correlation matrix (PH) should be structured. For this example, the error covariance matrix is diagonal (DI) and freely estimated (FR) and the inter-factor correlation matrix is standardized (i.e., it has 1's on the diagonal) and symmetric (ST). The factor-loading matrix is set to be full (FU) and fixed (FI) meaning there is a complete 18 by 3 loading matrix ($\mathbf{\Lambda}$), but none of the loadings are to be estimated. This is not the model we are interested in, but this is remedied in the next three lines. These lines, each of which begins with FR, indicate to LISREL which elements of the factor loading matrix are to be estimated. For instance, LX 3 1 is the factor loading for the third measured variable on the first factor, found in row 3, column 1 of $\mathbf{\Lambda}$. The last two lines indicate the output desired. The PD line produces a path diagram of the model being estimated, which is a convenient way to verify that the model being estimated is the desired model. The final line is an output line (OU), which defines the structure of the output file (RS prints residuals, ND = 2 sets the number of decimal places in the output file to two) and indicates which method of estimation (ME) should be used (ML indicates maximum likelihood).

There were no improper estimates such as negative variances, thus we proceed to evaluation of model fit. Though LISREL produces numerous global fit statistics, we followed Hu and Bentler's (1999) recommendations (described above) for selecting and evaluating a subset of them. The model fits very well (SRMR: .04; RMSEA: .00 with 90% CI: .00, .03; TLI: 1.00; CFI: 1.00). LISREL also provides a great deal of information about residuals which are differences between the sample covariance matrix and the model-implied covariance matrix (labeled the "fitted covariance matrix" in the output). Residuals are presented in both raw and standardized metrics, and plotted several ways. A model that fits the data well has mostly small residuals that do not show any particular pattern.

The estimated factor loadings, their SEs and the communalities (usually referred to as squared multiple correlations in a CFA context) are given in Table 3. Correlations among factors and their SEs were: $r_{12} = .43$ (.07), $r_{13} = .37$ (.07), and $r_{23} = .54$ (.06). The estimates match the true values reasonably well; accuracy improves with larger samples. LISREL provides t-statistics for testing whether each factor loading or inter-factor correlation is significantly different from 0. All the estimates were significant ($\alpha = .05$) for this example.

8.3. CFA with categorical MVs using Mplus

The data for this example were simulated using Mplus from a model with three correlated factors and 18 MVs ($N = 400$). As before, there were six indicators for each factor. The variables are binary (coded 0 or 1), thus each one has a single threshold parameter. The population thresholds, factor loadings and communalities are given in Table 4. Population correlations among factors were: $\rho_{12} = .3$, $\rho_{13} = .5$, and $\rho_{23} = .4$.

The Mplus syntax we used for the CFA is given in Appendix B. Following the title is the DATA line that specifies a path for the raw data file. The VARIABLE command specifies names for the variables. For the correct analysis, it is extremely important to indicate here that the MVs are categorical. The MODEL statement specifies the model. BY indicates a directional path and WITH requests estimation of a correlation or covariance. In the context of CFA, relationships between MVs and factors are directional paths; thus, "f1 BY y1-y6" indicates that factor 1 should load on MVs y1, y2, y3, y4, y5, and y6. An asterisk is used to override the default method for setting the scale (fixing the first factor loading for each factor to one) and the last three lines of the MODEL statement fix the factor

Table 3
Factor loadings and communalities for the CFA example

	Sample Estimates ($N = 200$)			
MV	$\hat{\lambda}_{j1}(SE)$	$\hat{\lambda}_{j2}(SE)$	$\hat{\lambda}_{j3}(SE)$	R_j^2
1	.60 (.07)	–	–	.36
2	.58 (.07)	–	–	.32
3	.57 (.07)	–	–	.31
4	.65 (.07)	–	–	.45
5	.66 (.07)	–	–	.41
6	.79 (.07)	–	–	.59
7	–	.75 (.06)	–	.56
8	–	.73 (.06)	–	.53
9	–	.79 (.07)	–	.56
10	–	.78 (.06)	–	.61
11	–	.91 (.06)	–	.69
12	–	.91 (.06)	–	.72
13	–	–	.58 (.07)	.35
14	–	–	.61 (.07)	.36
15	–	–	.64 (.07)	.42
16	–	–	.75 (.06)	.59
17	–	–	.81 (.06)	.64
18	–	–	.83 (.06)	.67

Note: MV, measured variable; –, loading was fixed to 0 (not estimated); $\hat{\lambda}_{jk}(SE)$, estimated factor loading for MV j on factor k, with its standard error; R_j^2, squared multiple correlation for MV j.

variances to 1. The ANALYSIS line specifies the estimation method; WLSMV is robust DWLS. Finally, the OUTPUT line controls elements of the output. For categorical MVs, thresholds are obtained by requesting sample statistics (SAMPSTAT).

There were no improper estimates such as negative variances and global model fit was very good (SRMR: .07; RMSEA: .02; TLI: .98; CFI: .98). The estimated

Table 4
Population parameters for the CFA example with categorical MVs

MV	τ_j	λ_{j1}	λ_{j2}	λ_{j3}	h_j^2
1	−.5	.5	0	0	.25
2	0	.5	0	0	.25
3	.5	.5	0	0	.25
4	−.5	.6	0	0	.36
5	0	.6	0	0	.36
6	.5	.6	0	0	.36
7	−.5	0	.6	0	.36
8	0	0	.6	0	.36
9	.5	0	.6	0	.36
10	−.5	0	.7	0	.49
11	0	0	.7	0	.49
12	.5	0	.7	0	.49
13	−.5	0	0	.5	.25
14	0	0	0	.5	.25
15	.5	0	0	.5	.25
16	−.5	0	0	.7	.49
17	0	0	0	.7	.49
18	.5	0	0	.7	.49

Note: MV, measured variable; τ_j, true threshold for MV j; λ_{jk}, true factor loading for MV j on factor k; h_j^2, true communality for MV j.

thresholds, factor loadings, their SEs, and the squared multiple correlations are given in Table 5. Correlations among factors and their SEs were: $r_{12} = .48$ (.08), $r_{13} = .48$ (.08), and $r_{23} = .41$ (.07). The estimates are fairly close to the generating values. All of the loadings and inter-factor correlations were significantly ($\alpha = .05$) different from 0 for this example.

For comparison, the analysis was redone using classic WLS (with a full weight matrix). The only change needed in the Mplus input file is the name of the estimator in the ANALYSIS statement. There were no improper estimates or other estimation difficulties, but global model fit declined quite a bit (SRMR: .12; RMSEA: .05; TLI: 88; CFI: .90) compared to the robust DWLS solution. WLS estimates of the thresholds, factor loadings, and communalities are given in Table 5. Correlations among factors and their SEs were: $r_{12} = .49$ (.05), $r_{13} = .55$ (.05), and $r_{23} = .49$ (.04). Two-thirds of the robust DWLS factor loadings are closer to the true values than the WLS estimates. This is consistent with Flora and Curran's (2004) finding that robust DWLS performs better than WLS in smaller (realistic) sample sizes.

9. Additional resources

This has been an introduction to EFA and CFA, with brief mention of the closely related procedures PCA and MIRT. For additional information, readers are referred to several textbooks on FA and related methods (Bartholomew and

Table 5
Factor loadings, thresholds, and communalities for the CFA example with categorical MVs

		Robust DWLS				WLS			
MV	$\hat{\tau}_j$	$\hat{\lambda}_{j1}(SE)$	$\hat{\lambda}_{j2}(SE)$	$\hat{\lambda}_{j3}(SE)$	R_j^2	$\hat{\lambda}_{j1}(SE)$	$\hat{\lambda}_{j2}(SE)$	$\hat{\lambda}_{j3}(SE)$	R_j^2
1	−.52	.45 (.08)	–	–	.20	.48 (.06)	–	–	.23
2	−.03	.49 (.07)	–	–	.24	.50 (.05)	–	–	.25
3	.38	.42 (.08)	–	–	.17	.62 (.06)	–	–	.38
4	−.55	.52 (.08)	–	–	.27	.59 (.05)	–	–	.35
5	−.01	.55 (.07)	–	–	.31	.64 (.05)	–	–	.41
6	.43	.64 (.08)	–	–	.41	.66 (.06)	–	–	.44
7	−.44	–	.67 (.06)	–	.45	–	.74 (.04)	–	.54
8	.06	–	.59 (.06)	–	.35	–	.57 (.04)	–	.33
9	.43	–	.71 (.06)	–	.51	–	.82 (.04)	–	.67
10	−.62	–	.65 (.06)	–	.43	–	.79 (.04)	–	.62
11	.04	–	.77 (.05)	–	.59	–	.84 (.03)	–	.70
12	.52	–	.78 (.06)	–	.61	–	.74 (.04)	–	.54
13	−.46	–	–	.61 (.06)	.37	–	–	.66 (.04)	.43
14	−.01	–	–	.58 (.06)	.34	–	–	.73 (.04)	.53
15	.53	–	–	.53 (.08)	.28	–	–	.57 (.05)	.32
16	−.57	–	–	.59 (.06)	.35	–	–	.72 (.04)	.52
17	−.01	–	–	.73 (.05)	.54	–	–	.89 (.03)	.80
18	.53	–	–	.69 (.07)	.48	–	–	.86 (.04)	.74

Note: MV, measured variable; $\hat{\tau}_j$, estimated threshold for MV j; $\hat{\lambda}_{jk}(SE)$, estimated factor loading for MV j on factor k, with its standard error; R_j^2, squared multiple correlation for MV j.

Knott, 1999; Bollen, 1989; Brown, 2006; Comrey and Lee, 1992; Gorsuch, 1983; McDonald, 1985; Thissen and Wainer, 2001). Many special issues in FA were not mentioned here, such as multiple group analyses, hierarchical FA, and missing data. Some of these topics are covered in the texts listed above, but developments are ongoing and the methodological literature should be consulted for the most current developments in FA.

Appendix A:. PRELIS and LISREL code for the CFA example with continuous MVs

PRELIS Code

```
PRELIS code to get covariance matrix for
FA chapter continuous CFA example
DA NI = 18 NO = 200 FI = '***insert your directory here***/conFA-2.dat'
OU CM = conFA-2.cm
```

LISREL Code

```
TI FA chapter continuous CFA example
DA NI = 18 NO = 200 NG = 1 MA = CM
CM = conFA-2.cm
MO NX = 18 NK = 3 LX = FU,FI TD = DI,FR PH = ST
FR LX 1 1 LX 2 1 LX 3 1 LX 4 1 LX 5 1 LX 6 1
FR LX 7 2 LX 8 2 LX 9 2 LX 10 2 LX 11 2 LX 12 2
FR LX 13 3 LX 14 3 LX 15 3 LX 16 3 LX 17 3 LX 18 3
PD
OU RS ND = 2 ME = ML
```

Appendix B:. Mplus code for CFA example with categorical MVs

```
TITLE: CFA with categorial measured variables in Mplus
DATA: FILE IS catFA.dat;
VARIABLE: NAMES ARE y1-y18;
    CATEGORICAL ARE y1-y18;
MODEL: f1 BY y1-y6;
    f2 BY y7-y12;
    f3 BY y13-y18;
    f1 WITH f2 f3;
    f2 WITH f3;
    f1 BY y1*.5;
    f2 BY y7*.5;
    f3 BY y13*.5;
    f1@1;
    f2@1;
    f3@1;
!ANALYSIS: ESTIMATOR = WLS;
ANALYSIS: ESTIMATOR = WLSMV;
OUTPUT: SAMPSTAT;
```

References

Bartholomew, D.J., Knott, M. (1999). *Latent Variable Models and Factor Analysis*, 2nd ed. Oxford University Press, New York.

Bartlett, M.S. (1950). Tests of significance in factor analysis. *British Journal of Psychology: Statistical Section* **3**, 77–85.

Bentler, P.M. (1989). *EQS: Structural Equations Program Manual.* BMDP Statistical Software, Los Angeles.

Bentler, P.M. (1990). Comparative fit indices in structural models. *Psychological Bulletin* **107**, 238–246.

Bentler, P.M. (1995). *EQS Structural Equations Program Manual.* Multivariate Software, Encino, CA.

Bentler, P.M., Bonett, D.G. (1980). Significance tests and goodness-of-fit in the analysis of covariance structures. *Psychological Bulletin* **88**, 588–606.

Bock, R.D., Aitkin, M. (1981). Marginal maximum likelihood estimation of item parameters: An application of the EM algorithm. *Psychometrika* **46**, 443–459.

Bock, R.D., Gibbons, R., Muraki, E.J. (1988). Full information item factor analysis. *Applied Psychological Measurement* **12**, 261–280.

Bock, R.D., Gibbons, R., Schilling, S.G., Muraki, E., Wilson, D.T., Wood, R. (2002). *TESTFACT 4 [Computer Software].* Scientific Software International, Inc., Chicago, IL.

Bollen, K. (1988). *A new incremental fit index for general structural equation models.* Paper presented at Southern Sociological Society Meeting, Nashville, TN.

Bollen, K. (1989). *Structural Equations with Latent Variables.* Wiley, New York.

Brown, T.A. (2006). *Confirmatory Factor Analysis for Applied Research.* Guilford Press, New York.

Browne, M.W. (1982). Covariance structures. In: Hawkins, D.M. (Ed.), *Topics in Applied Multivariate Analysis.* Cambridge University Press, Cambridge, pp. 72–141.

Browne, M.W. (1984). Asymptotic distribution free methods in the analysis of covariance structures. *British Journal of Mathematical and Statistical Psychology* **37**, 127–141.

Browne, M.W. (2001). An overview of analytic rotation in exploratory factor analysis. *Multivariate Behavioral Research* **21**, 230–258.

Browne, M.W., Cudeck, R. (1993). Alternative ways of assessing model fit. In: Bollen, K.A., Long, J.S. (Eds.), *Testing Structural Equation Models.* Sage, Newbury Park, CA, pp. 136–162.

Browne, M.W., Cudeck, R., Tateneni, K., Mels, G. (2004). CEFA: Comprehensive Exploratory Factor Analysis, Version 2.00 [Computer software and manual]. Retreived from http://faculty.psy.ohio-state.edu/browne/software.php.

Browne, M.W., Mels, G., Coward, M. (1994). Path analysis: RAMONA. In: Wilkinson, L., Hill, M.A. (Eds.), *Systat: Advanced Applications.* SYSTAT, Evanston, IL, pp. 163–224.

Cattell, R.B. (1966). The scree test for the number of factors. *Multivariate Behavioral Research* **1**, 245–276.

Cattell, R.B. (1978). *The Scientific Use of Factor Analysis.* Plenum, New York.

Chou, C.P., Bentler, P.M., Satorra, A. (1991). Scaled test statistic and robust standard errors for non-normal data in covariance structure analysis: A Monte Carlo study. *British Journal of Mathematical and Statistical Psychology* **44**, 347–357.

Comrey, A.L., Lee, H.B. (1992). *A First Course in Factor Analysis.* Erlbaum, Hillsdale, NJ.

Crawford, C.B., Ferguson, G.A. (1970). A general rotation criterion and its use in orthogonal rotation. *Psychometrika* **35**, 321–332.

Cudeck, R. (1989). Analysis of correlation matrices using covariance structure models. *Psychological Bulletin* **105**, 317–327.

Cudeck, R. (1991). Noniterative factor analysis estimators with algorithms for subset and instrumental variable selection. *Journal of Educational Statistics* **16**, 35–52.

Curran, P.J., Bollen, K.A., Chen, F., Paxton, P., Kirby, J.B. (2003). Finite sampling properties of the point estimators and confidence intervals of the RMSEA. *Sociological Methods and Research* **32**, 208–252.

Curran, P.J., West, S.G., Finch, J.F. (1996). The robustness of test statistics to nonnormality and specification error in confirmatory factor analysis. *Psychological Methods* **1**, 16–29.

DiStefano, C. (2002). The impact of categorization with confirmatory factor analysis. *Structural Equation Modeling* **9**, 327–346.

Embretson, S.E., Reise, S.P. (2000). *Item Response Theory for Psychologists.* Lawrence Erlbaum Associates, Mahwah, NJ.

Edwards, M.C. (2006). *A Markov chain Monte Carlo approach to confirmatory item factor analysis.* Unpublished doctoral dissertation, University of North Carolina at Chapel Hill, Chapel Hill, NC.

Flora, D.B., Curran, P.J. (2004). An empirical evaluation of alternative methods of estimation for confirmatory factor analysis with ordinal data. *Psychological Methods* **9**, 466–491.

Fornell, C., Larcker, D.F. (1981). Evaluating structural equation models with unobservable variables and measurement error. *Journal of Marketing Research* **18**, 39–50.

Gibbons, R.D., Hedeker, D.R. (1992). Full-information item bi-factor analysis. *Psychometrika* **57**, 423–436.

Gorsuch, R. (1983). *Factor Analysis*, 2nd ed. Erlbaum, Hillsdale, NJ.

Guilford, J.P. (1954). *Psychometric Methods*, 2nd ed. McGraw-Hill, New York.

Guttman, L. (1940). Multiple rectilinear prediction and the resolution into components. *Psychometrika* **5**, 75–99.

Hatcher, L. (1994). *A Step-by-Step Approach to Using SAS for Factor Analysis and Structural Equation Modeling*. SAS, Cary, NC.

Hendrikson, A.E., White, P.O. (1964). PROMAX: A quick method for rotation to oblique simple structure. *British Journal of Statistical Psychology* **17**, 65–70.

Holzinger, K.J., Swineford, F. (1937). The bi-factor model. *Psychometrika* **2**, 41–54.

Horn, J.L. (1965). A rationale and test for the number of factors in factor analysis. *Psychometrika* **30**, 179–185.

Hu, L., Bentler, P.M. (1998). Fit indices in covariance structure modeling: Sensitivity to underparameterized model misspecification. *Psychological Methods* **3**, 424–453.

Hu, L., Bentler, P.M. (1999). Cutoff criteria for fit indexes in covariance structure analysis: Conventional criteria versus new alternatives. *Structural Equation Modeling* **6**, 1–55.

Hu, L., Bentler, P.M., Kano, Y. (1992). Can test statistics in covariance structure analysis be trusted? *Psychological Bulletin* **112**, 351–362.

Insightful Corporation (2005). *S-PLUS Version 7.0 for Windows (Computer Software)*. Insightful Corporation, Seattle, Washington.

Jennrich, R.I., Sampson, P.F. (1966). Rotation for simple loadings. *Psychometrika* **31**, 313–323.

Jöreskog, K.G., Sörbom, D. (1981). *LISREL V: Analysis of linear structural relationships by the method of maximum likelihood*. National Educational Resources, Chicago.

Jöreskog, K.G., Sörbom, D. (1986). *LISREL VI: Analysis of linear structural relationships by maximum likelihood and least square methods*. Scientific Software International, Inc., Mooresville, IN.

Jöreskog, K.G., Sörbom, D. (2001). *LISREL 8: User's Reference Guide*. Scientific Software International, Inc., Lincolnwood, IL.

Jöreskog, K.G., Sörbom, D. (2005). *LISREL (Version 8.72) [Computer Software]*. Scientific Software International, Inc, Lincolnwood, IL.

Kaiser, H.F. (1958). The varimax criterion for analytic rotation in factor analysis. *Psychometrika* **23**, 187–200.

Kline, P. (1979). *Psychometrics and Psychology*. Academic Press, London.

MacCallum, R.C., Widaman, K.F., Zhang, S., Hong, S. (1999). Sample size in factor analysis. *Psychological Methods* **4**, 84–99.

MacCallum, R.C., Tucker, L.R. (1991). Representing sources of error in factor analysis: Implications for theory and practice. *Psychological Bulletin* **109**, 502–511.

MacCallum, R.C., Widaman, K.F., Preacher, K.J., Hong, S. (2001). Sample size in factor analysis: The role of model error. *Multivariate Behavioral Research* **36**, 611–637.

Mardia, K.V. (1970). Measures of multivariate skewness and kurtosis with applications. *Biometrika* **57**, 519–530.

McDonald, R.P. (1985). *Factor Analysis and Related Methods*. Erlbaum, Hillsdale, NJ.

McLeod, L.D., Swygert, K.A., Thissen, D. (2001). Factor analysis for items scored in two categories. In: Thissen, D., Wainer, H. (Eds.), *Test scoring*. Lawrence Erlbaum Associates, Inc., Mahwah, NH, pp. 189–216.

Muraki, E.J. (1993). *POLYFACT [Computer Program]*. Educational Testing Service, Princeton, NJ.

Muraki, E.J., Carlson, J.E. (1995). Full-information factor analysis for polytomous item responses. *Applied Psychological Measurement* **19**, 73–90.

Muthén, L.K., Muthén, B.O. (2006). *Mplus: Statistical Analysis with Latent Variables (Version 4.1) [Computer Software]*. Muthén & Muthén, Los Angeles, CA.

O'Connor, B.P. (2000). SPSS and SAS programs for determining the number of components using parallel analysis and Velicer's MAP test. *Behavior Research Methods, Instrumentation, and Computers* **32**, 396–402.

Olsson, U. (1979). Maximum likelihood estimation of the polychoric correlation coefficient. *Psychometrika* **44**, 443–460.

Potthast, M.J. (1993). Confirmatory factor analysis of ordered categorical variables with large models. *British Journal of Mathematical and Statistical Psychology* **46**, 273–286.

R Development Core Team. (2005). *R: A Language and Environment for Statistical Computing*. R Foundation for Statistical Computing, Vienna, Austria. ISBN 3-900051-07-0, URL http://www.R-project.org.

Rizopoulos, D. (2006). *ltm: Latent Trait Models under IRT, Version 0.5-1*. Retrieved from http://cran.r-project.org/src/contrib/Descriptions/ltm.html.

SAS Institute. (2006). *SAS/STAT Computer Software*. Cary, NC.

Satorra, A. (1990). Robustness issues in structural equation modeling: A review of recent developments. *Quality & Quantity* **24**, 367–386.

Satorra, A., Bentler, P.M. (1988). Scaling corrections for chi-square statistics in covariance structure analysis. *ASA Proceedings of the Business and Economics Section*, 308–313.

SPSS Incorporated. (2006). *SPSS Base 15.0 Computer Software*. Chicago, IL.

Steiger, J.H. (1990). Structural model evaluation and modification: An interval estimation approach. *Multivariate Behavioral Research* **25**, 173–180.

Steiger, J.H., Lind, J.M. (1980). *Statistically-based tests for the number of common factors*. Paper presented at the annual meeting of the Psychometric Society, May,Iowa City, IA.

Takane, Y., de Leeuw, J. (1987). On the relationship between item response theory and factor analysis of discretized variables. *Psychometrika* **52**, 393–408.

Thissen, D., Wainer, H. (eds.) (2001). Test Scoring. Lawrence Erlbaum Associates, Inc., Mahwah, NJ.

Thurstone, L.L. (1947). *Multiple Factor Analysis*. University of Chicago Press, Chicago.

Tucker, L.R., Lewis, C. (1973). A reliability coefficient for maximum likelihood factor analysis. *Psychometrika* **38**, 1–10.

West, S.G., Finch, J.F., Curran, P.J. (1995). Structural equation models with nonnormal variables: Problems and remedies. In: Hoyle, R.H. (Ed.), *Structural Equation Modeling: Concepts, Issues, and Applications*. Sage, Thousand Oaks, CA, pp. 56–75.

Yuan, K., Bentler, P.M., Zhang, W. (2005). The effect of skewness and kurtosis on mean and covariance structure analysis. *Sociological Methods and Research* **34**, 240–258.

Handbook of Statistics, Vol. 27
ISSN: 0169-7161

DOI: 10.1016/S0169-7161(07)27013-0

13

Structural Equation Modeling

Kentaro Hayashi, Peter M. Bentler and Ke-Hai Yuan

Abstract

Structural equation modeling (SEM) is a multivariate statistical technique for testing hypotheses about the influences of sets of variables on other variables. Hypotheses can involve correlational and regression-like relations among observed variables as well as latent variables. The adequacy of such hypotheses is evaluated by modeling the mean and covariance structures of the observed variables. After an introduction, we present the statistical model. Then we discuss estimation methods and hypothesis tests with an emphasis on the maximum likelihood method based on the assumption of multivariate normal data, including the issues of model (parameter) identification and regularity conditions. We also discuss estimation and testing with non-normal data and with misspecified models, as well as power analysis. To supplement model testing, fit indices have been developed to measure the degree of fit for a SEM model. We describe the major ones. When an initial model does not fit well, Lagrange Multiplier (score) and Wald tests can be used to identify how an initial model might be modified. In addition to these standard topics, we discuss extensions of the model to multiple groups, to repeated observations (growth curve SEM), to data with a hierarchical structure (multi-level SEM), and to nonlinear relationships between latent variables. We also discuss more practical topics such as treatment of missing data, categorical dependent variables, and software information.

1. Models and identification

1.1. Introduction

Structural equation modeling (SEM) is a multivariate statistical technique designed to model the structure of a covariance matrix (sometimes the structure of a mean vector as well) with a relatively few parameters, and to test the adequacy of such a hypothesized covariance (mean) structure in its ability to reproduce sample covariances (means). An interesting model would be well motivated substantively and provide a parsimonious and adequate representation of the data. SEM emerged from several different modeling traditions, e.g., multiple regression, path analysis, exploratory factor analysis (Lawley and Maxwell, 1971), confirmatory factor analysis (Jöreskog, 1969), and simultaneous equation models in econometrics. It is meant to be a unifying methodology that can handle these various models as special cases, as well as generalized models that are hard or impossible to handle with earlier methods. Initially, SEM was developed in the social sciences, especially in psychology and sociology, where it is still popular (e.g., MacCallum and Austin, 2000). However, it has become employed as a useful research tool in a variety of other disciplines such as education and marketing to more medically oriented fields such as epidemiology, imaging, and other biological sciences (see e.g., Batista-Foguet et al., 2001; Bentler and Stein, 1992; Davis et al., 2000; Dishman et al., 2002; Duncan et al., 1998; Hays et al., 2005; Peek, 2000; Penny et al., 2004; Shipley, 2000; van den Oord, 2000).

Numerous texts have been written on SEM. Introductory-level textbooks include Byrne (2006), Dunn et al. (1993), Kline (2005), Loehlin (2004), Maruyama (1998), Raykov and Marcoulides (2006). The most well-known intermediate-level text is Bollen (1989). Two more advanced overviews are those of Bartholomew and Knott (1999) and Skrondal and Rabe-Hesketh (2004). Some collections of articles on a variety of topics related to SEM can be found in Berkane (1997), Marcoulides and Schumacker (1996, 2001), and Schumacker and Marcoulides (1998). The most complete and somewhat technical overview is given by the 18 chapters in Lee's (2007) *Handbook of Structural Equation Models*.

Structural models are often represented by a path diagram in which squares represent observed variables, ovals represent hypothesized latent variables, unidirectional arrows represent regression-type coefficients, and bidirectional arrows represent unanalyzed correlations or covariances. Any such diagram is precisely synonymous with a set of equations and variance and covariance specifications (see e.g., Raykov and Marcoulides, 2006 (Chapter 1) for more details). In this section we concentrate on the algebraic and statistical representation.

1.2. Structural equation models

By late 1970s, full SEM formulations were given by several authors. The earliest and most widely known is the factor analytic simultaneous equation model based on the work of Jöreskog, Keesling, and Wiley (see Bentler, 1986 for a history). It is widely known as the Lisrel model, after Jöreskog and Sörbom's (1979, 1981) computer program. Another approach is the Bentler–Weeks model (Bentler and Weeks, 1980). These models are formally equivalent, though differing in apparent mathematical structure. We start with the Bentler–Weeks structure. Let $\boldsymbol{\xi}$ be a vector of independent variables and $\boldsymbol{\eta}$ be a vector of dependent variables, where "independent" variables may be correlated but, unlike dependent variables, are not explicit functions of other variables. The structural equation that relates these variables is

$$\boldsymbol{\eta} = \boldsymbol{L}\boldsymbol{\eta} + \boldsymbol{M}\boldsymbol{\xi}, \tag{1}$$

where $\boldsymbol{L}$ and $\boldsymbol{M}$ are coefficient matrices. Elements of these matrices are known as path coefficients, and would be shown as unidirectional arrows in a diagram. Note that this allows dependent variables to be influenced not only by independent variables, as in regression and linear models in general, but also by other dependent variables. Let us denote $\boldsymbol{B} = \begin{pmatrix} \boldsymbol{L} & \boldsymbol{0} \\ \boldsymbol{0} & \boldsymbol{0} \end{pmatrix}$, $\boldsymbol{\Gamma} = \begin{pmatrix} \boldsymbol{M} \\ \boldsymbol{I} \end{pmatrix}$, and $\boldsymbol{v} = \begin{pmatrix} \eta \\ \xi \end{pmatrix}$, where I is the identity matrix of an appropriate order. Then (1) can be expressed in an alternative form

$$\boldsymbol{v} = \boldsymbol{B}\boldsymbol{v} + \boldsymbol{\Gamma}\xi. \tag{2}$$

Now assume that $\boldsymbol{I}$–$\boldsymbol{B}$ is non-singular so that the inverse of $\boldsymbol{I}$–$\boldsymbol{B}$ exists, then

$$\boldsymbol{v} = (\boldsymbol{I} - \boldsymbol{B})^{-1}\boldsymbol{\Gamma}\xi. \tag{3}$$

This gives an expression of all the variables as a linear combination of the independent variables. For generality, we allow both independent and dependent variables to be observed variables, in the data file, as well as hypothesized latent variables such as factors, residuals, and so on. Thus, we introduce the matrix $\boldsymbol{G}$ whose components are either 1 or 0 which connects $\boldsymbol{v}$ to the observed variables $\boldsymbol{x}$ such that $\boldsymbol{x} = \boldsymbol{G}\boldsymbol{v}$. Let $\boldsymbol{\mu} = E(\boldsymbol{x})$, $\boldsymbol{\mu}_\xi = E(\xi)$, $\boldsymbol{\Sigma} = Cov(\boldsymbol{x})$, and $\boldsymbol{\Phi} = Cov(\xi)$. Various covariances ϕ_{ij} are shown as two-way arrows in path diagrams. The full mean and covariance structure analysis model (MCSA) follows as:

$$\text{Mean structure :} \qquad \boldsymbol{\mu} = \boldsymbol{G}(\boldsymbol{I} - \boldsymbol{B})^{-1}\boldsymbol{\Gamma}\boldsymbol{\mu}_\xi \tag{4}$$

$$\text{Covariance structure :} \ \boldsymbol{\Sigma} = \boldsymbol{G}(\boldsymbol{I} - \boldsymbol{B})^{-1}\boldsymbol{\Gamma}\boldsymbol{\Phi}\boldsymbol{\Gamma}'(\boldsymbol{I} - \boldsymbol{B})^{-1'}\boldsymbol{G}'. \tag{5}$$

When the mean structure is saturated, i.e., $\boldsymbol{\mu}$ does not have a structure as given by (4), then we may consider only the covariance structure (5). This explains the name covariance structure analysis (CSA) as another generic name for SEM in which means are ignored.

In the above, there is no obvious use of latent variables. Bollen (2002) provides a review of several definitions of such variables. Among these, Bentler's (1982) approach (see also Bentler and Weeks, 1980) is the clearest to differentiate a latent variable model from a measured variable model. In this approach, the ranks or dimensionality of $\boldsymbol{\Phi}$ and $\boldsymbol{\Sigma}$ are compared. If $dim(\boldsymbol{\Phi}) > dim(\boldsymbol{\Sigma})$, i.e., the dimensionality of the independent variables exceeds that of the data variables, the model is a latent variable model. This means that the measured variables $\boldsymbol{x}$ may be generated by the ξ, but the ξ cannot be generated by the $\boldsymbol{x}$. This clarifies some traditional controversies in the field, e.g., it follows immediately that principal components analysis is not a latent variable model, since the principal components exist in the space of measured variables; and similarly that factor analysis, although typically talked about as a dimension-reducing method, actually is a dimension-inducing method since the space of factors is at least the number of variables plus one.

In a simple variant of the factor analytic simultaneous equation model, the measurement model, a factor analysis model, relates observed to latent variables via

$$\boldsymbol{x} = \boldsymbol{\mu} + \boldsymbol{\Lambda}\boldsymbol{\xi} + \boldsymbol{\varepsilon}. \tag{6}$$

Here $\boldsymbol{\Lambda}$ is a matrix of factor loadings, $\boldsymbol{\xi}$ a vector of factors, and $\boldsymbol{\varepsilon}$ a vector of residuals often known as unique variates. The simultaneous equation model relates the latent variables to each other via

$$\boldsymbol{\xi} = \boldsymbol{B}\boldsymbol{\xi} + \boldsymbol{\zeta}, \tag{7}$$

where $\boldsymbol{B}$ is a coefficient matrix and $\boldsymbol{\zeta}$ a vector of residuals. Equation (7) allows any factor ξ_i to be regressed on any other factorξ_j. Assuming no correlations between $\boldsymbol{\xi}$, $\boldsymbol{\zeta}$, $\boldsymbol{\varepsilon}$, and a full rank $(\boldsymbol{I}-\boldsymbol{B})$, we can rewrite

$$\boldsymbol{\xi} = (\boldsymbol{I} - \boldsymbol{B})^{-1}\boldsymbol{\zeta}, \tag{8}$$

$$\boldsymbol{x} = \boldsymbol{\mu} + \boldsymbol{\Lambda}(\boldsymbol{I} - \boldsymbol{B})^{-1}\boldsymbol{\zeta} + \boldsymbol{\varepsilon}. \tag{9}$$

If the means are unstructured, $\boldsymbol{\mu} = E(\boldsymbol{x})$. With a structure, we take $\boldsymbol{\mu} = \boldsymbol{0}$ in (9) and let $\boldsymbol{\mu}_\zeta = E(\boldsymbol{\zeta})$, and with the covariance matrix of the $\boldsymbol{\zeta}$ and the $\boldsymbol{\varepsilon}$ given as $\boldsymbol{\Phi}_\zeta$ and $\boldsymbol{\Psi}$, respectively, the mean and covariance structure of the model are given as:

$$\boldsymbol{\mu} = \boldsymbol{\Lambda}(\boldsymbol{I} - \boldsymbol{B})^{-1}\boldsymbol{\mu}_\zeta, \tag{10}$$

$$\boldsymbol{\Sigma} = \boldsymbol{\Lambda}(\boldsymbol{I} - \boldsymbol{B})^{-1}\boldsymbol{\Phi}_\zeta\{(\boldsymbol{I} - \boldsymbol{B})^{-1}\}'\boldsymbol{\Lambda}' + \boldsymbol{\Psi}. \tag{11}$$

This representation makes it easy to show that the confirmatory factor analysis model

$$\boldsymbol{\Sigma} = \boldsymbol{\Lambda}\boldsymbol{\Phi}_\zeta\boldsymbol{\Lambda}' + \boldsymbol{\Psi} \tag{12}$$

can be obtained as a special case by setting $\boldsymbol{B} = \boldsymbol{0}$.

These two representation systems can also be made even more abstract. Considering the elements of the matrices in (4)–(5) or (10)–(11) as generic parameters arranged in the vector $\boldsymbol{\theta}$, we may write the SEM null hypothesis as $\boldsymbol{\mu} = \boldsymbol{\mu}(\boldsymbol{\theta})$ and $\boldsymbol{\Sigma} = \boldsymbol{\Sigma}(\boldsymbol{\theta})$. The statistical problem is one of estimating the unknown parameters in $\boldsymbol{\theta}$, and evaluating whether the population means $\boldsymbol{\mu}$ and covariances $\boldsymbol{\Sigma}$ are consistent with the null hypothesis or whether $\boldsymbol{\mu} \neq \boldsymbol{\mu}(\boldsymbol{\theta})$ and/or $\boldsymbol{\Sigma} \neq \boldsymbol{\Sigma}(\boldsymbol{\theta})$. This notation can be made even more compact by arranging $\boldsymbol{\beta} = \{\boldsymbol{\mu}', vech(\boldsymbol{\Sigma})'\}'$, where $vech(\boldsymbol{A})$ vectorizes the lower or upper triangle of a symmetric matrix $\boldsymbol{A}$, and writing $\boldsymbol{\beta} = \boldsymbol{\beta}(\boldsymbol{\theta})$. When only a covariance structure is of interest, we may write $\boldsymbol{\sigma} = \boldsymbol{\sigma}(\boldsymbol{\theta})$, where $\boldsymbol{\sigma} = vech(\boldsymbol{\Sigma})$. We use this notation extensively.

1.3. Model identification

Clearly SEM models can have many parameters, and hence, the identification of parameters in the model is an important issue. Model identification is discussed in detail in Bollen (1989) and especially in Bekker et al. (1994). The concept of model degrees of freedom is essential to understand identification. Let p be the number of observed variables. The number of non-redundant elements in the mean vector and covariance matrix is $p+p(p+1)/2$. Then the degrees of freedom in SEM is given by $df=p(p+1)/2+p-q_1$ for MCSA; $df=p(p+1)/2-q_2$ for CSA, where q_1 and q_2 are the number of parameters to be estimated. When the model df is positive, that is, when the number of non-redundant elements in the means and covariance matrix exceed the number of parameters, the model is said to be *over-identified*; when the model df is negative, the model is said to be *under-identified*; and when the model df is exactly zero, the model is said to be *just-identified*. Here, note that over-identification does not necessarily guarantee that the model can be identified. Over-identified models, if identified, are testable; under-identified models cannot be tested; and just-identified models also cannot be tested but simply represent a mapping of the data into an equivalent model structure.

Generic necessary conditions for model identification are given in many introductory textbooks (e.g., Raykov and Marcoulides, 2006). These are as follows:

(i) There are constraints to determine the scale of each of independent latent variables, which is typically done by either setting one of the coefficients to a fixed constant for each latent independent variable, or setting the variance of each to a fixed constant.
(ii) df needs to be non-negative ($df \geq 0$, that is, the model is not under-identified).
(iii) There are at least two (sometimes three) observed variables for each latent variable.

Note that the above three generic conditions are necessary but not sufficient conditions. Therefore, satisfying these conditions does not necessarily guarantee model identification. As we discuss next, identification serves as one of the regularity conditions for estimation of parameters.

2. Estimation and evaluation

2.1. *Regularity conditions*

The following regularity conditions are typical.

(i) *Compactness*: The true parameter vector $\boldsymbol{\theta}_0$ belongs to a compact subset of the multi-dimensional (q-dimensional) Euclidian space, where q is the number of parameters; $\boldsymbol{\theta}_0 \in \boldsymbol{\Theta} \subset \boldsymbol{R}^q$.
(ii) *Identification*: The model structure is identified; $\boldsymbol{\beta}(\boldsymbol{\theta}) = \boldsymbol{\beta}(\boldsymbol{\theta}_0)$ implies $\boldsymbol{\theta} = \boldsymbol{\theta}_0$.
(iii) *Differentiability*: $\boldsymbol{\beta}(\boldsymbol{\theta})$ is twice continuously differentiable.
(iv) *Rank condition 1*: The matrix of partial derivatives $\dot{\boldsymbol{\beta}} = \partial\boldsymbol{\beta}(\boldsymbol{\theta})/\partial\boldsymbol{\theta}'$ is of full rank.
(v) *Rank condition 2*: The covariance matrix of $(\boldsymbol{x}_i' \; \{vech((\boldsymbol{x}_i-\boldsymbol{\mu}_0)(\boldsymbol{x}_i-\boldsymbol{\mu}_0)')\}')'$ is of full rank.

Note that (1) Conditions (i) and (ii) are required for the consistency of the parameter estimates; (2) Conditions (iii) and (iv) are required for asymptotic normality; (3) Condition (v) is needed for the parameter estimates or the test statistics for the overall model to have proper asymptotic distributions; and (4) Condition (v) is typically satisfied in real data unless there are artificial dependencies among variables. These conditions imply that the information matrix is positive definite. In practice, rank deficiency in the estimated information matrix provides a clue as to lack of identification of the model (see e.g., Browne, 1984; Shapiro, 1984; Kano, 1986; Yuan and Bentler, 1997a for further discussions on regularity conditions in SEM).

2.2. Estimation methods and the corresponding fit functions

(1) *Estimation methods*: Based on a sample of size n, we may estimate the unstructured population mean vector and covariance matrix by $\bar{\boldsymbol{x}}$ and $\boldsymbol{S}$. Currently, there are four major estimation methods in SEM based on these unstructured estimates. They are: (i) LS (least squares), (ii) GLS (generalized least squares), (iii) ML (maximum likelihood), and (iv) ADF (asymptotic distribution free) (Browne, 1984). The first three are variants of methods routinely used in other areas of statistics such as multiple regression. The LS method is distribution free. The GLS and ML method are based on the assumption of multivariate normality of the variables to be analyzed. The ADF method, a minimum χ^2 method (see Ferguson, 1958, 1996), was developed to provide correct statistics regardless of the distribution of variables.

(2) *Fit functions*: For each estimation method there is a so-called fit function or discrepancy function to be minimized using some algorithm. The fit functions for MCSA are:
  - (i) LS : $F_{\text{LS}} = (\bar{x} - \boldsymbol{\mu}(\boldsymbol{\theta}))'(\bar{x} - \boldsymbol{\mu}(\boldsymbol{\theta})) + (1/2)tr(\boldsymbol{S} - \boldsymbol{\Sigma}(\boldsymbol{\theta}))^2$, where $tr(\boldsymbol{A})$ is the trace operator of a square matrix $\boldsymbol{A}$.
  - (ii) GLS : $F_{\text{GLS}} = (\bar{x} - \boldsymbol{\mu}(\boldsymbol{\theta}))'\boldsymbol{S}^{-1}(\bar{x} - \boldsymbol{\mu}(\boldsymbol{\theta})) + (1/2)tr(\boldsymbol{\Sigma}(\boldsymbol{\theta})\boldsymbol{S}^{-1} - \boldsymbol{I}_{\text{p}})^2$;
  - (iii) ML : $F_{\text{ML}} = (\bar{\boldsymbol{x}} - \boldsymbol{\mu}(\boldsymbol{\theta}))'\boldsymbol{\Sigma}(\boldsymbol{\theta})^{-1}(\bar{\boldsymbol{x}} - \boldsymbol{\mu}(\boldsymbol{\theta})) + tr(\boldsymbol{S}\boldsymbol{\Sigma}(\boldsymbol{\theta})^{-1}) - \log|\boldsymbol{S}\boldsymbol{\Sigma}(\boldsymbol{\theta})^{-1}| - p$, where $|\boldsymbol{A}|$ is the determinant of a matrix $\boldsymbol{A}$.
  - (iv) ADF : $F_{\text{ADF}} = (\boldsymbol{t} - \boldsymbol{\beta}(\boldsymbol{\theta}))'\hat{\boldsymbol{V}}^{-1}(\boldsymbol{t} - \boldsymbol{\beta}(\boldsymbol{\theta}))$,

where $t = (\bar{\boldsymbol{x}}', \boldsymbol{s}')', \boldsymbol{s} = vech(\boldsymbol{S})$, and $\boldsymbol{V}$ is the asymptotic covariance matrix of $\boldsymbol{t}$ which is expressed as a partitioned matrix $\begin{pmatrix} \boldsymbol{V}_1 & \boldsymbol{V}_{12} \\ \boldsymbol{V}_{21} & \boldsymbol{V}_2 \end{pmatrix}$, where $\boldsymbol{V}_1 = \boldsymbol{\Sigma}$, the elements of $\boldsymbol{V}_{12}$ are $E\{(x_i - \mu_i)(x_j - \mu_j)(x_k - \mu_k)\}$, $\boldsymbol{V}_{21} = \boldsymbol{V}_{12}'$, and the elements of $\boldsymbol{V}_2$ are $E\{(x_i - \mu_i)(x_j - \mu_j)(x_k - \mu_k)(x_l - \mu_l)\} - \sigma_{ij}\sigma_{kl}$ (cf., Bentler, 1995, pp. 211–212). Clearly, the ADF method assumes the existence of the finite fourth-order moments. Since these may be hard to estimate, the use of ADF requires a huge sample size (see e.g. Hu et al., 1992).

Clearly these fit functions simplify in CSA without a mean structure. For (i)–(iii), in CSA the first term can be dropped, since with a "saturated" mean structure, $\hat{\boldsymbol{\mu}} = \bar{\boldsymbol{x}}$. In CSA with ADF, the fit function in (iv) is reduced to $F_{\text{ADF}} = (\boldsymbol{s} - \boldsymbol{\sigma}(\boldsymbol{\theta}))'\hat{\boldsymbol{V}}_2^{-1}(\boldsymbol{s} - \boldsymbol{\sigma}(\boldsymbol{\theta}))$.

2.3. Maximum likelihood estimation with normal data

Because a maximum likelihood estimator (MLE) is known to have some good properties, we further discuss parameter estimation and model evaluation by ML. First, we summarize the results for ML with normal data. Under the null hypothesis of correct model structure:

(i) *Test statistic*: The test statistic

$$T_{\mathrm{ML}} = (n-1)F_{\mathrm{ML}} \tag{13}$$

is known to converge in distribution to a χ^2 distribution with $df = p(p+1)/2 + p - q_1$ for MCSA and with $df = p(p+1)/2 - q_2$ for CSA, where n is the sample size.

(ii) *Asymptotic normality*: When the data are from a multivariate normal distribution with true population mean vector and true population covariance matrix, the estimators are *consistent* and *asymptotic normal*, that is,

$$\sqrt{n}(\hat{\boldsymbol{\theta}} - \boldsymbol{\theta}_0) \to N(\mathbf{0}, \boldsymbol{\Omega}_{\mathrm{ML}}), \tag{14}$$

where the covariance matrix is $\boldsymbol{\Omega}_{\mathrm{ML}} = (\dot{\boldsymbol{\beta}}' \boldsymbol{W}^* \dot{\boldsymbol{\beta}})^{-1}$ with the weight matrix $\boldsymbol{W}^* = \begin{pmatrix} \boldsymbol{\Sigma}^{-1} & 0 \\ 0 & \boldsymbol{W} \end{pmatrix}$ with $\boldsymbol{W} = (1/2)\boldsymbol{D}'_{\mathrm{p}}(\boldsymbol{\Sigma}^{-1} \otimes \boldsymbol{\Sigma}^{-1})\boldsymbol{D}_{\mathrm{p}}$, where the duplication matrix $\boldsymbol{D}_p$ (Magnus and Neudecker, 1999) is defined such that $\mathrm{vec}(\boldsymbol{\Sigma}) = \boldsymbol{D}_p \mathrm{vech}(\boldsymbol{\Sigma})$. To compute MLEs we need to employ some algorithm for optimization, see e.g., Lee and Jennrich (1979) and Yuan and Bentler (2000b), among others.

Test statistics based on the other estimation methods are also possible. The simplest case is with GLS, where $T_{\mathrm{GLS}} = (n-1)F_{\mathrm{GLS}}$. Browne (1974) showed that for CSA with normal data, T_{GLS} and T_{ML} are asymptotically equivalent. This was extended to the MCSA by Yuan and Chan (2005), who showed that the asymptotic equivalence of T_{GLS} and T_{ML} does not depend on the distribution of data but on the correctness of the model structure. That is, the asymptotic equivalence holds for MCSA as long as the model is specified correctly. Similarly, the estimators $\hat{\boldsymbol{\theta}}_{\mathrm{ML}}$ and $\hat{\boldsymbol{\theta}}_{\mathrm{GLS}}$ are asymptotically equivalent.

2.4. Maximum likelihood estimation with non-normal data

(1) *Consistency and asymptotic normality*: It is natural to question whether ML is still valid if the data are not from a multivariate normal distribution. It has been shown that:

   (i) *Consistency*: The parameter estimates are still consistent as long as $\boldsymbol{\beta}(\boldsymbol{\theta})$ is identified and correctly specified.

   (ii) *Asymptotic normality*: With non-normal data, asymptotic normality still holds with a modified covariance matrix of the estimator as follows:

$$\sqrt{n}(\hat{\boldsymbol{\theta}} - \boldsymbol{\theta}_0) \to N(\mathbf{0}, \boldsymbol{\Omega}_{\mathrm{SW}}), \tag{15}$$

with the sandwich-type covariance matrix

$$\boldsymbol{\Omega}_{\mathrm{SW}} = (\dot{\boldsymbol{\beta}}' \boldsymbol{W}^* \dot{\boldsymbol{\beta}})^{-1} (\dot{\boldsymbol{\beta}}' \boldsymbol{W}^* \boldsymbol{V} \boldsymbol{W}^* \dot{\boldsymbol{\beta}}) (\dot{\boldsymbol{\beta}}' \boldsymbol{W}^* \dot{\boldsymbol{\beta}})^{-1}, \tag{16}$$

where $\boldsymbol{V}$ and $\boldsymbol{W}^*$ were defined above. The sandwich-type covariance matrix was originated in Huber (1967) and it has been used in SEM by many researchers (e.g., Bentler, 1983; Bentler and Dijkstra, 1985; Browne, 1984; Browne and Arminger, 1995; Satorra and Bentler, 1994; Shapiro, 1983; Yuan and Bentler, 1997b). Note that when the data are from a multivariate normal distribution, $\boldsymbol{W}^* = \boldsymbol{V}^{-1}$ in Eq. (16) and $\boldsymbol{\Omega}_{\mathrm{SW}}$ is reduced to $\boldsymbol{\Omega}_{\mathrm{ML}}$ in Eq. (14).

(2) *Satorra–Bentler rescaled statistic*: For CSA (i.e., with saturated means) with correctly specified models, T_{ML} can be approximated by a weighted sum of independent χ^2 distributions with 1 degree of freedom, that is

$$T_{\mathrm{ML}} \to \sum_{i=1}^{df} \kappa_i \chi^2_{i(1)} \quad \text{as} \quad n \to \infty, \tag{17}$$

where κ_i's are the nonzero eigenvalues of $\boldsymbol{U}\boldsymbol{V}_2$, with

$$\boldsymbol{U} = \boldsymbol{W} - \boldsymbol{W}\dot{\boldsymbol{\sigma}}(\dot{\boldsymbol{\sigma}}' \boldsymbol{W} \dot{\boldsymbol{\sigma}})^{-1} \dot{\boldsymbol{\sigma}}' \boldsymbol{W}, \tag{18}$$

(cf. e.g. the appendix of Yuan et al., 2002). When data are normal, the weights κ_i's are all 1 and T_{ML} approaches a χ^2 distribution with $df = p(p+1)/2 - q_2$. For CSA, Satorra and Bentler (1988, 1994, 2001) observed the relation $tr(\boldsymbol{U}\boldsymbol{V}_2) = \sum_{i=1}^{df} \kappa_i$ and proposed

$$T_{RML} = T_{\mathrm{ML}}/\hat{\kappa} \qquad \text{with} \qquad \hat{\kappa} = tr(\hat{\boldsymbol{U}}\hat{\boldsymbol{V}}_2)/df, \tag{19}$$

which is known as the *Satorra–Bentler rescaled statistic*. Simulation studies (Curran et al., 1996; Hu et al., 1992; Yuan and Bentler, 1998a) have shown that this rescaled statistic works quite well under a variety of conditions. Technically, however, the Satorra–Bentler rescaled statistic only corrects the scaling such that the expected ML test statistic matches the degrees of freedom of the model, i.e., $E(T_{\mathrm{ML}}) = df$. It does not correct the distributional shape to that of χ^2 (Yuan and Bentler, 1998a; Bentler and Yuan, 1999). Satorra and Bentler also proposed an adjusted statistic that corrects the variance in addition to the mean.

Similarly to CSA, for MCSA with correctly specified models, T_{ML} can be approximated by the weighted sum of independent χ^2 distributions with 1 degree of freedom, with the weights being the nonzero eigenvalues of $\boldsymbol{U}^*\boldsymbol{V}$ where

$$\boldsymbol{U}^* = \boldsymbol{W}^* - \boldsymbol{W}^*\dot{\boldsymbol{\beta}}(\dot{\boldsymbol{\beta}}' \boldsymbol{W}^* \dot{\boldsymbol{\beta}})^{-1} \dot{\boldsymbol{\beta}}' \boldsymbol{W}^* \tag{20}$$

(Yuan and Bentler, 2006). Thus the Satorra–Bentler rescaled statistic for MCSA can be defined as a simple extension of that for CSA, that is, $T_{ML} = T_{\mathrm{ML}}/\hat{\kappa}^*$ with $\hat{\kappa}^* = tr(\hat{\boldsymbol{U}}^*\hat{\boldsymbol{V}})/df$ with $df = p(p+1)/2 + p - q_1$. Clearly this is of the same form as in CSA.

(3) *Corrected ADF and F-statistics*: With normal distribution-based MLE from non-normal data, Browne (1984) proposed a residual-based ADF statistic in the context of CSA. Unlike the Satorra–Bentler rescaled statistic, the residual-based ADF statistic asymptotically follows a χ^2 distribution regardless of the distribution form of the data. However, like the ADF statistic, the residual-based ADF statistic needs a huge sample size to have its behavior described by a χ^2 distribution. In the context of MCSA, a corrected ADF statistic and an F-statistic were developed by Yuan and Bentler (1997a) and Yuan and Bentler (1999c), respectively. Their residual-based versions were given in Yuan and Bentler (1998a). All the four statistics are asymptotically distribution free and also perform well with finite sample sizes that are commonly encountered in practice (Bentler and Yuan, 1999).

(4) *Finite mixtures*: When the distribution is very different from normality, use of finite mixtures may be appropriate. See e.g., Yung (1997) and Hoshino (2001) on this point. Finite mixture SEMs have become very popular (e.g., Lubke and Muthén, 2005), but they are problematic to use and can falsely discover typologies when none exist (Bauer and Curran, 2003, 2004).

2.5. *Robustness*

Although we made a distinction between methods based on normal distribution theory and distribution-free methods, there are times where normal theory statistics can be used because they are robust to violation of distributional assumptions. Anderson and Amemiya (1988) and Amemiya and Anderson (1990) established the asymptotic robustness of SEM in the factor analysis context, namely that when (i) factors and error vector are independent and (ii) the elements of the error vector are also independent, then T_{ML} asymptotically follows a χ^2 distribution and information-based standard errors for factor loadings will be correct. The results were generalized in various direction by Browne and Shapiro (1988), Kano (1992), Mooijaart and Bentler (1991), Satorra (1992, 2002), Satorra and Bentler (1990), and Yuan and Bentler (1999a, 1999b). Unfortunately, there are two problems in applications. It is hard to know whether these independence conditions are met in any real data situation. Also, this is an asymptotic theory, and it is hard to know when it will work with moderate sample sizes.

Another approach to estimation with non-normal data is to employ a method that does not make a strong assumption such as multivariate normality. Historically, elliptical distributions provided the first generalization of non-normality used in SEM (e.g., Bentler and Berkane, 1985; Browne and Shapiro, 1988; Kano et al., 1993; Shapiro and Browne, 1987; Tyler, 1983; see Fang et al., 1990, on elliptical distributions). Elliptical distributions include heavy-tailed distributions with different degrees of multivariate kurtosis (Mardia, 1970) such as the multivariate t-distribution, however, they have a drawback of not allowing any skewed distributions. A more general distribution that allows heterogeneous kurtosis parameters also has been developed for CSA (Kano et al., 1990).

In classical statistics, case weighting to achieve robust statistics has a long history (see e.g. Huber, 1964, 1981; Hampel et al., 1986). This methodology has been extended to SEM (Yuan and Bentler, 1998c). A promising approach to robust procedures in SEM is based on M-estimators. Maronna (1976) obtained the properties of the M-estimators for the population mean vector and covariance matrix. The two commonly used weight functions for the M-estimators are (i) Huber-type weights and (ii) weights based on multivariate t-distribution. The robust transformation by Yuan et al. (2000) is a useful robust procedure based on the M-estimator approach that can be applied to SEM (see also Yuan et al., 2004, and the appendix of Yuan, 2005). Their robust transformation can be used in a variety of situations (e.g., Hayashi and Yuan, 2003). Concretely speaking the M-estimators are defined as follows: Let

$$d(\boldsymbol{x}_i, \boldsymbol{\mu}, \boldsymbol{\Sigma}) = [(\boldsymbol{x}_i - \boldsymbol{\mu})'\boldsymbol{\Sigma}^{-1}(\boldsymbol{x}_i - \boldsymbol{\mu})]^{1/2}, \tag{21}$$

with

$$\boldsymbol{\mu} = \sum_{i=1}^{n} u_1(d_i)x_i / \sum_{i=1}^{n} u_1(d_i), \tag{22}$$

$$\boldsymbol{\Sigma} = \sum_{i=1}^{n} u_2(d_i^2)(\boldsymbol{x}_i - \boldsymbol{\mu})(\boldsymbol{x}_i - \boldsymbol{\mu})'/n. \tag{23}$$

The weight functions are defined through a tuning parameter ρ that gives the percentage of influential cases we want to control, and r is a constant determined through $P(\chi_p^2 > r^2) = \rho$. Then the weight functions u_1 and u_2 are given by

$$u_1(d_i) = \begin{cases} 1 & \text{if} \quad d_i \leq r, \\ r/d_i & \text{if} \quad d_i > r, \end{cases} \tag{24}$$

$$u_2(d_i) = \{u_1(d_i)\}^2/\varphi, \tag{25}$$

where φ is a constant determined by ρ through $E\{\chi_p^2 u_2(\chi_p^2)\} = p$. Note that equations (22) and (23) can be solved by iteration, and let $\hat{\mu}$ and $\hat{\Sigma}$ be the solution of (22) and (23), respectively. Yuan et al. (2004) proposed to choose ρ based on empirical efficiency by applying the bootstrap to the transformed sample (Yuan et al., 2000)

$$\boldsymbol{x}_i^{(p)} = \sqrt{u_{2i}}(\boldsymbol{x}_i - \hat{\boldsymbol{\mu}}), \tag{26}$$

where $u_{2i} = u_2\{d_2(\boldsymbol{x}_i, \hat{\boldsymbol{\mu}}, \hat{\boldsymbol{\Sigma}})\}$; the optimal ρ corresponds to the most efficient parameter estimates. Yuan et al. (2000) and Yuan and Hayashi (2003) proposed alternative rationales for choosing ρ. Other approaches to robust SEM are developed in Yuan and Bentler (1998b, 2000b) and Yuan et al. (2004). For other forms of M-estimator, see e.g., Campbell (1980).

2.6. *Misspecification and power*

(1) *Model misspecification*: Any model is only an approximation to the truth. This implies that we inevitably encounter misspecified models in SEM. Misspecified models are known to create: (i) biases to parameter estimates; (ii) inconsistent standard errors; and (iii) an invalid asymptotic distribution of the χ^2 test statistic (White, 1982). A brief summary of research on model misspecification in SEM is as follows:

(i) *Consistency*: Many parameter estimates in CSA and MCSA are still consistent even when the model is misspecified (Yuan et al., 2003; Yuan and Bentler, 2006).

(ii) *Convergence in distribution*: The test statistics under misspecified models can be approximated by the non-central χ^2 distribution. However, a problem in this approximation is that it requires the assumption of a sequence of local alternative hypotheses, which may not be realistic in practice. Alternatively, we can employ the asymptotic normal distribution (Vuong, 1989; Yanagihara et al., 2005; Yuan et al., 2007). Based on the approach by Vuong (1989), Yuan et al. (2007) derived the following normal approximation:

$$\sqrt{n}(T_{\text{ML}}/n - \mu) \to N(0, \omega_{\text{ML}}^2), \tag{27}$$

where $\mu = F_{\text{ML}} + tr(\boldsymbol{U}_* \boldsymbol{V})/n$ and ω_{ML}^2 is quite involved; the formulas for $\boldsymbol{U}_*$ and ω_{ML}^2 are given in Yuan et al. (in press). Here, note that the second term $tr(\boldsymbol{U}_* \boldsymbol{V})/n$ substantially improves the normal approximation. For additional recent research, see Li and Bentler (2006).

(2) *Power*: Misspecification of the model means that the null hypothesis $\beta = \beta(\theta)$ on the mean and covariance structure is wrong. Thus, it is tightly connected with the concept of power. There are two main approaches to obtaining power in SEM:

(i) *Non-central χ^2 distribution*: Among the approaches to obtain power, the most common approach is based on a non-central χ^2 distribution. The references include Satorra and Saris (1985); Saris and Satorra (1993); Kim (2005); MacCallum et al. (1996); Hancock (2001). The Satorra and Saris (1985) approach requires a specification of the model under the alternative hypothesis, which can be quite complicated in a heavily parameterized model. Later they relaxed the requirement (Saris and Satorra, 1993). MacCallum et al. (1996) developed an approach where the degree of misspecification can be measured by the RMSEA fit index (see below), which does not require specification of specific alternative values for various parameters. In addition to testing the standard exact fit null hypothesis, they also discussed assessment of "close" fit. Statistical justifications for such approach are only recently being developed (Li and Bentler, 2006).

(ii) *Bootstrap approach*: A problem in using the non-central χ^2 distribution to evaluate power is that the meaning of a non-centrality parameter is not clear when the behavior of the test statistic cannot be described by a χ^2 variates (Yuan and Marshall, 2004). Because of its flexibility, the bootstrap has frequently been used in SEM (Beran and Srivastava, 1985; Bollen and Stine, 1993; Yung and Bentler, 1996; Yuan and Hayashi, 2006), and recently, it has been used to develop a promising approach to power (Yuan and Hayashi, 2003). On the bootstrap in general, see e.g., Beran (1986) or Davison and Hinkley (1997). According to Yuan and Hayashi (2003), for data sets with heavy tails, the bootstrap can be applied to a transformed sample by a downweighting procedure as in (26) (Yuan et al., 2000), which has the advantage of not requiring the assumption that the data come from a multivariate normal distribution.

Besides methods based on the non-central χ^2 distribution or the bootstrap, there are other approaches to power such as simulation (see e.g., Muthén and Muthén, 2002, and Mooijaart, 2003).

2.7. *Fit indices*

Besides the test statistics T, there exist numerous so-called fit indices to measure the degree of overall fit of a model to data. χ^2 tests inherently have the following two major problems in practice. The first problem is that $T = (n-1)F$ increases as n increases. As a result, any model structure null hypothesis such as (12) will tend to be rejected when the sample size n gets large enough, yet the model may be good enough for practical purposes. Another problem is that in SEM, the role of null and alternative hypothesis is reversed compared to classical hypothesis testing. As the positer of a model (such as (12)), we hope to retain the null hypothesis. Because of these shortcomings, fit indices based on test statistics have been developed. The statistical properties of some fit indices are known (e.g., Ogasawara, 2001), and simulation studies are needed to fully understand the behaviors of various fit indices (see e.g., Hu and Bentler, 1998, 1999). While many fit indices have been proposed, only a few are frequently used (McDonald and Ho, 2002) and we limit our discussion to those.

There are several ways to classify fit indices (e.g., Tanaka, 1993). Recently, Yuan (2005) classified fit indices based on their distributional assumptions. For convenience, we classify fit indices into the following four categories: (i) residual-based; (ii) independence-model-based; (iii) root mean square error of approximation; and (iv) information-criterion-based fit indices. The first two types are only appropriate to covariance structures.

(1) *Residual-based fit indices* (see e.g., Jöreskog and Sörbom, 1981*)*: The following three are all the functions of the residuals $\boldsymbol{S} - \boldsymbol{\Sigma}(\hat{\boldsymbol{\theta}})$.

  (i) *Standardized root mean square residual* (*SRMR*): As the name shows, SRMR is the square root of the sum of squares of the residuals in a correlation metric. SRMR is given by

$$\mathrm{SRMR} = \sqrt{\frac{2}{p(p+1)}\sum_{i\leq j}\{s_{ij} - \sigma_{ij}(\hat{\boldsymbol{\theta}})\}^2/s_{ii}s_{jj}}, \tag{28}$$

where $\sigma_{ij}(\hat{\boldsymbol{\theta}})$ is the (i, j) element of $\boldsymbol{\Sigma}(\hat{\boldsymbol{\theta}})$. Obviously, when the value of SRMR is small and close to zero, the fit is good.

(ii) *Goodness of fit index* (*GFI*): GFI has been compared to a squared multiple correlation in multiple regression. GFI is given by

$$\mathrm{GFI} = 1 - \frac{tr[\{\boldsymbol{\Sigma}(\hat{\boldsymbol{\theta}})^{-1}(\boldsymbol{S} - \boldsymbol{\Sigma}(\hat{\boldsymbol{\theta}}))\}^2]}{tr[\{\boldsymbol{\Sigma}(\hat{\boldsymbol{\theta}})^{-1}\boldsymbol{S}\}^2]}. \tag{29}$$

When the value of GFI is close to 1, the fit is good.

(iii) *Adjusted goodness of fit index* (*AGFI*): AGFI corresponds to the squared multiple correlation adjusted for degrees of freedom. AGFI is given by

$$\mathrm{AGFI} = 1 - \frac{p(p+1)(1 - GFI)}{p(p+1) - 2q_2}. \tag{30}$$

When the value of AGFI is close to 1, the fit is good. AGFI is always less than or equal to GFI.

(2) *Independence-model-based fit indices*: The independence model is defined as model in which the covariance structure is diagonal: $\boldsymbol{\Sigma}_{\mathrm{I}} = \mathrm{diag}(\sigma_{11}, \ldots, \sigma_{pp})$. Clearly the independence model is the smallest (i.e., most constrained) model in SEM. In contrast, the largest model is the saturated model (Bentler and Bonett, 1980). The idea of these 0–1 fit indices is to locate the current model along a line between the independence model and the saturated model, where 0 is a model no better than the independence model and 1 is a model as good as the saturated model. Let T_{M} and T_{I} be the test statistics under the current model and the independence model, respectively, and let df_{M} and df_{I} be the associated degrees of freedom.

(i) *Normed fit index* (*NFI;* Bentler and Bonett, 1980): NFI is given by the relative location of the current model between the saturated model with $T_{\mathrm{S}} = 0$ and the independence model T_{I}:

$$\mathrm{NFI} = 1 - \frac{T_{\mathrm{M}}}{T_{\mathrm{I}}}. \tag{31}$$

NFI ranges between 0 and 1, and a value of NFI close to 1 means a good fit. An advantage of this index is that it can be defined even if T is only a descriptive statistic that has no known distribution.

(ii) *Non-normed fit index* (*NNFI;* Bentler and Bonett, 1980; Tucker and Lewis, 1973): Originally, Tucker and Lewis (1973) proposed what is now called the Tucker–Lewis index (TLI) in the context of exploratory factor analysis. NNFI is an extension of TLI to SEM. When the sample size n is not large, NFI is known to have a drawback of not approaching 1 even if the current model is correct. NNFI corrects this drawback by introducing the model degrees of freedom, as follows:

$$\mathrm{NNFI} = 1 - \frac{(T_{\mathrm{M}}/d_{\mathrm{M}}) - 1}{(T_{\mathrm{I}}/d_{\mathrm{I}}) - 1}. \tag{32}$$

When the current model is correct, the expected value of T_{M} should be close to its degrees of freedom df_{M}. Thus, $T_{\mathrm{M}}/df_{\mathrm{M}}$ should be close to 1. However, NNFI can exceed 1.

(iii) *Comparative fit index* (*CFI;* Bentler, 1990): Bentler (1990) proposed to use population non-centrality parameters to define an index like (31):

$$\mathrm{CFI} = 1 - \frac{\tau_{\mathrm{M}}}{\tau_{\mathrm{I}}}. \tag{33}$$

In practice, CFI is estimated using $\hat{\tau}_{\mathrm{M}} = \max\{T_{\mathrm{M}} - df_{\mathrm{M}}, 0\}$ and $\hat{\tau}_{\mathrm{I}} = \max\{T_{\mathrm{M}} - df_{\mathrm{M}}, T_{\mathrm{I}} - df_{\mathrm{I}}, 0\}$. Obviously, CFI is always between zero and 1. It avoids the underestimation of NFI and the overestimation of NNFI. In this category of fit indices, CFI is the most frequently reported one.

(3) *Root mean square error of approximation* (*RMSEA*; Steiger and Lind, 1980; Browne and Cudeck, 1993): First introduced by Steiger and Lind (1980) for exploratory factor analysis, the RMSEA became popular due to Browne and Cudeck (1993). As a population index it is given as

$$\mathrm{RMSEA}_{\mathrm{pop}} = \sqrt{\tau_{\mathrm{M}}/df}, \tag{34}$$

which can be interpreted as the square root of population misfit per degree of freedom. When the value of RMSEA is small, the fit is good, and for the same degree of misfit as measured by τ_{M}, models with higher df fit better. In practice, RMSEA is computed as

$$\mathrm{RMSEA} = \sqrt{\max\{(T_{\mathrm{M}} - df_{\mathrm{M}})/(n \cdot df_{\mathrm{M}}), 0\}}. \tag{35}$$

Yuan (2005) pointed out that an implicit assumption in RMSEA is that T_{M} under the alternative hypothesis is distributed as a non-central χ^2 with the non-centrality parameter τ_{M} equal to the sample size n times the value measured by the fit function. For this to be true, we need to assume that the concept of a sequence of local alternative hypotheses makes sense. However, this holds only when the true population covariance matrix is sufficiently close to the hypothesis $\boldsymbol{\Sigma}(\boldsymbol{\theta})$. According to Yuan (2005), the distribution of the sample RMSEA is unknown in general. Any probability or confidence interval attached to RMSEA, as printed out in software, has little justification for real data or even simulated data from a normal distribution. Nonetheless, applied researchers keep using it in practice to assess the fit of their model.

(4) *Information-criterion-based fit indices*: The goodness of fit of several different models can be compared with the information criteria AIC (e.g., Akaike, 1974, 1987), CAIC (Bozdogan, 1987), and BIC (Schwarz, 1978), defined as follows:

$$\mathrm{AIC} = T_{\mathrm{ML}} + 2q, \tag{36}$$

$$\mathrm{CAIC} = T_{\mathrm{ML}} + (1 + \log n)q, \tag{37}$$

$$\text{BIC} = T_{\text{ML}} + (\log n)q, \tag{38}$$

respectively, where q is the number of parameters (either q_1 or q_2 depending on the model). Assuming that the model makes sense theoretically, the model with the smallest information criterion may be chosen.

2.8. *Modification of the model*

When an initial model has a poor fit, it may be desirable to modify the model to improve the fit. In principle, for nested models this can be accomplished by a model comparison procedure based on the χ^2 difference test such as $T_{\text{D}} = T_{\text{ML1}} - T_{\text{ML2}}$, where T_{ML1} is the test statistic for a more restricted model and T_{ML2} is the test for a more general model. However, this would require specifying various pairs of models and estimating both models in a pair. In SEM, two types of well-known tests, the Lagrange Multiplier (LM) or score test and the Wald test, are frequently used in addition or instead of a difference test. They only require estimation of one model, either the more restricted model in the case of the LM test, or the more general model in case of the Wald test. More importantly, both tests are available in an exploratory methodology where a search procedure can be used to find alternative parameters that may influence model fit (see e.g., Lee and Bentler, 1980; Bentler and Dijkstra, 1985; Lee, 1985; Bentler, 1986; Satorra, 1989; Chou and Bentler, 1990, 2002).

(1) *LM test or Score test*: When we would like to know which paths may be added to improve the fit of a model, i.e., which restricted parameters in a model should perhaps be freed and estimated, we can employ the score test (Rao, 1947, 1973) or its equivalent, the LM test (Aitchison and Silvey, 1958). When considering a single parameter to free, asymptotically the LM test follows a χ^2 distribution with 1 *df* (Satorra, 1989). A large χ^2 indicates that the restriction is not consistent with the data, that a better model most likely can be obtained when the parameter is freed, and that the model test statistic (e.g., T_{ML}) then would decrease by an amount approximately equal to the LM test value. Then the model can be re-estimated, and the procedure repeated. However, the tests can also be applied sequentially before re-estimating the model. In this way it is a multivariate LM test with *df* equal to the number of restrictions being tested. The multivariate test can be implemented in a forward stepwise procedure where the parameter making the biggest improvement in fit is added first, a next parameter is added that yields the largest increment in fit after controlling the influence of the first, etc. (Bentler, in press). For a comparison of these two approaches, see e.g., Green et al. (1999). In some SEM software, the LM test is called the modification index (Sörbom, 1989). Under the null hypothesis that the model differentiating parameters are zero in the population, LM tests are asymptotically χ^2 distributed, but this may not be true when applied in a search methodology. In small samples, parameters may be chosen that capitalize on chance, i.e., the method may identify restrictions to

release that do not hold up well in cross-validation (e.g., MacCallum et al., 1992).

(2) *Wald test*: If we have a model that fits but seems to have unnecessary parameters, standard errors can be used to find and eliminate particular nonsignificant parameters. The Wald test (Wald, 1943) is a multivariate generalization that allows testing a set of parameters simultaneously to see if they are sufficiently unimportant that they could be eliminated. Again this methodology has been implemented in a search fashion. The procedure corresponds to backward elimination in multiple regression, that is, the least significant parameter is removed first, residuals are computed, then next least significant parameter is removed, and so on until a set is obtained that is simultaneously not significant. This implies that removal of those parameters from the model may increase the test statistic (e.g., T_{ML}), but only by a small amount. Like the LM test, under the null hypothesis that the model parameters are zero in the population, and with an *a priori* selection of parameters to test, the Wald test asymptotically follows the χ^2 distribution with either 1 *df* or as many *df*'s as there are parameters being tested (see e.g., Satorra, 1989). Again, however, this test procedure can be misleading in small samples when used empirically to search for unimportant parameters.

(3) *A word of caution*: The asymptotic distribution of the difference test T_{D} in SEM was studied theoretically by Steiger et al. (1985). In theory, the more general model need not be true for the distribution of T_{D} to be asymptotically χ^2. However, recent research has shown that when the more general model is false, tests such as T_{D} perform very badly in small to medium sized samples and cannot be relied upon (Yuan and Bentler, 2004a; Maydeu-Olivares and Cai, 2006). Clearly the same caution should be used with LM and Wald tests. This is not a trivial matter because in practice, even the best model may not fit statistically (see fit indices above).

3. Extensions of SEM

3.1. Extensions

So far, we have discussed SEM for the simplest case of only linear latent variable models for one standard sample from a population. However, the SEM paradigm has been extended in many different directions so that more complicated model and data structures can be handled effectively. This includes the ability to handle incomplete data, nonlinear relations among latent variables, multiple samples, hierarchical data structures, categorical variables, and so on. Here we just give a flavor of some of these developments.

3.2. Multi-group SEM

The most typical extension of SEM is to the multiple-group case, where parts of models or entire models may be held to be equal across groups in order to determine similarities or differences among samples or populations. A typical example is the two-group case, where males vs. females may be compared. Multi-group SEM was originated by Jöreskog (1971) and Sörbom (1974), and has been further developed by Bentler et al. (1987), Lee and Tsui (1982), and Muthén (1989a, 1989b). Yuan and Bentler (2001) gave a unified approach to multi-group SEM under non-normality and with missing data. Thus, we follow their notation.

(1) *Test statistic and fit function*: Suppose we have m groups with sample sizes n_j, $j = 1, \ldots, m$. Let $N = n_1 + \cdots + n_m$ be the total sample size including all the m groups. The parameters from the m groups can be arranged as $\boldsymbol{\theta} = (\boldsymbol{\theta}_1', \ldots, \boldsymbol{\theta}_m')'$. Then the test statistics is given by

$$T^m_{\text{ML}} = N \cdot F^m_{\text{ML}}, \tag{39}$$

where

$$\begin{aligned} F^m_{\text{ML}} = \sum_{j=1}^{m} \frac{n_j}{N} &([\hat{\boldsymbol{\mu}}_j - \boldsymbol{\mu}_j(\boldsymbol{\theta}_j)]' \boldsymbol{\Sigma}_j^{-1}(\boldsymbol{\theta}_j)[\hat{\boldsymbol{\mu}}_j - \boldsymbol{\mu}_j(\boldsymbol{\theta}_j)]) \\ &+ tr[\hat{\boldsymbol{\Sigma}}_j \boldsymbol{\Sigma}_j^{-1}(\boldsymbol{\theta}_j)] - \log|\hat{\boldsymbol{\Sigma}}_j \boldsymbol{\Sigma}_j^{-1}(\boldsymbol{\theta}_j)| - p) \end{aligned} \tag{40}$$

is a weighted sum of the fit functions from each group. Obviously, when there are no constraints on parameters, the degrees of freedom is m times the degrees of freedom for the model for each group. More typically, the fit function will be optimized under r constraints in the form of $\boldsymbol{h}(\boldsymbol{\theta}) = \mathbf{0}$, and the *df* will be adjusted accordingly. In addition to likelihood ratio tests of nested models, multi-group version of the Satorra–Bentler rescaled statistic (Satorra, 2000) and the sandwich-type covariance matrix exist to handle distributional violations. In addition, normal theory or generalized LM tests can be used to test the significance of the constraints.

(2) *Constraints and invariance*: As noted, multi-group SEM typically will involve constraints on the parameters because it is natural to evaluate whether path coefficients are the same among m groups. If we can assume the existence of the same latent variable(s) among the groups in the populations, we say that factorial invariance exists in the populations (see e.g., Meredith, 1993, and Millsap, 1997, on factorial invariance). However, there are different levels of factorial invariance (Horn et al., 1983). For example, when the test using the test statistic of the form (39) (without any equality constraints among the groups) is not rejected, we say that we could not reject *configural* invariance. When the structure of path coefficients is identical across groups in the populations, we say that *metric* invariance holds. We can put equality constraints also on the residual variances and/or factor correlations among the groups and can test for the factorial invariance under stronger conditions. A concrete example of these ideas is the confirmatory factor model, where each group has a structure such as (12). If the structure of factor loadings is equal across groups, we have metric invariance even if the remaining parameter matrices differ. Equality of the factorial structure implies that the same latent factors are measured in each group.

(3) *Mean structure*: When considering a factor model such as (6) for each group, it is possible to fix $\boldsymbol{\mu}$ and $\boldsymbol{\Lambda}$ as common across all groups, but to have $E(\xi) = \boldsymbol{\mu}_\xi$ differ across groups. This implies that the same latent factors are being measured in the groups, but that they differ in their level on the trait. For example, a natural question to ask might be whether there is any significant difference in factor means between males vs. females. Because factor means can have any location unit, one group's vector of factor means $\boldsymbol{\mu}_\xi$ is set to zero. Without such a constraint, the model is usually non-identified.

3.3. Growth curve models

In medical and epidemiological research, many research designs are longitudinal in nature and the consistency or change of individuals across time is a key focus. We can imagine a line or curve connecting all the repeated observations of a given individual across time, and dozens or hundreds of such lines or curves to represent the entire sample. When the repeated measures are obtained a few to a dozen times, such data can be analyzed using SEM as a procedure to characterize mean trends in these curves as well as individual differences and their antecedents, correlates, or consequences. In this field, the methodology is known as growth curve modeling, see e.g., Bentler (2005) or Stoel (2003) for summaries, or Bollen and Curran (2006) and Duncan et al. (2006) for text-length treatments. In the simplest model setup, this methodology represents a special case of (4)–(5) or (6)–(11) and it amounts to an application of MCSA. For example, we may take $\boldsymbol{x} = \boldsymbol{\mu} + \boldsymbol{\Lambda}\xi + \varepsilon$, but consider $\boldsymbol{\mu} = \boldsymbol{0}$ so that the mean information is carried by $\boldsymbol{\mu}_\xi$. Then there are some features unique to growth curve SEM that are worth noting.

(1) The $\boldsymbol{x}_i$ will represent a quantitative variable repeatedly measured across time, and the latent factors ξ are interpreted as representing important features of the shapes of the growth curves across time. There are many ways to code shapes, but a standard one is to consider the starting point or "intercept," the linear trend (commonly referred to as "slope"), or a higher order curve feature such as a "quadratic" trend. When the repeatedly measured variable represents a substantive construct (such as "depression"), the factors represent time trends in that construct (e.g., "depression").
(2) A given latent factor, say the slope ξ_j, has scores for every individual in the sample. Each of those scores represents the given trend in scores for that individual, e.g., for slope it can be considered to be a coefficient to represent that person's linear trend across time. Some persons may be growing rapidly, and others not at all, and these individual differences show up in the variance of ξ_j. The corresponding factor mean $\boldsymbol{\mu}_{\xi(j)}$ represents the average trend in the data, e.g., it would be the group average slope or linear trend. Predictors, correlates, and consequences of ξ_j can also be determined.
(3) Since factor loadings are weights attached to the factors to predict a variable, those for a given factor, such as the jth column of $\boldsymbol{\Lambda}$, contains weights that represent time. Unlike standard factor analysis, the coefficients in $\boldsymbol{\Lambda}$ are taken

to be known *a priori* in accord with the coding of time. Different factors code different aspects of time, such as the starting point, or linear or quadratic changes across time. In particular, (i) the path coefficients from the intercept factor to the observed variables are set to an equal constant, typically to 1; (ii) the factor loadings for the linear slope factor are set proportional to time elapsed. For example, if the time differences are equal among the observed variables, the path to the initial measure may take the value of 0, that to the second measure the value of 1, that to the third measure gets the value of 2, etc.; (iii) likewise, paths from the quadratic factor may be coded as $(0^2, 1^2, 2^2, \ldots) = (0, 1, 4, \ldots)$; (iv) because raw polynomial coefficients become very large as time elapses and as the degree of polynomials increase, standardized coefficients can be used. For example, for three equally spaced observed variables, the coefficients from the intercept, linear, and quadratic factors are (0.577, 0.557, 0.555), (−0.707, 0, 0.707), and (0.408, −0.816, 0.408), respectively. This is one example of orthogonal polynomials (see e.g., Maxwell and Delaney, 2004, Chapter 6); (v) alternative approaches to the linear slope factor exist, such as spline factors by Meredith and Tisak (1990) and the piecewise linear model (Raudenbush and Bryk, 2002, p. 178). Also, since a model with fixed nonzero factor loadings may be hard to fit, researchers sometimes free these loadings. This leads to a different interpretation of time trends, and thus needs to be done with caution (see e.g., Bentler, 2005).

3.4. Multilevel SEM

Multilevel analysis, also called hierarchical linear modeling, is a statistical technique for analyzing data collected from a hierarchical sampling scheme such as level-1 observations (e.g., students) nested within level-2 observations (e.g., classes). The number of levels can be extended, though a large sample size at the highest level is required for stable estimation. Most multi-level analyses are two-level. Some general references for multi-level analysis include Goldstein (2003), Raudenbush and Bryk (2002), and Reise and Duan (2003). SEM can be used to estimate parameters for multi-level data, and this approach is especially useful when latent variables are involved, e.g., Bentler and Liang (2003), Bentler et al. (2005), du Toit and du Toit (2002), Goldstein and McDonald (1988), McDonald and Goldstein (1989), Lee (1990), Lee and Poon (1998), Lee et al. (1995), Lee and Shi (2001), Lee and Song (2001), Liang and Bentler (2004), Muthén (1994, 1997), Poon and Lee (1994), and Yuan and Bentler (2002, 2003, 2004b).

According to Liang and Bentler (2004) and Bentler et al. (2005), two-level SEM can be formulated as

$$\begin{pmatrix} \mathbf{z}_g \\ \mathbf{y}_{gi} \end{pmatrix} = \begin{pmatrix} \mathbf{z}_g \\ \mathbf{v}_g \end{pmatrix} + \begin{pmatrix} \mathbf{0} \\ \mathbf{v}_{gi} \end{pmatrix}, \tag{41}$$

where $\mathbf{z}_g$ $(p_2 \times 1)$ is a vector of *i.i.d.* level-2 observations $(g = 1, \ldots, G)$, and $\mathbf{y}_{gi}$ $(p_1 \times 1)$ is a vector of level-1 observations $(i = 1, \ldots, N_g)$ from the same cluster or group (level-2 unit), and $p = p_1 + p_2$. Under the model, the observed $\mathbf{y}_{gi}$ are decomposed into a part exhibiting between-cluster variation $\mathbf{v}_g$ and a part exhibiting within-cluster variation $\mathbf{v}_{gi}$.

Note that for a fixed group g, $\mathbf{y}_{gi}$ are *i.i.d.*, while for all i's and g's, $\mathbf{y}_{gi}$ are not independent. In Eq. (41), we typically assume: (i) $\mathbf{z}_g$ and $\mathbf{v}_g$ are independent of $\mathbf{v}_{gi}$; (ii) $\mathbf{z}_g$ and $\mathbf{v}_g$ are correlated. Let us introduce further notation: $\boldsymbol{\mu}_z = E(\mathbf{z}_g)$, $\boldsymbol{\mu}_y = E(\mathbf{y}_{gi}) = E(\mathbf{v}_g)$, $\boldsymbol{\Sigma}_{zz} = Cov(\mathbf{z}_g)$, $\boldsymbol{\Sigma}_B = Cov(\mathbf{v}_g)$, $\boldsymbol{\Sigma}_{Wi} = Cov(\mathbf{v}_{gi})$ typically assumed to be homogeneous across clusters with $\boldsymbol{\Sigma}_{Wi} = \boldsymbol{\Sigma}_W$, and $\boldsymbol{\Sigma}_{zy} = Cov(\mathbf{z}_g, \mathbf{y}_{gi}) = Cov(\mathbf{z}_g, \mathbf{v}_g)$. Under a SEM structure, we can further structure the within-cluster covariance matrix, for example, as a confirmatory factor model (see (12)) as in:

$$\boldsymbol{\Sigma}_w = \boldsymbol{\Lambda}_W \boldsymbol{\Phi}_W \boldsymbol{\Lambda}_W' + \boldsymbol{\Psi}_W. \tag{42}$$

More generally, the means and covariances in multi-level SEM are $\boldsymbol{\mu} = \begin{pmatrix} \boldsymbol{\mu}_z \\ \boldsymbol{\mu}_y \end{pmatrix}$, $\tilde{\boldsymbol{\Sigma}}_B = \begin{pmatrix} \boldsymbol{\Sigma}_{zz} & \boldsymbol{\Sigma}_{zy} \\ \boldsymbol{\Sigma}_{yz} & \boldsymbol{\Sigma}_B \end{pmatrix}$, and $\boldsymbol{\Sigma}_W$, and any of these vectors and matrices can be further structured as in (4)–(5) or (10)–(11).

Parameter estimation methods such as ML have been developed for multilevel SEM. For ML estimation based on Gauss–Newton or Fisher scoring algorithms, see du Toit and du Toit (2002), Goldstein and McDonald (1988), Lee (1990), and McDonald and Goldstein (1989). Muthén (1994, 1997) proposed an approximate ML estimator commonly called Muthén's ML, or MUML. MUML has the advantage of easier calculation and faster convergence than full ML estimation. When level-1 samples are equal in size, MUML is equivalent to full ML estimation. Yuan and Hayashi (2005) analytically studied the statistical properties of MUML and identified further conditions for MUML to be close to ML. The EM algorithm (Dempster et al., 1977) also has been applied by Raudenbush (1995) and Lee and Poon (1998). The approach of Lee and Poon (1998) was further extended by Bentler and Liang (2003) and Liang and Bentler (2004). Finally, just as ML test statistics in simple SEM can lead to distorted χ^2 tests and standard error estimates under non-normality, the same can occur if level-1 or level-2 observations are not multivariate normal. Corrected test statistics for this situation, and the study of robustness of multilevel SEM can be found in Yuan and Bentler (2003, 2004b, 2005a, 2005b).

3.5. Nonlinear SEM

In multiple regression, the dependent variable can be a nonlinear function of the independent variables by the use of polynomial and/or interaction terms. This is straightforward. On the contrary, in SEM it has been a difficult task to connect a dependent latent variable with independent latent variables in a nonlinear fashion. Efforts to construct and estimate a nonlinear SEM have been made for the last 20 years. Early works include Kenny and Judd (1984), Bentler (1983), Mooijaart (1985), and Mooijaart and Bentler (1986). The Kenny–Judd model, a particular simple nonlinear model that includes an interaction term, has been intensively studied. More recent works include Bollen (1996), Bollen and Paxton (1998), Jöreskog and Yang (1996), Klein and Moosbrugger (2000), Lee et al. (2004), Lee and Zhu (2000, 2002), Marsh et al. (2004), Wall and Amemiya (2000, 2001, 2003), Yang Jonsson (1998). The Bollen–Paxton and Klein–Moosbrugger approaches seem to be especially attractive. The Wall–Amemiya approach seems to be the most theoretically defensible under a wide range of conditions, since it yields consistent estimates under distributional violations. The Bayesian approaches of Lee and his colleagues are the most promising for small samples. However, to the best of the authors' knowledge, no general SEM software incorporates the Wall–Amemiya or Lee approaches.

4. Some practical issues

4.1. Treatment of missing data

Missing data are encountered frequently in data analysis, and this problem certainly also arises in the context of SEM. Rubin (1976) and Little and Rubin (2002) are general references on the missing data problem, while Allison (2002) provides a non-technical account. It is useful to discuss this topic by considering Rubin's (1976) missing data mechanisms: (1) *MCAR* (missing completely at random): Missingness of the data is independent of both the observed and the missing values; (2) *MAR* (missing at random): Missingness of the data is independent of the missing values but can depend on the observed values; (3) *NMAR* (not missing at random): Misssingness depends on the missing values themselves. While unprincipled methods such as listwise deletion require MCAR data for appropriate inference, most methodological developments on missing data in SEM focus on the normal theory ML procedure because it allows the weaker MAR mechanism. When the data are from a multivariate normal distribution and the missing data mechanism is either MCAR or MAR, the MLE is consistent and asymptotically normal. However, note that MAR mechanism may not be ignorable when using the wrong density to perform the ML estimation. Yuan (2006) employed the normal density to model a non-normal distribution with missing data and gave sufficient conditions under which consistent MLE will be guaranteed when data are MAR.

The references on missing data related to ML include Arbuckle (1996), Jamshidian and Bentler (1999), Lee (1986), Muthén et al. (1987), and Tang and Bentler (1998). When missingness occurs in the context of non-normal data, the classical ML methodology has to be extended to provide corrections to test statistics and standard errors. References include Arminger and Sobel (1990), Savalei and Bentler (2005), Yuan and Bentler (2000a), and Yuan (2006) mentioned above.

Because of its importance in the missing data context, we describe one approach using the EM algorithm (Dempster et al., 1977) to obtaining MLE in this context. Let $\boldsymbol{x}_i$ be the ith case including both observed variables $\boldsymbol{x}_{io}$ and missing variables $\boldsymbol{x}_{im}$. That is, $\boldsymbol{x}_i = (\boldsymbol{x}_{io}', \boldsymbol{x}_{im}')'$. Corresponding to the partition of

$\boldsymbol{x}_i$, let $\boldsymbol{\mu} = (\boldsymbol{\mu}_o', \boldsymbol{\mu}_m')'$ and $\boldsymbol{\Sigma} = \begin{pmatrix} \boldsymbol{\Sigma}_{oo} & \boldsymbol{\Sigma}_{om} \\ \boldsymbol{\Sigma}_{mo} & \boldsymbol{\Sigma}_{mm} \end{pmatrix}$ be the partitioned population mean vector and the covariance matrix.

(1) *E-step*: Then, under the normal distribution assumption, the conditional expectation of $E(\boldsymbol{x}_{im}|\boldsymbol{x}_{io})$ and $E(\boldsymbol{x}_{im}\boldsymbol{x}_{im}'|\boldsymbol{x}_{io})$ are given by:

$$E(\boldsymbol{x}_{im}|\boldsymbol{x}_{io}) = \boldsymbol{\mu}_m + \boldsymbol{\Sigma}_{mo}\boldsymbol{\Sigma}_{oo}^{-1}(\boldsymbol{x}_{io} - \boldsymbol{\mu}_o), \tag{43}$$

$$E(\boldsymbol{x}_{im}\boldsymbol{x}_{im}'|\boldsymbol{x}_{io}) = (\boldsymbol{\Sigma}_{mm} - \boldsymbol{\Sigma}_{mo}\boldsymbol{\Sigma}_{oo}^{-1}\boldsymbol{\Sigma}_{om}) + E(\boldsymbol{x}_{im}|\boldsymbol{x}_{io})E(\boldsymbol{x}_{im}|\boldsymbol{x}_{io})'. \tag{44}$$

These Eqs (43) and (44) are incorporated in

$$E(\boldsymbol{x}_i|\boldsymbol{x}_{io}) = (\boldsymbol{x}_{io}', E(\boldsymbol{x}_{im}|\boldsymbol{x}_{io})')', \tag{45}$$

$$E(\boldsymbol{x}_i\boldsymbol{x}_i'|\boldsymbol{x}_{io}) = \begin{pmatrix} \boldsymbol{x}_{io}\boldsymbol{x}_{io}' & \boldsymbol{x}_{io}E(\boldsymbol{x}_{im}|\boldsymbol{x}_{io})' \\ E(\boldsymbol{x}_{im}|\boldsymbol{x}_{io})\boldsymbol{x}_{io}' & E(\boldsymbol{x}_{im}\boldsymbol{x}_{im}'|\boldsymbol{x}_{io}) \end{pmatrix}, \tag{46}$$

respectively.

(2) *M-step*: Let $\bar{\boldsymbol{x}} = (1/n)\sum_{i=1}^{n} E(\boldsymbol{x}_i|\boldsymbol{x}_{io})$ and $\boldsymbol{S} = (1/n)\sum_{i=1}^{n} E(\boldsymbol{x}_i\boldsymbol{x}_i'|\boldsymbol{x}_{io}) - \bar{\boldsymbol{x}}\,\bar{\boldsymbol{x}}'$. Then the M-step consists of minimizing the ML fit function:

$$F_{\text{ML}} = (\bar{x} - \mu(\theta))'\Sigma(\theta)^{-1}(\bar{x} - \mu(\theta)) + tr(S\Sigma(\theta)^{-1}) - \log|S\Sigma(\theta)^{-1}| - p \tag{47}$$

with respect to $\boldsymbol{\theta}$. Further details can be found in Jamshidian and Bentler (1999). More general methods based on Markov chain Monte Carlo (MCMC) methods (e.g., Lee et al., 2003; Song and Lee, 2002) hold promise for improved inference in small samples. Robert and Casella (2004) provide an overview of MCMC methods.

It would be desirable to be able to evaluate whether data are MCAR, MAR, or NMAR. With regard to MCAR, it is possible to evaluate whether the various patterns of missing data are consistent with sampling from a single normal population. This can be done by testing homogeneity of means, covariances, or homogeneity of both means and covariances (Kim and Bentler, 2002). It is difficult to find general approaches to testing MAR and NMAR, although specific models for NMAR have been proposed and evaluated (Tang and Lee, 1998; Lee and Tang, 2006).

4.2. Treatment of categorical dependent variables

So far, we have assumed that the observed variables are continuous. This may not always hold true in practice. Categorical variables are frequently used in medical and epidemiological research. First of all, note that no special methods are needed if the categorical variables are independent variables. It is common that independent variables are categorical in multiple regression, and SEM can handle such variables by dummy coding as is done in multiple regression. Second, if a dependent categorical variable is ordered and has at least 4 or 5 categories as in a typical Likert scale, treating it as a continuous variable will create few serious problems (e.g., Bentler and Chou, 1987). The remaining case is when a dependent categorical variable is either binary or with three categories. Even three-category data treated continuously can perform well enough (Coenders et al., 1997), but we do not recommend it as routine practice. General accounts on how to treat such dependent categorical variables in the context of exploratory factor analysis, and hence to SEM more generally, are given by Flora and Curran (2004), Jöreskog and Moustaki (2001), and Moustaki (2001). Approaches can be categorized into two major types (see Jöreskog and Moustaki, 2001).

(1) *Underlying variable approach*: The idea that the observed correlation between categorical variables does not optimally represent the correlation between continuous latent variables that may have given rise to the observed categories is about a century old. The tetrachoric correlation was developed to describe the correlation between two underlying continuous normal variables that are categorized into binary variables. Extensions of tetrachorics to polychoric and polyserial correlations (see Poon and Lee, 1987) provided the foundation for an SEM approach (Muthén, 1978, 1984). In this approach either a sample polychoric or polyserial correlation between variables is computed from bivariate marginal likelihoods for given thresholds, which are estimated from the univariate marginal distribution. After polychoric or polyserial correlations have been computed, their asymptotic covariance matrix is computed and used in an ADF-type estimation method to estimate the covariance structure. Because ADF requires large sample sizes, inefficient estimates such as least squares estimates can be computed, and the results corrected for misspecification using Satorra–Bentler type procedures. Related approaches were given by Jöreskog (1994), Lee et al. (1990, 1992, 1995), and Lee and Song (2003). This methodology is implemented in most major SEM software.
(2) *Generalized latent variable model approach*: This approach stems from the models for educational tests called the item response theory (Baker and Kim, 2004). In this approach, conditional on the latent variables, the response model is identical to a generalized linear model (McCullagh and Nelder, 1989). The linear latent predictors are then connected with a dependent variable via a link function, which takes care of the categorical nature of the dependent variable. References on this approach include Bartholomew and Knott (1999), Maydeu-Olivares (2001, 2005), and Skrondal and Rabe-Hesketh (2004).

4.3. Further practical information

(1) *Software*: Finally, we provide some practical information. Because of the complexity of optimization algorithm(s) required in SEM, we recommend that applied researchers use existing SEM software such as Amos (http://www.spss.com/amos/), EQS (Bentler, in press; http://www.mvsoft.com/), Lisrel (Jöreskog and Sörbom, 2001; http://www.ssicentral.com/), Mplus (Muthén

and Muthén, 2001; http://www.statmodel.com/), or SAS Proc Calis (http://www.sas.com/). It is possible to learn to use the software of choice from the associated program manuals or from some textbooks mentioned in the introduction. Both sources provide many examples of worked problems. Amos and EQS are especially easy to learn to use due to their graphical interface that allows model specification via path diagrams.

(2) *Computational difficulties*: We do not want to overemphasize the ease of use of SEM. A well thought-out model with many variables can be difficult to fit because such a model may be misspecified in hundreds of ways. When a model is complex, and starting values are poor, the iterative calculations may not be able to optimize the statistical function involved, i.e., non-convergence may occur. Also, a related practical problem may be that one or more residual variances may be estimated negatively or held to a zero boundary, called an improper solution (or a Heywood case; see e.g., Boomsma, 1985, Chen et al., 2001, Kano, 1998, Rindskopf, 1984, or van Driel, 1978). In these situations, simplifying the model, improving start values, or other strategies such as fitting submodels may be needed to provide meaningful as well as statistically adequate solutions. In general, SEM modeling will require subject-matter experts to cooperate with statistical experts.

Acknowledgement

This work was supported in part by grants P01 DA01070 and K05 DA00017 from the National Institute on Drug Abuse awarded to Peter Bentler and also by NSF grant DMS04-37167 awarded to Ke-Hai Yuan.

References

Aitchison, J., Silvey, S.D. (1958). Maximum likelihood estimation of parameters subject to restraints. *Annals of Mathematical Statistics* **29**, 813–828.

Akaike, H. (1974). A new look at the statistical model identification. *IEEE Transactions on Automatic Control* **19**, 716–723.

Akaike, H. (1987). Factor analysis and AIC. *Psychometrika* **52**, 317–332.

Allison, P.D. (2002). *Missing Data*. Sage, Thousand Oaks, CA.

Amemiya, Y., Anderson, T.W. (1990). Asymptotic chi-square tests for a large class of factor analysis models. *Annals of Statistics* **18**, 1453–1463.

Anderson, T.W., Amemiya, Y. (1988). The asymptotic normal distribution of estimators in factor analysis under general conditions. *Annals of Statistics* **16**, 759–771.

Arbuckle, J.L. (1996). Full information estimation in the presence of incomplete data. In: Marcoulides, G.A., Schumacker, R.E. (Eds.), *Advanced Structural Equation Modeling: Issues and Techniques*. Erlbaum, Mahwah, NJ, pp. 243–277.

Arminger, G., Sobel, M.E. (1990). Pseudo-maximum likelihood estimation of mean and covariance structures with missing data. *Journal of the American Statistical Association* **85**, 195–203.

Baker, F.B., Kim, S-H. (2004). *Item Response Theory: Parameter Estimation Techniques*, 2nd ed. Marcel Dekker, New York.

Bartholomew, D.J., Knott, M. (1999). *Latent Variable Models and Factor Analysis*, 2nd ed. Arnold, London.

Batista-Foguet, J.M., Coenders, G., Ferragud, M.A. (2001). Using structural equation models to evaluate the magnitude of measurement error in blood pressure. *Statistics in Medicine* **20**, 2351–2368.

Bauer, D.J., Curran, P.J. (2003). Distributional assumptions of growth mixture models: Implications for overextraction of latent trajectory classes. *Psychological Methods* **8**, 338–363.

Bauer, D.J., Curran, P.J. (2004). The integration of continuous and discrete latent variable models: Potential problems and promising opportunities. *Psychological Methods* **9**, 3–29.

Bekker, P.A., Merckens, A., Wansbeek, T.J. (1994). *Identification, Equivalent Models, and Computer Algebra*. Academic Press, Boston.

Bentler, P.M. (1982). Linear systems with multiple levels and types of latent variables. In: Jöreskog, K.G., Wold, H. (Eds.), *Systems Under Indirect Observation: Causality, Structure, Prediction*. North-Holland, Amsterdam, pp. 101–130.

Bentler, P.M. (1983). Some contributions to efficient statistics in structural models: Specification and estimation of moment structures. *Psychometrika* **48**, 493–517.

Bentler, P.M. (1986). *Lagrange Multiplier and Wald tests for EQS and EQS/PC*. BMDP Statistical Software, Los Angeles.

Bentler, P.M. (1990). Comparative fit indexes in structural models. *Psychological Bulletin* **107**, 238–246.

Bentler, P.M. (1995). *EQS Structural Equation Program Manual*. Multivariate Software, Inc, Encino, CA.

Bentler, P.M. (2005). Latent growth curves. In: Werner, J. (Ed.), *Zeitreihenanalysen*. Logos, Berlin, pp. 13–36.

Bentler, P.M. (in press). EQS 6 *Structural Equations Program Manual*. Multivariate Software, Encino, CA.

Bentler, P.M., Berkane, M. (1985). Developments in the elliptical theory generalization of normal multivariate analysis. *Proceedings of the Social Statistics Section, American Statistical Association*. Alexandria, VA, 291–295.

Bentler, P.M., Bonett, D.G. (1980). Significance tests and goodness of fit in the analysis of covariance structures. *Psychological Bulletin* **88**, 588–606.

Bentler, P.M., Chou, C-P. (1987). Practical issues in structural modeling. *Sociological Methods and Research* **16**, 78–117.

Bentler, P.M., Dijkstra, T. (1985). Efficient estimation via linearization in structural models. In: Krishnaiah, P.R. (Ed.), *Multivariate Analysis VI*. North-Holland, Amsterdam, pp. 9–42.

Bentler, P.M., Lee, S-Y., Weng, L-J. (1987). Multiple population covariance structure analysis under arbitrary distribution theory. *Communication in Statistics – Theory and Method* **16**, 1951–1964.

Bentler, P.M., Liang, J. (2003). Two-level mean and covariance structures: Maximum likelihood via an EM algorithm. In: Reise, S.P., Duan, N. (Eds.), *Multilevel Modeling: Methodological Advances, Issues, and Applications*. Erlbaum, Mahwah, NJ, pp. 53–70.

Bentler, P.M., Liang, J., Yuan, K-H. (2005). Some recent advances in two-level structural equation models: Estimation, testing, and robustness. In: Fan, J., Li, G. (Eds.), *Contemporary Multivariate Analysis and Experimental Designs – in Celebration of Professor Kai-Tai Fang's 65th Birthday*. World Scientific, Hackensack, NJ, pp. 99–120.

Bentler, P.M., Stein, J.A. (1992). Structural equation models in medical research. *Statistical Methods in Medical Research* **1**, 159–181.

Bentler, P.M., Weeks, D.G. (1980). Linear structural equations with latent variables. *Psychometrika* **45**, 289–308.

Bentler, P.M., Yuan, K-H. (1999). Structural equation modeling with small samples: Test statistics. *Multivariate Behavioral Research*. NewYork **34**, 181–197.

Beran, R. (1986). Simulated power functions. *Annals of Statistics* **14**, 151–173.

Beran, R., Srivastava, M.S. (1985). Bootstrap tests and confidence regions for functions of a covariance matrix. *Annals of Statistics* **13**, 95–115.

Berkane, M. (Ed.) (1997). Latent Variable Modeling and Applications to Causality. Springer, New York.

Bollen, K.A. (1989). *Structural Equations with Latent Variables*. Wiley, New York.

Bollen, K.A. (1996). An alternative two stage least squares (2SLS) estimator for latent variable equations. *Psychometrika* **61**, 109–121.

Bollen, K.A. (2002). Latent variables in psychology and the social sciences. *Annual Review of Psychology* **53**, 605–634.

Bollen, K.A., Curran, P.J. (2006). *Latent Curve Models: A Structural Equation Approach*. Wiley, New York.

Bollen, K.A., Paxton, P. (1998). Two-stage least squares estimation of interaction effects. In: Schumacker, R.E., Marcoulides, G.A. (Eds.), *Interaction and Nonlinear Effects in Structural Equation Modeling*. Erlbaum, Mahwah, NJ, pp. 125–151.

Bollen, K.A., Stine, R. (1993). Bootstrapping goodness of fit measures in structural equation models. In: Bollen, K.A., Long, J.S. (Eds.), *Testing Structural Equation Models*. Sage, Newbury Park, CA, pp. 111–135.

Boomsma, A. (1985). Nonconvergence, improper solutions, and starting values in LISREL maximum likelihood estimation. *Psychometrika* **50**, 229–242.

Bozdogan, H. (1987). Model selection and Akaike's information criteria (AIC): The general theory and its analytical extensions. *Psychometrika* **52**, 345–370.

Browne, M.W. (1974). Generalized least-squares estimators in the analysis of covariance structures. *South African Statistical Journal* **8**, 1–24.

Browne, M.W. (1984). Asymptotic distribution-free methods for the analysis of covariance structures. *British Journal of Mathematical and Statistical Psychology* **37**, 62–83.

Browne, M.W., Arminger, G. (1995). Specification and estimation of mean and covariance structure models. In: Arminger, G., Clogg, C.C., Sobel, M.E. (Eds.), *Handbook of Statistical Modeling for the Social and Behavioral Sciences*. Plenum, New York, pp. 185–249.

Browne, M.W., Cudeck, R. (1993). Alternative ways of assessing model fit. In: Bollen, K.A., Long, J.S. (Eds.), *Testing Structural Equation Models*. Sage, Newbury Park, CA, pp. 136–162.

Browne, M.W., Shapiro, A. (1988). Robustness of normal theory methods in the analysis of linear latent variate models. *British Journal of Mathematical and Statistical Psychology* **41**, 193–208.

Byrne, B.M. (2006). *Structural Equation Modeling with EQS: Basic Concepts, Applications, and Programming*, 2nd ed. Erlbaum, Mahwah, NJ.

Campbell, N.A. (1980). Robust procedures in multivariate analysis I: Robust covariance estimation. *Applied Statistics* **29**, 231–237.

Chen, F., Bollen, K.A., Paxton, P., Curran, P.J., Kirby, J.B. (2001). Improper solutions in structural equation models: Causes, consequences, and strategies. *Sociological Methods and Research* **29**, 468–508.

Chou, C-P., Bentler, P.M. (1990). Model modification in covariance structure modeling: A comparison among likelihood ratio, Lagrange multiplier, and Wald tests. *Multivariate Behavioral Research* **25**, 115–136.

Chou, C-P., Bentler, P.M. (2002). Model modification in structural equation modeling by imposing constraints. *Computational Statistics and Data Analysis* **41**, 271–287.

Coenders, G., Satorra, A., Saris, W.E. (1997). Alternative approaches to structural modeling of ordinal data: A Monte Carlo study. *Structural Equation Modeling* **4**, 261–282.

Curran, P.J., West, S.G., Finch, J.F. (1996). The robustness of test statistics to nonnormality and specification error in confirmatory factor analysis. *Psychological Methods* **1**, 16–29.

Davis, P.J., Reeves, J.L., Hastie, B.A., Graff-Radford, S.B., Naliboff, B.D. (2000). Depression determines illness conviction and pain impact: A structural equation modeling analysis. *Pain Medicine* **1**, 238–246.

Davison, A.C., Hinkley, D.V. (1997). *Bootstrap Methods and their Application*. Cambridge University Press, New York.

Dempster, A.P., Laird, N.M., Rubin, D.B. (1977). Maximum likelihood estimation from incomplete data via the EM algorithm (with discussion). *Journal of the Royal Statistical Society B* **39**, 1–38.

Dishman, R.K., Motl, R.W., Saunders, R.P., Dowda, M., Felton, G., Ward, D.S., Pate, R.R. (2002). Factorial invariance and latent mean structure of questionnaires measuring social-cognitive determinants of physical activity among black and white adolescent girls. *Preventive Medicine* **34**, 100–108.

Duncan, S.C., Duncan, T.E., Hops, H. (1998). Progressions of alcohol, cigarette, and marijuana use in adolescence. *Journal of Behavioral Medicine* **21**, 375–388.

Duncan, T.E., Duncan, S.C., Strycker, L.A. (2006). *An Introduction to Latent Variable Growth Curve Modeling*, 2nd ed. Erlbaum, Mahwah, NJ.

Dunn, G., Everitt, B., Pickles, A. (1993). *Modelling Covariances and Latent Variables Using EQS*. Chapman and Hall, London.

du Toit, S.H.C., du Toit, M. (2002). Multilevel structural equation modeling. In: de Leeuw, J., Kreft, I.G.G. (Eds.), *Handbook of Quantitative Multilevel Analysis*. Kluwer Academic, Boston.

Fang, K-T., Kotz, S., Ng., K.W. (1990). *Symmetric Multivariate and Related Distributions*. Chapman and Hall, London.

Ferguson, T. (1958). A method of generating best asymptotically normal estimates with application to estimation of bacterial densities. *Annals of Mathematical Statistics* **29**, 1046–1062.

Ferguson, T. (1996). *A Course in Large Sample Theory*. Chapman and Hall, London.

Flora, D.B., Curran, P.J. (2004). An empirical evaluation of alternative methods of estimation for confirmatory factor analysis with ordinal data. *Psychological Methods* **9**, 466–491.

Goldstein, H. (2003). *Multilevel Statistical Models*, 3rd ed. Arnold, London.

Goldstein, H., McDonald, R.P. (1988). A general model for the analysis of multilevel data. *Psychometrika* **53**, 435–467.

Green, S.B., Thompson, M.S., Poirier, J. (1999). Exploratory analyses to improve model fit: Errors due to misspecification and strategy to reduce their occurrence. *Structural Equation Modeling* **6**, 113–126.

Hampel, F.R., Ronchetti, E.M., Rousseeuw, P.J., Stahel, W.A. (1986). *Robust Statistics: The Approach Based on Influence Functions*. Wiley, New York.

Hancock, G.R. (2001). Effect size, power, and sample size determination for structured means modeling and MIMIC approaches to between-groups hypothesis testing of means on a single latent construct. *Psychometrika* **66**, 373–388.

Hayashi, K., Yuan, K-H. (2003). Robust Bayesian factor analysis. *Structural Equation Modeling* **10**, 525–533.

Hays, R.D., Revicki, D., Coyne, K. (2005). Application of structural equation modeling to health outcomes research. *Evaluation and the Health Professions* **28**, 295–309.

Horn, J.L., McArdle, J., Mason, R. (1983). When is invariance not invariant: A practical scientist's look at the ethereal concept of factor invariance. *Southern Psychologist* **1**, 179–188.

Hoshino, T. (2001). Bayesian inference for finite mixtures in confirmatory factor analysis. *Behaviormetrika* **28**, 37–63.

Hu, L.T., Bentler, P.M. (1998). Fit indices in covariance structure modeling: Sensitivity to underparameterized model misspecification. *Psychological Methods* **3**, 424–453.

Hu, L.T., Bentler, P.M. (1999). Cutoff criteria for fit indexes in covariance structure analysis: Conventional criteria versus new alternatives. *Structural Equation Modeling* **6**, 1–55.

Hu, L.T., Bentler, P.M., Kano, Y. (1992). Can test statistics in covariance structure analysis be trusted? *Psychological Bulletin* **112**, 351–362.

Huber, P.J. (1964). Robust estimation of a location parameter. *Annals of Mathematical Statistics* **35**, 73–101.

Huber, P.J. (1967). The behavior of maximum likelihood estimates under nonstandard conditions. In: *Proceedings of the Fifth Berkeley Symposium on Mathematical Statistics and Probability*. University of California Press, Berkeley, CA, pp. 221–233.

Huber, P.J. (1981). *Robust Statistics*. Wiley, New York.

Jamshidian, M., Bentler, P.M. (1999). Using complete data routines for ML estimation of mean and covariance structures with missing data. *Journal Educational and Behavioral Statistics* **23**, 21–41.

Jöreskog, K.G. (1969). A general approach to confirmatory maximum likelihood factor analysis. *Psychometrika* **34**, 183–202.

Jöreskog, K.G. (1971). Simultaneous factor analysis in several populations. *Psychometrika* **36**, 409–426.

Jöreskog, K.G. (1994). On the estimation of polychoric correlations and their asymptotic covariance matrix. *Psychometrika* **59**, 381–389.

Jöreskog, K.G., Moustaki, I. (2001). Factor analysis of ordinal variables: A comparison of three approaches. *Multivariate Behavioral Research* **36**, 347–387.

Jöreskog, K.G., Sörbom, D. (1979). *Advances in Factor Analysis and Structural Equation Models*. Abt Books, Cambridge, MA.

Jöreskog, K.G., Sörbom, D. (1981). *LISREL 5: Analysis of linear structural relationships by maximum likelihood and least squares methods*. Research report 81–8, Department of Statistics, University of Uppsala, Uppsala, Sweden.

Jöreskog, K.G., Sörbom, D. (2001). *LISREL 8 User's Reference Guide*. Scientific Software International, Lincolnwood, IL.

Jöreskog, K.G., Yang, F. (1996). Nonlinear structural equation models: The Kenny–Judd model with interaction effects. In: Marcoulides, G.A., Schumacker, R.E. (Eds.), *Advanced Structural Equation Modeling: Issues and Techniques*. Erlbaum, Mahwah, NJ, pp. 57–88.

Kano, Y. (1986). Conditions on consistency of estimators in covariance structure model. *Journal of the Japan Statistical Society* **16**, 75–80.

Kano, Y. (1992). Robust statistics for test-of-independence and related structural models. *Statistics and Probability Letters* **15**, 21–26.

Kano, Y. (1998). Improper solutions in exploratory factor analysis: Causes and treatments. In: Rizzi, A., Vichi, M., Bock, H. (Eds.), *Advances in Data Sciences and Classification*. Springer-Verlag, Berlin, pp. 375–382.

Kano, Y., Berkane, M., Bentler, P.M. (1990). Covariance structure analysis with heterogeneous kurtosis parameters. *Biometrika* **77**, 575–585.

Kano, Y., Berkane, M., Bentler, P.M. (1993). Statistical inference based on pseudo-maximum likelihood estimators in elliptical populations. *Journal of the American Statistical Association* **88**, 135–143.

Kenny, D.A., Judd, C.M. (1984). Estimating the nonlinear and interactive effects of latent variables. *Psychological Bulletin* **96**, 201–210.

Kim, K. (2005). The relationship among fit indexes, power, and sample size in structural equation modeling. *Structural Equation Modeling* **12**, 368–390.

Kim, K.H., Bentler, P.M. (2002). Tests of homogeneity of means and covariance matrices for multivariate incomplete data. *Psychometrika* **67**, 609–624.

Klein, A., Moosbrugger, H. (2000). Maximum likelihood estimation of latent interaction effects with the LMS method. *Psychometrika* **65**, 457–474.

Kline, R.B. (2005). *Principles and Practice of Structural Equation Modeling*, 2nd ed. Guilford Press, New York.

Lawley, D.N., Maxwell, A.E. (1971). *Factor Analysis as a Statistical Method*, 2nd ed. American Elsevier, New York.

Lee, S-Y. (1985). On testing functional constraints in structural equation models. *Biometrika* **72**, 125–131.

Lee, S-Y. (1986). Estimation for structural equation models with missing data. *Psychometrika* **51**, 93–99.

Lee, S-Y. (1990). Multilevel analysis of structural equation models. *Biometrika* **77**, 763–772.

Lee, S-Y. (Ed.) (2007). Handbook of Latent Variable and Related Models. Elsevier, Amsterdam.

Lee, S-Y., Bentler, P.M. (1980). Some asymptotic properties of constrained generalized least squares estimation in covariance structure models. *South African Statistical Journal* **14**, 121–136.

Lee, S-Y., Jennrich, R.I. (1979). A study of algorithms for covariance structure analysis with specific comparisons using factor analysis. *Psychometrika* **44**, 99–113.

Lee, S-Y., Poon, W.Y. (1998). Analysis of two-level structural equation models via EM type algorithms. *Statistica Sinica* **8**, 749–766.

Lee, S-Y., Poon, W.Y., Bentler, P.M. (1990). Full maximum likelihood analysis of structural equation models with polytomous variables. *Statistics and Probability Letters* **9**, 91–97.

Lee, S-Y., Poon, W.Y., Bentler, P.M. (1992). Structural equation models with continuous and polytomous variables. *Psychometrika* **57**, 89–106.
Lee, S-Y., Poon, W.Y., Bentler, P.M. (1995). A two-stage estimation of structural equation models with continuous and polytomous variables. *British Journal of Mathematical and Statistical Psychology* **48**, 339–358.
Lee, S-Y., Shi, J.Q. (2001). Maximum likelihood estimation of two-level latent variables model with mixed continuous and polytomous data. *Biometrics* **57**, 787–794.
Lee, S-Y., Song, X.Y. (2001). Hypothesis testing and model comparison in two-level structural equation models. *Multivariate Behavioral Research* **36**, 639–655.
Lee, S-Y., Song, X.Y. (2003). Maximum likelihood estimation and model comparison of nonlinear structural equation models with continuous and polytomous variables. *Computational Statistics and Data Analysis* **44**, 125–142.
Lee, S-Y., Song, X.Y., Lee, J.C.K. (2003). Maximum likelihood estimation of nonlinear structural equation models with ignorable missing data. *Journal of Educational and Behavioral Statistics* **28**, 111–124.
Lee, S-Y., Song, X.Y., Poon, W.Y. (2004). Comparison of approaches in estimating interaction and quadratic effects of latent variables. *Multivariate Behavioral Research* **39**, 37–67.
Lee, S-Y., Tang, N-S. (2006). Bayesian analysis of nonlinear structural equation models with non-ignorable missing data. *Psychometrika* **71**, 541–564.
Lee, S-Y., Tsui, K.L. (1982). Covariance structure analysis in several populations. *Psychometrika* **47**, 297–308.
Lee, S-Y., Zhu, H.T. (2000). Statistical analysis of nonlinear structural equation models with continuous and polytomous data. *British Journal of Mathematical and Statistical Psychology* **53**, 209–232.
Lee, S-Y., Zhu, H.T. (2002). Maximum likelihood estimation of nonlinear structural equation models. *Psychometrika* **67**, 189–210.
Li, L., Bentler, P.M. (2006). Robust statistical tests for evaluating the hypothesis of close fit of misspecified mean and covariance structural models. *UCLA Statistics Preprint No. 494* (http://preprints.stat.ucla.edu/).
Liang, J., Bentler, P.M. (2004). A new EM algorithm for fitting two-level structural equation models. *Psychometrika* **69**, 101–122.
Little, R.J.A., Rubin, D.B. (2002). *Statistical Analysis with Missing Data*, 2nd ed. Wiley, New York.
Loehlin, J.C. (2004). *Latent Variable Models: An Introduction to Factor, Path, and Structural Equation Analysis*, 4th ed. Erlbaum, Mahwah, NJ.
Lubke, G., Muthén, B. (2005). Investigating population heterogeneity with factor mixture models. *Psychological Methods* **10**, 21–39.
MacCallum, R.C., Austin, J.T. (2000). Applications of structural equation modeling in psychological research. *Annual Review of Psychology* **51**, 201–226.
MacCallum, R.C., Browne, M.W., Sugawara, H.M. (1996). Power analysis and determination of sample size for covariance structure modeling. *Psychological Methods* **1**, 130–149.
MacCallum, R.C., Roznowski, M., Necowitz, L.B. (1992). Model modifications in covariance structure analysis: The problem of capitalization on chance. *Psychological Bulletin* **111**, 490–504.
Magnus, J.R., Neudecker, H. (1999). *Matrix Differential Calculus with Applications in Statistics and Econometrics*, revised ed. Wiley, New York.
Marcoulides, G.A., Schumacker, R.E. (eds.) (1996). Advanced Structural Equation Modeling: Issues and Techniques. Erlbaum, Mahwah, NJ.
Marcoulides, G.A., Schumacker, R.E. (eds.) (2001). New Developments and Techniques in Structural Equation Modeling. Erlbaum, Mahwah, NJ.
Mardia, K.V. (1970). Measures of multivariate skewness and kurtosis with applications. *Biometrika* **57**, 519–530.
Maronna, R.A. (1976). Robust M-estimators of multivariate location and scatter. *Annals of Statistics* **4**, 51–67.
Marsh, H.W., Wen, Z., Hau, K.T. (2004). Structural equation models of latent interactions: Evaluation of alternative estimation strategies and indicator construction. *Psychological Methods* **9**, 275–300.

Maruyama, G.M. (1998). *Basics of Structural Equation Modeling*. Sage, Thousand Oaks, CA.
Maxwell, S.E., Delaney, H.D. (2004). *Designing Experiments and Analyzing Data: A Model Comparison Perspective*, 2nd ed. Erlbaum, Mahwah, NJ.
Maydeu-Olivares, A. (2001). Multidimensional item response theory modeling of binary data: Large sample properties of NOHARM estimates. *Journal of Educational and Behavioral Statistics* **26**, 51–71.
Maydeu-Olivares, A. (2005). Linear IRT, nonlinear IRT, and factor analysis: A unified framework. In: Maydeu-Olivares, A., McArdle, J.J. (Eds.), *Contemporary Psychometrics*. Erlbaum, Mahwah, NJ.
Maydeu-Olivares, A., Cai, L. (2006). A cautionary note on using G^2(dif) to assess relative model fit in categorical data analysis. *Multivariate Behavioral Research* **41**, 55–64.
McCullagh, P., Nelder, J.A. (1989). *Generalized Linear Models*, 2nd ed. Chapman and Hall, London.
McDonald, R.P., Goldstein, H. (1989). Balanced versus unbalanced designs for linear structural relations in two-level data. *British Journal of Mathematical and Statistical Psychology* **42**, 215–232.
McDonald, R.P., Ho, R.M. (2002). Principles and practice in reporting structural equation analyses. *Psychological Methods* **7**, 64–82.
Meredith, W. (1993). Measurement invariance, factor analysis and factorial invariance. *Psychometrika* **58**, 525–543.
Meredith, W., Tisak, J. (1990). Latent curve analysis. *Psychometrika* **55**, 107–122.
Millsap, R.E. (1997). Invariance in measurement and prediction: Their relationship in the single-factor case. *Psychological Methods* **2**, 248–260.
Mooijaart, A. (1985). Factor analysis for non-normal variables. *Psychometrika* **50**, 323–342.
Mooijaart, A. (2003). Estimating the statistical power in small samples by empirical distributions. In: Yanai, H., Okada, A., Shigemasu, K., Kano, Y., Meulman, J.J. (Eds.), *New Development in Psychometrics*. Springer-Verlag, Tokyo, pp. 149–156.
Mooijaart, A., Bentler, P.M. (1986). Random polynomial factor analysis. In: Diday, E., Escoufier, Y., Lebart, L., Pages, J., Schektman, Y., Tomassone, R. (Eds.), *Data Analysis and Informatics IV*. Elsevier Science, Amsterdam, pp. 241–250.
Mooijaart, A., Bentler, P.M. (1991). Robustness of normal theory statistics in structural equation models. *Statistica Neerlandica* **45**, 159–171.
Moustaki, I. (2001). A review of exploratory factor analysis for ordinal categorical data. In: Cudeck, R., du Toit, S., Sörbom, D. (Eds.), *Structual Equation Modeling: Present and Future*. Scientific Software International, Lincolnwood, IL.
Muthén, B. (1978). Contributions to factor analysis of dichotomous variables. *Psychometrika* **43**, 551–560.
Muthén, B. (1984). A general structural equation model with dichotomous, ordered categorical, and continuous latent variable indicators. *Psychometrika* **49**, 115–132.
Muthén, B. (1989a). Multiple group structural modelling with nonnormal continuous variables. *British Journal of Mathematical and Statistical Psychology* **42**, 55–62.
Muthén, B. (1989b). Latent variable modeling in heterogeneous populations. *Psychometrika* **54**, 557–585.
Muthén, B. (1994). Multilevel covariance structure analysis. *Sociological Methods and Research* **22**, 376–398.
Muthén, B. (1997). Latent variable modeling of longitudinal and multilevel data. In: Raftery, A. (Ed.), *Sociological Methodology 1997*. Blackwell Publishers, Boston, pp. 453–480.
Muthén, B., Kaplan, D., Hollis, M. (1987). On structural equation modeling with data that are not missing completely at random. *Psychometrika* **52**, 431–462.
Muthén, L.K., Muthén, B. (2001). *Mplus User's Guide*, 2nd ed. Muthen & Muthen, Los Angeles, CA.
Muthén, L.K., Muthén, B. (2002). How to use a Monte Carlo study to decide on sample size and determine power. *Structural Equation Modeling* **9**, 599–620.
Ogasawara, H. (2001). Approximations to the distributions of fit indices for misspecified structural equation models. *Structural Equation Modeling* **8**, 556–574.
Peek, M.K. (2000). Structural equation modeling and rehabilitation research. *American Journal of Physical Medicine and Rehabilitation* **79**, 301–309.

Penny, W.D., Stephan, K.E., Mechelli, A., Friston, K.J. (2004). Comparing dynamic causal models. *NeuroImage* **22**, 1157–1172.

Poon, W.Y., Lee, S-Y. (1987). Maximum likelihood estimation of multivariate polyserial and polychoric correlation coefficient. *Psychometrika* **52**, 409–430.

Poon, W.Y., Lee, S-Y. (1994). A distribution free approach for analysis of two-level structural equation model. *Computational Statistics and Data Analysis* **17**, 265–275.

Rao, C.R. (1947). Large sample tests of statistical hypotheses concerning several parameters with applications to problems of estimation. *Proceedings of the Cambridge Philosophical Society* **44**, 50–57.

Rao, C.R. (1973). *Linear Statistical Inference and Its Applications*, 2nd ed. Wiley, New York.

Raudenbush, S.W. (1995). Maximum likelihood estimation for unbalanced multilevel covariance structure models via the EM algorithm. *British Journal of Mathematical and Statistical Psychology* **48**, 359–370.

Raudenbush, S.W., Bryk, A.S. (2002). *Hierarchical Linear Models*, 2nd ed. Sage, Newbury Park, CA.

Raykov, T., Marcoulides, G.A. (2006). *A First Course in Structural Equation Modeling*, 2nd ed. Erlbaum, Mahwah, NJ.

Reise, S.P., Duan, N. (Eds.) (2003). *Multilevel Modeling: Methodological Advances, Issues, and Applications*. Erlbaum, Mahwah, NJ.

Rindskopf, D. (1984). Structural equation models: Empirical identification, Heywood cases, and related problems. *Sociological Methods and Research* **13**, 109–119.

Robert, C.P., Casella, G. (2004). *Monte Carlo Statistical Methods*, 2nd ed. Springer, New York.

Rubin, D.B. (1976). Inference and missing data (with discussions). *Biometrika* **63**, 581–592.

Saris, W.E., Satorra, A. (1993). Power evaluations in structural equation models. In: Bollen, K.A., Long, J.S. (Eds.), *Testing Structural Equation Models*. Sage, Newbury Park, CA, pp. 181–204.

Satorra, A. (1989). Alternative test criteria in covariance structure analysis: A unified approach. *Psychometrika* **54**, 131–151.

Satorra, A. (1992). Asymptotic robust inferences in the analysis of mean and covariance structures. *Sociological Methodology* **22**, 249–278.

Satorra, A. (2000). Scaled and adjusted restricted tests in multi-sample analysis of moment structures. In: Heijmans, D.D.H., Pollock, D.S.G., Satorra, A. (Eds.), *Innovations in Multivariate Statistical Analysis: A Festschrift for Heinz Neudecker*. Kluwer Academic, Dordrecht, pp. 233–247.

Satorra, A. (2002). Asymptotic robustness in multiple group linear-latent variable models. *Econometric Theory* **18**, 297–312.

Satorra, A., Bentler, P.M. (1988). Scaling corrections for chi-square statistics in covariance structure analysis. In: *American Statistical Association 1988 Proceedings of Business and Economics Sections*. American Statistical Association, Alexandria, VA, pp. 308–313.

Satorra, A., Bentler, P.M. (1990). Model conditions for asymptotic robustness in the analysis of linear relations. *Computational Statistics and Data Analysis* **10**, 235–249.

Satorra, A., Bentler, P.M. (1994). Corrections to test statistics and standard errors in covariance structure analysis. In: von Eye, A., Clogg, C.C. (Eds.), *Latent Variables Analysis: Applications for Developmental Research*. Sage, Thousand Oaks, CA, pp. 399–419.

Satorra, A., Bentler, P.M. (2001). A scaled difference chi-square test statistic for moment structure analysis. *Psychometrika* **66**, 507–514.

Satorra, A., Saris, W. (1985). Power of the likelihood ratio test in covariance structure analysis. *Psychometrika* **50**, 83–90.

Savalei, V., Bentler, P.M. (2005). A statistically justified pairwise ML method for incomplete nonnormal data: A comparison with direct ML and pairwise ADF. *Structural Equation Modeling* **12**, 183–214.

Schumacker, R.E., Marcoulides, G.A. (Eds.) (1998). *Interaction and Nonlinear Effects in Structural Equation Modeling*. Erlbaum, Mahwah, NJ.

Schwarz, G. (1978). Estimating the dimension of a model. *Annals of Statistics* **6**, 461–464.

Shapiro, A. (1983). Asymptotic distribution theory in the analysis of covariance structures (a unified approach). *South African Statistical Journal* **17**, 33–81.

Shapiro, A. (1984). A note on the consistency of estimators in the analysis of moment structures. *British Journal of Mathematical and Statistical Psychology* **37**, 84–88.

Shapiro, A., Browne, M.W. (1987). Analysis of covariance structures under elliptical distributions. *Journal of the American Statistical Association* **82**, 1092–1097.

Shipley, B. (2000). *Cause and Correlation in Biology*. Cambridge University Press, New York.

Skrondal, A., Rabe-Hesketh, S. (2004). *Generalized Latent Variable Modeling: Multilevel, Longitudinal, and Structural Equation Models*. Chapman & Hall, London.

Song, X.Y., Lee, S-Y. (2002). Analysis of structural equation model with ignorable missing continuous and polytomous data. *Psychometrika* **67**, 261–288.

Sörbom, D. (1974). A general method for studying differences in factor means and factor structures between groups. *British Journal of Mathematical and Statistical Psychology* **27**, 229–239.

Sörbom, D. (1989). Model modification. *Psychometrika* **54**, 371–384.

Steiger, J.H., Lind, J.M. (1980). Statistically based tests for the number of common factors. Paper presented at the Annual Meeting of the Psychometric Society. Iowa City, IA.

Steiger, J.H., Shapiro, A., Browne, M.W. (1985). On the multivariate asymptotic distribution of sequential chi-square statistics. *Psychometrika* **50**, 253–264.

Stoel, R.D. (2003). *Issues in Growth Curve Modeling*. TT-Publikaties, Amsterdam.

Tanaka, J.S. (1993). Multifaceted conceptions of fit in structural equation models. In: Bollen, K.A., Long, J.S. (Eds.), *Testing Structural Equation Models*. Sage, Newbury Park, CA, pp. 10–39.

Tang, M.L., Bentler, P.M. (1998). Theory and method for constrained estimation in structural equation models with incomplete data. *Computational Statistics and Data Analysis* **27**, 257–270.

Tang, M.L., Lee, S-Y. (1998). Analysis of structural equation model with non-ignorable missing data. *Computational Statistics and Data Analysis* **27**, 33–46.

Tucker, L.R., Lewis, C. (1973). A reliability coefficient for maximum likelihood factor analysis. *Psychometrika* **38**, 1–10.

Tyler, D.E. (1983). Robustness and efficiency properties of scatter matrices. *Biometrika* **70**, 411–420.

van den Oord, E.J. (2000). Framework for identifying quantitative trait loci in association studies using structural equation modeling. *Genetic Epidemiology* **18**, 341–359.

van Driel, O.P. (1978). On various causes of improper solutions in maximum likelihood factor analysis. *Psychometrika* **43**, 225–243.

Vuong, Q.H. (1989). Likelihood ratio tests for model selection and nonnested hypotheses. *Econometrica* **57**, 307–333.

Wald, A. (1943). Tests of statistical hypotheses concerning several parameters when the number of observations is large. *Transactions of the American Mathematical Society* **54**, 426–482.

Wall, M.M., Amemiya, Y. (2000). Estimation for polynomial structural equation models. *Journal of the American Statistical Association* **95**, 920–940.

Wall, M.M., Amemiya, Y. (2001). Generalized appended product indicator procedure for nonlinear structural equation analysis. *Journal of Educational and Behavioral Statistics* **26**, 1–29.

Wall, M.M., Amemiya, Y. (2003). A method of moments technique for fitting interaction effects in structural equation models. *British Journal of Mathematical and Statistical Psychology* **56**, 47–64.

White, H. (1982). Maximum likelihood estimation of misspecified models. *Econometrica* **50**, 1–25.

Yanagihara, H., Tonda, T., Matsumoto, C. (2005). The effects of nonnormality on asymptotic distributions of some likelihood ratio criteria for testing covariance structures under normal assumption. *Journal of Multivariate Analysis* **96**, 237–264.

Yang Jonsson, F. (1998). Modeling interaction and nonlinear effects: A step-by-step Lisrel example. In: Schmacker, R.E., Marcoulides, G.A. (Eds.), *Interaction and Nonlinear Effects in Structural Equation Modeling*. Erlbaum, Mahwah, NJ, pp. 17–42.

Yuan, K-H. (2005). Fit indices versus test statistics. *Multivariate Behavior Research* **40**, 115–148.

Yuan, K-H. (2006). Normal theory ML for missing data with violation of distribution assumptions (Under review).

Yuan, K-H., Bentler, P.M. (1997a). Mean and covariance structure analysis: Theoretical and practical improvements. *Journal of the American Statistical Association* **92**, 767–774.

Yuan, K-H., Bentler, P.M. (1997b). Improving parameter tests in covariance structure analysis. *Computational Statistics and Data Analysis* **26**, 177–198.

Yuan, K-H., Bentler, P.M. (1998a). Normal theory based test statistics in structural equation modeling. *British Journal of Mathematical and Statistical Psychology* **51**, 289–309.

Yuan, K-H., Bentler, P.M. (1998b). Robust mean and covariance structure analysis. *British Journal of Mathematical and Statistical Psychology* **51**, 63–88.

Yuan, K-H., Bentler, P.M. (1998c). Structural equation modeling with robust covariances. *Sociological Methodology* **28**, 363–396.

Yuan, K-H., Bentler, P.M. (1999a). On normal theory and associated test statistics in covariance structure analysis under two classes of nonnormal distributions. *Statistica Sinica* **9**, 831–853.

Yuan, K-H., Bentler, P.M. (1999b). On asymptotic distributions of normal theory MLE in covariance structure analysis under some nonnormal distributions. *Statistics and Probability Letters* **42**, 107–113.

Yuan, K-H., Bentler, P.M. (1999c). F-tests for mean and covariance structure analysis. *Journal of Educational and Behavioral Statistics* **24**, 225–243.

Yuan, K-H., Bentler, P.M. (2000a). Three likelihood-based methods for mean and covariance structure analysis with nonnormal missing data. *Sociological Methodology* **30**, 167–202.

Yuan, K-H., Bentler, P.M. (2000b). Robust mean and covariance structure analysis through iteratively reweighted least squares. *Psychometrika* **65**, 43–58.

Yuan, K-H., Bentler, P.M. (2001). A unified approach to multigroup structural equation modeling with nonstandard samples. In: Marcoulides, G.A., Schumacker, R.E. (Eds.), *Advanced Structural Equation Modeling: New Developments and Techniques*. Erlbaum, Mahwah, NJ, pp. 35–56.

Yuan, K-H., Bentler, P.M. (2002). On normal theory based inference for multilevel models with distributional violations. *Psychometrika* **67**, 539–561.

Yuan, K-H., Bentler, P.M. (2003). Eight test statistics for multilevel structural equation models. *Computational Statistics and Data Analysis* **44**, 89–107.

Yuan, K-H., Bentler, P.M. (2004a). On chi-square difference and z-tests in mean and covariance structure analysis when the base model is misspecified. *Educational and Psychological Measurement* **64**, 737–757.

Yuan, K-H., Bentler, P.M. (2004b). On the asymptotic distributions of two statistics for two-level covariance structure models within the class of elliptical distributions. *Psychometrika* **69**, 437–457.

Yuan, K-H., Bentler, P.M. (2005a). Asymptotic robustness of the normal theory likelihood ratio statistic for two-level covariance structure models. *Journal of Multivariate Analysis* **94**, 328–343.

Yuan, K-H., Bentler, P.M. (2005b). Asymptotic robustness of standard errors in multilevel structural equation models. *Journal of Multivariate Analysis* **94**, 328–343.

Yuan, K-H., Bentler, P.M. (2006). Mean comparison: Manifest variable versus latent variable. *Psychometrika* **71**, 139–159.

Yuan, K-H., Bentler, P.M., Chan, W. (2004). Structural equation modeling with heavy tailed distributions. *Psychometrika* **69**, 421–436.

Yuan, K-H., Chan, W. (2005). On nonequivalence of several procedures of structural equation modeling. *Psychometrika* **70**, 791–798.

Yuan, K-H., Chan, W., Bentler, P.M. (2000). Robust transformation with applications to structural equation modeling. *British Journal of Mathematical and Statistical Psychology* **53**, 31–50.

Yuan, K-H., Fung, W.K., Reise, S. (2004). Three Mahalanobis-distances and their role in assessing unidimensionality. *British Journal of Mathematical and Statistical Psychology* **57**, 151–165.

Yuan, K-H., Hayashi, K. (2003). Bootstrap approach to inference and power analysis based on three statistics for covariance structure models. *British Journal of Mathematical and Statistical Psychology* **56**, 93–110.

Yuan, K-H., Hayashi, K. (2006). Standard errors in covariance structure models: Asymptotics versus bootstrap. *British Journal of Mathematical and Statistical Psychology* **59**, 397–417.

Yuan, K-H., Hayashi, K. (2005). On Muthen's maximum likelihood for two-level covariance structure models. *Psychometrika* **70**, 147–167.

Yuan, K-H., Hayashi, K., Bentler, P.M. (2007). Normal theory likelihood ratio statistic for mean and covariance structure analysis under alternative hypotheses. *Journal of Multivariate Analysis* **98**, 1262–1282.

Yuan, K-H., Marshall, L.L. (2004). A new measure of misfit for covariance structure models. *Behaviormetrika* **31**, 67–90.

Yuan, K-H., Marshall, L.L., Bentler, P.M. (2002). A unified approach to exploratory factor analysis with missing data, nonnormal data, and in the presence of outliers. *Psychometrika* **67**, 95–122.

Yuan, K-H., Marshall, L.L., Bentler, P.M. (2003). Assessing the effect of model misspecifications on parameter estimates in structural equation models. *Sociological Methodology* **33**, 241–265.

Yung, Y-F. (1997). Finite mixtures in confirmatory factor-analysis models. *Psychometrika* **62**, 297–330.

Yung, Y-F., Bentler, P.M. (1996). Bootstrapping techniques in analysis of mean and covariance structures. In: Marcoulides, G.A., Schumacker, R.E. (Eds.), *Advanced Structural Equation Modeling: Techniques and Issues*. Erlbaum, Hillsdale, NJ, pp. 195–226.

Handbook of Statistics, Vol. 27
ISSN: 0169-7161

DOI: 10.1016/S0169-7161(07)27014-2

14

Statistical Modeling in Biomedical Research: Longitudinal Data Analysis

Chengjie Xiong, Kejun Zhu, Kai Yu and J. Philip Miller

Abstract

This chapter discusses some major statistical methods for longitudinal data analysis in biomedical research. We have provided a detailed review to some of the most used statistical models for the analyses of longitudinal data and relevant design issues based on these models. Our focus is on the conceptualization of longitudinal statistical models, the assumptions associated with them, and the interpretations of model parameters. It is not our intention to present the detailed theory on statistical estimations and inferences for these models in this chapter. Instead, we have presented the implementations for some of these basic longitudinal models in SAS through real-world applications.

1. Introduction

Why should longitudinal studies in biomedical research be conducted? The answer to this question depends on the study objectives in biomedical research. There is a fundamental difference between a longitudinal study and a cross-sectional study. Cross-sectional studies are those in which individuals are observed only once. Most surveys are cross-sectional, as are studies to construct reference ranges. Longitudinal studies, however, are those that investigate changes over time, possibly in relation to an intervention. Therefore, the primary characteristic of a longitudinal study is that study subjects are measured repeatedly through time. The major advantage of a longitudinal study is its capacity to separate what in the context of population studies are called *cohort* and *age* effects (Diggle et al., 2002). Outcome variables in the longitudinal studies may be continuous measurements, counts, dichotomous, or categorical indicators, and in many cases, outcomes may even be multivariate as well. Covariates in the longitudinal studies may also be continuous measurements, counts, dichotomous, or categorical indicators, and in many cases, covariate may be time varying as well. As an example, in the study of healthy ageing and Alzheimer's disease (AD), the understanding of natural history of AD requires a longitudinal design and the corresponding appropriate analysis. One of the primary objectives in these studies is to model the cognitive function as a function of baseline age, the time lapse from the baseline, the disease status, and other possible risk factors. For the purpose of demonstration, we consider a simple case and let $Y(a,t)$ be the cognitive function at time lapse t from the baseline (i.e., $t = 0$ at baseline) for a subject whose baseline age is a. Assume that the expected value of $Y(a,t)$ is a linear function of both baseline age a and the time lapse t from the baseline, i.e.,

$$EY(a,t) = \beta_0 + \beta_1 a + \beta_2 t.$$

The standard interpretation of β_1 is the expected change of cognitive function at the baseline (or at the same time t during the longitudinal course) for two subjects whose baseline age is 1 year apart. The standard interpretation of β_2 is the expected change of cognitive function per time unit for the same subject during the longitudinal course of the study. The crucial difference between β_1 and β_2 is that β_1 measures a between-subject or a cross-sectional change, whereas β_2 measures a within-subject or a longitudinal change. If only cross-sectional cognitive measures are available, i.e., the study is measured only at baseline, then $t = 0$ and $EY(a,t) = \beta_0 + \beta_1 a$. Therefore, any statistical inferences from the cross-sectional data can only be made on β_1, i.e., the cross-sectional rate of change. On the other hand, if longitudinal cognitive measures are available, then statistical inferences can be made on both β_1 and β_2. Therefore, longitudinal studies enable not only the estimation of cross-sectional rate of change based on baseline age, but also the estimation of the rate of intra-individual change based on the time lapse in the study.

Another main study objective for a longitudinal study is to relate intra-subject rate of change over time to individual characteristics (e.g., exposure, age, etc.), or to an experimental condition. In the above example, studying the healthy ageing and AD, many potential risk factors in addition to baseline age could affect not only the cognitive status of subjects at baseline but also the rate of cognitive decline after the baseline. These risk factors range from demographics such as gender and education to genetic status (i.e., Apolipoprotein E genotypes) and to relevant biomarkers and imaging markers. In addition, the stage or the severity of AD could also be an important factor affecting the rate of further cognitive decline. In general, therapeutic trials of AD are longitudinal, and the most crucial scientific question to be addressed in these trials is whether the therapeutic treatment is efficacious in slowing the cognitive and functional decline of AD patients. Therefore, the rate of cognitive decline in AD clinical trials is modeled as a function of treatment received. More specifically, let β_2^{t} be the expected rate of cognitive decline over time for subjects randomly assigned to receive a therapeutic treatment, and let β_2^{c} be the expected rate of cognitive decline over time for control subjects. The longitudinal nature of the study allows the statistical test on whether β_2^{t} is the same as $\beta_2^{\mathrm{c}}$and the statistical estimation on the difference between these two rates of cognitive decline.

As in all biomedical studies, there are two major statistical components in longitudinal studies: statistical design and statistical analysis. This chapter will review some of the most used statistical models for the analyses of longitudinal data and relevant design issues based on these models. Throughout this chapter, we will focus on the conceptualization of basic longitudinal statistical models, the basic assumptions these models are based on, and the interpretations of model parameters. It is not our intention to present the detailed theory on statistical estimations and inferences based on these models. Instead, we will present the implementations for some of these basic longitudinal models in SAS through real-world applications. For detailed statistical theory on the parameter estimation and inferences from these models, readers are referred to some of the excellent references in longitudinal statistical methods such as Diggle et al. (2002), Fitzmaurice et al. (2004), Verbeke and Molenberghs (2000), and Singer and Willett (2003).

2. Analysis of longitudinal data

The defining characteristic of longitudinal data analysis is the fact that the response variable or variables are repeatedly measured on the same individuals over time and therefore the resulting responses on the same individuals are statistically correlated. Whereas much of the focus in the analysis of longitudinal data is on the mean response over time, the correlation among the repeated measures plays a crucial role and cannot be ignored. Generally, there are two approaches for modeling the mean response over time. The first approach is the analysis of response profile in which repeated measures analysis of variance or covariance serves as special examples. The important feature of analysis of response profile is that it allows for an unstructured pattern of mean response over time, i.e., no specific time trend is assumed. Because the analysis of response profile treats times of measurements as levels of a discrete study factor, it is especially useful when the objective of the study is to make statistical inferences at individual times or to compare mean responses among different time points. On the other hand, this approach to the analysis of longitudinal data is generally only applicable to the case when all individuals under study are measured at the same set of time points and the number of time points is usually small compared to the sample size.

Another common approach to analyze longitudinal data is based on a parametric growth curve for the mean response over time. Because this approach assumes a parametric function of time, it generally has the advantage of a much smaller number of parameters in the model as compared to the analysis of response profile and provides a very parsimonious summary of trend over time in the mean response, and therefore is especially useful when the objective of the study is to make statistical inferences on certain parameters from the parametric curve. As an example, if a linear trend is appropriate to model the mean response over time, two parameters, the intercept and the slope over time, completely characterize the entire mean response over time. Because the slope parameter measures the rate of change in mean response over time, it could be the primary interest in the statistical inference. In contrast to the analysis of response profile, the longitudinal analysis based on a parametric or semi-parametric growth curve does not require the study subjects be measured at the same set of time points, nor even the same number of repeated measures among different subjects.

2.1. Analysis of response profiles

When all individuals under study are measured at the same set of time points, the vector of longitudinal means over time is usually called the mean response profile. The analysis of response profiles is especially useful when there is a one-way treatment structure and when there is no pilot information on the mean response profiles over time among different treatment groups. This method assumes no specific structure on the mean response profile and nor on the covariance structure of the repeated measures.

Assume a longitudinal study in which the treatment factor has a total of u levels and the response variable Y is measured at each of the v time points. For the ith treatment group, $i = 1,2, \ldots, u$ and kth time point, $i = 1,2, \ldots, v$, let μ_{ik} be the mean of the response variable. Let $\mu^i = (\mu_{i1}, \mu_{i2}, \ldots, \mu_{iv})^t$ (superscript t stands for the matrix transpose) be the response profile for the ith treatment group. In general, the most important question in this type of longitudinal study is whether the response profiles are parallel among different treatment groups, which are the same as whether there exists an interaction between the treatment factor and the time factor. Mathematically, let $d^i = \mu^i - \mu^1 = (d_{i1}, d_{i2}, \ldots, d_{iv})^t$ be the vector of mean difference profile between the ith treatment group and the first treatment group (i.e., the reference group). If there is no interaction between the treatment factor and the time factor, then the hypothesis $H_0 : d_{i1} = d_{i2} = \cdots = d_{iv}$ holds for $i = 2, 3, \ldots, u$. The test of this hypothesis has a degree of freedom equal to $(u-1)(v-1)$. Notice that the null hypothesis of no interaction between the treatment factor and the time factor is equivalent to

$$H_0 : \Delta = (\delta_{22}, \delta_{23}, \ldots, \delta_{2v}, \delta_{32}, \delta_{33}, \ldots, \delta_{3v}, \ldots, \delta_{u2}, .\delta_{u3}, \ldots, \delta_{uv})^t = 0,$$

where $\delta_{ik} = d_{ik} - d_{i1}$, $i = 2, 3, \ldots, u$, and $k = 2, 3, \ldots, v$.

When analyzing response profiles, it is generally assumed that the response vector $Y_j = (y_1, y_2, \ldots, y_v)^t$ follows a multivariate normal distribution (Graybill, 1976) and that the covariance matrix of response vector $Y_j = (y_i, y_2, \ldots, y_v)^t$ is unstructured, although it is required to be symmetric and positive-definite. When longitudinal data are observed, the maximum likelihood (ML) estimates or the restricted maximum likelihood (REML) estimates $\hat{\Delta} = (\hat{\delta}_{22}, \hat{\delta}_{23}, \ldots, \hat{\delta}_{2v}, \hat{\delta}_{32}, \hat{\delta}_{33}, \ldots, \hat{\delta}_{3v}, \ldots, \hat{\delta}_{u2}, .\hat{\delta}_{u3}, \ldots, \hat{\delta}_{uv})^t$ can then be obtained (Diggle et al., 2002). Further, assume that the covariance matrix of $\hat{\Delta}$ can be estimated by $\hat{\Sigma}_{\hat{\Delta}}$. Then the test of interaction effect between the treatment factor and the time factor can be carried out through the standard Wald test by computing

$$\chi^2 = \hat{\Delta}^t \left(\hat{\sum}_{\hat{\Delta}} \right)^{-1} \hat{\Delta}.$$

At a significance level of $\alpha(0<\alpha<1)$, this test rejects the null hypothesis when $\chi^2>\chi^2_\alpha((u-1)(v-1))$, where $\chi^2_\alpha((u-1)(v-1))$ is the upper 100α% percentile of the χ^2 distribution with $(u-1)(v-1)$ degrees of freedom.

Likelihood-ratio test can also be used to test the interaction effect between the treatment factor and the time factor. This requires fitting two models with and without the constraint of the null hypothesis. Without the constraint (also called the full model), this amounts to the standard sampling theory of multivariate normal distributions, and the likelihood function L_{full} can be readily computed through the standard ML estimates of mean response vector and covariance matrices. Under the null hypothesis (also called the reduced model), another maximization procedure is needed to find the ML estimates of mean response vector and covariance matrices, and the likelihood function L_{reduced} under the null hypothesis can be obtained. Finally, the likelihood-ratio test of interaction effect between the treatment factor and the time factor can be carried out by computing

$$\text{LRT} = 2\log(L_{\text{full}}) - 2\log(L_{\text{reduced}}),$$

and further by comparing it to the upper 100α% percentile of the χ^2 distribution with $(u-1)(v-1)$ degrees of freedom. Depending on the results from the statistical test on the interaction effect between the treatment factor and the time factor, one can proceed to test the main effects for both the treatment factor and the time factor, as well as the pairwise comparisons between different levels of the treatment factor at given time points and between different levels of the time factor at given treatment levels.

An analysis of response profiles can be implemented in SAS through the following codes, where TREATMENT is the classification variable of the treatment factor, TIME is the classification variable for the time factor, and ID is the identification for subjects under the study:

```
PROC MIXED DATA = ; CLASSES ID TREATMENT TIME;
MODEL Y = TREATMENT TIME TREATMENT*TIME;
REPEATED TIME/TYPE = UN SUBJECT = ID R RCORR;
LSMEANS TREATMENT TIME TREATMENT*TIME/PDIFF;
RUN;
```

When the number of time points is relatively large, the omnibus test with $(u-1)(v-1)$ degrees of freedom on the interaction effect might become rather insensitive to the specific departures from parallelism and therefore have a rather low statistical power to detect the treatment differences. There are several different ways that more powerful tests on the interaction effect could be derived. In a two-arm randomized clinical trial consisting of a novel therapeutic treatment and a placebo, by the nature of randomization, the treated group and the placebo group should have the same mean response at the baseline. Therefore, it might make sense to examine the treatment difference by comparing the difference between the mean response over all time points beyond the baseline and the mean response at the baseline. More specifically, if there are 6 time points used in the study (coded as 1,2,3,4,5,6 with 1 = baseline), one would assess the effect of the novel treatment (coded as 2) as compared to the placebo (coded as 1) by testing $\mathrm{H}_0 : ((\mu_{22} + \mu_{23} + \mu_{24} + \mu_{25} + \mu_{26})/5) - \mu_{21} = ((\mu_{12} + \mu_{13} + \mu_{14} + \mu_{15} + \mu_{16})/5) - \mu_{11}$. This test has 1 degree of freedom and can be implemented by the following SAS codes with a CONTRAST statement. (The CONTRAST statement could differ depending on how these factors are coded in SAS, but option E should clearly indicate whether a correct CONTRAST statement was written (SAS Institute, Inc., 1999).)

```
PROC MIXED DATA = ; CLASSES ID TREATMENT TIME;
MODEL Y = TREATMENT*TIME/NOINT;
REPEATED TIME/TYPE = UN SUBJECT = ID R RCORR;
CONTRAST '1 DF INTERACTION TEST'
TREATMENT*TIME 1 -0.2 -0.2 -0.2 -0.2 -0.2 -1 0.2 0.2 0.2 0.2 0.2/E;
RUN;
```

In addition to the insensitivity of the general test with $(u-1)(v-1)$ degrees of freedom on the interaction effect to specific departures from the parallelism, the analysis of response profiles has other limitations in the analyses of longitudinal data despite the fact it is relatively simple to understand and easy to implement. The primary limitation of this approach is the requirement that all individuals under study be measured at the same set of time points, which prevents the use of the method in unbalanced and incomplete longitudinal studies. Another limitation is the fact that the analysis does not take into account of the time ordering of the repeated measurements from the same subjects, resulting in a possible loss of power in the analysis. Further, when the number of time points is relatively large, the analysis requires the estimation of a large covariance matrix, which also partly explains the fact the omnibus test with $(u-1)(v-1)$ degrees of freedom on the interaction effect has a rather low statistical power to detect the treatment differences.

2.2. *Repeated measures analysis of variance*

When a longitudinal study has a simple and classical design in which all subjects are measured at the same set of time points, and the only covariates which vary over time do so by design, the repeated measure analysis of variance can be used. The rationale for the repeated measures analysis of variance is to regard time as a within-subject factor in a hierarchical design which is generally referred to as a split-plot design in agricultural research. Unlike the analysis of response profiles in which the covariance matrix from the repeated measures from the same subjects are generally assumed unstructured, the repeated measures analysis of variance allows much simpler covariance matrix structure for the repeated measures over time. However, the usual randomization requirement in a standard split-plot design is not available in the longitudinal design because allocation of times to the multiple observations from the same subjects cannot be randomized. Therefore, it is necessary to assume an underlying model for the longitudinal data, which is essentially a special case of the general linear mixed models to be discussed in the next section.

Assume again that the covariate (i.e., the study conditions or treatments) takes a total of u possibilities and the response variable Y is measured at a total of v time points. The repeated measures analysis of variance models the response y_{ijk} for the jth subject at the ith study condition and the kth time point as

$$y_{ijk} = \mu_{ik} + p_{ij} + e_{ijk},$$

where μ_{ik} is the mean response for the ith study condition or treatment at the kth time point, p_{ij} represents the subject error, and e_{ijk} the time interval error. The standard assumptions made to this type of models are that p_{ij} are independent and identically distributed as $N(0, \sigma_p^2)$, e_{ijk} are independent and identically distributed as $N(0, \sigma_e^2)$, and that e_{ijk}'s and p_{ij}'s are statistically independent. Let $Y_{ij} = (y_{ij1}, y_{ij2}, \ldots, y_{ijv})$ be the vector of the repeated measures for the jth subject under the ith study condition. Under the above assumptions, it is straightforward to derive the covariance matrix of Y_{ij} as

$$\mathrm{Cov}(Y_{ij}) = \begin{pmatrix} \sigma_p^2 + \sigma_e^2 & \sigma_p^2 & \cdots & \sigma_p^2 \\ \sigma_p^2 & \sigma_p^2 + \sigma_e^2 & \cdots & \sigma_p^2 \\ \cdots & \cdots & \cdots & \cdots \\ \sigma_p^2 & \sigma_p^2 & \cdots & \sigma_p^2 + \sigma_e^2 \end{pmatrix}.$$

This covariance structure is called the structure of compound symmetry, which further implies that the correlation between any two repeated measures from the same subject j is $\mathrm{Corr}(Y_{ijk}, Y_{ijk'}) = \sigma_p^2/(\sigma_p^2 + \sigma_e^2)$.

The above assumptions on the variance components p_{ij} and e_{ijk} will guarantee that the usual F-tests from a standard two-way analysis of variance of a split-plot design are still valid to test the main effect of study conditions and the main effect of the time intervals, as well as the interaction effect between the study conditions and the time intervals. The more general assumptions required for the usual F-tests from a standard two-way analysis of variance to be valid requires certain forms of the covariance matrix of the measurement errors of the time intervals and of the covariance matrix of the error terms of the subjects assigned to a given study conditions. This form is called the Huynh–Feldt (H–F) condition (Huynh and Feldt, 1970). A covariance matrix Σ of dimension v by v satisfies the H–F condition if $\Sigma = \lambda I_v + \gamma J_v^t + J_v \gamma^t$, where I_v is the v by v identity matrix, J_v a v-dimensional column vector of 1's, λ an unknown constant, and γ a v-dimensional unknown column vector of parameters. The following SAS code can be used to fit the above model (where GROUP is the classification variable of study conditions):

```
PROC MIXED DATA = ; CLASS GROUP ID TIME;
MODEL Y = GROUP TIME GROUP*TIME;
RANDOM ID(GROUP);
RUN;
```

The covariance structure of compound symmetry may be inappropriate in longitudinal studies because of the constant correlation between any two repeated measures from the same subjects regardless of their time distance between the repeated measures. Many other covariance structures on the repeated measures have been proposed, most of which are motivated by the standard time series analyses and therefore might be more appropriate in longitudinal data. For example, in the following autoregressive error structure, the covariance matrix is proportional to

$$\sum = \begin{pmatrix} 1 & \rho & \dots & \rho^{v-1} \\ \rho & 1 & \dots & \rho^{v-2} \\ \dots & \dots & \dots & \dots \\ \rho^{v-1} & \rho^{v-2} & \dots & 1 \end{pmatrix}$$

for some $-1<\rho<+1$. This covariance matrix represents the fact that the more two repeated measures are apart in time, the less correlation are between them. Unfortunately, when such covariance matrix is assumed for the within-subject error terms on the repeated measures, the H–F condition generally no longer holds. When the H–F condition is not satisfied, the statistical comparison on the study conditions (i.e., the whole plot analysis in the standard two-way analysis of variance from a split-plot design) from the usual analysis of variance is still accurate and valid. The inferences from the within-subject comparisons, however, can only be approximated through various appropriate F-tests or t-tests. These are especially true for the tests of the main effect on time and the interactive effect between the study condition and the time factor. Multiple approximations to these tests can be used, for example, Box's correction method (Box, 1954), and those based on the Satterthwaite's approximation (Satterthwaite, 1946) to the denominator degrees of freedoms in F- and t-tests. Other types of covariance matrix on the errors of the time intervals can also be fitted to this model in SAS. SAS also provides several different options for approximating the degrees of freedoms when approximate F-tests are needed.

The following SAS code fits the repeated measures analysis of variance model with autoregressive within-subject error structure and the approximate F- and t-tests based on Satterthwaite's method:

```
PROC MIXED DATA = ; CLASS GROUP ID TIME;
MODEL Y = GROUP TIME GROUP*TIME/DDFM = SATTERTH;
RANDOM ID(GROUP);
REPEATED TIME/SUBJECT = ID TYPE = AR;
RUN;
```

2.3. *General linear models and general linear mixed models*

2.3.1. *General linear models for longitudinal data*

General linear models and general linear mixed models are statistical methodologies frequently used to analyze longitudinal data. These models recognize the likely correlation structure from the repeated measurements on same subjects over time. The general linear models are built on either explicit parametric models of the covariance structure of repeated measures over time whose validity can be checked against the available data or, where possible, to use methods of inference which are robust to misspecification of the covariance structure. Unlike the analysis of response profiles and repeated measures analysis of variance, the general linear models and general linear mixed models do not require that the longitudinal design be balanced or completed. In many cases, especially when the sample size is relatively small or moderate with many covariate variables, a parametric structure also need to be imposed on the covariance matrix of repeated measurements over time. Many different types of covariance structures have been used in the general linear models. In general, there are essentially two most popular ways to build a structure into a covariance matrix: using serial correlation models, and using random effects. The uniform correlation model assumes a positive correlation between any two measurements on the same subject. In contrast, the exponential correlation model (also called the first-order autoregressive model, Diggle, 1990) assumes an exponential decay toward 0 for the correlation between two measurements on the same subject as the time separation between the two measurements increases. The covariance structure of repeated measures based on random effects depends on the design matrix associated with the random effects.

Let $Y_j = (y_{j1}, y_{j2}, \ldots, y_{jk_j})^t$ be the vector of longitudinal observations for the variable of interest on the jth subject over k_j different time points $T_j = (t_{j1}, t_{j2}, \ldots, t_{jk_j})^t$. Notice that here we allow not only different numbers of time points but also different design vector over time among different subjects. Let $X_{jk} = (x_{jk1}, x_{jk2}, \ldots, x_{jkp})^t$ be the p by 1 vector of covariates associated with the kth measurement on the jth subject. Notice here that the vector of covariates could be time dependent. Let $X_j = (X_{j1}, X_{j2}, \ldots, X_{jk_j})^t$ be the design matrix of the jth subject. In longitudinal data analyses, it is generally assumed that X_j contains T_j itself and possibly some other covariates. The most general assumptions of a general linear model is

(1) $(Y_1, X_1), (Y_2, X_2), \ldots, (Y_n, X_n)$ are stochastically independent, which, in the case of fixed design matrix by design, is equivalent to $(Y_1, Y_2, \ldots, Y_n)$ that are independent, where n is the sample size of subjects under study;
(2) Given X_j, $EY_j = X_j\beta$, where β is a p by 1 column vector of regression coefficients, and $\text{cov}(Y_j) = \Sigma_j$.

2.3.2. Random effects models and general linear mixed models

A general way of introducing a covariance structure on repeated measurements is through the two-stage random effects models. When study subjects are sampled from a population, various aspects of their behavior may show stochastic variation between subjects. The simplest example of this is when the general level of the response profile varies between subjects, that is, some subjects are intrinsically high responders, others low responders. The two-stage random effect model (Diggle, 1988; Laird and Ware, 1982; Vonesh and Carter, 1992) allows the individual-specific response profile or 'growth curve' for each study subject at the first stage. The second stage of the two-stage random effects models introduces the between-subjects variation of the subject-specific effects and the population parameters of the subject-specific effects. The entire process leads to the development of the general linear mixed models. The ML estimates, the REML estimates, and the method-of-moment estimators are used to estimate the regression parameters in general linear mixed models. In addition, the general linear mixed models not only provide the best linear unbiased estimator (BLUE) (Graybill, 1976) for any estimable contrast of the regression parameters, but also estimate the subject-specific effects through the best linear unbiased predictor (BLUP) (Harville, 1977).

The major advantages of using random effects model is both to provide a way of modeling correlation among repeated measures from the same subjects and to derive good estimates to the subject-specific random effects. First, random effects are useful when strict measurements protocols in biomedical studies are not followed or when the design matrix on time was irregularly spaced and not consistent among subjects. Although many times biomedical studies are not designed this way, it can happen because of protocol deviation, bad timing, or missing data. Therefore the covariance matrix in the vector of longitudinal measurements might then depend on the individual subjects. Random effects model can handle this type of dependence in a very natural way. More specifically, the two-stage random effects models first assume that given the subject-specific design matrix Z_j of dimension $k_j \times q$ and the subject-specific regression coefficients β_j of dimension $q \times 1$,

$$Y_j = Z_j\beta_j + e_j,$$

where e_j follows a multivariate normal distribution with a mean vector of 0's and a covariance matrix equal to $\sigma^2 I_{k_j \times k_j}$ ($I_{k_j \times k_j}$ is the identity matrix of dimension k_j). At the second stage, given subject-level covariates A_j of dimension $q \times p$ and another set of regression coefficients β of dimension $p \times 1$, the variation among subject-specific regression coefficients β_j is modeled by another linear function of subject-level covariates as

$$\beta_j = A_j\beta + b_j,$$

where b_j follows another multivariate normal distribution with a mean vector of 0's and a covariance matrix D of dimension q. Other standard assumptions about the two-stage random effects model are that the vectors (Y_j, Z_j, A_j) are independent among a sample of size n, $j = 1, 2, \ldots, n$, and that e_j and b_j are statistically independent, $j = 1, 2, \ldots, n$. Notice that the design matrix A_j at the second stage is between-subjects and typically time independent, whereas the design matrix Z_j at the first stage is within-subjects and could be time dependent. In fact, Z_j usually specifies some type of growth curve model over time, such as linear or quadratic or spline functions.

An intuitive way to think of the two-stage random effects models in a longitudinal design is that each subject has his or her own 'growth curve' which is specified by the subject-specific regression coefficients β_j in the model from the first stage, and the population means of subject-specific regression coefficients β_j are given by the model at the second stage, which depends on the between-subjects covariates A_j. Combining the model from Stage 1 and that from Stage 2 in the two-stage random effects models, it follows that

$$Y_j = X_j(A_j\beta + b_j) + e_j,$$

i.e.,

$$Y_j = (X_jA_j)\beta + Z_jb_j + e_j.$$

This final model is a special case of the general linear mixed model formulation which has the following general form:

$$Y_j = W_j\beta + Z_jb_j + e_j,$$

where b_j follows a multivariate normal distribution with a mean vector of 0's and a covariance matrix D of dimension q, e_j follows another multivariate normal distribution with a mean vector of 0's and a covariance matrix R_j, W_j and Z_j are the design matrices associated with the fixed and random effects, respectively. Although R_j could assume different structures, it is generally assumed the diagonal matrix $\sigma^2 I_{k_j}$, where I_{k_j} is the identity matrix of dimension k_j. Under this assumption, e_{ji}'s could be interpreted as measurement errors. Other standard assumptions about the general linear mixed model are that, given W_j, e_j, and Y_j are statistically independent, $j = 1, 2, \ldots, n$. In the general linear mixed models, coefficients β are called the vector of fixed effects, which are assumed the same for all individuals and can be interpreted as the population parameters. In contrast to β, b_j are called random effects and are comprised of subject-specific regression coefficients, which, along with the fixed effects, describe the mean response for the jth subject as

$$E(Y_j|b_j) = W_j\beta + Z_jb_j.$$

It is also straightforward to derive that

$$E(Y_j) = W_j\beta,$$

and

$$\Sigma_j = \mathrm{Cov}(Y_j) = Z_jDZ_j^t + R_j.$$

Weighted least squares estimation and the ML or REML methods through the EM algorithm (Patterson and Thompson, 1971; Cullis and McGilchrist, 1990; Verbyla and Cullis, 1990; Tunnicliffe-Wilson, 1989; Dempster et al., 1977; Laird and Ware, 1982; Vonesh and Carter, 1992) are used to estimate the mean response and the covariance parameters. Software is readily available for ML and REML.

2.3.3. Predictions of random effects

In many longitudinal biomedical studies, subject-specific growth curve on repeated measures could be crucial information not only for investigators to understand the biological mechanism of the diseases under study, but also for clinicians to better predict the disease progression and eventually offer better care to the patients. Under the framework of the general linear mixed model, it is possible to obtain estimates to the subject-specific effects, b_j. The estimate to b_j, along with the estimates to the fixed effects, β, subsequently provides an estimate to the subject-specific longitudinal trajectories, $W_j\beta + Z_jb_j$.

The prediction of random effects can be best understood in the framework of Bayesian analysis when each random effect is treated as a random parameter whose prior is a multivariate normal distribution with a mean vector of 0's and a covariance matrix D. Given the vector of responses $Y_j = (y_{j1}, y_{j2}, \ldots, y_{jk_j})^t$, it is well known (Graybill, 1976) that the best predictor of b_j is the conditional expectation of the posterior distribution:

$$\hat{b}_j = E(b_j | Y_j).$$

The well-known Bayesian Theorem then implies that the conditional distribution of b_j, given $Y_j = (y_{j1}, y_{j2}, \ldots, y_{jk_j})^t$, is another normal distribution with mean

$$\hat{\mu}_{b_j} = DZ_j^t\Sigma_j^{-1}(Y_j - W_j\beta)$$

and covariance matrix

$$\Sigma_{b_j} = Cov(b_j | Y_j) = D - DZ_j^t\Sigma_j^{-1}Z_jD.$$

Because $\hat{\mu}_{b_j}$ is a linear function of the response vector $Y_j = (y_{j1}, y_{j2}, \ldots, y_{jk_j})^t$, and it can be shown that $\hat{\mu}_{b_j}$ is also an unbiased predictor to b_j and has the minimum variance in the class of unbiased linear predictors of b_j, $\hat{\mu}_{b_j}$ is therefore a BLUP of b_j. Because $\hat{\mu}_{b_j}$ is also a function of unknown parameters β, D, and Σ_j, the ML or REML estimates to these parameters can be used to obtain the empirical BLUP of b_j as

$$\hat{b}_j = \hat{D}Z_j^t\hat{\Sigma}_j^{-1}(Y_j - W_j\hat{\beta}).$$

Obtaining a valid estimate to the covariance matrix of the empirical BLUP $\hat{b}_j$ turns out to be more challenging. A simple replacement of unknown parameters by their estimates in Σ_{b_j} would underestimate the variability because of the ignorance to the uncertainty in the estimate of β. Notice that

$$\mathrm{Cov}(\hat{b}_j - b_j) = D - DZ_j^t\Sigma_j^{-1}Z_jD + DZ_j^t\Sigma_j^{-1}W_j \times \left(\sum_{j=1}^{n} W_j^t\Sigma_j^{-1}W_j\right)^{-1} W_j^t\Sigma_j^{-1}Z_jD.$$

The standard error of the empirical BLUP $\hat{b}_j$ can be obtained by substituting the ML or REML estimates for the unknown parameters in $\mathrm{Cov}(\hat{b}_j - b_j)$. Finally, the predicted growth curve for the jth subject is

$$\hat{Y}_j = W_j\hat{\beta} + Z_j\hat{b}_j,$$

which can be rewritten as

$$\hat{Y}_j = \left(\hat{R}_j\hat{\Sigma}_j^{-1}\right)W_j\hat{\beta} + \left(I_{k_j} - \hat{R}_j\hat{\Sigma}_j^{-1}\right)Y_j.$$

Therefore, the predictor of individual growth curve Y_j can be conceptualized as a weighted sum between the population mean growth curve $W_j\hat{\beta}$ and the observed growth curve $Y_j = (y_{j1}, y_{j2}, \ldots, y_{jk_j})^t$, which indicates some type of 'shrinkage' (James and Stein, 1961) for the predictor of individual growth curve Y_j toward the population mean growth curve $W_j\hat{\beta}$. The degree of 'shrinkage' that is reflected by the weights depends on R_j and Σ_j. In general, when the within-subject variability, R_j, is large relative to the between-subject variability, more weight is given to the population mean growth curve $W_j\hat{\beta}$ than to the individual growth curve $Y_j = (y_{j1}, y_{j2}, \ldots, y_{jk_j})^t$. On the other hand, when the between-subject variability is large relative to the within-subject variability, more weight is assigned to the individually observed growth curve than to the population mean growth curve $W_j\hat{\beta}$.

We now present some applications of general linear mixed models in biomedical applications, especially in the study of AD. AD is a neurodegenerative disease which is characterized by the loss of cognitive and functional ability. It is the most common of the degenerative dementias affecting up to 47% of the population over the age of 85 (Evans et al., 1989; Herbert et al., 1995; Crystal et al., 1988; Katzman et al., 1988; Morris et al., 1991). Many neuropsychological measures and staging instruments have been used to describe the longitudinal disease progression. For example, the severity of dementia can be staged by the clinical dementia rating (CDR) according to published rules (Morris, 1993). A global CDR is derived from individual ratings in multiple domains by an experienced clinician such that CDR 0 indicates no dementia and CDR 0.5, 1, 2, and 3 represent very mild, mild, moderate, and severe dementia, respectively. A major interest in longitudinal AD research is to estimate and compare the rate of cognitive decline as a function of disease severity and other possible risk factors such as age, education, and the number of Apolipoprotein E4 alleles.

Example 1. Random intercept and random slope model at different stages of AD.

Let $Y_j = (y_{j1}, y_{j2}, \ldots, y_{jk_j})^t$ be the vector of longitudinal observations for the cognitive function on the jth subject over k_j time points $T_j = (t_{j1}, t_{j2}, \ldots, t_{jk_j})^t$ (i.e., TIME). Suppose that the growth curve over time is approximately linear for each stage of the disease as measured by CDR and that subjects stayed at the same CDR stage during the longitudinal follow-up. At the first stage of the two-stage random effects model, a linear growth curve is assumed for each subject, i.e., given the subject-specific intercept and slope over time,

$$y_{jk} = \beta_{0j} + \beta_{1j}t_{jk} + e_{jk},$$

for $k = 1, 2, \ldots, k_j$, or $Y_j = A_j\beta_j + e_j$ in the matrix form, where $A_j = (J\ T_j), J$ is the column vector of 1's, $\beta_j = (\beta_{0j}\ \beta_{1j})$, and $e_j = (e_{j1}, e_{j2}, \ldots, e_{jk_j})^t$. At the second stage, the subject-specific intercept and slope are modeled as functions of possible subject-level covariates. Because it has been well established in the literature that the rate of cognitive decline in AD is associated with the disease severity at the baseline (Storandt et al., 2002), one such subject-level covariate could be the baseline disease severity as measured by CDR. Therefore, one can model the subject-specific intercept and slope separately as a function of CDR in a standard analysis of variance (ANOVA) model (Milliken and Johnson, 1992), i.e.,

$$\beta_{0j} = \beta^0_{\text{CDR}} + b_{0j},$$

$$\beta_{1j} = \beta^1_{\text{CDR}} + b_{1j}.$$

One difference between here and the standard ANOVA model is that two variables (the intercept and the slope) are conceptualized from the same subjects. Therefore a correlation structure is usually required to account for the possible correlation between the intercept and the slope from the same subjects. These are generally done by assuming that the error vector $b_j = (b_{0j}\ b_{1j})^t$ follows a normal distribution with mean vector of 0's and a covariance matrix D which could be assumed completely unstructured (i.e., specified by the option TYPE = UN) or with certain structured form. The above model can be easily implemented in SAS with the following codes:

```
PROC MIXED DATA = ; CLASSES ID CDR;
MODEL Y = CDR TIME CDR*TIME /DDFM = SATTERTH;
RANDOM INT TIME/SUBJECT = ID TYPE = UN;
RUN;
```

It is important to understand the hypothesis that each term in the model is testing. The term CDR*TIME is testing the hypothesis that the mean slopes are the same across all baseline CDR groups, whereas the term CDR is testing whether the mean intercepts at TIME = 0 (i.e., the baseline) are the same across the CDR groups. The term TIME is testing the main effect of the slope over time across the CDR groups, which can in general only be interpreted if the test on CDR*TIME is not statistically significant.

If the estimates to the mean intercepts and mean slopes for each CDR and subject-specific predictions to the random effects are needed, the following SAS code can be used:

```
PROC MIXED DATA = ; CLASSES ID CDR;
MODEL Y = CDR CDR*TIME/NOINT S DDFM = SATTERTH;
RANDOM INT TIME/SUBJECT = ID TYPE = UN SOLUTION;
RUN;
```

One needs to be careful about the interpretation of the output from this new set of codes. The term CDR*TIME is no longer testing the hypothesis that the mean slopes are the same across all CDR groups, but the hypothesis that all mean slopes across CDR groups are simultaneously equal to 0. Likewise, the term CDR is no longer testing whether the mean intercepts at TIME = 0 are the same across the CDR groups, but whether all the mean intercepts are simultaneously equal to 0. Some of these hypotheses tested by this new set of codes might not be scientifically interesting, but the set of codes does offer the valid estimates to the fixed effects and random effects.

Example 2. Random intercept and random slope model at different stages of AD adjusting for the baseline age.

In Example 1, a random intercept and random slope model was used to describe the growth curve of cognitive decline across different stages of AD. It is also well known that baseline age is an important risk factor for the cognitive decline. An extended two-stage random effects model can be used to describe the rate of cognitive decline as a function of both baseline CDR and baseline age (i.e., AGE). The first stage of this model will be the same as the first stage of the model introduced in Example 1. At the second stage, where the subject-specific intercept and slope are modeled as functions of possible subject-level covariates, one can conceptualize both the subject-specific intercept and subject-specific rate of cognitive decline for each CDR stage as a linear function of baseline age in a standard analysis of covariance (ANOCOVA) model (Milliken and Johnson, 2001), i.e.,

$$\beta_{0j} = \beta^0_{\text{CDR}} + \gamma^0_{\text{CDR}} * \text{AGE} + b_{0j},$$

$$\beta_{1j} = \beta^1_{\text{CDR}} + \gamma^1_{\text{CDR}} * \text{AGE} + b_{1j}.$$

Notice here β^0_{CDR}, γ^0_{CDR} are the intercept and slope of the subject-specific intercept as a linear function of AGE, and β^1_{CDR}, γ^1_{CDR} are the intercept and slope of the subject-specific longitudinal rate of cognitive decline as a linear function of AGE. Again, a correlation structure is usually required to account for the possible correlation between the intercept and the slope from the first-stage model by assuming that the error vector $b_j = (b_{0j}\ b_{1j})^t$ at the second stage of the model follows a normal distribution with mean vector of 0's and a covariance matrix D which could be assumed completely unstructured. The above model can be easily implemented in SAS by the following code:

```
PROC MIXED DATA = ; CLASSES ID CDR;
MODEL Y = CDR AGE CDR*AGE TIME AGETIME CDR*TIME
CDR*AGETIME /DDFM = SATTERTH;
RANDOM INT TIME/SUBJECT = ID TYPE = UN;
RUN;
```

In these codes, AGETIME is the variable created in the data set by multiplying TIME and AGE. All the terms CDR AGE CDR*AGE in the MODEL statement are modeling the intercept part of the cognitive function, whereas all the other terms in the MODEL statement are modeling the longitudinal rate of the cognitive function. More specifically, the term CDR*AGETIME here tests whether all γ^1_{CDR} are the same across different CDR levels, the term CDR*AGE tests whether all γ^0_{CDR} are the same across different CDR levels, and the term CDR*TIME tests whether all β^1_{CDR} are the same across different CDR levels.

Different variations and extensions to the above models can also be used. These include the cases when either the subject-specific intercepts or subject-specific slopes but not both are assumed random and the other cases when additional risk factors for AD such as education and the number of Apolipoprotein E4 alleles are also entered into the model. There are also cases that additional random effects need to be introduced into the model. For example, with a multicenter study, centers are usually treated as a random effect to account for the possible variation among centers and the possible correlation of the measures for subjects from the same centers.

Example 3. Piecewise random coefficients model in AD.

Piecewise linear growth curves are common in many biomedical applications. In AD research, it has been well recognized that the rate of cognitive decline depends on the disease severity at the baseline (Storandt et al., 2002). This further implies that a simple linear growth curve over time is inappropriate when subjects make conversions from lower CDR level to higher CDR levels. Again let $Y_j = (y_{j1}, y_{j2}, \ldots, y_{jk_j})^t$ be the vector of longitudinal observations for the cognitive function on the jth subject over k_j time points $T_j = (t_{j1}, t_{j2}, \ldots, t_{jk_j})^t$. Assume that the subject begins with CDR 0 and then converts into CDR 0.5 at time $t_{jk_j^{0.5}}$, $1 < k_j^{0.5} < k_j$, the subject goes on at CDR 0.5 and makes another conversion into CDR 1 at time $t_{jk_j^1}$, $1 \le k_j^{0.5} < k_j^1 \le k_j$. Suppose that the growth curve over time is approximately linear at each CDR level. Then at the first stage of a two-stage random effects model, a piecewise linear growth curve connected at the CDR conversion times is assumed for each subject, i.e., given the subject-specific intercept and slopes over time,

$$y_{jk} = \beta_{0j} + \beta_j^0 t_{jk} + \beta_j^{0.5} t_{jk}^{0.5} + \beta_j^1 t_{jk}^1 + e_{jk},$$

where $t_{jk}^{0.5} = t_{jk}$ when $k \ge k_j^{0.5}$, and $t_{jk}^{0.5} = 0$ when $k < k_j^{0.5}$; and $t_{jk}^1 = t_{jk}$ when $k \ge k_j^1$, and $t_{jk}^1 = 0$ when $k < k_j^1$. Notice that the parameters in this model indicate three different rates of cognitive decline at three different CDR levels during the longitudinal follow-up. β_j^0 represents the slope of cognitive decline at CDR 0, $\beta_j^0 + \beta_j^{0.5}$ represents the slope of cognitive decline at CDR 0.5, and $\beta_j^0 + \beta_j^{0.5} + \beta_j^1$ represents the slope of cognitive decline at CDR 1. Therefore, $\beta_j^{0.5}$ represents the difference on the slope of cognitive decline between CDR 0.5 and CDR 0, and β_j^1 represents the difference on the slope of cognitive decline between CDR 1 and CDR 0.5. At the second stage, the subject-specific intercept and slopes are again modeled as a function of possible subject-level covariates. Assume that the subject-specific slopes are to be compared between subjects with at least one Apolipoprotein E4 allele (i.e., E4 positive) and those without Apolipoprotein E4 alleles (i.e., E4 negative). One can then write four analysis of variance models as

$$\beta_{0j} = \beta_{0\mathrm{E4}} + b_{0j},$$

$$\beta_j^0 = \beta_{\mathrm{E4}}^0 + b_j^0,$$

$$\beta_j^{0.5} = \beta_{\mathrm{E4}}^{0.5} + b_j^{0.5},$$

and

$$\beta_j^1 = \beta_{\mathrm{E4}}^1 + b_j^1.$$

The variation among subject-specific parameters and the correlation for within-subject parameters are modeled by assuming $b_j = \left(b_{0j}\ b_j^0\ b_j^{0.5}\ b_j^1\right)^t$ follows a normal distribution with mean vector of 0's and a covariance matrix D which could be assumed completely unstructured. The above model could be implemented in SAS by the following codes:

```
PROC MIXED DATA = ; CLASSES ID E4;
MODEL Y = E4 T T^0.5 T^1 E4*T E4*T^0.5 E4*T^1;
RANDOM INT T T^0.5 T^1 /SUBJECT = ID TYPE = UN;
RUN;
```

In these codes, T, $\mathrm{T}^{0.5}$, and T^1 represent t_{jk}, $t_{jk}^{0.5}$, and t_{jk}^1, respectively. All terms in above model test specific hypotheses. For example, $\mathrm{E4*T}^{0.5}$ tests whether the difference on the rate of cognitive decline between CDR 0.5 and CDR 0 is the same between E4-positive and E4-negative subjects. The following SAS codes give estimates to the mean intercepts and mean slopes for each CDR level and subject-specific predictions to the random effects. (The ESTIMATE statement could differ depending on how these factors are coded in SAS, but option E should clearly indicate whether a correct ESTIMATE statement was written (SAS Institute, Inc., 1999.)

```
PROC MIXED DATA = ; CLASSES ID E4;
MODEL Y = E4 E4*T E4*T^0.5 E4*T^1/NOINT DDFM = SATTERTH
SOLUTION;
RANDOM INT T T^0.5 T^1 /SUBJECT = ID TYPE = UN SOLUTION;
ESTIMATE 'rate at CDR 0.5 for E4 +' E4*T 1 0 E4*T^0.5 1 0/E;
ESTIMATE 'rate difference by E4 at CDR 0.5' E4*T 1 -1 E4*T^0.5 1 -1/E;
RUN;
```

The first ESTIMATE statement gives the estimated mean rate of cognitive decline at CDR 0.5 for subjects with positive E4 (it could be for subjects with negative APOE4 depending on the code of APOE4, but the option E should indicate clearly which one is estimated). The second ESTIMATE statement estimates the mean difference on the mean rate of cognitive decline at CDR 0.5 between subjects with positive E4 and those with negative E4 and tests whether the difference is 0. Similar additional ESTIMATE statements can be written to estimate the rate of cognitive decline at CDR 1 and test whether a difference exists between E4-positive and E4-negative subjects.

2.4. Generalized linear models for longitudinal data

The generalized linear models for longitudinal data extend the techniques of general linear models. They are suited specifically for non-linear models with binary or discrete responses, such as logistic regression, in which the mean response is linked to the explanatory variables or covariates through a non-linear link function (McCullagh and Nelder, 1989; Liang and Zeger, 1986; Zeger and Liang, 1986). Several approaches have been proposed to model longitudinal data in the framework of generalized linear models. The marginal models for longitudinal data permit separate modeling of the regression of the response on explanatory variables, and the association among repeated observations of the response for each subject. They are appropriate when inferences about the population averages are the focus of the longitudinal studies. For example, in an AD treatment clinical trial, the average difference between control and treatment is the most important, not the difference for any single subject. Marginal models are also useful in AD epidemiological studies. It could help to address what the age-specific prevalence of AD is, whether the prevalence is greater in a specific sub-population, and how the association between a specific sub-population and the AD prevalence rate changes with time. The techniques of generalized estimating equations (GEEs) can be used to estimate the regression parameters in the marginal models (Liang and Zeger, 1986; Gourieroux et al., 1984; Prentice, 1988; Zhao and Prentice, 1990; Thall and Vail, 1990; Liang et al., 1992; Fitzmaurice et al., 1993). The approach of random effects models in the setup of generalized linear model allows the heterogeneity among subjects in a subset of the entire set of the regression parameters. Two general approaches of the estimation are used in the random effects models. One is to find the marginal means and variance of the response vector and then apply the technique of GEE (Zeger and Qaqish, 1988; Gilmore et al., 1985; Goldstein, 1991; Breslow and Clayton, 1993; Lipsitz et al., 1991). The other is the likelihood approach (Anderson and Aitkin, 1985; Hinde, 1982) or the penalized quasi-likelihood (PQL) approach (Green, 1987; Laird, 1978; Stiratelli et al., 1984; McGilchrist and Aisbett, 1991; Breslow and Clayton, 1993). Another generalized linear model is the transition model for which the conditional distribution of the response at a time given the history of longitudinal observations is assumed to depend only on the prior observations with a specified order through a Markov chain. Full ML estimation can be used to fit the Gaussian autoregressive models (Tsay, 1984), and the conditional ML estimation can be used to fit logistic and log-linear models (Korn and Whittemore, 1979; Stern and Coe, 1984; Zeger et al., 1985; Wong, 1986; Zeger and Qaqish, 1988). A comprehensive description of various models for discrete longitudinal data can be found in Molenberghs and Verbeke (2005).

2.4.1. Marginal models and generalized estimating equations

In many biomedical applications the longitudinal responses are not necessarily continuous, which imply that the general linear models and general linear mixed models might not apply. For example, the presence or absence of depression and the count of panic attacks during certain time interval are all likely response variables of scientific interest. When the longitudinal responses are discrete, generalized linear models are required to relate changes in the mean responses to covariates. In addition, another component is needed to introduce the within-subject associations among the vector of repeated responses. Marginal models are one of these choices.

We again let $Y_j = (y_{j1}, y_{j2}, \ldots, y_{jk_j})^t$ be the vector of longitudinal observations for the response variable on the jth subject over k_j time points $T_j = (t_{j1}, t_{j2}, \ldots, t_{jk_j})^t$. Let $X_{jk} = (x_{jk1}, x_{jk2}, \ldots, x_{jkp})^t$ be the p by 1 vector of covariates associated with the kth measurement on the jth subject. Notice here that the vector of covariates could be time dependent. Let $X_j = (X_{j1}, X_{j2}, \ldots, X_{jk_j})^t$ be the design matrix of the jth subject. A marginal model for longitudinal data specifies the following three components:

(1) The conditional expectation of Y_{jk}, given X_{jk}, is assumed to depend on the covariates through a given link function g, i.e.,

$$E(Y_{jk}|X_{jk}) = \mu_{jk}$$

and

$$g(\mu_{jk}) = X_{jk}^t \beta,$$

where β is a p by 1 vector of unknown regression parameters.

(2) The conditional variance of Y_{jk}, given X_{jk}, is assumed to depend on the mean according to some given 'variance function' V, i.e.,

$$\text{Var}(Y_{jk}|X_{jk}) = \phi V(\mu_{jk}),$$

where ϕ is an additional parameter.

(3) The conditional within-subject association among repeated responses, given the covariates, is assumed to depend on an additional set of parameters α, although it could also depend on the mean parameters.

The first two conditions in a marginal model are standard requirements from a generalized linear model (McCullagh and Nelder, 1989) relating the marginal means to a set of covariates at each individual time point. The third condition is in addition to the standard assumptions in generalized linear model, which makes the application of generalized linear model to longitudinal data possible. Notice that even if all three components are completely specified in a marginal model, the model still does not completely specify the joint distribution of the vector of repeated measures on the response variable. In fact, it will be clear later that such a complete specification of joint distribution is not needed to obtain valid asymptotic statistical inferences to the regression parameters β. The following are several examples of marginal models for longitudinal data.

Example 1: In the case of continuous response variables, the standard repeated measure analysis of variance models and the two-stage random effects models are special cases of marginal models. Here the link function is the simple identity function, i.e., $g(\mu_{jk}) = \mu_{jk}$, and the variance function is constant 1, i.e., $V = 1$. The conditional within-subject association is described by correlations among repeated measures of the response, which are independent of the mean parameters.

Example 2: In a longitudinal study to examine the longitudinal trend on the probability of depression and to relate this probability to other covariates such as gender and education, the occurrence of depression is longitudinally observed. Because Y_{jk} is binary and coded as 1 when depression occurs and 0 otherwise, the distribution of each Y_{jk} is Bernoulli which is traditionally modeled through a logit- or probit-link function, i.e., the conditional expectation of Y_{jk}, given X_{jk}, is $E(Y_{jk}|X_{jk}) = Pr(Y_{jk} = 1|X_{jk}) = \mu_{jk}$, and the logit-link function links μ_{jk} with covariates by

$$\ln\left(\frac{\mu_{jk}}{1-\mu_{jk}}\right) = X_{jk}^t\beta.$$

The conditional variance of Y_{jk}, given X_{jk}, is given by the 'variance function',

$$\mathrm{Var}(Y_{jk}|X_{jk}) = \mu_{jk}(1-\mu_{jk}),$$

i.e., $\phi = 1$. The conditional within-subject association among repeated responses, given the covariates, is usually specified by an unstructured pairwise odds ratio between two repeated responses,

$$\alpha_{k_1k_2} = \frac{Pr(Y_{jk_1} = 1, Y_{jk_2} = 1)Pr(Y_{jk_1} = 0, Y_{jk_2} = 0)}{Pr(Y_{jk_1} = 1, Y_{jk_2} = 0)Pr(Y_{jk_1} = 0, Y_{jk_2} = 1)}.$$

Example 3: In many studies of AD, psychometric tests are generally used to assess subjects' cognition longitudinally. One of these tests records the number of animals that the subject can name within a given period of time. This type of count data could be modeled by a Poisson distribution, using a log-link function. More specifically, the conditional expectation of Y_{jk}, given X_{jk}, is $E(Y_{jk}|X_{jk}) = \mu_{jk}$, and is assumed to depend on the covariates through the log-link function,

$$\ln(\mu_{jk}) = X_{jk}^t\beta.$$

The conditional variance of Y_{jk}, given X_{jk}, is given by the Poisson 'variance function',

$$\mathrm{Var}(Y_{jk}|X_{jk}) = \mu_{jk},$$

i.e., $\phi = 1$. The conditional within-subject association among repeated responses, given the covariates, is usually specified by unstructured pairwise correlations between two repeated responses,

$$\alpha_{k_1 k_2} = \mathrm{CORR}(Y_{jk_1}, Y_{jk_2}).$$

This marginal model is sometimes referred to a log-linear model.

When a marginal model is specified, the estimation of the model parameters is generally done through the GEE instead of the standard inferences based on the ML estimates. Part of the reason that a standard ML approach is not used here is that the marginal model fails to specify the joint distribution on the vector of repeated responses and therefore a likelihood function is not available. The basic idea of GEE is to find β that minimizes the following generalized sum of square (also called the objective function):

$$\sum_j [Y_j - \mu_j]^t V_j^{-1} [Y_j - \mu_j],$$

where μ_j is the vector of expectations of repeated responses for the jth subject which is a function of the regression parameters β. V_j is called the 'working' covariance matrix of Y_j and is given by

$$V_j = A_j^{1/2} \mathrm{CORR}(Y_j) A_j^{1/2},$$

where $A_j^{1/2}$ is the diagonal matrix such that $(A_j^{1/2})^2 = A_j$, and A_j the diagonal matrix consisting of the variance of Y_{jk}, and $\mathrm{CORR}(Y_j)$ the correlation matrix of Y_j depending on the set of parameters α's (also possibly β's). The reason that V_j is called the 'working' covariance matrix of Y_j is that it is not necessarily the same as the true covariance matrix of Y_j. The mathematical minimization of the above objective function is equivalent to finding β that solves the following GEEs:

$$\sum_j D_j^t V_j^{-1} [Y_j - \mu_j] = 0,$$

where

$$D_j = \begin{pmatrix} \partial\mu_{j1}/\partial\beta_1 & \partial\mu_{j1}/\partial\beta_2 & \dots & \partial\mu_{j1}/\partial\beta_p \\ \partial\mu_{j2}/\partial\beta_1 & \partial\mu_{j2}/\partial\beta_2 & \dots & \partial\mu_{j2}/\partial\beta_p \\ \dots & \dots & \dots & \dots \\ \partial\mu_{jk_j}/\partial\beta_1 & \partial\mu_{jk_j}/\partial\beta_2 & \dots & \partial\mu_{jk_j}/\partial\beta_p \end{pmatrix}$$

is called the derivative matrix of μ_j with respect to the regression parameters β. Notice that $\mu_{jk} = g^{-1}(X_{jk}^t \beta)$, where g^{-1} is the inverse of the link function g. Although the derivative matrix is only a function of the regression parameters, the GEEs involve not only the regression parameters β but also the parameters α and ϕ. The latter are usually called nuisance parameters because they generally are not the major interest in biomedical research, but they play important roles in the inferential process. In general, the GEEs have no closed form solutions with a non-linear link function, and therefore require an iterative algorithm to approximate the solutions. The standard two-stage iterative algorithms are available for these computations and can be found in the literature (Fitzmaurice et al., 2004). These iterative algorithms begin with some seed estimates to parameters α and ϕ, and then estimate regression parameters β by solving the system of GEEs at the first stage. At the second stage of the iterative algorithms, the current estimates of β's are used to update the estimates of α and ϕ. These two-stage processes are iterated until computational convergence is achieved. These algorithms are also implemented in many standard statistical software packages.

Assume that $\hat{\beta}$ is the final solution of β to the GEEs after the two-stage iterative algorithm converges. The most appealing part of a marginal model is the fact that $\hat{\beta}$ is a consistent estimator, i.e., when the sample size is sufficiently large, $\hat{\beta}$ approaches the true regression parameters β. This is true even when the within-subject associations have been incorrectly specified in the marginal model. In other words, as long as the mean component of the marginal model is correctly specified, $\hat{\beta}$ will provide valid statistical inferences. Another important appealing property of GEE estimate $\hat{\beta}$ is the fact that it is almost as efficient as the MLE estimate, especially in the generalized linear mixed models for continuous outcome variable under the assumption of multivariate normality over repeated measures. Similar to the standard asymptotic properties of ML estimates, when the sample size is sufficiently large, $\hat{\beta}$ follows an asymptotically multivariate normal distribution with mean β and a covariance matrix which can be estimated by the so-called 'sandwich' estimator

$$\hat{\Sigma} = \hat{B}^{-1}\hat{M}\hat{B}^{-1},$$

where $\hat{B} = \Sigma_j \hat{D}_j^t \hat{V}_j^{-1} \hat{D}_j$ and $\hat{M} = \Sigma_j \hat{D}_j^t \hat{V}_j^{-1} [Y_j - \hat{\mu}_j][Y_j - \hat{\mu}_j]^t \hat{V}_j^{-1} \hat{D}_j$, and the estimates $\hat{D}_j$, $\hat{V}_j$, and $\hat{\mu}_j$ are obtained by replacing β, α, and ϕ by their GEE estimates from D_j, V_j, and μ_j, respectively.

For the statistical inferences about the regression parameters β, valid standard errors can be obtained based on the above sandwich estimator $\hat{\Sigma} = \hat{B}^{-1}\hat{M}\hat{B}^{-1}$. In fact, both GEE estimate of β and the sandwich estimator to $\mathrm{Cov}(\hat{\beta})$ are robust in the sense that it is still valid even if the within-subject associations have been incorrectly specified in the marginal model. This does not imply that it is not necessary to try to specify correctly the within-subject associations in the marginal model. In fact, the correct modeling or approximation to the within-subject associations is important as far as the efficiency or the precision on the estimation of regression parameters β is concerned. It can be mathematically proved that the optimum efficiency in the estimation of regression parameters β can be obtained when the working matrix V_j is the same as the true within-subject association among repeated responses. On the other hand, the sandwich estimate is most appropriate when the study design is almost balanced and the number of subjects is relatively large and the number of repeated measures from the same subject is relatively small, especially when there are many replications on the response vectors associated with each distinct set of covariate values. When the longitudinal study designs severely deviate from these 'ideal' cases, the use of sandwich estimator for the statistical inferences might be problematic, in which case, the specification of the entire model over the repeated measures might be desired and therefore the effort to specify the correct covariance matrix become necessary.

The following is a SAS code to obtain GEE for Example 2 above in which the longitudinal trend on the probability of depression is modeled as a function of gender and time through the logit-link function. The occurrence of depression is treated as binary and longitudinally observed. The option LOGOR specifies the possible working covariance structure based on log odds ratio for the within-subject responses:

```
PROC GENMOD DESCENDING DATA = ;
CLASSES ID GENDER;
MODEL DEPRESSION = GENDER TIME GENDER*TIME/
DIST = BINOMIAL LINK = LOGIT;
REPEATED SUBJECT = ID/WITHINSUBJECT = TIME LOGOR = ;
RUN;
```

2.4.2. Generalized linear mixed effect models

The basic conceptualization of the generalized linear mixed effects models is quite similar to that of the general linear mixed effects models, although there are crucial differences in the parameter interpretations of these models. More specifically, a generalized linear mixed effects model for longitudinal data assumes the heterogeneity across subjects in the study in the entire set or a subset of the regression coefficients. In other words, the entire set or a subset of the subject-specific regression coefficients are assumed to be random variables across study subjects which follow a univariate or a multivariate normal distribution.

The generalized linear mixed effects models can also be thought of following a standard two-stage paradigm in which the first stage specifies a conditional distribution for each response Y_{jk}. More specifically, at the first stage, it is assumed that conditional on the subject-specific random effect b_j and covariates X_{jk}, the distribution of Y_{jk} belongs to a very wide family of distributions called the exponential family. The exponential family covers essentially all the important distributions used in biomedical applications. These distributions include, but are not limited to, the normal distribution, the binomial distribution, and the Poisson distribution. Let

$$\mu_{jk} = E(Y_{jk}|b_j, X_{jk}).$$

The conditional variance of Y_{jk} is given through some known variance function V

$$\mathrm{Var}(Y_{jk}|b_j, X_{jk}) = \phi V(\mu_{jk}).$$

Further, conditional on the random effect b_j and covariates X_{jk}, Y_{jk}'s are assumed independent. The conditional mean of Y_{jk} is linked to a linear predictor through a given link function g

$$g(\mu_{jk}) = X^t_{jk}\beta + Z^t_{jk}b_j.$$

The final assumption on generalized linear mixed models is about the distribution for the random effects. It is common to assume that b_j follows a multivariate normal distribution with a mean vector of 0's and a covariance matrix D and is independent of covariates X_{jk}.

The primary difference between a generalized linear mixed model and a marginal model is that the former completely specifies the distribution of Y_j while the latter does not. It is also clear that the general linear mixed model is a special case of the generalized linear mixed models. However, the interpretations of regression parameters are also different between the marginal models and the generalized linear mixed models. Because the mean response and the within-subject association are modeled separately, the regression parameters in a marginal model are not affected by the assumptions on the within-subject associations, and therefore can be interpreted as population averages, i.e., they describe the mean response in the population and its relations with covariates. As an example, a marginal model can be used in a longitudinal study to examine the longitudinal trend on the probability of depression and to relate this probability to other covariates such as gender. Because Y_{jk} is binary and coded as 1 when depression occurs and 0 otherwise, the distribution of each Y_{jk} can be modeled through a logit-link function, i.e., the conditional expectation of Y_{jk}, given time (i.e., t_{jk}) and gender (coded numerically as GENDER), is $E(Y_{jk}|X_{jk}) = Pr(Y_{jk} = 1|X_{jk}) = \mu_{jk}$, and

$$\ln\left(\frac{\mu_{jk}}{1-\mu_{jk}}\right) = \beta_0 + t_{jk}\beta_1 + \text{GENDER}^*\beta_2.$$

The parameter β's here have the standard population averaged interpretations. β_2 is the log odds ratio of depression between the two genders at a given time point, and β_1 is the log odds ratio of depression for each unit increase of time for a given gender. On the other hand, in a generalized linear mixed model with time (i.e., t_{jk}) and gender through the same logit link, assuming a random coefficient for the intercept and the regression coefficient (i.e., the slope) before time,

$$\ln\left(\frac{P(Y_{jk}=1|b_j,\text{GENDER})}{1-P(Y_{jk}=1|b_j,\text{GENDER})}\right) = \beta_0 + t_{jk}\beta_1 + \text{GENDER}^*\beta_2 + b_{0j} + t_{jk}b_{1j},$$

where $(b_{0j}, b_{1j})^t$ follows a bivariate normal distribution. The regression parameters β's now describe the subject-specific mean response and its association with covariates. β_1 is the subject-specific log odds ratio of depression for each unit increase of time because $(b_{0j}, b_{1j})^t$, the random effects from the individual, and gender are fixed for the subject. The interpretation of β_2 has to be extrapolated because gender is a between-subject covariate and it is impossible to change it within a subject. Therefore, β_2 can only be interpreted as the log odds ratio of depression between two subjects of different genders who happen to have exactly the same random effects $(b_{0j}, b_{1j})^t$. A SAS code to implement the above generalized linear mixed effects model is given below:

```
PROC GLIMMIX DATA = ; CLASSES ID GENDER;
MODEL DEPRESSION = GENDER TIME/DIST = BINOMIAL
LINK = LOGIT;
RANDOM INT TIME/SUBJECT = ID TYPE = UN;
RUN;
```

Much of the difference in the interpretation of the regression parameters between a marginal model and a generalized linear mixed effects model is due to the fact that the former directly specifies $E(Y_{jk}|X_{jk})$, whereas the latter specifies $E(Y_{jk}|X_{jk}, b_j)$ instead. When there is an identical link, both approaches become equivalent based on the fact $E(Y_{jk}|X_{jk}) = E_{b_j}[E(Y_{jk}|X_{jk}, b_j)]$, and the interpretation of regression parameters in the generalized linear mixed model can also be made in terms of population averages. When the link function is non-linear, however, the interpretations for the regression parameters in generalized linear mixed models are distinct from those in the marginal models. These distinctions allow different scientific questions to be addressed in longitudinal biomedical studies. Because of the subject-specific feature on the regression coefficients at least to within-subject covariates or time-varying covariates, the generalized linear mixed effects models are most useful when the primary scientific objective is to make inferences about individuals rather than the population averages in the longitudinal studies.

2.5. *Missing data issues*

Missing data arise in the analysis of longitudinal data whenever one or more of the sequences of measurements from subjects within the study are incomplete, in the sense that the intended measurements are not taken, are lost, or are otherwise unavailable. Missing data occur in almost all longitudinal studies, and they cause not only technical difficulties in the analysis of such data, but also deeper conceptual issues as one has to ask why the measurements are missing, and more specifically whether their being missing has any bearing on the practical and scientific objectives to be addressed by the data. A general treatment of statistical analysis with missing data along with a hierarchy of missing data mechanisms (MDM) has been proposed (Little and Rubin, 2002). MDM is classified as missing completely at random (MCAR), missing at random (MAR), or non-ignorable (NI). These are generally described in a designed study which calls for k planned observations on each subject but lesser than k are actually observed.

Let $Y_j = (y_{j1}, y_{j2}, \ldots, y_{jk})^t$ be the vector of planned longitudinal measurements for the variable of interest on the jth subject over k time points. Let $I_j = (I_{j1}, I_{j2}, \ldots, I_{jk})^t$ be the vector of indicators of observations with $I_{ji} = 1$ if the ith measurement is actually observed and $I_{ji}=0$ otherwise. Let X_j be the vector of covariates on the jth subject, and let $f(Y_j|X_j,\beta)$ be the conditional density of Y_j given X_j and a set of parameters β, and let $f(I_j|Y_j,X_j,\psi)$ be the conditional density of I_j given (Y_j,X_j,ψ), where ψ is the parameters associated with missing data. The missing responses are said to be MCAR if

$$f(I_j|Y_j,X_j,\psi)=f(I_j|X_j,\psi),$$

i.e., given the covariates X_j, the probability of missingness does not depend on $Y_j=(y_{j1},y_{j2},\ldots,y_{jk})^t$, observed or not. This simply implies that the missingness is the results of a chance mechanism that does not depend on either observed or unobserved components of $Y_j=(y_{j1},y_{j2},\ldots,y_{jk})^t$. With missing data MCAR, it can be mathematically proved that the joint distribution of these observed y_{ji}'s is the same as the ordinary marginal distribution of these observed from Y_j. This then implies that the observed y_{ji}'s are just random samples of y_{ji}'s, and thus essentially any method of analysis will yield valid statistical inferences as long as the distribution satisfies the assumptions under which the method is justified. In a longitudinal study, if dropout from the study is not related to any factors under study, the missingness is considered MCAR.

The missing responses are said to be MAR if

$$f(I_j|Y_j,X_j,\psi)=f(I_j|Y_j^{\mathrm{o}},X_j,\psi),$$

where Y_j^{o} is the observed vector of $Y_j=(y_{j1},y_{j2},\ldots,y_{jk})^t$. The MAR implies that given the covariates, the probability of missingness depends only on the observed y_{ji}'s, but not on the missing values. With missing data MAR, it is no longer true that the joint distribution of these observed y_{ji}'s is the same as the marginal distribution of these observed from Y_j. However, it can be concluded that the contribution of the jth subject to the full likelihood as a function of β is proportional to the ordinary marginal distribution of these observed from Y_j as long as β and ψ do not share any parameters, or in another word, are functionally distinct. The implication of this result is that, as far as the statistical inferences of β are concerned, any likelihood-based methods are still valid as long as the distribution satisfies the assumptions under which the method is justified. Examples of MAR include the cases when a study protocol requires that subjects be removed from the study once the value of an outcome variable falls outside of a normal range, which implies that the missingness is related to the observed components only. In summary, whether missing data are MCAR or MAR, standard likelihood procedures can be applied to the observed data without worrying about the effect of missing to the validity of the statistical inferences. It is in this sense that both MCAR and MAR are called ignorable.

The missing responses are said to be NI or not missing at random (NMAR) if $f(I_j|Y_j,X_j,\psi)$ depends on the missing data, although it may or may not depend on Y_j^{o}. In a longitudinal study of cognitive function for Alzheimer's patients, the missing responses are NI if patients are not able to complete the cognitive and psychometric tests because their cognition is severely impaired. Several other examples of NI can also be found in Diggle and Kenward (1994). With missing data NI, special attention should be paid to the case when non-likelihood-based statistical inferential procedures are used. Likelihood-based inferential procedures can still be used, but generally this can only be done with the specification of the MDM. The validity of such likelihood-based inference methods depends on the validity of these specifications of MDM, $f(I_j | Y_j, X_j, \psi)$, which are generally not verifiable based on the collected data. NI missingness is also sometimes called informative, indicating the crucial role of the MDM in the analyses of this type of missing data. Other approaches have also been available in the literature that tried to relax the requirement on the precise specification of MDM when missingness is NI. Little (1993) discussed pattern-mixture models, a broad class of models that do not require precise specification of the MDM. Little and Wang (1996) extended the simple pattern-mixture model developed in Little (1994) to repeated-measures data with covariates. Little (1995) developed a model-based framework for repeated-measures data with dropouts, and placed existing literature within this framework.

The details on the analyses of missing data can be found in Little and Rubin (2002). Little and Raghunathan (1999) compared ML and summary measures approaches to longitudinal data with dropouts in a simulation study. There is also an important distinction between intermittent missing and dropout in the analysis, where the latter refers only to missing all measurements after a certain time point. If the intermittent missing values arise from a known censoring mechanism, for example, if all values below a known threshold are missing, the EM algorithm (Dempster et al., 1977) provides a possible theoretical framework for the analysis, but practical implementation for a realistic range of longitudinal data seems to be rather difficult (Laird, 1988). When the intermittent missing values do not arise from censoring, it may be reasonable to assume that they arise from mechanisms unrelated to the measurement process, and therefore are MCAR or MAR. In such cases, all likelihood-based inferences would be valid. Dropouts do not arise as a result of censoring mechanism applied to individual measurements. Often a subject's withdrawal is for reasons directly or indirectly related to the measurement process. Methods are also proposed for the statistical test of MDM (Diggle, 1989; Ridout, 1991; Cochran, 1977; Barnard, 1963). The modeling of the dropout process (Diggle and Kenward, 1994; Wu and Carroll, 1988; Wu and Bailey, 1989) highlights the practical implications of the distinctions between MCAR, MAR, and informative dropouts and provides a possible framework for routine analysis of longitudinal data with dropouts. Although complete generality in dealing with missing values in longitudinal data is not available as yet, one should be very aware of the fact that in general likelihood-based inferences will no longer be valid when the MDM is NI. The sensitivity analysis has also been recommended as a necessary step to help the analysis of missing data.

3. Design issues of a longitudinal study

In this section we focus on the response variables which are of continuous type, although the case when the longitudinally measured response variable is binary or ordinal can be worked out in a similar fashion.

As stated earlier, the major objective of a longitudinal study is to study the rate of change over time on response variables. There are different designs that can be used when planning a longitudinal study. The determination of sample sizes and the corresponding statistical powers are some of the most important issues when designing a longitudinal study. The answers to these questions depend on several factors: the primary hypotheses/objectives of the study, the statistical models used for analyzing the longitudinal data, the significance level of the primary statistical test or the confidence level of the confidence interval estimate to the rate of change over time, the statistical power desired for a statistical test, or the degree of accuracy in the confidence interval estimate to the rate of change. Most of times, analysis of response profiles, repeated measures analysis of variance, and the general linear mixed models are the major statistical models used for determining the sample sizes of longitudinal studies when the primary outcome variable is of continuous type.

When no parametric forms are assumed for the mean response profiles which are estimated and compared based on the analysis of response profiles or the repeated measures analysis of variance, the methods of sample size determination can be based on the standard analysis of response profiles and repeated measures analysis of variance. In a longitudinal study to compare multiple treatment groups over time, if repeated measures analysis of variance is used under the assumption that the covariance matrices of the measurement errors of the time intervals and the error terms of the subjects assigned to a given study conditions satisfy the H–F condition (Huynh and Feldt, 1970), the sample size determination can be further based on the F-tests or t-tests from a standard two-way analysis of variance (Chow and Liu, 2003) based on appropriate statistical tests on the primary hypothesis of the study. We consider here several types of longitudinal studies which are analyzed by the general linear mixed effects models in which a linear growth curve over time is assumed, one is to estimate the rate of change over time, and the other is to compare two subject groups on the rate of change over time.

Case 1. Estimating a single rate of change over time.

The simplest longitudinal study design is an observational study for which study subjects are followed for a certain period of time. This type of longitudinal study can be used to estimate the rate of change for the outcome variable over a certain time period. In many of these observational studies, the most important objective is to achieve an accurate estimate to the rate of change over time on some important measures for a population of subjects. Suppose that a sample of size n will be used in the study for which each subject is planned to take k repeated measures of the response variable at time points $t_1, t_2, \ldots, t_k$. Let $Y_j = (y_{j1}, y_{j2}, \ldots, y_{jk})^t$ be the vector of longitudinal measurements of the jth subject. For simplicity, we assume that changes in the mean response can be modeled by a linear trend over time and therefore the slope over time can be used to describe the rate of change. The major objective here is to obtain an accurate confidence interval estimate to the mean slope over time for the population of subjects under study. Recall that the two-stage random effects model assumes an individual growth curve for each subject at Stage 1

$$Y_{ji} = \beta_{0j} + \beta_{1j}t_i + e_{ji},$$

where e_{ji}'s are assumed to be independent and identically distributed as a normal distribution with mean 0 and variance σ_e^2. At Stage 2, the subject-specific rates of change β_{1j}'s are assumed to follow another normal distribution with mean β_1 and variance σ_b^2 and are independent of e_{ji}'s (the distribution of β_{0j} need not be used here). The major interest is in the estimation of mean change of rate β_1 in the population. The simple least square estimate to the subject-specific rate of change for the jth subject is

$$\hat{\beta}_{1j} = \frac{\sum_{i=1}^{k}(t_i - \bar{t})Y_{ji}}{\sum_{i=1}^{k}(t_i - \bar{t})^2},$$

where $\bar{t} = \Sigma_{i=1}^{k} t_i/k$. Notice that $\hat{\beta}_{1j}$ follows a normal distribution with mean β_1 and variance σ^2, where

$$\sigma^2 = \sigma_e^2 \left\{ \sum_{i=1}^{k}(t_i - \bar{t})^2 \right\}^{-1} + \sigma_b^2.$$

Therefore a $100(1-\alpha)\%$ $(0<\alpha<1)$ confidence interval for β_1 based on a sample of size n is $\bar{\beta}_1 \pm z_{\alpha/2}(\sigma/\sqrt{n})$, where

$$\bar{\beta}_1 = \frac{\sum_{j=1}^{n} \hat{\beta}_{1j}}{n}.$$

This gives the sample size required for achieving a confidence interval estimate of β_1 with a margin of error $\pm\delta$ as

$$n = \frac{(z_{\alpha/2}\sigma)^2}{\delta^2}.$$

If the longitudinal study is unbalanced or incomplete in which different study subjects may have different design vectors of times or even different number of time points, similar sample size formula could be derived under certain convergence assumptions on the design vectors of times.

Case 2. Estimating the difference of two rates of change over time.

A comparative longitudinal study compares the longitudinal courses of one or more response variables over two or more techniques, treatments, or levels of a covariate. In many clinical trials that evaluate the efficacy of one or more therapeutic treatments for a disease such as AD, a comparative longitudinal design is likely used to compare the treatments with placebo on the rate of change over time for a primary endpoint. Here we consider estimating the difference on the rates of change for the primary endpoint between the treated group and the placebo. The random coefficients model in this case assumes that the subject-specific slope β_{1j} follows a normal distribution with mean β_t and variance σ_{bt}^2 when the subject belongs to the treated group and another normal distribution with mean β_c and variance σ_{bc}^2 when the subject belongs to the control group. Similar to Case 1, when the subject belongs to the treated group, $\hat{\beta}_{1j}$ follows a normal distribution with mean β_t and variance σ_t^2, where

$$\sigma_t^2 = \sigma_e^2 \left\{ \sum_{i=1}^{k} (t_i - \bar{t})^2 \right\}^{-1} + \sigma_{bt}^2.$$

When the subject belongs to the control group, $\hat{\beta}_{1j}$ follows another normal distribution with mean β_c and variance σ_c^2, where

$$\sigma_c^2 = \sigma_e^2 \left\{ \sum_{i=1}^{k} (t_i - \bar{t})^2 \right\}^{-1} + \sigma_{bc}^2.$$

Therefore a $100(1-\alpha)\%$ $(0<\alpha<1)$ confidence interval for the difference $\beta_t - \beta_c$ on the mean rates of change over time between the treated group and the control group is $\bar{\beta}_t - \bar{\beta}_c \pm z_{\alpha/2}\sqrt{(\sigma_t^2/n_t) + (\sigma_c^2/n_c)}$, where

$$\bar{\beta}_i = \frac{\sum_{j=1}^{n_i} \hat{\beta}_{1j}}{n_i}$$

for $i =$ t, c, and n_t, n_c are the sample size for the treated group and the control group, respectively. Let $\lambda = n_t/n_c$ be the sample size ratio between two subject groups. This confidence interval also yields the sample sizes for the two study groups required for achieving a confidence interval estimate of $\beta_t - \beta_c$ with a margin of error $\pm\delta$ as

$$n_c = \left(\frac{\sigma_t^2}{\lambda} + \sigma_c^2 \right) \left(\frac{z_{\alpha/2}}{\delta} \right)^2,$$

and $n_t = \lambda n_c$.

Case 3. Testing a hypothesis on the difference of two rates of change over time.

Along the similar arguments made in Case 2, the test statistic for testing $H_0 : \beta_t = \beta_c$ against $H_a : \beta_t - \beta_c = \Delta \neq 0$ is

$$z = \frac{\bar{\beta}_t - \bar{\beta}_c}{\sqrt{(\sigma_t^2/n_t) + (\sigma_c^2/n_c)}}.$$

The test statistic follows a standard normal distribution when the null hypothesis is true. The test therefore rejects the null hypothesis when $|z|>z_{\alpha/2}$ at a significance level of α $(0<\alpha<1)$. The power of the test, as a function of Δ is given by

$$P(\Delta) = 1 - \Phi\left(z_{\alpha/2} - \frac{\Delta}{\sqrt{(\sigma_{\rm t}^2/n_{\rm t}) + (\sigma_{\rm c}^2/n_{\rm c})}} \right) + \Phi\left(-z_{\alpha/2} - \frac{\Delta}{\sqrt{(\sigma_{\rm t}^2/n_{\rm t}) + (\sigma_{\rm c}^2/n_{\rm c})}} \right).$$

Therefore, the sample sizes required to achieve a statistical power of $(1-\gamma)(0<\gamma<1)$ is the solution to $n_{\rm t}$ and $n_{\rm c}$ such that

$$P(\Delta) = 1 - \gamma.$$

Notice that in all these sample size formulas, the length of the study, the number of repeated measures on the response variable, and the time spacing of the repeated measures all impact the statistical power through the quantity

$$f(t_1, t_2, \ldots, t_k) = \sum_{i=1}^{k} (t_i - \bar{t})^2.$$

Because this quantity is inversely related to the variance of the estimated subject-specific rate of change over time, the larger the quantity is, the smaller the variance for the estimated subject-specific slope is, the more accurate the confidence interval estimates to the mean slopes are, and the more powerful the statistical test is for comparing the two mean rates of changes over time between the treated group and the control group. Therefore, an optimal design should in theory maximize the quantity $f(t_1, t_2, \ldots, t_k)$ over the choice of $k, t_1, t_2, \ldots, t_k$. Notice that $t_k - t_1$ is the entire duration of the study. Although theoretically it should be chosen to maximize $f(t_1, t_2, \ldots, t_k)$, many economic and logistic and subject matters factors constrain the choice of $t_k - t_1$. In addition, the validity of the assumed statistical model also constrains the choice of $t_k - t_1$ in the sense that a linear growth over time might not be a reasonable assumption with a very long study duration, which is especially the case in the study of cognitive decline in Alzheimer's patients. Similarly, the number of repeated measures in a longitudinal study might also be constrained by many practical factors and cannot be freely chosen by the designers of the study. As a result, many longitudinal studies are restricted to relatively short duration with a predetermined number of repeated measures which is not chosen statistically based on an optimal design. Given that $t_k - t_1$ and k are typically chosen by some non-statistical reasons, the optimal design now relies on the choice of time spacing to maximize $f(t_1, t_2, \ldots, t_k)$. It can be mathematically proved that with an even k, $f(t_1, t_2, \ldots, t_k)$ is maximized when $k/2$ observations are taken at baseline t_1 and the other $k/2$ taken at the final time point t_k for each study subject. This mathematically optimal design, however, is not only impractical in many longitudinal studies but also completely erases the ability of verifying the validity of the linear growth curve based on the collected data. Therefore optimal longitudinal designs are sometimes based on further assumptions on the spacing of design vector of times. For example, if the researchers would want to design an equally spaced longitudinal study, then

$$f(t_1, t_2, \ldots, t_k) = \frac{(t_k - t_1)^2 k(k+1)}{12(k-1)}.$$

This function indicates the relevant influence of $t_k - t_1$ and k on the sample size computations. In general, if the linear growth curve is a valid statistical model and that the logistic and practical factors allow, an increase of either the study duration or the frequency of repeated measures will decrease the within-subject variability and improve the precision of parameter estimates or the statistical power in the test on the rate of change over time.

Missing data almost always happen in longitudinal studies. In general, the impact of missing data on sample size determination is difficult to quantify precisely because of the complexity in the patterns of missingness. The simplest conservative approach to account for the missing data in sample size determination is to first compute the sample sizes required assuming all subjects have the complete data, and then adjust the sample sizes based on an estimated rate of attrition accordingly.

Acknowledgements

The work was supported by National Institute on Aging grants AG 03991 and AG 05681 (for C.X. and J.P.M.) and AG 025189 (for C.X.). The work of K.Z. was supported by the National Natural Science Foundation, Grant # 70275101, of People's Republic of China.

References

Anderson, D.A., Aitkin, M. (1985). Variance component models with binary response: Interviewer variability. *Journal of the Royal Statistical Society, Series B* **47**, 203–210.

Barnard, G.A. (1963). Contribution to the discussion of professor Bartlett's paper. *Journal of the Royal Statistical Society, Series B* **25**, 294.

Box, G.E.P. (1954). Some theorems on quadratic forms applied in the study of analysis of variance problems. *Annals of Mathematical Statistics* **25**, 290–302.

Breslow, N.E., Clayton, D.G. (1993). Approximate inference in generalized linear mixed models. *Journal of the American Statistical Association* **88**, 9–25.

Chow, S.-C., Liu, J.-P. (2003). *Design and Analysis of Clinical Trials: Concepts and Methodologies*. Wiley, New York.

Cochran, W.G. (1977). *Sampling Techniques*. Wiley, New York.

Crystal, H., Dickson, D., Fuld, P., Masur, D., Scott, R., Mehler, M., Masdeu, J., Kawas, C., Aronson, M., Wolfson, L. (1988). Clinico-pathologic studies in dementia: Nondemented subjects with pathologically confirmed Alzheimer's disease. *Neurology* **38**, 1682–1687.

Cullis, B.R., McGilchrist, C.A. (1990). A model for the analysis of growth data from designed experiments. *Biometrics* **46**, 131–142.

Dempster, A.P., Laird, N.M., Rubin, D.B. (1977). Maximum likelihood from incomplete data via the EM algorithm (with discussion). *Journal of the Royal Statistical Society, Series B* **39**, 1–38.

Diggle, P.J. (1988). An approach to the analyses of repeated measures. *Biometrics* **44**, 959–971.

Diggle, P.J. (1989). Testing for random dropouts in repeated measurement data. *Biometrics* **45**, 1255–1258.

Diggle, P.J. (1990). *Time Series: A Biostatistical Introduction*. Oxford University Press, Oxford.

Diggle, P.J., Heagerty, P., Liang, K.-Y., Zeger, S.L. (2002). *Analysis of Longitudinal Data*, 2nd ed. Oxford University Press, New York.

Diggle, P.J., Kenward, M.G. (1994). Informative dropout in longitudinal data analysis (with discussion). *Applied Statistics* **43**, 49–93.

Evans, D.A., Funkenstein, H.H., Albert, M.S., Scheer, P.A., Cook, N.C., Chown, M.J., Hebert, L.E., Hennekens, C.H., Taylor, J.O. (1989). Prevalence of Alzheimer's disease in a community population of older persons: Higher than previously reported. *Journal of the American Medical Association* **262**, 2551–2556.

Fitzmaurice, G.M., Laird, N.M., Rotnitsky, A.G. (1993). Regression models for discrete longitudinal response (with discussion). *Statistical Science* **8**, 284–309.

Fitzmaurice, G.M., Laird, N.M., Ware, J.H. (2004). *Applied Longitudinal Analysis*. Wiley, Hoboken, NJ.

Gilmore, A.R., Anderson, R.D., Rae, A.L. (1985). The analysis of binomial data by a generalized linear mixed model. *Biometrika* **72**, 593–599.

Goldstein, H. (1991). Nonlinear likelihood approaches to variance component estimation and to related problems. *Journal of the American Statistical Association* **72**, 320–340.

Gourieroux, C., Monfort, A., Trognon, A. (1984). Pseudo-maximum likelihood methods: Theory. *Econometrica* **52**, 681–700.

Graybill, F.A. (1976). *Theory and Application of the Linear Model*. Wadsworth & Brooks, California.

Green, P.J. (1987). Penalized likelihood for general semi-parametric regression models. *International Statistical Review* **55**, 245–259.

Harville, D.A. (1977). Maximum likelihood approaches to variance component estimation and to related problems. *Journal of the American Statistical Association* **72**, 320–340.

Herbert, L.E., Scheer, P.A., Beckett, L.A., Albert, M.S., Pilgrim, D.M., Chown, M.J., Funkenstein, H.H., Evans, D.A. (1995). Age-specific incidence of Alzheimer's disease in a community population. *Journal of the American Medical Association* **273**, 1354–1359.

Hinde J. (1982). Compound Poisson regression models. In: Gilchrist R. (Ed.), *GLIM 82. Proceedings of the International Conference on Generalized Linear Models*. Springer, Berlin.

Huynh, H., Feldt, L.S. (1970). Conditions under which mean square ratios in repeated measures designs have exact F-distributions. *Journal of the American Statistical Association* **65**, 1582–1589.

James, W., Stein, C. (1961). Estimation with quadratic loss. *Proceedings of the Fourth Berkeley Symposium on Mathematical Statistics and Probability* **1**, 311–319.

Katzman, R., Terry, R., DeTeresa, R., Brown, T., Davies, P., Fuld, P., Renbing, X., Peck, A. (1988). Clinical, pathological and neurochemical changes in dementia: A subgroup with preserved mental status and numerous neocortical plaques. *Annals of Neurology* **23**, 138–144.

Korn, E.L., Whittemore, A.S. (1979). Methods for analyzing panel studies of acute health effects of air pollution. *Biometrics* **35**, 795–802.

Laird, N.M. (1978). Empirical Bayes methods for two-way tables. *Biometrika* **65**, 581–590.

Laird, N.M. (1988). Missing data in longitudinal studies. *Statistics in Medicine* **7**, 305–315.

Laird, N.M., Ware, J.H. (1982). Random-effects models for longitudinal data. *Biometrics* **38**, 963–974.

Liang, K.-Y., Zeger, S.L. (1986). Longitudinal data analysis using generalized linear models. *Biometrika* **73**, 13–22.

Liang, K.-Y., Zeger, S.L., Qaqish, B. (1992). Multivariate regression analyses for categorical data (with discussion). *Journal of the Royal Statistical Society, Series B* **54**, 3–40.

Lipsitz, S., Laird, N., Harrington, D. (1991). Generalized estimating equations for correlated binary data: Using odds ratios as a measure of association. *Biometrika* **78**, 153–160.

Little, R.J.A. (1993). Pattern-mixture models for multivariate incomplete data. *Journal of the American Statistical Association* **88**, 125–134.

Little, R.J.A. (1994). A class of pattern-mixture models for normal missing data. *Biometrika* **81**(3), 471–483.

Little, R.J.A. (1995). Modeling the drop-out mechanism in longitudinal studies. *Journal of the American Statistical Association* **90**, 1112–1121.

Little, R.J.A., Raghunathan, T.E. (1999). On summary-measures analysis of the linear mixed-effects model for repeated measures when data are not missing completely at random. *Statistics in Medicine* **18**, 2465–2478.

Little, R.J.A., Rubin, D.B. (2002). *Statistical Analysis with Missing Data*, 2nd ed. Wiley, New York.

Little, R.J.A., Wang, Y.-X. (1996). Pattern-mixture models for multivariate incomplete data with covariates. *Biometrics* **52**, 98–111.

McCullagh, P., Nelder, J.A. (1989). *Generalized Linear Models*, 2nd ed. Chapman & Hall, London.

McGilchrist, C.A., Aisbett, C.W. (1991). Restricted BLUP for mixed linear models. *Biometrical Journal* **33**, 131–141.

Milliken, G.A., Johnson, D.E. (1992). *Analysis of Messy Data, Volume 1: Designed Experiments*. Chapman & Hall/CRC, New York.

Milliken, G.A., Johnson, D.E. (2001). *Analysis of Messy Data, Volume 3: Analysis of Covariance*. Chapman & Hall/CRC, New York.

Molenberghs, G., Verbeke, G. (2005). *Models for Discrete Longitudinal Data*. Springer, New York.

Morris, J.C. (1993). The clinical dementia rating (CDR): Current version and scoring rules. *Neurology* **43**, 2412–2414.

Morris, J.C., MeKeel, D.W., Storandt, M., Rubin, E.H., Price, L., Grant, E.A., Ball, M.J., Berg, L. (1991). Very mild Alzheimer's disease: Informant-based clinical, psychometric and pathologic distinction from normal aging. *Neurology* **41**, 469–478.

Patterson, H.D., Thompson, R. (1971). Recovery of inter-block information when block sizes are unequal. *Biometrika* **58**, 545–554.

Prentice, R.L. (1988). Correlated binary regression with covariates specific to each binary observation. *Biometrics* **44**, 1033–1048.

Ridout, M. (1991). Testing for random dropouts in repeated measurement data. *Biometrics* **47**, 1617–1621.

SAS Institute, Inc. (1999). *SAS/STAT User's Guide, Version 8*, vols. 1–5. SAS Publishing, Cary, NC.

Satterthwaite, F.E. (1946). An approximate distribution of estimates of variance components. *Biometrics Bulletin* **2**, 110–114.

Singer, J.D., Willett, J.B. (2003). *Applied Longitudinal Data Analysis: Modeling Change and Event Occurrence*. Oxford University Press, New York.

Stern, R.D., Coe, R. (1984). A model fitting analysis of daily rainfall data (with discussion). *Journal of the Royal Statistical Society, Series A* **147**, 1–34.

Stiratelli, R., Laird, N.M., Ware, J.H. (1984). Random effects models for serial observations with dichotomous response. *Biometrics* **40**, 961–972.

Storandt, M., Grant, E.A., Miller, J.P., Morris, J.C. (2002). Rates of progression in mild cognitive impairment and early Alzheimer disease. *Neurology* **59**, 1034–1041.

Thall, P.F., Vail, S.C. (1990). Some covariance models for longitudinal count data with overdispersion. *Biometrics* **46**, 657–671.

Tsay, R. (1984). Regression models with time series errors. *Journal of the American Statistical Association* **79**, 118–124.

Tunnicliffe-Wilson, G. (1989). On the use of marginal likelihood in time series model estimation. *Journal of the Royal Statistical Society, Series B* **51**, 15–27.

Verbeke, G., Molenberghs, G. (2000). *Linear Mixed Models for Longitudinal Data*. Springer, New York.

Verbyla, A.O., Cullis, B.R. (1990). Modeling in repeated measures experiments. *Applied Statistics* **39**, 341–356.

Vonesh, E.F., Carter, R.L. (1992). Mixed effect nonlinear regression for unbalanced repeated measures. *Biometrics* **48**, 1–18.

Wong, W.H. (1986). Theory of partial likelihood. *Annals of Statistics* **14**, 88–123.

Wu, M.C., Bailey, K.R. (1989). Estimation and comparison of changes in the presence of informative right censoring: Conditional linear model. *Biometrics* **45**, 939–955.

Wu, M.C., Carroll, R.J. (1988). Estimation and comparison of changes in the presence of right censoring by modeling the censoring process. *Biometrics* **44**, 175–188.

Zeger, S.L., Liang, K.Y. (1986). Longitudinal data analysis for discrete and continuous outcomes. *Biometrics* **42**, 121–130.

Zeger, S.L., Liang, K.Y., Self, S.G. (1985). The analysis of binary longitudinal data with time-dependent covariates. *Biometrika* **72**, 31–38.

Zeger, S.L., Qaqish, B. (1988). Markov regression models for time series: A quasi-likelihood approach. *Biometrics* **44**, 1019–1031.

Zhao, L.P., Prentice, R.L. (1990). Correlated binary regression using a generalized quadratic model. *Biometrika* **77**, 642–648.

Handbook of Statistics, Vol. 27
ISSN: 0169-7161

DOI: 10.1016/S0169-7161(07)27015-4

15

Design and Analysis of Cross-Over Trials

Michael G. Kenward and Byron Jones

Abstract

This chapter provides an overview of recent developments in the design and analysis of cross-over trials. We first consider the analysis of the trial that compares two treatments, A and B, over two periods and where the subjects are randomized to the treatment sequences AB and BA. We make the distinction between fixed and random effects models and show how these models can easily be fitted using modern software. Issues with fitting and testing for a difference in carry-over effects are described and the use of baseline measurements is discussed. Simple methods for testing for a treatment difference when the data are binary are also described. Various designs with two or more treatments but with three or four periods are then described and compared. These include the balanced and partially balanced designs for three or more treatments and designs for factorial treatment combinations. Also described are nearly balanced and nearly strongly balanced designs. Random subject-effects models for the designs with two or more treatments are described and methods for analysing non-normal data are also given. The chapter concludes with a description of the use of cross-over designs in the testing of bioequivalence.

1. Introduction

In a completely randomized, or parallel group, trial, each experimental unit is randomized to receive one experimental treatment. Such experimental designs are the foundation of much research, particularly in medicine and the health sciences. A cross-over trial is distinguished from such a parallel group study by each unit, or subject, receiving a *sequence* of experimental treatments. Typically however the aim is still to compare the effects of individual treatments, not the sequences themselves. There are many possible sets of sequences that might be used in a design, depending on the number of treatments, the length of the sequences and the aims of the trial.

A cross-over trial allows the calculation of *within-subject* treatment comparisons and so is able to make such comparisons with comparatively high precision, provided the response being measured is at least moderately highly correlated within an individual subject. This potential gain in precision comes with a price however. Obviously such a design cannot be used with treatments that irreversibly change the subject, such as treatments that are curative. Once treatment has ceased, the subject must return to the original condition, at least approximately. Hence there is always the possibility when using such a design that some consequence of earlier treatment may still be influential later in the trial. In the cross-over context this is called a *carry-over* effect. This potential source of bias is akin to confounding in an epidemiological study and implies that to some extent the analysis of data from a cross-over trial will inevitably rely more on assumptions and modelling, and less directly on the randomization, than a conventional parallel group study.

This issue is particularly apparent in the so-called *two-period two-treatment* or 2×2 design. This is the simplest, and arguably the most commonly used design, in a clinical setting. In this design each subject receives two different treatments which we conventionally label as A and B. Half the subjects are randomized to receive A first and then, after a suitably chosen period of time, *cross over* to B. The remaining subjects receive B first and then cross over to A. Because this particular design is so commonly used, and because it raises very special issues in its own right, we devote the next section of this chapter specifically to it. There are many other so-called *higher-order* designs, with more than two periods, and/or treatments and/or sequences and we consider the choice of such designs and the analysis of continuous data from such designs in Section 3. Data from cross-over trials are examples of repeated measurements and so raise special issues when analysed with non-linear models, in particular those commonly used with binary and categorical data. This has not always been properly appreciated when alternative models have been used for analysing cross-over data, and when results are compared with those from parallel group studies. We consider the analysis of such non-normal data in Section 4, together with some issues surrounding this. Recent developments in the design of cross-over trials are addressed in Section 6. Two standard references for cross-over trials are Jones and Kenward (2003) and Senn (2002), and recent reviews are given in Kenward and Jones (1998) and Senn (1997, 2000).

Cross-over data are examples of repeated measurements. Consequently, a key concept in the design and analysis of cross-over trials is that of *between-subject* and *within-subject* information. This is most easily conceptualized for continuous responses. Between-subject information is that contained in the total (or mean) of the measurements from a subject, while within-subject information is that contained among all differences among measurements from a subject.

This is reflected in the use of *subject-effect models*. We introduce these now for use in later sections, and to set out the notation we will be using.

For a cross-over trial we will denote by t, p and s, respectively, the number of treatments, periods and sequences. So for example, in a trial in which each subject received three treatments A, B and C, in one of the six sequences: ABC, ACB,

BAC, BCA, CAB and CBA, we have $t = 3, p = 3$ and $s = 6$. In general, we denote by y_{ijk} the response observed on the kth subject in period j of sequence group i. It is assumed that n_i subjects are in sequence group i. To represent sums of observations we will use the dot notation, for example:

$$y_{ij.} = \sum_{k=1}^{n_i} y_{ijk}, \quad y_{i..} = \sum_{j=1}^{p} y_{ij.}, \quad y_{...} = \sum_{i=1}^{s} y_{i..}.$$

In a similar way, the corresponding mean values will be denoted, respectively as,

$$\bar{y}_{ij.} = \frac{1}{n_i}\sum_{k=1}^{n_i} y_{ijk}, \quad \bar{y}_{i..} = \frac{1}{pn_i}\sum_{j=1}^{p} y_{ij.}, \quad \bar{y}_{...} = \frac{1}{p\sum n_i}\sum_{i=1}^{s} y_{i..}.$$

To construct a statistical model we assume that y_{ijk} is the observed value of a random variable Y_{ijk}. For a continuous outcome we assume that Y_{ijk} can be represented by a linear model that, in its most basic form, can be written

$$Y_{ijk} = \mu + \pi_j + \tau_{d[i,j]} + s_{ik} + e_{ijk}, \tag{1}$$

where the terms in this model are:

μ, an intercept;
π_j, an effect associated with period j, $j = 1, \ldots, p$;
$\tau_{d[i,j]}$, a direct treatment effect associated with the treatment applied in period j of sequence i, $d[i,j] = 1, \ldots, t$;
s_{ik}, an effect associated with the kth subject on sequence i, $i = 1, \ldots, s$, $k = 1, \ldots, n_i$;
e_{ijk}, a random error term, with zero mean and variance σ^2.

Sometimes we need to represent a potential carry-over effect in the model. A simple first-order carry-over effect (that is, affecting the outcome in the following period only) will be represented by the term $\lambda_{d[i,j-1]}$ where it is assumed that $\lambda_{d[i,0]} = 0$. Additional terms such as second-order carry-over and direct treatment-by-period interaction effects can be added to this model, but such terms are rarely of much interest in practice.

An important distinction needs to be made between those models in which the subject effects (the s_{ik}) are assumed to be unknown fixed parameters and those in which they are assumed to be realizations of random variables, usually with zero mean and variance σ_s^2. The use of the former implies that the subsequent analysis will use information from within-subject comparisons only. This is appropriate for the majority of well-designed cross-over trials and has the advantage of keeping the analysis within the familiar setting of linear regression. There are circumstances, however, in which the subject totals contain relevant information and this can only be recovered if the subject effects are treated as random. Such a model is an example of a linear mixed model and the use of these introduces some additional issues: properties of estimators and inference procedures are asymptotic (possibly requiring small-sample adjustments), and an additional assumption is needed for the distribution of the random subject effects.

Model fitting and inference for fixed subject-effect models will follow conventional ordinary least squares (OLS) procedures and for random subject-effect models we will use the now well-established restricted maximum likelihood (REML) analyses for linear mixed models (see, for example, Verbeke and Molenberghs, 2000). These analyses can be done relatively simply in several widely available software packages, examples are SAS procs MIXED and GLIMMIX, Stata command xtmixed, Splus lme, MLwiN and, for Bayesian analysis, Win-BUGS (references for all of these are given at the end of this chapter). The two SAS procedures have the advantage of incorporating the small sample adjustments introduced by Kenward and Roger (1997). Cross-over trials can be very small in practice, and it is in such settings that small sample procedures may be relevant.

2. The two-period two-treatment cross-over trial

In this section, we consider the two-period two-treatment or so-called 2×2 cross-over trial. The simplicity of this design, and its relevance for trials with two treatments, has led to its widespread use in a clinical setting. This simplicity of design, however, does mask some important issues which discuss below.

2.1. An example

First, we introduce a comparatively simple illustrative example of such a trial which is taken from Jones and Kenward (2003, Chapter 2). This was a single-centre, randomized, placebo-controlled, double-blind study to evaluate the efficacy and safety of an inhaled drug (A) given twice daily via an inhaler in patients with chronic obstructive pulmonary disease (COPD). Patients who satisfied the initial entry criteria entered a two-week run-in period. Clinic Visit 1 is used to denote the start of this period. After 13 days they returned to the clinic for a histamine challenge test (Clinic Visit 2). On the following day (Clinic Visit 3) they returned to the clinic and following a methacholine challenge test, eligible patients were randomized to receive either Drug (A) or matching Placebo (B) twice daily for four weeks. The patients then switched over at Clinic Visit 5 to the alternative treatment for a further four weeks. The patients also returned to the clinic a day before the end of each treatment period (Clinic Visits 4 and 6) when repeat histamine challenge tests were performed. There was a final clinic visit two weeks after cessation of all treatment (Clinic Visit 8). Patients were instructed to attend the clinic at approximately the same time of day for each visit.

The primary comparison of efficacy was based on the mean morning expiratory flow rate (PEFR) obtained from data recorded on daily record cards. Each day patients took three measurements of PEFR on waking in the morning, and at bedtime, prior to taking any study medication. On each occasion the highest of the three readings was recorded.

Of a total of 77 patients recruited into the study, 66 were randomized to treatment (33 per sequence group). Ultimately, data on the mean morning PEFR

Table 1
Group 1(AB) mean morning PEFR (L/min)

Subject Number	Subject Label	Period 1	Period 2
1	7	121.9	116.7
2	8	218.5	200.5
3	9	235.0	217.1
4	13	250.0	196.4
5	14	186.2	185.5
6	15	231.6	221.8
7	17	443.2	420.5
8	21	198.4	207.7
9	22	270.5	213.2
10	28	360.5	384.0
11	35	229.7	188.2
12	36	159.1	221.9
13	37	255.9	253.6
14	38	279.0	267.6
15	41	160.6	163.0
16	44	172.1	182.4
17	58	267.0	313.0
18	66	230.7	211.1
19	71	271.2	257.6
20	76	276.2	222.1
21	79	398.7	404.0
22	80	67.8	70.3
23	81	195.0	223.2
24	82	325.0	306.7
25	86	368.1	362.5
26	89	228.9	227.9
27	90	236.7	220.0

Source: Table reproduced from Jones and Kenward (2003) with the permission of the publisher.

(over the treatment days in each period) from 56 patients were obtained: 27 in the AB group and 29 in the BA group. The data from the patients in the AB sequence group are given in Table 1, and the data from the BA sequence group are given in Table 2.

The corresponding group-by-period means are given in Table 3.

2.2. The direct treatment effect

We consider first the analysis of these data under the assumption that there is no carry-over effect, sequence effect or treatment-by-period interaction. Using the notation introduced earlier we can write a simple linear model for these data:

$$Y_{ijk} = \mu + \pi_j + \tau_{d[i,j]} + s_{ik} + e_{ijk}, \quad i = 1, 2; \quad j = 1, 2, \tag{2}$$

where $k = 1, \ldots, 27$ in group 1 (AB) and $k = 1, \ldots, 29$ in group 2 (BA). In this design, with this model, *all* the information on the treatment difference $\tau_d = \tau_1 - \tau_2$ is within-subject. This implies that it is irrelevant for the analysis whether we use

Table 2
Group 2(BA) mean morning PEFR (L/min)

Subject Number	Subject Label	Period 1	Period 2
1	3	138.3	138.6
2	10	225.0	256.2
3	11	392.9	381.4
4	16	190.0	233.3
5	18	191.4	228.0
6	23	226.2	267.1
7	24	201.9	193.5
8	26	134.3	128.9
9	27	238.0	248.5
10	29	159.5	140.0
11	30	232.7	276.6
12	32	172.3	170.0
13	33	266.0	305.0
14	39	171.3	186.3
15	43	194.7	191.4
16	47	200.0	222.6
17	51	146.7	183.8
18	52	208.0	241.7
19	55	208.7	218.8
20	59	271.4	225.0
21	68	143.8	188.5
22	70	104.4	135.2
23	74	145.2	152.9
24	77	215.4	240.5
25	78	306.0	288.3
26	83	160.5	150.5
27	84	353.8	369.0
28	85	293.9	308.1
29	99	371.2	404.8

Source: Table reproduced from Jones and Kenward (2003) with the permission of the publisher.

Table 3
The group-by-period means for the mean PEFR data

Group	Period 1	Period 2	Mean
1(AB) $n_1 = 27$	$\bar{y}_{11.} = 245.84$	$\bar{y}_{12.} = 239.20$	$\bar{y}_{1..} = 242.52$
2(BA) $n_2 = 29$	$\bar{y}_{21.} = 215.99$	$\bar{y}_{22.} = 230.16$	$\bar{y}_{2..} = 223.08$
Mean	$\bar{y}_{.1.} = 230.38$	$\bar{y}_{.2.} = 234.52$	$\bar{y}_{...} = 232.45$

Source: Table reproduced from Jones and Kenward (2003) with the permission of the publisher.

fixed or random subject effects. The least squares estimator of τ_d is

$$\hat{\tau}_d = \frac{1}{2}\left(\bar{y}_{11\cdot} - \bar{y}_{12\cdot} - \bar{y}_{21\cdot} + \bar{y}_{22\cdot}\right)$$

This is the treatment estimator adjusted for period effect. It is sometimes suggested that a simple unadjusted estimator can be used, possibly after testing for period effect. Given that the trial is designed to allow adjustment for period differences, and given that sequential testing procedures are best avoided where possible, such an approach is not recommended. The variance of the treatment estimator is

$$\mathrm{V}(\hat{\tau}_d) = \frac{\sigma_d^2}{4}\left(\frac{1}{27}+\frac{1}{29}\right)$$

for σ_d^2 the variance of a within subject difference $Y_{i1k}-Y_{i2k}$. That is, in terms of the earlier definitions, $\sigma_d^2 = 2\sigma^2$. This is estimated in the usual way from a regression residual mean square or pooled variance. Inference about τ_d then uses the conventional t based pivot

$$\frac{\tau_d - \hat{\tau}_d}{\sqrt{\hat{\mathrm{V}}(\hat{\tau}_d)}} \sim t_{54}.$$

In the present example we have $\hat{\tau}_d = 10.40$ and $\mathrm{V}(\hat{\tau}_d) = 11.66$. Hence a 95% confidence interval for the average treatment difference is given by

$$10.40 \pm \sqrt{11.66} \times 2.01 \quad \text{or} \quad (3.55,\ \ 17.25).$$

Such statistics are very simply calculated by applying standard t test and confidence interval calculations to the within-subject differences. As an aside, note that because this test can be formulated as a t test, conventional sample size calculations can be used in the 2×2 cross-over setting, provided the variance used corresponds to *within-subject* differences.

For the calculated confidence interval we see that there is some evidence that treatment A, the active drug, is producing greater average lung function.

2.3. Carry-over/treatment-by-period interaction

This analysis above is based on the important assumption that treatment-by-period interaction, carry-over and sequence effects are all negligible. The latter effect should be removed through randomization. The first two effects, while conceptually separate, cannot be distinguished in this design. Suppose that we introduce carry-over into the model. We might use the following extension of (2):

$$Y_{ijk} = \mu + \pi_j + \tau_{d[i,j]} + \lambda_{d[i,j-1]} + s_{ik} + e_{ijk}, \quad i = 1,2; \quad j = 1,2. \tag{3}$$

It is easily shown that the least squares estimator of the carry-over effect $\lambda = \lambda_1 - \lambda_2$ is then equal to the difference of the subject means:

$$\hat{\lambda} = \frac{1}{2}\left(\bar{y}_{11\cdot} + \bar{y}_{12\cdot} - \bar{y}_{21\cdot} - \bar{y}_{22\cdot}\right).$$

This is based wholly on *between-subject* information, so to derive this estimator it must be assumed that the subject effects are *random.* If instead in (3) a treatment-by-period interaction were introduced:

$$Y_{ijk} = \mu + \pi_j + \tau_{d[i,j]} + (\pi\tau)_{jd_{[i,j]}} + s_{ik} + e_{ijk}, \quad i = 1,2; \quad j = 1,2, \tag{4}$$

the least squares estimator of the interaction effect

$$\{(\pi\tau)_{11} - (\pi\tau)_{12} - (\pi\tau)_{21} + (\pi\tau)_{22}\}$$

would be proportional to $\hat{\lambda}$ above. Thus, the two quantities, carry-over and treatment-by-period interaction, are aliased in this particular design. This is not a general rule. In higher-order designs such effects may be partially aliased or separately estimable.

The variance of $\hat{\lambda}$ is

$$\mathrm{V}(\hat{\lambda}) = \sigma_B^2\left(\frac{1}{27} + \frac{1}{29}\right)$$

for σ_B^2 the variance of a *subject sum* $Y_{i1k} + Y_{i2k}$ or $2\sigma^2 + 4\sigma_s^2$. t-based inferences can be made as in the same way as for the treatment effect but based on the subject sums rather than the differences. Here we obtain a 95% confidence interval for λ of (−43.33, 121.17).

2.4. Preliminary testing and its problems

The existence of a test for the key assumption of carry-over/interaction led early users to suggest making a preliminary test for this before proceeding to the comparison of the direct treatment effects (Grizzle, 1965). The proposed procedure is as follows. Depending on the result of the carry-over test, one of two different estimates for a direct treatment difference is used. If the test for a carry-over difference is not significant, then the t-test above, based on the within-subject differences is used. If the carry-over test is significant, then the two treatments are compared using only the Period 1 data, as in a parallel groups design. That is, using a two-sample t-test comparing the mean of A in Period 1 with the mean of B in Period 1. This test uses between-subject information, and so negates the advantages of using a cross-over design.

A first objection to this procedure is the lack of power of the carry-over test. The ratio of variances of the carry-over and treatment estimators can be written

$$R = 2 + \frac{\rho}{1-\rho}$$

for ρ the within-subject (intraclass) correlation $\sigma_s^2/(\sigma^2 + \sigma_s^2)$. Cross-over trials are suited to settings in which this correlation is large and will typically be powered for the treatment comparison. The resulting power of the carry-over test will then be very low indeed. For example, in the COPD trial $\hat{\rho} = 0.945$, giving $\hat{R} = 19.2$, implying that the carry-over test is effectively useless. It has been suggested that because of the low power of this test, it should be made at a less stringent level, for example 10%. Not only is this typically insufficient to bring the power up to a worthwhile level, this whole sequential procedure has a more fundamental problem, as pointed out by Freeman (1989). Because of the dependence between the preliminary test for carry-over and the first period comparison, the sequential procedure leads to both bias in the resultant treatment estimator and increases the probability of making a Type I error. In other words, the actual significance level of the direct treatment test is higher than the nominal one chosen for the test. Although attempts have been made to circumvent this problem, there is no solution that does not involve introducing information about the carry-over/treatment-by-period interaction that is not contained in the data. Given that a cross-over trial will be powered for within-subject estimation of the treatment effect and so will *not* have the sensitivity to provide useful information on the carry-over/treatment-by-period interaction, arguably the best approach to the problem is to take all practical steps to avoid possible carry-over such as using wash-out periods of adequate length between the treatment periods and then assume that this effect is negligible in the analysis. This in turn requires a good working knowledge of the treatment effects, which will most likely be based on prior knowledge of the drugs under study, or ones known to have a similar action.

2.5. Use of baseline measurements

In many studies *baseline measurements* are collected at the end of the run-in and wash-out periods. Because of the within-subject nature of the analysis these baselines do not have the usual role familiar from parallel group studies. We label these X_1 and X_2, implying that there are now four measurements from each subject, i.e., from subject $(i,k):\{x_{i1k}, y_{i1k}, x_{i2k}, y_{i2k}\}$. In an obvious way we can write a simple model for the expectations of these variables:

Group 1 (AB)	Group 2(BA)
$E(X_{11k}) = \mu - \pi_1$	$E(X_{21k}) = \mu + \pi_1$
$E(Y_{11k}) = \mu - \pi_2 - \tau$	$E(Y_{21k}) = \mu + \pi_2 + \tau$
$E(X_{12k}) = \mu - \pi_3 - \theta$	$E(X_{22k}) = \mu + \pi_3 + \theta$
$E(Y_{12k}) = \mu - \pi_4 + \tau - \lambda$	$E(Y_{22k}) = \mu + \pi_4 - \tau + \lambda$

The parameters μ, π_j, τ and λ are as defined above. The final parameter θ represents carry-over from the treatment period that is apparent at the end of the wash-out period. In more general terms, θ represents any difference between groups of the second baseline means and λ any direct-by-period interaction, whether due to carry-over differences or not. There are many ways in which effects can arise which are aliased with these two parameters. Some authors set $\pi_1 = \pi_2$ and $\pi_3 = \pi_4$. Unless the treatment periods are very short compared with the wash-out period there seems little justification for this.

It is important at this point to distinguish two types of baseline. (1) The four measurements may be fairly evenly spaced in time with similar correlations between them. (2) Alternatively, the baselines may be made "close" to the response measurements, relative to the gap between the treatment periods, and change from these may even be defined as the primary response measurement. Given the choice of using or not using the baseline measurements, which route should be taken? This is most easily answered by considering the analysis of change from baseline, rather than full covariate adjustment. The question then becomes, under what circumstances is it more efficient to analyse change from baseline rather than the response (Y) observations only? The answer depends on the relative sizes of the correlations within periods and between periods.

We could postulate the following covariance matrix for the four measurements $\{X_1, Y_1, X_2, Y_2\}$:

$$\sigma^2 \begin{bmatrix} 1 & \rho_1 & \rho_3 & \rho_5 \\ \rho_1 & 1 & \rho_2 & \rho_4 \\ \rho_3 & \rho_2 & 1 & \rho_1 \\ \rho_5 & \rho_4 & \rho_1 & 1 \end{bmatrix}$$

Without using baselines, the variance of a within-subject difference is

$$V = \sigma^2(1 - \rho_4).$$

With baselines, the corresponding variance is

$$V_B = 4\sigma^2(2 - 2\rho_1 - \rho_4 - \rho_3 + \rho_2 + \rho_5).$$

If all the correlations were equal (to $\rho > 0$ say, as would be implied by a random subject effects model)

$$V_B = 4\sigma^2(1 - \rho) = 2V.$$

In other words introducing the baselines *doubles* the variance of the treatment estimator. To have smaller variance using the baselines we would need:

$$V > V_B$$

After some re-arranging, we see that this implies

$$2\rho_1 + \rho_3 > 1 + \rho_2 + \rho_5.$$

This will be true only when the correlations between response and preceding baseline (ρ_1) and between the two baselines (ρ_3) tend to be large relative to the other correlations, as in case (2) above.

Using the baselines as covariates will modify this conclusion to some extent, but the main picture does not alter. For a full discussion see for example Kenward and Jones (1987).

A simple rule therefore is to ignore baselines for estimating the direct treatment effect, unless we know that they will be particularly highly correlated with the associated response measurement (because of the timing of the baseline measurements for example). The reason we gain so little from baseline measurements in the cross-over setting is that we are already using within-subject information and so the baselines are not required to explain between-subject variation as in a parallel group trial. Further, the concept of presenting effects in terms of change from baseline is less meaningful here as the treatment estimator is already a within-subject comparison.

The baselines do provide additional information on the two carry-over parameters θ and λ however, in particular allowing the latter to be estimated using within-subject information. Details are given in Jones and Kenward (2003, Section 2.10). However, any attempt to use these in a sequential procedure is likely to run into the same difficulties as those seen earlier.

2.6. Analysis of binary data

A *binary observation* can take only two values, traditionally labelled 0 and 1; examples are no/yes, failure/success and no effect/effect. In keeping with standard practice we shall refer to the responses 1 and 0 as a success and a failure, respectively, and we shall refer to a 2×2 cross-over with binary data as a binary 2×2 cross-over. The design of the trial will take exactly the same form as before: the subjects are divided into Groups 1 and 2 (treatment orders AB and BA, respectively) and we assume that we have a single observation that takes the value 0 or 1 from each subject in each period.

Consider the following example of safety data from a trial on the disease cerebrovascular deficiency in which a placebo (A) and an active drug (B) were compared (Jones and Kenward, 2003, Section 2.13). A 2×2 design was used at each of two centres, with 33 and 67 subjects, respectively, at each centre. The response measured was binary and was defined according to whether an electrocardiogram was considered by a cardiologist to be normal (1) or abnormal (0). In such a trial each subject supplies a pair of observations (0,0), (0,1), (1,0) or (1,1) where *(a,b)* indicates a response *a* in Period 1 and *b* in Period 2. We can therefore summarize the data from one 2×2 trial in the form of a 2×4 contingency table as follows for centre 1:

Group	(0,0)	(0,1)	(1,0)	(1,1)	Total
1(AB)	6	2	1	7	16
2(BA)	4	2	3	8	17
Total	10	4	4	15	33

Table reproduced from Jones and Kenward (2003) with the permission of the publisher.

Several tests can be defined in terms of this table, here we focus on two: the analogues of the two *t*-tests presented earlier for direct treatment effect and for carry-over effect/treatment-by-period interaction. As before we first will make the assumption that the latter are negligible. We can associate with each entry in the 2×4 table a probability ρ_{ij}:

Group	(0,0)	(0,1)	(1,0)	(1,1)	Total
1(AB)	ρ_{11}	ρ_{12}	ρ_{13}	ρ_{14}	1
2(BA)	ρ_{21}	ρ_{22}	ρ_{23}	ρ_{24}	1
Total	$\rho_{.1}$	$\rho_{.2}$	$\rho_{.3}$	$\rho_{.4}$	2

The odds in favour of a (1,0) response in Group 1 as opposed to a (0,1) response is the ratio of probabilities ρ_{13}/ρ_{12}. If there were no carry-over difference or direct treatment effect we ought to get the same odds in Group 2, i.e., ρ_{23}/ρ_{22}. If these two odds were not equal this would indicate that there was a direct treatment effect. A natural way to express this effect is as the ratio of the odds

$$\phi_\tau = \frac{\rho_{23}/\rho_{22}}{\rho_{13}/\rho_{12}} = \frac{\rho_{12}\rho_{23}}{\rho_{13}\rho_{22}}.$$

This is just the odds-ratio in the 2×2 contingency table with probabilities proportional to these:

	(0,1)	(1,0)
Group 1	ρ_{12}	ρ_{13}
Group 2	ρ_{22}	ρ_{23}

In the absence of a direct treatment effect there should be no evidence of association in this table. This points to a test for the direct treatment effect in terms of the following 2×2 contingency table:

	(0,1)	(1,0)	Total
Group 1	n_{12}	n_{13}	m_1
Group 2	n_{22}	n_{23}	m_2
Total	$n_{.2}$	$n_{.2}$	$m.$

where $m_1 = n_{12}+n_{13}$ and $m_2 = n_{22}+n_{23}$. To test for this association we can apply the standard tests for a 2×2 contingency table to this table, where evidence of association indicates a direct treatment effect. This is known as the *Mainland–Gart* test. Mainland (1963, pp. 236–238) derived this test using a heuristic argument based on the randomization of subjects to groups, while Gart (1969) gave a rigorous derivation in which he conditioned on subject effects in a linear logistic model for each individual observation in each period. We return to this view later.

For centre 1 we have the following:

	(0,1)	(1,0)	Total
Group 1	2	1	3
Group 2	2	3	5
Total	4	4	8

Any conventional test for association can be used with such a table, but in the light of the very small numbers we might use *Fisher's exact test* for this particular example. Unsurprisingly, given the small numbers, the test for direct treatment effect is far from significant.

Omitting the derivation, which is less direct than for the Mainland–Gart test, the corresponding test for carry-over/treatment-by-period interaction is given by the test for association in the 2×2 table of *non-preference* responses:

	(0,0)	(1,1)	Total
Group 1	n_{11}	n_{14}	M_1
Group 2	n_{21}	n_{24}	M_2
Total	$n_{.3}$	$n_{.3}$	$M.$

As with a continuous response, such a test will typically have very low power for trials that are powered for the direct treatment effect.

Both these tests can be derived from a more general framework that we consider later when we present models and analyses for higher-order designs, which will also point the way to analyses for count, for ordinal and for nominal categorical data. The advantage of these two tests is their great simplicity.

3. Higher-order designs

3.1. Higher-order two-treatment designs

As seen in Section 2, the 2×2 design without baselines does not permit a within-subjects estimator of the carry-over/treatment-by-period interaction to be obtained. However, if additional sequences and/or periods are used then this deficiency can be remedied. For example, extending the design to three periods means that the following three alternative designs with two sequences may be used: ABB/BAA; ABA/BAB or AAB/BAA. Assuming the data from the trial are analysed using the linear model defined in (1) then all three designs are equivalent in the sense they all give the same estimator of the treatment difference. Suppose, however, that model (1) is extended to include the carry-over effects of the treatments given in periods $j = 2, 3, \ldots, p$, as follows:

$$Y_{ijk} = \mu + \pi_j + \tau_{d[i,j]} + \lambda_{d[i,j-1]} + s_{ik} + e_{ijk}, \tag{5}$$

where $\lambda_{d[i,j-1]}$ is the carry-over effect in period j of treatment $d[i,j-1]$ in period $j-1$.

Then the first design ABB/BAA is superior to the other two as it provides an estimator of the treatment difference with smallest variance (Jones and Kenward, 2003). Extending the design to four periods ultimately leads to a choice between the two equivalent designs (under model (1)): AABB/BBAA and ABBA/BAAB. The latter of these has the further advantage of allowing estimation of the second-order carry-over difference, although this is unlikely to be of importance in practice, when care has been taken to allow sufficient wash-out time between the periods. Both designs ABB/BAA and ABBA/BAAB are useful designs to use when testing for bioequivalence, as we will mention in Section 5. Other two-period designs with more than two sequences are described in some detail in Jones and Kenward (2003, Chapter 3).

Of course, the merits of the alternative designs depend on the model assumed for the carry-over effects. We have assumed a simple additive model. For a criticism of this simple model see Fleiss (1986, 1989). For further discussion see Senn and Lambrou (1998) and Senn (2002).

3.2. Higher-order designs with more than two treatments

When there are three or more treatments there will be more than one possible contrast between the treatment effects. The type and number of contrasts of interest will determine the choice of design that should be used. For example, suppose $t = 4$ and all six pairwise comparisons between the treatments are of interest. Then a variance-balanced design will be the ideal choice, because in such a design the variance of every estimated pairwise comparison is equal to the same constant value. Such a design is given in Table 4, which is an example of a so-called Williams design (Williams, 1949). To calculate the variance of a treatment contrast we assume here, and in the following, that the fixed-effects model (5) holds. It should be noted that all the designs considered in this section permit the treatment contrasts to be estimated using within-subject information and in the presence of differential carry-over effects. The Williams designs also possess combinatorial balance in the sense that every treatment follows every other treatment (except itself) the same number of times. Williams designs can be constructed for every value of t: when t is even the design contains t different treatment sequences and when t is odd the design contains $2t$ different sequences. Variance-balanced designs for odd t that contain only t different sequences exist for some values of t, e.g., $t = 9$, 15 and 27. A design is variance-balanced and strongly balanced in the combinatorial sense if every treatment follows every other treatment (including itself) the same number of times. A simple way to construct such designs is to repeat the last treatment of each sequence in a Williams design. An algorithm for constructing Williams designs was given by Sheehe and Bross (1961). Williams designs are special cases of sequentially counter balanced Latin squares and Isaac et al. (2001) describe a range of methods for constructing such designs.

Table 4
Williams design for four treatments

Subject	Period			
	1	2	3	4
1	A	D	B	C
2	B	A	C	D
3	C	B	D	A
4	D	C	A	B

Table 5
"Nearly" balanced latin square design for five treatments

Subject	Period				
	1	2	3	4	5
1	A	B	C	D	E
2	B	D	E	C	A
3	C	E	B	A	D
4	D	C	A	E	B
5	E	A	D	B	C

To fill the gap when sequentially counter balanced squares do not exist for odd t, Russell (1991) gave a method for constructing "nearly" sequentially counter balanced squares. In these squares each treatment is preceded by all but two treatments once, by one of the remaining two twice and not at all by the remaining treatment. An example of such a design for $t = 5$ is given in Table 5.

As already noted, William's designs for odd t require $2t$ sequences (except in a few special cases). To provide additional designs for odd t Newcombe (1996) gave designs for $3t$ sequences, made up of three $\times t$ Latin squares, such that the sequences formed a balanced design. Prescott (1999) later gave a systematic method of construction of these designs.

The above methods have filled in the gaps left by the Williams designs when the aim is to construct a balanced design. Bate and Jones (2006) described methods of constructing "nearly strongly balanced" designs to fill the gaps where no strongly balanced designs exist.

Often when t is bigger than 4 or 5, it will not be possible to use a design with p periods. In this situation it may be possible to use a variance-balanced (incomplete block) design. Jones and Kenward (2003, Chapter 4) provide a large table of variance-balanced designs for $3 < t < 9$, for $p < t$, $p = t$ and $p > t$.

When a variance-balanced design does not exist for given values of t, p and s, then a useful alternative may be to use a partially balanced design. In these designs the variances of the pairwise treatment comparisons are not all equal. There are various ways of constructing such designs and some of these are described by Jones and Kenward (2003, Chapter 4), who also provide a table of the most useful ones for $t < 9$.

Software to calculate the efficiency of an arbitrary cross-over trial has been given by Jones and Lane (2004).

When the treatment structure is such that not all pairwise comparisons are of interest more appropriate designs may exist. For example, control-balanced designs are suitable for the situation where one treatment (say a control) is to be compared to all the other treatments. Factorial designs are suitable when the treatments are structured and made up of the combinations of the levels of two or more factors. For example, the four treatments in a clinical trial may be made up of the combinations of the high and low doses of two different drugs. The

Table 6
Trial on intermittent claudication, design and LVET measurements (ms)

Subject	Sequence	Period			
		1	2	3	4
1	PBCA	590	440	500	443
2	ACPB	490	290	250	260
3	CABP	507	385	320	380
4	BPAC	323	300	440	340
5	PABC	250	330	300	290
6	ABCP	400	260	310	380
7	CPAB	460	365	350	300
8	BCPA	317	315	307	370
9	PBCA	430	330	300	370
10	CBAP	410	320	380	290
11	CAPB	390	393	280	280
12	ACBP	430	323	375	310
13	PBAC	365	333	340	350
14	APBC	355	310	295	330

Source: Table reproduced from Jones and Kenward (2003) with the permission of the publisher.

combination is of interest because there may be a synergistic effect when both drugs are used together.

Although, the theory of optimal design construction is well developed for the standard additive model (5) and a few variants (see Stufken, 1996; Afsarinejad and Hedayat, 2002), there are situations where the theory needs to be replaced by computer search algorithms. One useful example of such an algorithm has been described by John et al. (2004).

3.3. Simple analyses for higher-order designs

To illustrate the conventional least squares regression analysis of a design with four treatments we will use the data given in Table 6, which are taken from Jones and Kenward (2003). These data were obtained in a trial that compared the effects of three active drugs A, B, C and a placebo P on blood flow, cardiac output and an exercise test on subjects with intermittent claudication. The trial was a single-centre, double-blind trial in which each treatment period lasted a week and there was a 1-week wash-out period between the active periods. There was no run-in period. One of the observations taken at the end of each treatment period was left ventricular ejection time (LVET) and the values recorded on each subject are given in Table 6. Note that no sequence occurs more than once.

The results obtained from fitting the *fixed-effects model* (5) are given in Table 7. The conclusions that may be drawn are that B and C are no different to Placebo, but A gives a significant improvement over placebo.

3.4. Random subject effects models

One consequence of using fixed subjects effects, as done in the previous section, is that all treatment information contained in the subject totals is discarded. For the

Table 7
Conventional analysis with fixed subject effects

Effect	Estimate	SE	DF	t	P
A–P	47.31	16.52	36	2.86	0.007
B–P	−18.70	16.70	36	−1.12	0.270
C–P	24.52	16.52	36	1.48	0.147

Source of Variation	NDF	DDF	F-test	P
Subjects	13	36	4.65	<0.001
Period	3	36	7.87	<0.001
Treatment	3	36	6.02	0.002

typical well-designed higher-order trial there will be little information lost and so this is usually a sensible route to take. To recover the information in the subject totals we need to introduce random subject effects. Because such analyses introduce extra assumptions and the use of approximations in the inference procedures as well, we need to be sure that this extra step is worthwhile, i.e., it should be considered only when a substantial amount of information is contained in the subject totals and this will be true, for example, for incomplete designs in which $p < t$. The 2×2 design is an extreme example in which *all* the information on carry-over effects is contained in the subject totals.

Recall that the model for random subject effects is identical to that introduced earlier (5):

$$Y_{ijk} = \mu + \pi_j + \tau_{d[i,j]} + s_{ik} + e_{ijk},$$

with the exception that the subject effects s_{ik} are now assumed to be random draws from some distribution, typically the normal, with variance σ_s^2 say. For this random subjects model

$$V(Y_{ijk}) = \sigma^2 + \sigma_s^2$$

and

$$\mathrm{Cov}(Y_{ijk}, Y_{ij'k}) = \sigma_s^2, \quad \text{for all} \quad j \neq j'.$$

In other words, assuming a *random subjects model* is equivalent to imposing a specific covariance structure on the set of measurements from one subject:

$$V\begin{bmatrix} Y_{i1k} \\ Y_{i2k} \\ \vdots \\ Y_{ipk} \end{bmatrix} = \begin{bmatrix} \sigma^2 + \sigma_s^2 & \sigma_s^2 & \cdots & \sigma_s^2 \\ \sigma_s^2 & \sigma^2 + \sigma_s^2 & \cdots & \sigma_s^2 \\ \vdots & \vdots & \ddots & \vdots \\ \sigma_s^2 & \sigma_s^2 & \cdots & \sigma^2 + \sigma_s^2 \end{bmatrix}.$$

This is called a *uniform, compound symmetry* or *exchangeable* covariance structure.

The introduction of the random effects means that this is no longer an example of a simple linear regression model, and ordinary least squares estimation and standard least squares theory no longer apply. Instead, a modified version of maximum likelihood is used for estimation, called *restricted maximum likelihood (REML)* (Patterson and Thompson, 1971). This can be thought of as a two stage procedure in which the variance components (σ^2 and σ_s^2) are first estimated from a marginal likelihood that does not depend on the fixed effects (period, treatment, etc.). The fixed effects are then estimated using generalized least squares with the covariance matrix constructed from the estimated variance components. In matrix terms, if $\mathbf{Y}$ is the vector of observations, with covariance matrix Σ and expectation

$$\mathrm{E}(\mathbf{Y}) = \mathbf{X}\boldsymbol{\beta}$$

for $\mathbf{X}$ the design matrix and $\boldsymbol{\beta}$ the vector of fixed effects, then the REML estimator of $\boldsymbol{\beta}$ is

$$\tilde{\boldsymbol{\beta}} = \left(\mathbf{X}^T\hat{\boldsymbol{\Sigma}}^{-1}\mathbf{X}\right)^{-1}\mathbf{X}^T\hat{\boldsymbol{\Sigma}}^{-1}\mathbf{Y}$$

where $\hat{\Sigma} = \Sigma(\hat{\sigma}^2, \hat{\sigma}_s^2)$, for $\hat{\sigma}^2$ and $\hat{\sigma}_s^2$ the REML estimators of σ^2 and σ_s^2. Asymptotically, as the number of subjects increases,

$$\tilde{\boldsymbol{\beta}} \sim \mathrm{N}[\boldsymbol{\beta}, (\mathbf{X}^T\boldsymbol{\Sigma}^{-1}\mathbf{X})^{-1}].$$

These random subject analyses are examples of the *recovery of interblock information.* In such an analysis a weighted average is implicitly used that combines between- and within-subject estimates. The weights are equal to the inverse of the covariance matrices of the two vectors of estimates. If there is little information in the subject totals, recovery of this information is not worth the effort, and the amount of such information will depend on two things: the size of the between-subject variance (σ_s^2) relative to the within-subject variance (σ^2), often measured by the intraclass correlation, and the efficiency of the design. We need an inefficient design, a moderately small intraclass correlation and a sufficiently large number of subjects to make the procedure worthwhile. Otherwise it may even be counter-productive because the need to estimate the weights introduces extra variation into the combined estimate. In a very small trial these weights will be poorly estimated. Also, the simpler fixed subjects analysis is more robust as it does not require distributional assumptions for the random effects, and moving to the random effects analysis means moving from small sample inference based on exact distribution theory to methods of inference based on distributional approximations such as those in Kenward and Roger (1997). In conclusion, recovery of interblock information through random subject effects models should be considered *only* when there is likely to be a substantial benefit.

A further step in generalizing the assumptions underlying the dependence structure of the repeated measurements in a cross-over trial is to allow an *unstructured* covariance matrix. These ideas are developed in Jones and Kenward (Section 5.7). In small trials such analyses will typically be very inefficient and should be considered only when there are good reasons to expect large departures from homogeneity of variances and covariances in the repeated measurements. In a well-run trial this would be unusual, given that we are expecting as a basis for the treatment comparisons comparatively stable subject conditions throughout the period of the trial. It should also be noted that small trials do not provide much useful information of the assessment and comparison of covariance structures from the data. In the light of these points it is probably good practice in typical trials to assume a subject effects based model, with these either treated as random or fixed as appropriate.

Robust methods of analysis using permutation and bootstrap methods are also available, some examples are also given in Jones and Kenward (2003, Section 5.7).

4. Analysis with non-normal data

The analysis of *non-normal cross-over data* falls into the class of analyses of non-normal *clustered* or *dependent* data. Such analyses are much less straightforward than those for continuous data based on the linear model. There are two main reasons for this. First, there is no single "natural" choice of multivariate model in such settings to parallel the multivariate normal linear model. Second, for most problems in this class, it is appropriate to assume a *non-linear* relationship between the mean or expectation of an observation and the linear predictor with the various fixed effects (treatment, period, etc.). A recent treatment of the whole subject is given by Molenberghs and Verbeke (2005). Here we outline some common approaches to such analyses and draw attention to some of the key issues.

As in the analysis of continuous data, the aim of the analysis is to explain the variation in the observed responses in terms of period, treatment and possible other effects, such as carry-over. In the present setting we relate a linear model involving these effects to a function of the expectation of an observation. As before let Y_{ijk} be the response observed on subject k in group i in period j. We can write for a model with period and direct treatment effects

$$g\{\mathrm{E}(Y_{ijk})\} = \mu + \pi_j + \tau_{d[i,j]}. \tag{6}$$

The construction on the right-hand side of (6) is just the same as used earlier in Eq. (1) and the effects carry over their associations, although not their strict meanings.

The function relating the success probability to this linear component or *linear predictor* is represented by $g(\cdot)$. We term $g(\cdot)$ the link function, noting that some authors use this for its inverse. Typically the expectation will be a probability or rate. The use of the identity function would imply that the expectations are modelled directly on a linear scale. This is usually avoided in practice because it is typically not sensible to expect treatment or other effects to act additively across the whole range of such expectations. Common choices of the function for probabilities are the logit and probit which have a form for which the inverse is sigmoid in shape or the natural logarithm for rates.

To fix ideas we now consider the common and important example of a *binary* outcome, in which the expectation is a probability. The commonly used link functions have the added advantage of mapping values of the linear predictor to the appropriate (0,1) interval for probabilities. In other words, any calculable linear predictor will correspond to a genuine probability. This is not true when the probabilities are modelled on the linear scale. We note in passing that these sigmoid functions are fairly linear for probabilities between about 0.2 and 0.8, and if, for a particular example, the observed probabilities lie in this range then there is often little to choose between an analysis on the linear and transformed scales. Given the typical small size of cross-over trials there is also usually little practical difference among the functions mentioned above, and we will use the logit function almost exclusively in the following, pointing out where necessary if there is any restriction on the choice of link function for a particular analysis. Thus, the logit version of (6) can be written

$$\operatorname{logit}\{P(Y_{ijk}=1)\} = \ln\left\{\frac{P(Y_{ijk}=1)}{1-P(Y_{ijk}=1)}\right\} = \mu + \pi_j + \tau_{d[i,j]}$$

or equivalently,

$$E[Y_{ijk}] = P(Y_{ijk}=1) = \frac{e^{\mu+\pi_j+\tau_{d[i,j]}}}{1+e^{\mu+\pi_j+\tau_{d[i,j]}}}.$$

Effects in this model are *log odds-ratios*. To see this let $\pi_{d,j}$ be the probability that a randomly chosen subject responds with a 1 in period j under treatment d. Then the treatment effect $\tau_a - \tau_b$ can expressed as the log odds-ratio

$$\tau_a - \tau_b = \ln\left\{\frac{\pi_{a,j}/(1-\pi_{a,j})}{\pi_{b,j}/(1-\pi_{b,j})}\right\}. \tag{7}$$

This type of model has been termed *marginal* or *population averaged* (Zeger et al., 1988). The model determines the average success probability over all individuals from the population under consideration for the given covariate values (treatment, period and so on). It is marginal with respect to the observations in other periods. That is, the same model for the marginal probabilities would be used if different subjects were used in different periods (albeit without the need to allow for within-subject dependence as well). Such a model might be regarded as appropriate if, for example, we wished to present treatment effects in terms of such population averaged quantities. One objection to the use of such models in a *trial setting* is that the subjects rarely represent a random sample from any well-defined population and so the idea of averaging over this population, or making random draws from it, lacks credibility.

It turns out that likelihoods are difficult to construct for such marginal models in typical non-normal settings and in practice it is much easier to use non-likelihood methods. In particular methods based on *Generalized Estimating Equations* (Zeger and Liang, 1986; Liang and Zeger, 1986) are widely implemented in computer packages and commonly used.

The marginal model as presented above is not a complete one for the observations: it does not define the form of within-subject dependence. Hence, the marginal model cannot tell us the whole story about the comparative behaviour of one individual on different treatments, and this is particularly relevant if subgroups of individuals have quite different patterns of behaviour across the treatments in the trial. The marginal model would simply average over this behaviour and, when the link function is not the identity, the resulting marginal model can misrepresent the average behaviour in each subgroup. The likelihood of this actually occurring in practice depends on the particular setting, but does require rather large differences in the behaviour among the subgroups to have substantial impact. Models that directly address individual patterns of behaviour are termed *subject-specific*. A very simple subject-specific model that is often used in practice parallels the subject effects model used for continuous data (1) is as follows:

$$\text{logit}\{P(Y_{ijk} = 1|s_{ik})\} = \mu + \pi_j + \tau_{d[i,j]} + s_{ik}, \tag{8}$$

for s_{ik} an effect associated with the (ik)th subject. It is assumed that the observations from a subject are conditionally independent given the subject effect. Again is usually assumed that the subject effects follow a normal distribution. This is an example of a *generalized linear mixed model.* Such models are comparatively easy to fit using maximum likelihood. Although calculation of the likelihood requires integration over the distribution of the subject effects, this is relatively easy to accomplish in the cross-over setting using numerical integration, and a number of computer packages have facilities for fitting such models.

These two modelling approaches, *marginal* and *subject-specific*, are not the only ones available for the cross-over setting with non-normal data, but they are by far the most widely used in practice. Given the widespread use of both approaches it is important to understand the fundamental differences between them and between such methods and models for normally distributed outcomes. In the conventional linear model for which the expectation and linear predictor are on the same scale the parameters in both the marginal and subject-specific models have the same interpretation. The extra terms have implications for the error structure. With a non-identity link function this is no longer necessarily true and the corresponding parameters in (6) and (8) do not in general represent equivalent quantities. This also underlies the problem of averaging over disparate subgroups mentioned above in the context of marginal models. The parameters in the subject-specific model modify a particular subject's underlying probability, determined by s_{ik}. This does not mean, however, that functions of these subject-specific parameters cannot have an interpretation that applies globally. For example, within-subject odds-ratios will be the same for all subjects with common covariates. Extending the earlier notation, let $\pi_{a,j,s}$ be the probability that a subject with effect s under treatment a in period j responds with a 1. Then from (8)

$$\tau_a - \tau_b = \ln\left\{\frac{\pi_{a,j,s}/(1-\pi_{a,j,s})}{\pi_{b,j,s}/(1-\pi_{b,j,s})}\right\}, \tag{9}$$

which is the same for all s. But we do emphasize that this is not the same quantity as the marginal log odds-ratio in (7).

Marginal probabilities can be obtained from subject-specific ones by taking expectations over the distribution of the subject effects. In general, however, the model structure (linear additive model on a logit scale, for example) on which the subject-specific probabilities are based will not carry over to the resulting marginal probabilities. There are exceptions to this, and if normally distributed subject effects are used, then, to a close approximation for the logit link and exactly for the probit link, the marginal model will have the same structure with the parameters scaled downwards in absolute size. Neuhaus et al. (1991) show more generally that for any distribution of the subject effects there is a sense in which parameters are attenuated in the marginal model. Good discussions of the distinction between population-averaged and subject-specific models can be found in Diggle et al. (2002) and Molenberghs and Verbeke (2005) and Carlin et al. (2001) explore some issues with the conventional interpretation of subject-specific models for binary data.

An important implication of this is that we should not in general expect parameter estimates from analogous marginal and subject-specific models to coincide. This means that particular care needs to be taken when results are combined or compared from sets of trials containing a mix of parallel group and cross-over designs. A brief discussion of this in the context of meta-analyses is given by Elbourne et al. (2002).

5. Other application areas

An important area where cross-over trials are used is in the early phases of drug development within the pharmaceutical industry and in testing for bioequivalence of two drug formulations. Patterson and Jones (2006) give a comprehensive account of the use of cross-over designs in bioequivalence testing and in the following areas: clinical pharmacology safety studies, QTc assessment, clinical pharmacology safety studies and population pharmacokinetics. Here we will briefly describe and illustrate the use of bioequivalence trials.

During the development of a drug its formulation will change as it moves forward through the different phases of its development. In Phase I trials escalating doses of a drug are evaluated using healthy volunteers, and are often undertaken to establish the maximum tolerated dose. Once a safe range of doses has been established the drug moves into Phase II trials using small numbers of patients. Then, finally, once a safe and efficacious dose has been established the drug is tested in large numbers of patients in Phase III confirmatory trials. It is important that if changes are made to the formulation of a drug, the effect of a given dose using the new formulation is not different to that of the effect of the same dose using the previous formulation. The bioavailability of a drug is used as a surrogate for its effect. This is measured for a given dose by giving a healthy volunteer a dose of the formulation and taking blood samples at a number of time points after dosing. Each blood sample is assayed to determine the concentration of drug in the sample and the resulting concentrations are plotted against their corresponding sampling times. The area under this curve (the AUC) is taken as a surrogate for the amount of exposure or bioavailability of the drug in the body. Two different formulations are considered bioequivalent if they have similar bioavailability values. Often the marketed formulation of a drug is not the same as that used in the Phase III trials that were used to gain regulatory approval to market the drug. The formulation change is usually required in order to mass produce the drug in a commercially acceptable form, e.g., a tablet. To gain approval to market the drug the regulator must be convinced that the marketed dose is as efficacious and safe as the one used in the Phase III trial. This is typically done using a 2×2 cross-over trial with a small number of volunteers in each sequence group. Another important use of bioequivalence trials is when regulatory approval is sought for the sale of a generic version of an existing marketed drug. The generic must be shown to be bioequivalent to the original.

Suppose, for illustration, we consider the situation where the formulation used in a Phase III trial is to be compared to the formulation used in the marketed version of the drug. In order to gain regulatory approval that the two formulations are bioequivalent, equivalence has to be shown on two metrics: the AUC as already described and $C_{\max}$, the maximum concentration of drug in the blood (i.e., the peak of the concentration curve). To better satisfy the assumption that the analysed data are normally distributed, it is standard practice to analyse the transformed values, log(AUC) and $\log(C_{\max})$, rather than the original values. Similarity, or equivalence, for each of these metrics is defined by the United States Food and Drug Administration (FDA) as follows. Let μ_T denote the mean of log(AUC) of the Test formulation (i.e., the to-be-marketed formulation) and μ_R denote the mean of the Reference formulation (i.e., the formulation used in the Phase III trial). The two formulations are compared using the *TOST (two one-sided tests)* procedure in which each of the following two hypotheses is tested at the 5% level (Schuirmann, 1987). If both are rejected the two formulations are considered equivalent (on log(AUC) in this case).

$$H_{01} : \mu_T - \mu_R \leq -\Delta \tag{10}$$

versus the alternative

$$H_{11} : \mu_T - \mu_R > -\Delta$$

and

$$H_{02} : \mu_T - \mu_R \geq \Delta \tag{11}$$

versus the alternative

$$H_{02} : \mu_T - \mu_R < \Delta$$

where, for example, the FDA has set $\Delta = \log(1.25) = 0.2231$.

This would be repeated for $\log(C_{\max})$ and if the formulations were declared equivalent on both metrics they would be considered bioequivalent by the FDA.

As an illustrative example we consider Example 3.2 from Patterson and Jones (2006). There were 24 subjects who received the Reference (R) and Test (T) formulations in the order RT and 25 who received them in the reverse order TR. Only subjects that had data in both periods have been included in the bioequivalence analysis described here. See Patterson Jones (2006) for the analysis of all the data. The group-by-period means are given in Table 8.

It can be shown that an equivalent way of implementing the TOST procedure is to calculate a 90% two-sided confidence interval for $\mu_T - \mu_R$ for each metric. If both confidence intervals are entirely within the limits $(-\Delta, \Delta)$ then bioequivalence is declared. The results of doing this for our example are given in Table 9, where we have fitted model (1) and included only those subjects that had a data value in both periods. It can be seen that for $\log C_{\max}$ the confidence interval lies entirely within $(-\Delta, \Delta)$ but for log AUC the upper limit of the confidence interval is above Δ. Consequently T and R cannot be declared bioequivalent.

As mentioned in Section 3.1, three-period cross-over designs for two treatments are useful when testing for bioequivalence. This is in the situation where the drugs are highly variable and extra replication is needed to reduce the sample size

Table 8
Groups-by-periods means (sample size in brackets)

Group	Period 1	Period 2	Mean
log AUC			
1(RT)	$\bar{y}_{11.} = 4.55(22)$	$\bar{y}_{12.} = 4.60(22)$	$\bar{y}_{1..} = 4.57$
2(TR)	$\bar{y}_{21.} - 4.43(23)$	$y_{22.} = 4.28(23)$	$\bar{y}_{2..} = 4.35$
Mean	$\bar{y}_{.1.} = 4.49$	$\bar{y}_{.2.} = 4.43$	$\bar{y}_{...} = 4.46$
$\log C_{\max}$			
1(RT)	$\bar{y}_{11.} = 1.33(23)$	$\bar{y}_{12.} = 1.36(23)$	$\bar{y}_{1..} = 1.34$
2(TR)	$\bar{y}_{21.} = 1.27(24)$	$\bar{y}_{22.} = 1.19(24)$	$\bar{y}_{2..} = 1.23$
Mean	$\bar{y}_{.1.} = 1.30$	$\bar{y}_{.2.} = 1.27$	$\bar{y}_{...} = 1.29$

Table 9
TOST procedure results-log scale

Endpoint	$\hat{\mu}_T - \hat{\mu}_R$	90% Confidence Interval
log AUC	0.0970	(−0.0610, 0.2550)
$\log C_{\max}$	0.0508	(−0.0871, 0.1887)

Source: Table reproduced from Patterson and Jones (2006) with the permission of the publisher.

Table 10
RTT/TRR design: groups-by-periods means (sample size in brackets)

Group	Period 1	Period 2	Period 3	Mean
log AUC				
1(RTT)	$\bar{y}_{11.} = 4.35(46)$	$\bar{y}_{12.} = 4.36(45)$	$\bar{y}_{13.} = 4.60(43)$	$\bar{y}_{1..} = 4.43$
2(TRR)	$\bar{y}_{21.} = 4.66(47)$	$\bar{y}_{22.} = 4.88(47)$	$\bar{y}_{23.} = 4.92(47)$	$\bar{y}_{2..} = 4.82$
Mean	$\bar{y}_{.1.} = 4.51$	$\bar{y}_{.2.} = 4.63$	$\bar{y}_{.3.} = 4.77$	$\bar{y}_{...} = 4.63$
log C_{max}				
1(RTT)	$\bar{y}_{11.} = 1.18(47)$	$\bar{y}_{12.} = 1.10(47)$	$\bar{y}_{13.} = 1.46(45)$	$\bar{y}_{1..} = 1.24$
2(TRR)	$\bar{y}_{21.} = 1.39(48)$	$\bar{y}_{22.} = 1.60(48)$	$\bar{y}_{23.}. = 1.64(48)$	$\bar{y}_{2..} = 1.54$
Mean	$\bar{y}_{.1.} = 1.29$	$\bar{y}_{.2.} = 1.35$	$\bar{y}_{.3.} = 1.55$	$\bar{y}_{...} = 1.40$

Source: Table reproduced from Patterson and Jones (2006) with the permission of the publisher.

Table 11
Example 4.1: TOST procedure result for RTT/TRR design

	log Scale	
Endpoint	$\hat{\mu}_T - \hat{\mu}_R$	90% Confidence Interval
log AUC	−0.0270	(−0.1395, 0.0855)
log C_{max}	−0.0557	(−0.1697, 0.0583)

Source: Table reproduced from Patterson and Jones (2006) with the permission of the publisher.

to a manageable level. Patterson and Jones (2006) describe the analysis of data from a bioequivalence trial that used the design with sequences RTT and TRR. There were 47 subjects on the sequence RTT and 48 subjects on the sequence TRR. The group-by-period means are given in Table 10. As in the previous example not all subjects had a data value in all three periods.

The analysis proceeds as for the RT/TR design using the TOST procedure. The results are given in Table 11. It can be seen that T and R are bioequivalent as both confidence limits are within the regulatory bounds.

In conclusion, we note that cross-over trials are widely used in experimental research in a range of disciplines. Jones and Deppe (2000), for instance, give examples of the use of cross-over designs in psychology, pharmacokinetics and sensory testing.

6. Computer software

MLwiN: Centre for Multilevel Modelling, Institute of Education, 20 Bedford Way, London WC1 H 0AL, UK.

SAS: SAS Institute Inc., SAS Campus Drive, Cary, North Carolina 27513, USA.

Splus 6.1 for Windows: Insightful Corporation, 1700 Westlake Avenue N, Suite 500, Seattle, Washington 98109, USA.

Stata: Stata Corporation, 702 University Drive East, College Station, Texas 77840, USA.

WinBUGS: MRC Biostatistics Unit, Institute of Public Health, University Forvie Site, Robinson Way, Cambridge CB2 2SR, UK.

References

Afsarinejad, K., Hedayat, A.S. (2002). Repeated measurements designs for a model with self and simple mixed carryover effects. *Journal of Statistical Planning and Inference* **106**, 449–459.

Bate, S.T., Jones, B. (2006). The construction of nearly balanced and nearly strongly balanced uniform cross-over designs. *Journal of Statistical Planning and Inference* **136**, 3248–3267.

Carlin, J.B., Wolfe, R., Brown, C.H., Gelman, A. (2001). A case study on the choice interpretation and checking of multilevel models for longitudinal binary outcomes. *Biostatistics* **2**, 397–416.

Diggle, P.J., Heagerty, P., Liang, K.-Y., Zeger, S.L. (2002). *Analysis of Longitudinal Data*, 2nd ed. Oxford University Press, Oxford.

Elbourne, D.R., Altman, D.G., Higgins, J.P.T., Curtin, F., Worthington, H.V., Vail, A. (2002). Meta-analyses involving cross-over trials: Methodological issues. *International Journal of Epidemiology* **31**, 140–149.

Fleiss, J.L. (1986). Letter to the editor. *Biometrics* **42**, 449.

Fleiss, J.L. (1989). A critique of recent research on the two-treatment cross-over design. *Controlled Clinical Trials* **10**, 237.

Freeman, P. (1989). The performance of the two-stage analysis of two treatment, two period crossover trials. *Statistics in Medicine* **8**, 421–1432.

Gart, J.J. (1969). An exact test for comparing matched proportions in crossover designs. *Biometrika* **56**, 75–80.

Grizzle, J.E. (1965). The two-period change-over design and its use in clinical trials. *Biometrics* **21**, 467–480.

Isaac, P.D., Dean, A.M., Ostrom, T. (2001). Generating pairwise balanced Latin Squares. *Statistics and Applications* **3**, 25–46.

Jones, B., Deppe, C. (2000). Recent developments in the design of cross-over trials: A brief review and bibliography. *Proceedings of the Conference on Recent Developments in the Design of Experiments and Related Topics*, Nova Science.

Jones, B., Kenward, M.G. (2003). *Design and Analysis of Cross-Over Trials*, 2nd ed. Chapman & Hall/CRC, London.

Jones, B., Lane, P.W. (2004). Procedure XOEFFICIECY (Calculates efficiency of effects in cross-over designs). GenStat Release 7.1 Reference Manual, Part 3: Procedure Library PL15, VSN International, Oxford.

John, J.A., Russell, K.G., Whitaker, D. (2004). Crossover: An algorithm for the construction of efficient cross-over designs. *Statistics in Medicine* **23**, 2645–2658.

Kenward, M.G., Jones, B. (1987). The analysis of data from 2×2 cross-over trials with baseline measurements. *Statistics in Medicine* **6**, 911–926.

Kenward, M.G., Jones, B. (1998). Cross-over trials. In: Kotz, S., Banks, D.L., Read, C.B. (Eds.), *The Encyclopedia of Statistical Sciences*, Update, vol. II. Wiley, Chichester.

Kenward, M.G., Roger, J.H. (1997). Small sample inference for fixed effects estimators from restricted maximum likelihood. *Biometrics* **53**, 983–997.

Liang, K.-Y., Zeger, S.L. (1986). Longitudinal data analysis using generalized linear models. *Biometrika* **73**, 13–22.

Mainland, D. (1963). *Elementary Medical Statistics*, 2nd ed. Saunders, Philadelphia.

Molenberghs, G., Verbeke, G. (2005). *Models for Discrete Longitudinal Data*. Springer, New York.

Newcombe, R.G. (1996). Sequentially balanced three-squares cross-over designs. *Statistics in Medicine* **15**, 2143–2147.

Neuhaus, J.M., Kalbfleisch, J.D., Hauck, W.W. (1991). A comparison of cluster-specific and population-averaged approaches for analyzing correlated binary data. *International Statistical Review* **59**, 25–35.

Patterson, H.D., Thompson, R. (1971). Recovery of interblock information when block sizes are unequal. *Biometrika* **58**, 545–554.

Patterson, S.D., Jones, B. (2006). *Bioequivalence and Statistics on Clinical Pharmacology*. Chapman & Hall/CRC, Boca Raton.

Prescott, P. (1999). Construction of sequentially counterbalanced designs formed from two latin squares. *Utilitas Mathematica* **55**, 135–152.

Russell, K.G. (1991). The construction of good change-over designs when there are fewer units than treatments. *Biometrika* **78**, 305–313.

Schuirmann, D.J. (1987). A comparison of the two one sided tests procedure and the power approach for assessing the equivalence of average bioavailability. *Journal of Pharmacokinetics and Biopharmaceutics* **15**, 657–680.

Senn, S.J. (1997). Cross-over trials. In: Ar-mitage, P., Colton, T. (Eds.),**vol. 2** *Encyclopedia in Biostatistics*. Wiley, New York.

Senn, S.J. (2000). Crossover design. In: Chow, S.C. (Ed.), *Encyclopedia of Biopharmaceutical Statistics*. Marcel Dekker, New York.

Senn, S.J. (2002). *Cross-over Trials in Clinical Research*, 2nd ed. Wiley, Chichester.

Senn, S.J., Lambrou, D. (1998). Robust and realistic approaches to carry-over. *Statistics in Medicine* **17**, 2849–2864.

Sheehe, P.R., Bross, I.D.J. (1961). Latin squares to balance immediate residual and other effects. *Biometrics* **17**, 405–414.

Stufken, J. (1996). Optimal Crossover Designs. In: Gosh, S., Rao, C.R. (Eds.), *Handbook of Statistics 13: Design and Analysis of Experiments*. Amsterdam, North-Holland, pp. 63–90.

Verbeke, G., Molenberghs, G. (2000). *Linear Mixed Models in Practice*. Springer, New York.

Williams, E.J. (1949). Experimental designs balanced for the estimation of residual effects of treatments. *Australian Journal of Scientific Research* **2**, 149–168.

Zeger, S.L., Liang, K.-Y. (1986). Longitudinal data analysis for discrete and continuous. *Biometrics* **42**, 121–130.

Zeger, S.L., Liang, K.Y., Albert, P.S. (1988). Models for longitudinal data: A generalized estimating equation approach. *Biometrics* **44**, 1049–1060.

Handbook of Statistics, Vol. 27
ISSN: 0169-7161

DOI: 10.1016/S0169-7161(07)27016-6

16

Sequential and Group Sequential Designs in Clinical Trials: Guidelines for Practitioners

Madhu Mazumdar and Heejung Bang

Abstract

In a classical fixed sample design, the sample size is set in advance of collecting any data. The main design focus is choosing the sample size that allows the clinical trial to discriminate between the null hypothesis of no difference and the alternative hypothesis of a specified difference of scientific interest. A disadvantage of fixed sample design is that the same number of subjects will always be used regardless of whether the true treatment effect is extremely beneficial, marginal, or truly harmful relative to the control arm. Often, it is difficult to justify because of ethical concerns and/or economic reasons. Thus, specific early termination procedures have been developed to allow repeated statistical analyses to be performed on accumulating data and to stop the trial as soon as the information is sufficient to conclude. However, repeated analyses inflate the false positive error to an unacceptable level. To avoid this problem, many approaches of group sequential methods have been developed. Although there is an increase in the planned sample size under these designs, due to the sequential nature, substantial sample size reductions compared with the single-stage design is also possible not only in the case of clear efficacy but also in the case of complete lack of efficacy of the new treatment. This feature provides an advantage in utilization of patient resource. These approaches are methodologically complex but advancement in software packages had made the planning, monitoring, and analysis of comparative clinical trials according to these approaches quite simple. Despite this simplicity, the carrying on of a trial under group sequential design requires efficient logistics with dedicated team of data manager, study coordinator, biostatistician, and clinician. Good collaboration, rigorous monitoring, and guidance offered by an independent data safety monitoring committee are all indispensable pieces for its successful implementation.

In this chapter, we provide a review of sequential designs and discuss the underlying premise of all current methods. We present a recent example and an historical example to illustrate the methods discussed and to provide a flavor of the variety and complexity in decision making. A comprehensive list of softwares is provided for easy implementation along with practical guidelines. Few areas with potential for future research are also identified.

1. Introduction

Randomized clinical trial (RCT) is regarded as the gold standard for assessing the relative effectiveness/efficacy of an experimental intervention, as it minimizes selection bias and threats to validity by estimating average causal effects. There are two general approaches for designing RCT: (1) fixed sample design (FSD) and (2) group sequential design (GSD). In FSD, a predetermined number of patients (ensuring a particular power for proving a given hypothesis) are accrued, and the study outcome is assessed at the end of the trial. In contrast, a design where analyses are performed at regular intervals after a group of patients are accrued is called GSD. In comparative therapeutic trials with sequential patient entry, FSDs are often unjustified on ethical and economic grounds, and GSDs are preferred for their flexibility (Geller et al., 1987; Fleming and Watelet, 1989). Currently used methods can be classified into three categories: group sequential methods for repeated significance testing; stochastic curtailment or conditional power (Lan et al., 1982; Pepe and Anderson, 1992; Betensky, 1997) and Bayesian sequential methods (Spiegelhalter and Freedman, 1994; Fayers et al., 1997). While no single approach addresses all the issues, they do provide useful guidance in assessing the emerging trends for safety and benefit.

Trials using GSDs are common in published literature and the advantage of this kind of design is self evident by their impact (Gausche et al., 2000; Kelly et al., 2001; Sacco et al., 2001). One example of its successful use is a trial reported by Frustaci et al., where 190 sarcoma patients (a rare form of cancer) were to be accrued in order to detect a 20% difference in 2-year disease-free survival (60% on the adjuvant chemotherapy treatment arm versus 40% in the control arm undergoing observation alone) (Frustaci et al., 2001). An interim analysis was planned after half of the patients were accrued with stopping rule in terms of adjusted p-value. The trial was stopped as this criterion was met thereby saving 50% of the planned patient accrual. The observed difference was found to be 27% (72% on the treatment arm versus 45% on the control arm), 7% higher than what was hypothesized initially at the design stage. Therefore, the risk of treating additional patients with suboptimal therapy was greatly reduced.

Independent data safety monitoring committee (DSMC) with responsibilities of (1) safeguarding the interests of study patients, (2) preserving the integrity and credibility of the trial in order to ensure that future patients be treated optimally, and (3) ensuring that definitive and reliable results be available in a timely manner to the medical community has been mandated for all comparative therapeutic clinical trials sponsored by national institutes (URL: http://cancertrials.nci.nih.gov; Ellenberg, 2001). GSD provides an excellent aid to the DSMC for decision making. Other names utilized for this kind of committees playing virtually the same role are data or patient safety monitoring board (DSMB or PSMB), data monitoring and ethics committees (DMEC), and policy and data monitoring board (PDMB).

In this chapter, we start with a historical account of sequential methods and provide introduction to the underlying concept and approaches to the commonly utilized methods of inflation factor (IF) for sample size calculation and alpha spending function for monitoring the trials for early stopping. A listing of softwares is provided that has the capabilities of accommodating all of the methods discussed. A table of IF for sample size calculation of GSD is provided for quick assessment of feasibility of a trial (in regard to sample size) even before acquiring any special software for GSD. One current example is presented with standard template of a biostatistical consideration for writing study protocol, details of a stopping boundary utilized, items to be included in an interim analysis reports presented to the DSMC, and the substance included in the statistical section write-up for final dissemination in published literature. Another historical example (the BHAT trial) is discussed to highlight that the DSMC's decision to stop early was based not only on statistical group sequential boundary point, but also on a variety of other subjective considerations.

Several review papers and books from various perspectives are recommended to those who wish to learn about further details (Fleming and DeMets, 1993; Jennison and Turnbull, 2000; Sebille and Bellissant, 2003; Proschan et al., 2006).

2. Historical background of sequential procedures

The first strictly sequential method, the sequential probability ratio test, was developed during the Second World War (Wald, 1947). As its main application was the quality control of manufactured materials, its publication was only authorized after the end of the war, in 1947. Another class of sequential test is based on triangular continuation regions (Anderson, 1960). The basic idea on which these methods rely is to constantly use the available information to determine whether the data are compatible with null hypothesis, with alternative hypothesis, or insufficient to choose between these two hypotheses. In the first two cases, the trial is stopped and the conclusion is obtained whereas in the third case the trial continues. The trial is further processed until the data allows a legitimate (or per-protocol) decision between the two hypotheses. An example of a completely sequential trial can be found in Jones et al. (1982).

Armitage (1954) and Bross (1952) pioneered the concept of group sequential methods in medical field (Bross, 1952; Armitage, 1954). At first, these plans were fully sequential and did not gain widespread acceptance perhaps due to the inconvenience in their application. The problems discussed included the fact that response needs to be available soon after the treatment is started and that there would be organizational problems, such as coordination in multicenter trials and a much greater amount of work for the statistician. The shift to group sequential methods for clinical trials did not occur until the 1970s. Elfring and Schultz (1973) specifically used the term 'group sequential design' to describe their procedure for comparing two treatments with binary response (Elfring et al., 1973).

McPherson (1974) suggested that the repeated significance tests of Armitage et al. (1969) might be used to analyze clinical trial data at a small number of interim analyses (Armitage et al., 1969; McPherson, 1974). Canner (1977) used Monte Carlo simulation to find critical values of a test statistic for a study with periodic analyses of survival endpoint (Canner, 1977). However, Pocock (1977) was the first to provide clear guidelines for the implementation of the GSD attaining particular operating characteristics of type I error and power (Pocock, 1977). He made the case that most investigators do not want to evaluate results every time a couple of new patients are accrued but do want to understand the comparative merit every few months to assess if the trial is worth the time and effort and that continual monitoring does not have a remarkable benefit. More specifically, only a minor improvement is expected with more than five interim looks. A more comprehensive account of this history can be read from the excellent book by Jennison and Turnbull (2000).

3. Group sequential procedures for randomized trials

A primary difficulty in performing repeated analyses over time is the confusion about the proper interpretation of strength of evidence obtained from such evaluations. Suppose that only a single data analysis is performed after data collection has been fully completed for a trial. Then a two-sided (or one-sided if justified, e.g., non-inferiority design) significance value of $p \leq 0.05$, obtained from a test of hypothesis of no difference between an experimental therapy and a control, is usually interpreted as providing strong enough evidence that the new therapy provides an advantage. The interpretation is justified by the willingness of investigators to accept up to five false-positive conclusions in every 100 trials of regimens that, in truth, have equivalent efficacy. Unfortunately, even when a new treatment truly provides no advantage over a standard therapy, performing repeated analyses can greatly increase the chance of obtaining positive conclusions when this $p \leq 0.05$ guideline is repeatedly used.

As such, interim data safety reports pose well-recognized statistical problems related to the multiplicity of statistical tests to be conducted on the accumulating set of data. The basic problem is well known and is referred to as "sampling to a foregone conclusion" (Cornfield, 1966) and has been illustrated mathematically, pictorially or through simulations by many researchers (Fleming and Green, 1984). Specifically, in a simulation of 100 typical clinical trials of two interventions with truly equivalent efficacy that called for up to four periodic evaluations, 17 (rather than five) trials yielded false-positive conclusions (i.e. $p \leq 0.05$) in at least one analysis. The rate of false-positives continues to rise as the frequency of interim analyses rises. This serious increase in the likelihood of reaching false-positive conclusions due to misinterpretation of the strength of evidence when repeated analyses are conducted over time partly explains why many published claims of therapeutic advances have been false leads and provides the motivation for development of GSD.

A GSD first provides a schedule that relates patient accrual to when the interim analyses will occur. This schedule is conveniently expressed in terms of the proportion of the maximal possible number of patients that the trial could accrue. Second, such designs give a sequence of statistics used to test the null hypothesis, and third, they give a stopping rule defined in terms of a monotone increasing sequence of nominal significance levels at which each test will be conducted. This sequence of significance levels is carefully chosen to maintain the overall type I error at some desired level (e.g., 0.05 or 0.10) using one- or two-sided hypothesis. Either the number or the time of analyses is prespecified or the rate at which the overall significance level is "used up" is fixed in advance. Thus, undertaking group sequential trials assumes that hypothesis testing at nominal significance levels less than a prestated overall significance level will be performed, and that if results are ever extreme enough to exceed prespecified thresholds, the trial should be stopped. While such group sequential procedures differ in detail, they have certain common features.

The two commonly discussed pioneering mechanisms in GSD are given by Pocock (Pocock, 1977) and O'Brien and Fleming (OBF) (O'Brien and Fleming, 1979). Pocock adapted the idea of a repeated significance test at a constant nominal significance level to analyze accumulating data at a relatively small number of times over the course of the study. Patient entry was divided into equally sized groups and the data are analyzed after each group of observations has been collected. As an alternative, OBF proposed a test in which the nominal significance levels needed to reject the null hypothesis at sequential analyses increase as the study progresses, thus, making it more difficult to reject the null hypothesis at the earliest analysis but easier later on. Other variations to these schemes have also been developed but OBF is the most commonly utilized GSD as it fits well with the wishes of clinical trialists who do not want to stop a trial prematurely with insufficient evidence based on less reliable or unrepresentative data. There are other reasons for this preference. Historically, most clinical trials fail to show a significant treatment difference, hence from a global perspective, it is more cost-effective to use conservative designs. Indeed, even a conservative design such as OBF often shows a dramatic reduction in the average sample number (ASN or expected sample size) under the alternative hypothesis, H_A, compared to a FSD (see Table 1 for brief overview). Moreover, psychologically, it is preferable to have a nominal p-value at the end of the study for rejecting the null hypothesis, H_0, which is close to 0.05 in order to avoid the embarrassing situation where, say, a p-value of 0.03 at the final analysis would be declared non-significant.

Table 1
General properties of monitoring designs

Design	General	ASN (under H_0)	ASN (under H_A)
Fixed	Most conservative	Low	Large
OBF	Conservative, hard to stop early	Mid	Mid
Pocock	Most liberal, early stopping properties	Large	Low

Later, Wang et al. (1987) proposed a class of generalized formulation that encompasses Pocock and OBF methods as two extreme members.

Although the formulation of GSD started with binary outcomes, a generalized formulation has helped establish the wide applicability of the large sample theory for multivariate normal random variables with independent increments (i.e., standardized partial sums) to group sequential testing (Jennison and Turnbull, 1997; Scharfstein et al., 1997). This structure applies to the limiting distribution of test statistics which are fully efficient in parametric and semiparametric models, including generalized linear models and proportional hazards models (Tsiatis et al., 1995). It applies to all normal linear models, including mixed-effects models (Lee and Demets, 1991; Reboussin et al., 1992). Gange and Demets showed its applicability to the generalized estimating equation setting and Mazumdar and Liu showed the derivation for the comparative diagnostic test setting where area under the receiver operating characteristic curve is the endpoint (Mazumdar and Liu, 2003; Mazumdar, 2004). In short, almost any statistic likely to be used to summarize treatment differences in a clinical trial will justify group sequential testing with this basic structure and common mathematical formulation (Jennison and Turnbull, 2000).

3.1. Power and sample size calculation using inflation factor

Sample size computation in GSD setting involves the size of the treatment effect under some non-null hypothesis, the standard error of the estimated treatment effect at the end of the trial, and the drift of the underlying Brownian motion used to model the sequentially computed test statistics. The appropriate drift is determined by multiple factors such as the group sequential boundaries, type I error, and desired power. The theoretical background for design of group sequential trials has been discussed elsewhere (Kim and DeMets, 1992; Lan and Zucker, 1993) but the drift of commonly used GSDs can be easily translated into the corresponding IFs, provided in Table 2. The sample size approximation for a GSD in any setting is simply obtained by multiplying the sample size under the corresponding FSD by the IF provided in this table for the features of the specific GSD chosen. It is easy to note that the sample size inflation under OBF is minimal.

3.2. Monitoring boundaries using alpha spending functions

The earlier publications for group sequential boundaries required that the number and timing of interim analyses be fixed in advance. However, while monitoring data for real clinical trials, it was felt that more flexibility in being able to look at the data at time points dictated by the emerging beneficial or harmful trend is desired. To accommodate this capability, Lan and Demets proposed a more flexible implementation of the group sequential boundaries through an innovative 'alpha spending function' (Lan and Demets, 1983; Lan and DeMets, 1989). The spending function controls how much of the false-positive error (or false-negative error when testing to rule out benefit) can be used at each interim analysis as a function of the proportion (t^*, range 0 (study start)–1 (study

Table 2
Inflation Factors for Pocock and O'Brien–Fleming alpha spending functions for different total numbers of looks (K) under equal-sized increments

$\alpha = 0.05$ (Two-sided)					$\alpha = 0.01$ (Two-sided)				
K	Spending function	Power $(1-\beta)$			K	Spending function	Power $(1-\beta)$		
		0.80	0.90	0.95			0.80	0.90	0.95
2	Pocock	1.11	1.10	1.09	2	Pocock	1.09	1.08	1.08
2	OBF	1.01	1.01	1.01	2	OBF	1.00	1.00	1.00
3	Pocock	1.17	1.15	1.14	3	Pocock	1.14	1.12	1.12
3	OBF	1.02	1.02	1.02	3	OBF	1.01	1.01	1.01
4	Pocock	1.20	1.18	1.17	4	Pocock	1.17	1.15	1.14
4	OBF	1.02	1.02	1.02	4	OBF	1.01	1.01	1.01
5	Pocock	1.23	1.21	1.19	5	Pocock	1.19	1.17	1.16
5	OBF	1.03	1.03	1.02	5	OBF	1.02	1.01	1.01

end)) of total information observed. In many applications, t^* may be estimated as the fraction of patients recruited (for dichotomous outcomes) or the fraction of events observed (for time to event outcomes) out of the respective total expected. The alpha spending functions underlying OBF GSD correspond to

$$\alpha_1(t^*) = 2 - 2\Phi\left[\frac{Z_{1-(\alpha/2)}}{(t^*)^{1/2}}\right],$$

whereas the one for Pocock is described by

$$\alpha_2(t^*) = \alpha \ln[1 + (e - 1)t^*].$$

The advantage of the alpha spending function is that neither the number nor the exact timing of the interim analyses needs to be specified in advance. Only the particular spending function needs to be specified. It is useful to note that the nominal significance levels utilized in any GSD will always add up to more than the overall significance level, because with multiple significance testing the probability of rejecting the null hypothesis does not accumulate additively due to positive correlations among test statistics.

Following is a sample 'Biostatistical Consideration' write-up for a clinical trial in Germ Cell Tumor (GCT) utilizing GSD with OBF boundaries. IF approach with three total looks ($K = 3$) was chosen at design stage and a series of boundaries and sequence of significance level were computed accordingly. The option of utilizing spending function approach was also kept open, which is often the case in practice.

3.3. Design of a phase 3 study with OBF GSD: A sample template

3.3.1. Biostatistical considerations

1. *Objective and background*: The objective of this study is to compare in a prospective randomized manner the efficacy of an experimental combination

regimen versus the standard regimen in previously untreated 'poor' risk GCT patients. The poor risk criterion helps identify patients who are expected to have high probability of worse outcome. It is described in the protocol and roughly depends on the primary site, histology, and specific blood markers being high. For this kind of cancer, a patient's prognosis is considered to be favorable if their tumor completely disappears and does not come back at least for a year. The response of these patients is called durable complete responder (DCR) at one year. In the institutional database at Memorial Sloan–Kettering Cancer Center (MSKCC) of size 796 patients treated by standard therapy, the proportion of patients remaining DCR at one year for the poor risk group ($n = 141$) is 30% with a 95% confidence interval (Cl) of 22.2–37.3%.

2. *Primary endpoint, power and significance level*: The major endpoint for this trial is DCR at one year where the time is computed from the day a patient is defined responder. This study is planned to detect a 20% absolute difference from the currently observed rate of 30% (30% versus 50%). We are expecting an accrual of 50 patients per year. The sample size calculation based on log-rank test for an FSD with 80% power and 5% level of significance, 195 patients will be needed. To incorporate two interim looks and a final look (so total $K = 3$) at the end of full accrual, an IF of 1.02 was multiplied to 195 requiring 199 patients ($= 1.02 \times 195$) using OBF method (O'Brien and Fleming 1979). Rounding it off to 200 patients (100 per arm), we decide to place the two interim looks at the end of second and third year and the final look at the end of fourth year as the accrual rate of 50 patients makes the length of study to be four years.
3. *Randomization*: After eligibility is established, patients will be randomized via a telephone call to the coordinating center at MSKCC clinical trial office (Phone number: XXX-XX-XXXX; 9:00 am to 5:00pm Monday through Friday). Randomization will be accomplished by the method of stratified random permuted block, where patient institution (MSKCC versus ECOG versus SWOG versus remaining participating institutions) was adopted for stratification, where ECOG denotes Eastern Cooperative Oncology Group and SWOG denotes Southwest Oncology Group.
4. *Data safety monitoring committee and interim analyses*: The data will be reviewed at designated intervals by an independent DSMC. This committee was formed with two independent oncologists and one independent biostatistician. The committee will be presented with the data summary on accrual rates, demographics and bio-chemical markers etc. and comparative analysis (using Fisher's exact test) on toxicity and DCR proportion by the principal investigator (PI) and the biostatistician on study. Survival and progression-free survival curves will be estimated only if there is an enough number of events that governs statistical power. Semi-annual reports on toxicity will be disseminated to all the participating groups.

Normalized z-statistics according to the OBF boundary to be used for stopping early if the experimental regimen looks promising are ± 3.471, ± 2.454, ± 2.004, where the corresponding sequence of nominal significance levels are 0.001, 0.014, and 0.036, respectively (East, Cytel Statistical Software). If situation emerges where these time points are not the most convenient or desirable, Lan–Demets spending function utilizing OBF boundaries will be used to compute the corresponding z-statistics and significance level. The committee is expected to use the statistical stopping rules as a guideline in addition to both medical judgment and the relevant emerging data in the literature, especially ones obtained from similar trials.

5. *Final analysis*: All toxicities will be evaluated based on the NCI common toxicity criteria and tabulated by their frequencies and proportions. Fisher's exact test will be used to compare the toxicities and adverse events by the two arms. The primary analysis, DCR-free survival curves will be estimated using Kaplan–Meier method and with appropriate follow-up, comparisons will be made using log-rank test (Kaplan and Meier, 1958; Mantel, 1966). Once the trial stops (either at interim look or at final look), standard statistical estimation and inference will be undertaken for the observed treatment difference.

3.4. *Analyses following group sequential test*

Analysis following a group sequential test consists of two scenarios: The first is upon conclusion of the trial after the test statistic has crossed a stopping boundary and the second is when an interval estimate of the treatment difference is desired whether the design calls for a termination or not. Tsiatis et al. (1984) have shown that in both situation, it is inappropriate to compute a 'naïve' CI, treating the data as if they had been obtained in a fixed sample size experiment. They estimated naïve CI following a five-stage Pocock's test with 5% level of significance and found their coverage to vary between 84.6% and 92.9%, depending on the true parameter value.

For the first scenario, Tsiatis et al. suggested a numerical method for calculating an exact CIs following group sequential tests with Pocock (1977) or O'Brien and Fleming (1979) boundaries based on ordering the sample space in a specific manner. They derived the CIs based on normal distribution theory, which pull the naive CIs toward zero and are no longer symmetric about the sample mean. They also commented that their method is applicable to any (asymptotically) normal test statistic which has uncorrelated increments and for which the variance can be estimated consistently. Whitehead (1986) suggested an approach for adjusting the maximum likelihood estimate as the point estimate by subtracting an estimate of the bias. Wang and Leung (1997) proposed a parametric bootstrap method for finding a bias-adjusted estimate, whereas Emerson and Fleming (1990) provide a formulation of uniformly minimum variance unbiased estimator calculated by Rao–Blackwell technique.

For the second scenario, the multiple-looks problem affects the construction of CIs just as it affects significance levels of hypothesis tests. Repeated CIs for a parameter θ are defined as a sequence of intervals I_k, $k = 1, \ldots, K$, for which a simultaneous coverage probability is maintained at some level, say, $1-\alpha$. The defining property of a $(1-\alpha)$-level sequence of repeated CIs for θ is $P[\theta \in I_k \text{ for all } k = 1, \ldots, K] = 1-\alpha$ for all θ (Jennison and Turnbull, 1983,

1984, 1985). The interval I_k, $k = 1, \ldots, K$, provides a statistical summary of the information about the parameter θ at the kth analysis, automatically adjusted to compensate for repeated looks at the accumulating data. As a result, repeated CIs instead of group sequential testing can be used for monitoring clinical trials (Jennison and Turnbull, 1989).

Most conventional trials are designed to have a high probability of detecting a predefined treatment effect if such an effect truly exists. That probability is called the power of the trial. Most trials use power in the range of 0.8–0.95 for a plausible range of alternatives of interest and the sample size of the study is calculated to achieve that power. The concept of 'conditional power' comes into play when supporting evidence is sought to decide the power midstream.

3.5. Stochastic curtailment

Once the trial starts and data become available, the probability that a treatment effect will ultimately be detected can be recalculated (Halperin et al., 1982; Lan et al., 1982; Lan and Wittes, 1988). An emerging trend in favor of the treatment increases the probability that the trial will detect a beneficial effect, while an unfavorable trend decreases the probability of establishing benefit. The term 'conditional power' is often used to describe this evolving probability. The term 'power' is used because it is the probability of claiming a treatment difference at the end of the trial, but it is 'conditional' because it takes into consideration the data already observed that will be part of the final analysis. Conditional power can be calculated for a variety of scenarios including a positive beneficial trend, a negative harmful trend, or no trend at all. However, these calculations are frequently made when interim data are viewed to be unfavorable. For this scenario, it represents the probability that the current unfavorable trend would improve sufficiently to yield statistically significant evidence of benefit by the scheduled end of the trial. This probability is usually computed under the assumption that the remainder of the data will be generated from a setting in which the true treatment effect was as large as the originally hypothesized in the study protocol.

When an unfavorable trend is observed at the interim analysis, the conditional probability of achieving a statistically significant beneficial effect is much less than the initial power of the trial. If the conditional power is low for a wide range of reasonable assumed treatment effect, including those originally assumed in the protocol, this might suggest to the DSMC that there is little reason to continue the trial since the treatment is highly unlikely to show benefit. Of course, this conditional power calculation does increase the chance of missing a real benefit (false-negative or type II error) since termination eliminates any chance of recovery by the intervention. However, if the conditional power under these scenarios is less than 0.2 compared to the hypothesis for which the trial originally provided power of 0.85–0.9, the increase in the rate of false-negative error is negligible. There is no concern with false-positive error in this situation since there is no consideration of claiming a positive result. An example of its use will follow in the Beta-Blocker Heart Attack Trial (BHAT) trial description later in this chapter.

3.6. Bayesian monitoring

The Bayesian approach for monitoring accumulating data considers unknown parameters to be random and to follow probability distributions (Spiegelhalter et al., 1986; Freedman et al., 1994; Parmar et al., 1994; Fayers et al., 1997). The investigators specify a prior distribution(s) describing the uncertainty in the treatment effect and other relevant parameters. These prior distributions are developed based on previous data and beliefs. It is quantified through a distribution of possible values and is referred to as the prior distribution. The observed accumulating data are used to modify the prior distribution and produce a posterior distribution, a distribution that reflects the most current information on the treatment effect, taking into account the specified prior as well as the accumulated data. This posterior distribution can then be used to compute a variety of summaries including the predictive probability that the treatment is effective. In 1966, Cornfield introduced the idea of Bayesian approach to monitoring clinical trial (Cornfield, 1966). Although, interest has recently increased in its use (Kpozehouen et al., 2005) and availability of computational tools have made it more feasible to use, these methods are still not widely utilized.

3.7. Available softwares

Softwares for implementing GSDs have been developed and commercialized since the early 1990s. Extended descriptions of these softwares are available through their user's guide and some review papers (Emerson, 1996; Wassmer and Vandemeulebroecke, 2006). Most of the computational tools employ the recursive numerical integration technique that takes advantage of a quadrature rule of replacing integral by a weighted sum for probabilistic computations (Armitage et al., 1969; Jennison and Turnbull, 2000).

Here, we provide a comprehensive listing of appropriate links for free self-executable softwares as well as codes written in FORTRAN, SAS, Splus, and R languages. FORTRAN source code used in the textbook by Jennison and Turnbull (2000) can be downloaded from Dr. Jennison's homepage on http://people.bath.ac.uk/mascj/book/programs/general. The code provides continuation regions and exit probabilities for classical GSDs including those proposed by Pocock (1977), O'Brien and Fleming (1979), Wang and Tsiatis (1987) and Pampallona and Tsiatis (1994). In addition, the spending function approach according to Lan and Demets (1983) is implemented. Another implementation in FORTRAN of the spending function approach is available for use under UNIX and MS-DOS. It can be downloaded from http://www.biostat.wisc.edu/landemets/ as a stand-alone program with a graphical user interface, while details of methodologies and algorithms are found in Reboussin et al. (2000). These codes provide computation of boundaries and exit probabilities for any trial based on normally or asymptotic normally distributed test statistics with independent increments, including those in which patients give a single continuous or binary response, survival studies, and certain longitudinal designs. Interim analyses need not be equally spaced, and their number need not be specified in advance via flexible alpha spending mechanism. In addition to boundaries, power computations, probabilities associated with a given set of boundaries, and CIs can also be computed.

The IML (Interactive Matrix Language) module of SAS® features the calls SEQ, SEQSCALE, and SEQSHIFT that perform computations for group sequential tests. SEQ calculates the exit probabilities for a set of successive continuation intervals. SEQSCALE scales these continuation regions to achieve a specified overall significance level and also returns the corresponding exit probabilities. SEQSHIFT computes the non-centrality parameter for a given power.

S-PLUS that is commercially available provides a package for designing, monitoring, and analyzing group sequential trials through its S+SeqTrial™ module. It makes use of the unifying formulation by Kittelson et al. (Kittelson and Emerson, 1999), including all classical GSDs, triangular tests (Whitehead, 1997), and the spending function approach. It offers the calculation of continuation regions, exit probabilities, power, sample size distributions, overall p-values and adjusted point estimates and CIs, for a variety of distributional assumptions. It comes with a graphical user interface and very good documentation, which can be downloaded from http://www.insightful.com/products/seqtrial/default.asp.

In R (http://www.r-project.org/), cumulative exit probabilities of GSDs can be computed by the function seqmon. It implements an algorithm proposed by Schoenfeld (2001) and the documentation and packages are freely downloadable at http://www.maths.lth.se/help/R/.R/library/seqmon/html/seqmon.html.

PEST, version 4 offers a wide range of scenarios, including binary, normal, and survival endpoints, and different types of design. The main focus of PEST is the implementation of triangular designs. Sequential designs from outside PEST can also be entered and analyzed. Besides the planning tools, the software offers a number of analysis tools including interim monitoring and adjusted p-values, CIs, and point estimates for the final analysis. An important and unique feature of PEST is that interim and final data can be optionally read from SAS data sets. More information about the software can be found at http://www.rdg.ac.uk/mps/mps_home/software/software.htm#PEST%204.

East of Cytel Statistical Software and Services (http://www.cytel.com/Products/East/) is the most comprehensive package for planning and analyzing group sequential trials. The software provides a variety of capabilities of advanced clinical trial design, simulation and monitoring, and comes with extensive documentation including many real data examples. Tutorial sessions for East are frequently offered during various statistical meetings and conferences and educational settings.

"PASS 2005 Power Analysis and Sample Size" is distributed by NCSS Inc. This software supplies the critical regions and the necessary sample sizes but it is not yet possible to apply a sequential test to real data in the sense of performing an adjusted analysis (point estimates, CIs, and p-values). Documentation and a free download are available on http://www.ncss.com./passsequence.html.

"ADDPLAN Adaptive Designs-Plans and Analyses" (http://www.addplan.com/) is designed for the purpose of planning and conducting a clinical trial based on an adaptive group sequential test design. New adaptive (flexible) study designs allow for correct data-driven re-estimation of the sample size while controlling the type I error rate. Redesigning the sample size in an interim analysis based on the results observed so far considerably improves the power of the trial since the best available information at hand is used for the sample size adjustment. The simulation capabilities for specific adaptation rules are also provided.

The choice of software is based on the users' need and the complexity of design. The freely available softwares are often enough to implement basic functions to be used in standard or popular designs and to perform associated data analyses outlined in this chapter unless special features are required.

3.8. Data safety monitoring committee

Early in the development of modern clinical trial methodology, some investigators recognized that, despite the compelling ethical needs to monitor the accumulating results, repeated review of interim data raised some problems. It was recognized that knowledge of the pattern of the accumulating data on the part of investigators, sponsors, or trial participants, could affect the course of the trial and the validity of the results. For example, if investigators were aware that the interim trial results were favoring one of the treatment groups, they might be reluctant to continue to encourage adherence to all regimens in the trial, or to continue to enter patients in the trial, or they may alter the types of patients they would consider accrual. Furthermore, influenced by financial or scientific conflicts of interest, investigators, or the sponsor might take actions that could diminish the integrity and credibility of the trial. A natural and practical approach to dealing with this problem is to assign sole responsibility for interim monitoring of data on safety and efficacy to a committee whose members have no involvement in the trial, no vested interest in the trial results, and sufficient understanding of the trial design, conduct, and data-analytical issues to interpret interim analyses with appropriate caution. These DSMCs consisting of members from variety of background (clinical, statistical, ethical, etc.) have become critical components of virtually all clinical trials.

For the above example, an independent DSMC consisting of three members with background in oncology (one from community hospital and one from specialized center) and biostatistics met every year to discuss the progress of the trial. The outcome comparison was only presented when an interim analysis with OBF was allowed. Below we present a list of items that were included in the interim report for this trial. This is a typical template for a clinical trial and could be useful in other scenarios.

Items included in the interim report:

1. Brief outline of the study design
2. Major protocol amendments with dates (or summary) if applicable
3. Enrollment by arm and year and center (preferably, updated within a month of the DSMC meeting date)
4. Information on eligibility criterion violation or crossover patients
5. Summary statistics (e.g., mean/median) on follow-up times of patients
6. Frequency tables of baseline characteristics (demographics, toxicity, and

adverse event summary, laboratory test summary, precious treatment) of the full cohort

7. Comparative analysis of primary and secondary endpoints (when data mature)
8. Subgroup analyses and analyses adjusted for baseline characteristics (and some secondary outcomes data, if any)
9. Comparative analysis of adverse event and toxicity data
10. Comparative analysis of longitudinal lab values.

The GCT study referred above struggled with accrual of patients and remained open for 10 years instead of the four years planned initially. To improve accrual rate, new centers were added and the patient eligibility was expanded. DSMC met annually and approved these actions. The first DSMC meeting where outcome data were compared was at 6th year after study start instead of the 2nd year. Lan–Demets with OBF boundary was utilized to compute the appropriate boundary but the boundary was not crossed. DSMC deliberations continued with concern for the accrual rate but since the experimental regimen utilizing autologus bone marrow transplant was quite a novel and unique approach and it was added to the standard therapy, the DSMC did not feel any harm to patients and decided to keep the trial open. More assertive accrual plans were adopted but when many of these plans failed to improve accrual, the study was at last closed at 219 patients (in contrast, $N = 270$ in the original plan).

3.8.1. Details included in the final paper (on design and primary analysis)

The final write-up or summary report needs to include as much details as possible about the original design (including sample size/power calculation), modifications, rationale for modification, decisions by DSMC, and conclusions. Here's part of the 'Statistical Methods' section from the final paper related to the GCT study (Motzer et al., 2007):

> The trial was designed with the proportion of patients with durable complete response (DCR) at one year from entry onto the trial as the primary endpoint. The original study population to be enrolled on this study was poor-risk GCT patients only. We had planned to accrue 200 patients (100 per arm) to detect a 20% difference in DCR rate at one year (an improvement from 30% to 50%) with a 5% level of significance and 80% power. However, as the trial progressed, the accrual rate was far lower than our expectation of 50 poor-risk patients per year. Also during this time, an international effort brought along a newly developed but broadly accepted risk group classification and it was felt that the intermediate-risk group patients with poor markers (lactate dehydrogenase greater than 3 times upper limit of normal) would benefit from the treatment under investigation. Therefore it was decided to extend the study to this modified intermediate risk group from the poor risk classification utilized before. Based on a historical one-year DCR rate of 45% in the poor and intermediate risk groups combined, we then modified our target accrual to 218 patients to detect an improvement of 20% with the same level and power.

A final modification to the study was implemented in 2002 after a new center CALGB was added to the study and accrual at that center began. At that point, it was our hope to be able to address the original question of interest in the poor-risk group of patients. We planned to accrue 270 patients, consisting of 216 poor-risk patients (200 per original calculation +16 to account for withdrawals) and 54 intermediate-risk patients. However, as accrual did not meet our expectations even with the additional cooperative group participating, the study was closed in August of 2003. The data were reviewed annually by an independent DSMC. Initially, the design included an O'Brien and Fleming stopping rule with the sequence of nominal significance levels of 0.001, 0.014, and 0.036 for the two interim analyses and the final analysis, respectively. A formal comparative interim analysis on DCR proportion and overall survival was presented in May 2000 based on a recalculated boundary utilizing Lan–Demets spending function. The decision was to continue the trial as the boundary was not crossed and no ethical conflict was found since the experimental regimen was an autologus bone marrow transplant regimen on top of the standard therapy. The study was at last stopped in 2003 due to not being able to improve accrual rate.

3.9. Historical example of GSD use

It is always educational to look back on the trials that were planned with GSD and benefited from it. Two excellent books by DeMets et al., 2006 and Ellenberg et al., 2006 provide essential and in-depth reading materials for clinical trialists starting in this field. An example considered by these books and many other publications is described below to show the multifaceted decision process that goes into the deliberation of DSMB.

The BHAT compared the beta-blocker propranolol against placebo in patients who had a myocardial infarction recently. The statistical design called for enrollment of 4,020 patients, aged 30–69 years, who had a myocardial infarction 5–21 days prior to randomization. The primary objective of the study was to determine if long-term administration of propranolol would result in a difference in all-cause mortality. The design utilized O'Brien–Fleming boundary with alpha level set at two-tailed 0.05, 90% power, and three-year average follow-up. The attempt was to detect a 21.25% relative change in mortality, from a three-year rate of 17.46% in the control (placebo) group to 13.75% in the intervention group, which were obtained from earlier studies (Furberg and Friedwald, 1978; Anderson et al., 1979) after taking non-adherence into account (Byington, 1984).

Enrollment began in 1978 and a total of 3,837 participants were accrued instead of the planned 4,020. This reduced the power slightly from the planned 90% to 89%. The PDMB first reviewed the data in May 1979. Subsequent data reviews were to occur approximately every six months, until the scheduled end of the trial in June 1982. At the *October, 1979* meeting of the PDMB, the log-rank z-value exceeded the conventional 1.96 critical value for a nominal p of 0.05 but was far from significance due to the conservative nature of the O'Brien–Fleming boundaries early in the study. PDMB recommended continuation of the trial.

At the meeting in *April 1981*, the PDMB reviewed not only the accumulating BHAT data but the results of the timolol trial that had just been published. This trial of 1,884 survivors of an acute myocardial infarction showed a statistically significant reduction in all-cause mortality, from 16.2% to 10.4%, during a mean follow-up of 17 months. At this point, BHAT was no longer enrolling patients, but follow-up was continuing. The PDMB recommended that BHAT continues, primarily because, despite the timolol findings, the BHAT data did not show convincing evidence of benefit. Not only had the monitoring boundary not been crossed, but the long-term effect on mortality and possible adverse events was unknown. Importantly, all patients in BHAT had been in the trial for at least six months post-infarction, and there was no evidence that beta-blockers started after that time produced benefit. Thus, there was not an ethical concern about leaving the participants on placebo. The PDMB advised that the study investigators be informed of the timolol results. However, it also advised that because there had been conflicting results from other beta-blocker trials, the positive results of the timolol trial should not preclude the continuation of BHAT. Furthermore, timolol was not available for sale in the United States then. At its *October 1981* data review, the PDMB noted that the upper OBF boundary had been crossed. The normalized log-rank statistic was then 2.82, which exceeded the boundary value of 2.23. In addition to the monitoring boundaries, the PDMB considered a number of factors in its recommendation to stop early:

> 1) Conditional power calculations indicated that there was little likelihood that the conclusions of the study would be changed if follow-up were to continue; 2) The gain in precision of the estimated results for the first two years would be tiny, and only modest for the third year; 3) The results were consistent with those of another beta-blocker trial; 4) There would be potential medical benefits to both study participants on placebo and to heart attack patients outside the study; 5) Other characteristics, such as subgroup examinations and baseline comparability, confirmed the validity of the findings; 6) The consent form clearly called for the study to end when benefit was known. Following points in favor of continuing until the scheduled end were considered but were not found to weigh enough in favor of not stopping: 1) Even though slight, there remained a chance that the conclusions could change; 2) Because therapy would be continued indefinitely, it would be important to obtain more long-term (4 year) data; 3) It would be important to obtain more data on subgroups and secondary outcomes; 4) The results of a study that stopped early would not be as persuasive to the medical community as would results from a fully powered study that went to completion, particularly given the mixed results from previous trials.

> Lessons learnt from these experiences are that 1) O'Brien-Fleming approach to sequential boundaries could prove very helpful in fostering a cautious attitude with regard to claiming significance prematurely. Even though conventional significance was seen early in the study, the use of sequential boundaries gave the study added credibility and probably helped make it persuasive to the practicing medical community; 2) The use of conditional power added to the

persuasiveness of the results, by showing the extremely low likelihood that the conclusions would change if the trial were to continue to its scheduled end; 3) The decision-making process involves many factors, only some of which are statistical (Friedman et al., 2003).

4. Steps for GSD design and analysis

4.1. Classical design

Step 1: Decide the number of maximum looks (or groups) K and the choice of boundary (that can be indexed by shape parameter, Δ (Wang and Tsiatis, 1987).

Remark:

a) The gain in ASN is most dramatic when going from $K = 1$ (i.e., the fixed sample size design) to $K = 2$. Beyond $K = 5$, there is relatively little change in ASN.
b) The choice of K may be dictated by some practicality such as the frequency of the DSMC meetings that is feasible.
c) $\Delta = 0$ for OBF and $\Delta = 0.5$ for Pocock.

Step 2: Compute the sample size for fixed design as you would ordinarily do (using significance level, power, and effect size). Multiply by the appropriate IF.

Step 3: After computing the maximum sample size, divide it into K equal group sizes and conduct interim analyses after each group. Reject H_0 at the first interim analysis where the test statistic using all the accumulated data exceeds the boundary values computed. Alternatively, we can translate the boundaries to the corresponding nominal p-values at each look and conduct the test using p-values.

4.2. Information-based design

Step 1: Specify level of significance, power, K and alternative of interest (γ).

Remark:

You specify K at the design stage but you may deviate from this at the time of analysis.

Step 2: Choose a spending function and stopping boundary (Lan and DeMets spending function with OBF or Pocock or other boundaries).

Step 3: Compute maximum information (MI) required to have a specific power as $\text{MI} = (z_{1-\alpha/2} + z_{1-\beta}/\gamma)^2$ X IF.

Step 4: The first time the data are monitored, say, at time t_1, compute the proportion of information compared to MI. Then find the first boundary value. If the test statistic exceeds the boundary computed, stop and reject H_0. If not, continue to next monitoring time.

Step 5: At time t_2, compute the ratio of observed information and MI. Then perform the testing.

Step 6: Continue in this fashion, if necessary, until the final analysis, at which point you use up the remaining significance level.

Remark:

With this strategy, you are guaranteed a level alpha test regardless of how often or when you look at the data prior to obtaining MI.

5. Discussion

In RCTs designed to assess the efficacy and safety of medical interventions, evolving data are typically reviewed on a periodic basis during the conduct of the study. These interim reviews are especially important in trials conducted in the setting of diseases that are life-threatening or result in irreversible major morbidity. Such reviews have many purposes. They may identify unacceptably slow rates of accrual or high rates of ineligibility determined after randomization, protocol violations that suggest that clarification of or changes to the study protocol are needed or unexpectedly high dropout rates that threaten the trial's ability to produce unbiased results. The most important purpose, however, is to ensure that the trial remains appropriate and safe for the individuals who have been or are still to be enrolled. Efficacy results must also be monitored to enable benefit-to-risk assessments to be made. Repeated statistical testing of the primary efficacy endpoint was seen to increase the chance of false-positive rate. The methods of adjusting the significance levels at each interim analysis so that the overall false-positive rate stays at an acceptable level gave rise to GSDs. The field has been developing for past 30 years and is now quite mature with various methods with well-studied operating characteristics and availability of an array of user-friendly software.

One new field of applications has been cluster-randomized trials (CRTs). CRTs have been used increasingly over the past two decades to measure the effects of health interventions applied at the community level. Excellent reviews and books are written by Donner et al. and Murray (Donner and Brown, 1990; Murray, 1998; Donner and Klar, 2000). Recently, Zou et al. (2005) developed group sequential methods that can be applied to CRT. Although the design aspect is well characterized and related computer program is available upon request, effect estimation following this group sequential test remains a topic of future research. This method is not yet used prospectively on a clinical trial. Development of methodology for novel design such as the split-cluster design could also be a useful addition to this field (Donner and Klar, 2004).

Adaptive designs in the context of group sequential testing allow modifications of particular aspects of the trials (such as inappropriate assumptions, excessive cost, or saving in time) after its initiation without undermining the validity and integrity of the trial. Some developments have been made to combine the advantages of adaptive and of classical group sequential approaches. Although research has been ongoing in this field, it still remains a field of research priority (Tsiatis and Mehta, 2003; Jennison and Turnbull, 2005; Kuehn, 2006; Wassmer, 2006).

There are some settings where GSDs may not be appropriate. For example, when the endpoint assessment time is lengthy relative to the recruitment period, there might be enough interim results to perform an analysis only after all or most subjects have been recruited and treated, thereby potentially rendering the GSD irrelevant. Most other large studies will benefit from having planned look at the data as trial progresses. Quite surprisingly, we found that many large trials follow FSD (Cooper et al., 2006; Cotton et al., 2006; Nicholls et al., 2006). A systematic literature search to assess the percentage of studies that would benefit from GSD but is not currently planning to use it would be interesting. This effort could also identify additional areas for further research or need for expanded exposure of these designs among practitioners.

Acknowledgement

We thank Ms. Anita Mesi for her excellent help with the published literature management using endnote software and past collaborators, Dr. Robert Motzer, and Ms. Jennifer Bacik, for many discussions on this topic. Partial support for this work came from the following grants: CERTs (AHRQ RFA-HS-05-14), CIPRA (NIAID U01 AI058257), R25 CA105012, and Cornell Institute of Clinical Research (supported by Tolly Vinik Trust).

References

Anderson, M., Bechgaard, P., Frederiksen, J. (1979). Effect of Alprenolol on mortality among patients with definite or suspected acute myocardial infarction: Preliminary results. *Lancet* **2**, 865–868.

Anderson, T. (1960). A modification of the sequential probability ratio test to reduce the sample size. *Ann Math Stat* **31**, 165–197.

Armitage, P. (1954). Sequential tests in prophylactic and therapeutic trials. *Quarterly Journal of Medicine* **23**, 255–274.

Armitage, P., McPherson, C.K., Rowe, B.C. (1969). Repeated significance tests on accumulating data. *Journal of Royal Statistical Society. Series A* **132**, 235–244.

Betensky, R.A. (1997). Early stopping to accept H(o) based on conditional power: Approximations and comparisons. *Biometrics* **53**(3), 794–806.

Bross, I. (1952). Sequential medical plans. *Biometrics* **8**, 188–205.

Byington, R. (1984). Beta-Blocker Heart Attack Trial: Design, methods, and baseline results. *Controlled Clinical Trials* **5**, 382–437.

Canner, P.L. (1977). Monitoring treatment differences in long-term clinical trials. *Biometrics* **33**(4), 603–615.

Cooper, C.J., Murphy, T.P. et al. (2006). Stent revascularization for the prevention of cardiovascular and renal events among patients with renal artery stenosis and systolic hypertension: Rationale and design of the CORAL trial. *American Heart Journal* **152**(1), 59–66.

Cornfield, J. (1966). A Bayesian test of some classical hypotheses – with application to sequential clinical trials. *Journal of the American Statistical Association* **61**, 577–594.

Cotton, S.C., Sharp, L. et al. (2006). Trial of management of borderline and other low-grade abnormal smears (TOMBOLA): Trial design. *Contemporary Clinical Trials* **27**(5), 449–471.

DeMets, D., Furberg, C. et al. (2006). *Data Monitoring in Clinical Trials: A Case Studies Approach*. Springer, New York.

Donner, A., Brown, K. (1990). A methodological review of non-therapeutic inter vention trials employing cluster randomization. *International Journal of Epidemiology* **19**(4), 795–800.

Donner, A., Klar, N. (2000). *Design and Analysis of Cluster Randomization Trials in Health Research*. Arnold, London.

Donner, A., Klar, N. (2004). Methods for statistical analysis of binary data in split-cluster designs. *Biometrics* **60**(4), 919–925.

Elfring, G.L., Schultz, J.R. et al. (1973). Group sequential designs for clinical trials. *Biometrics* **29**(3), 471–477.

Ellenberg, S.S. (2001). Independent monitoring committees: Rationale, operations, and controversies. *Statistics in Medicine* **20**, 2573–2583.

Ellenberg, S.S., Fleming, T. et al. (2006). *Data Monitoring Committees in Clinical Trials: A Practical Perspective*. Wiley, London.

Emerson, S. (1996). Statistical packages for group sequential methods. *The American Statistician* **50**, 183–192.

Emerson, S., Fleming, T. (1990). Parameter estimation following group sequential hypothesis testing. *Biometrika* **77**, 875–892.

Fayers, P.M., Ashby, D. et al. (1997). Tutorial in biostatistics: Bayesian data monitoring in clinical trials. *Statistics in Medicine* **16**, 1413–1430.

Fleming, T., DeMets, D. (1993). Monitoring of clinical trials: Issues and recommendations. *Controlled Clinical Trials* **14**(3), 183–197.

Fleming, T.R., Green, S. (1984). Considerations for monitoring and evaluating treatment effect in clinical trials. *Controlled Clinical Trials* **5**, 55–66.

Fleming, T.R., Watelet, L.F. (1989). Approaches to monitoring clinical trials. *Journal of the National Cancer Institute* **81**, 188–193.

Freedman, L., Spiegelhalter, D. et al. (1994). The what, why, and how of Bayesian clinical trials monitoring. *Statistics in Medicine* **13**, 1371–1383.

Friedman, L., Demets, D., et al. (2003). Data and safety monitoring in the Beta-Blocker Heart Attach Trial: Early experience in formal monitoring methods.

Frustaci, S., Gherlinzoni, F. et al. (2001). Adjuvant chemotherapy for adult soft tissue sarcomas of the extremities and girdles: Results of the Italian randomized cooperative trial. *Journal of Clinical Oncology* **19**, 1238–1247.

Furberg, C., Friedwald, W. (Eds.) (1978). Effects of chronic administration of beta-blockade on long-term survival following myocardial infarction. *Beta-Adrenergic Blockade: A New Era in Cardiovascular Medicine*. Excerpta Medica, Amsterdam.

Gausche, M., Lewis, R.J. et al. (2000). Effect of out-of-hospital pediatric endotracheal intubation on survival and neurological outcome. *The Journal of the American Medical Association* **283**(6), 783–790.

Geller, N.L., Pocock, S.J. et al. (1987). Interim analyses in randomized clinical trials: Ramifications and guidelines for practitioners. *Biometrics* **43**(1), 213–223.

Halperin, M., Lan, K. et al. (1982). An aid to data monitoring in long-term clinical trials. *Controlled Clinical Trials* **3**, 311–323.

Jennison, D., Turnbull, B. (1983). Confidence interval for a bionomial parameter following a multistage test with application to MIL-STD 105D and medical trials. *Technometrics* **25**, 49–63.

Jennison, C., Turnbull, B. (1984). Repeated confidence intervals for group sequential clinical trials. *Controlled Clinical Trials* **5**, 33–45.

Jennison, C., Turnbull, B. (1985). Repeated confidence intervals for the median survival time. *Biometrika* **72**, 619–625.

Jennison, C., Turnbull, B. (1989). Interim Analyses: The repeated confidence interval approach (with discussion). *Journal of Royal Statistical Society. Series B* **51**, 305–361.

Jennison, C., Turnbull, B.W. (1997). Group sequential analysis incorporating covariate information. *Journal of the American Statistical Association* **92**, 1330–1341.

Jennison, C., Turnbull, B.W. (2000). *Group Sequential Methods with Application to Clinical Trials*. Chapman & Hall.

Jennison, C., Turnbull, B.W. et al. (2005). Meta-analyses and adaptive group sequential designs in the clinical development process. *Journal of Biopharmaceutical Statistics* **15**(4), 537–558.

Jones, D., Newman, C. et al. (1982). The design of a sequential clinical trial for the comparison of two lung cancer treatments. *Statistics in Medicine* **1**(1), 73–82.

Kaplan, E., Meier, P. (1958). Nonparametric estimation from incomplete observations. *Journal of American Statistical Association* **53**, 457–481.

Kelly, K., Crowley, J. et al. (2001). Randomized phase III trial of paclitaxel plus carboplatin versus vinorelbine plus cisplatin in the treatment of patients with advanced non–small-cell lung cancer: A southwest oncology group trial. *Journal of Clinical Oncology* **19**, 3210–3218.

Kim, K., DeMets, D. (1992). Sample size determination for group sequential clinical trials with immediate response. *Statistics in Medicine* **11**(10), 1391–1399.

Kittelson, J., Emerson, S. (1999). A unifying family of group sequential test designs. *Biometrics* **55**, 874–882.

Kpozehouen, A., Alioum, A. et al. (2005). Use of a Bayesian approach to decide when to stop a therapeutic trial: The case of a chemoprophylaxis trial in human immunodeficiency virus infection. *American Journal of Epidemiology,* **161**(6), 595–603, (see comment).

Kuehn, B. (2006). Industry, FDA warm to "Adaptive" trials. *The Journal of the American Medical Association* **296**(16), 1955–1971.

Lan, K., DeMets, D.L. (1989). Group sequential procedures: Calendar versus information time. *Statistics in Medicine* **8**, 1191–1198.

Lan, K., Demets, D. (1983). Discrete sequential boundaries for clinical trials. *Biometrika* **70**, 659–663.

Lan, K., Simon, R. et al. (1982). Stochastically curtailed tests in long-term clinical trials. *Communications in Statistics C* **1**, 207–219.

Lan, K., Wittes, J. (1988). The B-value: A tool for monitoring data. *Biometrics* **44**, 579–585.

Lan, K., Zucker, D. (1993). Sequential monitoring of clinical trials: The role of information and Brownian motion. *Statistics in Medicine* **12**, 753–765.

Lee, J., Demets, D. (1991). Sequential comparison of changes with repeated measurement data. *Journal of American Statistical Association* **86**, 757–762.

Mantel, N. (1966). Evaluation of survival data and two new rank order statistics arising in its consideration. *Cancer Chemotherapy Reports* **50**, 163–170.

Mazumdar, M. (2004). Group sequential design for comparative diagnostic accuracy studies: Implications and guidelines for practitioners. *Medical Decision Making: An International Journal of the Society for Medical Decision Making* **24**(5), 525–533.

Mazumdar, M., Liu, A. (2003). Group sequential design for comparative diagnostic accuracy studies. *Statistics in Medicine* **22**(5), 727–739.

McPherson, K. (1974). Statistics: The problem of examining accumulating data more than once. *New England Journal of Medicine* **290**, 501–502.

Motzer, R., Nichols, C. et al. (2007). Phase III randomized trial of conventional-dose chemotherapy with or without high-dose chemotherapy and autologous hematopoietic stem-cell rescue as first-line treatment for patients with poor-prognosis metastatic germ cell tumors. *Journal of Clinical Oncology* **25**(3), 247–256.

Murray, D.M. (1998). *Design and Analysis of Group-randomized Trials*. Oxford University Press, New York.

Nicholls, S.J., Sipahi, I. et al. (2006). Intravascular ultrasound assessment of novel antiatherosclerotic therapies: Rationale and design of the Acyl-CoA:Cholesterol Acyltransferase Intravascular Atherosclerosis Treatment Evaluation (ACTIVATE) Study. *American Heart Journal* **152**(1), 67–74.

O'Brien, P., Fleming, T. (1979). A multiple testing procedure for clinical trials. *Biometrics* **35**, 549–556.

Pampallona, S., Tsiatis, A. (1994). Group sequential designs for one-sided and two-sided hypothesis testing with provision for early stopping in favor of null hypothesis. *Journal of Statistical Planning and Inference* **42**, 19–35.

Parmar, M., Spiegelhalter, D. et al. (1994). The CHART trials: Bayesian design and monitoring in practice. *Statistics in Medicine* **13**, 1297–1312.

Pepe, M., Anderson, G. (1992). Two-stage experimental designs: Early stopping with a negative result. *Applied Statistics* **41**(1), 181–190.

Pocock, S.J. (1977). Group sequential methods in the design and analysis of clinical trials. *Biometrika* **64**, 191–199.

Proschan, M., Lan, K. et al. (2006). *Statistical Monitoring of Clinical Trials: A Unified Approach.* Springer.

Reboussin, D., Lan, K. et al. (1992). Group Sequential Testing of Longitudinal Data. Tech Report No. 72, Department of Biostatistics, University of Wisconsin.

Reboussin, D.M., DeMets, D.L. et al. (2000). Computations for group sequential boundaries using the Lan–DeMets spending function method. *Controlled Clinical Trials* **21**(3), 190–207.

Sacco, R.L., DeRosa, J.T. et al. (2001). Glycine antagonist in neuroprotection for patients with acute stroke: GAIN Americas – a randomized controlled trial. *The Journal of the American Medical Association* **285**(13), 1719–1728.

Scharfstein, D., Tsiatis, A. et al. (1997). Semiparametric efficiency and its implication on the design and analysis of group-sequential studies. *Journal of the American Statistical Association* **92**, 1342–1350.

Schoenfeld, D.A. (2001). A simple algorithm for designing group sequential clinical trials. *Biometrics* **57**(3), 972–974.

Sebille, V., Bellissant, E. (2003). Sequential methods and group sequential designs for comparative clinical trials. *Fundamental and Clinical Pharmacology* **17**(5), 505–516.

Spiegelhalter, D., Freedman, L. et al. (1994). Bayesian approaches to clinical trials (with discussion). *Journal of Royal Statistics Society Association* **157**, 357–416.

Spiegelhalter, D., Freedman, L. et al. (1986). Monitoring clinical trials: Conditional or predictive power? *Controlled Clinical Trials* **7**, 8–17.

Tsiatis, A., Boucher, H. et al. (1995). Sequential methods for parametric survival models. *Biometrics* **82**, 165–173.

Tsiatis, A., Rosner, G. et al. (1984). Exact confidence intervals following a group sequential test. *Biometrics* **40**, 797–803.

Tsiatis, A.A., Mehta, C.R. (2003). On the inefficiency of the adaptive design for monitoring clinical trials. *Biometrika* **90**(2), 367–378.

URL: http://cancertrials.nci.nih.gov Policy of the National Cancer Institute for Data and Safety Monitoring of Clinical Trials.

Wald, A. (1947). *Sequential Analysis*. Wiley, New York.

Wang, S.K., Tsiatis, A.A. et al. (1987). Approximately optimal one-parameter boundaries for group sequential trials. *Biometrics* **43**(1), 193–199.

Wang, Y., Leung, D. (1997). Bias reduction via resampling for estimation following sequential tests. *Sequential Analysis* **16**, 298–340.

Wassmer, G. (2006). Planning and analyzing adaptive group sequential survival trials. *Biometrical Journal* **48**(4), 714–729.

Wassmer, G., Vandemeulebroecke, M. (2006). A brief review on software developments for group sequential and adaptive designs. *Biometrical Journal* **48**(4), 732–737.

Whitehead, J. (1986). On the bias of maximum likelihood estimation following a sequential test. *Biometrika* **73**, 573–581.

Whitehead, J. (1997). *The Design and Analysis of Sequential Clinical Trials*. Wiley, Chichester.

Zou, G.Y., Donner, A. et al. (2005). Group sequential methods for cluster randomization trials with binary outcomes. *Clinical Trials* **2**(6), 479–487.

Handbook of Statistics, Vol. 27
ISSN: 0169-7161

DOI: 10.1016/S0169-7161(07)27017-8

17

Early Phase Clinical Trials: Phases I and II

Feng Gao, Kathryn Trinkaus and J. Philip Miller

Abstract

A clinical trial is a planned experiment on human subjects to assess one or more potentially beneficial therapies. A central problem in early phase clinical trials is the limited knowledge on the new treatment of interest. As a consequence, extreme caution needs to be taken in study designs to minimize the risk of participants while maximizing the benefit. This chapter provides an overview of the recent advances in statistical designs of early phase clinical trials. Since formal statistical methods for phase I and II trials have been mostly developed for cancer drugs, a considerable portion of this chapter addresses statistical issues in this particular setting.

1. Introduction

Clinical trials, usually classified as phases I, II, III, and IV, are true experiments on human beings to assess one or more potentially beneficial therapies. The primary objective of phase I trials is to characterize the safety profile of a new regimen and to determine the best dose for subsequent clinical evaluation of its efficacy. The purpose of phase II trials is to assess the therapeutic efficacy of a regimen in a well-defined patient population and to further evaluate its toxicity profile. Phase III trials are conducted in a randomized controlled manner to provide more definitive results regarding the benefits and risks associated with a new treatment as compared to the standard therapy. Phase IV trials carry out post-marketing surveillance of treatment effects with long-term follow-up in a broader clinical setting (i.e., to examine issues of quality of life) or for goals other than clinical benefits (i.e., for marketing purposes). This chapter is devoted to the recent development of statistical designs in early phase clinical trials. Since many formal statistical methods for phase I and II trials have been developed to evaluate cytotoxic drug development in oncology studies, a considerable portion of this chapter addresses statistical issues in this particular setting.

In Section 2, a variety of innovative designs in phase I trials is presented. A common feature shared by these designs is to seek the highest dose associated with a tolerable level of toxicity, the maximum tolerated dose (MTD). The strategy for identifying the MTD is one of the key features that differentiate these designs. Section 2.1 describes the *conventional* 3 + 3 *design* and its modifications. Section 2.2 presents *up-and-down designs* that are based on a random walk concept and allow dose escalation or de-escalation based on the occurrence of dose limiting toxicity (DLT) among previous patients. *Accelerated titration designs* are presented in Section 2.3, where a two-stage process of escalation and de-escalation rules is used to shorten the trial and treat fewer patients at subtherapeutic doses. Section 2.4 introduces the *continuous reassessment method* (*CRM*) and Section 2.5 presents the *dose escalation with overdose control* (*EWOC*), both of which take a Bayesian modeling approach and treat MTD as a parameter of the model. Sections 2.6 outlines some complex innovative phase I designs and Section 2.7 explores the integration of phase I and II trials.

Section 3 presents recent advances beyond conventional single-arm phase II trials. Though nowadays small randomized phase II trials are not uncommon, a typical phase II trial is conducted without concurrent controls. It usually considers efficacy (often measured as a binary variable based on tumor shrinkage) as the solely primary endpoint and treats a relatively homogenous patient population (Geller, 1984; Retain et al., 1993). Estey and Thall (2003) recently have given an excellent review of the problems with current phase II trials and proposed some practical alternatives. In Section 3.1, we describe *phase II trials with multiple stages* that allow early stopping due to inactivity of regimen. *Phase II trials with multiple endpoints* are introduced in Section 3.2, including trials that simultaneously consider toxicity and efficacy as well as trials that distinguish the relative importance of complete response (CR) versus partial response (PR). Section 3.3 presents *covariate-adjusted phase II trials* that estimate efficacy in the presence of patient heterogeneity, and Section 3.4 introduces *randomized phase II trials* that aim to select the best regimen among several experimental therapies. Some miscellaneous innovations in phase II designs are also discussed in Section 3.5. These include *adaptive designs* that allow investigators to re-adjust the sample size based on information accumulated during the first stage, *three-outcome trials* that allow rejection of the null hypothesis (H_0), rejection of the alternative hypothesis (H_a), or rejecting of neither, as well as *flexible designs* that permit the actual size achieved at each stage to deviate slightly from the exact design. Finally, Section 3.6 deals with some issues of transition from a phase II trial to phase III.

A short summary in Section 4 compares the different developmental strategies used for cytotoxic and non-cytotoxic agents. Several useful websites and free available software to implement some of the published methods are also presented in Section 4.

2. Phase I designs

The first use of a drug or device ("treatment") in humans or in a new disease setting usually takes place in conditions of uncertainty. The treatment may be entirely new, or its effect may be as yet unexplored in a combination of treatments or in a new disease setting. Phase I trial designs provide a structure for these first steps. They typically involve few patients, are relatively quickly completed and gather specific, limited information. Participants are often either healthy volunteers or patients whose treatment options have been exhausted, so they are not representative of the population in which the treatment, if successful, will be used. Patients are recruited in small cohorts, often 1–3 in each, into a single-arm, uncontrolled study. The primary goal of phase I treatment trials is to identify highest dose that can be tolerated without excessive toxicity or other adverse effects (MTD). Adverse effects are monitored and described, as are any indications of efficacy, although neither can be observed with great precision. Phase I studies are not intended to stand alone, however. The goal is to identify ethically acceptable treatments so that further efficacy testing can take place, while exposing the smallest possible number of patients to ineffective and possibly harmful treatments.

Planning a phase I trial requires definition of a starting dose and of the dose levels, or the range of acceptable doses, to be tested. These are based on an explicit or implicit dose–toxicity model and on a prior estimate of the MTD. The design further specifies the sample size at each dose level, a rule for dose escalation, a rule identifying DLT, and clear criteria for stopping the trial. Given these parameters, simulation studies are commonly used to compare alternative designs while planning a trial, especially to estimate the total sample size, the rate of DLT, the duration of the trial, and the number of patients treated at sub-optimal doses.

The phase I framework described above emphasizes single-treatment trials associated with substantial toxicity, which has been the standard for some years. The development of targeted therapies requires different strategies for testing, as the effects of such therapies may not be dose dependent, and some have low toxicity. There is also a need to anticipate differences in patient subgroups, defined by quantities measured prior to or updated continuously during the trial, and to accommodate trials with multiple agents and outcomes. Extensive reviews of the statistical basis of phase I designs can be found in the statistical literature (Chevret, 2006; Edler, 2001; Rosenberger and Haines, 2002; O'Quigley, 1999, 2002; Ahn, 1998). Horstmann et al. (2005) provide a comprehensive summary of the conduct and outcomes of 460 completed phase I trials, representing a complete survey of adult oncology trials conducted by the Cancer Therapy Evaluation Program (CTEP) between 1991 and 2002. The focus here is on new models and refinements of existing models made within the past 5 years. A review of software and websites, with code samples for developing phase I monitoring applications, can be found in Chevret (2006).

2.1. Traditional 3+3 and generalized A+B designs

Cohort designs rely on simple, rule-based algorithms to make decisions concerning dose escalation and trial continuation. Such algorithms are popular in practice because they are straightforward to carry out in complex clinical settings. The target sample size can be specified in advance, but the final trial size is not known at the outset. The resulting estimates of MTDs and DLTs are generally imprecise but may be adequate as a basis for further testing, especially when the underlying assumptions concerning dose escalation steps and toxicity rates are appropriate (Christian and Korn, 1994).

The simplest of rule-based algorithms accrue a fixed number of patients per cohort and escalate or de-escalate doses in fixed, pre-specified steps. The traditional 3 + 3 design uses cohorts of three patients each. Dose escalation occurs between cohorts, rather than within single patients, and the experience of the previous cohort usually is fully observed before proceeding to the next cohort.

The initial dose is chosen to cause little or no toxicity in humans. An acceptable initial dose may be specified using information from use of the experimental treatment in another multi-drug combination or a different disease setting. If no information is available on the treatment's activity in humans, the initial dose may be based on animal studies, e.g., 10% of the lethal dose in 10% of another species. Modified Fibonacci designs use dose multipliers such as 1.0, 2.0 (+100%), 3.3 (+65%), 5.0 (+52%), 7.0 (+49%), 9.0 (+33%), 12.0 (+33%), etc. (Edler, 2001; Lin and Shih, 2001).

An example of a traditional 3 + 3 design is

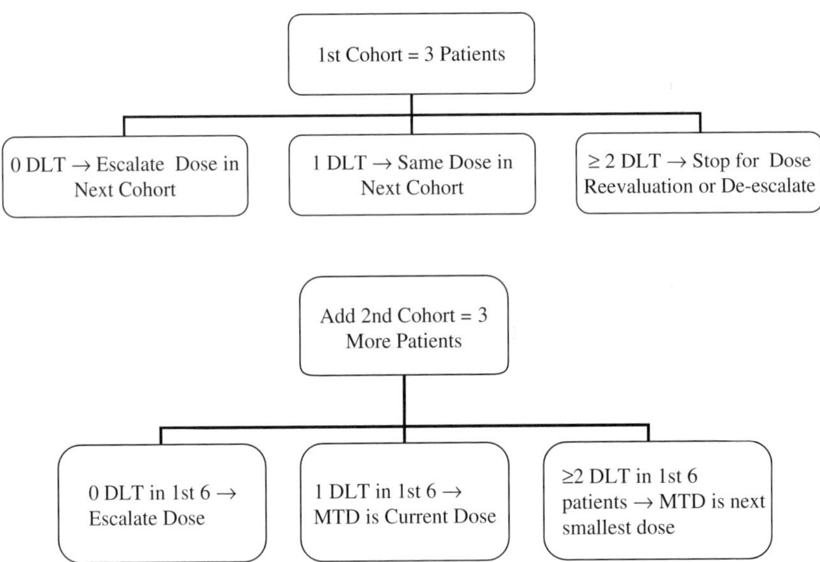

The trial continues until a pre-specified number of DLTs is observed and the MTD is determined. The number of cohorts may be specified in advance if there is a maximum dose that cannot be exceeded. In this case, the maximum trial size is known in advance.

The structure outlined above can be generalized to cohorts of varying size in an A + B design (Korn et al., 1994; Ivanova, 2006; Kang and Ahn, 2002). Properties used in designing an A + B trial with and without dose de-escalation can be found in Lin and Shih (2001). The simple case without de-escalation is described below.

Given $A = \sharp$ DLTs in the first cohort, $B = \sharp$ patients in the 1st cohort, $C = \sharp$ DLTs in the second (or both) cohorts, $D = \sharp$ patients in the second cohort, $E = \sharp$ DLTs in A + B, $n =$ the pre-specified number of dose levels, and $p_i =$ probability of DLT at dose level i, an A + B trial with dose de-escalation and $1 \leq j \leq n$, then the probability of $< C$ DLTs in cohort A is

$$P_0^j = \sum_{k=0}^{C-1} \binom{A}{k} p_j^k (1 - p_j)^{(A-k)}.$$

The probability of $\geq C$ but $\leq D$ DLTs in cohort A and $\leq E$ DLTs in cohorts (A + B) is

$$Q_0^j = \sum_{k=C}^{D} \sum_{m=0}^{E-k} \binom{A}{k} p_j^k (1 - p_j)^{A-k} \binom{B}{m} p_j^m (1 - p_j)^{B-m}.$$

Thus, for $1 \leq I < n$, the MTD falls at dose I if there is escalation at dose $\leq i$ and escalation stops at dose $(i + 1)$:

$$P(\text{MTD} = \text{dose}_i) = (1 - P_0^{i+1} - Q_0^{i+1}) \prod_{j=1}^{i} (P_0^j + Q_0^j).$$

The final sample size is not known in advance, primarily because the number of levels from the initial dose to the first DLT is unknown. The expected number of patients at each dose level can be estimated. If the probability of $\geq C$ but $\leq D$ DLTs in cohort A at dose level j is

$$P_1^j = \sum_{k=C}^{D} \binom{A}{k} p_j^k (1 - p_j)^{A-k}$$

and X_j is the number of patients to be treated at dose level j, then

$$E(X_i) = \sum_{i=0}^{n} E(X_j | \text{MTD} = \text{dose}_i) P(\text{MTD} = \text{dose}_i),$$

where

$$\begin{aligned} E(X_j | \text{MTD} = \text{dose}_i) &= \left\{ \frac{AP_0^j + (A + B)Q_0^j}{P_0^j + Q_0^j}, \quad j \leq i \right. \\ &= \left\{ \frac{A(1 - P_0^j - P_1^j) + (A + B)(P_1^j - Q_0^j)}{1 - P_0^j - Q_0^j}, \quad j = i + 1 \right. \\ &= \{0, j > i + 1. \end{aligned}$$

These designs are simple to describe and to apply, and they are among the simplest to monitor as they have relatively few rules. Estimates of the MTD are discontinuous and usually imprecise, but they cannot fall outside the pre-specified dose levels. The probability of unexpected, short-term toxicity is limited to a single cohort, as the experience of each cohort is observed before starting the next. In practice, there is often pressure to enroll as quickly as possible, so long-term toxicity must be monitored separately and may affect a larger number of patients. A trial with a very low starting dose or one that does not observe a DLT may be very long, exposing too many patients to toxicity at sub-therapeutic doses. The widespread use and intuitive appeal of these designs have motivated attempts to improve their precision and unpredictable length.

2.2. Up-and-down designs

Up-and-down designs are based on a random walk concept, allowing dose escalation or de-escalation to occur within single patients or small cohorts based on the occurrence of DLT among previous patients. A simple Markovian random walk would assign subsequent doses on the basis of the previous patient's experience, escalating the dose in the absence of DLT and de-escalating it if a DLT is observed at the previous dose. The probability of underdosing or overdosing can be high, which has prompted several reformulations (O'Quigley and Chevret, 1991; Durham et al., 1997).

Biased coin allocation designs use the maximum allowable probability of DLT ($P_{\max}$) to weight the probability of dose escalation. For example, if a DLT is observed, then the subsequent dose is de-escalated. If there is no DLT, then the subsequent dose is escalated only if a binary random variable with $P(X = 1) = P_{\max}/(1 - P_{\max})$ takes the value 1. Otherwise, the next patient is treated at the same dose.

Using the experience of more than one previous patient is possible using a k-in-a-row rule or moving average rule. Storer (1989) suggested escalating the dose only if the two consecutive previous patients were without DLT. Ivanova et al. (2003) describe a more general k-in-a-row rule which de-escalates from dose level j to level $j-1$ if the most recent patient experienced a DLT at level j, escalates from dose level j to $j+1$ if the previous, consecutive k patients have received dose level j without DLT, and remains at the same dose otherwise. A related, moving average rule, escalates to dose level $j+1$ if the previous, consecutive k patients have been treated at dose level j without DLT and de-escalates otherwise. The probability of DLT at the MTD is defined as $P_{\max} = 1 - (0.5)^{1/k}$, where $k = 1, 2, 3$. There is no provision for remaining at the same dose.

Up-and-down designs may be group sequential, treating cohorts of more than one patient (Storer, 1989). Such designs are similar to the A + B concept. The dose would be escalated if there are no DLTs in the first cohort, maintained at the same level in three additional patients if there is one DLT, and de-escalated if there is more than one DLT (see also Edler, 2001). An up-and-down stage can be added to the initial cohorts of an A + B design without de-escalation to move rapidly through sub-therapeutic doses and progress by slower steps once a DLT has occurred (Gatsonis and Greenhouse, 1992; O'Quigley and Chevret, 1991).

The primary disadvantage of up-and-down designs is that they can escalate or de-escalate too rapidly. In the first case, the patients are placed at undue risk. In the second case, the first stage may be lengthened or fail to reach an active dose. If toxicity is severe, up-and-down designs may be better suited to treatments with small dosing steps than to those with large gaps due to the nature of the treatment or its delivery.

Several studies have shown that isotonic regression estimators can be efficient at estimating the MTD within a set of ordinal toxicity categories (Ivanova et al., 2003; Stylianou and Flournoy, 2002). Greater efficiency means that fewer patients are treated before reaching the MTD and that, in at least one case (Paul et al., 2004), the MTD is reached with fewer DLTs.

2.3. Accelerated titration designs

Accelerated titration designs (Simon et al., 1997; Eisenhauer et al., 2000) build on A + B and up-and-down concepts by using a two-stage process with escalation and de-escalation rules to shorten the trial and treat fewer patients at sub-therapeutic doses. In general, these designs begin with one patient per cohort, using pre-clinical information to determine the starting dose. Doses are escalated within or between patients until one DLT or two grade 2 toxicities are observed. Early dose escalation steps are large, e.g., adding 40–100% of the current dose as the expected toxicity profile of the treatment allows. In the second stage, patients are treated in small cohorts. Dose determination may follow an A + B design, or it may escalate the dose in 40% increments in a standard A + B design. The cost of shortening the trial and treating fewer patients at lower doses is a greater risk of more severe toxicity. Simulation and consideration of real-world trials indicate that a standard A + B design may have up to three times as many patients whose worst toxicity is none or mild (grade I by the NCI Common Toxicity Criteria) as does an accelerated design. An accelerated design may have 1.5–3.0 times as many patients with grade 4 (potentially life-threatening) toxicity (Simon et al., 1997).

Titrating doses, or altering doses up or down, within patients yield information about intra-patient variability which simpler designs lack, as well as an estimate of toxicity at lower levels than DLT. The trial can produce estimates of between-patient variability in probability of toxicity, as well as of the probability of cumulative toxicity. The magnitude of worst toxicity is described by

$$y_{ij} = \log(d_{ij} + \alpha D_{ij}) + \beta_i + \varepsilon_{ij},$$

where $i = 1, \ldots, n$ is the number of patients, $j = 1, 2, 3 \ldots$ the number of the dose level, d_j the dose at the jth dose level, and D_{ij} the total dose received by the ith patient up to but not including the jth dose level. α is the cumulative toxicity of doses D_{ij}, β_i represents patient-specific sensitivity to toxicity, and ε_{ij} measures intra-patient variability in experience of toxicity at a given dose level j.

The probability of grades 2–4 toxicity in a single course of treatment may be computed over the range of specified dose levels D as

$$\Phi\left(\frac{\log(d + \alpha D) + \mu_\beta - Kj}{\sqrt{\sigma_\beta^2 + \sigma_\alpha^2}}\right),$$

where Φ is the cumulative standard normal distribution function, K = 1, 2, 3, ... a set of constants defining critical toxicity categories, such that $y_{ij}<K_1$ indicates that patient i experienced less than grade 2 toxicity at dose level d_j, $K_1<y_{ij}<K_2$ indicates that patient 1 experienced grade 2 toxicity, $K_2<y_{ij}<K_3$ indicates DLT, and $y_{ij}\geq K_3$ indicates unacceptably severe toxicity. Using this definition of K, the probability of grade $j+$ toxicity at dose D and cumulative toxicity over previous doses D is

$$\Phi\left(\frac{\log(d+\alpha D)+\beta_i-K_{j-1}}{\sigma_\varepsilon}\right).$$

In practice, the risk of toxicity can be controlled by careful definition of the level considered dose limiting, as well as the level of toxicity considered sufficiently mild to permit intra-patient dose escalation, with reference to a given disease setting and patient population. First phase dose escalation steps can be smaller than 100%, if desirable. The second phase design is also flexible, taking any form that provides the required toxicity control features.

2.4. *Continuous reassessment method*

The CRM was proposed by O'Quigley et al. (1990) as a Bayesian strategy for estimation of the MTD as a parameter of a model, rather than a fixed quantity. Using prior information about the treatment, disease setting and patient population, a working dose–response function Ψ(d,a) is specified, where d is the dose level from a pre-specified range of possible doses $D_J=\{d_1,\ldots,d_J\}$ and a is a parameter vector to be estimated. The goal is to find a unique solution corresponding to the MTD such that $\Psi(\text{MTD}, a)=\theta$. The curve is refit as observations are taken from each patient or cohort as the trial progresses. After observing the result of treatment for the ith patient, $i=1,\ldots,N$, a new dose is chosen to minimize the difference between θ, the value of the dose–toxicity function at the MTD, and θ_{ij}, the observed value for the ith patient at the jth dose. That is, the current dose is determined from the most recent estimate of the MTD, rather than being fixed in advance.

Given the dose–toxicity function Ψ(d,a), information about the dose–toxicity relationship observed from patients 1 to $i-1=\Omega(y_1,\ldots,y_{i-1})$, and the prior density of the parameter a, $f(a,\Omega_i)$, the new estimate of the MTD is the probability of DLT at dose level j

$$P(d_j,a)=\int_0^\infty \Psi(d_j,a)f(a,\Omega_i)da=\theta_{ij}.$$

Once the toxicity at dose level j is known, the posterior density can be derived using the prior density and the likelihood of toxicity for the ith patient (Edler, 2001; O'Quigley, 2001):

$$L(y_i,d_{ij},a)=\Psi(d_{ij},a)^{y_i}[(1-\Psi(d_{ij},a))]^{1-y_i}.$$

By means of Bayes Theorem,

$$f(a, \Omega_{i+1}) = \frac{L(y_i, d_{ij}, a) f(a, \Omega_i)}{\int_0^\infty L(y_i, d_{ij}, u) f(u, \Omega_i) du}.$$

In principle, dose D_j is equal to the most recently estimated MTD, although, in practice, early estimates of the MTD may be imprecise. Very high estimates of the MTD may occur, which would result in large increases in dose from one patient to the next, and wide swings in the estimated MTD may increase the number of patients needed to achieve a stable estimate of the MTD. Overly high estimates of the MTD pose an unacceptable danger to patients, so a variety of modifications have been proposed to contain dose escalation within pre-specified limits. For example, the dose may be escalated by one level when the estimated MTD exceeds the current dose level, or it may be escalated by one level only if no DLT has been observed at the previous dose level. A maximum value of MTD may be pre-specified or derived from the prior dose–toxicity function, providing a cap for dose escalation. Treating more than one patient at each dose level also provides substantial improvement in the estimate of MTD, reducing the number of patients treated and decreasing the trial duration (Edler, 2001). Storer (2001) has shown that, although the precision of a CRM design may be lessened by the need to use fixed, rather than continuous, dose levels, precision can be improved by adding a model-fitting step after data collection is complete. Post-trial modeling treats dosing as continuous and incorporates all information collected by the trial.

CRM design can be used to identify levels of toxicity lower than DLT. This is a useful feature, as the cumulative effect of lower level toxicity can have severe consequences for the patient (Korn et al., 1994). To prevent unexpected DLT at the first dose level, Korn et al. (1994) suggested using a pre-specified initial dose level. The authors used a one-variable logistic model with an exponential prior and a maximum of six patients at any one dose level to estimate the MTD, concluding that there was little increase in safety or efficiency over rule-based approaches. Gatsonis and Greenhouse (1992) suggest estimating the MTD directly and propose escalation steps from these estimates. The need to protect against both overdosing and underdosing is addressed using a modified CRM design by Heyd and Carlin (1999). The authors propose modifying the CRM strategy to allow early stopping when the posterior 95% probability interval for the MTD reaches a pre-specified width. The authors review several alternative rules under a variety of erroneous prior information conditions, and conclude that trial size can be reduced and patient protection from overdosing and underdosing can be improved by these means. Their discussion is particularly interesting for the consideration of alternative dose–toxicity relationships and the inclusion of an additional parameter indicating the level of risk attached to a patient, for example, due to the presence or absence of a genotype or gene signature.

Observations such as these have prompted formulation of a modified, practical form of CRM (mCRM). This method defines the starting dose in the traditional fashion, based on pre-clinical or clinical information, and enrolls three patients at the starting dose. An initial estimate of sample size is made, as this information is needed for practical planning of the trial. The MTD, its posterior distribution, and a dose–toxicity curve are estimated at each step. Beyond this point, mCRM differs from the initial definition of CRM chiefly in the flexibility with which it accommodates disease, treatment, response, and toxicity characteristics of individual trials. A summary of the decision parameters can be found in Eisenhauer et al. (2000).

A good general discussion of the theoretical basis for optimal Bayesian design can be found in Haines et al. (2003). Although formulated as a Bayesian method, continuous reassessment can be carried out using maximum likelihood estimation as well (O'Quigley, 2002). Defining patient outcomes (primarily toxicity) as generalized to time-to-event endpoints (TITE–CRM, Braun, 2006) offers an alternative means of including information from patients who have not yet completed treatment. This extension also allows estimation of the incidence of late-onset toxicity. Dose–toxicity models can be stratified in order to take into account heterogeneity in MTDs in the designated patient population. Given significantly different responses to treatment, estimates of both average and patient-specific MTDs are often desirable (Legedza and Ibrahim, 2001; Whitehead, 2002). The critique that CRM may lead to exceeding the true MTD has led to a decision theoretic method to estimate the highest dose not exceeding a pre-specified toxicity risk, rather than the dose "closest to" that risk (Leung and Wang, 2002). TITE–CRM has also been modified to allow inclusion of late-onset toxicities, a useful feature when the agents involve are known to have lingering effects (Cheung and Chappell, 2000).

Software for CRM trials and other practical considerations are presented by Zohar et al. (2003) and Piantadosi et al. (1998).

2.5. Dose escalation with overdose control

A more formal approach to overdose control in CRM studies has been proposed by Babb et al. (1998), treating the probability of exceeding the MTD as a parameter to be estimated. The probability of overdose (dose > MTD) is limited to a pre-specified amount, the feasibility bound α, while minimizing the amount by which each patient is underdosed (= MTD–dose received). The first patient receives a starting dose, the minimum known to be safe in humans. All successive patients are assigned doses based on the posterior cumulative distribution function (CDF) of the MTD, $\pi_i(\gamma)$, or the probability that the MTD is exceeded by the dose d_i assigned to the ith patient, given prior information on doses received, toxicity administered, and any other clinically relevant covariates. That is, for all patients i, $i = 2, \ldots, N$, the dose chosen has $\pi_i(d_i) = \alpha$, or probability α of exceeding the MTD. The dose, then, satisfies $d_i = \pi_{i-1}^{-1}(\alpha)$. If dose levels are discontinuous, as if often the case, subsequent dose levels will differ from those derived from the posterior CDF of the MTD. If the pre-specified levels are $D_j = \{D_1, \ldots, D_J\}$, then the next dose is chosen to be the maximum of the D_j which meets two conditions: the difference between the actual and the calculated dose, $d_j - D_j$, does not exceed a pre-specified tolerance, and the difference between the probability of overdose at the calculated d_j and the maximum probability of overdose, $\pi_j(d_j)-\alpha$, does not exceed a second, pre-specified tolerance. This method converges efficiently toward MTD from below, while controlling the probability of a DL. It also provides a confidence interval for the MTD (Eisenhauer et al., 2000).

An extension of the EWOC method by Tighiouart et al. (2005) has shown that efficient estimation of the MTD using the EWOC method can improve the safety profile of the trial as a whole by assuming a prior negative correlation structure for the two primary parameters of the dose–toxicity model, the probability of DLT at the initial dose and the MTD. The EWOC framework shares the strengths of CRM strategies, including the use of any available prior information on clinically significant covariates and the ability to include treatment data from patients who have not yet completed therapy (early-onset toxicity) or from those who have been followed after completion of therapy (late-onset toxicity). Additional information and study planning tools are available at this writing at http://www.sph.emory.edu/BRI-WCI/ewoc.html.

2.6. More complex designs

2.6.1. Bivariate dose–toxicity designs

The potential for poor decision making involved in using purely algorithm-driven or purely CRM approaches has been a subject of comment for some years (Storer, 1989, 2001; Korn et al., 1994; Gatsonis and Greenhouse, 1992). There are clear advantages to combining the robustness of algorithm-driven designs, which protect patients from dosing extremes, and model driven approaches, which estimate the MTD more precisely and are more efficient in making use of available information. In addition to the combination of rule-based and CRM methods proposed by Storer (2001), Potter (2002) suggests a three-patient cohort design with a rule-based first stage, in which doses are escalated by 50% up to the first DLT. After this point a bivariate logistic dose–toxicity model is used to estimate the MTD, and subsequent patients are assigned a dose as close as possible to the estimated MTD. Initial settings of proportions at which 10% and 90% of patients would experience DLT can be customized to the patient population and disease setting in question. Alternative stopping rules are also described.

Bayesian methods offer several alternative designs incorporating a positive (efficacy) and a negative outcome (toxicity). Whitehead et al. (2006) propose a bivariate cohort design with two primary outcomes observed for each patient, a desirable outcome (DO) and a dose-limiting event (DLE). The goal is to define a "therapeutic window" of doses that optimizes both outcomes for each patient. Safety is given more weight than efficacy, so presence of toxicity is considered a single outcome, whether or not benefit is present. The other possible outcomes are benefit without toxicity and lack of benefit without toxicity. A prior joint distribution of benefit and toxicity is required. The outcomes are modeled using two logistic regression models with binary outcomes. A means of maximizing a gain function is proposed to identify the therapeutic window.

A similar model described by Loke et al. (2006) also treats toxicity and efficacy as binary endpoints. Using a Dirichlet prior, the authors define a utility for each possible decision that can be made at each dose level. The expected utility is maximized under the observed bivariate posterior distribution to identify the optimum dose.

Ivanova (2003) proposes an optimal Bayesian solution to choice between three outcomes: toxicity (with or without response, response without toxicity, and a neutral outcome (no response and no toxicity)). This design maximizes the probability of the response–no toxicity outcome for all doses with toxicity below the maximum tolerable level.

Zhang et al. (2006) propose a flexible continuation-ratio model with optimal dose selection criteria (TriCRM). Both toxicity and efficacy data are used, and information from all patients is used to determine successive dose levels. This method can incorporate several forms of monotonic dose–toxicity relationships, as well as an increasing–decreasing relationship with a single mode. The outcome is a biologically optimal dose defined by both efficacy and toxicity, where efficacy can be the effect on a molecular target. The inclusion of an efficacy endpoint measurable in small numbers of patients makes this design less reliant on toxicity, so it is suitable for biologic agents that may have low toxicity. Ishizuka and Ohashi (2001) have also proposed a method of monitoring toxicity and efficacy separately, which allow a natural expansion of a phase I trial into a phase II trial.

2.6.2. *Lagged designs*

Phase I designs generally require that outcomes be measured from each patient, or from all members of a cohort, before the subsequent patient or cohort can be treated. Considerable delays can result if the outcomes are not immediately observable. Several designs deal with this problem in a Bayesian framework that estimates subsequent doses at specified stages of the trial (Thall et al., 1999; Hüsing et al., 2001). Subsequent doses are estimated using all information available at the time, including information from patients who have not yet completed treatment. These generally specify a rule for assessing the inclusion of a new patient and result in a decision to continue or to wait for more information.

2.6.3. *Stratified designs*

Phase I trials have been criticized in the past for excessive simplicity, as they omit from consideration many features of the patients, their disease state, and the standard treatment. Patients enrolled in a phase I trial may differ from one another in age, gender, or other personal characteristics. They may not be uniform in disease subtype, severity, or prior treatment. They may be receiving concurrently a variety of standard treatments for the disease under consideration or for a co-morbid condition. Stratification is one way to adjust for systematic heterogeneity in the patient sample. Ivanova and Wang (2006) propose a bivariate isotonic design for estimation of separate MTDs in an ordered pair of patient subgroups with different probabilities of DLT. Using information on the probability of toxicity in each subgroup, a matrix of toxicity probabilities at each dose level is estimated using data from all patients and estimating from a different starting probability in each subgroup. Escalation stops separately in each subgroup when a pre-defined threshold is exceeded. Continuous reassessment provides a parametric approach to stratified studies using a two-parameter working model. O'Quigley et al. (2002) suggest an initial stage in which escalation occurs until one patient with DLT and one patient without DLT have been observed in each subgroup. After this point, the two-parameter model is fit, using either maximum likelihood or Bayesian methods, and the toxicity probability vector is updated with each observation. Low doses can be skipped in the subgroup less likely to experience toxicity. The occurrence of toxicity in one group can be used to inform decisions about the other, offering an advantage over entirely separate, parallel trials. The initial stage of the trial also can be used to explore the relative probability of toxicity if the ordering of subgroups is not already known.

2.6.4. Multiple treatments and/or multiple patient subgroups

Oncology treatments often involve more than one agent used concurrently, sequentially, or partially overlapping in time. The complementary, synergistic or antagonistic action of multiple drugs is often in need of investigation. Estimates of an MTD obtained from trials of monotherapy are unrepresentative at best and may be ethically impossible to carry out. There is an obvious benefit to simultaneous estimation of MTDs where two drugs are to be used in concert. In this situation, Ivanova and Wang (2004) have proposed a non-parametric method for estimating the MTD with respect to two drugs administered simultaneously. The authors assume that the dose ranges and levels of each drug are fixed in advance. The method is non-parametric in the sense that the dose–toxicity relationship of each drug is assumed to be non-decreasing at each fixed level of the other. Estimation of the MTD is based on the set of all possible dose combinations.

Kramar et al. (1999) have developed a maximum likelihood-based approach to CRM in order to monitor simultaneously two drugs with different toxicity profiles.

Still more complex situations may require assessment of multiple drugs or treatments in more than one subgroup of patients. In a review of both Bayesian and maximum likelihood approaches, He et al. (2006) propose a model-based approach that estimates effects for more than one treatment in more than one subgroup. Conaway et al. (2004) present a method of evaluating toxicity in multiple agents when the joint dose–toxicity relationship is poorly understood. Rather than requiring a fully ordered dose–response at the outset, the method accommodates partial orders, in which the relative probability of toxicity is initially unknown within pairs of treatments.

2.6.5. Multiple outcomes

Response has been the most common endpoint used to represent benefit in phase I trials, although many other aspects of biologic function may be equally as important in addition to toxicity. To deal with multiple outcomes, Fan and Wang (2006) propose a Bayesian decision-theoretic design for estimation of a single MTD based on multiple criteria. The authors propose a computationally compromised method of MTD estimation that is feasible, given commonly available computing resources, and that contains safeguards against overdosing by restricting the number of dose levels that can be escalated in a single step. An initial distribution for the dose–toxicity curve is assumed, and the curve is refit after each patient in a fashion similar to CRM. The degree of precision can be specified in advance and can be increased by more extensive computing.

Modeling biomarker expression level with toxicity is particularly complex because of the correlation between discrete (binary or ordinal) and continuous outcomes. Bekele and Shen (2005) present an adaptive Bayesian design for continuous monitoring of toxicity in phase I or phase II biomarker studies.

2.7. Phase I/II trials

If a substantial amount of information is available about the affect of a treatment, perhaps from clinical studies in another disease setting, and documented toxicity is low, there may be a need to progress rapidly from phase I dose-finding to documentation of toxicity and efficacy in a larger phase II study. The continuous reassessment framework offers the possibility of seamless progression from a small phase I trial with small dose steps to a larger phase II trial. Zohar and Chevret (2001) point out that CRM-based calculation of the MTD extends naturally in a larger trial to estimation of the minimum effective dose. The authors propose alternative decision rules based on posterior or predictive probabilities of both DLT and a predetermined level of efficacy. Since response, or other measure of efficacy, is monitored simultaneously, efficacy becomes the focus of the trial as it expands. Ishizuka and Ohashi (2001) have proposed using the posterior density function describing the probability of DLT, as this is readily interpreted by non-statisticians. The authors also suggest starting at the lowest dose level when the prior distribution of DLT is poorly defined, and terminating the trial when the posterior densities at each dose level are well separated. Bekele and Shen's (2005) adaptive design for monitoring a continuous biomarker and a discrete measure of toxicity also extends from a phase I to a phase II setting.

The single-drug focus of phase I trials is a handicap for disease settings in which multiple agents is the norm. Huang et al. (2007) suggest identifying the combination doses of possible interest and carrying out parallel phase I CRM trials to measure the safety and preliminary efficacy of each combination. Combinations with high toxicity can then be dropped. An adaptive randomization scheme is used to direct more patients to phase II trials of combinations with high efficacy and fewer to the combination doses with lower efficacy, based on Bayesian posterior probabilities.

3. Phase II designs

Once the dose and schedule of an agent has been set as a result of a phase I trial, the regimen is ready for a phase II trial. The primary goal of a classical phase II trial is to screen new regimens based on their efficacy. Unlike phase I trials where a problem of estimation is addressed, phase II trials inherently deal with a problem of hypothesis testing even though usually there is often no concurrent control arm in the trial. Let p_0 denote the maximum unacceptable probability of response and p_1 be the minimum acceptable probability of response ($p_0<p_1$), then the problem can be formulated as testing the null hypothesis H_0 versus the alternative H_a

$$H_0 : p \leq p_0 \text{ versus } H_a : p \geq p_1,$$

where p is the response rate.

The design of a typical phase II trial is based on a one-sample binomial distribution with the probability of success being the probability of achieving an objective response. In planning a trial, investigators choose a sample size (N) and a boundary value of response (r) to guarantee that the type I error α (i.e., the probability that we accept the new therapy when its true response rate is p_0) and type II error β (i.e., the probability that we reject the new therapy when its true response rate is p_1) are controlled under some pre-specified levels,

$$B(r; p_0, N) = \sum_{x=0}^{r} b(x; p_0, N) \geq 1 - \alpha,$$

$$B(r; p_1, N) = \sum_{x=0}^{r} b(x; p_1, N) \leq \beta,$$

$$b(x; p, N) = \binom{N}{x} p^x (1 - p)^{N-x},$$

$$b(x; p, N) = \binom{N}{x} p^x (1 - p)^{N-x},$$

where $b(x; p, N)$ and $B(x; p, N)$ denote the probability mass function and cumulative function for binomial distribution with probability of success p and number of trials N. That is, we want to reject the experimental treatment with a very high probability ($\geq 1-\alpha$) given a true H_0 and to reject the experimental treatment with a very low probability ($\leq \beta$) if H_1 is true. For a trial with (p_0, p_1, α, β) = (0.05, 0.20, 0.05, 0.10), for example, a minimum of 38 patients are required with a boundary value of 4 for rejecting H_0. There is approximately 95% chance ($\alpha = 0.05$) that four or less responders will be observed given an ineffective regimen ($p_0 = 5\%$) and there is 90% chance ($\beta = 0.10$) to observe five or more responses if the true response is 20% or above.

3.1. Phase II trials with multiple stages

Since phase I trials generally treat only three to six patients per dose level, such trials provide limited information regarding anti-tumor activity. It is important, both for ethical reasons and for the purpose of allocating limited resources, to minimize the number of patients exposed to drugs with poor activity. A variety of designs have been proposed to allow early stopping due to inactivity of the regimen, and the most popular one is Simon's two-stage design (Simon, 1989). A two-stage design can be described as follows. At first stage, N_1 patients will be treated. If the number of responders is not larger than a boundary r_1, the trial is terminated due to lack of treatment efficacy. Otherwise, additional N_2 patients will be accrued. If the accumulated number of responders is not larger than the boundary r, the trial will be claimed as lack of sufficient evidence to warrant further study.

Let $R(p)$ denote the probability of rejecting the treatment (or equivalently, accepting the null hypothesis H_0: $p \le p_0$),

$$R(p) = B(r_1; p, N_1) + \sum_{x=r_1+1}^{\min(r,N_1)} b(x; p, N_1)B(r - x; p, N_2)$$

For a given set of parameters (p_0, p_1, α, β), the sample sizes (N_1, $N = N_1+N_2$) and boundaries (r_1, r) can be searched by enumeration using exact binomial probabilities with constraints such that $R(p_0) \ge 1-\alpha$ and $R(p_1) \le \beta$. It is anticipated that many designs (N_1, N, r_1, r) can satisfy such α and β requirements. Simon's two-stage designs impose one more constraint that either minimizes the expected sample size (EN) when $p = p_0$ (the so-called optimal design) or minimizes the maximum number of patients N (the so-called minimax design). Sometimes, a choice between optimal and minimax designs can be difficult, especially when the optimal design has a much smaller EN but much large N than the minimax design. The size of the first stage is also a concern. Optimal designs often require fewer patients in the first stage, and so are suitable when the probability of severe toxicity is high or unknown. To this end, Jung et al. (2001) propose a heuristic graphical method to search for a good design that is a compromise between the optimal and minimax designs. Jung et al. (2004) also develop a family of two-stage designs that are admissible according to a Bayesian decision-theoretic criterion based on an ethically justifiable loss function. These admissible designs include Simon's optimal and minimax designs as special cases and thus facilitate investigators choosing trials with more appealing operational features.

Although two-stage designs are preferable to single-stage ones, they still suffer from the fact that in any cases a trial cannot be stopped until all patients in stage 1 have finished the experimental therapy, even if the true response rate is a value substantively inferior to the standard therapy ($p << p_0$). In order to protect patients from very poor regimens, some investigators place greater emphasis on minimizing the initial cohort of patients. Chen (1997) extends Simon's two-stage designs to three stages, with the overall probability of rejecting the treatment being

$$\begin{aligned} R(p) = {} & B(r_1; p, N_1) + \sum_{x=r_1+1}^{\min(r_2,N_1)} b(x; p, N_1)B(r_2 - x; p, N_2) \\ & + \sum_{x_1=r_1+1}^{\min(r_3,N_1)} \cdot \sum_{x=r_1+1}^{\min(r_3-x_1,N_2)} b(x_1; p, N_1)b(x_2; p, N_2) \\ & \times B(r_3 - x_1 - x_2; p, N_3). \end{aligned}$$

Similar to Simon's designs, the parameters for three-stage design (N_1, N_2, N, r_1, r_2, r_3) are searched such that the expected sample size (EN) is minimized when $p = p_0$ (three-stage optimal design), or the maximum sample size $N = N_1+N_2+N_3$ is minimized (three-stage minimax design). Comparing to two-stage designs, in average, the three-stage trials can reduce the expected sample size by 10% when the treatment is ineffective. For the same concern, Hanfelt et al. (1999) modify Simon's optimal design to minimize the median sample size rather than the expected sample size. As comparing with the optimal two-stage design, the modified design tends to have a smaller initial cohort of patients (N_1) and has a slightly larger expected sample size. Both of the above designs suffer from a potential drawback that there is a greater risk to reject a promising experimental therapy, especially when there is a substantial heterogeneity in the patient population. One possible solution to this issue is to limit the eligibility to a relative homogeneous population for patients entering the first stage.

Theoretically, the more stages in a multi-stage design, the better the performance in terms of sample-size gain under null hypothesis. However, the largest gain is actually seen when moving from one-stage to two-stage designs. In addition, designs with more than two stages can create an onerous administrative burden, especially for trials conducted in co-operative groups or multi-institute settings. Thus, Simon's two-stage designs remain the most popular designs in practice.

3.2. *Phase II trials with multiple endpoints*

3.2.1. *Designs incorporating both safety and efficacy*

Although the primary goal of a phase II trial is to assess the clinical efficacy, toxicity could affect the course of treatment and sometimes evaluation of toxicity may be equal in importance to the assessment of efficacy. In most clinical protocols for phase II trials, the study designs are based on a single "primary" outcome associated with treatment efficacy while ignoring the safety issues. Rather, the adverse events of treatment are "monitored" using early stopping rules derived from sequential probability ratio test (SPRT) or Bayesian methods. That is, two tests are carried out separately – one for side effects and one for treatment efficacy. This double testing will affect the operating characteristics of both tests, but the problem is ignored in a typical design. In addition, such a strategy is incapable of identifying experimental regimens that have substantially low adverse events but have nearly the same efficacy comparing with the standard therapy.

With these considerations in mind, a variety of phase II designs based on multiple outcomes have been developed. Bryant and Day (1995) propose a two-stage design to evaluate both clinical response and toxicity, where the trial is terminated after the first stage if either the observed toxicity rate is too high or the response rate is too low. In analogy to Simon's two-stage design, let p_{r_0} and p_{r_1} denote the maximum unacceptable and the minimum acceptable probabilities of *response* ($p_{\mathrm{r}_0} < p_{\mathrm{r}_1}$), let p_{t_0} and p_{t_1} be the maximum unacceptable and the minimum acceptable probabilities of *non-toxicity* ($p_{\mathrm{t}_0} < p_{\mathrm{t}_1}$), let p_{r} denote probability of response, and let p_{t} be the probability of *not experiencing* toxicity. The proposed design can be formulated as testing the hypotheses

$$\mathrm{H}_0 : p_\mathrm{r} \le p_{\mathrm{r}_0} \text{ or } p_\mathrm{t} \le p_{\mathrm{t}_0} \quad \text{versus } \mathrm{H}_\mathrm{a} : p_\mathrm{r} \ge p_{\mathrm{r}_1} \text{ and } p_\mathrm{t} \ge p_{\mathrm{t}_1}.$$

The trial will be terminated after stage 1 if either less than rr_1 responders or less than rt_1 *non-toxicity* patients are observed. At the completion of study, the experimental regimen will be concluded effective if the number of responders and the number of non-toxicity exceed rr and rt simultaneously. These design parameters (rr_1, rt_1, N_1, rr, rt, N) are chosen such that the following error bounds are satisfied: α_r is an upper bound on the probability of erroneously accepting a regimen whose toxicity rate is acceptable ($p_\mathrm{t} \ge p_{\mathrm{t}_1}$) but with inadequate response rate ($p_\mathrm{r} \le p_{\mathrm{r}_0}$); α_t is an upper bound on the probability of erroneously accepting a regimen whose response rate is acceptable ($p_\mathrm{r} \ge p_{\mathrm{r}_1}$) but with excess toxicity ($p_\mathrm{t} \le p_{\mathrm{t}_0}$); and β is a bound on the probability of failing to recommend a regimen that is acceptable with respect to both response and toxicity ($p_\mathrm{r} \ge p_{\mathrm{r}_1}$ and $p_\mathrm{t} \ge p_{\mathrm{t}_1}$). These design parameters also depend on the values of potential associations between response and toxicity. To search for an optimal design, Bryant and Day apply the above error constraints uniformly over all possible correlations between toxicity and response. They have shown that the design is very insensitive to the misspecification of correlations as long as a small-to-moderate β is specified ($\beta \le 0.15$, say).

Similar designs are proposed by other investigators for joint modeling of safety and efficacy. Conaway and Petroni (1995) propose two- and three-stage designs based on response and toxicity, taking the same strategy as Bryant and Day while allowing the associations between response and toxicity to be explicitly specified. Conaway and Petroni (1996) further propose a design allowing trade-offs between toxicity and response. That is, the design allows more patients with toxicity when the response rate is high, and vice versa. The trade-offs between toxicity and response are quantified by a so-called "I-divergence" statistics, which in some sense measures the distance from p to H_0. Thall and Cheng (2001) extend Simon's two-stage design to randomized trials based on a two-dimensional test. The parameters (i.e., efficacy and safety) are defined as the difference between experimental and control regimens so that all the effects are in the same scale. If the endpoints are binary variables such as response rate, for example, an arcsine difference transformation $\Delta = (\sin^{-1}\sqrt{p_1} - \sin^{-1}\sqrt{p_0})$ will make the variance of Δ independent of p_1 or p_0, approximately with $\mathrm{var}(\Delta) \approx 1/4n$. One attractive feature of the proposed design is its adaptability to many different situations. The design accommodates both continuous and discrete outcomes, applies to both randomized and single-arm trials, and also allows one to test for an improvement in one dimension while maintaining the null level in the other. In contrast, the designs by Bryant and Day (1995) and Conaway and Petroni (1995, 1996) require that the alternative hypothesis specifies improvements in both toxicity and response.

3.2.2. Designs distinguishing complete response from partial response

A most commonly used measure of efficacy in phase II oncology trials is response rate. It is standard practice to further classify responders as either complete response (CR) or partial response (PR). CR is consistently characterized as the complete disappearance of measurable lesions for a fixed minimal time period without appearance of new lesions. Usually PR is defined as 50% reduction of the target lesions though the definition can vary from one protocol to another (Geller, 1984). For many trials, an increase in the number of CR will be more impressive because CR is rare in many tumors, and a presence of CR usually indicates a substantial improvement in patient survival. Thus, a regimen that shows a significant improvement in CR may be also of interest to clinicians even if the improvement in total response (TR = CR + PR) does not achieve its goal. The conventional phase II designs such as Simon's, however, are based on a binary indicator of TR without differentiating CR versus PR.

In recognizing the relative importance of CR versus PR, a variety of alternative designs have been proposed in recent years. Lu et al. (2005) propose to add CR as an additional efficacy endpoint to a conventional study. The proposed design can be expressed as testing the hypotheses

$$\mathrm{H}_0 : p_{\mathrm{tr}} \leq p_{\mathrm{tr}_0} \text{ and } p_{\mathrm{cr}} \leq p_{\mathrm{cr}_0} \text{ versus } \mathrm{H}_{\mathrm{a}} : p_{\mathrm{tr}} \geq p_{\mathrm{tr}_1} \text{ or } p_{\mathrm{cr}} \geq p_{\mathrm{cr}_1},$$

where p_{tr_0} and p_{tr_1} denote the maximum unacceptable and the minimum acceptable probabilities of TR as usual ($p_{\mathrm{tr}_0} < p_{\mathrm{tr}_1}$), p_{cr_0} and p_{cr_1} are the maximum unacceptable and the minimum acceptable probabilities of CR ($p_{\mathrm{cr}_0} < p_{\mathrm{cr}_1}$), and p_{tr} and p_{cr} are the probabilities of TR and CR, respectively. That is, the objective of the trial is to seek a regimen that shows significant improvements in either TR or CR (or both). To design a trial with proper sample sizes and cutoff values, the following three error bounds are specified: a type I error α for erroneously accepting a regimen ineffective in both TR and CR, a marginal type II error β_{tr} for erroneously rejecting a regimen effective in TR, and a marginal type II error β_{cr} for erroneously rejecting a regimen effective in CR. Depending on the relative importance of TR and CR, β_{tr} and β_{cr} do not have to be the same. Owing to the hierarchical structure of TR and CR (TR = CR + PR), it has been shown that the marginal power functions of TR and PR are the lower bounds of the joint power,

$$Pr(\text{reject } \mathrm{H}_0 | p_{\mathrm{tr}_1} \text{ and } p_{\mathrm{cr}_1}) \geq \max(1 - \beta_{\mathrm{tr}}, 1 - \beta_{\mathrm{cr}}).$$

The optimal design is chosen as the one that produces a minimum sample size among those trials satisfying above error bounds. Because of the multivariate nature of the problem, it is possible that more than one solution can be obtained. If this happens, one more constraint will be imposed and the optimal design is sought until the joint power of TR and CR is maximized.

Similar designs are also proposed by Lin and Chen (2000) to differentiate the importance of CR versus PR. Their method combines CR and PR information using a weighted linear score based on the relative importance, and the optimum design is constructed with a likelihood-ratio test. Panageas et al. (2002) propose a similar design where the optimization is performed by a direct search based on enumerating exact trinomial probabilities, but sometimes the computation for such a direct search can be prohibitively intensive. Both of the above designs use the information on CR and PR separately. In contrast, Lu et al. (2005) treat CR

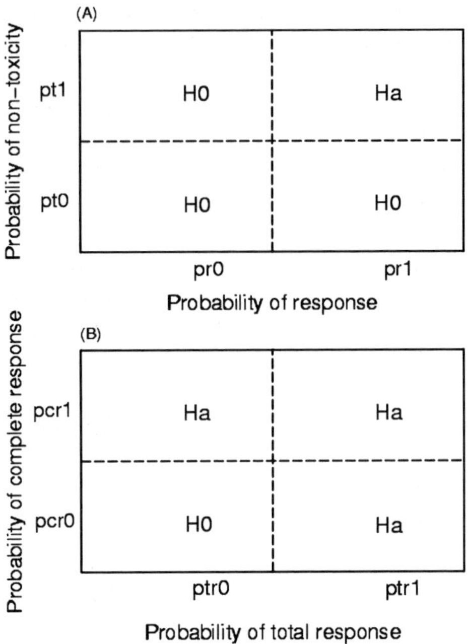

Fig. 1. Null and alternative regions for designs with multiple endpoints: (A) Designs incorporate toxicity and response simultaneously (Bryant and Day, 1995). (B) Designs distinguish the relative importance of complete response (CR) versus partial response (PR) (Lu et al., 2005).

as additional information and thus makes the design more consistent with conventional practice. The design by Lu et al. also permits rejection regions to be searched for under marginal power functions, thus allowing investigators to specify separate powers for TR and CR according to their clinical importance.

Note that the trials with multiple efficacy endpoints address a research question different from designs simultaneously considering efficacy and toxicity. The main objective of trials with multiple efficacy endpoints is to seek a new regimen that shows improvement in either of the endpoints, and thus the specification of its alternative hypothesis will be different from design such as Bryant and Day (1995) that aims to meet both safety and efficacy criteria. The null and alternative regions for both types of designs are displayed in Fig. 1. Comparing to conventional Simon's designs, trials with multiple endpoints share a common complexity that additional parameters must be prospectively specified. The communication of the design characteristics to clinicians who actually conduct the trial can be a challenge. A graphical presentation, analogous to Jung et al. (2001), of the operational characteristics of candidate trials may provide a useful tool for such a purpose.

3.3. *Covariate-adjusted phase II trials*

To increase the chance of detecting treatment activity and to minimize the possibility of rejecting a potentially promising regimen, phase II trials usually are conducted in a selected well-defined patient group. However, patient heterogeneity is inevitable in many clinical trials and sometimes this can raise challenges for study planning. In the treatment of ER/PR positive metastatic breast cancer patients, for example, it has been shown that letrozole alone can result in a clinical benefit (CR + PR) of 50% as a first-line therapy, but the response rate is only 25% in those refractory patients. Conventional phase II trials take two rather extreme strategies to handle the problem of patient heterogeneity. One approach is simply ignoring the existence of heterogeneity, and the drawback of this approach is apparent. An ideal approach is to conduct a series of independent phase II trials within each homogeneous patient group, but sometimes this becomes infeasible due to limited number of patients or prohibitively high cost. The second approach also turns out to be inefficient and wasteful of resources because it fails to "borrow strength" for the information carried among these separate trials. That is, if an improvement is seen in the refractory patients, this can provide evidence that an improvement is also more likely in newly diagnosed untreated patients, and vice versa. The so-called covariate-adjusted designs provide a more desirable approach for this situation.

London and Chang (2005) propose an algorithm to design stratified phase II trials. Their designs are based on a global one-sample test that is analogous to the stratified log-rank test for time-to-event data

$$T = \frac{\sum_{i=1}^{k} r_i - \sum_{i=1}^{k} N_i p_{i0}}{\sqrt{N \sum_{i=1}^{k} P_i p_{i0}(1 - p_{i0})}},$$

where (r_i, p_{i0}, N_i) are the number of responders, response rate, and number of patients in stratum i with $N = \Sigma_i^k N_i$, and the proportion of patients in stratum i is denoted as P_i which is assumed to be known. The optimal sample size (N) and critical value (t_0) will be searched via simulations such that the constraints on significance level and power are satisfied:

$$Pr(T > t_0 | N, p_i = p_{i0}, i = 1, ..., k) \leq \alpha$$

and

$$Pr(T > t_0 | N, p_i = p_{i0} + \Delta_i, i = 1, ..., k) \geq 1 - \beta,$$

where Δ_i is the treatment effect which can be different across strata. In the case where the true proportions of patients for each stratum is unknown, the design will be selected with following test instead:

$$T = \frac{\sum_{i=1}^{k} r_i - \sum_{i=1}^{k} N_i p_{i0}}{\sqrt{\sum_{i=1}^{k} N_i p_{i0}(1 - p_{i0})}}.$$

Taking the demonstrating example on relapsed neuroblastoma patients by London and Chang (2005) with three age strata (<1 year, 1–4 years, ≥ 5 years) which account for 10, 60, and 30% of patients, respectively. It is well known that younger patients have a better outcome, with the anticipated response rates under null hypothesis being 35, 20, and 15%, respectively. If an individual single-stage trial is planned within each stratum, a total number of 91 patients (37, 29, and 25 for the three strata, respectively) will be required to detect a 20% improvement with 80% power and at 0.05 type I error. In contrast, the stratified design requires only 30 patients when the true proportion of the patients in each stratum is known or 33 patients when the proportions need to be estimated.

A'Hern (2004) proposes a method based on an arcsine transformation of response rates. Instead of testing the usual hypotheses H_0: $p \leq p_0$ versus H_a: $p \geq p_1$, the proposed method re-parameterizes the new hypotheses as H_0: $B = 0$ versus H_a: $B \geq b$, where B is an arcsine difference transformation with $b = (\sin^{-1}\sqrt{p_1} - \sin^{-1}\sqrt{p_0})$. To account for patient heterogeneity, the method allows response rates to vary across patients (or more accurately, strata of patients), i.e., $b_i = (\sin^{-1}\sqrt{p_{1i}} - \sin^{-1}\sqrt{p_{0i}})$. A unique feature of an arcsine difference transformation is that its variance is approximately independent of actual response rates, with $\mathrm{var}(B) \approx 1/4n$, implying that all patients sharing a common b can enter into the same trial. For the same situation, Thall et al. (2003) use a hierarchical Bayesian approach to account for the heterogeneity of disease with multiple subtypes.

3.4. Randomized phase II trials

When making inferences from a single-arm phase II trial, one compares the new regimen based on a current series of patients to a historical control based on a group of patients with potentially different characteristics. One inherent problem in such a single-arm trial is the existence of "treatment-trial" confounding. That is, the observed improvement in efficacy actually is a mixture of two effects – the differences because of true treatment effect and the differences simply due to presence of different prognostic factors in the two trials. Examples of such prognostic factors can be supportive cares, skills of physicians or nurses, different institutions, subtypes of patients enrolled and other patient characteristics, and some of these factors can be even unobservable (Estey and Thall, 2003).

The rationale for randomized phase II trials has long been recognized (Simon et al., 1985), and an increasing number of randomized phase II trials (the so-called "selection design") have been conducted in recent years. However, the goal of a randomized phase II trial is quite different from that in a phase III study. The purpose of a phase II trial is to select a promising treatment for further evaluation. In this framework, the study is not designed to ensure that the best treatment is definitely selected (such a decision would be more appropriate for a phase III trial). Rather, the design is to ensure that an inferior treatment would have a low probability of being selected. In the other words, a randomized phase II trial would allow a rather large false-positive (type I) error α. A typical selection design intends to select the best treatment among competing candidates regardless of the magnitude of difference in response rates. Such a design will require fewer patients than conventional single-arm phase II designs. However, some potential problems related to the selection designs include that (a) a selection has to be made even if all the arms are poorly performed, (b) increasing type I error may raise an ethical consideration if there is no standard treatment available, and (c) the inclusion of a standard treatment into trial can endanger the selection process because investigators may be tempted to interpret the results as coming from definitive phase III trials. Liu (2001) provides a thorough discussion on issues regarding selection designs.

As an extension, Sargent and Goldberg (2001) propose a flexible design for multiple armed screening trials. The proposed design first prospectively specifies a cutoff value for the differences among response rates. Then, the design allows the selection to depend on factors other than response when the observed difference in response rates is deemed "small". Inoue et al. (2002) propose another innovative randomized phase II designs, intending to achieve a seamlessly transition from phase II to phase III trials. Instead of assuming that response rate Y is a surrogate of survival-based outcome T, the proposed design considers both Y and T as the efficacy endpoints. It specifies a parametric model for $\Pr(T|Y)$ and $\Pr(Y)$, and then also assumes that Y may affect T through the mixture model

$$Pr(T) = \sum_{y} Pr(T|Y = y)Pr(Y = y).$$

The proposed design will be conducted in a multi-stage manner and patients will be randomized throughout the trial. At each planned interim analysis, the decision will be made to stop the trial due to futility, continue the trial as a phase II study, or expand the trial to a phase III study via inclusion of more participation centers when the treatment deems promising. As comparing to a conventional phase III design, this design can fully utilize the information at phase II portion when a phase III study is completed, thus substantially reducing sample size and trial duration. A similar randomized design combining phase II and III has also been proposed recently via a two-stage adaptive design, i.e., allowing the sample size and dose being adjusted at the second stage given the information accumulated in stage 1 (Liu and Pledger, 2005).

3.5. *Miscellaneous innovations on phase II designs*

3.5.1. *Adaptive phase II designs*

Recently, there has been an increasing interest in applying the concept of adaptive designs, also known as "sample size re-estimation" (SSR) in blinded trials or "internal pilot" for unblinded studies, to two-stage phase II trials (Lin and Shih, 2004; Banerjee and Tsiatis, 2006; Shih, 2006). In a broader sense, all these multi-stage trials described in Section 3.1 are also adaptive in nature because the future course of a trial is dependent on the interim outcome. However, the interim analyses for usual multi-stage sequential designs and adaptive designs are performed to serve different, though sometimes overlapped, purposes. For the multi-stage sequential designs, interim data are mainly examined for ethical reasons to seek an early stopping due to either excess toxicity or overwhelm evidence of efficacy. In adaptive designs, on the other hand, the purpose of an interim analysis is to update the knowledge based on accumulated data and to re-estimate the sample size if necessary.

Lin and Shih (2004) propose an adaptive two-stage design for single-arm phase IIA cancer clinical trials. Instead of testing the hypotheses H_0: $p \leq p_0$ versus H_a: $p \geq p_1$ with error bounds α and β as in Simon's designs, the proposed design aims to test either H_0: $p \leq p_0$ versus H_{a1}: $p \geq p_1$ with error bounds α and β_1, or H_0: $p \leq p_0$ versus H_{a2}: $p \geq p_2$ with error bounds α and β_2 (preferably with $\beta_1 \geq \beta_2$), depending on the observed response rate at the first stage. Note that, in classical adaptive designs, the treatment effect is "re-estimated" based on interim data and then, if needed, the sample size will be re-adjusted based on updated estimates. In the proposed design, however, both p_1 and p_2 (as well as β_1 and β_2) are prospectively specified, and the interim data are used to guide the choice of a proper alternative hypothesis.

Banerjee and Tsiatis (2006) derive an optimum adaptive two-stage design taking Bayesian decision-theoretic approach to minimize the expected sample size under null hypothesis. They show that, as comparing to Simon's designs, only a small-to-moderate gain can be achieved (3–5% reduction of expected sample size given a true H_0). An adaptive design allows investigators the flexibility to re-adjust the subsequent sample size if needed. However, a drawback is that the sample size for second stage is unknown at the initiation of a trial, and this makes it difficult to allocate resources, especially for trials conducted at co-operative group setting. In addition, due to the nature of small sample size in phase II designs, the information accumulated in the first stage is limited and usually results in imprecise estimates. The usefulness of adaptive design in phase II trial setting remains unclear.

3.5.2. Three-outcome phase II trials

Phase II trails are typically designed under the hypothesis-testing framework that will have two possible outcomes: either rejecting the null hypothesis H_0 or rejecting the alternative hypothesis H_a. In contrast, a three-outcome design (Storer, 1992; Sargent et al., 2001) allows three possible outcomes: rejecting H_0, rejecting H_a, or rejecting neither.

It is not uncommon in practice that a larger than affordable sample size is obtained based on given H_0 versus H_a with standard error bounds ($\alpha = 0.05$ and $\beta = 0.10$, say). To counteract the problem of large sample size, certain adjustment in either error bounds or target effects must be taken. However, the availability of three-outcome designs provides an alternative strategy that allows investigators quantifying the size of uncertainty with the achievable sample size. For a single-stage design, for example, a three-outcome design can result in three possible outcomes:

(a) accepting the new treatment if r or more responses are observed,
(b) rejecting the new treatment if s or less responses are observed, and
(c) inconclusive otherwise.

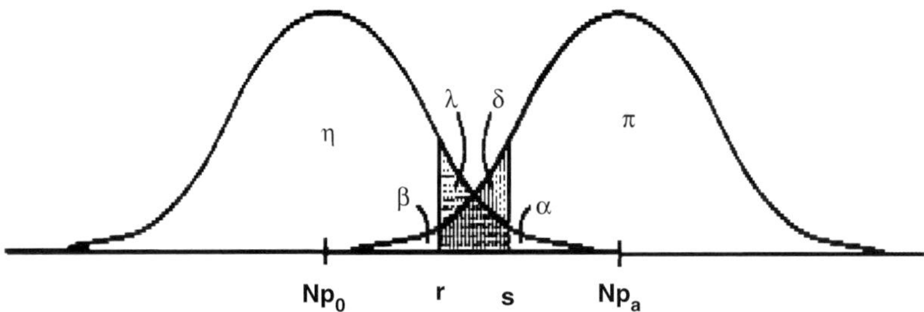

Fig. 2. Probabilities for a three-outcome design based on a normal approximation, where (a) α and β are the usual error bounds; (b) λ and δ are the probabilities of uncertainty under H_0 and H_a, respectively; (c) $\pi = 1-\beta-\delta$ is the probability of rejecting H_0 under H_a (the typical statistical power); and (d) $\eta = 1-\alpha-\lambda$ is the probability of rejecting H_0 given a true H_0 (from Sargent et al., 2001).

Such a design will require fewer patients than conventional designs. Taking as an example of a one-stage design with $(p_0, p_1, \alpha, \beta) = (0.05, 0.20, 0.05, 0.10)$, a standard single-stage design will end up with $(r, N) = (4, 38)$, while a three-outcome design will be $(s, r, N) = (2, 4, 27)$. The reason for the gain in sample size is that, as depicted in Fig. 2, two more error bounds besides the usual α and β are also defined in a three-outcome design. One (denoted as λ) reflects the uncertainty under H_0 and the other (denoted as δ) represents the uncertainty under H_a. Thus, the probability of rejecting H_0 under H_a (the typical statistical power) will be $1-\beta-\delta$ rather than $1-\beta$, and probability of rejecting H_0 given a true H_0 will be $1-\alpha-\lambda$ rather than $1-\alpha$.

3.5.3. Flexible phase II designs

A typical phase II trial is designed in a fixed sample size. In real applications, however, it is difficult for a trial to reach the planned sample exactly, especially for trials conducted in co-operative groups or multi-center settings. In a multi-center study, for example, investigators would not turn away patients who have already approached for participation just because the number of patients needed has been met. It is reasonable to have a grace period before the official suspension of accrual and thus allow the actual number at each stage to deviate slightly from what is planned. Green and Dahlberg (1992) propose a flexible design that adapts the stopping rules when the attained sample size is not the same as planned. For a two-stage trial, for example, suppose n is the planned size for stage 1 and N is the total size. In consideration to the factor that over accrual is more common, the flexible design allows the actual sample sizes a range of $(n-2, n+5)$ for stage 1 and $(N-2, N+5)$ for total sample sizes, respectively. This will lead to a total number of 64 possible designs, and the optimal rejection regions will be searched among all these possible combination, under the assumption that the occurrence of any of these trials is equal to 1/64. Chen and Ng (1998) take a similar approach for flexible designs, primarily focusing on the extension of Simon's optimal design. They also explore the robustness of the resultant flexible designs to the uniform assumption regarding the probability of attainable trials.

3.6. Transition from phase II to phase III trials

Phase II and III trials have different operation characteristics in many aspects. For example, the objectives of a phase II trial are quite different from those of a phase III study. Despite the fact that phase II trials are formulated as formal hypothesis test and decision rules, they are not designed to give definitive results regarding treatment efficacy. Rather, the goal of a phase II trial is to select promising regimens within a short time period based on limited resources. Phase II and III trials are also different in patient selection, study endpoints as well as on how the studies are conducted. In many cases, patients enrolled in phase II trials are markedly different from those of phase III trials. Phase II trials are based on relatively homogeneous patients in order to minimize the chance of rejecting promising treatment. However, results based on selected patients may not provide the most appropriate information for designing a phase III study. Since a phase III trial usually requires a large number of patients and takes many years to complete, it is desirable to release some eligibility restrictions and make the patients more resemble between phase II and III trials. In addition, due to time and sample size constraints, most oncology phase II trials use tumor response (i.e., tumor shrinkage) rather than clinical benefits such as survival-based outcomes to evaluate the treatment efficacy. Tumor shrinkage as a surrogate measurement to survival is sustainable for a cytotoxic agent that works by killing tumor cells, but it is usually problematic for some new agents such as anti-angiogensis factors or cancer vaccines that work by modulating tumor environments and delaying tumor progression. Another pitfall in conventional phase II trial is the presence of "treatment-trial" confounding that imposes an inherent difficulty for the interpretation of phase II trials. To this consideration, Fazzari et al. (2000) propose a modified phase II trial that has a phase III flavor, namely, with relatively heterogeneous patients and including survival-based endpoints. Though such a design considerably enriches the information required for planning a phase III study, it suffers from some constraints. The design requires relative large sample size, and the design is only applicable to advanced-stage disease where survival-based endpoints can be obtained in a relatively short time period. Some other examples of combining features of phase II and III trials include the randomized phase II designs by Inoue et al. (2002) to achieve a seamlessly transition from phase II to phase III trials, as well as the adaptive randomized phase II designs by Liu and Pledger (2005) to allow sample size re-adjustment during the middle course of a trial.

Some authors further classify phase II trials into sub-classes of IIA and IIB. Usually, a phase IIA trial is performed on a single agent and the typical objective is to determine whether the experimental regimen has any anti-disease activity as measured by binary variable such as response rate. In contrast, phase IIB trials are conducted on combination regimens to determine whether the anti-disease activity is sufficiently high to warrant further evaluation by a phase III study, and some survival-based endpoints usually need to be considered. In summary, it is a rather complex decision to advance a treatment from phase II to phase III design.

4. Summary

Many of the above methods are proposed exclusively for cytotoxic agents based on an implicit assumption that both toxicity and efficacy are monotone functions of the therapeutic dose. However, this may not be true for non-cytotoxic agents or non-pharmacological therapies. In this section, we first compare the differences in developmental strategies for cytotoxic and non-cytotoxic agents, taking therapeutic cancer vaccines as an example. We also outline the unique features of another type of early phase studies, translational clinical trials, which serve as a bridge between the therapeutic ideas emerging from laboratory works and traditional clinical development. Finally, several useful websites and free available software to implement some of the aforementioned methods are presented.

4.1. Early clinical development on therapeutic cancer vaccines

A cytotoxic agent works by killing existing cancer cells and/or by interfering with the generation of new cancer cells. Since it is generally assumed that the activity of a cytotoxic agent increases with dose, toxicity is a prerequisite for anti-tumor activity in cytotoxic agents. In contrast, non-cytotoxic agents such as anti-angiogensis factors, growth modulators, or cancer vaccines, usually selectively work on molecular targets to modulate tumor environment and thus associated with a minimum toxicity. Clinical benefit based on tumor shrinkage is no longer an appropriate efficacy endpoint for early vaccine studies. Patient selection can also be different. Those incurable or otherwise untreatable patients, the target population for usual phase I trials, are less likely to benefit from a cancer vaccine due to lack of intact immune systems. Therefore, quite different strategies are taken for the early development of therapeutic cancer vaccines (Simon et al., 2001; Casadei et al., 2005). To determine the MTD in studies with molecular endpoints, Ivanova et al. (2003) have proposed a fully sequential Narayana rule for calculating the probability of toxicity for each patient based on a pre-specified number of previous patients. The rule is particularly slow to escalate in the early stages of the trial when the probability of toxicity is based on few patients. Such conservatism may lengthen the trial, but it is ethically preferable to rapid overshooting of the MTD. Babb and Rogatko (2001) have proposed using clinical characteristics of the patient, such as the pretreatment level of an antibody, to determine the initial dose. Each patient is monitored and the dose adjusted if necessary; however, no dose–response relationship is assumed. In the absence of a pretreatment marker, Hunsberger et al. (2005) propose a binary endpoint measuring the effect of the vaccine on its molecular target. An initial low dose is chosen in the expectation of a low response rate. The dose is increased with high probability until the rate of effect on the molecular target rises, or until evidence of toxicity appears. Since therapeutic cancer vaccines often use well-defined purified tumor-specific and tumor-associated antigens intending to achieve biologic control of cancer, a phase I safety study usually is not necessary (Simon et al., 2001). Consequently, the boundaries between phase I and II trials in such a setting become blurred. Table 1 compares the differences in early development of

Table 1
Differences between studies in early development of cytotoxic agents and therapeutic cancer vaccines

Study Features	Phase I Trials on Cytotoxic Agents	Phase II Trials on Cytotoxic Agents	Phase I Trials on Cancer Vaccines	Phase II Trials on Cancer Vaccines
Primary objective	To determine an optimal dose for subsequent study	To evaluate the preliminary anti-tumor activity	To determine an optimal dose for subsequent study	To evaluate the immunologic activity and/or anti-tumor activity
Patient selection	End-stage metastatic cancer patients who are otherwise untreatable	Well-defined disease- and stage-specific patient population, thus providing consistent results for larger trials	Normal volunteers or less-advanced cancer patients who have intact immune systems	Less-advanced cancer patients who have intact immune systems
Primary endpoints	Dose limiting toxicity (DLT)	Response based on tumor shrinkage	Immunologic endpoints or clinical benefit endpoints such as time-to-tumor progression	Immunologic endpoints or clinical benefit endpoints such as time-to-tumor progression
Typical design	Single-arm dose-escalation design, with 3–6 patients per dose cohort	Single-arm two-stage design, at a fixed dose determined during phase I stage	Single-arm or randomized design, with 10–15 patients per dose level which is determined by pre-clinical studies	Single-arm or randomized design, at fixed dose level(s) determined by either phase I studies or pre-clinical studies

cytotoxic agents and cancer vaccines in terms of study objectives, patient selection, primary endpoints as well as on how the studies are conducted.

4.2. Translational clinical trials

Translational clinical trials are small studies of therapies emerging from laboratory researches. Though it is often said that "phase I" study is the first application of a new regimen in human subjects, actually it is the translational clinical trials that serve as a bridge between the therapeutic ideas emerging from laboratories and traditional clinical development. The major difference between traditional phase I and translational studies lies in their objectives (Piantadosi, 2005). A phase I trial is usually conducted to characterize the relationship between dose and safety, and its interest mainly focuses on potential clinical benefit. In contrast, a translational clinical trial is used to guide the further experiments in the laboratory or clinic, to inform subsequent treatment modifications, or to validate the treatment effect on a biologic target. Owing to recent progression in molecular biology, translational studies have become an essential tool to the screening of numerous target-based therapies including inhibitors for signal transduction, cyclin-dependent kinase, gene therapy, therapeutic cancer vaccines, etc. Saijo (2002) gives an excellent review of translational studies in cancer research and proposes strategies to incorporate translational studies into the traditional early phase (I and II) clinical trials. In a recent work by Piantadosi (2005), a formal definition for translational clinical trials is given following a thorough reviewing on the purpose of study, the uniqueness of its outcomes, and how the study is designed, conducted, and interpreted. An entropy-based approach is also proposed to guide the sample size consideration for planning translational clinical trials.

4.3. Some useful websites and software

The development and application of innovative designs on early clinical trials have been, and will be, greatly facilitated by continued expansion in the number of easily accessible computational tools. Next, we first present a free-download program that serves general purpose of study design. Then several links to software that implements some of innovative designs covered in this chapter are also given.

- DSTPLAN (http://biostatistics.mdanderson.org/SoftwareDownload/) is a general-purpose program and provides power, sample size, and related calculations to plan a variety of studies.
- CRM (http://biostatistics.mdanderson.org/SoftwareDownload/) implements the continual reassessment method (CRM) for dose-finding in phase I clinical trials (O'Quigley et al., 1990). A simplified version of the CRM (*CRM Simulator*) is also available in the same website.
- EWOC (http://www.sph.emory.edu/BRI-WCI/ewoc.html) implements the phase I design of escalation with over dose control (Babb et al., 1998).
- A web-based calculator is provided by following link to find Simon's two stage Optimal/MiniMax phase II designs (Simon, 1989): http://biostat.hitchcock.org/BSR/Analytics/OptimalMiniMax.asp.
- CRTR2Stage (http://gnome.ucsf.edu:8080/crtr2stage.html) designs two-stage phase II trials using both total response (TR) and complete response (CR) as the efficacy endpoints (Lu et al., 2005).
- A web-based calculator is provided by following link to implement the bivariate two-stage phase II design proposed by Bryant and Day (1995): http://biostats.upci.pitt.edu/biostats/ClinicalStudyDesign/Phase2BryantDay.html.

References

A'Hern, R.P. (2004). Widening eligibility to phase II trials: Constant arcsine difference phase II trials. *Controlled Clinical Trials* **25**, 251–264.

Ahn, C. (1998). An evaluation of phase I cancer clinical trial designs. *Statistics in Medicine* **17**, 1537–1549.

Babb, J.S., Rogatko, A. (2001). Patient specific dosing in a cancer phase I clinical trial. *Statistics in Medicine* **20**, 2079–2090.

Babb, J.C., Rogatko, A., Zacks, S. (1998). Cancer phase I clinical trials: Efficient dose escalation with overdose control. *Statistics in Medicine* **17**, 1103–1120.

Banerjee, A., Tsiatis, A. (2006). Adaptive two-stage designs in phase II clinical trials. *Statistics in Medicine* **25**, 3382–3395.

Bekele, B.N., Shen, Y. (2005). A Bayesian approach to jointly modeling toxicity and biomarker expression in a phase I/II dose-finding trial. *Biometrics* **61**, 344–354.

Braun, T.M. (2006). Generalizing the TITE-CRM to adapt for early- and late-onset toxicities. *Statistics in Medicine* **25**, 2071–2083.

Bryant, J., Day, R. (1995). Incorporating toxicity considerations into the design of two-stage phase II clinical trials. *Biometrics* **51**, 1372–1383.

Casadei, J., Streicher, H.Z., Greenblett, J.J. (2005). Clinical trial design and regulatory issues for therapeutic cancer vaccines. In: Khleif, S. (Ed.), *Tumor Immunology and Cancer Vaccines*. Kluwer Academic Publishers, Norwell, MA, pp. 351–368.

Chen, T.T. (1997). Optimal three-stage designs for phase II cancer clinical trials. *Statistics in Medicine* **16**, 2701–2711.

Chen, T.T., Ng, T.H. (1998). Optimal flexible designs in phase II clinical trials. *Statistics in Medicine* **17**, 2301–2312.

Cheung, Y.K., Chappell, R. (2000). Sequential designs for phase I clinical trials with late-onset toxicities. *Biometrics* **56**, 1177–1182.

Chevret, S. (2006). *Statistical Methods for Dose-Finding Experiments*. Wiley, New York.

Christian, M.C., Korn, E.L. (1994). The limited precision of phase I trials. *Journal of the National Cancer Institute* **86**, 1662–1663.

Conaway, M.R., Dunbar, S., Peddada, S.D. (2004). Designs for single- or multiple-agent phase I clinical trials. *Biometrics* **60**, 661–669.

Conaway, M.R., Petroni, G.R. (1995). Bivariate sequential designs for phase II trials. *Biometrics* **51**, 656–664.

Conaway, M.R., Petroni, G.R. (1996). Designs for phase II trials allowing for a trade-off between response and toxicity. *Biometrics* **52**, 1375–1386.

Durham, S.D., Flournoy, N., Rosenberger, W.F. (1997). A random walk rule for phase I clinical trials. *Biometrics* **53**, 745–760.

Edler, L. (2001). Overview of phase I trials. In: Crowley, J. (Ed.), *Handbook of Statistics in Clinical Oncology*. Dekker, New York, pp. 1–34.

Eisenhauer, E.A., O'Dwyer, P.J., Christian, M., Humphrey, J.S. (2000). Phase I clinical trial design in cancer drug development. *Journal of Clinical Oncology* **18**, 684–692.

Estey, E.H., Thall, P.F. (2003). New design for phase 2 clinical trials. *Blood*, 442–448.

Fan, S.K., Wang, Y.-G. (2006). Decision-theoretic designs for dose-finding clinical trials with multiple outcomes. *Statistics in Medicine* **25**, 1699–1714.

Fazzari, M., Heller, G., Scher, H.I. (2000). The phase II/III transition: Toward the proof of efficacy in cancer clinical trials. *Controlled Clinical Trials* **21**, 360–368.

Gatsonis, C., Greenhouse, J.B. (1992). Bayesian methods for phase I clinical trials. *Statistics in Medicine* **11**, 1377–1389.

Geller, N.L. (1984). Design of phase I and II clinical trials in cancer: A statistician's view. *Cancer Investigation* **2**, 483–491.

Green, S.J., Dahlberg, S. (1992). Planned versus attained design in phase II clinical trials. *Statistics in Medicine* **11**, 853–862.

Haines, L.M., Perevozskaya, I., Rosenberger, W.F. (2003). Bayesian optimal designs for phase I. *Biometrics* **59**, 591–600.

Hanfelt, J.J., Slack, R.S., Gehan, E.A. (1999). A modification of Simon's optimal design for phase II trials when the criterion is median sample size. *Controlled Clinical trials* **20**, 555–566.

He, W., Liu, J., Binkowitz, B., Quan, H. (2006). A model-based approach in the estimation of the maximum tolerated dose in phase I cancer clinical trials. *Statistics in Medicine* **25**, 2027–2042.

Heyd, J.M., Carlin, B. (1999). Adaptive design improvements in the continual reassessment method for phase I studies. *Statistics in Medicine* **18**, 1307–1321.
Horstmann, E., McCabe, M.S., Grochow, L., Yamamoto, S., Rubinstein, L., Budd, T., Shoemaker, D., Emanuel, E.J., Grady, C. (2005). Risks and benefits of phase 1 oncology trials, 1991 through 2002. *New England Journal of Medicine* **352**, 895–904.
Huang, X., Biswas, S., Oki, Y., Issa, J.-P., Berry, D. (2007). A parallel phase I/II trial design for combination therapies. *Biometrics* **63**, published online 12/7/2006.
Hunsberger, S., Rubinstein, L.V., Dancey, J., Korm, E.L. (2005). Dose escalation designs based on a molecularly targeted endpoint. *Statistics in Medicine* **24**, 2171–2181.
Hüsing, J., Sauerwein, W., Hideghéty, K., Jöckel, K.-H. (2001). A scheme for a dose-escalation study when the event is lagged. *Statistics in Medicine* **20**, 3323–3334.
Inoue, L.Y.T., Thall, P.F., Berry, D.A. (2002). Seamlessly expanding a randomized phase II trials to phase III. *Biometrics* **58**, 823–831.
Ishizuka, Ohashi (2001). The continual reassessment method and its applications: A Bayesian methodology for phase I cancer clinical trials. *Statistics in Medicine* **20**, 2661–2681.
Ivanova, A. (2003). A new dose-finding design for bivariate outcomes. *Biometrics* **59**, 1001–1007.
Ivanova, A. (2006). Escalation, group and A + B designs for dose-finding trials. *Statistics in Medicine* **25**, 3668–3678.
Ivanova, A., Montazer-Haghighi, A., Mohanty, S.G., Durham, S.D. (2003). Improved up-and-down designs for phase I trials. *Statistics in Medicine* **22**, 69–82.
Ivanova, A., Wang, K. (2004). A non-parametric approach to the design and analysis of two-dimensional dose-finding trials. *Statistics in Medicine* **23**, 1861–1870.
Ivanova, A., Wang, K. (2006). Bivariate isotonic design for dose-finding with ordered groups. *Statistics in Medicine* **25**, 2018–2026.
Jung, S.H., Carey, M., Kim, K.M. (2001). Graphical search for two-stage designs for phase II clinical trials. *Controlled Clinical Trials* **22**, 367–372.
Jung, S.H., Lee, T., Kim, K.M., George, S.L. (2004). Admissible two-stage designs for phase II cancer clinical trials. *Statistics in Medicine* **23**, 561–569.
Kang, S., Ahn, C. (2002). An investigation of the traditional algorithm-base designs for phase I cancer clinical trials. *Drug Information Journal* **36**, 865–873.
Korn, E.L., Mithune, D., Chen, T.T., Rubinstein, L.V., Christian, M.C., Simon, R.M. (1994). A comparison of two phase I trial designs. *Statistics in Medicine* **13**, 1799–1806.
Kramar, A., Lebecq, A., Candalh, E. (1999). Continual reassessment methods in phase I trials of the combination of two drugs in oncology. *Statistics in Medicine* **18**, 1849–1864.
Legedza, A.T.R., Ibrahim, J.G. (2001). Heterogeneity in phase I clinical trials: Prior elicitation and computation using the continual reassessment method. *Statistics in Medicine* **20**, 867–882.
Leung, D.H.-Y., Wang, Y.-G. (2002). An extension of the continual reassessment method using decision theoretic theory. *Statistics in Medicine* **21**, 51–63.
Lin, S.P., Chen, T.T. (2000). Optimal two-stage designs for phase II trials with differentiation of complete and partial responses. *Communications in Statistics, Part A – Theory and Methods* **29**, 923–940.
Lin, Y., Shih, W.J. (2001). Statistical properties of the traditional algorithm-based design for phase I cancer trials. *Biostatistics* **2**, 203–215.
Lin, Y., Shih, W.J. (2004). Adaptive two-stage designs for single-arm phase IIA cancer clinical trials. *Biometrics* **60**, 482–490.
Liu, P.Y. (2001). Phase II selection designs. In: Crowley, J. (Ed.), *Handbook of Statistics in Clinical Oncology*. Dekker, New York, pp. 119–127.
Liu, Q., Pledger, G.W. (2005). Phase 2 and 3 combination designs to accelerate drug development. *Journal of American Statistical Association* **100**, 493–502.
Loke, Y.-C., Tan, S.-B., Cai, Y., Machin, D. (2006). A Bayesian dose-finding design for dual endpoint phase I trials. *Statistics in Medicine* **25**, 3–22.
London, W.B., Chang, M.N. (2005). One and two-stage designs for stratified phase II clinical trials. *Statistics in Medicine* **24**, 2597–2611.
Lu, Y., Jin, H., Lamborn, K.R. (2005). A design of phase II cancer trials using total and complete response endpoints. *Statistics in Medicine* **24**, 3155–3170.

O'Quigley, J. (1999). Another look at two phase I clinical trial designs. *Statistics in Medicine* **18**, 2683–2690.
O'Quigley, J. (2001). Dose-finding designs using continuous reassessment. In: Crowley, J. (Ed.), *Handbook of Statistics in Clinical Oncology*. Dekker, New York, pp. 35–72.
O'Quigley, J. (2002). Continuous reassessment with early termination. *Biostatistics* **3**, 87–99.
O'Quigley, J., Chevret, S. (1991). Methods for dose finding studies in cancer clinical trials: A review and results of a Monte Carlo study. *Statistics in Medicine* **10**, 1647–1884.
O'Quigley, J., Paoletti, X., Maccario, J. (2002). Non-parametric optimal design in dose finding studies. *Biostatistics* **3**, 51–56.
O'Quigley, J., Pepe, M., Fisher, M. (1990). Continual reassessment method: A practical design for phase I clinical trials in cancer. *Biometrics* **46**, 33–48.
Panageas, K.S., Smith, A.S., Gonen, M., Chapman, P.B. (2002). An optimal two-stage phase II design utilizing complete and partial information separately. *Controlled Clinical Trials* **23**, 367–379.
Paul, R.K., Rosenberger, W.F., Flournoy, H. (2004). Quantile estimation following non-parametric phase I clinical trials with ordinal response. *Statistics in Medicine* **23**, 2483–2495.
Piantadosi, S. (2005). Translational clinical trials: An entropy-based approach to sample size. *Clinical Trials* **2**, 182–192.
Piantadosi, S., Fisher, J.D., Grossman, S. (1998). Practical implementation of a modified continual reassessment method for dose-finding trials. *Cancer Chemotherapy and Pharmacology* **41**, 429–436.
Potter, D.M. (2002). Adaptive dose-finding for phase I clinical trials of drugs used for chemotherapy of cancer. *Statistics in Medicine* **21**, 1805–1823.
Ratain, M.J., Mick, R., Schilsky, R.L., Siegler, M. (1993). Statistical and ethical issues in the design and conduct of phase I and II clinical trials of new anticancer agents. *Journal of the National Cancer Institute* **85**, 1637–1643.
Rosenberger, W.F., Haines, L.M. (2002). Competing designs for phase I clinical trials: A review. *Statistics in Medicine* **21**, 2757–2770.
Saijo, N. (2002). Translational study in cancer research. *Internal Medicine* **41**, 770–773.
Sargent, D.J., Chan, V., Goldberg, R.M. (2001). A three-outcome design for phase II clinical trials. *Controlled Clinical Trials* **22**, 117–125.
Sargent, D.J., Goldberg, R.M. (2001). A flexible design for multiple armed screening trials. *Statistics in Medicine* **20**, 1051–1060.
Shih, W.J. (2006). Group sequential, sample size re-estimation and two-stage adaptive designs in clinical trials: A comparison. *Statistics in Medicine* **25**, 933–941.
Simon, R., Freidlin, B., Rubinstein, L., Arbuck, S.G., Collins, J., Christian, M.C. (1997). Accelerated titration designs for phase I clinical trials in oncology. *Journal of the National Cancer Institute* **89**, 1138–1147.
Simon, R.M. (1989). Optimal two-stage designs for phase II clinical trials. *Controlled Clinical trials* **10**, 1–10.
Simon, R.M., Steinberg, S.M., Hamilton, M., Hildesheim, A., Khleif, S., Kwak, L.W., Mackall, C.L., Schlom, J., Topalian, S.L., Berzofsky, J.A. (2001). Clinical trial designs for the early clinical development of therapeutic cancer vaccines. *Journal of Clinical Oncology* **19**, 1848–1854.
Simon, R.M., Wittes, R.E., Ellenberg, S.S. (1985). Randomized phase II clinical trials. *Cancer Treatment Report* **69**, 1375–1381.
Storer, B.E. (1989). Design and analysis of phase I clinical trials. *Biometrics* **45**, 925–937.
Storer, B.E. (1992). A class of phase II designs with three possible outcomes. *Biometrics* **48**, 55–60.
Storer, B.E. (2001). An evaluation of phase I clinical trials designs in the continuous dose-response setting. *Statistics in Medicine* **20**, 2399–2408.
Stylianou, M., Flournoy, N. (2002). Dose finding using the biased coin up-and-down design and isotonic regression. *Biometrics* **58**, 171–177.
Thall, P.F., Cheng, S.C. (2001). Optimal two-stage designs for clinical trials based on safety and efficacy. *Statistics in Medicine* **20**, 1023–1032.
Thall, P.F., Lee, J.J., Tseng, C.-H., Estey, E.H. (1999). Accrual strategies for phase I trials with delayed patient outcome. *Statistics in Medicine* **18**, 1155–1169.

Thall, P.F., Wathen, J.K., Bekele, B.N., Champlin, R.E., Baker, L.H., Benjamin, R.S. (2003). Hierarchical Bayesian approaches to phase II trials in disease with multiple subtypes. *Statistics in Medicine* **22**, 763–780.

Tighiouart, M., Rogatko, A., Babb, J.C. (2005). Flexible Bayesian methods for cancer phase I clinical trials: Dose escalation with overdose control. *Statistics in Medicine* **24**, 2183–2196.

Whitehead, J. (2002). Heterogeneity in phase I clinical trials: Prior elicitation and computation using the continual reassessment method by A. Legedza and J.G. Ibrahim. *Statistics in Medicine* **20**, 867–882 (Letter to the Editor). *Statistics in Medicine* **21**, 1172.

Whitehead, J., Zhou, Y., Stevens, J., Blakey, G., Price, J., Leadbetter, J. (2006). Bayesian decision procedures for dose-escalation based on evidence of undesirable events and therapeutic benefit. *Statistics in Medicine* **25**, 37–53.

Zhang, W., Sargent, D.J., Mandrekar, S. (2006). An adaptive dose-finding design incorporating both toxicity and efficacy. *Statistics in Medicine* **25**, 2365–2383.

Zohar, S., Chevret, S. (2001). The continuous reassessment method: Comparison of Bayesian stopping rules for dose-ranging studies. *Statistics in Medicine* **20**, 2827–2843.

Zohar, S., Latouche, A., Taconnet, M., Chevret, S. (2003). Software to compute and conduct sequential Bayesian phase I or II dose-ranging clinical trials with stopping rules. *Computer Methods and Programs in Biomedicine* **72**, 117–125.

Handbook of Statistics, Vol. 27
ISSN: 0169-7161

DOI: 10.1016/S0169-7161(07)27018-X

18

Definitive Phase III and Phase IV Clinical Trials

Barry R. Davis and Sarah Baraniuk

Abstract

This chapter provides an overview of current practices in phase III and IV clinical trials, including a brief summary of the major topics and principles considered when executing such clinical trials. The topics covered include basic definitions, classic questions and their requisite response variables, randomization, blinding, recruitment, sample size issues, data analysis, data quality and control, data monitoring, and dissemination. Relevant examples from many clinical trials are presented.

1. Introduction

A clinical trial is a prospective comparative study conducted in human beings to evaluate the effect of an intervention on an outcome. This type of study provides the most compelling evidence of a causal relationship between treatment and effect. Commonly performed clinical trials evaluate new drugs, medical devices, biologics, or other interventions in patients. They are designed to assess the safety and efficacy of an experimental therapy, whether a new intervention is better than standard therapy, or the efficacy of two standard interventions.

The purpose of this chapter is to give an overview of phase III and IV clinical trials, and some critical issues, key examples, and further questions about these studies. There are many useful high-quality books about clinical trials and we refer the reader to these to obtain more details (Friedman et al., 1998; Piantadosi, 2005; Meinert and Tonascia, 1986; Pocock, 1984; Chow and Liu, 2003). Also, there are journals specifically devoted to clinical trials methodology (Controlled Clinical Trials, Clinical Trials – The Journal of the Society for Clinical Trials).

1.1. Clinical trial phases

Drug clinical trials are commonly classified into four phases, and the drug development process usually proceeds through all stages over many years. Device and biologics trials may also include these phases. If the drug successfully passes through the first three phases, it will usually be approved for use in the general population.

1.2. Phase I

Phase I trials are the first stage of testing in human subjects (Ahn, 1998). Usually, a small (20–80) group of healthy volunteers will be selected although for some diseases, e.g., cancer, patients are used. This phase includes trials designed to assess the safety, tolerability, pharmacokinetics, and pharmacodynamics of a therapy. Phase I trials are usually dose-finding studies wherein the tested range will be a small fraction of the dose that causes harm in animal testing.

1.3. Phase II

Once the initial safety of the therapy has been confirmed in phase I trials, phase II trials are performed on larger groups (100–300) and are designed to assess clinical efficacy of the therapy (Kramar et al, 1996; Lee and Feng, 2005). This phase typically involves randomization and a control group but extracting new information about the efficacy of treatment remains the primary goal of this study design (Meinert and Tonascia, 1986). The development process for a new drug commonly fails during phase II trials due to lack of efficacy or toxic effects.

1.4. Phase III

A phase III trial is a prospectively defined experiment used to test the efficacy and safety of a randomly assigned treatment in patients. Phase III trials can evaluate drugs, surgery, behavioral (diet/exercise) interventions, devices, complementary and alternative medicine (CAM), and screening procedures (e.g., mammography to detect breast cancer).

Trials can be labeled as superiority (prove one treatment is better than another), equivalence (prove the treatments are equivalent within some predefined metric), or non-inferiority (prove one treatment is as good as or better than another).

A definitive phase III clinical trial is one that evaluates the efficacy of an intervention and whose results will be used to decide on approval for use of that intervention in practice. A definitive clinical trial should have the following elements – (1) a relevant, timely and clearly posed question, (2) a well-defined clinical endpoint, (3) requisite statistical power to answer the question, and (4) the necessary structure and components for a well-executed design.

Phase III studies are usually large double-blind randomized controlled trials on sizeable patient groups (1000–3000 or more) and are aimed at being the definitive assessment of the efficacy of the new therapy, especially in comparison with currently available alternatives. Phase III trials are the most expensive, time-consuming and difficult studies to design and run, especially in therapies for chronic conditions.

1.5. Phase IV

A phase IV trial is concerned with the long-term safety and efficacy of a drug post-Food and Drug Administration (FDA) approval. They may be mandated by regulatory authorities or may be undertaken by the sponsoring company for competitive or other reasons. Safety surveillance is designed to detect any rare or long-term adverse effects over a much larger patient population and timescale than was possible during the initial clinical trials. Such adverse effects detected by phase IV trials may result in the withdrawal or restriction of a drug – recent examples include cerivastatin (SoRelle, 2001) (brand names Baycol and Lipobay), troglitazone (Faich and Moseley, 2001) (brand name Rezulin), and rofecoxib (Bresalier et al., 2005) (brand name Vioxx).

2. Questions

2.1. Primary and secondary questions

A clinical trial must have a primary question about a treatment effect on a specific outcome. This question will serve as the basis for the study design and sample size and needs to be stated in advance. It should be very specific and be posed in the form of testing a hypothesis. A specific example might be "Does treatment A when compared to placebo reduce the five-year risk of total mortality by 20% or more in persons with disease X?"

The trial can and will usually have several secondary questions. These arise from possible treatment effects on other outcomes. These should also be stated in advance and a rationale provided for them. Multiple comparisons can be an issue (Davis, 1997; O'Neill, 1997; Pocock, 1997).

2.2. Subgroup questions

Many trials also consider subgroup questions (Yusuf et al., 1991; DeMets, 2004). These are questions about effect of therapy in a subpopulation of subjects entered into the trial. They are most often used to assess internal consistency of results, and can confirm prior hypotheses or generate new hypotheses. These types of questions should be pre-specified.

Analyses of a trial by subgroups result in separate statistical tests for each subgroup. As a result the probability of false positive conclusions increases and the greater the number of subgroups analyzed separately, the larger this probability will be. Tests for interaction are also usually performed to see if there are any subgroup differences in treatment effect. Interactions are of two types – (a) qualitative wherein the treatment effect is different in direction in two subgroups and (b) quantitative wherein the treatment effect is of same direction but of different magnitude. Interaction tests are model dependent, and are not very powerful. Even if such a test is statistically significant, its result should be interpreted with caution.

2.3. Other questions

Other questions that arise in clinical trials include natural history questions, ancillary questions, and exploratory ones. A natural history question is not related to the intervention. For example, the placebo group of a trial may be used to assess what factors are predictive of a clinical outcome (Davis et al., 1998).

Ancillary questions are not related to the primary and secondary questions but still may be of scientific interest. An example is the Genetics of Hypertension Associated Treatment (GenHAT) study which is determining whether variants in hypertension susceptibility genes interact with antihypertensive medication to modify coronary heart disease (CHD) risk in hypertensive individuals (Arnett et al., 2002). GenHAT is an ancillary study of the Antihypertensive and Lipid-Lowering Treatment to Prevent Heart Attack Trial (ALLHAT). ALLHAT was a double-blind, randomized trial of 42,418 hypertensives, 55 years of age or older, with systolic or diastolic hypertension and one or more risk factors for cardiovascular disease, designed to determine if the incidence of CHD is lower with treatment with any of the three newer antihypertensive drug classes: a calcium channel blocker (amlodipine), an ACE inhibitor (lisinopril), and an alpha-adrenergic blocker (doxazosin) each compared to treatment with a diuretic (chlorthalidone) (ALLHAT Collaborative Research Group, 2002). GenHAT is typing variants in hypertension genes to permit analyses of gene-treatment interactions in relation to outcomes include CHD, stroke, heart failure, and blood pressure (BP) lowering.

Exploratory questions arise from trying to address why things happened in a trial. These are usually based on unanticipated results and are used to help explain certain findings. However, they must be treated with caution. For example, in most randomized clinical trials not all patients adhere to the therapy to which they were randomly assigned. Instead, they may receive the therapy assigned to another treatment group, or a therapy different from any prescribed in the protocol. When non-adherence occurs, problems occur with the analysis comparing the treatments under study. However, there are several biases associated with methods other than intent-to-treat analyses (Peduzzi et al., 1993).

2.4. Response variables

Response variables are outcomes measured during the course of the trial and are used to answer the primary, secondary, and other questions. These outcomes should be well defined, ascertainable, and specific to the questions. A definitive clinical trial will most often have a clinical primary outcome rather than a physiologic-based one. Clinical outcomes (i.e., mortality or morbidity) are ones that seriously affect the health and well-being of an individual. These include myocardial infarctions, strokes, cancer, blindness, visual impairment, infection, mobility, pain, etc. Physiologic-based outcomes are usually measures, or surrogates, for clinical outcomes. These include BP, cholesterol levels, glucose levels, CD4 counts, electrocardiogram abnormalities, bone density measurements, etc. Many drugs are approved solely on the basis of these surrogate outcomes without showing their effect of clinical outcomes. However, surrogates do not consistently predict treatment effect on clinical outcome and reliance on them should be minimized (De Gruttola et al., 2001).

3. Randomization

Random allocation or randomization of patients to treatment or control is a key element of a phase III clinical trial that requires proper execution for successful completion and reliable results. The randomization process assures with a reasonable amount of certainty that the groups will be comparable, thus removing the possibility of investigator bias (Friedman et al., 1998). Ethical issues have been raised with regard to randomization in clinical studies (Royall, 1991) and adjustments in study design have tried to alleviate this conflict (crossover designs, historical controls, etc.), but these are not always applicable. The randomized clinical trial still remains the gold standard when considering the available study designs. For a detailed presentation of randomization in clinical trials, see Rosenberger and Lachin (2002).

3.1. Fixed allocation

Fixed allocation, the most common type of randomization procedure, assigns interventions to patients with a pre-specified probability that is not altered during the study. A classic example of this is when participants are randomly allocated in a set ratio (usually 1:1) to two different treatments. The most elementary form is simple randomization wherein participants are assigned treatments using software that uses a random number generating algorithm (such as PROC PLAN in SAS (SAS, 2003)).

3.2. Blocked and stratified randomization

A drawback with simple randomization is that treatment groups may not be comparable in size especially when the total sample size is not large. Blocked randomization assures that at no time during the randomization process will an imbalance be large and that at certain points the number of participants in each group will be equal. Essentially blocked randomization creates small fixed size sets of randomly generated balanced patterns. For example, for size $n = 4$, and two treatment groups there are six possible patterns – AABB, ABAB, BAAB, BABA, BBAA, and ABBA. Over a designated amount of time we will have equal numbers of individuals in each group. This is particularly helpful when we are doing interim analyses (see Section 8.2).

Stratified randomization makes assignments in such a way that the resulting randomized groups have comparable numbers of individuals of a certain covariate. For example when we stratify randomization based on gender, we expect that there will be equal numbers of men and women in each group. One of the most common uses of stratified randomization is to assure equal allocation to treatment assignments within a center of a multi-site trial thus eliminating the potential bias of a center effect.

3.3. Adaptive randomization

In contrast to fixed allocation, adaptive randomization changes the allocation procedure as the study progresses. There are two types – baseline adaptive and response adaptive. The classic baseline adaptive procedure is Efron's biased coin design (Efron, 1971). The main purpose of this design is to achieve an equal number of subjects in each group. The probability of assignment to a group depends on the balance between the groups wherein the group with the smaller number of subjects is assigned a larger assignment probability. The classic adaptive response designs are play the winner (Zelen, 1969) and the two-armed bandit strategy (Robbins, 1952). The play the winner strategy starts with a random assignment to treatment or control and if the response of this subject is successful the subsequent participant is assigned to the same group, if not the subject is assigned to the other group. This procedure requires that we be able to assess the response quickly enough so as not to delay the treatment assignment of newly enrolled participants. The two-armed bandit strategy works under the same premise. However assignment probability is linked with success proportion as results become known. There are situations where this method of treatment assignment may be justified as we may find a need to randomize based on variables assessed at baseline or randomize based on the responses of participants to their treatment.

3.4. Blinding

Blinding or masking is "A condition imposed on an individual (or group of individuals) from knowing or learning of some fact or observation, such as treatment assignment" (Meinert and Tonascia, 1986). Blinding prevents bias that can result from participants and investigators knowing treatment assignment thus reducing the possibility that they will change their behavior and/or decisions regarding endpoint ascertainment. Regardless of which procedure is used to enact the blind this does not resolve the issue of guessing which treatment a patient is on. Often assessing the blind at the trial's end can be reassuring

There are four types of blinding in a trial – (a) unblinded trials (patient and investigators are aware of the treatment assignment), (b) single-blind trials (only the patient is not informed), (c) double-blind trials (patient and investigator are blind), and (d) triple-blind trials (patient, investigator, and the Data and Safety Monitoring Board (DSMB), see Section 8.1, are blind). The last type is not recommended (Meinert, 1998) as it may prevent the DSMB from making informed decisions regarding interruptions to the trial. The choice of whom and how to blind in a trial is subject to the type of intervention being measured and logistics, and in the event that it is impossible or impractical to enforce a blind other tactics can be implemented. For example during the Ocular Hypertension Treatment Study (OHTS) (Kass, 1994), the fundus photographs were read at a central reading center by individuals masked to treatment. Unblinding can occur during a trial either accidentally or intentionally. In the event that a patient needs to be removed from a trial, there should be a prospectively stated procedure for unblinding the patient.

4. Recruitment

Recruitment is a critical component of clinical trials that needs to be accomplished in a timely manner. Poor recruitment can affect the feasibility of a trial and affects its timeline. Any extension of the recruitment period can result in increased cost, increased effort, and possibly decreased power if there is no concomitant increase in the follow-up period.

The main issue of recruitment is getting enough patients, but this varies depending on the intervention in question. Solutions to this problem may involve adding more clinical centers (in a multi-center clinical trial situation), extension of the recruitment period, or changes to the exclusion/inclusion criteria. Trials may encounter problems stemming from competing for patients, possibly overestimating the rate of prevalence of the condition or disease in population or simply the public (specifically the medical community) is unaware of ongoing clinical trials and physicians do not refer patients.

Much effort has been expended in trying to profile the type of individual who would participate in a clinical study, however, many of the reasons why an individual would participate in a trial is not as well discussed. In many cases patients believe they may receive more or better care (Mattson et al., 1985), and it is generally the case that they are seen more often. Clinical trials offer a "second opinion" of their health status they may otherwise not have access to. However, too many visits or even the process of getting to visits may discourage participation as well as simply not feeling comfortable with perceived risks.

5. Adherence/sample size/power

Adherence and compliance refer to the level of participation of an individual during a trial. Adherence usually is used with reference to all protocol matters (visits, procedures, etc.) whereas compliance usually refers to the intervention itself, e.g., taking medications, staying on a diet, etc. In general, some non-compliance is expected and this is reflected in accounting for crossovers (drop-ins and drop-outs to treatment) when calculating the sample size. Monitoring of adherence and compliance is important, because this can affect the feasibility of continuing the trial as well as the validity of the trial's results.

An intention to treat analysis should always be the primary one as it is based upon the randomized cohort. However, in the case where non-adherence is measured in a reliable way and tracked throughout the trial it may be of interest to do a secondary, explanatory analysis based on which patients actually received the intervention. Of course, such on-treatment analyses are fraught with potential biases and must be assessed in context.

The calculation of sample size needed to properly execute a clinical trial is often based on a basic formula (Chow et al., 2003). However there are situations where sample sizes are estimated by simulation, such as in the Amblyopia Treatment Study (Pediatric Eye Disease Investigator Group, 2002). The formulas are determined by the nature of the primary endpoint of interest. There are formulas for continuous, binary, time to event and repeated measures/longitudinal endpoints.

All the formulas begin with the prospectively defined type I error (the α level), type II error (or β), and the effect size (δ). The type I error is the probability of rejecting the null hypothesis when in fact it is true and this is usually set at 0.05.

The type II error is the probability of accepting the null hypothesis when it is false, and this usually is around 0.10, but can reasonably range between 0.20 and 0.10. The power to detect the difference is $1-\beta$. For comparing outcome occurrences, an effect size can be proposed by specifying event rates for each group. Let p_c be the event rate in the control group and p_t the event rate in the treatment group. We could define the effect size as the minimal detectable difference, which would be just $\delta = p_c - p_t$, or we could express the effect size as a relative measure and calculate $\delta = (p_c - p_t)/p_c$.

For dichotomous outcome measures, the basic formula is:

$$N = \frac{2(Z_\alpha + Z_\beta)^2(p_c + p_t)}{(p_c - p_t)^2},$$

where N is the total sample size, and Z_α and Z_β are the critical values from the standard normal distribution. Typical critical values are $Z_\alpha = 1.96$ (for a two-sided test at the 0.05 level) and $Z_\beta = 1.645$ for 90% power. Note that this formula assumes equal allocation between n_t, the number in the treatment group and n_c the number in the control group and $N = n_t + n_c$.

For continuous outcomes, the basic formula is:

$$N = \frac{2(Z_\alpha + Z_\beta)^2(\sigma^2)}{(\mu_c - \mu_t)^2}$$

where N, Z_α, and Z_β are the same as defined above, but now the effect size is expressed in terms of the means (μ) for each group.

For time to event data, the basic formula is:

$$N = \frac{2(Z_\alpha + Z_\beta)^2}{(\ln(\lambda_c/\lambda_t))^2}$$

where λ_c represent the hazard rate in the control group and λ_t is the hazard rate in the treatment group.

For repeated measures/longitudinal data, the formula involves a calculation of the intraclass correlation coefficient in the case of continuous response variables and the kappa coefficient for binary response variables. The intraclass correlation coefficient, usually denoted by ρ, is calculated by a ratio of the within cluster variance (w) and the variance between clusters (b), so $\rho = \sigma_b^2/\sigma_b^2 + \sigma_w^2$. Assuming we have r clusters we calculate the sample size to be $N_{\text{adjusted}} = N(1 + (r-1)\rho)$.

The kappa coefficient is a function of the rate of the event in control group, and in particular the proportion of concordant clusters in the control group, $p_{\text{concordant}}$. The kappa coefficient is defined as $\kappa = p_{\text{concordant}} - (p_c^r + (1 - p_c)^r)/1 - (p_c^r + (1 - p_c)^r)$ and affects the sample size in a similar way as the intraclass correlation coefficient, $N_{\text{adjusted}} = N(1 + (r-1)\kappa)$.

Each of these formulas can be adapted to adjust for multiple arms (factorial design), differences in allocation ratios and drop-ins and drop-outs. In the case of multiple arms, say for example three arms, the formula for the total sample size would include not just n_c and n_t but n_c, n_{t1}, and n_{t2}. It is possible that each of these arms would have unequal allocations and then the appropriate constant is matched with the respective arm. The case where there is equal allocation to each of the three arms results in a formula simplified to include just n_c and $2n_t$.

Assuming the rate of drop-ins (R_{IN}) and drop-outs (R_{OUT}) are known. The sample size calculation for the case where no crossovers exist can be adjusted by a factor of $1/(1 - R_{\mathrm{IN}} - R_{\mathrm{OUT}})^2$.

In the case of multiple endpoints unless the correlation between the arms is known, and often times it is not, each endpoint's sample size is calculated. Then, to be conservative, the largest of the sample sizes is used.

6. Data analysis

There are many items to consider in choosing a data analysis. However, a data analysis plan needs to be written and agreed to before the trial begins and can only be changed according to strict guidelines with the full consent of all parties involved and not after looking at blinded data.

Good clinical practice requires that the study protocol describe the methods of data analysis that will be employed at the end of the study. The data analysis section of a protocol should distinguish the primary endpoints of the study from other outcome measures, and should describe any plans to exclude certain treated patients from the analysis, to conduct comparisons among subgroups, or to carry out interim analyses of patient data. In all cases, the protocol should describe the specific statistical tests to be used.

Where several endpoints will be analyzed to determine the success of the clinical study, the data analysis plan should also address the issue of multiple comparisons. When several statistical tests are performed, it is more likely that some will be significant by chance alone. Thus, if multiple endpoints are evaluated, statistical adjustment or increased sample size should be contemplated by the analysis plan.

A data analysis plan should also encompass a data closeout plan including when the study is to end for each patient and what events will or will not be counted. This should include a date by which events are to be reported in order to close and lock the database and begin the predefined statistical analyses. All this needs to be done prior to the study end. In order for the results of clinical trials to be valid, analyses must be performed according to a predetermined plan that is not changed once the randomization code is broken and the study unblinded. Otherwise, bias is introduced and the validity of the results comes into question. According to the intention to treat principle all participants allocated to a treatment group should be followed up, assessed, and analyzed as members of that group irrespective of their compliance with the planned course of treatment. All patients should have a final visit for complete outcome assessment and transition to post-trial therapy. It is essential that all missing and lost to follow-up patients be found if possible. Plans should be made for notification of trial results and data archiving, as well as for transitioning patient care, clinic staff, and support centers.

Most definitive clinical trials will examine a clinical outcome that is meaningful to a patient – e.g., death stroke, loss of vision, etc. This primary outcome can be

Table 1
Summary table of typical data analyses by type of outcome

Type of Outcome	Type of Analysis
Continuous	
Two or more samples with underlying normal assumptions	Two sample t-test (equal or unequal variances), paired t-test, F-tests, simple linear regression, or multiple linear regression
Categorical	
Binary or >2 categories	Fisher's exact, Chi square, binomial proportions test, contingency tables, Mantel Haenszel, Kruskal–Wallis, logistic regression, multinomial logistic regression, ordinal logistic regression
Time to event	Logrank test, Kaplan–Meier curves, Cox Proportional Hazards, Cox Proportional Hazards with time dependent covariates.
Count data	Poisson regression, Poisson processes (used with very low event rates)

viewed as a dichotomous one in a short-term trial with complete follow-up, or can best be viewed as a time to event to provide more power. The usual method of analysis is to calculate Kaplan–Meier curves and to compare using a logrank procedure or a variation. Cox proportional hazards models can be used to provide an estimate of the hazard ratio (or relative risk) of one arm of the trial to another (e.g., active vs. placebo). A summary (Table 1) of the typical methods for analysis subject to the endpoint of interest is provided.

6.1. Categorical data

Major clinical trials can have a categorical data endpoint as their primary outcome. Usually the outcome is binary but it can encompass more than two categories. One example of this type of analysis comes from the Cryotherapy for Retinopathy of Prematurity (CRYO-ROP) trial (Cryotherapy for retinopathy of prematurity cooperative group, 1988). In this trial, investigators applied cryotherapy (essentially destroying tissue by the use of very cold temperature) to the retina in one randomly selected eye of a pair where there was retinopathy or prematurity. ROP is an eye disease of premature infants characterized by increased vasculature of the retina potentially leading to blindness. The trial showed that an unfavorable outcome (essentially retinal detachment and blindness) at 3 months was significantly less frequent in the eyes undergoing cryotherapy (21.8%) compared with the untreated eyes (43%). The data supported the efficacy of cryotherapy in reducing by approximately one half the risk of an unfavorable outcome in ROP.

6.2. Continuous measure

Some clinical trials utilize a continuous measure as a primary outcome. An example of this comes from another eye trial performed by the Pediatric Eye Disease

Investigator Group (Pediatric Eye Disease Investigator Group, 2002). In this study, investigators compared patching and atropine as treatments for moderate amblyopia ("lazy eye") in children younger than 7 years. After 6 months, the difference in visual acuity between treatment groups was small and clinically inconsequential (mean difference, 0.034 logMAR (Minimum Angle of Resolution) units; 95% confidence interval, 0.005–0.064 logMAR units). The trial showed that atropine and patching produced improvement of similar magnitude, and both are appropriate modalities for the initial treatment of amblyopia in children 3–7 years old.

Another trial utilized a multivariate longitudinal continuous outcome. The Casa Pia Study of the Health Effects of Dental Amalgams in Children was a randomized clinical trial designed to assess the safety of low-level mercury exposure from dental amalgam restorations in children (DeRouen et al., 2002). Since the goal of the trial was to assess the safety of a treatment currently in use, rather than the efficacy of an experimental treatment, unique design issues came into play. The identification of a primary study outcome measure around which to design the trial was problematic, since there was little evidence to indicate how health effects from such low-level exposure would be manifested. The solution involved the use of multiple outcomes over time.

6.3. Time to event outcomes

An example of a time to event outcome analysis comes from the Hypertension Detection and Follow-up Program (HDFP), a community-based, randomized controlled trial involving 10,940 persons with high BP (Hypertension detection and follow-up program cooperative group, 1979). The trial compared the effects on 5-year mortality of a systematic antihypertensive treatment program (Stepped Care (SC)) and referral to community medical therapy (Referred Care, RC). Five-year mortality from all causes was 17% lower for the SC group compared to the RC group (6.4 vs. 7.7 per 100, $p<0.01$) The findings of the HDFP indicated that the systematic effective management of hypertension had a great potential for reducing mortality for the large numbers of people with high BP in the population.

Another example of a time to even outcome analysis comes from the Systolic Hypertension in the Elderly Program (SHEP) (SHEP cooperative research group, 1991). This trial was designed to assess the ability of antihypertensive drug treatment to reduce the risk of stroke in isolated systolic hypertension. Persons aged 60 years and above were randomized to active (using the diuretic chlorthalidone) or placebo antihypertensive treatment. Systolic BP ranged from 160 to 219 mm Hg and diastolic BP was <90 mm Hg. Antihypertensive stepped-care drug treatment with chlorthalidone reduced the incidence of total stroke by 36%, and major cardiovascular events were also reduced.

6.4. Multiple approaches

Clinical trials often involve a variety of clinical and laboratory measures that are used as endpoints and sometimes two of these measures are combined in one endpoint. One such solution is to utilize a so-called combined endpoint. When the individual components of such a combined endpoint are time to event measurements, the analysis is straightforward. However, the analysis of the combined endpoint is more difficult when one component of the endpoint is time to event and the other is a continuous measure. There are proposed solutions to this. One example comes from the Survival and Ventricular Enlargement (SAVE) trial (Moye et al., 1992), which investigated whether the ACE inhibitor, captopril, could reduce morbidity and mortality in patients with left ventricular dysfunction after a myocardial infarction. A combined endpoint of mortality or a nine-unit decrease in left ventricular ejection fraction was significantly reduced in the captopril group with $p = 0.016$. Long-term administration of captopril was associated with an improvement in survival and reduced morbidity and mortality due to major cardiovascular events (Pfeffer et al., 1992).

6.5. *Other issues*

Other issues to consider in data analysis include missing data and measuring safety versus efficacy (Wood et al., 2004). There is a wealth of missing data techniques (Little and Rubin, 2002) that can be applied to the analysis of clinical trials. However, the paramount issue might be why the data are missing. Missingness could be related to the treatment and this can severely affect the ability to assess the data. Other points to consider are whether the analysis should focus solely on efficacy with safety as a secondary issue or whether safety should also have primary outcome status (Cook and Farewell, 1994; Jennison and Turnbull, 1993; Todd, 2003).

6.6. *Bayesian approaches*

Another approach to the analysis of clinical trials involves Bayesian statistics (Berry, 2006; Multiple authors, 2005). The Bayesian approach to statistical analysis makes explicit and quantitative use of external evidence in the design, analysis, and interpretation of data from clinical trials. Bayesian methods have the flexibility and capacity to integrate data from multiple sources. Freedman (1996) provides a brief description of the differences between Bayesian and conventional ("frequentist") methods – "Frequentist analysis may conclude that treatment A is superior because there is a low probability that such an extreme difference would have been observed when the treatments were in fact equivalent. Bayesian analysis begins with the observed difference and asks how likely is it that treatment A is in fact superior to B".

Like classical statistics, the Bayes method is applicable to problems of parameter estimation and hypothesis testing. However, there are several important differences between the Bayesian and frequentist approach. One is that the Bayesian formulation is based on the likelihood principle. The likelihood principle states that a decision should have its foundation in what has occurred, not in what has not happened. In addition, although Bayesians like frequentists are interested in parameter estimation and hypothesis testing, Bayesians do not believe that the parameter θ of a distribution is constant, but rather has a probability distribution, called the prior distribution, or $\pi(\theta)$.

Once the prior distribution is identified, the Bayesian uses the probability distribution of the data given the value of the parameter. This conditional distribution (because it is the distribution of the data conditional on the value of the unknown parameter) is denoted as $f(x_1, x_2, x_3, \ldots, x_n|\theta)$. The Bayes process continues by combining the prior distribution with this conditional distribution to create a posterior distribution, or the distribution of the parameter θ given the observed sample, denoted as $\pi(\theta|x_1, x_2, x_3, \ldots, x_n)$.

From the Bayes' perspective, the prior distribution reflects knowledge about the location and behavior of θ before the experiment is carried out. The execution of the experiment provides new information that is combined with the prior information to obtain a new estimate of θ. To help in interpreting the posterior distribution, some Bayesians will construct a loss function that identifies the penalty to pay for underestimating or overestimating the population parameter. Bayesian hypothesis testing is based on the posterior distribution. However, the requirement of a realistic specification of the prior distribution can be a burden if there is no information about the parameter to be estimated. Similarly, the choice of the loss function can be difficult to justify from a clinical perspective.

Bayesian analysis can be computer intensive. We are seeing more computational software becoming available to perform Bayesian analysis now that powerful and inexpensive computers are widely available. Raftery and colleagues at the University of Washington (www.stat.washington.edu/raftery/) have developed programs that can be run in SPlus (Insightful, 2006) to perform a variety of Bayesian analyses. Similarly, Albert at Bowling Green State University (www.math.bgsu.edu/~albert/) has developed Matlab (Mathworks, 2006) programs for Bayesian analysis.

7. Data quality and control/data management

Data quality and data management are extremely important facets in the conduct of a clinical trial (McFadden, 1997). A clinical trial is only as good as the data that is collected. Quality control begins with the protocol and the manual of operations. The protocol serves as the overall plan for the conduct of the trial. The manual of operations provides the details for every aspect of running the trial.

Quality control procedures should be put in place for all aspect of the trial and data collection should be as simple as possible to carry out the essential questions of the trial. Data editing of forms should include checking for missing data, allowable ranges of data, and consistency within forms or across forms. Online submission of information improves the efficiency of checking (in most cases immediately) for the information captured from case report forms (Winget et al., 2005).

8. Data monitoring

Investigators engaging in clinical trial must make accommodations for monitoring the outcomes, recruitment, participation, various logistic elements of conducting a trial (usually involving data quality and control), and above all the safety of the trial participants. How the monitoring proceeds is detailed in the trial protocol and is often subject to the guidelines of the funding agency (such as NIH guidelines for data monitoring). A Data and Safety Monitoring Board (DSMB) is essential for almost all definitive phase III clinical trials.

8.1. Data and safety monitoring boards

The DSMB has a long tradition in clinical trials dating back over 40 years. It has many names (Policy Advisory Board (or Committee) Data and Safety Monitoring Board (or Committee), Data Monitoring Board (or Committee), Independent Data and Safety Monitoring Committee). There is an excellent book that deals in detail with the policies and procedures of such a committee and another book that highlights many important cases studies that DSMB's face (Ellenberg et al., 2002; DeMets et al., 2005). The purpose of a DSMB is to provide oversight to the trial by monitor the accumulating data. Issues that the Board has to deal with include whether recruitment is going as planned, whether there are protocol violations, whether there are safety concerns, and whether the accumulating efficacy data warrant an early stopping of the trial for efficacy or futility. The DSMB should agree to a charter before the trial begins. Such a charter should include a brief description of the trial, DSMB members and affiliations, frequency of meetings, how often data are reviewed in the course of the trial, content of reports, stopping rules and stopping logistics for the trial, and how DSMB deliberations are communicated to the trial's sponsor leadership.

8.2. Stopping guideline

The statistical evidence brought to the DSMB is only one of many elements to the decision-making regarding stopping a trial. Stopping a trial can happen when there is evidence of harm, overwhelming benefit or if the trial will not return clear results (futility). Three basic types of procedures are used in interim monitoring (a) group sequential, (b) conditional power, and (c) Bayesian methods (see Section 6.6).

8.2.1. Group sequential procedures

Repeated analyses of accumulating data increase the type I error. For example if we wish to reject a null hypothesis of no treatment difference using a statistical test based on the standard normal distribution, i.e., where $|Z| > 1.96$, then five interim looks at the data can lead to a type I error of 0.14 and for 10 looks, it is 0.20.

The idea behind group sequential boundaries is to use a more conservative critical value of Z such that for a given number of looks the total type I error at the end of the study will be 0.05. A summary statistic is computed at each interim analysis, based on additional groups of new subjects (or events) and this is compared to a conservative critical value. Various methods have been proposed (Jennison and Turnbull, 2000; Haybittle, 1971; Peto et al., 1976; Pocock, 1977; O'Brien and Fleming, 1979).

In classical group sequential analysis, the intervals between looks are prespecified. For example, analyses are performed after each of k groups of $2n$ subjects are entered, and then the same critical value is used at each analysis. If the statistic is greater than the critical value, then the trial may be stopped. If not, then it is continued. As the stopping rules are really a guideline, a trial can continue even if a stopping boundary is crossed. In this case, one may buy back the previously spent type I error to be re-spent or re-distributed at future looks (Lan et al., 2003).

O'Brien and Fleming (OBF) (O'Brien and Fleming, 1979) modified the constant conservative critical value procedure to allow decreasing critical values. This made it much more difficult for early stopping. Lan–DeMets (Lan and DeMets, 1983) modified this procedure even further by not having to specify the number of analyses in advance nor equally spaced interim analyses. They defined an alpha-spending function, $\alpha^*(t)$, such that $\alpha^*(t)$ defines rate at which type I error is used where t (information time) is proportion of total information accumulated by the end of the study $(0 \leq t \leq 1)$. Therefore, $\alpha^*(t)$ is increasing, $\alpha^*(0) = 0$, and $\alpha^*(1) = \alpha$ (our usual type I error). For immediate response trials $t = n/N$, where n is the number of subjects accrued and N the total sample size. For time to event trials $t = d/D$, where d is the number of events accrued and D the total expected number of events.

Some examples of $\alpha^*(t)$ are

1. $\alpha_1{}^*(t) = 2\{1-\Phi(z_{\alpha/2}/t^{1/2})\}$ (approximately equivalent to OBF (O'Brien and Fleming, 1979) procedure)
2. $\alpha_2{}^*(t) = \alpha \ln\{1+(e-1)t\}$ (approximately equivalent to Pocock (1977) procedure)
3. $\alpha_3{}^*(t) = \alpha t$.

As an example, we show the comparison of the critical values for five equally spaced intervals using the above spending functions and their counterparts with $\alpha = 0.025$.

Method	Intervals				
	1	2	3	4	5
OBF	4.56	3.23	2.63	2.28	2.04
$\alpha_1{}^*(t)$	4.90	3.35	2.68	2.29	2.03
Pocock	2.41	2.41	2.41	2.41	2.41
$\alpha_2{}^*(t)$	2.44	2.43	2.41	2.40	2.38
$\alpha_3{}^*(t)$	2.58	2.49	2.41	2.34	2.28

8.2.2. Conditional power

The concept of futility has been used to also monitor trials. Futility is generally considered as the inability of a trial to meet its primary goal. The most popular method for assessing futility is conditional power, which assesses the likelihood of achieving a statistically significant result at the trial conclusion. This is done by computing the probability of rejecting the null hypothesis at the trial's conclusion, given the current result and some assumed effect for the remaining portion of the trial (Lan et al., 1982; Lan and Wittes, 1988). Typically, conditional power is computed for a series of assumed effects, e.g., the observed effect to date, the protocol defined effect, the null effect, and effects in between. Trials have been stopped for futility (Lachin and Lan, 1992; Davis and Cutler, 2005).

As an example, Table 2 and Fig. 1 demonstrate the calculations performed to monitor the ALLHAT trial (ALLHAT Collaborative Research Group, 2002; Davis and Cutler, 2005) (see Section 2.3). The Lan–DeMets version of the O'Brien–Fleming group sequential boundaries was used to assess treatment group differences for the primary outcome (CHD), and conditional power was used to assess futility. The doxazosin arm was terminated early because of futility for finding a primary outcome difference and an increased incidence of cardiovascular disease, especially heart failure, relative to chlorthalidone. The likelihood of observing a significant difference for the primary outcome by the scheduled end of the trial was very low (only 2%) for the protocol-specified reduction of 16% for doxazosin compared with chlorthalidone.

Software to facilitate the statistical analysis required to implement the above-described methods exist such as S+SeqTrial (Insightful C, 2005), and the Lan–DeMets program (Reboussin et al., 2003).

8.3. Tracking adverse effects

Ideally, any intervention should result in more benefit than harm. However, AEs do occur and are not always easy to specify in advance. An adverse event is "any undesirable clinical outcome that has the added dimensions of physical findings, complaints and lab results". These "adverse effects can be both objective measures and subjective responses" (Friedman et al., 1998). Tracking such effects is a critical task in monitoring clinical trials but serious adverse events defined as death, an irreversible event, or an event that requires hospitalization need to be reported to regulatory agencies and institutional review boards.

The severity of adverse events as well as their frequency over time should be considered before stopping treatment for an individual participant or before changing the protocol or procedures of a trial include terminating an arm or stopping the trial (Pressel et al., 2001). Included in tracking adverse effects are any reasons for removing a participant from a trial, reducing their dosage or exposure to the intervention and group levels of frequency of the event. The way in which these are assessed (labs, clinical exams, etc.) should also be recorded.

It is very likely that we will see some adverse effects in a clinical study. Some effects may be expected (known effects from the intervention). However, we must be prepared for unexpected effects and methods for reporting must be available. This can be achieved by allowing participants to volunteer effects they believe are adverse.

Challenges of monitoring adverse effects include whether they are short- or long-term and whether long-term follow-up may show additional ones. Some rare

Table 2
ALLHAT interim data for the primary outcome (CHD)

		CHD Events – n, rate per 100 (SE)			Group Sequential Boundaries[a]	
DSMB Meeting Date	Information Time	Chlorthalidone ($N = 15{,}255$)	Doxazosin ($N = 9{,}061$)	Logrank	Z_L	Z_U
3/12/98	0.22	224 Year 3 – 2.9 (0.2)	140 2.8 (0.3)	0.46	−5.46	5.46
12/10/98	0.37	366 Year 4 – 3.4 (0.2)	226 3.5 (0.3)	0.45	−4.16	4.16
6/28/99	0.50	498 Year 4 – 6.4 (0.4)	310 6.3(0.5)	0.86	−3.53	3.53
1/6/00	0.59	608 Year 4 – 6.3 (0.4)	365 6.3(0.3)	0.38	−3.24	3.24

[a] Goup sequential boundaries are based on a Dunnett multiple (3–1) comparison procedure (Davis and Cutler, 2005).

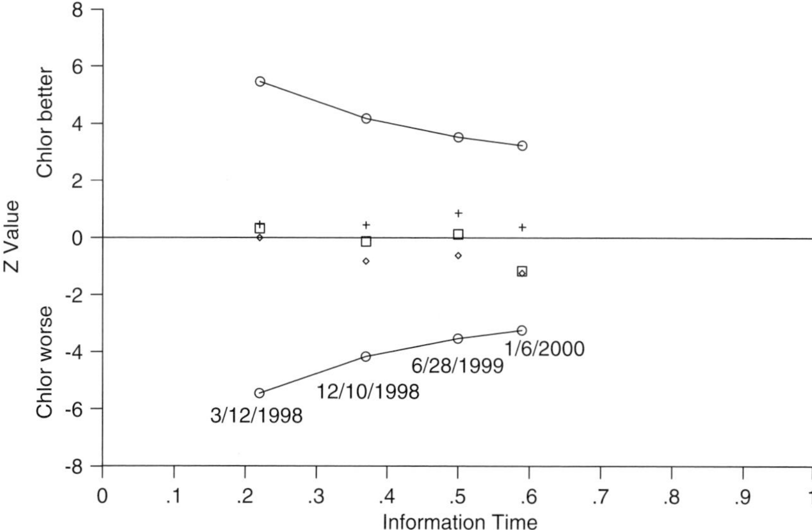

Fig. 1. ALLHAT group sequential boundaries (○) for the primary endpoint (CHD). The values of the logrank statistics for the comparison of the newer treatments (amlodipine [◇], lisinopril [□], doxazosin [+]) group versus the standard treatment (chlorthalidone) are plotted.

adverse effects may be seen only with very large numbers of exposed patients and long-term follow-up. This is a compelling reason for doing phase IV trials.

9. Phase IV trials

A phase IV trial occurs after the FDA has approved the drug/device for use. There may be several goals in a phase IV trial. These include specifying new indications for use, expanding the safety profile, gathering new information about the therapy, educating clinical researchers, and fulfiling a regulatory edict (Friedman et al., 1998). Cost effectiveness may also be explored. A phase IV trial may also be a pilot study for other potential product indications. It may be conducted at single or multiple sites and last months to several years. There is usually no control group and the number of subjects varies depending on the objective. The participants may be as few as those in a phase I trial or as many in a phase III trial (Liang, 2002).

One example of a phase IV trial was conducted on patients who had received intravenous tissue plasminogen activator (t-PA) for acute ischemic stroke (Chiu et al., 1998). The study examined the feasibility, safety, and efficacy of t-PA in the first year after the FDA had approved the use of the drug for this patient population. Thirty patients with acute ischemic stroke from three sites were included. Findings confirmed the safety and efficacy of t-PA were comparable to the previous National Institute of Neurological Disorders and Stroke Phase III t-PA study (The National Institute of Neurological Disorders and Stroke rt-PA Stroke Study Group, 1995).

10. Dissemination – trial reporting and beyond

Dissemination of clinical trial results is usually accomplished solely through scientific publications and presentations. However, there is a general lack of success translating research results into medical practice. In the 2003 Shattuck lecture, Dr. Claude Lenfant, former director of the National Heart, Lung, and Blood Institute (NHLBI), pointed out that despite clinical trials demonstrating the importance of several treatments in preventing serious outcomes, the health care system is not applying what is known (Lenfant, 2003). Three examples in cardiovascular disease illustrate the problem. In 1996, 15 years after the Beta-Blocker Heart Attack Trial demonstrated the benefits of a beta-blocker for patients who had a myocardial infarction (β-Blocker Heart Attack Study Group, 1981), only 62.5% of these patients were prescribed such medication (National Committee for Quality Assurance, 1999). Numerous studies have shown the benefits of cholesterol-lowering in patients with CHD; yet only 50–75% of such patients were screened for elevated serum cholesterol let alone prescribed such medication (National Committee for Quality Assurance, 1997). BP control (<140/90 mm Hg) rates for hypertension fall far short of the U.S. national goal of 50% or more. However, the recent ALLHAT demonstrated that BP could be controlled in two-thirds of a multiethnic hypertensive population in diverse practice settings (Cushman et al., 2002).

In an effort to address issues of translation of knowledge into practice, the NHLBI created a new policy on dissemination activities, which evolved and was finalized during the ALLHAT trial (Pressel et al., 2005). The policy requires a detailed dissemination plan, including evaluation, for trials with potential for immediate public health applicability. The rationale for this program was well summarized by a member of the ALLHAT Steering Committee. "People do a wonderful press conference, publish in prestigious journals, present at important meetings – and nothing happens. Publishing your data will not get doctors to change their practice" (McCarthy, 2003).

At the conclusion of the ALLHAT trial, a joint dissemination project of ALLHAT and the National High Blood Pressure Education Program was implemented. This project planned to further the traditional approaches of dissemination by utilizing press release/press conferences, media coverage, presentation at scientific meetings, and publications in peer-reviewed journals by applying novel approaches based on intervention mapping theory (Bartholomew et al., 1998, 2000) to include health care provider persuasion (academic detailing) (Soumerai and Avorn, 1990), influencing formulary systems and reaching out to patients.

Thus, the lessons of ALLHAT can serve as a guide to other clinical trials. If researchers want their findings to be disseminated and to change clinical practice, plans should be in place from the beginning for doing more than reporting results. There should be attempts at reaching physicians, patients, formularies, and health practices through concerted efforts to spread the word about the importance and significance of the trial's results (Pressel et al., 2005).

11. Conclusions

Randomized clinical trials are considered the gold standard of human studies. New methods in both statistics and clinical trials operations are continuing to be developed that improve the efficiency of these studies. Novel technologies in genomics, nanotechnology, and stem cells will require clinical trials to assess their utility. Trials are important in proving the effect of new drugs, new devices, and new biological interventions. Although these studies cannot always be done because of resources and ethical issues, treatment guidelines for human diseases and conditions need to be based on such evidence.

References

Ahn, C. (1998). An evaluation of phase I cancer clinical trial designs. *Statistics in Medicine* **17**, 1537–1549.

ALLHAT Officers and Coordinators for the ALLHAT Collaborative Research Group. The Antihypertensive and Lipid-Lowering Treatment to Prevent Heart Attack Trial (2002). Major outcomes in high-risk hypertensive patients randomized to angiotensin-converting enzyme inhibitor or calcium channel blocker vs diuretic: The antihypertensive and lipid-lowering treatment to prevent heart attack trial (ALLHAT). *Journal of the American Medical Association* **288**, 2981–2997.

Arnett, D.K., Boerwinkle, E., Davis, B.R., Eckfeldt, J., Ford, C.E., Black, H. (2002). Pharmacogenetic approaches to hypertension therapy: Design and rationale for the genetics of hypertension associated treatment (GenHAT) study. *Pharmacogenomics Journal* **2**, 309–317.

Bartholomew, L.K., Parcel, G.S., Kok, G. (1998). Intervention mapping: A process for developing theory- and evidence-based health education programs. *Health Education & Behavior* **25**(5), 545–563.

Bartholomew, L.K., Parcel, G.S., Kok, G., Gottlieb, N.H. (2000). *Intervention Mapping: Designing Theory- and Evidence-Based Health Promotion Programs*. Mayfield Publishing, Thousand Oaks, CA.

Berry, D.A. (2006). Bayesian clinical trials. *Nature Reviews Drug Discovery* **5**, 27–36.

β-Blocker Heart Attack Study Group (1981). The β-blocker heart attack trial. *Journal of the American Medical Association* **246**, 2073–2074.

Bresalier, R.S., Sandler, R.S., Quan, H., Bolognese, J.A., Oxenius, B., Horgan, K., Lines, C., Riddell, R., Morton, D., Lanas, A., Konstam, M.A., Baron, J.A., for Adenomatous Polyp Prevention on Vioxx (APPROVe) Trial Investigators. (2005). Cardiovascular events associated with rofecoxib in a colorectal adenoma chemoprevention trial. *New England Journal of Medicine* **352**, 1092–1102 (see comment).

Chiu, D., Krieger, D., Villar-Cordova, C. et al. (1998). Intravenous tissue plasminogen activator for acute ischemic stroke: Feasibility, safety, and efficacy in the first year of clinical practice. *Stroke* **29**, 18–22, (see comment).

Chow, S., Liu, J. (2003). *Design and Analysis of Clinical Trials: Concepts and Methodologies*, 2nd ed. Wiley-Interscience Inc., New York.

Chow, S., Shao, J., Wang, H. (2003). *Sample Size Calculations in Clinical Research*. Marcel Dekker, Inc., New York, NY.

Cook, R.J., Farewell, V.T. (1994). Guidelines for monitoring efficacy and toxicity responses in clinical trials. *Biometrics* **50**, 1146–1152.

Cryotherapy for retinopathy of prematurity cooperative group (1988). Multicenter trial of cryotherapy for retinopathy of prematurity: Preliminary results. *Archives of Ophthalmology* **106**, 471–479.

Cushman, W.C., Ford, C.E., Cutler, J.A. et al. (2002). Success and predictors of blood pressure control in diverse North American settings: The antihypertensive and lipid-lowering treatment to prevent heart attack trial (ALLHAT). *Journal of Clinical Hypertension* **4**, 393–405.

Davis, B., Cutler, J. (2005). The data monitoring experience in the antihypertensive and lipid-lowering treatment to prevent heart attack trial (ALLHAT): Early termination of the doxazosin treatment arm. In: DeMets, D., Furberg, C., Friedman, L. (Eds.), *Data Monitoring in Clinical Trials: A Case Studies Approach*. Springer, New York.

Davis, B.R., Vogt, T., Frost, P.H., et al., for Systolic Hypertension in the Elderly Program Cooperative Research group. (1998). Risk factors for stroke and type of stroke in persons with isolated systolic hypertension. *Stroke* **29**, 1333–1340.

Davis, C.E. (1997). Secondary endpoints can be validly analyzed, even if the primary endpoint does not provide clear statistical significance. *Controlled Clinical Trials* **18**, 557–560.

De Gruttola, V.G., Clax, P., DeMets, D.L. et al. (2001). Considerations in the evaluation of surrogate endpoints in clinical trials: Summary of a national institutes of health workshop. *Controlled Clinical Trials* **22**, 485–502.

DeMets, D., Furberg, C., Friedman, L. (eds.) (2005). Data Monitoring in Clinical Trials: A Case Studies Approach. Springer, New York.

DeMets, D.L. (2004). Statistical issues in interpreting clinical trials. *Journal of Internal Medicine* **255**, 529–537.

DeRouen, T.A., Leroux, B.G., Martin, M.D. et al. (2002). Issues in design and analysis of a randomized clinical trial to assess the safety of dental amalgam restorations in children. *Controlled Clinical Trials* **23**, 301–320.

Efron, B. (1971). Forcing a sequential experiment to be balanced. *Biometrika* **58**, 403–417.

Ellenberg, S., Fleming, T., DeMets, D. (2002). *Data Monitoring Committees in Clinical Trials: A Practical Perspective*. Wiley, Chichester, West Sussex.

Faich, G.A., Moseley, R.H. (2001). Troglitazone (rezulin) and hepatic injury. *Pharmacoepidemiology and Drug Safety* **10**, 537–547.

Freedman, L. (1996). Bayesian statistical methods. *BMJ* **313**, 569–570.

Friedman, L.M., Furberg, C., Demets, D.L. (1998). *Fundamentals of Clinical Trials*, 3rd ed. Springer, New York.

Haybittle, J.L. (1971). Repeated assessment of results in clinical trials of cancer treatment. *British Journal of Radiology* **44**, 793–797.

Hypertension detection and follow-up program cooperative group (1979). Five-year findings of the hypertension detection and follow-up program. I. Reduction in mortality of persons with high blood pressure, including mild hypertension. *Journal of the American Medical Association* **242**, 2562.

Insightful C. S + SEQTRIAL. (2005). Seattle, Washington.

Insightful C. S-plus. (2006). Seattle, Washington.

Jennison, C., Turnbull, B.W. (2000). *Group Sequential Methods with Applications to Clinical Trials*. Chapman & Hall/CRC, Boca Raton.

Jennison, C., Turnbull, B.W. (1993). Group sequential tests for bivariate response: Interim analyses of clinical trials with both efficacy and safety endpoints. *Biometrics* **49**, 741–752.

Kass, M.A. (1994). The ocular hypertension treatment study. *Journal of Glaucoma* **3**, 97–100.

Kramar, A., Potvin, D., Hill, C. (1996). Multistage designs for phase II clinical trials: Statistical issues in cancer research. *British Journal of Cancer* **74**, 1317–1320.

Lan, K.K.G., Demets, D.L. (1983). Discrete sequential boundaries for clinical trials. *Biometrika* **70**, 659–663.

Lachin, J.M., Lan, S.P. (1992). Termination of a clinical trial with no treatment group difference: The lupus nephritis collaborative study. *Controlled Clinical Trials* **13**, 62–79.

Lan, K.K., Lachin, J.M., Bautista, O. (2003). Over-ruling a group sequential boundary – a stopping rule versus a guideline. *Statistics in Medicine* **22**, 3347–3355.

Lan, K.K.G., Simon, R., Halperin, M. (1982). Stochastically curtailed tests in long-term clinical trials. *Sequential Analysis* **1**, 207–219.

Lan, K.K.G., Wittes, J. (1988). The B-value: A tool for monitoring data. *Biometrics* **44**, 579–585.

Lee, J.J., Feng, L. (2005). Randomized phase II designs in cancer clinical trials: Current status and future directions. *Journal of Clinical Oncology* **23**, 4450–4457.

Lenfant, C. (2003). Shattuck lecture: Clinical research to clinical practice – lost in translation? *New England Journal of Medicine* **349**, 868–874.

Liang, B. (2002). The drug development process III: Phase IV clinical trials. *Hospital Physician* **38**, 42.

Little, R.J.A., Rubin, D.B. (2002). *Statistical Analysis with Missing Data*, 2nd ed. Wiley-Interscience, New York.

Mattson, M.E., Curb, J.D., McArdle, R. (1985). Participation in a clinical trial: The patients' point of view. *Controlled Clinical Trials* **6**, 156–167.

McCarthy, M. (2003). Researchers try marketing techniques to sell their results: Trial investigators say publishing results not enough to change practice. *The Lancet* **362**, 1204–1205.

McFadden, E. (1997). *Management of Data in Clinical Trials*. Wiley-Interscience, New York.

Meinert, C.L., Tonascia, S. (1986). *Clinical Trials: Design, Conduct, and Analysis*. Oxford University Press, Oxford.

Meinert, C.L. (1998). Masked monitoring in clinical trials – blind stupidity? *New England Journal of Medicine* **338**, 1381–1382.

Moye, L., Davis, B., Hawkins, C. (1992). Analysis of a clinical trial involving a combined mortality and adherence dependent interval censored endpoint. *Statistics in Medicine* **11**, 1705–1717.

Multiple authors (2005). An entire issue devoted to Bayesian methods in clinical trials. *Clinical Trials* **2**, 271–378.

National Committee for Quality Assurance. (1997). The state of managed care quality. Washington, DC.

National Committee for Quality Assurance. (1999). The state of managed care quality. Washington, DC.

O'Brien, P.C., Fleming, T.R. (1979). A multiple testing procedure for clinical trials. *Biometrics* **35**, 549–556.

O'Neill, R.T. (1997). Secondary endpoints cannot be validly analyzed if the primary endpoint does not demonstrate clear statistical significance. *Controlled Clinical Trials* **18**, 550–556.

Pediatric Eye Disease Investigator Group (2002). A randomized trial of atropine vs. patching for treatment of moderate amblyopia in children. *Archives of Ophthalmology* **120**, 268–278, (see comment).

Peduzzi, P., Wittes, J., Detre, K., Holford, T. (1993). Analysis as-randomized and the problem of non-adherence: An example from the veteran's affairs randomized trial of coronary artery bypass surgery. *Statistics in Medicine* **12**, 1185–1195.

Peto, R., Pike, M.C., Armitage, P. et al. (1976). Design and analysis of randomized clinical trials requiring prolonged observation of each patient Introduction and design. *British Journal of Cancer* **34**, 585–612.

Pfeffer, M., Braunwald, E., Moye, L. et al. (1992). Effect of captopril on mortality and morbidity in patients with left ventricular dysfunction after myocardial infarction: Results of the survival and ventricular enlargement trial. *New England Journal of Medicine* **327**, 669–677.

Piantadosi, S. (2005). *Clinical Trials: A Methodologic Approach*, 2nd ed. Wiley-Interscience, New York.

Pocock, S. (1984). *Clinical Trials – A Practical Approach*. Wiley, New York.

Pocock, S.J. (1977). Group sequential methods in the design and analysis of clinical trials. *Biometrika* **64**, 191–200.

Pocock, S.J. (1997). Clinical trials with multiple outcomes: A statistical perspective on their design, analysis, and interpretation. *Controlled Clinical Trials* **18**, 530–545.

Pressel, S., Davis, B., Bartholomew, L., Cushman, W., Whelton, P., Nwachuku, C. (2005). Disseminating clinical trial tesults: Case study from the antihypertensive and lipid-lowering treatment to prevent heart attack trial (ALLHAT). *Clinical Trials* **2**(Suppl. 1), S37.

Pressel, S.L., Davis, B.R., Wright, J.T. et al. (2001). Operational aspects of terminating the doxazosin arm of the antihypertensive and lipid lowering treatment to prevent heart attack trial (ALLHAT). *Controlled Clinical Trials* **22**, 29–41.

Reboussin, D., DeMets, D., KyungMann, K., Lan, K. (2003). Programs for Computing Group Sequential Boundaries Using the Lan-DeMets Method, Version 2. Available at: http://www.biostat.wisc.edu/landemets/.

Robbins, H. (1952). Some aspects of the sequential design of experiments. *Bulletin of the American Mathematical Society* **58**, 527–535.

Rosenberger, W.F., Lachin, J.M. (2002). *Randomization in Clinical Trials: Theory and Practice*. Wiley-Interscience, New York.

Royall, R.M. (1991). Ethics and statistics in randomized clinical trials. *Statistical Science* **6**, 52–62.

SAS Institute Inc. (2003). Cary, NC, USA.: 9.1.

SHEP Cooperative Research Group (1991). Prevention of stroke by antihypertensive drug treatment in older persons with isolated systolic hypertension. Final results of the systolic hypertension in the elderly program (SHEP). *Journal of the American Medical Association* **265**, 3255–3264, (see comment).

SoRelle, R. (2001). Baycol withdrawn from market. *Circulation* 2001, **104**, E9015–E9016.

Soumerai, S.B., Avorn, J. (1990). Principles of educational outreach ('academic detailing') to improve clinical decision making. *Journal of the American Medical Association* **263**(4), 549–556.

The MathWorks. (2006). I. MATLAB. Natick, MA.

The National Institute of Neurological Disorders and Stroke rt-PA Stroke Study Group. (1995). Tissue plasminogen activator for acute ischemic stroke. *New England Journal of Medicine* **333**(24), 1581–1587.

Todd, S. (2003). An adaptive approach to implementing bivariate group sequential clinical trial designs. *Journal of Biopharmaceutical Statistics* **13**, 605–619.

Winget, M., Kincaid, H., Lin, P., Li, L., Kelly, S., Thornquist, M. (2005). A web-based system for managing and co-ordinating multiple multisite studies. *Clinical Trials* **2**, 42–49.

Wood, A.M., White, I.R., Thompson, S.G. (2004). Are missing outcome data adequately handled? A review of published randomized controlled trials in major medical journals. *Clinical Trials* **1**, 368–376.

Yusuf, S., Wittes, J., Probstfield, J., Tyroler, H.A. (1991). Analysis and interpretation of treatment effects in subgroups of patients in randomized clinical trials. *Journal of the American Medical Association* **266**, 93–98.

Zelen, M. (1969). Play the winner rule and the controlled clinical trial. *Journal of the American Statistical Association* **64**, 131–146.

Handbook of Statistics, Vol. 27
ISSN: 0169-7161

DOI: 10.1016/S0169-7161(07)27019-1

19

Incomplete Data in Epidemiology and Medical Statistics

Susanne Rässler, Donald B. Rubin and Elizabeth R. Zell☆

Abstract

Missing data are a common problem in most epidemiological and medical studies, including surveys and clinical trials. Imputation, or filling in the missing values, is an intuitive and flexible way to handle the incomplete data sets that arise because of such missing data. Here, in addition to imputation, including multiple imputation (MI), we discuss several other strategies and their theoretical background, as well as present some examples and advice on computation. Our focus is on MI, which is a statistically valid strategy for handling missing data, although we review other less sound methods, as well as direct maximum likelihood and Bayesian methods for estimating parameters, which are also valid approaches. The analysis of a multiply-imputed data set is now relatively standard using readily available statistical software. The creation of multiply-imputed data sets is more challenging than their analysis but still straightforward relative to other valid methods of handling missing data, and we discuss available software for doing so. Ad hoc methods, including using singly-imputed data sets, almost always lead to invalid inferences and should be eschewed, especially when the focus is on valid interval estimation or testing hypotheses.

1. Introduction

Missing data are a common problem with large databases in general and with epidemiological, medical, and health-care databases in particular. Missing data also occur in clinical trials when subjects fail to provide data at one or more time points or drop out, for reasons including lack of interest or untoward side effects. Data may also be "missing" due to death, although the methods described here

☆ The findings and conclusions in this chapter are those of the author and do not necessarily represent the views of the Centers for Disease Control and Prevention.

are generally not appropriate for such situations because such values are not really missing (see Little and Rubin, 2002, Example 1.7; Zhang and Rubin, 2003; Rubin, 2006).

Epidemiological and medical databases nearly always have missing data. Unit nonresponse occurs when a selected unit (e.g., patient, doctor, hospital) does not provide any of the information being sought. Item nonresponse occurs when a unit responds to some items but not to others. Discussions of many issues related to missing data are contained in the three volumes produced by the Panel on Incomplete Data of the Committee on National Statistics in 1983 (Madow et al., 1983a, 1983b; Madow and Olkin, 1983), as well as in the volume stimulated by the 1999 International Conference on Survey Nonresponse (Groves et al., 2002).

A classical textbook on analysis with missing data (Little and Rubin, 1987, 2002) categorizes methods for analyzing incomplete data into four main groups. The first group comprises simple procedures such as complete-case analysis (also known as "listwise deletion") and available-case analysis, which discards the units with incomplete data in different ways. Although these simple methods are relatively easy to implement, they can often lead to inefficient and biased estimates. The second group of methods comprises weighting procedures, which deals with unit nonresponse by increasing the survey weights for responding units in an attempt to account for the nonrespondents, who are dropped from further analysis. The third group comprises imputation-based procedures, a standard approach for handling item nonresponse, especially in databases that are to be shared by many users. Imputation methods fill in values that are missing, and the resultant completed data are then analyzed as if there never were any missing values.

Of particular interest, multiple imputation (MI) is a method for reflecting the added uncertainty due to the fact that imputed values are not actual values, and yet still allows using complete-data methods to analyze each data set completed by imputation. The final group of methods comprises direct analyses using model-based procedures, in which models are specified for the observed data, and inferences are based on likelihood or Bayesian analyses. In general, only MI and direct analysis can lead to valid inferences. By valid inferences we mean ones that satisfy three criteria:

(a) approximately unbiased estimates of population estimates (e.g., means, correlation coefficients),
(b) interval estimates with at least their nominal coverage (e.g., 95% intervals for a population mean should cover the true population mean at least 95% of the time), and
(c) tests of significance should reject at their nominal level or less frequently when the null hypothesis is true (e.g., a 5% test of a zero population correlation should reject at most 5% of the time when the population correlation is zero).

Resampling methods, such as the bootstrap and jackknife, can satisfy criteria (b) and (c) asymptotically, but give no guidance on how to satisfy criterion (a) in the presence of missing data, but rather implicitly assume that estimates satisfying (a) have already been obtained (see Efron, 1994 and the discussion by Rubin,

1994). Such methods are only briefly discussed in Section 4.2 because they do not represent a complete approach to the problem of missing data.

This chapter reviews these four classes of approaches to handling missing data, with a focus on MI, which we believe is the most generally useful approach for medical and epidemiological databases. Before presenting our review of approaches, we start with a basic discussion of missing-data mechanisms, i.e., the processes that govern why certain values are missing and others are observed.

2. Missing-data mechanisms and ignorability

When data are missing, it is important to distinguish various missing-data mechanisms, which describe to what extent missingness depends on the observed and/or unobserved data values. Many simple methods for dealing with missing data are based, either implicitly or explicitly, on the assumption of a particularly simple missing-data mechanism, and these methods' behavior can be influenced strongly by differences between the assumed and the true mechanisms. More formally, let Y represent the $N \times P$ matrix of complete data, and let R represent the $N \times P$ matrix of indicator values for observed and missing values in Y. Then, the missing-data mechanism gives the probability of the matrix of indicator variables, R, given Y and possible parameters governing this process, $\xi : p(R|Y, \xi)$.

Key concepts about missing-data mechanisms were formalized by Rubin (1976), and following this work, subsequent statistical literature (e.g., Little and Rubin, 2002, p. 12) distinguishes three cases: missing completely at random (MCAR), missing at random (MAR), and not missing at random (NMAR). This language was chosen to be consistent with much older terminology in classical experimental design for completely randomized, randomized, and not randomized studies.

MCAR refers to missing data for which missingness does not depend on any of the data values, missing or observed. Thus, the probability that units provide data on a particular variable does not depend on the value of that variable or the value of any other variable: $p(R|Y, \xi) = p(R|\xi)$. The MCAR assumption can be unrealistically restrictive and can be contradicted by the observed data, for example, when men are observed to have a higher rate of missing data on postoperative blood pressure than women.

Often, it is plausible to assume that missingness can be explained by the observed values in the data set. For example, in an epidemiological survey, the missingness for certain medical variables might depend on completely observed variables such as gender, age group, health conditions, social status, etc. If the probability of units responding to items depends only on such observed values but not on any missing values, then the missing data are MAR, but not necessarily MCAR because of the following possible dependence: $p(R|Y, \xi) = p(R|Y_{\text{obs}}, \xi)$, where Y_{obs} are observed values in Y, $Y = (Y_{\text{obs}}, Y_{\text{mis}})$, Y_{mis} being the missing values in Y. Thus, if the value of blood pressure at the end of a clinical trial is more likely to be missing when some previously observed values of blood pressure are high, and given these, the probability of missingness is independent of the value of blood pressure at the end of the trial, the missingness mechanism is MAR.

If, even given the observed values, missingness still depends on data values that are missing, the missing data are NMAR. This could be the case, for example, with final blood pressure, if people with higher final blood pressure tend to be less likely to provide their blood pressure than people with lower final blood pressure, even though they have the exact same observed values of race, education, all previous blood pressure measurements, etc. Obviously, the richer the data set in terms of observed variables, the more plausible the MAR assumption becomes.

In addition to defining formally the concepts underlying MCAR, MAR, and NMAR, Rubin (1976) defined the concept of ignorability. Suppose that, in a situation with missing data, parametric models have been specified for: (1) the distribution of the data that would occur in the absence of missing value, $p(Y|\psi)$, and (2) the missing-data mechanism, $p(R|Y,\xi)$. Rubin (1976) showed that if the missing data are MAR and the parameters of the data distribution, ψ, and the missing-data mechanism, ξ, are distinct (which means, in disjoint parameter spaces and, if Bayesian models are used, a priori independent), then valid inferences about the distribution of the data can be obtained using a likelihood function that does not contain a factor for the missing-data mechanism and is simply proportional to $p(Y_{\text{obs}}|\psi) = \int p(Y|\psi)dY_{\text{mis}}$. In this situation, the missing-data mechanism may be "ignored" for likelihood or Bayesian inferences.

In many cases, it is reasonable to assume that the parameters of the data distribution and the missing-data mechanism are distinct, so that the practical question of whether the missing-data mechanism is ignorable often reduces to a question of whether the missing data are MAR. This argument requires some care, however, when using random parameter models, where there can exist ambiguity between unknown parameters and missing data (see Shih, 1992). Also, even when the parameters are not distinct, if the missing data are MAR, then inferences based on the likelihood ignoring the missing-data mechanism are still potentially valid in the sense of satisfying criteria (a)–(c) of Section 1, but may not be fully efficient. Thus, the MAR condition is typically regarded as the more important one in considerations of ignorability. Little and Rubin (2002, Section 6.2) include further discussion of these ideas, as does Rubin (1978b) in a very simple but instructive artificial example.

It is common to make the ignorability assumption in analyses of incomplete data even when it is not known to be correct, and it can be advantageous to do so for a variety of reasons. First, it can simplify analyses greatly. Second, the MAR assumption is often reasonable, especially when there are fully observed covariates available in the analysis to "explain" the reasons for the missingness; further, MAR cannot be contradicted by the observed data without the incorporation of external assumptions such as exact normality of variables. Third, even when the missing data are NMAR, an analysis based on the assumption of MAR can be helpful in reducing bias by effectively imputing missing data using relationships that are observed. Finally, even if the missing data are NMAR, it is usually not at all easy to specify a correct nonignorable model, for the simple reason that any evidence concerning the relationship of missingness to the missing values is absent because the missing values are, by definition, not observed (for example, see Rubin et al., 1995).

3. Simple approaches to handling missing data

3.1. Complete-case analysis

The simplest analysis with incomplete data is to delete all units (cases) with at least one missing variable, i.e., to use "complete-case" analysis (sometimes called listwise deletion). This approach is generally biased unless the missing data are MCAR; the degree of bias depends on (a) the amount of the missing data, (b) the degree to which the assumption of MCAR is violated, and (c) the particular analysis being implemented. Even when complete-case analysis is unbiased, it can be highly inefficient, especially with multivariate data sets. For example, consider a data set with 20 variables, each of which has probability of being missing of .05, and suppose that missingness on each variable is independent of missingness on the other variables. Then, the probability of a unit having complete data is $(.95)^{20} = .36$, so that complete-case analysis would be expected to include only 36% of the units, and many of the discarded units have a large fraction of their values observed.

3.2. Available-case analysis

A simple alternative to the complete-case method is to include all units that have complete data on the variables that are needed for the analysis being considered. This approach, "available-case" analysis, can be regarded as "complete-case analysis restricted to the variables of interest." Available-case analysis retains at least as many of the data values as does complete-case analysis. However, it can be problematic when more than one quantity is estimated and the different estimates are compared or combined, because the sample base generally changes from one estimated quantity to the next. For example, if summaries of different variables are to be compared, the set of units for which each variable is summarized can differ across variables, and the summaries can be incomparable if the missing data are not MCAR; an extreme artificial illustration of incomparable estimation using available-case analyses would occur if last year's mean cholesterol were based on males because it was not collected for females, and this year's were based on females because it was not collected for males. As an extreme example in the context of combining estimates, if the covariance of two variables and their individual standard deviations have been estimated using available-case analyses, when these estimates are combined to estimate the correlation between the two variables, the resulting estimated correlation can lie outside the range $[-1, 1]$.

Complete-case analysis and available-case analysis were often the default treatments of missing data in older software packages, and they are simple to implement, which is undeniably attractive. However, as just discussed, they can have serious deficiencies, which can be avoided when using more modern and more appropriate methods.

3.3. Weighting adjustments

For the case of unit nonresponse in surveys, a modification of complete-case analysis that can help to remove bias when the missing data are not MCAR is to weight the complete cases (i.e., the respondents) based on background information that is available for all of the units in the survey. For example, when a nonrespondent matches a respondent with respect to background variables that are observed for both, the nonrespondent's weight is simply added to the matching respondent's weight, and the nonrespondent is discarded. Because the match is defined by observed variables, such adjustments implicitly assume MAR.

A weighting procedure was used, for example, in the National Health Interview Survey (Botman et al., 2000). Typically, even if there were no adjustments for unit nonresponse in a survey, each sampled unit would already be weighted by the inverse of its probability of its selection, so that unbiased estimates of certain population quantities, such as totals, under repeated sampling could be calculated using those weights. The basic idea underlying a weighting adjustment for unit nonresponse is to treat unit nonresponse as an extra layer of sampling, which is accurate assuming ignorability, and then to weight each responding unit by the inverse of its estimated probability of both selection *and* response. For dealing with item nonresponse, the use of weighting adjustments is nearly always problematic, in large part because discarding the incomplete cases discards additional observed data that are not used in creating the weighting adjustment. Therefore, the standard method for handling item nonresponse in surveys is imputation, discussed in the next two sections. For further discussion of weighting procedures for nonresponse in general, see Bethlehem (2002), Gelman and Carlin (2002), and Little and Rubin (2002, Section 3.3).

4. Single imputation

Single imputation refers to imputing one value for each missing datum. Singly imputed data sets are straightforward to analyze using standard complete-data methods, which is again an undeniably attractive feature. Little and Rubin (2002, p. 72) offer the following guidelines for creating imputations. They should be: (1) conditional on observed variables; (2) multivariate, to reflect associations among missing variables; and (3) randomly drawn from predictive distributions rather than set equal to means, to ensure that correct variability is reflected. Methods for single imputation typically assume ignorability, and for simplicity, we concentrate discussion on the ignorable case.

4.1. Simple imputation methods

Unconditional mean imputation, which replaces each missing value with the mean of the observed values of that variable, meets none of the three guidelines listed above. Regression imputation can satisfy the first two guidelines by replacing the missing values for each variable with the values predicted from a regression (e.g., least squares, logistic) of that variable on other variables. Replacing missing values of each variable with the mean of that variable calculated within cells defined by categorical variables is a special case of regression imputation. Stochastic regression imputation adds random noise to the value predicted by the regression model, and when done properly can meet all three guidelines for single imputation.

Hot-deck imputation replaces each missing value with a random draw from a "donor pool" consisting of values of that variable observed on units similar to the unit with the missing value. Donor pools are selected, for example, by choosing units with complete data who have "similar" observed values to the unit with missing data, e.g., by exact matching on their observed values or using a distance measure (metric) on observed variables to define "similar." When the distance is defined as the difference between units on the predicted value of the variable to be imputed (Rubin, 1986), the imputation procedure is termed "predictive mean matching imputation" (Little, 1988). Hot-deck imputation, when done properly, can also satisfy all three of the guidelines listed above for single imputation.

Suppose that single imputations have been created following the three guidelines of Little and Rubin (2002) mentioned above. Then, analyzing such a singly imputed data set with standard complete-data techniques is straightforward and can lead to approximately unbiased point estimates under ignorability. This approach then satisfies criterion (a) of Section 1. However, the resulting analyses will nearly always result in estimated standard errors that are too small, confidence intervals that are too narrow, and p-values for hypothesis tests that are too significant, regardless of how the imputations were created, thus failing to satisfy criteria (b) and (c). The reason is that imputed data are treated by standard complete-data analyses as if they were known with no uncertainty. Thus, single imputation followed by a complete-data analysis that does not distinguish between real and imputed values is almost always statistically invalid.

4.2. Interval estimation after single imputation

Special methods for variance estimation following single imputation have been developed for specific imputation procedures and estimation problems; see, for example, Schafer and Schenker (2000) and Lee et al. (2002). However, such techniques need to be customized to the imputation method used and to the analysis methods at hand, and they often require the user to have information from the imputation model that is not typically available in shared data sets. A more broadly applicable but computationally intensive approach with singly imputed data is to use a replication technique such as balanced repeated replication, the jackknife, or the bootstrap for variance estimation, with the imputation procedure repeated separately for each replicate; see, for example, Efron (1994) and Shao (2002). But, again, such replication methods assume criterion (a) has been satisfied by the single imputation method.

Multiple imputation (MI), described in Section 5, is a generally valid approach (i.e., satisfying criteria (a)–(c)), that is broadly applicable but less computationally intensive than the replication approach just mentioned, and it is thus particularly useful in the context of creating data sets to be shared by many users. MI simply involves repeating the drawing of single imputations several times, but its exact validity requires that the imputations are "proper" (Rubin, 1987), or more generally "confidence proper" (Rubin, 1996), both of which satisfy the three criteria of Little and Rubin (2002) for imputation.

4.3. Properly drawn single imputations

For notational simplicity, assume ignorability of the missing-data mechanism, even though the ignorability assumption is not necessary for MI to be appropriate. A proper imputation is often most easily obtained as a random draw from the "posterior predictive distribution" of the missing data given the observed data, which formally can be written as: $p(Y_{\text{mis}}|Y_{\text{obs}}) = \int p(Y_{\text{mis}}, \psi|Y_{\text{obs}})d\psi = \int p(Y_{\text{mis}}|Y_{\text{obs}}, \psi)p(\psi|Y_{\text{obs}})d\psi$. This expression effectively gives the distribution of the missing values, Y_{mis}, given the observed values, Y_{obs}, under a model for Y governed by ψ, $p(Y|\psi)p(\psi)$, where $p(\psi)$ is the prior distribution on ψ. The distribution $p(Y_{\text{mis}}|Y_{\text{obs}})$ is called "posterior" because it is conditional on the observed Y_{obs}, and it is called "predictive" because it predicts the missing Y_{mis}. It can be proper" because it reflects all uncertainty, including in parameter estimation, by taking draws of ψ from its posterior distribution, $p(\psi|Y_{\text{obs}})$, before using ψ to impute the missing data, Y_{mis}, from $p(Y_{\text{mis}}|Y_{\text{obs}}, \psi)$. More details are given in Sections 4.4 and 4.5.

Rubin (1987, Chapter 4) labeled imputation methods that do not account for all sources of variability as "improper." Thus, for example, fixing ψ at a point estimate $\hat{\psi}$, and then drawing m imputations for Y_{mis} independently with density $p(Y_{\text{mis}}|Y_{\text{obs}}, \hat{\psi})$, would constitute an improper MI procedure.

For simple patterns of missing data, such as with only one variable subject to missingness, the two-step paradigm of drawing ψ from $p(\psi|Y_{\text{obs}})$ and then drawing Y_{mis} from $p(Y_{\text{mis}}|Y_{\text{obs}}, \psi)$ is relatively straightforward to implement. For a simple example, Rubin and Schenker (1987) described its use in the context of fully parametric imputation involving logistic regression models. These steps can also incorporate more nonparametric analogs. The simple hot-deck procedure that randomly draws imputations for incomplete cases from matching complete cases is not proper because it ignores the sampling variability due to the fact that the population distribution of complete cases is not known, but rather it is estimated from the complete cases in the sample. Rubin and Schenker (1986, 1991) described a two-step procedure, termed "approximate Bayesian bootstrap imputation," which draws a bootstrap sample from the complete cases and then draws imputations randomly from the bootstrap sample. The initial bootstrap step is a nonparametric analog to the process of drawing a value ψ^* with density $p(\psi|Y_{\text{obs}})$, and the subsequent hot-deck step is a nonparametric analog to the process of drawing a value of Y_{mis} with density $p(Y_{\text{mis}}|Y_{\text{obs}}, \psi^*)$. Dorey et al. (1993) combined an initial bootstrap step with a fully parametric second step, whereas Schenker and Taylor (1996) combined a fully parametric first step with predictive mean matching imputation at the second step. Finally, Heitjan and Little (1991) combined an initial bootstrap step with bivariate predictive mean matching imputation at the second step.

4.4. Properly drawing imputations with monotone missingness

If the missing data follow a monotone pattern, it is straightforward to draw random samples from $p(Y_{\text{mis}}|Y_{\text{obs}})$. When the missing data are not monotone, iterative computational methods are generally necessary, as described in Section 4.5. A missing-data pattern is monotone if the rows and columns of the data matrix can be sorted so that an irregular staircase separates Y_{obs} and Y_{mis}. Figure 1 illustrate monotone missing-data patterns. Missing data in clinical trials are often monotone or nearly monotone when data are missing due to patient dropout, where once a patient drops out, the patient never returns. Similarly some longitudinal surveys have monotone or nearly monotone missingness patterns when people who drop out never return.

Let Y_0 represent fully observed variables, Y_1 the incompletely observed variable with the fewest missing values, Y_2 the variable with the second fewest missing values, and so on, and assume a monotone pattern of missingness. Proper imputation with a monotone missing data pattern begins by fitting an appropriate model to predict Y_1 from Y_0 and then using this model to impute the missing values in Y_1. For example, fit a least squares regression of Y_1 on Y_0 using the units with Y_1 observed, draw the regression parameters of this model from their posterior distribution, and then draw the missing values of Y_1 given these drawn parameters and the observed values of Y_0. Next impute the missing values for Y_2 using Y_0 and the observed and imputed values of Y_1; for example, if Y_2 is dichotomous, use a logistic regression model for Y_2 given (Y_0, Y_1). Continue to impute the next most complete variable until all missing values have been imputed. The collection of imputed values is a proper imputation of the missing data, Y_{mis}, under this model, and the collection of univariate prediction models defines the implied full imputation model, $p(Y_{\text{mis}}|Y_{\text{obs}})$. When missing data are not monotone, this method of imputation as described cannot be used directly to define $p(Y_{\text{mis}}|Y_{\text{obs}})$.

4.5. Properly drawing imputations with nonmonotone missingness

Creating imputations when the missing-data pattern is nonmonotone generally involves iteration because the distribution $p(Y_{\text{mis}}|Y_{\text{obs}})$ is often difficult to draw from directly. However, the Data-Augmentation algorithm (DA; Tanner and Wong, 1987), a stochastic version of the Expectation-Maximization algorithm (EM; Dempster et al., 1977), is often straightforward to implement. Briefly, DA involves iterating between randomly sampling missing data given a current draw of the model parameters and randomly sampling model parameters given a current draw of the missing data. The draws of Y_{mis} form a Markov Chain whose stationary distribution is $p(Y_{\text{mis}}|Y_{\text{obs}})$.

Thus, once the Markov Chain has reached effective convergence, a draw of Y_{mis} obtained by DA is effectively a single proper imputation of the missing data from the correct target distribution $p(Y_{mis}|Y_{obs})$, the posterior predictive distribution of Y_{mis}. Many of the programs discussed in Section 5.3 use DA or variants of DA to impute missing values. Other algorithms that use Markov Chain Monte Carlo methods for imputing missing values include the Gibbs sampler (Geman and Geman, 1984) and the Metropolis–Hastings algorithm (Metropolis and Ulam, 1949; Hastings, 1970). See, e.g., Gelman et al. (2003) for more details for these algorithms in general, and Schafer (1997) for the application of DA for imputation. This general approach is also discussed in Section 6.

An alternative to doing imputation under one specified model is to do imputation under potentially incompatible models, e.g., a potentially incompatible Gibbs sampler. These iterative simulation methods run a regression (e.g., least squares, logistic) on each variable with some missing data on all other variables using previously imputed values for these other variables, and then cycle through each variable with missing data. In fact, such regression imputation methods that are not necessarily derived from a joint distribution for all of the data have been more extensively developed recently, and they provide very flexible tools for creating imputations. As we will see in Section 5, such methods have gained prominence for the creation of MIs in recent years, although they have a relatively long history of application (e.g., Kennickell, 1991; Van Buuren and Oudshoorn, 2000; Raghunathan et al., 2001; Münnich and Rässler, 2005; Van Buuren et al., 2006). Further research should lead to greater understanding of the theoretical properties of such methods as well as to refinements of the methods in practice.

5. Multiple imputation

Multiple imputation (MI) was introduced by Rubin (1978a) and discussed in detail in Rubin (1987, 2004a, 2004b); it is an approach that retains the advantages of single imputation while allowing the uncertainty due to the process of imputation to be assessed directly and included to create valid inferences in many situations. MI is a simulation technique that replaces the missing values Y_{mis} with $m>1$ plausible values, and therefore reveals and quantifies uncertainty in the imputed values. Each set of imputations (i.e., each single imputation Y_{mis}) thus creates a completed data set, thereby creating m "completed" data sets: $Y^{(1)}, \ldots, Y^{(l)}, \ldots, Y^{(m)}$, where $Y^{(l)} = (Y_{obs}, Y_{mis}^{(l)})$. Typically m is fairly small; $m = 5$ is a standard number of imputations to use. Each of the m completed data sets is then analyzed as if there were no missing data, just as with single imputation, and the results of the m analyses are combined using simple rules described shortly.

Obtaining proper multiple-imputations is no more difficult than obtaining a single proper imputation because the process for obtaining a proper single imputation is simply repeated independently m times. Schafer (1997) is an excellent source for computational guidance on creating multiple-imputations under a variety of models for the data Y. Multiple-imputations can be created under both ignorable and nonignorable models for missingness, although the use of ignorable models has been the norm, in part based on considerations of the type discussed at the conclusion of Section 2.

5.1. *Combining rules for proper multiple imputation – scalar point estimates*

Let θ represent the scalar estimand of interest (e.g., the mean of a variable, a relative risk, the intention-to-treat effect, etc.), let $\hat{\theta}$ represent the standard complete-data estimator of θ (i.e., the quantity calculated treating all imputed values of Y_{mis} as observed data), and let $\hat{V}(\hat{\theta})$ represent the standard complete-data estimated variance of $\hat{\theta}$.

Suppose MI has been used to create m completed data sets. A standard complete-data analysis of each will produce m completed data sets, each associated with completed-data statistics, say $\hat{\theta}_l$ and $\hat{V}_l = \hat{V}(\hat{\theta})_l$, $l = 1, \ldots, m$. The m sets of statistics are combined to produce the final point estimate $\hat{\theta}_{\mathrm{MI}} = m^{-1}\Sigma_{l=1}^{m}\hat{\theta}_l$ and its estimated variance $T = W + (1 + m^{-1})B$, where $W = m^{-1}\Sigma_{l=1}^{m}\hat{V}_l$ is the "within-imputation" variance, $B = (m-1)^{-1}\Sigma_{l=1}^{m}(\hat{\theta}_l - \hat{\theta}_{\mathrm{MI}})^2$ is the "between-imputation" variance, and the factor $(1 + m^{-1})$ reflects the fact that only a finite number of completed-data estimates $\hat{\theta}_l$, $l = 1, \ldots, m$, are averaged together to obtain the final point estimate. The quantity $\hat{\gamma} = (1 + m^{-1})B/T$ estimates the fraction of information about θ that is missing due to the missing data.

Inferences from multiply imputed data are based on $\hat{\theta}_{\mathrm{MI}}$, T, and a Student's t reference distribution. Thus, for example, interval estimates for θ have the form $\hat{\theta}_{\mathrm{MI}} \pm t(1-\alpha/2)\sqrt{T}$, where $t(1-\alpha/2)$ is the $(1-\alpha/2)$ quantile of the t distribution. Rubin and Schenker (1986) provided the approximate value $\upsilon_{\mathrm{RS}} = (m-1)\hat{\gamma}^{-2}$ for the degrees of freedom of the t distribution, under the assumption that with complete data, a normal reference distribution would have been appropriate (i.e., the complete data would have had large degrees of freedom). Barnard and Rubin (1999) relaxed the assumption of Rubin and Schenker (1986) to allow for a t reference distribution with complete data, and proposed the value $\upsilon_{\mathrm{BR}} = (\upsilon_{\mathrm{RS}}^{-1} + \hat{\upsilon}_{\mathrm{obs}}^{-1})^{-1}$ for the degrees of freedom in the MI analysis, where $\hat{\upsilon}_{\mathrm{obs}} = (1-\hat{\gamma})(\upsilon_{\mathrm{com}})(\upsilon_{\mathrm{com}} + 1)(\upsilon_{\mathrm{com}} + 3)$, and υ_{com} is the complete-data degrees of freedom.

See Rubin and Schenker (1991) for additional methods for combining vector-valued estimates, significance levels, and likelihood ratio statistics; also see Little and Rubin (2002, Section 10.2). These sources summarize work done in Meng and Rubin (1992) and Li et al. (1991).

5.2. *Discussion of MI in practice*

A feature of imputation, either single or multiple, that gives such procedures great inherent flexibility and is especially attractive in the context of data sets that are shared by many users, is that the implicit or explicit model used for imputation, i.e., that leads to $p(Y_{\mathrm{mis}}|Y_{\mathrm{obs}})$, need not be the same as the explicit or implicit model used in subsequent analyses of the completed data. Thus, for example, an organization distributing public-use data can do its best job at imputing missing data, and then secondary analysts are free to explore a variety of models for analyzing the completed data. The formal derivation of procedures for analyzing multiply imputed data, however, is based on the assumption that the imputer's and analyst's models are compatible, in the sense that the imputation model is proper or confidence proper. Formally, the imputer's and analyst's models must be "congenial" (Meng, 1994) for the resulting analyses to be fully valid. Such congeniality can be enforced more easily when the imputer and analyst are the same entity or communicate with each other. In the context of shared data sets, however, to promote near-congeniality of the imputer's and user's implicit models, so that analyses based on multiply imputed data will be at least approximately valid, the imputer should include as rich a set of variables in the imputation model as possible in order to accommodate the variety of analyses that might be carried out by secondary analysts. For example, when the data come from a complex sample survey, variables reflecting features of the sample design should be included as well (e.g., variables used to determine sampling weights, these weights themselves, stratification indicators); this was done, for instance, when NHANES III was multiply imputed (Ezzati-Rice et al., 1993) as well as when NMES was multiply imputed (Rubin, 2003).

This advice to include as many variables as possible in an MI model was present from the beginning (e.g., Rubin, 1987). Especially important is to include variables used in the design of the data collection, such as variables used to derive sampling weights, or the sampling weights themselves. Also critical is to include domain indicators when domain estimates are to be obtained by subsequent users. There are some criticisms of MI's sampling variance estimation equations in situations when such critical variables are excluded from the MI model (e.g., Kim et al., 2006). Obviously, if a statistical method is implemented in a way that does not even approximate its correct use, resulting answers cannot be valid in general. Although the focus in these criticisms has been on sampling variance estimation, even the point estimates based on an imputation model that excludes weights or domain indicators will be biased in general, so the issue of biased sampling variance estimation becomes secondary.

5.3. Software for multiple imputation

Many standard statistical software packages now have built-in or add-on functions for creating and analyzing multiply-imputed data sets. Routines for creating such data sets include, for example, the S-plus libraries NORM, CAT, MIX, and PAN, for multiply imputing normal, categorical, mixed, and panel data, respectively, which are freely available (see http://www.stat.psu.edu/~jls/misoftwa.html). NORM is also available as a stand-alone version, as is MICE–MI by chained equations (see http://web.inter.nl.net/users/S.van.Buuren/mi/hmtl/mice.htm). In addition, IVEware is very flexible and freely available; it can be called using SAS or can be run as a stand-alone version (http://www.isr.umich.edu/src/smp/ive/). SAS now has procedures PROC MI and PROC MIANALYZE making the analysis of multiply imputed data sets easy. Other software packages have been developed specifically for creating multiply-imputed data sets, for example, the commercially available SOLAS (http://www.statsol.ie/solas/solas.htm), which has been available for years, is most appropriate for data sets with a monotone or nearly monotone pattern of missing data. Additionally, STATA provides MI routines based on the chained equation approach and supports analyses of multiply-imputed data sets. For more information, see www.multiple-imputation.com or for some historical perspective, see Horton and Lipsitz (2001).

6. Direct analysis using model-based procedures

Direct analyses of the incomplete data can be implemented by specifying a model for the complete data and then basing inferences on the likelihood or posterior distribution under that model. In its full generality, modeling the incomplete data is accomplished by simultaneously modeling both Y and R, as explicitly introduced in Rubin (1976). Selection models (e.g., Heckman, 1976) specify the marginal distribution of Y as well as how the distribution of R depends on Y, as follows:

$$p(Y, R|\psi, \xi) = p(Y|\psi)p(R|Y, \xi), \tag{1}$$

where ψ and ξ are unknown parameters. In contrast, pattern-mixture models (e.g., Rubin, 1977, 1978a; Little, 1993) specify the distribution of Y for each pattern of missing data (implied by R) as well as the probability of the various patterns occurring, as follows:

$$p(Y, R|\phi, \pi) = p(Y|R, \phi)p(R|\pi),$$

where ϕ and π are unknown parameters. When R is independent of Y, the missing data are MCAR, and the selection and pattern-mixture specifications are equivalent when $\psi = \phi$ and $\xi = \pi$, i.e., the implied models are the same. When the missing data are not MCAR, the two specifications generally differ.

Little and Rubin (2002, Chapter 15) discuss the use of selection and pattern-mixture approaches in the context of nonignorable missingness for a variety of types of data. As discussed earlier, the correct specification of nonignorable models is usually difficult due to lack of information in the data about the relationship between the missing-data mechanism and the missing values themselves. For this reason, selection models and pattern-mixture models for nonignorable missing data tend to depend strongly on assumptions about specific distributions. Thus, although they offer different and interesting approaches to modeling nonignorable missing data, it is suggested that they be used primarily for sensitivity analyses; as in Rubin (1977) and Little (1993), with a baseline analysis under ignorability being used as a primary point of comparison.

Consider now the situation of ignorable missing data. The observed data are Y_{obs} and R, and under the selection model specification given by expression (1), the likelihood function based on the observed data is

$$L(\psi, \xi | Y_{\text{obs}}, R) \propto \int p(Y_{\text{obs}}, Y_{\text{mis}} | \psi) p(R | Y_{\text{obs}}, Y_{\text{mis}}, \xi) dY_{\text{mis}}. \tag{2}$$

As shown by Rubin (1976) and discussed previously, if the missing data are MAR (i.e., $p(R | Y_{\text{obs}}, Y_{\text{mis}}, \xi) = p(R | Y_{\text{obs}}, \xi)$), and if ψ and ξ are distinct, then inferences for ψ based on expression (2) are equivalent to inferences for ψ based on the likelihood for ψ ignoring the missing-data mechanism

$$L(\psi | Y_{\text{obs}}) \propto \int p(Y_{\text{obs}}, Y_{\text{mis}} | \psi) dY_{\text{mis}}, \tag{3}$$

because (2) factors into (3) and a factor that is free of ψ. Articles have appeared in the literature describing analyses of incomplete data under the assumption of ignorable missingness for a vast number of different analytic problems. Little and Rubin (2002, Chapters 11–14) review several such examples.

The remainder of this section describes two general techniques: (1) the EM algorithm (Dempster et al., 1977) and its extensions for maximum likelihood estimation of ψ, and (2) DA (Tanner and Wong, 1987) and its extensions for Bayesian posterior simulation. These techniques can be applied in the context of nonignorable missing data as well as that of ignorable missing data, but the presentation here is in the latter context for simplicity.

In many missing-data problems, even the observed-data likelihood (3) is complicated, and explicit expressions for maximum likelihood estimation of ψ are difficult to derive. The EM algorithm, a technique for computing maximum likelihood estimates iteratively, takes advantage of the facts that: (1) if ψ were known, it would be relatively easy to estimate many functions of Y_{mis}, and (2) if the data were complete, computation of maximum likelihood estimates would be relatively simple. Starting with an initial estimate of ψ, the EM algorithm iterates between two steps, an E-step (E for expectation) and an M-step (M for maximization), until convergence. Given the estimate of ψ at iteration t, $\psi^{(t)}$, the E-step computes the expected value of the complete-data log-likelihood given Y_{obs} and $\psi = \psi^{(t)}$, $Q(\psi | \psi^{(t)}) = \int \log L(\psi | Y) p(Y_{\text{mis}} | Y_{\text{obs}}, \psi = \psi^{(t)}) dY_{\text{mis}}$; this step often involves computing the expected values of the complete-data sufficient statistics, which are linear in the data for exponential family distributions. Then, the M-step determines $\psi^{(t+1)}$ by maximizing the expected complete-data log-likelihood $Q(\psi | \psi^{(t)})$. For discussions of the theoretical properties of the EM algorithm, examples of its use, methods for obtaining standard errors based on the algorithm, and extensions, see Dempster et al. (1977), McLachlan and Krishnan (1997), Schafer (1997), and Little and Rubin (2002, Chapters 8, 9, and 11–15). Extensions of EM include the ECM (Meng and Rubin, 1993), ECME (Liu and Rubin, 1994), AECM (Meng and van Dyk, 1997), and PXEM (Liu et al., 1998) algorithms.

Bayesian inferences for ψ are based on the observed-data posterior distribution with density $p(\psi | Y_{\text{obs}}) \propto p(\psi) L(\psi | Y_{\text{obs}})$, where $p(\psi)$ is the prior density for ψ.

As is the case with maximum likelihood estimation, working explicitly with the observed-data posterior distribution can be difficult. DA, introduced in Section 4.5, facilitates the creation of draws of ψ from density $p(\psi|Y_{\text{obs}})$ using steps that are analogous to those of the EM algorithm but that involve simulation. In a simple version, DA begins with an initial approximation to $p(\psi|Y_{\text{obs}})$ and then iterates between two steps, an I-step, which imputes an updated value for Y_{mis}, and a P-step, which draws a value from an updated conditional posterior distribution for ψ, until convergence of the distribution of draws of Y_{mis} and ψ. Specifically, given the drawn value of ψ at iteration t, $\psi^{(t)}$, the I-step draws a value $Y_{\text{mis}}^{(t+1)}$ from density $p(Y_{\text{mis}}|Y_{\text{obs}}, \psi^{(t)})$, and then the P-step draws a value $\psi^{(t+1)}$ from density $p(\psi|Y_{\text{obs}}, Y_{\text{mis}}^{(t+1)})$. As t increases, the draws $(Y_{\text{mis}}^{(t)}, \psi^{(t)})$ converge in distribution to draws from joint density $p(Y_{\text{mis}}, \psi|Y_{\text{obs}})$, and thus the draws $\psi^{(t)}$ converge in distribution to draws from density $p(\psi|Y_{\text{obs}})$. The empirical distribution of such multiple draws of ψ can be used to approximate the observed-data posterior distribution of ψ. The draws at successive iterations are serially correlated, however. Therefore, to obtain multiple independent draws from the observed-data posterior distribution of ψ, it is standard practice either to independently repeat the entire iterative procedure until convergence multiple times to generate multiple draws or to implement the iterative procedure once until convergence and then take every kth draw thereafter, with k chosen large enough to achieve approximate independence. For discussions of theoretical properties, extensions of DA, and examples of the use of Bayesian iterative simulation methods, see Tanner and Wong (1987), Gelfand and Smith (1990), Schafer (1997), and Little and Rubin (2002, Chapters 10–14). Gelman et al. (2003) is a good reference for related MCMC methods such as the Gibbs sampler and the Metropolis–Hastings algorithm.

For a specific problem, if the sample is large, likelihood-based analyses and Bayesian analyses under diffuse prior distributions are expected to give similar results, because the likelihood would be expected to dominate the prior distribution. For small samples, however, Bayesian analyses have the advantage of avoiding the assumption of asymptotic normality of the likelihood that is typically made. Moreover, results under various prior assumptions can be compared.

7. Examples

The examples we present here are from a randomized clinical trial and epidemiological databases. All use MI to address missing data rather than any of the ad hoc methods described at the start of this chapter or methods of direct analysis just described. We believe this emphasis is generally appropriate in epidemiology and medical statistics. In special cases, of course, methods other than MI can also be appropriate or even more appropriate.

7.1. Missing data in Genzyme's Randomized Trial of Fabrazyme®

Fabrazyme® is a synthetic enzyme developed by Genzyme Corporation to treat Fabry's disease, a rare and serious X-linked recessive genetic disorder that occurs due to an inability to metabolize creatinine. Preliminary results from a randomized trial of Fabrazyme® versus placebo revealed that the Fabrazyme® appeared to work well in patients in their 30s, who were not yet severely ill, in the sense that it lowered their serum creatinine substantially. A similar randomized clinical trial involved older patients who were more seriously ill. Since there was no other fully competitive treatment, it was desired to make Fabrazyme® commercially available earlier than initially planned, a decision that would allow patients randomized to placebo to begin taking Fabrazyme®, but would create missing $Y(0)$ outcome data among placebo patients once they began taking Fabrazyme®. The study had staggered enrollment because of the rareness of the condition, so that the number of monthly observations of serum creatinine for each placebo patient depended on the time of entry into the study. Figure 1 illustrates the general pattern of monotone missing data with the same length follow-up intended for each patient. Again, X represents baseline covariates, $Y(0)$ represents the repeated measures of serum creatinine for placebo patients, and $Y(1)$ represents the repeated measures of serum creatinine for Fabrazyme® patients.

In order to impute the missing outcomes under placebo, a complex hierarchical Bayesian model was developed for the progression of serum creatinine in untreated Fabry patients. In this model, inverse serum creatinine varies linearly and quadratically in time, and the prior distribution for the quadratic trend in placebo patients is obtained from the posterior distribution of the quadratic trend in an analogous model fit to a historical database of untreated Fabry patients. Thus, the historical patients' data only influence the imputations of the placebo patients' data rather subtly – via the prior distribution on the quadratic trend parameters.

Although the model fitting algorithm is complex, it is straightforward to use the algorithm to draw ψ from $p(\psi|Y_{\text{obs}})$ for the placebo patients, and then draw Y_{mis} in the placebo group conditional on the drawn value of ψ, where, as earlier, ψ represents all model parameters. Drawing the missing values in this way creates a sample from $p(Y_{\text{mis}}|Y_{\text{obs}})$ and thus an imputation for the missing values in the placebo group.

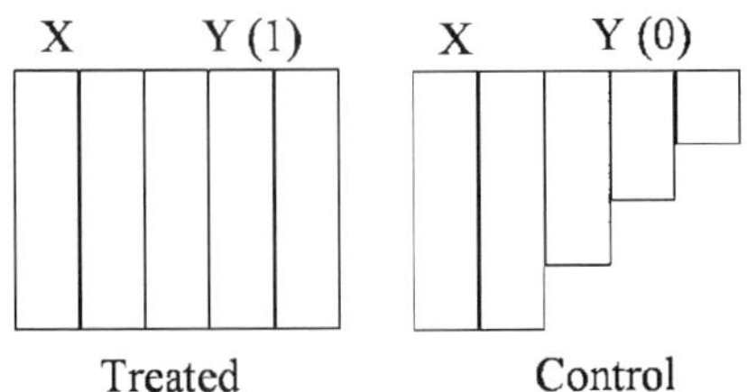

Fig. 1. Pattern of missing data for Genzyme trial.

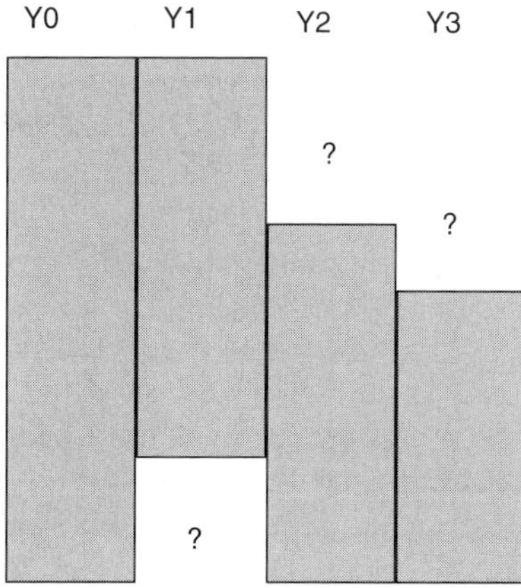

Fig. 2. Illustrative display for type of pattern of missing data in NMES.

7.2. Missing Data in NMES

The NMES collects data on a random sample of approximately 30,000 members of the US population, including hundreds of measurements of medical expenditures, background information, and demographic information. MI for NMES was more complicated than in the previous two examples because the missing-data pattern was not monotone. Figure 2 depicts a tremendous simplification of the missing-data pattern for NMES, where, if *Y*1 were fully observed, the missing-data pattern would be monotone.

Rubin (2003) imputed the missing data in NMES by capitalizing on the simplicity of imputation for monotone missing data by first imputing the missing values that destroyed the monotone pattern (the "nonmonotone missing values") and then proceeding as if the missing-data pattern were in fact monotone, and then iterating this process. More specifically, after choosing starting values for the missing data, iterate between the following two steps. (1) Regress each variable with any nonmonotone missing values (i.e., *Y*1), on all the other variables (i.e., *Y*0, *Y*2, *Y*3), treating the current imputations as true values, but use this regression to impute only the nonmonotone missing values. (2) Impute the remaining missing values in the monotone pattern; first impute the variable with the fewest missing values (*Y*2 in Fig. 2), then the variable with the second fewest missing values (*Y*3 in Fig. 2), and so on, treating the nonmonotone missing values inputed in Step 1 as known. This process was repeated five times to create five sets of imputations in the NMES example.

7.3. Missing data in the ABCs, a disease surveillance system

The Active Bacterial Core surveillance (ABCs) system is population-based and laboratory-based surveillance network. Five bacterial pathogens are monitored through the ABCs. These pathogens are: group A streptococcus, group B streptococcus, *Streptococcus pneumoniae*, *Haemophilus influenzae*, and *Neisseria*

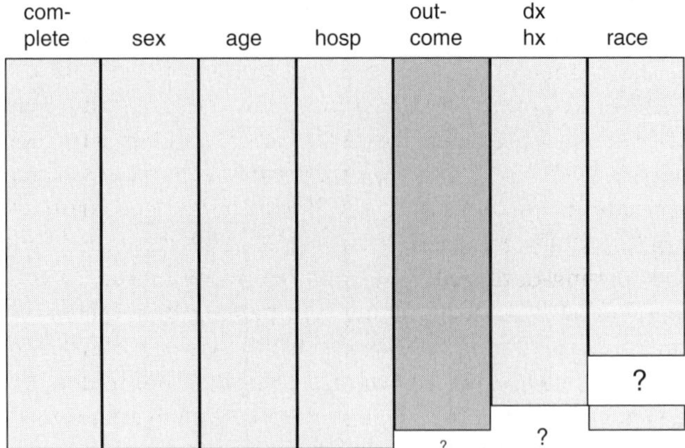

Fig. 3. Pattern of missing data in ABCs 2002.

meningitidis (Schuchat et al., 2001). A case of invasive disease is identified through bacteria isolated from a normally sterile site from an individual residing within the defined surveillance areas for each pathogen. Cases are identified through active contact with clinical laboratories – hence the label "active surveillance." Chart reviews are conducted to obtain demographic, clinical, and risk factor information. Additional susceptibility testing and serotyping is completed for ABCs pathogens at reference laboratories. Chart reviews generally suffer from missing data because not all information, particularly demographic data, are recorded in the medical record.

Multiple imputation (MI) ($m = 5$) was used to complete the data using a sequential regression multivariate approach (Raghunathan et al., 2001) implemented with IVEware (Raghunathan et al., 2002). This approach allows a model that accounts for the categorical and continuous nature of the variables in the database. It also allows for skip patterns, which are important because surveillance systems evolve over time with the case report forms adding or modifying variables. Different sites have implemented these changes to the case report form at different times. Also, for example, one site by law cannot report on a specific underlying disease. The missingness in this data set is close to monotone, as shown in Fig. 3.

8. Literature review for epidemiology and medical studies

Over the last decade, there has been increasing use of MI for databases in many areas of public health, clinical research, and epidemiology. Examples include cross-sectional survey data, longitudinal studies, clinical trials, surveillance systems, case–control studies, etc. These databases address quality of care, descriptive health statistics, AIDS-related studies, cancer mortality and survival rates, comparison of health-related costs and outcomes across countries, prognostic factors for cancer survival, and many other epidemiological, medically and clinically important questions. An intensive literature search and review brought up at least 40 articles using MI, as summarized in Appendix A.

There also have been many articles comparing, evaluating, and reviewing approaches to deal with missing data in many disciplines. For example, articles dealing with longitudinal studies have often compared "last observation carried forward" to MI techniques with the primary recommendation that MI is preferable to last observation carried forward. Others studies have compared complete-case analysis with MI and have found clear advantages when using MI to retain all observations for data analysis. There have been many review articles across different disciplines in health care (e.g., nursing) on the importance of addressing the missing-data problem correctly. A common theme when MI is used is the ease of data analysis using complete-data methods of analysis on multiply-imputed data sets, and the ease of creating multiply-imputed data sets using readily available statistical software packages. More than a hundred articles can be found very easily regarding the comparison and evaluation of missing-data techniques, as summarized in Appendix B.

9. Summary and discussion

Missing values are a common problem in medical and epidemiological databases. This entry has discussed concepts regarding mechanisms that create missing data, as well as strengths and weaknesses of commonly used approaches. Simple approaches, such as complete-case analysis and available-case analysis, are generally valid only when the missing data are MCAR. Even then, such approaches can be problematic.

Multiple imputation (MI) is especially useful in the context of data sets to be shared by many users, because of its general applicability and flexibility, as well as the fact that it allows the data producer to create one "adjustment" for missing data that can be used by all secondary data analysts. MI is also a useful technique in the context of designed missing data, such as when split questionnaire designs (also known as matrix sampling designs) are used to reduce costs and respondent burden (e.g., Raghunathan and Grizzle, 1995). Moreover, it offers potential for new analyses, e.g., in the context of censored data (see Gartner and Rässler, 2005 or Jensen et al., 2006).

For specific analyses problems in the presence of missing data, especially when the data producer and data analyst are the same entity, direct analyses of the incomplete data can be conducted. Techniques such as the EM and DA algorithms and their extensions are useful for handling the complexities created by missing data. MI has the advantage of flexibility over direct analyses, in the sense that the imputer can use one model to fill in the missing data, whereas the analyst can use a different model to draw inferences from the completed data. However, incompatibility of the two models can degrade the approximations underlying MI methods somewhat, although many evaluations in practice suggest that this degradation is often quite limited.

Because of uncertainties about correct models in the presence of missing data, it is useful to conduct sensitivity analyses under different modeling assumptions. In fact, this was one of the original motivations for MI. Rubin (1978a, 1987,

Chapter 1) recommended the creation of imputations under multiple models for purposes of sensitivity analysis, in addition to the creation of repeated imputations under a single model for assessments of variability due to missing data under that model. For examples of such sensitivity analyses, see Rubin (1977, 1986) and Rässler (2002).

Many of the approaches discussed herein can be applied under the assumption of either ignorable or nonignorable missing data. The assumption of ignorability cannot be contradicted directly by the observed data, and procedures that assume ignorability typically lead to at least partial corrections for bias due to missing data. Nonignorable models can be very difficult to specify, and their performance can be quite sensitive to modeling assumptions. Therefore, a sensible approach is to use ignorability as a "baseline" assumption, and to conduct additional sensitivity analyses using nonignorable models. For comparisons of the performance of ignorable and nonignorable models, see Glynn et al. (1986), Rubin et al. (1995), and Baker et al. (2003).

For interested readers, some recent books containing further discussion of topics covered in this chapter, as well as related topics, include Robert and Casella (1999), Groves et al. (2002), Little and Rubin (2002), and Gelman and Meng (2004).

Acknowledgements

This chapter borrows in places from two previous reviews written with other combinations of coauthors, and we thank them for their generosity. These two other articles are presented in the publications by Cook and Rubin (2005) and Rässler et al. (2007).

Appendix A

Boshuizen, H.C., Viet, A.L., Picavet, H.S.J., Botterweck, A., van Loon, A.J.M. (2006). Non-response in a survey of cardiovascular risk factors in the Dutch population: Determinants and resulting biases. *Public Health* **120**(4), 297–308.

Brancato, G., Pezzotti, P., Rapiti, E., Perucci, C.A., Abeni, D., Babbalacchio, A., Rezza, G. (1997). Multiple imputation method for estimating incidence of HIV infection. The Multicenter Prospective HIV Study. *International Journal of Epidemiology* **26**(5), 1107–1114.

Burd, R.S., Jang, T.S., Nair, S.S. (2006). Predicting hospital mortality among injured children using a national trauma database. *Journal of Trauma-Injury Infection & Critical Care* **60**(4), 792–801.

Choe, J.H., Koepsell, T.D., Heagerty, P.J., Taylor, V.M. (2005). Colorectal cancer among Asians and Pacific Islanders in the U.S.: Survival disadvantage for the foreign-born. *Cancer Detection & Prevention* **29**(4), 361–368.

Clark, T.G., Stewart, M.E., Altman, D.G., Gabra, H., Smyth, J.F. (2001). A prognostic model for ovarian cancer. *British Journal of Cancer* **85**(7), 944–952.

Clarke, A.E., Petri, M., Manzi, S., Isenberg, D.A., Gordon, C., Senecal, J.L., Penrod, J., Joseph, L., St. Pierre, Y., Fortin, P.R., Sutcliffe, N., Richard Goulet, J., Choquette, D., Grodzicky, T., Esdaile, J.M., Tri-Nation Study Group. (2004). The systemic lupus erythematosus Tri-Nation Study: Absence of a link between health resource use and health outcome. *Rheumatology* **43**(8), 1016–1024.

De Roos, A.J., Hartge, P., Lubin, J.H., Colt, J.S., Davis, S., Cerhan, J.R., Severson, R.K., Cozen, W., Patterson Jr., D.G., Needham, L.L., Rothman, N. (2005). Persistent organochlorine chemicals in plasma and risk of non-Hodgkin's lymphoma. *Cancer Research* **65**(23), 11214–11226.

European Collaborative Study. (1994). Caesarean section and risk of vertical transmission of HIV-1 infection. *Lancet* **343**, 1464–1467.

Fitten, L.J., Perryman, K.M., Wilkinson, C.J., Little, R.J., Burns, M.M., Pachana, N., Mervis, J.R., Malmgren, R., Siembieda, D.W., Ganzell, S. (1995). Alzheimer and vascular dementias and driving – A prospective road and laboratory study. *Journal of the American Medical Association* **273**, 1360–1365.

Fitzgerald, A.P., DeGruttola, V.G., Vaida, F. (2002). Modelling HIV viral rebound using non-linear mixed effects models. *Statistics in Medicine* **21**(14), 2093–2108.

Foshee, V.A., Bauman, K.E., Ennett, S.T., Suchindran, C., Benefield, T., Linder, G.F. (2005). Assessing the effects of the dating violence prevention program "safe dates" using random coefficient regression modeling. *Prevention Science* **6**(3), 245–258.

Freedman, V.A., Wolf, D.A. (1995). A case study on the use of multiple imputation. *Demography* **32**(3), 459–470.

Garfield, R., Leu, C.S. (2000). A multivariate method for estimating mortality rates among children under 5 years from health and social indicators in Iraq. *International Journal of Epidemiology* **29**(3), 510–515.

Hediger, M.L., Overpeck, M.D., McGlynn, A., Kuczmarski, R.J., Maurer, K.R., Davis, W.W. (1999). Growth and fatness at three to six years of age of children born small- or large-for-gestational age. *Pediatrics* **104**(3), e33.

Hennekens, C.H., Lee, I.-M., Cook, N.R., Hebert, P.R., Karlson, E.W., LaMotte, F., Mason, J.E., Buring, J.E. (1996). Self-reported breast implants and connective-tissue diseases in female health professionals. *Journal of the American Medical Association* **275**(8), 616.

Heo, M., Leibel, R.L., Boyer, B.B., Chung, W.K., Koulu, M., Karvonen, M.K., Pesonen, U., Rissanen, A., Laakso, M., Uusitupa, M.I., Chagnon, Y., Bouchard, C., Donohoue, P.A., Burns, T.L., Shuldiner, A.R., Silver, K., Andersen, R.E., Pedersen, O., Echwald, S., Sorensen, T.I., Behn, P., Permutt, M.A., Jacobs, K.B., Elston, R.C., Hoffman, D.J., Allison, D.B. (2001). Pooling analysis of genetic data: The association of leptin receptor (LEPR) polymorphisms with variables related to human adiposity. *Genetics* **159**(3), 1163–1178.

Hill, J.L., Waldfogel, J., Brooks-Gunn, J., Han, W.J. (2005). Maternal employment and child development: A fresh look using newer methods. *Developmental Psychology* **41**(6), 833–850.

Hopman, W.M., Berger, C., Joseph, L., Towheed, T., Van den Kerkhof, E., Anastassiades, T., Adachi, J.D., Ioannidis, G., Brown, J.P., Hanley, D.A.,

Papadimitropoulos, E.A., CaMos Research Group. (2006). The natural progression of health-related quality of life: Results of a five-year prospective study of SF-36 scores in a normative population. *Quality of Life Research* **15**(3), 527–536.

Hopman, W.M., Berger, C., Joseph, L., Towheed, T., Van den Kerkhof, E., Anastassiades, T., Cranney, A., Adachi, J.D., Loannidis, G., Poliquin, S., Brown, J.P., Murray, T.M., Hanley, D.A., Papadimitropoulos, E.A., Tenenhouse, A., CaMos Research Group. (2004). Stability of normative data for the SF-36: Results of a three-year prospective study in middle-aged Canadians. *Canadian Journal of Public Health-Revue Canadienne de Sante Publique* **95**(5), 387–391.

Huo, D., Lauderdale, D.S., Li, L. (2003). Influence of reproductive factors on hip fracture risk in Chinese women. *Osteoporosis International* **14**(8), 694–700.

Jackson, L.W., Schisterman, E.F., Dey-Rao, R., Browne, R., Armstrong, D. (2005). Oxidative stress and endometriosis. *Human Reproduction* **20**(7), 2014–2020.

Jiang, Y., Hesser, J.E. (2006). Associations between health-related quality of life and demographics and health risks. Results from Rhode Island's 2002 behavioral risk factor survey. *Health & Quality of Life Outcomes* **4**, 14.

Kagan, R.S., Joseph, L., Dufresne, C., Gray-Donald, K., Turnbull, E., St. Pierre, Y., Clarke, A.E. (2003). Prevalence of peanut allergy in primary-school children in Montreal, Canada. *Journal of Allergy & Clinical Immunology* **112**(6), 1223–1228.

Kessler, R.C., Adler, L., Barkley, R., Biederman, J., Conners, C.K., Demler, O., Faraone, S.V., Greenhill, L.L., Howes, M.J., Secnik, K., Spencer, T., Ustun, T.B., Walters, E.E., Zaslavsky, A.M. (2006). The prevalence and correlates of adult ADHD in the United States: Results from the National Comorbidity Survey Replication. *American Journal of Psychiatry* **163**(4), 716–723.

Kessler, R.C., Adler, L.A., Barkley, R., Biederman, J., Conners, C.K., Faraone, S.V., Greenhill, L.L., Jaeger, S., Secnik, K., Spencer, T., Ustun, T.B., Zaslavsky, A.M. (2005). Patterns and predictors of attention-deficit/hyperactivity disorder persistence into adulthood: Results from the National Comorbidity Survey Replication. Biological *Psychiatry* **57**(11), 1442–1451.

Kessler, R.C., Birnbaum, H., Demler, O., Falloon, I.R.H., Gagnon, E., Guyer, M., Howes, M.J., Kendler, K.S., Shi, L., Walters, E., Wu, E.Q. (2005). The prevalence and correlates of nonaffective psychosis in the National Comorbidity Survey Replication (NCS-R). *Biological Psychiatry* **58**(8), 668–676.

Lento, J., Glynn, S., Shetty, V., Asarnow, J., Wang, J., Belin, T.R. (2004). Psychologic functioning and needs of indigent patients with facial injury: A prospective controlled study. *Journal of Oral & Maxillofacial Surgery* **62**(8), 925–932.

Lu, M., Ma, C. (2002). Consistency in performance evaluation reports and medical records. *The Journal of Mental Health Policy & Economics* **5**(4), 141–152.

McCleary, L. (2002). Using multiple imputation for analysis of incomplete data in clinical research. *Nursing Research* **51**(5), 339–343.

Powers, J.R., Mishra, G., Young, A.F. (2005). Differences in mail and telephone responses to self-rated health: Use of multiple imputation in correcting for response bias. *Australian & New Zealand Journal of Public Health* **29**(2), 149–154.

Salvan, A., Thomaseth, K., Bortot, P., Sartori, N. (2001). Use of a toxicokinetic model in the analysis of cancer mortality in relation to the estimated absorbed dose of dioxin (2,3,7,8-tetrachlorodibenzo-*p*-dioxin, TCDD). *Science of the Total Environment* **274**(1–3), 21–35.

Sbarra, D.A., Emery, R.E. (2005). Coparenting conflict, nonacceptance, and depression among divorced adults: Results from a 12-year follow-up study of child custody mediation using multiple imputation. *American Journal of Orthopsychiatry* **75**(1), 63–75.

Serrat, C., Gomez, G., Garcia de Olalla, P., Cayla, J.A. (1998). CD4+ lymphocytes and tuberculin skin test as survival predictors in pulmonary tuberculosis HIV-infected patients. *International Journal of Epidemiology* **27**(4), 703–712.

Sheppard, L., Levy, D., Norris, G., Larson, T.V., Koenig, J.Q. (1999). Effects of ambient air pollution on nonelderly asthma hospital admissions in Seattle, Washington, 1987–1994. *Epidemiology* **10**(1), 23–30 (see Comment in *Epidemiology*, 1999, **10**(1), 1–4, PMID: 9888271; Comment in *Epidemiology*, 2000, **11**(3), 367–368, PMID: 10784265).

Stadler, W.M., Huo, D., George, C., Yang, X., Ryan, C.W., Karrison, T., Zimmerman, T.M., Vogelzang, N.J. (2003). Prognostic factors for survival with gemcitabine plus 5-fluorouracil based regimens for metastatic renal cancer. *Journal of Urology* **170**(4 Pt 1), 1141–1145.

Stefan, V.H. (2004). Assessing intrasample variation: Analysis of Rapa Nui (Easter Island) museum cranial collections example. *American Journal of Physical Anthropology* **124**(1), 45–58.

Taylor, J.M.G., Cooper, K.L., Wei, J.T., Sarma, A.V., Raghunathan, T.E., Heeringa, S.G. (2002). Use of multiple imputation to correct for nonresponse bias in a survey of urologic symptoms among African-American men. *American Journal of Epidemiology* **156**(8), 774–782.

Taylor, J.M., Munoz, A., Bass, S.M., Saah, A.J., Chmiel, J.S., Kingsley, L.A. (1990). Estimating the distribution of times from HIV seroconversion to AIDS using multiple imputation. Multicentre AIDS Cohort Study. *Statistics in Medicine* **9**(5), 505–514.

van Dijk, M.R., Steyerberg, E.W., Stenning, S.P., Habbema, J., Dik, F. (2006). Survival estimates of a prognostic classification depended more on year of treatment than on imputation of missing values. *Journal of Clinical Epidemiology* **59**(3), 246–253 (Review, 25 refs.).

Weinfurt, K.P., Castel, L.D., Li, Y., Sulmasy, D.P., Balshem, A.M., Benson 3rd, A.B., Burnett, C.B., Gaskin, D.J., Marshall, J.L., Slater, E.F., Schulman, K.A., Meropol, N.J. (2003). The correlation between patient characteristics and expectations of benefit from Phase I clinical trials. *Cancer* **98**(1), 166–175.

Weisfelt, M., van de Beek, D., Spanjaard, L., Reitsma, J.B., de Gans, J. (2006). Clinical features, complications, and outcome in adults with pneumococcal meningitis: A prospective case series. *Lancet Neurology* **5**(2), 123–129 (see Comment in *Lancet Neurology*, 2006, **5**(2), 104–105, PMID: 16426981).

Appendix B

Ali, M.W., Siddiqui, O. (2000). Multiple imputation compared with some informative dropout procedures in the estimation and comparison of rates of change in longitudinal clinical trials with dropouts. *Journal of Biopharmaceutical Statistics* **10**(2), 165–181.

Allison, P.D. (2003). Missing data techniques for structural equation modeling. *Journal of Abnormal Psychology* **112**(4), 545–557.

Arnold, A.M., Kronmal, R.A. (2003). Multiple imputation of baseline data in the cardiovascular health study. *American Journal of Epidemiology* **157**(1), 74–84.

Baccarelli, A., Pfeiffer, R., Consonni, D., Pesatori, A.C., Bonzini, M., Patterson Jr., D.G, Bertazzi, P.A., Landi, M.T. (2005). Handling of dioxin measurement data in the presence of non-detectable values: Overview of available methods and their application in the Seveso chloracne study. *Chemosphere* **60**(7), 898–906.

Barnard, J., Meng, X.L. (1999). Applications of multiple imputation in medical studies: From AIDS to NHANES. *Statistical Methods in Medical Research* **8**(1), 17–36 (Review, 44 refs.).

Barnes, S.A., Lindborg, S.R., Seaman Jr., J.W. (2006). Multiple imputation techniques in small sample clinical trials. *Statistics in Medicine* **25**(2), 233–245.

Barzi, F., Woodward, M. (2004). Imputations of missing values in practice: Results from imputations of serum cholesterol in 28 cohort studies. *American Journal of Epidemiology* **160**(1), 34–45.

Bebchuk, J.D., Betensky, R.A. (2000). Multiple imputation for simple estimation of the hazard function based on interval censored data. *Statistics in Medicine* **19**(3), 405–419.

Bechger, T.M., Boomsma, D.I., Koning, H. (2002). A limited dependent variable model for heritability estimation with non-random ascertained samples. *Behavior Genetics* **32**(2), 145–151.

Beunckens, C., Molenberghs, G., Kenward, M.G. (2005). Direct likelihood analysis versus simple forms of imputation for missing data in randomized clinical trials. *Clinical Trials* **2**(5), 379–386.

Carabin, H., Gyorkos, T.W., Joseph, L., Payment, P., Soto, J.C. (2001). Comparison of methods to analyse imprecise faecal coliform count data from environmental samples. *Epidemiology & Infection* **126**(2), 181–190.

Catellier, D.J., Hannan, P.J., Murray, D.M., Addy, C.L., Conway, T.L., Yang, S., Rice, J.C. (2005). Imputation of missing data when measuring physical activity by accelerometry. *Medicine & Science in Sports & Exercise* **37**(11 Suppl.), S555–S562.

Cheung, Y.B. (2002). Early origins and adult correlates of psychosomatic distress. *Social Science & Medicine* **55**(6), 937–948.

Choi, Y.J., Nam, C.M., Kwak, M.J. (2004). Multiple imputation technique applied to appropriateness ratings in cataract surgery. *Yonsei Medical Journal* **45**(5), 829–837.

Clark, T.G., Altman, D.G. (2003). Developing a prognostic model in the presence of missing data: An ovarian cancer case study. *Journal of Clinical Epidemiology* **56**(1), 28–37.

Collins, L.M., Schafer, J.L., Kam, C.M. (2001). A comparison of inclusive and restrictive strategies in modern missing data procedures. *Psychological Methods* **6**(4), 330–351.

Cook, N.R. (1997). An imputation method for non-ignorable missing data in studies of blood pressure. *Statistics in Medicine* **16**(23), 2713–2728.

Cordell, H.J. (2006). Estimation and testing of genotype and haplotype effects in case–control studies: Comparison of weighted regression and multiple imputation procedures. *Genetic Epidemiology* **30**(3), 259–275.

Croy, C.D., Novins, D.K. (2005). Methods for addressing missing data in psychiatric and developmental research. *Journal of the American Academy of Child & Adolescent Psychiatry* **44**(12), 1230–1240.

Demirtas, H. (2005). Multiple imputation under Bayesianly smoothed pattern-mixture models for non-ignorable drop-out. *Statistics in Medicine* **24**(15), 2345–2363.

Dorey, F.J., Little, R.J., Schenker, N. (1993). Multiple imputation for threshold-crossing data with interval censoring. *Statistics in Medicine* **12**(17), 1589–1603.

Faris, P.D., Ghali, W.A., Brant, R., Norris, C.M., Galbraith, P.D., Knudtson, M.L. (2002). Multiple imputation versus data enhancement for dealing with missing data in observational health care outcome analyses. *Journal of Clinical Epidemiology* **55**(2), 184–191.

Faucett, C.L., Schenker, N., Taylor, J.M.G. (2002). Survival analysis using auxiliary variables via multiple imputation, with application to AIDS clinical trial data. *Biometrics* **58**(1), 37–47.

Foster, E.M., Fang, G.Y., Conduct Problems Research Group. (2004). Alternative methods for handling attrition: An illustration using data from the fast track evaluation. *Evaluation Review* **28**(5), 434–464.

Fox-Wasylyshyn, S.M., El-Masri, M.M. (2005). Handling missing data in self-report measures. *Research in Nursing & Health* **28**(6), 488–495 (Review, 29 refs.).

Fridley, B., Rabe, K., de Andrade, M. (2003). Imputation methods for missing data for polygenic models. *BMC Genetics* **4**(Suppl. 1), S42.

Gauderman, W.J., Thomas, D.C. (2001). The role of interacting determinants in the localization of genes. *Advances in Genetics* **42**, 393–412 (Review, 63 refs.).

Geskus, R B. (2001). Methods for estimating the AIDS incubation time distribution when date of seroconversion is censored. *Statistics in Medicine* **20**(5), 795–812.

Goetghebeur, E., Ryan, L. (2000). Semiparametric regression analysis of interval-censored data. *Biometrics* **56**(4), 1139–1144.

Graham, J.W., Hofer, S.M., Piccinin, A.M. (1994). Analysis with missing data in drug prevention research. *NIDA Research Monograph* **142**, 13–63 (Review, 27 refs.).

Greenland, S., Finkle, W.D. (1995). A critical look at methods for handling missing covariates in epidemiologic regression analyses. *American Journal of Epidemiology* **142**(12), 1255–1264 (Review, 26 refs.).

Herrchen, B., Gould, J.B., Nesbitt, T.S. (1997). Vital statistics linked birth/infant death and hospital discharge record linkage for epidemiological studies. *Computers & Biomedical Research* **30**(4), 290–305.

Hopke, P.K., Liu, C., Rubin, D.B. (2001). Multiple imputation for multivariate data with missing and below-threshold measurements: Time-series concentrations of pollutants in the Arctic. *Biometrics* **57**(1), 22–33.

Houck, P.R., Mazumdar, S., Koru-Sengul, T., Tang, G.M, Benoit H., Pollock, B.G., Reynolds 3rd, C.F. (2004). Estimating treatment effects from longitudinal clinical trial data with missing values: Comparative analyses using different methods. *Psychiatry Research* **129**(2), 209–215.

Hunsberger, S., Murray, D., Davis, C.E., Fabsitz, R.R. (2001). Imputation strategies for missing data in a school-based multi-centre study: The Pathways study. *Statistics in Medicine* **20**(2), 305–316.

Joseph, L., Belisle, P., Tamim, H., Sampalis, J.S. (2004). Selection bias found in interpreting analyses with missing data for the prehospital index for trauma. *Journal of Clinical Epidemiology* **57**(2), 147–153.

Kang, T., Kraft, P., Gauderman, W.J., Thomas, D., Framingham Heart Study. (2003). Multiple imputation methods for longitudinal blood pressure measurements from the Framingham Heart Study. *BMC Genetics* **4**(Suppl. 1), S43.

Kim, K.Y., Kim, B.J., Yi, G.S. (2004). Reuse of imputed data in microarray analysis increases imputation efficiency. *BMC Bioinformatics* **5**, 160.

Kistner, E.O., Weinberg, C.R. (2005). A method for identifying genes related to a quantitative trait, incorporating multiple siblings and missing parents. *Genetic Epidemiology* **29**(2), 155–165.

Kmetic, A., Joseph, L., Berger, C., Tenenhouse, A. (2002). Multiple imputation to account for missing data in a survey: Estimating the prevalence of osteoporosis. *Epidemiology* **13**(4), 437–444.

Kneipp, S.M., McIntosh, M. (2001). Handling missing data in nursing research with multiple imputation. *Nursing Research* **50**(6), 384–389 (Review, 12 refs.).

Kosorok, M.R., Wei, W.H., Farrell, P.M. (1996). The incidence of cystic fibrosis. *Statistics in Medicine* **15**(5), 449–462.

Kraft, P., Cox, D.G., Paynter, R.A., Hunter, D., De Vivo, I. (2005). Accounting for haplotype uncertainty in matched association studies: A comparison of simple and flexible techniques. *Genetic Epidemiology* **28**(3), 261–272.

Kristman, V.L., Manno, M., Cote, P. (2005). Methods to account for attrition in longitudinal data: Do they work? A simulation study. *European Journal of Epidemiology* **20**(8), 657–662.

Lam, K.F., Fong, D.Y.T., Tang, O.Y. (2005). Estimating the proportion of cured patients in a censored sample. *Statistics in Medicine* **24**(12), 1865–1879.

Lavori, P.W., Dawson, R., Shera, D. (1995). A multiple imputation strategy for clinical trials with truncation of patient data. *Statistics in Medicine* **14**(17), 1913–1925.

Lipsitz, S.R., Molenberghs, G., Fitzmaurice, G.M., Ibrahim, J. (2000). GEE with Gaussian estimation of the correlations when data are incomplete. *Biometrics* **56**(2), 528–536.

Little, R., Yau, L. (1996). Intent-to-treat analysis for longitudinal studies with drop-outs. *Biometrics* **52**(4), 1324–1333.

Liu, G., Gould, A.L. (2002). Comparison of alternative strategies for analysis of longitudinal trials with dropouts. *Journal of Biopharmaceutical Statistics* **12**(2), 207–226.

Liu, M., Taylor, J.M., Belin, T.R. (2000). Multiple imputation and posterior simulation for multivariate missing data in longitudinal studies. *Biometrics* **56**(4), 1157–1163.

Longford, N.T. (2001). Multilevel analysis with messy data. *Statistical Methods in Medical Research* **10**(6), 429–444.

Lu, K., Tsiatis, A.A. (2001). Multiple imputation methods for estimating regression coefficients in the competing risks model with missing cause of failure. *Biometrics* **57**(4), 1191–1197.

Lubin, J.H., Colt, J.S., Camann, D., Davis, S., Cerhan, J.R., Severson, R.K., Bernstein, L., Hartge, P. (2004). Epidemiologic evaluation of measurement data in the presence of detection limits. *Environmental Health Perspectives* **112**(17), 1691–1696.

Lyles, R.H., Fan, D., Chuachoowong, R. (2001). Correlation coefficient estimation involving a left censored laboratory assay variable. *Statistics in Medicine* **20**(19), 2921–2933.

Lynn, H.S. (2001). Maximum likelihood inference for left-censored HIV RNA data. *Statistics in Medicine* **20**(1), 33–45.

Manca, A., Palmer, S. (2005). Handling missing data in patient-level cost-effectiveness analysis alongside randomised clinical trials. *Applied Health Economics & Health Policy* **4**(2), 65–75.

Mishra, G.D., Dobson, A.J. (2004). Multiple imputation for body mass index: Lessons from the Australian Longitudinal Study on Women's Health. *Statistics in Medicine* **23**(19), 3077–3087.

Molenberghs, G., Williams, P.L., Lipsitz, S. (2002). Prediction of survival and opportunistic infections in HIV-infected patients: A comparison of imputation methods of incomplete CD4 counts. *Statistics in Medicine* **21**(10), 1387–1408.

Moore, L., Lavoie, A., LeSage, N., Liberman, M., Sampalis, J.S., Bergeron, E., Abdous, B. (2005). Multiple imputation of the Glasgow Coma Score. *Journal of Trauma-Injury Infection & Critical Care* **59**(3), 698–704.

Morita, S., Kobayashi, K., Eguchi, K., Matsumoto, T., Shibuya, M., Yamaji, Y., Ohashi, Y. (2005). Analysis of incomplete quality of life data in advanced stage cancer: A practical application of multiple imputation. *Quality of Life Research* **14**(6), 1533–1544.

Munoz, A., Carey, V., Taylor, J.M., Chmiel, J.S., Kingsley, L., Van Raden, M., Hoover, D.R. (1992). Estimation of time since exposure for a prevalent cohort. *Statistics in Medicine* **11**(7), 939–952.

Naeim, A., Keeler, E.B., Mangione, C.M. (2005). Options for handling missing data in the Health Utilities Index Mark 3. *Medical Decision Making* **25**(2), 186–198.

Newgard, C.D. (2006). The validity of using multiple imputation for missing out-of-hospital data in a state trauma registry. *Academic Emergency Medicine* **13**(3), 314–324.

Nixon, R.M., Duffy, S.W., Fender, G.R.K. (2003). Imputation of a true endpoint from a surrogate: Application to a cluster randomized controlled trial with partial information on the true endpoint. *BMC Medical Research Methodology* **3**, 17.

Oostenbrink, J.B., Al, M.J. (2005). The analysis of incomplete cost data due to dropout. *Health Economics* **14**(8), 763–776.

Oostenbrink, J.B., Al, M.J., Rutten-van Molken, M.P.M.H. (2003). Methods to analyse cost data of patients who withdraw in a clinical trial setting. *Pharmacoeconomics* **21**(15), 1103–1112.

Paik, M.C. (1997). Multiple imputation for the Cox proportional hazards model with missing covariates. *Lifetime Data Analysis* **3**(3), 289–298.

Pan, W. (2000a). A multiple imputation approach to Cox regression with interval-censored data. *Biometrics* **56**(1), 199–203.

Pan, W. (2000b). A two-sample test with interval censored data via multiple imputation. *Statistics in Medicine* **19**(1), 1–11.

Pan, W. (2001). A multiple imputation approach to regression analysis for doubly censored data with application to AIDS studies. *Biometrics* **57**(4), 1245–1250.

Pan, W., Kooperberg, C. (1999). Linear regression for bivariate censored data via multiple imputation. *Statistics in Medicine* **18**(22), 3111–3121.

Patrician, P.A. (2002). Multiple imputation for missing data. *Research in Nursing & Health* **25**(1), 76–84 (Review, 24 refs.).

Penny, K.I., Jolliffe, I.T. (1999). Multivariate outlier detection applied to multiply imputed laboratory data. *Statistics in Medicine* **18**(14), 1879–1895 (discussion 1897).

Perez, A., Dennis, R.J., Gil, J.F.A., Rondon, M.A., Lopez, A. (2002). Use of the mean, hot deck and multiple imputation techniques to predict outcome in intensive care unit patients in Colombia. *Statistics in Medicine* **21**(24), 3885–3896.

Pinnaduwage, D., Beyene, J., Fallah, S. (2003). Genome-wide linkage analysis of systolic blood pressure slope using the Genetic Analysis Workshop 13 data sets. *BMC Genetics* **4**(Suppl. 1), S86.

Raghunathan, T.E. (2004). What do we do with missing data? Some options for analysis of incomplete data. *Annual Review of Public Health* **25**, 99–117.

Ratcliffe, J., Young, T., Longworth, L., Buxton, M. (2005). An assessment of the impact of informative dropout and nonresponse in measuring health-related quality of life using the EuroQol (EQ-5D) descriptive system. *Value in Health* **8**(1), 53–58.

Richardson, B.A., Flack, V.F. (1996). The analysis of incomplete data in the three-period two-treatment cross-over design for clinical trials. *Statistics in Medicine* **15**(2), 127–143.

Rubin, D.B., Schenker, N. (1991). Multiple imputation in health-care databases: An overview and some applications. *Statistics in Medicine* **10**(4), 585–598 (Review, 26 refs.).

Schafer, J.L. (1999). Multiple imputation: A primer. *Statistical Methods in Medical Research* **8**(1), 3–15 (Review, 29 refs.).

Schafer, J.L., Graham, J.W. (2002). Missing data: Our view of the state of the art. *Psychological Methods* **7**(2), 147–177.

Schiattino, I., Villegas, R., Cruzat, A., Cuenca, J., Salazar, L., Aravena, O., Pesce, B., Catalan, D., Llanos, C., Cuchacovich, M., Aguillon, J.C. (2005). Multiple imputation procedures allow the rescue of missing data: An application to determine serum tumor necrosis factor (TNF) concentration values during the treatment of rheumatoid arthritis patients with anti-TNF therapy. *Biological Research* **38**(1), 7–12.

Sinharay, S., Stern, H.S., Russell, D. (2001). The use of multiple imputation for the analysis of missing data. *Psychological Methods* **6**(4), 317–329 (Review, 31 refs.).

Souverein, O.W., Zwinderman, A.H., Tanck, M.W.T. (2006). Multiple imputation of missing genotype data for unrelated individuals. *Annals of Human Genetics* **70**(Pt 3), 372–381.

Stadler, W.M., Huo, D., George, C., Yang, X., Ryan, C.W., Karrison, T., Zimmerman, T.M., Vogelzang, N.J. (2003). Prognostic factors for survival with gemcitabine plus 5-fluorouracil based regimens for metastatic renal cancer. *Journal of Urology* **170**(4 Pt 1), 1141–1145.

Streiner, D.L. (2002). The case of the missing data: Methods of dealing with dropouts and other research vagaries. *Canadian Journal of Psychiatry-Revue Canadienne de Psychiatrie* **47**(1), 68–75.

Stuck, A.E., Aronow, H.U., Steiner, A., Alessi, C.A., Büla, C.J., Gold, M.N., Yuhas, K.E., Nisenbaum, R., Rubenstein, L.Z., Beck, J.C. (1995). A trial of annual in-home comprehensive geriatric assessments for elderly people living in the community. *The New England Journal of Medicine* **333**, 1184–1189.

Tang, L., Song, J., Belin, T.R., Unutzer, J. (2005). A comparison of imputation methods in a longitudinal randomized clinical trial. *Statistics in Medicine* **24**(14), 2111–2128.

Touloumi, G., Babiker, A.G., Kenward, M.G., Pocock, S.J., Darbyshire, J.H. (2003). A comparison of two methods for the estimation of precision with incomplete longitudinal data, jointly modelled with a time-to-event outcome. *Statistics in Medicine* **22**(20), 3161–3175.

Twisk, J., de Vente, W. (2002). Attrition in longitudinal studies. How to deal with missing data. *Journal of Clinical Epidemiology* **55**(4), 329–337.

Van Beijsterveldt, C.E.M., van Boxtel, M.P.J., Bosma, H., Houx, P.J., Buntinx, F., Jolles, J. (2002). Predictors of attrition in a longitudinal cognitive aging study: The Maastricht Aging Study (MAAS). *Journal of Clinical Epidemiology* **55**(3), 216–223.

Van Buuren, S., Boshuizen, H.C., Knook, D.L. (1999). Multiple imputation of missing blood pressure covariates in survival analysis. *Statistics in Medicine* **18**(6), 681–694.

Wang, C.Y., Anderson, G.L., Prentice, R.L. (1999). Estimation of the correlation between nutrient intake measures under restricted sampling. *Biometrics* **55**(3), 711–717.

Wood, A.M., White, I.R., Hillsdon, M., Carpenter, J. (2005). Comparison of imputation and modelling methods in the analysis of a physical activity trial with missing outcomes. *International Journal of Epidemiology* **34**(1), 89–99.

Wu, H., Wu, L. (2001). A multiple imputation method for missing covariates in non-linear mixed-effects models with application to HIV dynamics. *Statistics in Medicine* **20**(12), 1755–1769.

Wu, H., Wu, L. (2002). Identification of significant host factors for HIV dynamics modeled by non-linear mixed-effects models. *Statistics in Medicine* **21**(5), 753–771.

Xie, F., Paik, M.C. (1997). Multiple imputation methods for the missing covariates in generalized estimating equation. *Biometrics* **53**(4), 1538–1546.

Xue, X., Shore, R.E., Ye, X., Kim, M.Y. (2004). Estimating the dose response relationship for occupational radiation exposure measured with minimum detection level. *Health Physics* **87**(4), 397–404.

Zhou, X.H., Eckert, G.J., Tierney, W.M. (2001). Multiple imputation in public health research. *Statistics in Medicine* **20**(9–10), 1541–1549.

References

Baker, S.G., Ko, C.-W., Graubard, B.I. (2003). A sensitivity analysis for nonrandomly missing categorical data arising from a national health disability survey. *Biostatistics* **4**, 41–56.

Barnard, J., Rubin, D.B. (1999). Small-sample degrees of freedom with multiple imputation. *Biometrika* **86**, 948–955.

Bethlehem, J.G. (2002). Weighting nonresponse adjustments based on auxiliary information. In: Groves, R.M., Dillman, D.A., Eltinge, J.L., Little, R.J.A. (Eds.), *Survey Nonresponse*. Wiley, New York, pp. 275–287.

Botman, S.L., Moore, T.F., Moriarity, C.L., Parsons, V.L. (2000). Design and estimation for the National Health Interview Survey, 1995–2004. *Vital and Health Statistics*, Series 2, No. 130. National Center for Health Statistics, Hyattsville, MD.

Cook, S.R., Rubin, D.B. (2005). Multiple imputation in designing medical device trials. In: Becker, K.M., Whyte, J.J. (Eds.), *Clinical Evaluation of Medical Devices*. Humana Press, Washington, DC.

Dempster, A.P., Laird, N.M., Rubin, D.B. (1977). Maximum likelihood estimation from incomplete data via the EM algorithm. *Journal of the Royal Statistical Society B* **39**, 1–38, (with discussion).

Dorey, F.J., Little, R.J.A., Schenker, N. (1993). Multiple imputation for threshold-crossing data with interval censoring. *Statistics in Medicine* **12**, 1589–1603.

Efron, B. (1994). Missing data, imputation, and the bootstrap. *Journal of the American Statistical Association* **89**, 463–479.

Ezzati-Rice, T.M., Fahimi, M., Judkins, D., Khare, M. (1993). Serial imputation of NHANES III with mixed regression and hot-deck techniques. *American Statistical Association Proceedings of the Section on Survey Research Methods* **1**, 292–296.

Gartner, H., Rässler, S. (2005). Analyzing the changing gender wage gap based on multiply imputed right censored wages, *IAB Discussion Paper* 5/2005.

Gelfand, A.E., Smith, A.F.M. (1990). Sampling-based approaches to calculating marginal densities. *Journal of the American Statistical Association* **85**, 398–409.

Gelman, A., Carlin, J.B. (2002). Poststratification and weighting adjustment. In: Groves, R.M., Dillman, D.A., Eltinge, J.L., Little, R.J.A. (Eds.), *Survey Nonresponse*. Wiley, New York, pp. 289–302.

Gelman, A., Carlin, J.B., Stern, H.S., Rubin, D.B. (2003). *Bayesian Data Analysis*, 2nd ed. Chapman & Hall, London.

Gelman, A., Meng, X.L. (2004). *Applied Bayesian Modeling and Causal Inference from Incomplete-Data Perspectives*. Wiley, New York.

Geman, S., Geman, D. (1984). Stochastic Relaxation, Gibbs Distributions, and the Bayesian Restoration of Images. *IEEE Trans. Pattern Analysis and Machine Intelligence* **6**, 721–741.

Glynn, R., Laird, N.M., Rubin, D.B. (1986). Selection modeling versus mixture modeling with non-ignorable nonresponse. In: Wainer, H. (Ed.), *Drawing Inferences from Self-Selected Samples*. Springer, New York, pp. 119–146.

Groves, R.M., Dillman, D.A., Eltinge, J.L., Little, R.J.A. (2002). *Survey Nonresponse*. Wiley, New York.

Hastings, W.K. (1970). Monte Carlo sampling methods using Markov Chains and their applications. *Biometrika* **57**, 97–109.

Heckman, J.J. (1976). The common structure of statistical models of truncation, sample selection and limited dependent variables and a simple estimator for such models. *Annals of Economic and Social Measurement* **5**, 475–492.

Heitjan, D.F., Little, R.J.A. (1991). Multiple imputation for the fatal accident reporting system. *Journal of the Royal Statistical Society C* **40**, 13–29.

Horton, N.J., Lipsitz, S.R. (2001). Multiple imputation in practice. Comparison of software packages for regression models with missing variables. *The American Statistician* **55**, 244–254.

Jensen, U., Gartner, H., Rässler, S. (2006). Measuring overeducation with earnings frontiers and multiply imputed censored income data, *IAB Discussion Paper* 11/2006.

Kennickell, A.B. (1991). Imputation of the 1989 survey of consumer finances: Stochastic relaxation and multiple imputation. *American Statistical Association Proceedings of the Section on Survey Research Methods*, 1–10, (discussion 21–23).

Kim, J.K., Brick, J.M., Fuller, W.A., Kalton, G. (2006). On the bias of the multiple-imputation variance estimator in survey sampling. *Journal of the Royal Statistical Society, Series B (Statistical Methodology)* **68**, 509–521.

Lee, H., Rancourt, E., Särndal, C.E. (2002). Variance estimation for survey data under single imputation. In: Groves, R.M., Dillman, D.A., Eltinge, J.L., Little, R.J.A. (Eds.), *Survey Nonresponse*. Wiley, New York, pp. 315–328.

Li, K.H., Meng, X.L., Raghunathan, T.E., Rubin, D.B. (1991). Significance levels from repeated p-values with multiply-imputed data. *Statistica Sinica* **1**, 65–92.

Little, R.J.A. (1988). Adjustments in large surveys. *Journal of Business & Economic Statistics* **6**(3), 287–296.

Little, R.J.A. (1993). Pattern-mixture models for multivariate incomplete data. *Journal of the American Statistical Association* **88**, 125–134.

Little, R.J.A., Rubin, D.B. (1987). *Statistical Analysis with Missing Data*. Wiley, New York.

Little, R.J.A., Rubin, D.B. (2002). *Statistical Analysis with Missing Data*, 2nd ed. Wiley, Hoboken.

Liu, C., Rubin, D.B. (1994). The ECME algorithm: A simple extension of EM and ECM with faster monotone convergence. *Biometrika* **81**, 633–648.

Liu, C., Rubin, D.B., Wu, Y.N. (1998). Parameter expansion to accelerate EM: The PX-EM algorithm. *Biometrika* **85**, 755–770.

Madow, W.G., Nisselson, H., Olkin, I. (1983a). *Incomplete Data in Sample Surveys, Volume 1: Report and Case Studies*. Academic Press, New York.

Madow, W.G., Olkin, I. (1983). *Incomplete Data in Sample Surveys, Volume 3: Proceedings of the Symposium*. Academic Press, New York.

Madow, W.G., Olkin, I., Rubin, D.B. (1983b). *Incomplete Data in Sample Surveys, Volume 2: Theory and Bibliographies*. Academic Press, New York.

McLachlan, G.J., Krishnan, T. (1997). *The EM Algorithm and Extensions*. Wiley, New York.

Meng, X.-L. (1994). Multiple-imputation inferences with uncongenial sources of input. *Statistical Science* **9**, 538–573, (with discussion).

Meng, X.L., Rubin, D.B. (1992). Performing likelihood ratio tests with multiply-imputed data sets. *Biometrika* **79**, 103–111.

Meng, X.L., Rubin, D.B. (1993). Maximum likelihood estimation via the ECM algorithm: A general framework. *Biometrika* **80**, 267–278.

Meng, X.-L., van Dyk, D. (1997). The EM algorithm – An old folk-song sung to a fast new tune. *Journal of the Royal Statistical Society, Series B (Methodological)* **59**, 511–567.

Metropolis, N., Ulam, S. (1949). The Monte Carlo method. *Journal of the American Statistical Association* **49**, 335–341.

Münnich, R., Rässler, S. (2005). PRIMA: A new multiple imputation procedure for binary variables. *Journal of Official Statistics* **21**, 325–341.

Raghunathan, T.E., Grizzle, J.E. (1995). A split questionnaire survey design. *Journal of the American Statistical Association* **90**, 54–63.

Raghunathan, T.E., Lepkowski, J.M., Van Hoewyk, J., Solenberger, P. (2001). A multivariate technique for multiply imputing missing values using a sequence of regression models. *Survey Methodology* **27**, 85–95.

Raghunathan, T.E., Solenberger, P., Van Hoewyk, J. (2002). *IVEware: Imputation and Variance Estimation Software – User Guide. Survey Methodology Program.* Survey Research Center, Institute for Social Research, University of Michigan, Ann Arbor, MI.

Rässler, S. (2002). Statistical matching: A frequentist theory, practical applications, and alternative Bayesian approaches. In: *Lecture Notes in Statistics*, 168. Springer, New York.

Rässler, S., Rubin, D.B., Schenker, N. (2007). Incomplete data: Diagnosis, imputation, and estimation. In: de Leeuw, E., Hox, J., Dillman, D. (Eds.), *The International Handbook of Survey Research Methodology*. Sage, Thousand Oaks, in press.

Robert, C.P., Casella, G. (1999). *Monte Carlo Statistical Methods*. Springer, New York.

Rubin, D.B. (1976). Inference and missing data. *Biometrika* **63**, 581–590.

Rubin, D.B. (1977). Formalizing subjective notions about the effect of nonrespondents in sample surveys. *Journal of the American Statistical Association* **72**, 538–543.

Rubin, D.B. (1978a). Multiple imputation in sample surveys – A phenomenological Bayesian approach to nonresponse. *American Statistical Association Proceedings of the Section on Survey Research Methods*, 20–40.

Rubin, D.B. (1978b). A note on Bayesian, likelihood, and sampling distribution inferences. *The Journal of Educational Statistics* **3**, 189–201.

Rubin, D.B. (1986). Statistical matching using file concatenation with adjusted weights and multiple imputations. *Journal of Business and Economic Statistics* **4**, 87–95.

Rubin, D.B. (1987). *Multiple Imputation for Nonresponse in Surveys*. Wiley, New York.

Rubin, D.B. (1994). Comments on "Missing data, imputation, and the bootstrap" by Bradley Efron. *Journal of the American Statistical Association* **89**, 475–478.

Rubin, D.B. (1996). Multiple imputation after 18+ years. *Journal of the American Statistical Association* **91**, 473–489.

Rubin, D.B. (2003). Nested multiple imputation of NMES via partially incompatible MCMC. *Statistica Neerlandica* **57**, 3–18.

Rubin, D.B. (2004a). *Multiple Imputation for Nonresponse in Surveys*, 2nd ed. Wiley, New York, 1987.

Rubin, D.B. (2004b). The design of a general and flexible system for handling nonresponse in sample surveys. *The American Statistician* **58**, 298–302, (first appeared in unpublished form in 1977, prepared under contract for the U.S. Social Security Administration).

Rubin, D.B. (2006). Causal inference through potential outcomes and principal stratification: Application to studies with "censoring" due to death. *Statistical Science* **21**, 299–309.

Rubin, D.B., Schenker, N. (1986). Multiple imputation for interval estimation from simple random samples with ignorable nonresponse. *Journal of the American Statistical Association* **81**, 366–374.

Rubin, D.B., Schenker, N. (1987). Interval estimation from multiply imputed data: A case study using census agriculture industry codes. *Journal of Official Statistics* **3**, 375–387.

Rubin, D.B., Schenker, N. (1991). Multiple imputation in health-care databases: An overview and some applications. *Statistics in Medicine* **10**, 585–598.

Rubin, D.B., Stern, H., Vehovar, V. (1995). Handling "don't know" survey responses: The case of the Slovenian plebiscite. *Journal of the American Statistical Association* **90**, 822–828.

Schafer, J.L. (1997). *Analysis of Incomplete Multivariate Data.* Chapman and Hall, New York.

Schafer, J.L., Schenker, N. (2000). Inference with imputed conditional means. *Journal of the American Statistical Association* **95**, 144–154.

Schenker, N., Taylor, J.M.G. (1996). Partially parametric techniques for multiple imputation. *Computational Statistics & Data Analysis* **22**, 425–446.

Schuchat, A., Hilger, T., Zell, E., Farley, M.M., Reingold, A., Harrison, L., Lefkowitz, L., Danila, R., Stefonek, K., Barrett, N., Morse, D., Pinner, R. (2001). Active bacterial core surveillance of the emerging infections program network. *Emerging Infectious Diseases* **7**(1), 92–99.

Shao, J. (2002). Replication methods for variance estimation in complex sample surveys with imputed data. In: Groves, R.M., Dillman, D.A., Eltinge, J.L., Little, R.J.A. (Eds.), *Survey Nonresponse.* Wiley, New York, pp. 303–314.

Shih, W.J. (1992). On informative and random dropouts in longitudinal studies. *Biometrics* **48**, 970–972.

Tanner, M.A., Wong, W.H. (1987). The calculation of posterior distributions by data augmentation. *Journal of the American Statistical Association* **82**, 528–540.

Van Buuren, S., Brand, J.P.L., Oudshoorn, C.G.M., Rubin, D.B. (2006). Fully conditional specification in multivariate imputation. *Statistics in Medicine* **76**, 1049–1064.

Van Buuren, S., Oudshoorn C.G.M. (2000). Multivariate imputation by chained equations: MICE V1.0 user's manual. Report PG/VGZ/00.038. Leiden: TNO Preventie en Gezondheid.

Zhang, J.L., Rubin, D.B. (2003). Estimation of causal effects via principal stratification when some outcomes are truncated by "death". *Journal of Educational and Behavioral Statistics* **28**, 353–368.

Handbook of Statistics, Vol. 27
ISSN: 0169-7161

DOI: 10.1016/S0169-7161(07)27020-8

20

Meta-Analysis

Edward L. Spitznagel Jr.

Abstract

This chapter provides an overview of modern meta-analysis, a statistical method for combining the results of both published and unpublished studies involving a method of treatment, a source of illness, a protective factor, or any other aspect that has been repeatedly studied. Both fixed and random effects models are discussed. Forest plots as a reporting standard are introduced. The problem of publication bias, which is the tendency for results that are not statistically significant either not to be published or to appear in less accessible locations, is discussed, along with possible remedies. Finally, the important contribution of the Cochrane Collaboration to meta-analysis is described.

1. Introduction

The PubMed service of the U.S. National Library of Medicine currently indexes over 16,000,000 publications. For any common disease, there are many publications that study the effect of the same treatment on different subjects. These studies may vary from double-blind randomized controlled clinical trials to simple observational reports. Their conclusions may disagree, from a finding that a new treatment is superior to the standard, that no evidence for a difference exists, to the new treatment being inferior to the standard.

Combining the information from these studies into a state-of-our-knowledge summary is the province of meta-analysis. Meta-analysis can be considered a special case of a "systematic review." A systematic review has been defined (Egger and Davey Smith, 1997) as "any review of a body of data that uses clearly defined methods and criteria." In the case of meta-analysis, the methods and criteria are fully quantitative in nature, with the ultimate goal being not just to establish that an effect exists, but also to estimate the size of the effect.

Meta-analysis is used to combine information about treatment effects, but it is also used to combine information about risk and protective factors in epidemiology. Because treatment effects are estimated from randomized controlled trials, meta-analysis of them is fairly straightforward.

By contrast, a meta-analysis of the effects of second-hand smoke from epidemiologic data typically involves both prospective and retrospective information, with the possibility of there being different dosage levels in each study. (The tobacco companies know this and have used it aggressively in their legal defense.) Nevertheless, a subject such as the relationship between smoking and health is so important that the information should be combined, with care taken to avoid pitfalls, and any caveats remaining stated clearly.

2. History

The prefix "meta" is Greek for "after" or "beyond." It is part of the title of a work of Aristotle, *Metaphysics*, which was a philosophical work on existence. Aristotle, however, did not coin the term. An editor, in ordering Aristotle's works, placed those writings immediately after the writings on physics, and dubbed them metaphysics, meaning "beyond physics." Later philosophers took the prefix "meta" to imply being higher, on another plane, and that is how many words beginning with "meta" came into being. In meta-analysis the results of other studies are treated as data which the meta-analysis operates on or summarizes.

The term meta-analysis is fairly recent (Glass, 1976) but the idea itself goes back more than 100 years. Pearson (1904) investigated the relationship between inoculation and disease for "enteric fever," known to us as typhoid fever, in British soldiers in Africa and India. He calculated tetrachoric correlations for a number of subgroups, both for disease incidence and mortality, finding most of them to be statistically significant, but neither as high nor as uniform as the correlations between smallpox vaccination and mortality. The correlations for inoculation with disease incidence ranged from 0.100 to 0.445 across five groups. For smallpox, he noted that the correlations for inoculation and mortality were very uniform and all on the order of 0.6. Because of the nonuniformity of the correlations and the fact that inoculation was voluntary, he suggested that a study be done in which a list of volunteers be made with every other volunteer receiving inoculation. (This suggestion for selection of a control group was fairly common before randomization became adopted as a gold standard. Note that it would have been an "open label" study, not even single-blinded.)

In *Statistical Methods for Research Workers*, Fisher (1932) gave an easy-to-use method for combining P-values from several different studies through the chi-square distribution. For any single study in which the null hypothesis is true, $-2\ln(P)$ will have a chi-square distribution with 2 degrees of freedom (df). For a set of n studies in each of which the null hypothesis is true, $-2\Sigma\ln(P_i)$ will have a chi-square distribution with $2n$ df. For example, suppose three studies comparing the effectiveness of a new treatment for asthma with standard treatment have been performed, and that their P-values are 0.061, 0.033, and 0.020. The chi-square value combining these individual results is:

$$-2(\ln(0.061) + \ln(0.003) + \ln(0.020)) = -2(-2.797 - 3.411 - 3.912) \\ = 20.240.$$

The df are 6, and the corresponding P-value is 0.0025. Thus, the weak results from the three separate studies combine into a single very strong conclusion.

Fisher undoubtedly chose to use chi-squares with 2 df because of the simple relationship between the P-value and the distribution function. Chi-square with 2 df follows an exponential distribution, so all that is needed to go from the P-value to the distribution function is a table of natural logarithms, easily available at the time.

Fisher's method represents an important step beyond what Pearson did. In Pearson's example, most of the individual 2×2 tables were already statistically significant, so it was not so necessary to obtain an overall P-value. Most meta-analyses do not deal with such overwhelming evidence, making it very important to combine the evidence into an overall assessment of statistical significance.

However, Fisher's method does not attempt to make an overall estimate of effect size. Also, it does not address the possibility that the effect size might vary greatly from one site or study to another, as Pearson noticed with inoculation to prevent typhoid. Finally, because chi-square does not address directionality of effects, his method could wind up computing overall significance of effects that are in opposite directions. Fisher did address this last point (Mosteller and Fisher, 1948) by suggesting that all tests could be done one-tailed, and then double the final P-value.

3. The Cochran–Mantel–Haenszel test

Cochran (1954) provided the next important contribution, a way of computing a test for association that controls for the different sources of information. Shortly thereafter, Mantel and Haenszel (1959) developed an equivalent approach, which included a method for obtaining a combined estimate of the odds ratio. We know this approach today as the Cochran–Mantel–Haenszel test. The setting is that a set of 2×2 tables has been obtained, from different sources or by stratification within a single source. Collapsing these 2×2 tables into a single one can induce a spurious relation or reduce the strength of relations that were present in the individual tables (Yule, 1903; Simpson, 1951). The Cochran–Mantel–Haenszel approach avoids this pitfall, commonly known as Simpson's Paradox.

As an illustration of the Cochran–Mantel–Haenszel test we will examine the meta-analysis of three studies comparing two types of three-layer bandages, elastic and inelastic, for healing of venous leg ulcers (Fletcher et al., 1997). The results of the three separate studies are shown in Table 1.

The test can be done by hand, but it probably is best done with statistical software. Regardless of the number of individual studies, it produces a chi-square with 1 df. In our case, we obtain $\chi^2 = 11.237$, $P = 0.0008$. Thus, the combined information from the three studies yields a more convincing result than the best of the single studies.

While the chi-square is somewhat intricate to hand-calculate, the combined odds ratio is very easy to do by hand. Let the symbols A_i, B_i, C_i, and D_i represent the frequencies$_{123}$ from each study as shown in Table 2, and let $N_i = A_i + B_i + C_i + D_i$ be the sample size from each study.

Table 1
Frequencies from three studies of the effect of bandage type on the healing of leg ulcers

Study	Northeast et al.		Callam et al.		Gould et al.	
Outcome	Healed	Not Healed	Healed	Not Healed	Healed	Not Healed
Elastic Bandage	31	26	35	19	11	7
Inelastic Bandage	18	26	30	48	9	13
Odds Ratios	1.722		2.947		2.270	
Significance Tests	$\chi^2 = 1.806$, $P = 0.179$		$\chi^2 = 8.866$, $P = 0.003$		$\chi^2 = 1.616$, $P = 0.204$	

Table 2
Symbols for the frequencies used in the Cochran-Mantel-Haenszel estimate of the odds ratio

Study	Northeast et al.		Callam et al.		Gould et al.	
Outcome	Healed	Not Healed	Healed	Not Healed	Healed	Not Healed
Elastic Bandage	A_1	B_1	A_2	B_2	A_3	B_3
Inelastic Bandage	C_1	D_1	C_2	D_2	C_3	D_3

Then the combined odds ratio estimate is:

$$\mathrm{OR} = \frac{\sum A_i D_i / N_i}{\sum B_i C_i / N_i} = \frac{24.282}{10.527} = 2.307.$$

This value lies roughly in the middle of the three individual studies' odds ratios, 1.722, 2.270, and 2.947. This estimate makes sense if one believes that there is a common odds ratio across all trials, with each trial producing an estimate of that odds ratio. This would be described as a *fixed effects* model. The alternative to this assumption is that odds ratios differ across trials, with the goal being to estimate the center of the population of possible odds ratios. This would be described as a *random effects* model. As we will see, both kinds of models are amenable to meta-analysis.

A test for interaction, such as the Breslow–Day test, can help in determining whether a fixed effects or a random effects model is more appropriate. In our case, the Breslow–Day chi-square is 0.964, with 2 df, and *P*-value 0.617. Therefore, we have no evidence for the fixed effects model being incorrect.

The calculations above were performed using the SAS FREQ procedure, whose output is given below:

The FREQ procedure
Summary statistics for status by bandage controlling for study
Cochran–Mantel–Haenszel statistics (based on table scores)

Statistic	Alternative Hypothesis	df	Value	Probability
1	Nonzero correlation	1	11.2367	0.0008
2	Row mean scores differ	1	11.2367	0.0008
3	General association	1	11.2367	0.0008

Estimates of the common relative risk (row 1/row 2)

Type of Study	Method	Value	95%	Confidence limits
Case–control	Mantel–Haenszel	2.3067	1.4119	3.7685
(Odds ratio)	Logit	2.3065	1.4093	3.7749
Cohort	Mantel–Haenszel	1.5401	1.1900	1.9931
(Col 1 risk)	Logit	1.4875	1.1533	1.9187
Cohort	Mantel–Haenszel	0.6782	0.5373	0.8562
(Col 2 risk)	Logit	0.6740	0.5347	0.8495

Breslow–Day test for homogeneity of the odds ratios

Chi-square	0.9643
df	2
Probability > chi-square	0.6175

Total sample size = 273

The output gives six different estimates of association, of which the one we have discussed is the Cochran–Mantel–Haenszel estimate of the odds ratio. The other estimate of the odds ratio is calculated from a weighted mean of log-odds ratios. It comes out practically the same as the Mantel–Haenszel estimate. The Mantel–Haenszel odds ratio has the advantage of being computable even if one of the stratified tables contains a frequency of zero, while the other estimate is not.

The remaining four estimates of association are risk ratios, rather than odds ratios. The odds ratio has a special advantage in meta-analysis in that it can be estimated from a mixture of clinical trials, cohort studies, and case–control studies. Risk ratios cannot be estimated if there are any case–control studies in the mix.

4. Glass's proposal for meta-analysis

Glass (1976) appears to have been the first person to use the term *meta-analysis* in the published literature. He states, "I use it to refer to the statistical analysis of a large collection of analysis results from individual studies. It connotes a rigorous alternative to the casual, narrative discussions of research studies which typify our attempts to make sense of the rapidly expanding research literature." While not describing specific protocols for meta-analysis, he called for it to be statistical analysis just as rigorous as the statistics in the research being reviewed.

Although Glass's (1976) article did not give concrete details, Smith and Glass (1977) give a good illustration of what he had in mind: "Results of nearly 400 controlled evaluations of psychotherapy and counseling were coded and integrated statistically." Their conclusions were that psychotherapy is effective, but that essentially no differences among the many types of therapy were evident.

Modern meta-analyses, at least within the medical literature, focus on more modest numbers of studies, at most a few dozen. They do exclude studies based on lack of rigor, whereas Glass (1976) felt that studies should be included regardless of level of rigor: "... my experience over the past two years with a body of literature on which I will report in a few minutes leads me to wonder whether well-designed and poorly designed experiments give very different findings. At any rate, I believe the difference to be so small that to integrate research results by eliminating the "poorly done" studies is to discard a vast amount of important data."

A search of PubMed returned 7605 articles containing "meta-analysis" in the title and 14,387 articles with "meta-analysis" as publication type. Clearly, meta-analysis has become an important tool in the medical literature.

5. Random effects models

The Cochran–Mantel–Haenszel method has proved to be an important tool in meta-analysis. However, it makes the assumption that there is a common odds ratio across all studies. This would be described as a fixed effects model. In many practical settings, this assumption is not justified, and must be replaced with a random effects model. For example, in case–control studies of the relationship of occupational asbestos exposure to lung cancer, exposure to asbestos may only be available as a binary yes-or-no variable, rather than amount of exposure. The odds ratio from these studies then becomes random, and the goal of the meta-analysis is to estimate the "typical" odds ratio as some measure of the center of the distribution of all possible odds ratios.

DerSimonian and Laird (1986) developed a method for dealing with meta-analysis of random effects, which has become the standard. We will illustrate it by using the STATA user-contributed *metan* command to perform a meta-analysis of the venous leg ulcer data which we analyzed earlier. The *metan* command has the option to do both fixed and random effects meta-analyses. First, here is the result of using it to do the fixed effects meta-analysis:

Study	OR	[95% Confidence Interval]		% Weight
Northeast	1.722	0.777	3.816	44.02
Callam	2.947	1.433	6.062	41.02
Gould	2.270	0.636	8.106	14.96
M–H pooled OR	2.307	1.412	3.769	100.00

Heterogeneity chi-squared = 0.96 (df = 2), $P = 0.618$
I-squared (variation in OR attributable to heterogeneity) = 0.0%
Test of OR = 1: $z = 3.34$, $P = 0.001$

As indicated by the label "M–H pooled OR," this result is equivalent to the Cochran–Mantel–Haenszel results from the SAS FREQ procedure given earlier.

Second, here is the result of using it to do the random effects meta-analysis:

Study	OR	[95% Confidence	Interval]	% Weight
Northeast	1.722	0.777	3.816	38.35
Callam	2.947	1.433	6.062	46.67
Gould	2.270	0.636	8.106	14.98
D+L pooled OR	2.306	1.409	3.775	100.00

Heterogeneity chi-squared = 0.96 (df = 2), P = 0.618
I-squared (variation in OR attributable to heterogeneity) = 0.0%
Estimate of between-study variance Tau-squared = 0.0000
Test of OR = 1: z = 3.32, P = 0.001

The label "D + L pooled OR" refers to the method being that of DerSimonian and Laird. Note that the odds ratio and its confidence limits are almost identical with those from the Cochran–Mantel–Haenszel fixed effects analysis. Furthermore, the measures of heterogeneity give no evidence for favoring the random effects model over the fixed effects model.

For a demonstration of an appreciable difference between the two methods, let us return to the data from Pearson's (1904) study. He had noticed that, although all correlations between inoculation and disease incidence were positive, they were highly variable. Although he used tetrachoric correlations, the same is true of the odds ratios. First, let us examine the results of doing a fixed effects analysis:

Study	OR	[95% Confidence	Interval]	% Weight
Hospital staffs	0.328	0.209	0.516	7.60
Ladysmith Garrison	0.127	0.091	0.179	44.77
Methuen's column	0.432	0.288	0.649	10.51
Single regiments	0.931	0.671	1.290	8.23
Army in India	0.575	0.461	0.717	28.90
M–H pooled OR	0.370	0.322	0.425	100.00

Heterogeneity chi-squared = 84.79 (df = 4), $P = 0.000$
I-squared (variation in OR attributable to heterogeneity) = 95.3%
Test of OR = 1: $z = 14.04$, $P = 0.000$

The first four odds ratios are from South African units, while the last is from India. The measures of heterogeneity give strong evidence for favoring the random effects model over the fixed effects model. The five odds ratios themselves vary from 0.931 down to 0.127. (They are all less than 1, indicating that those who were inoculated had lower risk of contracting typhoid.) The Cochran–Mantel–Haenszel pooled estimate of the odds ratio is 0.370. However, since the test for heterogeneity of the odds ratios is significant, this pooling is inappropriate, and the DerSimonian–Laird estimate should be used in its stead. Here, then, are the results of fitting the random effects model:

Study	OR	[95% Confidence Interval]		% Weight
Hospital staffs	0.328	0.209	0.516	19.36
Ladysmith Garrison	0.127	0.091	0.179	20.10
Methuen's column	0.432	0.288	0.649	19.68
Single regiments	0.931	0.671	1.290	20.17
Army in India	0.575	0.461	0.717	20.69
D+L pooled OR	0.397	0.200	0.787	100.0

Heterogeneity chi-squared = 84.79 (df = 4), $P = 0.000$
I-squared (variation in OR attributable to heterogeneity) = 95.3%
Estimate of between-study variance Tau-squared = 0.5759
Test of OR = 1: $z = 2.65$, $P = 0.008$

The pooled estimate of the odds ratio is now 0.397, larger than the value 0.370 from the fixed effects analysis. In addition, its confidence interval is considerably larger, and while it is still significantly different from 1, its Z-value of 2.65 is much smaller than the value 14.04 from the fixed effects analysis. Thus, we have evidence that inoculation overall is effective, but due to the variations from one stratum to another, the evidence is not nearly as strong as it would have been had the odds ratios been homogeneous.

By combining our experience from these two examples, we conclude that in both cases it is safe to use the DerSimonian–Laird procedure. In the first case, of homogeneous odds ratios, it produces essentially the same results as Cochran–Mantel–Haenszel and therefore can be used in place of Cochran–Mantel–Haenszel. In the second case, of heterogeneous odds ratios, it gives very different results and therefore must be used.

6. The forest plot

The information given in the tables above can be graphed in a *forest plot*. The forest plot has come to be regarded as a standard for reporting meta-analysis results. In fact, the Cochrane Collaboration, to be described in Section 8, has adopted as its logo a forest plot contained in a circle made up of two opposing letters "C."

In Figure 1 is the forest plot for the Cochran–Mantel–Haenszel meta-analysis of the venous leg ulcer data. Three lines represent the odds ratios and confidence intervals for the individual studies. The box at the center of each line represents the point estimate of the odds ratio, and its size represents the weight given to the odds ratio in estimating the pooled odds ratio. Since the precision of estimate is related to the sample size, typically, the larger the box, the smaller is the

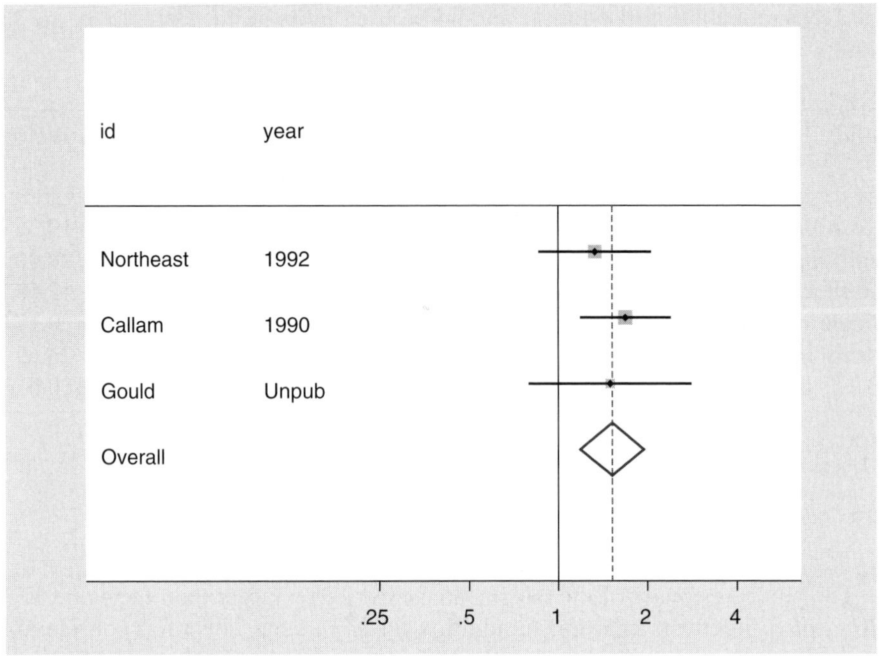

Fig. 1. Forest plot for the meta-analysis of three studies of the effect of bandage type on the healing of leg ulcers. A fixed effects model was used.

confidence interval. The center of the diamond represents the pooled point estimate of the odds ratio. The left and right vertices of the diamond represent the confidence interval for the pooled odds ratio.

Two vertical lines represent the null hypothesis OR = 1 (solid line) and the pooled point estimate of the odds ratio (dashed line). If the diamond does not overlap the solid line, we have rejected the null hypothesis of no treatment effect. Additional diagnostic information can be gleaned from whether the individual study confidence intervals overlap the dashed line. In our example, all three do. A confidence interval that does not overlap the dashed line indicates the corresponding study is inconsistent with the pooled estimate of the odds ratio. That would not be expected in a fixed effects meta-analysis, but would be perfectly reasonable in a random effects meta-analysis. In fact, in Figure 2, the forest plot from the DerSimonian–Laird meta-analysis of Pearson's typhoid data, two of the five confidence intervals do not overlap the dashed line.

7. Publication bias

In most fields of research, there is a tendency for studies to be published based on their results. This is known as *publication bias*. A meta-analysis that relies only on published results runs the risk of incorporating this bias into its own findings.

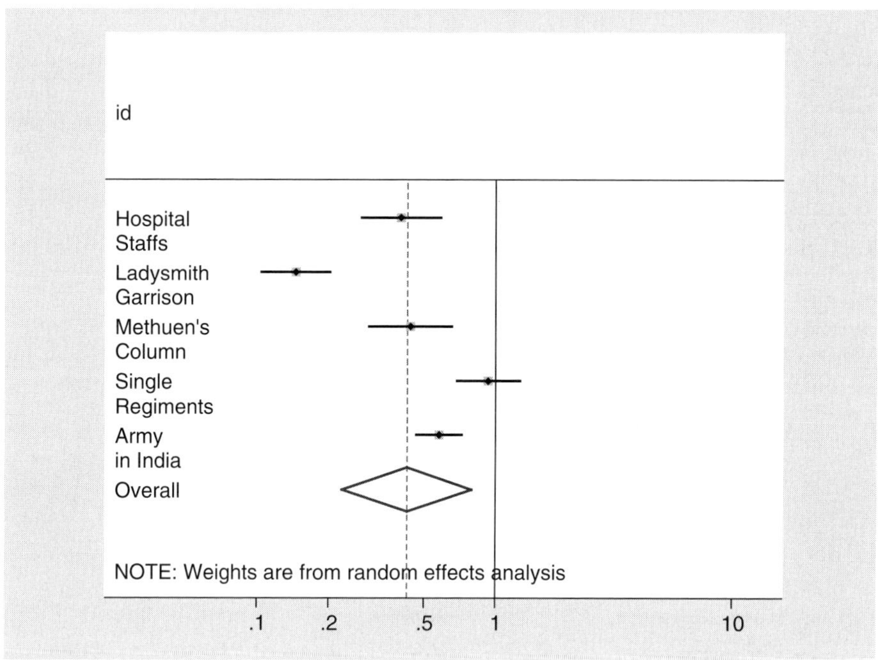

Fig. 2. Forest plot for the meta-analysis of Pearson's data on the effect of typhoid inoculation. A random effects model was used.

Experience suggests that this bias is most likely to be in whichever is the positive direction.

Egger and Davey Smith (1995) gave eight examples, four in which meta-analyses were corroborated by large randomized controlled trials, and the other four in which no effect was found in an RCT. One of the four in which no effect was found in the RCT was treatment with magnesium for reducing the risk of death following myocardial infarction.

Following is the result of a random effects meta-analysis on all studies uncovered by Sterne et al. (2001) up to the time of the ISIS-4 definitive study of 1995. The forest plot is given in Figure 3.

Study	OR	[95% Confidence	Interval]	% Weight
Morton (1984)	0.436	0.038	5.022	2.32
Rasmussen (1986)	0.348	0.154	0.783	12.08
Smith (1986)	0.278	0.057	1.357	4.91
Abraham (1987)	0.957	0.058	15.773	1.81
Feldstedt (1988)	1.250	0.479	3.261	10.02
Schechter (1989)	0.090	0.011	0.736	3.04
Ceremuzynski (1989)	0.278	0.027	2.883	2.51
Bertschat (1989)	0.304	0.012	7.880	1.36

Singh (1990)	0.499	0.174	1.426	8.94
Pereira (1990)	0.110	0.012	0.967	2.86
Schechter 1 (1991)	0.130	0.028	0.602	5.19
Golf (1991)	0.427	0.127	1.436	7.36
Thogersen (1991)	0.452	0.133	1.543	7.24
LIMIT-2 (1992)	0.741	0.556	0.988	22.18
Schechter 2 (1995)	0.208	0.067	0.640	8.16
D + L pooled OR	0.425	0.287	0.628	100.00

Heterogeneity chi-squared = 21.15 (df = 14), $P = 0.098$
I-squared (variation in OR attributable to heterogeneity) = 33.8%
Estimate of between-study variance Tau-squared = 0.1580
Test of OR = 1: $z = 4.29$, $P = 0.000$

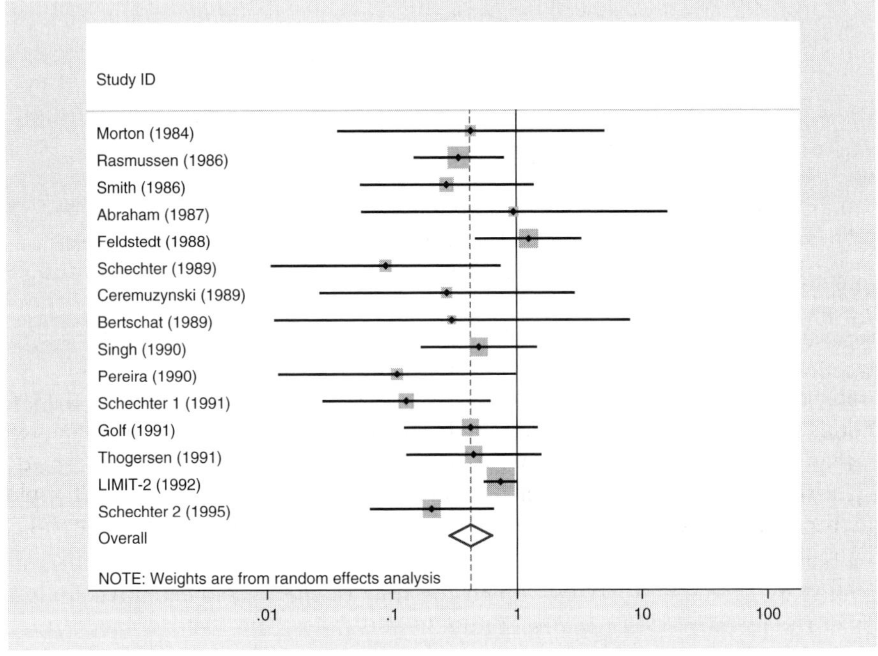

Fig. 3. Forest plot for 15 studies of treatment with magnesium following myocardial infarction. A random effects model was used.

The pooled odds ratio from these 15 studies is 0.425, representing a reduction in risk of greater than 50% associated with magnesium. Only one study (Feldstedt, 1988) had an odds ratio of greater than 1. The overall Z-value for the meta-analysis is 4.29, significant with P-value less than 0.0001. Yet the ISIS-4 study, based on a sample size of 58,050, resulted in a nonsignificant result, with odds ratio of 1.055 and confidence interval (0.991, 1.122). Clearly some form of publication bias occurred, with 14 of 15 studies of a noneffective treatment going

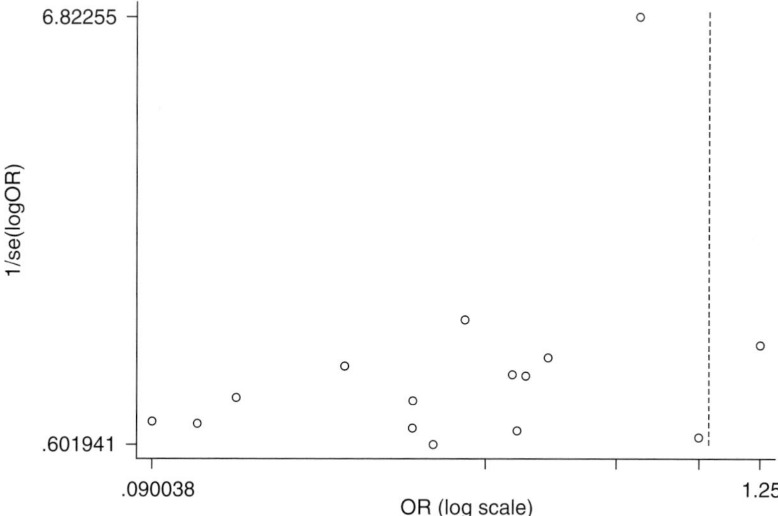

Fig. 4. Funnel plot for 15 studies of treatment with magnesium following myocardial infarction.

in the positive direction. Furthermore, 6 of the 15 had confidence intervals excluding 1 and therefore were statistically significant.

The question then arises as to whether we can tell from studies we have at hand whether there might be publication bias. Egger et al. (1997) recommend a graphical technique called a *funnel plot*. A funnel plot is a scatterplot of studies in which the estimated effect size is plotted on the horizontal axis and the reciprocal of the standard error (*precision*) of the estimate is plotted on the vertical axis. In the case of odds ratios, ln(OR) is plotted on the horizontal axis, and SE(ln(OR)) is plotted on the vertical axis. If there is no publication bias, the plot should be symmetric left-to-right, looking like an inverted funnel. If there is publication bias, the plot can be expected to be asymmetric. A funnel plot of these studies appears in Figure 4.

The plot is clearly asymmetric, with a very large tail of low-precision, high effect size studies to the left, but no tail whatsoever to the right. The one study with high precision, LIMIT-2, ought to be at the "spout" of the funnel, with roughly the same number of studies to its left and to its right. Instead we find it to be almost at the right edge of the scatterplot, with only two studies beyond it.

There are two formal tests for symmetry of the funnel plot (Begg and Mazumdar, 1994; Egger et al., 1997). There is also a technique called *trim and fill* (Duval and Tweedie, 2000) for adding studies to a funnel plot until it becomes symmetric. In the trim phase, studies are removed if they lie beyond 95% confidence limits for what the funnel is estimated to be. In the case of Figure 4, seven studies were removed. With these studies removed, a new estimate of the pooled OR is made. Those omitted studies are then returned to the meta-analysis along with mirror image counterparts. Based on Figure 4, it would seem that more than seven studies should have been trimmed and filled. Perhaps the method did not work due to the very large number of (apparently) missing studies.

An alternative to attempting to infer the results of unpublished studies is to become extremely aggressive about searching for such studies. For example, Cochrane Collaboration studies (discussed further in Section 8) typically involve searching three electronic databases, Medline, EMBASE, and CENTRAL (Cochrane Central Register of Controlled Trials) as well as the "gray literature," such as presentations at meetings that were never published and therefore not likely to be indexed in electronic databases.

8. The Cochrane Collaboration

The Cochrane Centre was founded in 1992 and became the Cochrane Collaboration a year later in 1993. It is named in honor of the British epidemiologist Archie Cochrane (1909–1988), who was instrumental in encouraging registry of all randomized controlled trials, beginning with the *Oxford Database of Perinatal Trials*.

As of mid-2005, 13,047 people from 100 different countries were listed as members of the Collaboration, as advisors, editors, translators, reviewers, and referees. As of early 2007, Medline indexes 4294 Cochrane Collaboration meta-analytic reviews of controlled clinical trials. (They may be found by searching PubMed for the string "*Cochrane Database Syst Rev*" [Journal].)

In addition to publishing reviews, the Cochrane Collaboration also maintains a searchable registry of randomized controlled trials. As of early 2007, this database listed 489,167 randomized clinical trials.

A Cochrane review must first go through a protocol stage in which the authors list background, objectives, consideration criteria for studies, search methods, methods to be used in the review, minimum methodological quality for study inclusion, and potential conflicts of interest. Only after the protocol has been approved can the actual review be undertaken. Most reviews will eventually be subject to revision based on availability of future studies.

While meta-analysis can be used for studies other than controlled clinical trials, the Cochrane Collaboration serves as an excellent example of the quality and methodology that can be used in systematic reviews.

References

Begg, C.B., Mazumdar, M. (1994). Operating characteristics of a rank correlation test for publication bias. *Biometrics* **50**, 1088–1101.

Cochran, W.G. (1954). Some methods for strengthening the common χ^2 tests. *Biometrics* **10**, 417–451.

DerSimonian, R., Laird, N. (1986). Meta-analysis in clinical trials. *Controlled Clinical Trials* **7**, 177–188.

Duval, S.J., Tweedie, R.L. (2000). Trim and fill: A simple funnel plot based method of testing and adjusting publication bias in meta-analysis. *Biometrics* **95**, 89–98.

Egger, M., Davey Smith, G. (1995). Misleading meta-analysis: Lessons from "an effective, safe, simple" intervention that wasn't. *BMJ* **310**, 752–754.

Egger, M., Davey Smith, G. (1997). Meta-analysis: Potentials and promise. *BMJ* **315**, 1371–1374.

Egger, M., Davey Smith, G., Schneider, M., Minder, C. (1997). Bias in meta-analysis detected by a simple graphical test. *BMJ* **315**, 629–634.

Fisher, R.A. (1932). *Statistical Methods for Research Workers*, 4th ed. Oliver and Boyd, London.

Fletcher, A., Cullum, N., Sheldon, T. (1997). A systematic review of compression treatment for venous leg ulcers. *BMJ* **315**, 576–580.

Glass, G.V. (1976). Primary, secondary, and meta-analysis of research. *Educational Research* **5**, 3–8.

Mantel, N., Haenszel, W. (1959). Statistical aspects of the analysis of data from retrospective studies of disease. *Journal of the National Cancer Institute* **22**, 719–748.

Mosteller, F., Fisher, R.A. (1948). Questions and answers, question 14. *American Statistician* **2**, 30–31.

Pearson, K. (1904). Report on certain enteric fever inoculation statistics. *BMJ* **3**, 1243–1246.

Simpson, E.H. (1951). The interpretation of interaction in contingency tables. *Journal of the Royal Statistical Society, Series B* **13**, 238–241.

Smith, M.L., Glass, G.V. (1977). Meta-analysis of psychotherapy outcome studies. *American Psychologist* **32**, 752–760.

Sterne, J.A.C., Bradburn, M.J., Egger, M. (2001). Meta-analysis in STATA^{TM}. In: Egger M., Davey Smith G., Altman D.G. (Eds.), *Systematic Reviews in Health Care*, 2nd ed. BMJ Publishing Group, London (Chapter 18).

Yule, G.U. (1903). Note on the theory of association of attributes in statistics. *Biometrika* **2**, 121–134.

Handbook of Statistics, Vol. 27
ISSN: 0169-7161

DOI: 10.1016/S0169-7161(07)27021-X

21

The Multiple Comparison Issue in Health Care Research

Lemuel A. Moyé

Abstract

Multiple analyses in clinical trials comprise the execution and interpretation of numerous statistical hypotheses within a single clinical research effort. These analyses appear in many guises, e.g., the effect of therapy on multiple endpoints, the assessment of a subgroup analysis, and the evaluation of a dose–response relationship. Both the research and medical communities are frequently exposed to the results of these analyses, and common forums for their dissemination are the presentation of clinical trial results at meetings; the appearance of these results in the peer-reviewed, scientific literature; and discussions before regulatory agencies that are considering the approval of a new intervention. Unfortunately, the result of these analyses is commonly confusing and not illuminating. This chapter provides a useful context in to interpret these sometimes complex results.

1. Introduction

The multiple comparison problem focuses on the best interpretation of significance testing in the multiple analysis setting. Since type I error is accrued with each statistical hypothesis test, the occurrence of multiple events increases the likelihood that a type I error has occurred. The correction for multiple comparisons is the process by which type I error is distributed across multiple statistical hypothesis tests in sample-based research. The multiple comparison issue has expanded to include multiple evaluations of the same endpoint over time, and in some cases, multiple comparisons of the same endpoint at the same point in time using different statistical procedures.

Accepted as a useful tool in health care investigations by biostatisticians, epidemiology has nevertheless retained important concerns, sometimes rising to crisis levels, over the strategy of allocating type I error in a clinical investigation. These issues have arisen because of the historical difficulties many epidemiologists retain with the *raison dêtre* of multiple comparisons, i.e., the use of significance testing in health care research. These historical concerns have identified important weaknesses in the strategy of relying on significance testing as the sole arbiter of a research effort's results. These limitations are well founded, and must inhabit the ensuring discussions of multiple comparison strategies.

After a brief discussion of the role of significance testing, this chapter will review the justification for multiple comparisons, commonly used corrections for multiple comparisons, and recent advances in the field including sequential rejective procedures, re-sampling algorithms, and the use of dependent hypothesis testing. The later will be applied to commonly used analyses (combined end-points, and subgroup evaluations) in health care research.

2. Concerns for significance testing

Ronald A Fisher's seminal manuscripts on field experimentation appeared in the first edition of his 1925 book *Statistical Methods for Research Workers* (Fisher, 1925) and in a short 1926 paper entitled "The arrangement of field experiments" (Fisher, 1926). This work contained many of Fisher's principal ideas on the planning of experiments, including the idea of significance testing. It is here that the notion of a 5% level of significance first appeared.

Fisher's example to motivate the use of significance testing was the assessment of manure's influence on crop yield. In this circumstance, the yields of two neighboring acres of land, one treated with manure and the other without were to be compared. Fisher concluded that if there was only one in twenty chance that the play of chance would produce a 10% difference in crop yield then,

> "... the evidence would have reached a point which may be called the verge of significance; for it is convenient to draw the line at about the level at which we can say 'Either there is something in the treatment or a coincidence has occurred such as does not occur more than once in twenty trials.' This level, which we may call the 5 per cent level point, would be indicated, though very roughly, by the greatest chance deviation observed in twenty successive trials." (Fisher, 1926).

The development of the null and alternative hypotheses, confidence intervals rapidly followed (Neyman and Peason, 1933; Pytkowsi, 1932; Neyman, 1937).

However, concerns about significance testing and its role in health care were raised at once (Edwards, 1972; Berkson, 1942a, b). The concerns were threefold. First, significance testing, with its emphasis on rejection or non-rejection of the null hypothesis, focused on the scientific thesis that the investigator did not believe (Fisher named the null hypothesis to indicate that it was the hypothesis to be nullified by the data). This was a change in the paradigm of a generation of scientists schooled to build a scientific case to affirm their concept of the research question, not to reject a hypothesis that they did not believe. Second, rejection of the null hypothesis did not mean that the null hypothesis was wrong. To many critics, a small p-value should alter the level of belief in the null hypothesis, but should not lead to its outright rejection, since the null hypothesis may still be true. Finally, many workers believed Fisher was equating small p-values with a causality argument (i.e., a small p-value was the *sine qua non* of a causal relationship).

These concerns were refuted by Fisher and others to the satisfaction of many in the research community, and significance testing became an accepted tool in science. The dramatic expansion of its use in health care was fueled by the explosive growth in medical research in the 1940s and 1950s, with grant reviews and journal editors turning to the p-value as a way to identify research that was both fundable and publishable (Goodman, 1999; Fisher, 1925).

It is not necessarily tragic that the use of p-values accelerated; however, it is unfortunate that they began to take on a new, subsuming, and inappropriate meaning in the medical research community. Despite Bradford Hill's attempts to relegate them to merely supportive (Hill, 1965)], other writing continued to coronate these measures (Anonymous, 1988), demonstrating that extreme, sometimes irrational conclusions were being based solely on the p-value. The critical concern expressed in epidemiology was that workers were now replacing their own thoughtful review of a research effort with the simple evaluation of the p-value (Poole, 1987). It was inevitable that some scientist would actively resist this degradation in the scientific thought process, with epidemiologists actively resisting the use of p-values (Walker, 1986a, b; Fleiss, 1986a, b, c), confusing statistical significance with clinical importance. Specifically, he feared that many workers now assumed that a finding of statistical significance was synonymous with clinical significance and the reverse, i.e., statistically insignificant effects were clinically insignificant. The sharp debates at the Federal Food and Drug Administration (FDA) over whether the heart failure drug carvedilol should be approved, revealed the confusion over the true role of p-values in health care research (Packer et al., 1996; Moyé and Abernethy, 1996; Fisher, 1999, Moyé, 1999).

3. Appropriate use of significance testing

If statisticians and epidemiologists are to have a shared role in research interpretation, then the appropriate role of significance testing in research efforts has to be identified. It perhaps might be found in the following line of reasoning.

It is undeniable that sampling error must be addressed in sample-based research. The compromise investigators make in selecting a sample (mandating that they give up the ability to answer the research question with certainty) injects sample-to-sample variability in their work. The tendency of a population with one effect size to produce different samples each with a different effect size presents an important obstacle to generalizing sample findings back to the population.

Both the confidence interval and p-value quantify the component of sampling error in a research effort's results. The confidence interval, by providing a range of values for the population parameter, gives an overt expression of this variability. Alternatively, by providing only one number, the p-value lends itself to dichotomous decisions regarding the strength of evidence that an analysis provides for a particular scientific hypothesis.

It is this final distillation that is one of the roots of difficulty with significance testing. The concentration of a research result down to a single number is the foundation of the *p*-value. The *p*-value is itself constructed from several components: (1) sample size, (2) effect size, (3) the precision of the estimate, and (4) a sampling error assessment. Each of these ingredients is important in the assessment of research interpretation.

However, by integrating them all into the *p*-value, investigators commonly succumb to the temptation of ignoring each of its component pieces. Instead, they withhold assessment of the research effort until these important components are mathematically integrated into the *p*-value, and then use the *p*-value to assess the research effort. Thus, they have permitted a multidimensional problem (made up of sample size, effect size, effect size precision, and sampling error) to be reduced to a one-dimensional problem (simply assessing the magnitude of the *p*-value). Like trying to understand a company by simply examining its yearly income tax bill, much useful information is lost in this dimensionality reduction (Lang et al., 1998).

Therefore, *p*-values can be fine descriptors of the role of sampling error. However, they are quite deficient in summarizing an analysis and must be supplemented by additional information, specifically research methodology, sample size, effect size, and effect size precision. The joint consideration of each of these is necessary in order for the study to have a fair and balanced interpretation.

The methodology of the research effort is an important, perhaps, the most important consideration in drawing conclusions from a research effort. If the research is poorly designed or is executed discordantly,[1] then statistical estimators are flawed. In this circumstance, effect size estimators, estimates of its variability, *p*-values, and confidence intervals are distorted. In this unfortunate set of circumstances, the research effort cannot be interpreted.

Multiple comparison procedures are most useful in the environment of a concordantly executed research program, where *p*-values are not interpreted in isolation, but jointly with an assessment of the research methodology, effect size, effect size variability, and the confidence interval. It is in this optimal research environment that the ensuring conversation of multiple comparison procedures should be interpreted.

4. Definition of multiple comparisons

Multiple comparisons (or multiple testing situations) are simply the collection of statistical hypothesis tests that are executed at the conclusion of a research effort. These include, but are not limited to dose–response analyses, the examination of

[1] Discordant execution is the process by which the study is not executed in accordance with its protocol, but meanders, changing its endpoints, and analyses based on the observed data. Concordant execution is a research effort, which follows its prospectively written protocol.

multiple endpoints, the use of subgroup analyses, and exploratory evaluations. In reality, these evaluations occur in complicated mixtures. For example, a clinical trial may compare the effect of a single dose intervention to a control group on several different endpoints, and in addition, examine the same effect in subgroups of interest. As another example, a clinical trial may assess the effect of the active intervention on total mortality, while dose–response information may be collected on a separate but related combined endpoint. In some circumstances, multiple comparisons include not just multiple endpoints, i.e., analyses of different endpoints, but also, multiple comparisons, using different procedures on the same endpoint (Moyé, 2003).

5. Rational for multiple comparisons

Significance testing focuses on decision-making; its original motivation was to draw a single conclusion concerning a single effect. In order to accomplish this, one experiment would be concordantly executed, producing one conclusion (such as therapy A yields a better clinical result on average than placebo). However, investigative circumstances have arisen in which the final results of the program involve not just one endpoint, but a collection of endpoints. For example, an observational study comparing the hospital stays of stroke patients versus patients with closed head injuries may choose to focus on duration of hospital stay. However, in reality, more than just one variable reflecting the outcome of a patient would be measured. Multiple comparisons are a natural byproduct of the complexity of these clinical research efforts. There are three motivations for conducting multiple comparisons. They are (1) to provide logistical efficiency, (2) to strengthen the causal argument, and (3) to explore new ideas and establish new relationships between risk (or beneficial) factors and disease. We will briefly discuss each of these in turn.

5.1. Efficiency

One of the motivations that generate multiple comparisons is the drive of both the investigator and the sponsor[2] for efficiency. Their natural expectation for the greatest return for resources invested translates into making the research effort as productive as possible, generating a full panoply of results in order to justify the commitment of the logistical and financial resources required for the research endeavor's execution.

Consider a controlled clinical trial, which involves randomizing patients to either the intervention group or the control group, following these patients until they have a fatal or nonfatal stroke, or the predefined follow-up period ends.

[2] The sponsor of the trial is the organization, which funds the study. It could be a government-funded study, underwritten by institutes, e.g., the National Eye Institute, or the National Institute of Environmental Health Services. Alternatively, the clinical trial could be funded by a private pharmaceutical company.

The investigators focus on this one measure of effectiveness. However, other competing measures are available. For example, the researchers might also measure the number of transient ischemic attacks (TIAs), duration of hospitalization, or cerebral blood flow studies. The incremental costs of these additional studies are relatively small given that the study is to be carried out to measure the impact of therapy on the fatal/nonfatal stroke rate. Thus, one can triple the number of endpoints and increase the number of statistical analyses (increasing the likelihood of a positive result on at least one), without tripling the cost of the experiment.

5.2. Epidemiologic strength

The careful selection of endpoints might be used to elicit further evidence from the data about the true nature of the relationship between exposure and disease (i.e., is it associative or causal?). Embedding an examination of the evidence that sheds light on Bradford Hill's causality tenets (Hill, 1965) (particularly those of dose–response, biologic plausibility, consistency, and coherency) could lead to their inclusion within the research enterprise; however, their incorporation would likely include additional endpoints in the study.

For example, an observational study that examines the relationship between the use of an anti-diabetic drug and liver failure may also focus on the relationship between exposure duration and the incidence of acute liver failure. This would require an odds ratio (with corresponding confidence interval and p-value) for each dose-duration category. In addition, one could measure the proportion of patients who have elevated liver enzymes. This collection of evaluations improves the quality of the assessment of the true nature of the exposure–disease relationship. However, each requires an additional analysis.

5.3. The need to explore

Confirmatory research executes a protocol that was designed to answer a prospectively asked scientific question. Exploratory research is the evaluation of a dataset for new and interesting relationships that were not anticipated. This will be covered in detail in the next section.

6. Multiple comparisons and analysis triage

Investigators will follow their nature, examining every endpoint with every analysis procedure they think will provide illumination. However, this intellectually and curiosity satisfying proclivity must be tempered with discipline so that sampling error can be managed and the research effort is interpretable.

One might integrate each of these actions by triaging analyses in accordance with some prospectively declared guidelines. This strategy of endpoint control permits the investigators the freedom to completely evaluate and analyze all of their endpoints measures; however, they must be clear about their plans for interpreting these.

The process is straightforward. The investigators should first identify each of the analyses that they wish to assess at the study's conclusion. Once this exhaustive process of analysis identification has completed, the investigators should then choose the small number of endpoints for which a type I error rate will be allocated. It is over this final subset of endpoints that the overall type I error level will be controlled. Other analyses that cannot be recognized prospectively will fall into the class of exploratory analyses.

6.1. Confirmatory versus exploratory analyses

Confirmatory analyses are those examinations that were prospectively selected by the researcher to answer the scientific questions that motivated the research effort. Exploratory evaluations were not anticipated by the researcher. Through their interrogation of the database, the investigators identify relationships that were not anticipated, but that the sample suggests are present. In exploratory analyses, the dataset suggests answers to questions that the researchers never prospectively thought to ask. As Miles (1993) points out "If the fishing expedition catches a boot, the fishermen should throw it back, not claim that they were fishing for boots."

The confirmatory evaluation provides the clearest measure of the magnitude of the effect of interest. Being chosen to answer the *a priori* research question, the sample is optimally selected and configured for the relationship that was suggested in the prospectively declared research protocol. Also, with the analysis fixed (i.e., the variable in which interest lies has been chosen prospectively and plans for its evaluation are already in place) the statistical estimators perform well, providing a reliable estimate of effect magnitude and the degree to which that magnitude may vary from sample-to-sample. Generalization from the sample to the population is strongest when it rests on a confirmatory finding.

Alternatively, exploratory analyses introduce two problems that make it difficult to generalize their sample-based results to the larger population. The first is that the sample was not chosen with the exploratory research question in mind. For example, the sample may be too small, or not have the most precise measure of the exploratory effect of interest. In addition, the usual sample statistical estimators are undermined because the assumption on which their accuracy is based is false (Moyé, 2003). Since the endpoints have been selected randomly (i.e., the dataset, containing sampling error, produced "endpoints" in an essentially random manner), the analysis has become random, the hallmark of random research (Moyé, 2003). These two influences combine to reduce the accuracy of any conclusions drawn from exploratory evaluations.

Certainly, investigators want to cover new ground, and commonly enjoy the exploration process. Exploratory analyses can evaluate the unanticipated, surprising effects of an exposure in an observational study, or a randomly allocated treatment in a controlled clinical trial. These evaluations are powerful motivation for multiple comparisons, and make valuable contributions if appropriately relegated to the hypothesis-generating arena.

6.2. Primary versus secondary analyses

If the analysis is prospectively determined, then the next step is to determine if the evaluation should be a primary or a secondary evaluation.

Primary analyses are the primary focus of the study. Their prospective declaration protects them from data driven changes during the course of the study's execution, thereby preserving the accuracy of the statistical estimators. In addition, since type I error is prospectively allocated to these primary endpoints in a way that controls the familywise error rates (FWERs), the analysis of these endpoints permits type I error conservation in accordance with community standards.

Secondary analyses are the prospectively declared evaluations that are assessed at the nominal 0.05 α level. They are not included in the calculations to control the overall α error level. These endpoints, being prospectively selected, produce trustworthy estimators of effect size, standard error, confidence intervals, and p-values, all of which measure the effect of the clinical trial's intervention. However, drawing confirmatory conclusions from these secondary endpoints is not permissible since conclusions based on these secondary endpoints will increase the overall type I error level above the prospectively declared acceptable levels. The role of secondary endpoints is simply to provide support for the study's conclusions drawn from the trial's primary analyses. For example, they can provide information about the mechanism of action by which an intervention works. Alternatively, they can provide useful data about the dose response relationship between the intervention and the clinical endpoint of interest.

7. Significance testing and multiple comparisons

The afore mentioned concerns of logistical efficiency, in concert with the need to build strong epidemiologic arguments, serve as solid motivation for conducting multiple comparisons in a modern health care research effort. However, since each of these analyses involves a statistical hypothesis test, and each hypothesis test produces a p-value, a relevant question is how should these p-values be interpreted?

This issue has been debated as statistical inference has matured. Some workers contend that many of these p-values should be ignored, (Nester, 1996; Rothman, 1990) allowing the reader to focus on the effect size. Others have argued that p-values should be interpreted as though the value of 0.05 is the cutoff point for statistical significance, regardless of how many p-values have been produced by the study. This is called using "nominal significance testing" or "marginal significance." Others have debated whether investigators should be able to analyze all of the data, and then choose the results they want to disseminate (Fisher, 1999; Moyé, 1999).

Commonly investigators do not prospectively state the analysis rule they will carry out during a research effort. The study results may suggest a multitude of

Table 1
Analysis of four endpoints and their *p*-values

Endpoint	Rel Risk	*p*-Value
P_1	0.81	0.015
P_2	0.82	0.049
P_3	0.79	0.025
P_4	0.83	0.076

ambiguous conclusions. The investigators believe they have the authority to choose the interpretation of the multiple findings in a way of their choosing. However, the resulting interpretation is problematic.

Consider, for example, four analyses from a randomized clinical trial designed to measure the effect of therapy of an intervention in patients with a propensity for gastrointestinal (GI) disease. Assume in this hypothetical example that the four endpoints are

P_1 – the effect of therapy on the cumulative total mortality rate.
P_2 – the effect of therapy on the cumulative incidence of upper GI bleeds.
P_3 – the effect of therapy on the cumulative incidence of upper GI obstructions.
P_4 – the effect of therapy on hospitalizations for upper GI illness.

The investigators make no prospective statement about which of these is the most important, but plan to use a nominal 0.05 level to determine significance. At the conclusion of the study, they report the results (Table 1).

Table 1 provides the relative risk and *p*-value for each of these evaluations. The relative risk reveals that the therapy has produced an effect that is beneficial in the sample. The investigators want to know which of these is positive.

One tempting approach would be to say that P_1, P_2, and P_3 are positive, accepting that any analysis that produces a *p*-value ≤ 0.05 is a positive one. This is the nominal approach to *p*-value assessment. The tack of interpreting each of several *p*-values from a single experiment, one at a time, based on whether they are greater or less than the traditional threshold of 0.05 may seem like a natural alternative to the *post hoc* decision structure. In fact, the nominal *p*-value approach is very alluring at first glance. The rule to use nominal *p*-values is easily stated prospectively at the beginning of the trial and is easy to apply at that trial's end.

However, there are unfortunate consequences of this approach. The acceptance of nominal *p*-values would require us to conclude that the population has not produced a misleading sample result for any of the total mortality, GI bleed, GI obstruction. How likely is this "triple positive result" to be true? The probability that no type I error occurs for any of these three evaluations, is easily computed[3] as

$$\text{no type I error} = (1 - 0.015)(1 - 0.049)(1 - 0.025) = 0.913.$$

[3] This computation assumes that the hypothesis tests are independent of each other.

The probability of at least 1 type I error is 1 – 0.913 = 0.087. Thus, the probability that the population has misled us just through a sampling error is 0.087, larger than the 0.05 level. We cannot accept the triple-veracity in this case because the likelihood of a type I error is too large.

However, the circumstances are even more perilous than that. Why did the investigators choose to focus only on analyses P_1, P_2, and P_3 as positive? Most likely because the p-values were all less than 0.05. If, for example, they had chosen P_4 as the most important analysis, the expended type I error would be too large. Thus, looking at the data, they excluded analysis P_4 from further consideration because its p-value was too large. Thus, they made their decision to focus on P_1, P_2, and P_3, based on the observed results, and not on a prospective statement declared before the data were collected.

The point is that with no prospective plan, the investigators are drawn to interpret the research endeavor in the most positive, attractive way they can. However, other investigators or readers would interpret the results differently. With no prospective plan to guide the community, every one falls into the temptation of using analysis rules for the study's interpretation that are based on the data. This is the hallmark of random research (Moyé, 2003).

8. Familywise error rate[4]

The calculation on the preceding section demonstrates how multiple statistical hypothesis tests propagate type I error rates. If there are two statistical analyses, one on the effect of the intervention on the total mortality rate and the second on the intervention's impact of the fatal and nonfatal stroke rate, then a type I error means that the population has produced (by chance alone) a sample that gives a false and misleading signal that the intervention reduced the cumulative total mortality incidence rate, the fatal/nonfatal stroke rate, or both. The key observation is that there are three errors of which we must now keep track when there are two endpoint analyses, and the misleading events of interest can occur in combination. A comprehensive method to track the magnitude of this combination of sampling errors is the FWER (Hochberg and Tamhane, 1987 ;Westfall and Young, 1993) and will be designated as ξ. This is simply the probability that at least one type I error has occurred across all of the analyses.

There is a critical difference between the standard type I error level for a single endpoint and ξ. The type I error probability for a single, individual endpoint focuses on the occurrence of a misleading positive result for a single analysis. This is the single test error level, or test-specific error level. The familywise error level focuses on the occurrence of at least one type I error in the entire collection of analyses.

A natural setting for multiple hypothesis testing where FWER control is essential is in analysis of variance, where several groups are evaluated. Tukey's

[4] The terms ***error probability***, ***error rate***, and ***error levels*** will be used interchangeably.

procedure, Duncan's test, and Student–Newman–Keuls procedures are commonly used. Also, a very useful procedure is that of Dunnett. In this setting each of several groups of data is compared to an overall control. A detailed discussion of these procedures is available.

9. The Bonferroni inequality

The previous section's discussion provides important motivation to control the type I error level in clinical trial hypothesis testing. One of the most important, easily used methods to accomplish this prospective control over type I error rate is through the use of the Bonferroni procedure (Miller, 1981).

Carlo Emilio Bonferroni was born on January 28, 1892, in Bergamo, Italy.[5] After studying the piano at the Conservatory in Torino, and completing a tour of duty in the Italian army engineers corps during World War I, he studied the mathematics of finance, writing two articles that established useful inequalities in his municipal and fiscal computations (Bonferroni, 1935; Bonferroni, 1936). This work contained the genesis of the idea that led to the inequality that now bears his name. The modern implementation of Bonferroni's inequality began with the rediscovery of his inequalities by Dunn (Dunn, 1959, 1961).

Its implementation is quite simple. Assume a research effort has K analyses, each analysis consisting of a hypothesis test. Assume also that each hypothesis test is to be carried out with a prospectively defined type I error probability of α; this is the test-specific type I error level or the test-specific α level. We will also make the simplifying assumption that the result of each of the hypothesis tests is independent of the others. This last assumption allows us to multiply type I error rates for the statistical hypothesis tests when we consider their possible joint results.

Our goal in this evaluation is to compute easily the familywise type I error level, ξ. This is simply the probability that there is a least one type I error among the K statistical hypothesis tests. Then ξ, the probability of the occurrence of at least one type I error, is one minus the probability of no type I error among any of the K tests, or

$$\xi = 1 - \prod_{j=1}^{K}(1-\alpha) = 1 - (1-\alpha)^K. \tag{1}$$

This is the precise estimate of type I error, in the setting of disjoint hypothesis tests. The exact value of ξ requires some computation. However, a simplification provided by Bonferroni demonstrates that $\xi \leq \sum_{i=1}^{K}\alpha_i$. If each of the test-specific type I error levels is the same value, α, this reduces to $\xi \leq K\alpha$, or $\alpha \leq \xi/K$. The conservatism of this computation is well recognized, and the correspondence

[5] The source of this material is a lecture given by Michael E. Dewey from the Trent Institute for Health Services Research, University of Nottingham. The lecture itself is posted at michael.dewey@nottingham.ac.uk, http://www.nottingham.ac.uk.~mhzmd/bonf.html.

between the Bonferroni approximation and the exact FWER is closest when the type I error for each individual test is very small.[6] Thus, a reasonable approximation for the α level for each of K hypothesis tests can be computed by dividing the familywise error level by the number of statistical hypothesis tests to be carried out. This is the most common method of applying the Bonferroni procedure.

Note that if a researcher wishes to keep ξ at less than 0.05, the number of analyses whose results can be controlled (i.e., the number of analyses that can be carried out and still keep the familywise error level ≤ 0.05) depends on the significance level at which the individual analyses are to be evaluated. For example, if each of the individual analyses is to be judged at the 0.05 level (i.e., the p-value resulting from the analyses must be less than 0.05 in order to claim the result is statistically significant), then only one analysis can be controlled, since the familywise error level for two analyses exceeds the 0.05 threshold. The researcher can control the familywise error level for three analyses if each is judged at the 0.0167 level. If each test is evaluated at the 0.005 level, then 10 independent hypothesis tests can be carried out.

Important criticism of tight control of ξ is commonly based on the fact that the type I error rate for any particular test must be too small in order to control the FWER. For example, if one were to conduct 20 hypothesis tests, the type I error threshold for each test must be $0.05/20 = 0.0025$, a uselessly small type I error rate threshold for many. However, a difficulty with this line of reason is the assumption that all statistical hypothesis tests are essential. In health care, pivotal research efforts result from well-considered literature reviews. This review and early discussion will commonly produce not 20, but two or three clinically relevant analyses among which type I error may be dispersed. Casting a wide net for a positive finding is the hallmark of exploratory, not confirmatory research work.

In addition, the main reason for controlling type I error rates in clinical research is that it represents the probability of a mistaken research conclusion for the treatment of a disease just due to sampling error. This sampling based error has important implications for the population of patients and the medical community. While sample-based research cannot remove the possibility of this mistake, the magnitude of this error rate must be accurately measured and discussed, so that the effectiveness of an exposure can be appropriately balanced against that exposure's risks.[7] This approach is very helpful for interpreting clinical trials designed to assess the risk–benefit ratio of a new therapy.

It is easy for the lay community to focus on the potential efficacy of new interventions for serious diseases (Adams, 2002). However, it is a truism in medicine that all therapies have risks ranging from mild to severe. Sometimes these risks can be identified in relatively small studies carried out before the invention is approved for use in larger populations. However, in addition to the occurrence of

[6] This is because the higher powers of α ($\alpha^2, \alpha^3, \ldots, \alpha^K$) become very small when α itself is small.

[7] We are setting aside the kinds of errors in clinical trial design that would produce a reproducible, systematic influence on the results. An example of such a bias would be a study in which compliance is so poor with the active therapy that patients do not receive the required exposure to see its anticipated beneficial effect.

specific, anticipated adverse events, there are circumstances in which serious adverse events are generated in large populations without warning. This occurs when the clinical studies (completed before regulatory approval of the compound was granted) are not able to discern the occurrence of these adverse events because the studies contained too few patients.

It is important to acknowledge that regardless of whether the drug is effective or not, the population will have to bear adverse events. Consider the following illustration: The background rate of primary pulmonary hypertension (PPH) is on the order of one case per 1,000,000 patients per year in the United States. Assume that a new drug being evaluated in a pre-FDA approved clinical trial increases this incidence by 20-fold, to one case per 50,000 patients exposed per year, representing a 20-fold increase in risk. However, in order to identify this effect, 50,000 patients would have to be exposed to the compound for one year to see one case of PPH. This is a cohort whose size dwarfs the size of studies that are conducted prior to the therapy's approval. The increased risk of PPH remains hidden, revealed only in the marketplace. If this drug were approved and released for general dispersal through the population for which the drug is indicated, patients would unknowingly be exposed to a devastating, unpredicted adverse event.

The fact that a research effort, not designed to detect an adverse effect, does not find the adverse effect is characterized by the saying "absence of evidence is not evidence of absence" (Senn, 1997). This summarizes the point that the absence of evidence within the clinical trial is not evidence that the compound has no serious side effect.

Thus, we expect adverse events to appear in the population regardless of whether the intervention demonstrates benefit or not. Some (perhaps the majority) of these adverse events are predictable; others may not be. In addition, the financial costs of these interventions are commonly considerable and must be weighed in the global risk–benefit assessment. Therefore, regardless of whether the medication is effective, the compound is assured to impose an adverse event and a financial/administrative burden on the patients who receive it. The occurrences of these events represent the risk side of the risk–benefit equation.

The use of the intervention is justified only by the expectation that its benefits outweigh these health and financial costs. The consequence of a type I error for efficacy in a clinical trial that is designed to measure the true risk–benefit balance of a randomly allocated intervention is the reverse of the Hippocratic Oath, succinctly summarized as "first do no harm."[8] In health care research, type I errors represent ethical issues as much as they do statistical concerns. In these studies, which are commonly the justification for the use of interventions in large populations, the familywise error level must be controlled within acceptable limits.

[8] This problem is exacerbated by the inability to measure type I error accurately, a situation generated by the random research paradigm.

An analogous line of reasoning is used in evaluating the relationship between an exposure that is believed to be dangerous and the occurrence of disease. The large number of evaluations carried out in these studies can commonly produce a plethora of *p*-values, and the occurrence of any positive *p*-value out of the collection can be used as evidence of harm. However, the possibility that sampling error has produced the small *p*-value must be overtly considered in concordant research; control of the FWER is a useful tool in this effort. Ethical considerations can require that the criteria for demonstrating harm be less stringent than the criteria for benefit; however, ethical considerations do not negate the need for prospectively declared assessment rules for controlling the FWER.

10. Alternative approaches

One of the many criticisms of the Bonferroni approximation is that it is too conservative. This conservatism leads to an unacceptably high possibility of missing a clinically important finding. There are several alternative approaches to the multiple analysis problem. Two of the most recent developments are sequential rejective procedures, and re-sampling *p*-values.

10.1. Sequentially rejective procedures

The sequential procedure approach is easy to apply. Assume that there are K statistical null hypotheses in a clinical trial and each statistical hypothesis generates a *p*-value. Let p_1 be the *p*-value for the first hypothesis test $H_{0,1}$, p_2 be the *p*-value for the second hypothesis test $H_{0,2}$, concluding with p_k as the *p*-value for the Kth and last hypothesis test $H_{0,K}$. These *p*-values must first be ranked from the smallest to largest. We will denote $p_{[1]}$ as the smallest of the K *p*-values, $p_{[2]}$ the next largest *p*-value ... to $p_{[K]}$ which is the maximum *p*-value of the K *p*-values from the clinical trial.

Once the *p*-values have been ranked, several evaluation procedures are available to draw a conclusion based on their values. One device proposed by Simes (1986) compares the jth smallest *p*-value, $p_{[j]}$ to $\xi j/K$. The procedure is as follows:

(1) Rank order the K *p*-values such that $p_{[1]} \leq p_{[2]} \leq p_{[3]} \leq \cdots \leq p_{[K]}$.
(2) Compare the smallest *p*-value, $p_{[1]}$ to the threshold ξ/K If $p_{[1]} \leq \xi/K$, then reject the null hypothesis for which $p_{[1]}$ is the *p*-value.
(3) Compare $p_{[2]}$ to $2\xi/K$. If $p_{[2]} \leq 2\xi/K$, then reject the null hypothesis for which $p_{[2]}$ is the *p*-value.
(4) Compare $p_{[3]}$ to $3\xi/K$. If $p_{[3]} \leq 3\xi/K$, then reject the null hypothesis for which $p_{[3]}$ is the *p*-value.
(5) Continue on, finally comparing $p_{[K]}$ to ξ. If $p_{[K]} \leq \xi$, then reject the null hypothesis for which $p_{[K]}$ is the *p*-value.

The procedure ceases at the first step for which the null hypothesis is not rejected. Thus, as j increases, *p*-values that are increasing are compared to significance levels, which are themselves increasing in a linear fashion. If the tests are independent one from another, then the familywise error level ξ is preserved. This procedure is more powerful than the Bonferroni procedure. Holm (1979), Hommel (1988), and Shaffer (1986) have developed similar procedures. It has been suggested that because these methods are easy to apply and less conservative than the classic Bonferroni procedure, they are preferable for hypothesis testing in which FWER control is critical (Zhang et al., 1997).

10.2. Re-sampling p-values

Another modern device to assist in the assessment of multiple comparisons is the use of re-sampling tools. This approach has been developed by Westfall et al. (Westfall and Young, 1993; Tukey et al., 1985; Dubey, 1985) and has figured prominently in the methodologic literature evaluating the multiple analysis issue. These workers focus on the smallest *p*-value obtained from a collection of hypothesis tests, using the re-sampling concept as their assessment tool.

Re-sampling is the process by which smaller samples of data are randomly selected from the research dataset. Essentially, this approach treats the research data sample as a "population" from which samples are obtained. Re-sampling is allowed to take place thousands of times, each time generating a new "sub-sample" and a new *p*-value from that sub-sample. Combining all of these *p*-values from these sub-samples produces, in the end, a distribution of *p*-values. The adjusted *p*-value measures how extreme a given *p*-value is, relative to the probability distribution of the most extreme *p*-value.

However, the new ingredient in this approach is that the investigator no longer sets the α threshold for each evaluation. Since the data determine the magnitude of the *p*-values, and therefore the rank ordering of the *p*-values, then the data must determine the order of hypotheses to be tested. We must also recognize that, as the significance level threshold varies from analysis to analysis, the link between the endpoint and the significance threshold is not set by the investigator but, again, is set by the data.

This latter point is of critical concern to the investigator. The collection of sequentially rejective significance testing rules and the family of procedures that fall under the *p*-value re-sampling provide increased statistical power when compared to the Bonferroni procedures. However, the clinical investigators lose the ability to determine the significance threshold for each of the analyses they wish to carry out. The requirement that each of the *p*-values be rank ordered essentially automates the significance testing procedures, locking the investigators out of choosing the type I error level thresholds for each analysis. Therefore, while sequentially rejective and re-sampling procedures might be useful in statistics in general, the fact that they take control of hypothesis testing away from the investigator could severely constrain their utility in health care research.

In addition, False Discovery Rate (FDR) offers a new and interesting perspective on the multiple comparisons problem. Instead of controlling the chance of *any* false positives (as Bonferroni does), the FDR controls the expected proportion of false positives among all tests (Benjamini and Hochberg, 1995;

Benjamini and Yekutieli, 2001) It is very useful in micro-array analyses in which thousands of significance tests are executed.

11. Dependent testing

Commonly in health care research statistical hypothesis tests are not independent. Analyses that are related to each other can produce some conservation of the type I error rate. This conservation can lead to an increase in test-specific α levels above those suggested by the strict application of the Bonferroni procedure.

Assume that investigators designing their clinical research settle on two primary endpoints, P_1 and P_2. The statistical hypothesis test for P_1 that will test the exposure at issue on P_1 is H_1. H_1 is assigned an *a priori* type I error level α_1. Analogously, the statistical hypothesis test for the effect of the intervention on the endpoint P_2 is H_2, and the type I error level for hypothesis test H_2 is α_2. What does "independent hypothesis testing" mean in this circumstance? Specifically, independence means that execution of hypothesis test H_1 neither educates us nor predicts for us the result of H_2. It would be useful to examine the nature of the relationship between H_1 and H_2 in terms of the type I error rate, since ultimately this is the error whose level we seek to control. In the end, we hope to learn the likelihood that we will commit a type I error in drawing conclusions from both H_1 and H_2 since this is the information that we need to control the familywise error level ξ.

If this is the investigator's goal, then, specifically, independence tells us that knowledge about the commission of a type I error for hypothesis test H_1 reveals nothing about the occurrence of a type I error for hypothesis test H_2; it does not inform us one way or the other about the commission of a type I error for the second hypothesis test. Before any hypothesis test proceeds, the best estimate of the likelihood of a type I error for H_2 is α_2. If H_1 and H_2 are truly independent, then after the evaluation of the hypothesis test for the primary endpoint P_1, our best estimate for the type I error level for the execution of H_2 remains α_2.

An adjustment that became popular for taking dependency between hypothesis tests into account was that recommended by Tukey et al. (1985). He suggested that an adjustment for dependence between hypothesis tests may be simply computed by calculating the test-specific type I error probability as α, where

$$\alpha = 1 - (1 - \xi)^{1/\sqrt{K}}. \tag{2}$$

This computation produces larger values of the type I error rate than that produced from the Bonferroni procedure.

One limitation of this approach is that the test-specific α is computed under the assumption that the test-specific α level is the same for each of the K primary hypothesis tests. In addition, it is difficult to see the degree of dependency between the endpoints from an examination of formula , i.e., Eq. (2).

The works of Dubey (1985) and of O'Brien (1984) have provided other related procedures for computing the test-specific α levels when the statistical hypothesis tests are correlated. If there are K hypothesis tests to be evaluated, each for a separate endpoint, then the calculation they suggest for the test-specific α level is

$$\alpha = 1 - (1 - \xi)^{1/m_k} \tag{3}$$

and

$$m_k = K^{1-r_k} \quad \text{and} \quad r_k = \frac{\sum_{j \neq k}^{K} r_{jk}}{K - 1}$$

where r_k is the average of the correlation coefficients reflecting the association between the K endpoints to be evaluated. An advantage of this method over Tukey's is that the actual correlations are built into the computation. However, in simulation analyses, Sankoh (Sankoh et al., 1997) points out that the Tukey procedure still works best when there are large numbers of highly correlated endpoints. Sankoh also noted that the procedure suggested by Dubey and O'Brien required additional adjustment at all correlation levels despite its specific inclusion of endpoint correlation.

Hochberg and Westfall discuss an important subset of multiplicity problems in biostatistics in general (Hochberg and Westfall, 2000). James uses multinomial probabilities when dealing with the issue of multiple endpoints in clinical trials (James, 1991). Neuhauser discusses an interesting application of multiple clinical endpoint evaluation in a trial studying patients with asthma (Neuhauser et al., 1999). Reitmeir and Wasmer (1996) discuss one-sided hypothesis testing and multiple endpoints, and Westfall, Ho, and Prillaman engage in a deeper discussion of multiple union–intersection tools in the evaluation of multiple endpoints in clinical trials (Westfall et al., 2001). Closed testing is discussed by Zhang (Westfall and Wolfinger, 2000). Weighted α-partitioning methods are available for the Simes' test as well (Hochberg and Liberman, 1994).

11.1. Multiple comparisons and the dependency parameter

An additional approach may be developed along the following lines. Assume that a research effort produces K prospectively declare primary hypothesis tests H_1, H_2, H_3, ... H_K. Let H_j denote the jth hypothesis test. For each of these K hypothesis tests, specify the prospectively specified type I error levels α_1, α_2, α_3, ... α_K. Define T_j for $j = 1, 2, 3, \ldots, K$ as a variable that captures whether a type I error has occurred for the jth hypothesis test, i.e., $T_j = 0$ if there is no type I error on the jth hypothesis test, and $T_j = 1$ if the jth hypothesis test produces a type I error. Thus, we can consider K pairs, (H_1, T_1), (H_2, T_2), (H_3, T_3), ..., (H_K, T_K), where H_j identifies the statistical hypothesis test and T_j denotes whether a type I error has occurred for that test, i.e., $P[T_j = 1] = \alpha_j$.

Using the customary definition of the familywise error as the event that there is at least one type I error among the K prospectively defined primary analyses (Hochberg and Tamhane, 1987; Westfall and Young, 1993) define ξ as the familywise error level, and T_ξ as the variable that denotes whether a familywise type I error level has occurred. Then $\xi = P[T_\xi = 1]$ and $P[T_\xi = 0]$ is the probability that there were no type I errors among the K hypothesis tests. Therefore,

$$P(T_\xi = 0) = P(\{T_1 = 0\} \cap \{T_2 = 0\} \cap \{T_3 = 0\} \cap \cdots \cap \{T_K = 0\}) \quad (4)$$

and

$$\begin{aligned} P(T_\xi = 1) &= 1 - P(\{T_1 = 0\} \cap \{T_2 = 0\} \cap \{T_3 = 0\} \cap \cdots \cap \{T_K = 0\}) \\ &= 1 - P\Big(\bigcap_{j=1}^{K} T_j = 0\Big). \end{aligned} \quad (5)$$

When the K individual hypotheses are independent of one another, then $P(\cap_{j=1}^{K} T_j = 0) = \prod_{j=1}^{K} P(T_j = 0) = \prod_{j=1}^{K}(1 - \alpha_j)$. However, if the K prospectively specified hypothesis tests are dependent, then the evaluation of the expression $P(\cap_{j=1}^{K} T_j = 0)$ becomes more complicated.

In the independence setting for $K = 2$, write

$$P[T_1 = 0 \cap T_2 = 0] = P[T_2 = 0 | T_1 = 0] P[T_1 = 0]. \quad (6)$$

This will be a useful equation for us as we develop the notion of dependency in hypothesis testing, since the key to computing the probability of a familywise error $P[T_\xi = 0]$ is the computation of the joint probability $P[T_1 = 0 \cap T_2 = 0]$. This calculation is straightforward in the independence scenario.

$$P[T_2 = 0 | T_1 = 0] = \frac{P[T_1 = 0 \cap T_2 = 0]}{P[T_1 = 0]} = \frac{(1 - \alpha_1)(1 - \alpha_2)}{(1 - \alpha_1)} = 1 - \alpha_2 \quad (7)$$

The opposite, extreme circumstance from that of dependence might be considered "perfect dependence." Perfect dependence denotes that state between two statistical hypothesis tests in which the occurrence of a type I error for H_1 automatically produces a type I error for statistical hypothesis test H_2. In this situation, the two tests are so intertwined that knowledge that a type I error occurred for the first hypothesis test guarantees that a type I error will occur for the second hypothesis test. Perfect dependence dictates that the conditional probability from Eq. (6) is one, i.e.,

$$P[T_2 = 0 | T_1 = 0] = 1. \quad (8)$$

Recalling that $\xi = 1 - P[T_1 = 0 \cap T_2 = 0]$, compute that

$$\begin{aligned} \xi &= 1 - P[T_1 = 0 \cap T_2 = 0] = 1 - P[T_2 = 0 | T_1 = 0] P[T_1 = 0] \\ &= 1 - (1)(1 - \alpha_1) = \alpha_1. \end{aligned} \quad (9)$$

Since the occurrence of a type I error on the first statistical hypothesis test implies that a type I error has occurred on the second hypothesis test, the joint occurrence of type I errors is determined by what occurs on H_1. We can, without any loss of generality, order these two hypothesis tests prospectively such that $\alpha_1 \geq \alpha_2$. In the setting of perfect dependence, one can execute two hypothesis tests and maintain ξ at its desired level by simply allowing α_2 to take any value such that $\alpha_2 \leq \alpha_1 = \xi$. As an example, consider the hypothetical case of a clinical trial in which there are two prospectively defined primary hypothesis tests H_1 and H_2 with associated test-specific α error levels α_1 and α_2. Choose $\alpha_1 = \alpha_2 = 0.05$. In the familiar case of independence, it is clear that $\xi =$ 1–(0.95)(0.95) = 0.0975. However, under the assumption of perfect dependence ξ remains at 0.05.

In clinical trials, rarely does one have either a collection of prospectively declared primary analyses that are completely independent of one another, or, a set of *a priori* analyses that are perfectly dependent. Our goal is to examine the range of dependency between these two extremes, and then compute ξ and α_2 as needed. Since these two extremes reflect the full range of dependence, write

$$1 - \alpha_2 \leq P[T_2 = 0 | T_1 = 0] \leq 1. \tag{10}$$

Let the measure D^2, reflect this level of dependence, $0 \leq D^2 \leq 1$, $D = 0$ corresponds to the condition of independence between the statistical hypothesis tests, and $D = 1$ denotes perfect dependence, i.e., the case in which the conditional probability of interest $P[T_2 = 0 | \mathrm{T}_1 = 0]$ attains its maximum value of one. If we are to choose a value of D that will have the aforementioned properties, then we can write D in terms of the conditional probability

$$D = \sqrt{1 - \frac{(1 - P[T_2 = 0 | T_1 = 0])}{\alpha_2}}. \tag{11}$$

In general, we will not use Eq. (11) to compute D. Our ultimate goal is to supply the value of D, and then write the familywise error level in terms of D^2.

$$\begin{aligned} P[T_2 = 0 | T_1 = 0] &= (1 - \alpha_2) + D^2[1 - (1 - \alpha_2)] \\ &= 1 - \alpha_2(1 - D^2). \end{aligned} \tag{12}$$

The familywise error level for the two statistical hypothesis tests H_1 and H_2 may be written as

$$\begin{aligned} \xi &= 1 - P[T_2 = 0 \cap T_1 = 0] \\ \xi &= 1 - P[T_2 = 0 | T_1 = 0] P[T_1 = 0] \\ &= 1 - [1 - \alpha_2(1 - D^2)](1 - \alpha_1). \end{aligned} \tag{13}$$

Therefore, the familywise error is formulated in terms involving the test-specific α error rates α_1, α_2 where $\alpha_1 \geq \alpha_2$, and the dependency parameter D.

During the design phase of the trial, as investigators work to select the appropriate levels of the test-specific α error levels for the study, they can first fix ξ, and then choose α_1 and D, moving on to compute the acceptable range of α_2. This is easily accomplished, recalling the assumption that the hypothesis tests are ordered so that $\alpha_1 \geq \alpha_2$.

$$\alpha_2(\max) = \min\left[\alpha_1, \frac{\xi - \alpha_1}{(1-\alpha_1)(1-D^2)}\right]. \tag{14}$$

Equation (14) provides the maximum value of α_2 that will preserve the familywise error. Denote this maximum value as $\alpha_2(\max)$.

The case for $K = 3$ is a straightforward generalization of the consideration for two endpoints and we can carry forward the same nomenclature developed above. In that circumstance, we find

$$D_{3|1,2} = \sqrt{1 - \frac{(1 - P[T_3 = 0 | T_1 = 0 \cap T_2 = 0])}{\alpha_3}}. \tag{15}$$

$D_{3|1,2}$ measures the degree of dependence between H_3 given knowledge of H_1 and H_2, and

$$\alpha_3(\max) = \min\left[\alpha_2, \frac{1 - \{(1-\xi)/[1-\alpha_1][1-\alpha_2(1-D^2_{2|1})]\}}{1 - D^2_{3|1,2}}\right]. \tag{16}$$

Results for the circumstance for $K > 3$ are available.

12. Multiple comparisons and combined endpoints

A particularly useful application of multiple comparisons in epidemiology is in its interpretation of combined endpoints. A combined endpoint is a clinically relevant endpoint that is constructed from combinations of other clinically relevant endpoints, termed *component endpoints* or *composite endpoints*. Two examples of component endpoints are (1) the cumulative incidence of stroke and (2) the cumulative incidence of TIAs. In this case, a patient experiences a combined endpoint if they have either a stroke, a TIA, or both.

Combined endpoints are an important component of clinical research design. Their use can improve the resolving ability of the clinical research effort, strengthening its capacity to pick out weaker signals of effect from the background noise of sampling error. For example, a well-designed clinical trial that prospectively embeds a combined endpoint into its primary analysis plan can be appropriately powered to measure clinically relevant but small effects. However, combined endpoints are double-edged swords. In some circumstances, the combined endpoint can be exceedingly difficult to analyze in a straightforward, comprehensible manner. In addition, the components of the endpoint, if not carefully chosen, may produce a conglomerate endpoint that measures different but relatively unrelated aspects of the same disease process. The medical community's resultant difficulty in understanding the meaning of this unbalanced combined endpoint can cast a shadow over the effect of the clinical trial's intervention.

12.1. Combined endpoint construction

In order to usefully and accurately depict the relationship between the exposure and the disease, a combined endpoint must be carefully constructed. The important properties of a combined endpoint can be described as (1) coherence, (2) endpoint equivalence, and (3) effect homogeneity.

Coherence means that the component endpoints from which the combined endpoint is constructed should measure the same underlying pathophysiology process and be consistent with the best understanding of the causes of the disease. Consideration of coherence requires an examination of the degree to which different component endpoints may measure related pathology. The components need not be mutually exclusive, nor should they be coincident, but should measure different but closely related manifestations of the same disease. An example would be the combined endpoint of congestive heart failure (CHF), death + CHF hospitalization.

The *equivalence assumption*, i.e., each of the component endpoints has the same set of clinical implications, while commonly clinically indefensible, must be considered in the construction of the combined endpoint. Its necessity arises from the absence of optimal analysis tools for combined endpoints. The state-of-the-art statistical analyses of component endpoints which are either continuous or dichotomous is well described and easily executed (Meinert, 1986; Piantadosi, 1997). However, the analysis for combinations of these endpoints is complex, commonly making untenable assumptions.

As an illustration, consider a clinical trial whose prospectively defined combined endpoint is assembled from two dichotomous component endpoints, death and hospitalization. The commonly accepted analysis in this setting is the duration of time until the first event. The patient is considered to have met the criteria for the combined endpoint (said to have "reached" the combined endpoint) if they have either died during the course of the trial, or the patient survived the trial but was hospitalized during the study. In the case of a patient who is hospitalized and then dies during the clinical trial, only the first endpoint is counted.

While this analysis is useful, it makes the explicit assumption that each of the two components of this combined endpoint is analytically equivalent to the other. This is the equivalence feature of the combined endpoint. Whether a patient meets the hospitalization part of the endpoint or the mortality part of the endpoint doesn't matter as far as the analysis is concerned. Nevertheless, hospitalization is in general not the same as death. This equivalence is a clinically troubling assumption and can complicate acceptability of the combined endpoint. Of course, there are alternative algorithms available that would provide different "weights" for the occurrence of the various component endpoints of a combined endpoint. For example, one might assume that for the combined endpoint of death or hospitalization, a death is w times as influential as a hospitalization. However, it is very difficult for investigators to reach a consensus on the correct weighting scheme to use, and any selection of weights that the investigators choose that is different from equal weighting of the components can be difficult to defend.

The analysis complexities deepen when continuous and dichotomous component endpoints are joined into a combined endpoint. Although complicated analysis procedures that address this issue have been developed (Moyé et al., 1992); these endpoints can be difficult to understand and their acceptance by the medical community is guarded at best (Transcript, 1993). Investigators are better off by choosing components whose clinical implications are as close to equivalence as possible.

The effect homogeneity concept addresses the purported relationship between the exposure and the combined endpoint. In general, it is assumed that the relationship between the exposure or intervention being assessed in the study and each component endpoint is the same.

12.2. Multiple comparisons and combined endpoints

An example of the incorporation of dependency between two prospectively declared statistical endpoints in a clinical trial could be embedded into its design is that of the CURE (Clopidogrel in Unstable Angina to Prevent Recurrent Events) trial (Trials Investigators, 2001). CURE examined the role of thienopyridine derivatives in preventing death and cardiovascular events in patients with unstable angina pectoris or acute coronary syndrome. To test the benefit of these thienopyridine derivatives, a clinical trial was designed to examine the effect of the oral anti-coagulation agent clopidogrel when compared to standard care for patients at risk of acute coronary syndrome.

CURE was a randomized, double-blind, placebo-controlled trial with two arms. Patients who had been hospitalized with acute coronary syndromes within 24 h of their symptoms but who did not demonstrate evidence of ST-segment elevation on their electrocardiograms were recruited. All of these patients received the standard care for this condition including the administration of aspirin. In addition, patients randomized to the active arm of the study received clopidogrel, while patients in the control group arm received placebo therapy.

The investigators prospectively designed this study for the analysis of two primary endpoints. The first primary endpoint was a combination of death from cardiovascular causes, or the occurrence of a nonfatal myocardial infarction (MI) or a nonfatal stroke. The second primary endpoint consisted of the first primary endpoint or the occurrence of refractory ischemia.[9] Thus, a patient meets the criteria for this second prospectively defined primary endpoint if (1) they meet the criteria for the first, or (2) they do not meet the criteria for the first primary endpoint, but they have refractory ischemia. Secondary outcomes included severe ischemia, heart failure, and the need for revascularization.

The idea of dependency between the two primary endpoints is an admissible one. However, the level of dependence requires some discussion. Certainly, if there are very few patients with recurrent ischemia, then the second primary endpoint is the same as the first, and we would expect strong dependence between

[9] Refractory ischemia was defined as recurrent chest pain lasting more than 5 min with new ischemic electrocardiographic changes while the patient was receiving "optimal" medical therapy.

the two hypothesis tests. However, if there are many patients who have recurrent ischemia, knowledge of a type I error for the first primary endpoint will provide less information about the probability of a type I error for the second primary endpoint, and the measure of dependency is reduced.[10]

The investigators in CURE utilized selected $\alpha_1 = 0.045$ and $\alpha_2 = 0.010$. Use of the Bonferroni approximation reveals that $\xi = 1-(1 - 0.045)(1-0.010) = 0.065$, suggesting that if the overall type I error was to be 0.05 then there was some conservation of the type I error through dependency. Apply formula, i.e., Eq. (13) and solving for the dependency parameter D, we find

$$D = \sqrt{1 - \frac{1}{\alpha_2}\left[1 - \frac{1-\xi}{1-\alpha_1}\right]}.$$

Using $\alpha_1 = 0.045$, $\alpha_2 = 0.010$, and $\xi = 0.05$, reveals $D = 0.69$. Thus, the CURE investigators assume a moderate level of dependency between the two primary endpoints for their study design. While the investigators do not tell us the degree of dependency between these two primary endpoint analyses, they do state that "partitioning the α maintains an overall level of 0.05 after adjustment for the overlap between the two sets of outcomes." An alternative analysis plan has also been provided in the literature (Berger, 2002).

As an example of how dependency might be used in the assessment of the effect of therapy for the evaluation of effect measures for a combined endpoint, consider the circumstances of investigators interested in assessing the effect of an intervention to reduce the occurrence of upper gastrointestinal (UGI) disease. They define the combined endpoint of the occurrence of UGI illness, consisting of either (1) fatal or nonfatal (UGI) bleed, or (2) fatal or nonfatal UGI obstruction. The investigators wish to assess the effect of the intervention on the rate of UGI illness as defined by these endpoints, allocating type I error across these three assessments in order to conserve the familywise error. During the design phase of the study, they carry out a simple sample size computation (Table 2).

Table 2 reports the cumulative control group events rates for the combined endpoint (Combined UGI illness) and each of its component endpoints. The size of the study would need to be at least 3867 patients if the investigators desire adequate power for each of the three analyses. However, the type I error has not been conserved across all three evaluations.

The investigators next conserve the FWER, applying a Bonferroni style adjustment (Table 3).

In this circumstance, the majority of the type I error is allocated for the first combined endpoint analysis, leaving a residual α error rate of 0.010 to be distributed among its two component endpoints (each of which is itself a combined

[10] For example, there could be a strong beneficial effect of therapy for the first primary endpoint. However, a large number of patients with recurrent ischemia and the absence of a beneficial effect of this therapy on recurrent ischemia could produce a different finding for this second primary endpoint. The occurrence of a type I error for the first primary endpoint would shed no light on the probability of the type I error for the second primary endpoint in this circumstance.

Table 2
Alpha allocation example for therapy effect on UGI illness: Scenario 1

Primary Analyses	Cumulative Control Group Event Rate	Efficacy	Alpha (two-tailed)	Power	Sample Size
Combined UGI illness	0.300	0.20	0.050	0.90	2291
Fatal/nonfatal bleed	0.200	0.20	0.050	0.90	3867
Fatal/nonfatal obstruction	0.200	0.20	0.050	0.90	3867

No attempt has been made to adjust the familywise error rate.

Table 3
Alpha allocation example for therapy effect on UGI illness: Scenario 2

Primary Analyses	Cumulative Control Group Event Rate	Efficacy	Alpha (two-tailed)	Power	Sample Size
Combined UGI illness	0.300	0.20	0.040	0.90	2425
Fatal/nonfatal bleed	0.200	0.20	0.005	0.90	6152
Fatal/nonfatal obstruction	0.200	0.20	0.005	0.90	6152

Bonferroni procedure has been applied, with a consequent increase in sample size.

endpoint). The reduction in the type I error rate for each specific test produces a dramatic increase in sample size.

However, the investigators recognize the dependency between the combined endpoint and each of its composite endpoints. They choose the measure of dependency between the evaluation of the fatal/nonfatal bleed and the combined UGI illness endpoint, $D_{2|1} = 0.80$, and the measure of dependency between these first two evaluations, and the third, $D_{3|1,2} = 0.90$. Using Eq. (14) they compute the maximum type I error available for the evaluation of the two component endpoints is 0.029. Of this they allocate 0.020 to the effect of therapy on the fatal/nonfatal bleed evaluation. Using Eq. (16) they have 0.017 type I error rate for the allocation of the effect of therapy on the cumulative incidence of fatal/nonfatal obstruction (Table 4).

From Table 4, we observe that the test-specific type I error levels are substantially higher for each of the three specific evaluations. In addition, the larger type I error rates decrease the required size of the study from 6152 to 4949, a 20% reduction. Thus, the direction incorporation of dependency within the statistical inference structure of the combined endpoint has produced a substantial reduction in sample size, in addition to the increased type I error levels for each of the combined endpoint's components.

12.3. Conclusions on combined endpoints

The implementation of combined endpoints in clinical trials holds both promise and danger. A carefully constructed combined endpoint can helpfully broaden the

Table 4
Alpha allocation example for therapy effect on UGI illness: Scenario 3

Primary Analyses	Cumulative Control Group Event Rate	Efficacy	Alpha (two-tailed)	Power	Sample Size
			$D = 0.050$		
Combined UGI illness	0.300	0.20	0.040	0.90	2425
			$D = 0.80$		
Fatal/nonfatal bleed	0.200	0.20	0.020	0.90	4790
			$D = 0.90$		
Fatal/nonfatal obstruction	0.200	0.20	0.017	0.90	4949

definition of a clinical endpoint when the disease being studied has different clinical consequences. This expansion commonly increases the incidence rate of the endpoint, reducing the sample size of the trial. Alternatively, if the larger sample size is maintained, the combined endpoint serves to decrease the sensitivity of the experiment to detect moderate levels of therapy effectiveness. However, if the combined endpoint is too broad it can become un-interpretable and ultimately meaningless to the medical and regulatory communities. Thus, the combined endpoint should be broad and simultaneously retain its interpretability. Additionally, there should be some experimental evidence or at least theoretical motivation justifying the expectation that the effect to be studied will have the same effect on each of the component endpoints of the combined endpoint.

These can be elaborated as a collection of principles, adapted from.

Principle 1. Both the combined endpoint and each of its component endpoints must be clinically relevant and prospectively specified in detail (*principle of prospective deployment*).

Principle 2. Each component of the combined endpoint must be carefully chosen to add coherence to the combined endpoint. The component endpoint that is under consideration must not be so similar to other components that it adds nothing new to the mixture of component endpoints make up the combined endpoint; yet, it should not be so dissimilar that it provides a measure which is customarily not clinically linked to the other component endpoints (*principle of coherence*).

Principle 3. The component endpoints that constitute the combined endpoint are commonly given the same weight in the statistical analysis of the clinical trial. Therefore, each of the component endpoints must be measured with the same scrupulous attention to detail. For each component endpoint, it is important to provide documentation not just that the endpoint occurred, but also to confirm the absence of the component endpoint (*principle of precision*).

Principle 4. The analysis of the effect of therapy on the combined endpoint should be accompanied by a tabulation of the effect of the therapy for each of the component endpoints. This allows the reader to determine if there has been any domination of the combined endpoint by any one of its components, or if the findings of the effect of therapy for component endpoints are not consistent (*principle of full disclosure*).

13. Multiple comparisons and subgroup analyses

Well-trained research investigators diligently work to identify every potentially valuable result. Having invested great time and effort in their studies, these scientists want and need to examine the data systematically and completely. They are well aware that interesting findings await them in non-prospectively declared analyses. Commonly, investigators believe that, like real gems, these tantalizing surprises lie just below the surface, hidden from view, waiting to be unearthed.

In addition, others can also raise intriguing questions concerning the investigators' analyses. In the process of publication, journal reviewers and editors will sometimes ask that additional analyses be carried out. These analyses can include considering the effect of the exposure in subsets of the data. Similar inquiries can come from the manuscript's readers.

The research program's cost-effectiveness and the investigator's desire for thoroughness require that all facets of a research effort's data be thoroughly examined. However, as we have seen, the need to protect the community from the dissemination of mistaken results from research programs can collide with the need to make maximum use of the data that has been so carefully collected. These problems are exemplified in subgroup analyses.

13.1. Definitions

A subgroup analysis is the evaluation of the exposure–disease relationship within a fraction of the recruited subjects. While the concept of subgroup analyses is straightforward, the terminology can sometimes be confusing.

A *subgroup* is the description of patient-based characteristic, e.g., gender that can be subdivided into categories. For example, if an investigator is interested in creating a gender subgroup, patients are classified into one of two groups – male or female. These groups are referred to as levels or *strata*. There is one stratum for each category.

The traditional subgroup analysis is an evaluation of the effect of therapy within each of the subgroup strata. In a gender-based subgroup, the subgroup analysis consists of an evaluation of the exposure for males and then for females. Thus, each stratum analysis generates its own effect size, standard error, confidence interval, and p-value.

A critical preliminary task in subgroup analysis is the proper classification of patients into each of the subgroup strata. Although membership determination may appear to be a trivial task, there are circumstances in which this classification is problematic. These concerns revolve around the timing of the subgroup membership determination.

There are two important possibilities for determination of the timing of subgroup membership. The first is the classification of patients into the correct subgroup stratum when the patients are randomized. The second choice is to classify patients into subgroup strata at some time during the execution of the study. While each has advantages, the determination of subgroup membership at the beginning of the study is preferred.

Determining subgroup membership at the beginning of the trial requires that not only must the subgroup be defined at the beginning of the study, but also subgroup strata membership should be defined prospectively as well. This is a straightforward procedure to apply to the gender subgroup with its two strata. However, for other subgroups of clinical interest, the process can be complex. For example, consider a clinical trial that assesses the effect of an agent that reduces cholesterol levels on stroke. In this case, it is relatively easy to evaluate the relationship between baseline cholesterol level strata (1) less than 175 mg/dl and (2) greater than or equal to 175 mg/dl and the cumulative incidence of stroke. However, the evaluation of these strata when they are based on follow-up levels of cholesterol is problematic.

The problems arise for two reasons. The first is that patients can change subgroup strata as the study progresses and their cholesterol levels fluctuate. By making it difficult to definitively and convincingly determine subgroup membership, the analysis can suffer from the observation that changing the subgroup membership of just a few patients can change the results of the subgroup analysis. Such brittle evaluations are unpersuasive.

Second, there are many influences that affect lipid measurements over time. If the exposure being evaluated reduces cholesterol levels, then patients with lower cholesterol levels are more likely to have received active therapy, and patients with the higher levels would have a greater chance of being in the control group. Thus, the evaluation of lipid levels will be confounded with exposure to the agents after the study was initiated, confusing the attribution of the observed effect on the endpoint.

There were many factors that influence baseline lipid levels. Race/ethnicity, gender, family history, prior treatment are but a few of them. However, the randomly assigned intervention did not influence baseline LDL-cholesterol levels. It is the absence of any relationship between the randomly allocated therapy and the baseline LDL-cholesterol level that allows a clear examination of the effect of LDL-cholesterol level on the relationship between the intervention and stroke. A subgroup whose strata membership criteria are based on baseline characteristics of the patient is called a *proper subgroup* (Yusuf et al., 1991). Improper subgroups are those whose strata membership can only be determined after the patient has been randomized. Because membership based on follow-up data can be influenced by the randomly allocated therapy, the interpretation of these results is complicated.

Despite the problems posed by improper subgroup evaluations, there are circumstances in which this type of analysis is nevertheless carried out. If the investigators are interested in an evaluation of the effect of lower blood pressure on the incidence of stroke, regardless of how the blood pressure was lowered, then analysis procedures are available.[11] However, these evaluations are exceedingly complicated and the results must be interpreted with great caution. Similar evaluations have examined the relationship between lipid lowering and atherosclerotic morbidity and mortality (Pedersen, 1998; West of Scotland, 1996; Sacks et al., 1998).

Finally, we will hold aside the issue of the analysis of a proper subgroup defined *post hoc*. In that circumstance, the subgroup criteria using baseline variables is defined at the end of the study. Since the subgroup analysis was planned after the data were examined, the analysis is exploratory.

13.2. "Intention-to-treat" versus "as treated"

The proper versus improper subgroup analyses frameworks adds another level of complication to the multiple analysis problem, complicating the result interpretation. Perhaps the most commonly occurring example of proper versus improper subgroup analyses in clinical trials is the distinction between "intention-to-treat" versus the "as treated" evaluations. Consider a clinical trial in which patients are randomized to receive an intervention to reduce the total mortality rate from end stage renal disease. At the inception of the study, patients are randomized to receive either control group therapy or the intervention. At the conclusion of the study, the investigators will compare the cumulative mortality rates of patients in each of the two treatment groups. However, at the end of the study, how will the investigators decide what patients should be assigned to each group in the final analysis? The commonly used approach is to assign treatment group membership simply as the group to which the patient was randomized. This is the "intention-to-treat" principle.

The "intention-to-treat" principle of analysis is the standard analysis procedure for the evaluation of clinical trial results. Undoubtedly, this analysis tends to be a conservative one, since not every patient is treated as they were "intended." For example, some patients randomized to the active group may not take their medication. These patients, although randomized to the active group, will have the control group experience and will therefore produce endpoints at rates similar to that of the control group. However, they would be included in the active group since they were randomized to and "intended to be treated" like active group patients. The inclusion of these patients in the active group for analysis purposes tends to make the active group experience look more like the control group experience, increasing the overall active group event rate.[12]

Similarly, patients who are randomized to the control group may nevertheless be exposed to active group medication. These patients will experience event rates similar to the rates of the active group, but since they are considered as part of the

[11] Cox hazard analysis with time dependent covariates has been one useful tool in this regard.

[12] There are occasional complications in an "intention-to-treat" analysis. In some cases, a patient is tested and randomized, but then, subsequent to the randomization the test result reveals that the patient is not eligible for the trial for a prospectively stated reason. In this case, there was no "intent" to randomize this patient when the test result was known, and the patient is removed from the study.

control group, the inclusion of these patients will produce an event rate for the control group that is closer to that of the active group.

Thus, the control group rate will approach that of the active group, while the cumulative event rate in the active group will be closer to that of the control group (described in the previous paragraph). This effect of these combined rate alterations reduces the magnitude of the treatment effect, thereby diminishing the power of the clinical trial.

An alternative analysis to the "intent to treat" principle is one that analyzes the endpoint results using an "as-treated" analysis. In this case, although patients are still randomized to receive either placebo or active therapy, they are classified for analysis purposes based on whether they actually took their medication or not. Since this is determined after the patient was randomized to the medication, and the effect (both perceived beneficial effects, and adverse effects) of the medication may determine whether the patient takes the medication, the "as-treated" evaluation is a confounded analysis. A clearly detailed examination of this issue is available (Peduzzi et al., 1993). The "as-treated" analysis complicates the subgroup analysis interpretation.

13.3. Interpretation difficulties

The analysis of subgroups is a popular, necessary, and controversial component of the complete evaluation of a research effort. Indeed, it is difficult to find a manuscript that reports the results of a large observational study or clinical trial that does not report findings within selected subgroups.

Subgroup analyses as currently utilized in clinical research are tantalizing and controversial. The results from subgroup assessments have traditionally been used to augment the persuasive power of a clinical research effort's overall results by demonstrating the uniform effect of the therapy in patients with different demographic and risk factor profiles. This uniformity leads to the development of easily understood and implemented rules to guide the use of therapy.[13] Some research efforts have reported these results in the manuscript announcing the trial's overall results (Pfeffer et al., 1992; Sacks et al., 1996; SHEP, 1991; LIPID Study Group, 1998). Others have separate manuscripts dealing exclusively with subgroup analyses (Moyé et al., 1994; Lewis et al., 1998a, b). Such subgroup analyses potentially provide new information about an unanticipated benefit (or hazard) of the exposure of interest on the effect measure.

However useful and provocative these results can be, it is well established that subgroup analyses are often misleading (Peto et al., 1995; MRFIT, 1982; ISIS, 1986; Lee et al., 1980). Assmann et al. (2000) has demonstrated how commonly subgroup analyses are misused, while others point out the dangers of accepting subgroup analyses as confirmatory (Bulpitt, 1988). A fine example of the

[13] The finding that a particular lipid lowering drug works better in women than in men can complicate the already complex decisions that practitioners must make as the number of available compounds increase.

misleading effects of subgroup analyses is in the PRAISE I and II clinical trials, in which a subgroup evaluation, raised to prominence (Packer et al., 1996) could not be confirmed (Packer, 2000).

Nevertheless, the medical community continues to be tantalized by spectacular subgroup findings from clinical trials. A recent example is the subgroup analysis-based suggestion that medication efficacy is a function of race; this has appeared in both peer-reviewed journals (Exner et al., 2001; Yancy et al., 2001) and the lay press (Stolberg, 2001).

13.4. Effect domination principle

The examination of individual subgroup strata effects in health care research can be misleading for reasons that have been elaborated. If we cannot believe the event rates that are present in the stratum are the best measures of that stratum's response to the exposure, then what is the best measure of the effect of an exposure on a subgroup stratum?

Some illumination is provided in the following example. An auditorium that can seat 300 people is divided down the middle into two sections of seats, with 150 on each of the left and right side of the room. Three hundred occupants seat themselves as they choose, distributing themselves in an unrestricted manner among all the seats in the auditorium. When all are seated, we measure the height of each person, finding that the average height is exactly 68 in. Does that mean that the average height of those seated on the left-hand side of the classroom will be 68 in? Because the 68 in measurement was produced from all 300 attendees in the room, not just the 150 on the left-hand side, we would expect the average height of those seated on the left side of the room would not be 68 in.

However, if the average height of the occupants on the left-hand side of the classroom is greater than 68 inches, then those seated on the right-hand side must have an average height less than 68 inches. Thus, those sitting on the left-hand side have a greater height than those on the right-hand side. While the fact is undeniable in this one auditorium during this one seating, it would of course be inappropriate to generalize this conclusion to the population at large. The random aggregation of observations has induced a subgroup effect that is based only on the play of chance here. Specifically, the "subgroup effect" was induced by selectively excluding individuals from the computation of the mean. The best predictor of the height of the occupants seated on the left side of the room is in general the average height of all attendees.

Allowing the overall measure of effect in the entire cohort to dominate the subgroup stratum effects can be termed the *effect domination principle* and is attributable to Yusuf et al. (1991).

This principle of effect domination is not very provocative, containing little of the excitement of exploratory analyses. However, it is far more reliable, given the general non-confirmatory analyses that the majority of subgroup analyses in health care results constitute.

13.5. Confirmatory subgroup analyses and multiple comparisons

Since subgroup analyses have and will, in all likelihood, continue to engender the interest of the medical community, it is logical to ask why there are not more confirmatory analyses involving subgroup evaluations. This is an especially interesting question since there are clear circumstances in which subgroup evaluations can produce confirmatory results of the therapy effect within (or across) subgroup strata. When executed, these confirmatory results stand on their own, separate and apart from the result of the effect of therapy in the overall cohort. The criteria for these evaluations are readily identified.

The first of these criteria for the development of confirmatory analyses in clinical trials is that the subgroup analysis must be prospectively designed and proper. This structure is required so that (1) the therapy effect size estimators that the subgroup analysis produces are trustworthy; and (2) that the effect of therapy to be evaluated in a subgroup is not confounded by (i.e., bound up with) post-randomization events. In general, there has been no difficulty with meeting this requirement of confirmatory subgroup analyses. Many clinical trials make statements in their protocols describing the plans of investigators to evaluate the effect of therapy within their subgroups of interest. These subgroups are, by and large, proper subgroups, e.g., demographic traits.

However, the final requirement for a confirmatory subgroup analysis is the prospective allocation of type I and type II error rates in the setting of adequate power. This last criterion has proved to be especially troublesome because of the severe sample size constraints this places on subgroup analyses. As we have pointed out earlier, the allocation of type I error rates for confirmatory testing must be such that the FWER, ξ, is conserved. This requires that statistical testing at the level of subgroup analyses will be governed by test-specific α error rates that are generally less than 0.05.

The difficulty of executing subgroup analyses in the presence of FWER control and adequate statistical power is not difficult to understand. In fact, resources are generally strained to the breaking point for the analysis of the effect of therapy in the overall cohort. This overall analysis is typically carried out with the minimum acceptable power (80%) because of either financial constraints or patient recruitment difficulties. By definition, subgroup analyses (and certainly within-stratum subgroup analyses) will involve a smaller number of patients; it is a daunting task to prospectively allocate type I and type II error rates at acceptable levels in a smaller number of patients, although the methodology for the accurate computation of sample size is available (Neyman, 1938). Thus, the growth of the use of subgroups as confirmatory tools has, to some extent, been stunted by the difficulty of constructing a prospective clinical trial with an embedded, prospectively defined proper subgroup for which tight statistical control is provided for type I and type II statistical errors.

13.6. Assessment of subgroup effects

The evaluation of subgroup effects in clinical trials focuses on the effect of the randomly allocated therapy on the subgroup of interest. However, this assessment can be carried out in two complementary manners. The first is the determination of a differential effect of therapy across subgroup strata. The second is the evaluation of the effect of therapy within a single subgroup stratum. Each approach, when prospectively planned and concordantly executed, can supplement the information provided by the evaluation of the main effect of a clinical trial.

We commonly think of the effect of the randomly allocated intervention in a clinical trial as an effect across the entire research cohort. The examination of a dataset for this effect, while complicated, has become a routine part of the evaluation of the randomly allocated therapy's influence in a clinical trial. The finding of both clinical and statistical significance for this analysis suggests that the effect of therapy is different for one subgroup stratum than for another.

This type of subgroup effect is commonly referred to as a *treatment by subgroup* interaction (exposure by subgroup interaction); a notable product of this analysis is the *p*-value for interaction. Typically, the analysis result is described as identifying how the subgroup strata interacts with the therapy to alter the occurrence of the endpoint, and the evaluation is called an *interaction analysis*. Alternatively, this approach is described as *effect modification*, i.e., it examines the degree to which the subgroup stratum modifies the effect of treatment on the endpoint.

We should not be surprised by the observation that statistically significant effect modification analyses in research are uncommon. The subgroup analyses involve an evaluation of an effect difference between smaller subsets of patients within the research cohort. Everything else being equal, the smaller sample sizes reduce the statistical power of the hypothesis tests. Since, the presence of a test statistic that does not fall in the critical region in a low power environment is not a null finding, but merely an uninformative one, many of these subgroup analyses are unhelpful and not generalizable.

13.7. Within-stratum effects

The evaluation of a subgroup-mediated effect modification may not directly address the question the investigators have raised about the subgroup. This is because the investigators' interest may not be in the entire subgroup, but only in selected subgroup strata. Specifically, the investigators may not ask whether the effect of therapy is the same across subgroup strata, but instead ask whether there is an explicit effect of the intervention in the prospectively defined subgroup stratum of interest. This is a different question than that addressed by an interaction analysis.

One such situation would be when the stratum is composed of patients who have a very different prognosis from that of patients in other strata of the subgroup. While investigators may be most interested in the effect of a new intervention on thyroid cancer, they may be particularly interested in the effect of the therapy in patients with an advanced stage of the disease. This interest does not require the investigators to ask whether the effect of therapy in patients with less advanced thyroid cancer is different from that of patients with advanced thyroid cancer; they simply desire confirmatory evidence that the therapy has explicit efficacy in patients with advanced thyroid cancer. Similarly, a new therapy for the treatment of CHF may hold promise for reducing mortality in all patients with CHF, but the investigator is motivated to demonstrate the effect of this therapy in patients with CHF whose etiology is non-ischemic. She is not interested in comparing or contrasting the efficacy of the intervention between ischemic versus non-ischemic etiologies of CHF. She is instead focused on two questions: (1) Is the therapy effective in the entire cohort and (2) Can the effect of this therapy be confirmed in the subcohort with CHF–non-ischemic etiology?

This approach begs the question of whether the therapy could be effective in the entire cohort but not the subcohort of interest. In order to address this, consider the possibility that the therapy in fact is effective for patients with CHF–ischemic etiology but ineffective for patients with a non-ischemic etiology for their CHF. Let the research sample primarily contain patients with CHF–ischemic etiology, with only a small number of patients who have a non-ischemic etiology for their heart failure. Since the research sample contains primarily those patients who will respond to the therapy, the result of the concordantly executed clinical trial will be positive (barring an effect that is driven by sampling error). The investigator will then argue that, since the trial is positive, this positive finding will apply to the CHF–non-ischemic subgroup as well. Essentially, the conclusion about the non-ischemic subcohort is based primarily on the findings of patients who are not in that subcohort at all. This is the consequence of the effect domination principle, in which the findings in the overall cohort devolve on each of the subgroup strata. In this example, the principle produces the wrong conclusion; nevertheless, it is the best conclusion available in the absence of a confirmatory subgroup analysis. In order to avoid this possibility, the investigator is interested in reaching a confirmatory conclusion about the population of patients with non-ischemic etiology for their CHF.

As another illustration of a circumstance in which prospectively specified, stratum-specific subgroup analyses can make an important contribution, consider the situation in which the adverse event profile of a therapy that is being studied in a controlled clinical trial is known to be different between women and men. As an illustration, consider a cholesterol-reducing drug that produces pre-malignant breast disease in women. In this circumstance, the risk–benefit profile of this drug is different for women than it is for men. Since women will be exposed to a greater risk with this therapy, it is reasonable to require investigators to produce a statistically valid demonstration of efficacy in women. The investigators are not disinterested in an effect in men; however, the relatively low risk of the drug in men allows the investigators to be satisfied with deducing the effect of the therapy in men from the effect of therapy in the overall cohort. It is the greater adverse event risk in women that requires an explicit demonstration of efficacy in them.

13.8. Multiple comparisons and designing confirmatory subgroup analyses

In designing confirmatory subgroup analyses, the investigators have several tools at their disposal. A common assumption in clinical research development is that the design parameters necessary for the computation for clinical trials are the same in all subgroup strata. However, the information is commonly available to the investigators that would lead to other conclusions. For example, event rate differences can be well established across subgroup strata. These differential event rates will have an important impact on the computed sample size.

Another design parameter that investigators have complete control over is efficacy. The investigators choose this measure of effect size, being guided by the twin concerns of research community standard and resource constraints for the execution of the clinical trial. However, the occurrence of serious adverse events at different frequencies across the subgroup strata affects the computation of efficacy. By shifting the level or risk in the risk–benefit calculation, the level of efficacy may need to be greater in the subgroup strata with the greatest adverse events.

Just as we recognized that the execution of prospectively defined analyses for a combined endpoint and its component endpoints was a research environment in which dependency between statistical hypothesis tests was very likely, we can easily see that this same concept of dependency can be applied to a collection of well-designed hypothesis tests carried out in both an entire cohort of patients as well as in a subgroup of them. Developments in dependent hypothesis testing can be employed in generating confirmatory subgroup analyses. We can write the dependency parameter D as $D = c$, where c is the proportion of patients in the entire cohort that are included in the subgroup stratum of interest.

These features can be used to compute the sample size required for a confirmatory analysis in each of the overall cohort and the subgroup of interest in the study, producing useful measures of within-stratum effects.

As an example of the use of these features, consider the circumstance of investigators interested in demonstrating the effect of a medication, which has anti-platelet activity in patients with essential hypertension. The investigators plan to recruit patients with essential hypertension, and then randomly assign them to one of two arms; the control arm or the active medication arm. Patients who are randomized to the control arm will receive instruction on adjustment of their lifestyle (including exercise, diet and sodium chloride control, smoking cessation, and stress management). They will then have their essential hypertension managed using a standard anti-hypertensive regimen. These control group subjects will also receive a placebo pill that they must take each day.

Patients who are randomized to the active treatment arm receive control group therapy plus, instead of the placebo, the anti-platelet agent which they must take every day for the duration of the trial. The trial designers believe that they will be able to recruit approximately 7000 patients for this trial.

The primary endpoint of this study will be the combined endpoint of fatal and nonfatal stroke. However, the anti-platelet agent is known to be associated with a different constellation of adverse events in elderly patients (including but not limited to bleeding). The investigators have a prospective interest in demonstrating that the benefits of anti-platelet therapy justify its use in this higher risk subcohort. Thus, they prospectively design two primary analyses in this study: (1) the effect of the anti-platelet agent on the cumulative incidence rate of fatal/nonfatal stroke in the entire cohort, and (2) the effect of the anti-platelet agent on the fatal/nonfatal stroke rate in the elderly cohort (Table 5).

The investigators have assumed a control group cumulative event rate of 12%. An initial examination of the efficacy issue in the total cohort leads the investigators to the assessment that the minimum clinical efficacy is 20%. For their first evaluation, the trial designers assume that the minimum clinical efficacy is the same for the elderly subcohort.

The sample size computation of Table 5 reveals that over 7020 patients are not only required for the evaluation of therapy effect in the total population, but 7020 patients are required for the evaluation in the elderly population as well. This is the classic conundrum of sample size computations in subgroups. In general, the investigators believe they will only be able to recruit 2500 elderly patients.

However, the researchers now bring several aspects of the subgroup characteristics to bear to plan for the prospective multiple analysis. The first is that the event rate is observed to be larger in the subgroup of elderly patients than in the overall cohort. Second, the investigators required a larger efficacy in the elderly patients to help offset the greater frequency of adverse events associated with the therapy. In addition, statistical dependency can be built into the structure of the evaluation. It is anticipated that 30% of the entire subcohort will be elderly. Thus, the dependency parameter is $D_s = 0.30$. In addition, the investigators have reduced the power of the elderly evaluation to 85%. (Table 6).

In this evaluation, a confirmatory evaluation is now available for the effect of therapy in each of the overall cohort, and the subgroup of the elderly.

Numerous examples and scenarios of the execution of subgroup stratum-specific analyses are available.

Table 5
Design paramters for stroke trial: Demonstration 1

Primary Analyses	Cohort	Cumulative Control Group Event Rate	Efficacy	Alpha (two-tailed)	Power	Sample Size
Fatal/nonfatal stroke	Total	0.120	0.20	0.050	0.90	7020
Fatal/nonfatal stroke	Elderly	0.120	0.20	0.050	0.90	7020

Table 6
Design paramters for stroke trial: Demonstration 1

Primary Analyses	Cohort	Cumulative Control Group Event Rate	Efficacy	Alpha (two-tailed)	Power	Sample Size
Fatal/nonfatal stroke	Total	0.120	0.20	0.035	0.90	7677
				$D = 0.300$		
Fatal/nonfatal stroke	Elderly	0.150	0.30	0.017	0.85	2562

14. Data dredging

Data dredging is the methodological examination of a database for all significant relationships. These database evaluations are thorough, and the analysis procedures are wide ranging, spanning the gamut from simple *t*-testing to more complex time-to-event evaluations, repeated measures assessments, and structure equation modeling. Typically, little thought is given to endpoint triage or the conservation of type I error rates across analyses.

The notion that, if they look hard enough, work long enough, and dig deep enough they will turn up something "significant" in the database drives the data dredger. Indeed, the investigators may identify a relationship that will ultimately be of great value to the medical community. However, while it is possible to discover a jewel in this strip mining operation, for every rare jewel identified, there will be many false finds, fakes, and shams. As Miles pointed out, datasets that are tortured long enough will provide the answers that the investigators seek, whether the answers are helpful, truthful, or not.

Unfortunately, many of the important principles of good experimental methodology are missing in the direct examination of interesting subgroups. Inadequate sample size, poorly performing estimators, low power, and the generation of multiple *p*-values combine to create an environment in which the findings of the data dredging operation are commonly not generalizable. Accepting the "significant" results of these data dredging activities can misdirect researchers into expending critical research resources in fruitless pursuits, a phenomenon described by Johnson. In his 1849 text *Experimental Agriculture*, Johnson stated that a badly conceived experiment was not only wasted time and money, but leads to both the adoption of incorrect results and the neglect of further research along more productive lines. It can therefore take tremendous effort for the medical and research community to sort out the wheat from the data-dredged chaff, often at great expense.

References

Adams, C. (2002). At FDA, approving cancer treatments can be an ordeal. *The Wall Street Journal* December 11, 1.

Anonymous (1988). Evidence of cause and effect relationship in major epidemiologic study disputed by judge. *Epidemiology Monitor* **9**, 1.

Assmann, S., Pocock, S., Enos, L., Kasten, L. (2000). Subgroup analysis and other (mis)uses of baseline data in clinical trials. *Lancet* **355**, 1064–1069.

Benjamini, Y., Hochberg, Y. (1995). Controlling the false discovery rate: A practical and powerful approach to multiple testing. *Journal of the Royal Statistical Society, Series B (Methodological)* **57**(1), 289–300.

Benjamini, Y., Yekutieli, D. (2001). The control of the false discovery rate in multiple testing under dependency. *The Annals of Statistics* **29**(4), 1165–1188.

Berger, V.W. (2002). Improving the information content of categorical clinical trial data. *Controlled Clinical Trials* **23**, 502–514.

Berkson, J. (1942a). Experiences with tests of significance. A reply to R.A. Fisher. *Journal of the American Statistical Association* **37**, 242–246.

Berkson, J. (1942b). Tests of significance considered as evidence. *Journal of the American Statistical Association* **37**, 335–345.

Bonferroni, C.E. (1935). Il calcolo delle assicurazioni su gruppi di teste. In *Studi in Onore del Professore Salvatore Ortu Carboni*. Rome, pp. 13–60.

Bonferroni, C.E. (1936). Teoria statistica delle classi e calcolo delle probabilità. *Pubblicazioni del R Istituto Superiore di Scienze Economiche e Commerciali di Firenze* **8**, 3–62.

Bulpitt, C. (1988). Subgroup Analysis. *Lancet* **2**, 31–34.

Dubey, S.D. (1985). Adjustment of *p*-values for multiplicities of intercorrelating symptoms. *Proceedings of the VIth International Society for Clinical Biostatisticians*, Germany.

Dunn, O.J. (1959). Confidence intervals for the means of dependent, normally distributed variables. *Journal of the American Statistical Association* **54**, 613–621.

Dunn, O.J. (1961). Multiple comparisons among means. *Journal of the American Statistical Association* **56**, 52–54.

Edwards, A. (1972). *Likelihood*. Cambridge University Press, Cambridge, UK.

Exner, D.V., Dreis, D.L., Domanski, M.J., Cohn, J.N. (2001). Lesser response to angiotensin–converting enzyme inhibitor therapy in black as compared to white patients with left ventricular dysfunction. *New England Journal of Medicine* **334**, 1351–1357.

Fisher, L. (1999). Carvedilol and the FDA approval process: The FDA paradigm and reflections upon hypotheses testing. *Controlled Clinical Trials* **20**, 16–39.

Fisher, R.A. (1925). *Statistical Methods for Research Workers*. Oliver and Boyd, Edinburg.

Fisher, R.A. (1926). The arrangement of field experiments. *Journal of the Ministry of Agriculture*(September), 503–513.

Fleiss, J.L. (1986a). Significance tests have a role in epidemiologic research; reactions to A.M. Walker. (Different views). *American Journal of Public Health* **76**, 559–560.

Fleiss, J.L. (1986b). Confidence intervals vs. significance tests: Quantitative interpretation. (Letter). *American Journal of Public Health* **76**, 587.

Fleiss, J.L. (1986c). Dr. Fleiss response (Letter). *American Journal of Public Health* **76**, 1033–1034.

Goodman, S.N. (1999). Toward evidence-based medical statistics. 1: The *p*-value fallacy. *Annals of Internal Medicine* **130**, 995–1004.

Hill, A.B. (1965). The environment and disease: Association or causation? *Proceedings of the Royal Society of Medicine* **58**, 295–300.

Hochberg, Y., Liberman, U. (1994). An extended Simes' test. *Statistics and Probability Letters* **21**, 101–105.

Hochberg, Y., Tamhane, A.C. (1987). *Multiple Comparison Procedures*. Wiley, New York.

Hochberg, Y., Westfall, P.H. (2000). On some multiplicity problems and multiple comparison procedures in biostatistics. In: Sen, P.K., Rao, C.R. (Eds.),**Vol. 18** *Handbook of Statistics*. Elsevier Sciences, pp. 75–113.

Holm, S. (1979). A simple sequentially rejective multiple test procedures. *Scandinavian Journal of Statistics* **6**, 65–70.

Hommel, G. (1988). A stepwise rejective multiple test procedure based on a modified Bonferroni test. *Biometrika* **75**, 383–386.

ISIS-1 Collaborative Group (1986). Randomized trial of intravenous atenolol among 16027 cases of suspected acute myocardial infarction–ISIS–1. *Lancet* **ii**, 57–66.

James, S. (1991). Approximate multinomial probabilities applied to correlated multiple endpoints in clinical trials. *Statistics in Medicine*, 1123–1135.

Lang, J.M., Rothman, K.J., Cann, D.I. (1998). That confounded *p*-value. *Epidemiology* **9**, 7–8.

Lee, K.L., McNeer, F., Starmer, C.F., Harris, P.J., Rosari, R.A. (1980). Clinical judgment and statistics. Lessons from a simulated randomized trial in coronary artery disease. *Circulation* **61**, 508–515.

Lewis, S.J., Moyé, L.A., Sacks, F.M., Johnstone, D.E., Timmis, G., Mitchell, J., Limacher, M., Kell, S., Glasser, S.P, Grant, J., Davis, B.R., Pfeffer, M.A., Braunwald, E. (1998a). Effect of pravastatin on cardiovascular events in older patients with myocardial infarction and cholesterol levels in the average range. Results of the cholesterol and recurrent events (CARE) trial. *Annals of Internal Medicine* **129**, 681–689.

Lewis, S.J., Sacks, F.M., Mitchell, J.S., East, C., Glasser, S., Kell, S., Letterer, R., Limacher, M., Moyé, L.A., Rouleau, J.L., Pfeffer, M.A., Braunwald, E. (1998b). Effect of pravastatin on cardiovascular events in women after myocardial infarction: The cholesterol and recurrent events (CARE) trial. *Journal of the American College of Cardiology* **32**, 140–146.

Meinert, C.L. (1986). *Clinical Trials Design, Conduct, and Analysis*. Oxford University Press, New York.

Miles, J.L. (1993). Data torturing. *New England Journal of Medicine* **329**, 1196–1199.

Miller, R.G. (1981). *Simultaneous Statistical Inference*, 2nd ed. Springer, New York.

Moyé, L.A. (1999). *p* value interpretation in clinical trials. The case for discipline. *Controlled Clinical Trials* **20**, 40–49.

Moyé, L.A. (2003). *Multiple Analyses in Clinical Trials: Fundamentals for Investigators*. Springer, New York.

Moyé, L.A., Abernethy, D. (1996). Carvedilol in patients with chronic heart failure (Letter). *New England Journal of Medicine* **335**, 1318–1319.

Moyé, L.A., Davis, B.R., Hawkins, C.M. (1992). Analysis of a clinical trial involving a combined mortality and adherence dependent interval censored endpoint. *Statistics in Medicine* **11**, 1705–1717.

Moyé, L.A., Pfeffer, M.A., Wun, C.C., Davis, B.R., Geltman, E., Hayes, D., Farnham, D.J., Randall, O.S., Dinh, H., Arnold, J.M.O., Kupersmith, J., Hager, D., Glasser, S.P., Biddle, T., Hawkins, C.M., Braunwald, E. (1994). Uniformity of captopril benefit in the post infarction population: Subgroup analysis in SAVE. *European Heart Journal* **15**(Supplement B), 2–8.

MRFIT Investigators (1982). Multiple risk factor intervention trial. *Journal of the American Medical Association* **248**, 1465–1477.

Nester, M.R. (1996). An applied statistician's creed. *Applied Statistics* **45**, 4401–4410.

Neuhauser, M., Steinijans, V.W., Bretz, F. (1999). The evaluation of multiple clinical endpoints with application to asthma. *Drug Information Journal* **33**, 471–477.

Neyman, J. (1937). Outline of a theory of statistical estimation based on the classical theory of probability. *Philosophical Transactions of the Royal Society (London), Series A* **236**, 333–380.

Neyman, J. (1938). L'estimation statistique traitée comme un problème classique de probabilité. *Actualités Scientifiques et Industrielles* **739**, 25–57.

Neyman, J., Peason, E.S. (1933). On the problem of the most efficient tests of statistical hypotheses. *Philosophical Transactions of the Royal Society (London), Series A* **231**, 289–337.

O'Brien, P.C. (1984). Procedures for comparing samples with multiple endpoints. *Biometrics* **40**, 1079–1089.

Packer, M. (2000). Presentation of the results of the Prospective Randomized Amlodipine Survival Evaluation-2 Trial (PRAISE-2) at the American College of Cardiology Scientific Sessions, Anaheim, California, March 15, 2000.

Packer, M., Cohn, J.N., Ccolucci, W.S. (1996). Response to Moyé and Abernethy. *New England Journal of Medicine* **335**, 1318–1319.

Packer, M., O'Connor, C.M., Ghali, J.K., Pressler, M.L., Carson, P.E., Belkin, R.N., Miller, R.P., Neuberg, G.W., Frid, D., Wertheimer, J.H., Cropp, A.B., DeMets, D.L., for the Prospective Randomized Amlodipine Survival Evaluation Study Group (1996). Effect of amlodipine on morbidity and mortality in severe chronic heart failure. *New England Journal of Medicine* **335**, 1107–1114.

Peduzzi, P., Wittes, J., Deter, K., Holford, T. (1993). Analysis as-randomized and the problem of non-adherence; an example from the veterans affairs randomized trial of coronary artery bypass surgery. *Statistics in Medicine* **12**, 1185–1195.

Pedersen, T.R., Olsson, A.G., Ole Færgeman, Kjekshus, J., Hans Wedel, H., Kåre Berg, K., Wilhelmsen, L., Haghfelt, T., Thorgeirsson, G., Pyörälä, K., Miettinen, T., Christophersen, B., Tobert, J.A., Musliner, T.A., Cook, T.J., for the Scandinavian Simvastatin Survival Study Group. (1998). Lipoprotein Changes and Reduction in the Incidence of Major Coronary Heart Disease Events in the Scandinavian Simvastatin Survival Study (4S) Circulation **97**, 1453–1460.

Peto, R., Collins, R., Gray, R. (1995). Large-scale randomized evidence: Large, simple trials and overviews of trials. *Journal of Clinical Epidemiology* **48**, 23–40.

Pfeffer, M.A., Braunwald, E., Moyé, L.A., Basta, L., Brown, E.J., Cuddy, T.E., Davis, B.R., Geltman, E.M., Goldman, S., Flaker, G.C., Klein, M., Lamas, G.A., Packer, M., Roleau, J., Routeau, J., Rutherford, J., Wertheimer, J.H., Hawkins, C.M. (1992). Effect of captopril on mortality and morbidity in patients with left ventricular dysfunction after myocardial infarction: Results of the survival and ventricular enlargement trial. *New England Journal of Medicine* **327**, 669–677.

Piantadosi, S. (1997). *Clinical Trials: A Methodologic Perspective*. Wiley, New York.

Poole, C. (1987). Beyond the confidence interval. *American Journal of Public Health* **77**, 195–199.

Pytkowsi, W. (1932). The dependence of the income in small farms upon their area, the outlay and the capital invested in cows, (Polish, English summaries), Monograph no. 31 of series Bioblioteka Pulawska, Publ. Agri. Res. Inst. Pulasy, Poland.

Reitmeir, P., Wassmer, G. (1996). One sided multiple endpoints testing in two-sample comparisons. *Communications in Statistics: Simulation and Computation* **25**, 99–117.

Rothman, R.J. (1990). No adjustments are needed for multiple comparisons. *Epidemiology* **1**, 43–46.

Sacks, F.M., Moyé, L.A., Davis, B.R., Cole, T.B., Rouleau, J.L., Nash, D., Pfeffer, M.A., Braunwald, E. (1998). Relationship between plasma LDL concentrations during treatment with pravastatin and recurrent coronary events in the cholesterol and recurrent events trial. *Circulation* **97**, 1446–1452.

Sacks, F.M., Pfeffer, M.A., Moyé, L.A., Rouleau, J.L., Rutherford, J.D., Cole, T.G., Brown, L., Warnica, J.W., Arnold, J.M., Wun, C.-C., Davis, B.R., Braunwald, E. (1996). The effect of pravastatin on coronary events after myocardial infarction in patients with average cholesterol levels. *New England Journal of Medicine* **335**, 1001–1009.

Sankoh, A.J., Huque, M.F., Dubey, S.D. (1997). Some comments on frequently used multiple endpoint adjustment methods in clinical trials. *Statistics in Medicine* **16**, 2229–2242.

Senn, S. (1997). *Statistical Issues in Drug Development*. Wiley, Chichester, Section 15.2.1.

Shaffer, J.P. (1986). Modified sequentially rejective multiple test procedures. *Journal of the American Statistical Association* **81**, 826–831.

Simes, R.J. (1986). An improved Bonferroni procedure for multiple tests of significance. *Biometrika* **73**, 819–827.

Stolberg, S.G. Should a pill be colorblind? New York Times. Week in Review. May 13, 2001, p. 1.

The Clopidogrel in Unstable Angina to Prevent Recurrent Events Trial Investigators (2001). Effects of clopidogrel in addition to aspirin in patients with acute coronary syndromes without ST-segment elevation. *New England Journal of Medicine* **345**, 494–502.

The Long-Term Intervention with Pravastatin in Ischaemic Disease (LIPID) Study Group (1998). Prevention of cardiovascular events and death with pravastatin in patients with CAD and a broad range of initial cholesterol levels. *New England Journal of Medicine* **339**, 1349–1357.

The SHEP Cooperative Research Group (1991). Prevention of stroke by antihypertensive drug therapy in older persons with isolated systolic hypertension: final results of the systolic hypertension in the elderly program (SHEP). *Journal of the American Medical Association* **265**, 3255–3264.

Transcript of the Cardiovascular and Renal Drugs Advisory Committee to the FDA Captopril. February 16, 1993.

Tukey, J.W., Ciminera, J.L., Heyse, J.F. (1985). Testing the statistical certainty of a response to increasing doses of a drug. *Biometrics* **41**, 295–301.

Wald, A. (1950). *Statistical Decision Functions*. Wiley, New York.

Walker, A.M. (1986a). Significance tests represent consensus and standard practice (Letter). *American Journal of Public Health* **76**, 1033. , (See also Journal erratum; **76**, 1087).

Walker, A.M. (1986b). Reporting the results of epidemiologic studies. *American Journal of Public Health* **76**, 556–558.

West of Scotland Coronary Prevention Study Group (1996). Influence of pravastatin and plasma lipids on clinical events in the West of Scotland Coronary Prevention Study (WOSCOPS). *Circulation* **97**, 1440–1445.

Westfall, P.H., Ho, S.Y., Prillaman, B.A. (2001). Properties of multiple intersection–union tests for multiple endpoints in combination therapy trials. *Journal of Biopharmaceutical Statistics* **11**, 125–138.

Westfall, P.H., Wolfinger, R.D. (2000). Closed Multiple Testing Procedures and PROC MULTITEST. SAS Observations, July 2000.

Westfall, P.H., Young, S.S. (1993). *Resampling Based Multiple Testing: Examples and Methods for P-Value Adjustment*. Wiley, New York.

Yancy, C.W., Fowler, M.B., Ccolucci, W.S., Gilber, E.M., Brisstow, M.R., Cohn, J.N., Luka, M.A., Young, S.T., Packer, M. for the US Carvedilol Heart Failure Study Group. (2001). Race and response to adrenergic blockade with carvedilol in patients with chronic heart failure. *New England Journal of Medicine* **334**, 1358–65.

Yusuf, S., Wittes, J., Probstfield, J., Tyroler, H.A. (1991). Analysis and interpretation of treatment effects in subgroups of patients in randomized clinical trials. *Journal of the American Medical Association* **266**, 93–98.

Zhang, J., Qwuan, H., Ng, J., Stapanavage, M.E. (1997). Some statistical methods for multiple end-points in clinical trials. *Controlled Clinical Trials* **18**, 204–221.

Handbook of Statistics, Vol. 27
ISSN: 0169-7161

DOI: 10.1016/S0169-7161(07)27022-1

22

Power: Establishing the Optimum Sample Size

Richard A. Zeller and Yan Yan

Abstract

This paper focuses on power, which is the probability that a real clinical pattern will be detected. Power depends on (a) the effect size, (b) the sample size, and (c) the significance level. But if the clinical researcher knew the size of the effect, there would be no reason to conduct the research! Researcher designers use power analysis to minimize the likelihood of both false positives and false negatives (Type I and Type II errors, respectively). Both software and simulation approaches to establishing power in research design are described in this paper. Basic software, such as SamplePower1.0, is effective for establishing power for means, proportions, ANOVA, correlation, and regression. Advanced softwares, such as UnifyPow and PASS, establish power for more complex designs. generalized estimating equations (GEEs) are designed for correlated data. Complex designs such as repeated measures ANOVA. Monte Carlo simulations provide an alternative and a validity check for software power analyses. Criteria for establishing sample sizes that are large enough, but not too large, are discussed.

1. Introduction

A crucial question faced by designers of clinical research is the determination of the sample size. How many observations should the clinical researcher seek to make? The sample should be large enough to reliably establish the clinical pattern. But the sample should not be so large as to waste precious research time, energy, money, and resources. In order to establish an optimal sample size, statisticians use the statistical tool of the null hypothesis.

A *null hypothesis* is a statement of no relationship. Traditionally, the null hypothesis has been used as the criterion for reliably establishing a clinical pattern. When a researcher establishes that the probability that "no reliable pattern exists" is less than .05, the researcher then claims that the clinical pattern has been reliably established. A Type I error is the rejection of a null hypothesis when, in fact, the null hypothesis is true. The *significance level* is the probability of making a Type I error when conducting a null hypothesis test.

Not wanting to find "false positives," the clinical researcher would like to have a low likelihood of making a Type I error. How low should the significance level be? It is standard protocol to set the significance level at the low probability of .05. This sets the probability of making a "false positive" Type I error at 5 chances in 100.

Null hypotheses are almost always false. An infinitesimal proportion of elections are ties. In elections, 50% + 1 vote is sufficient to win the election. But in clinical research the difference between 50% + 1 and 50% − 1 is trivial. Clinical researchers want to find *important* clinical patterns. But statistical theory focuses on the principle of falsification. This principle argues that we cannot prove anything to be true, but we can prove something to be false. The logical basis of the null hypotheses is that, if the null hypothesis is false, something else has to be true. That "something else" is the "clinical pattern."

The null hypothesis focuses on the lack of a clinical pattern, but the clinical researcher is not interested in *the lack of a clinical pattern*! Instead, the clinical researcher is interested in *establishing an important clinical pattern*! Instead of asking: "How likely is it that no relationship is not so?", the clinical researcher wants to ask: "Is there an important relationship?" More specifically, the clinical researcher wants to know, in advance, the likelihood of a research design detecting a real and important clinical effect. In asking this question, the clinical researcher is posing a question of statistical power.

The *power* of a significance test is the probability that a real clinical pattern will be detected. A *Type II error* is the failure to reject a null hypothesis when, in fact, there *is* a relationship between our variables in the population. Thus

$$\text{Power} = 1 - \text{Probability of a Type II error.}$$

The clinical researcher wants to know how powerful the research design is. Specifically, the clinical researcher wants to know how likely it is that a research design with a specific sample size will detect a real, important clinical effect. That is, the researcher would like to have a research design in which the odds of detecting the effect are high. Not wanting to waste time, energy, and resources to find "false negatives," the clinical researcher would like to have a low likelihood of making a Type II error. How high should power be? It is standard protocol to set power at the high probability of .80. This sets the probability of correctly inferring the effect at .80. It makes the odds of making a "false-negative" Type II error into 20 chances in 100.

The power of a significance test to detect a real pattern is based on

- the effect size,
- the sample size, and
- the significance level.

But if the clinical researcher knew the size of the effect, there would be no reason to conduct the research! *In order to conduct power analyses, the researcher must guess at the size of the effect before the study is conducted!* There are ways to make this guess reasonable. What does the literature say? What does the researcher's clinical experience suggest? What does a pretest indicate? Sometimes this estimated effect size comes from how big the effect must be to be "clinically important." However, the fact remains that *in order for a researcher to establish the power of the sample size for a research design, the researcher must estimate in advance the effect size!*

2. Illustrating power

Consider an illustration of power analysis. You specify the following parameters for a two-group, independent observations comparison:

- the effect size is equal to one fourth of a standard deviation unit (.25z),
- the sample size equals 100 cases ($N = 100$), and
- the significance level equals 1 chance in 20 of a Type I error ($\alpha = .05$).

What is the likelihood that a clinical trials random assignment experiment with these parameters will detect this effect? Alternatively asked: What is the power of this study? The answer, derived from the formulas of power analysis, is .70. If a researcher conducted an infinite number of studies with the above parameters, 70% of those studies would result a statistically significant outcome, whereas 30% would not. We know this because statisticians, such as Cohen (1977) and Cohen and Cohen (1983, pp. 59–61, 116–119), have gone to great lengths to solve for formulas that result in that 70% power rate.

But suppose that you are skeptical. Suppose that you want to see it to believe it. In one sense, we cannot satisfy your skepticism. We cannot conduct an infinite number of studies with the above parameters. However, we can conduct a large number of such studies and examine what percentage of those studies detect the effect. If we are unsuccessful at doing this, your skepticism is warranted. If, on the other hand, we successfully do this, your skepticism about power formulas should dissipate. The purpose of this section is to conduct a large number of studies with the above parameters. The result of this exercise will be to evaluate the degree to which the .70 power indicated by the formulas is also indicated by the illustration.

In order to conduct this illustration, we needed many thousands of random numbers. Prior to the widespread use of digital computers, statisticians had to select random outcomes one at a time. That made illustrations such as this one difficult to do. Today, however, we can create hundreds of thousands of random numbers in seconds. For example, we can create 100,000 random numbers using Microsoft Excel as follows:

- in cell A1, type: = rand(),
- copy cell A1,
- paste the copied material into an area of 10 columns by 10,000 rows.

Just like that, you have produced 100,000 random numbers between .0000 and .9999.

Table 1
Descriptive statistics for 10 variables of $N = 10{,}000$ random numbers

	N	Minimum	Maximum	Mean	Standard Deviation
R1	10000	.00	1.00	*.4945*	.2898
R2	10000	.00	1.00	*.5056*	*.2873*
R3	10000	.00	1.00	.5020	.2896
R4	10000	.00	1.00	.5016	.2889
R5	10000	.00	1.00	.5022	.2876
R6	10000	.00	1.00	.4992	.2892
R7	10000	.00	1.00	.5001	*.2904*
R8	10000	.00	1.00	.5010	.2886
R9	10000	.00	1.00	.4979	.2891
R10	10000	.00	1.00	.5010	.2895
Valid *N* (listwise)	10000				

For this illustration to be effective, the skeptic must be satisfied that the numbers are "really random." In the universe, the mean of each variable $= .500$ and each standard deviation $= .2887$. Table 1 presents the analysis of means and standard deviations for the 10 variables of $N = 10{,}000$ "population" created above. The means in Table 1 should be quite close to .5000 and the standard deviation quite close to .2887. The results of this analysis are presented in Table 1. An examination of Table 1 reveals that the means hover closely around .5000; these means range from $\bar{X} = .4945$ to $\bar{X} = .5056$. Moreover, the standard deviations hover closely around .2887; these standard deviations vary from $s = .2873$ to $s = .2904$.

But, the skeptic quite properly points out, the important thing is the lack of correlation between the variables, not the means and standard deviations. Each variable should have a sample correlation with each other variable quite close to .0000. The results of this analysis are presented in Table 2. An examination of Table 2 reveals that the correlations hover closely around .0000; these correlations range from $r = -.024$ to $r = .020$. They have a mean correlation of .0004 and a standard deviation of .0102.

The standard deviation of these sample correlations are called the standard error. Thus, the estimates of the standard error of correlations generated from the above "simulation" are quite low. Thus, our population of $N = 10{,}000$ is consistent with a universe of 10 variables composed of random numbers. Based on these analyses, a reasonable skeptic should be satisfied that these numbers are "really random."

The value of matrices of random numbers to power analysis is that we can conduct both simple and complex Monte Carlo simulations of power analyses *where the effect sizes in the universe are known.* That is, some combinations of variables will give us large populations that approximate universes where we know that the null hypothesis is true (i.e., that the effect size is zero); other combinations of variables will give us large populations that approximate universes where we know that the null hypothesis is false (i.e., that the effect size is not zero). More importantly, these populations will have *known* effect sizes. When we know the

Table 2
Correlation matrix among 10 variables of $N = 10{,}000$ random numbers

		R1	R2	R3	R4	R5	R6	R7	R8	R9	R10
R1	*R*	1	−.010	.013	−.006	.006	−.006	−.006	−.004	−.004	.005
	Significance		.326	.207	.530	.567	.557	.558	.703	.711	.587
R2	*R*	−.010	1	−.008	.003	−.016	.003	.017	.005	.002	−.006
	Significance	.326		.413	.746	.099	.789	.092	.586	.833	.546
R3	*R*	.013	−.008	1	−.011	.008	−.002	−.001	−.011	.013	.003
	Significance	.207	.413		.258	.409	.854	.919	.268	.210	.766
R4	*R*	−.006	.003	−.011	1	.005	−.009	−.006	−.011	−.007	*−.024**
	Significance	.530	.746	.258		.630	.353	.570	.261	.511	*.018*
R5	*R*	.006	−.016	.008	.005	1	.008	−.005	.016	.006	.012
	Significance	.567	.099	.409	.630		.398	.638	.119	.525	.236
R6	*R*	−.006	.003	−.002	−.009	.008	1	.007	−.017	−.009	−.001
	Significance	.557	.789	.854	.353	.398		.501	.091	.380	.900
R7	*R*	−.006	.017	−.001	−.006	−.005	.007	1	.001	−.011	.015
	Significance	.558	.092	.919	.570	.638	.501		.957	.293	.136
R8	*R*	−.004	.005	−.011	−.011	.016	−.017	.001	1	*.020**	.017
	Significance	.703	.586	.268	.261	.119	.091	.957		*.041*	.098
R9	*R*	−.004	.002	.013	−.007	.006	−.009	−.011	*.020**	1	−.012
	Significance	.711	.833	.210	.511	.525	.380	.293	*.041*		.225
R10	*R*	.005	−.006	.003	*−.024**	.012	−.001	.015	.017	−.012	1
	Significance	.587	.546	.766	*.018*	.236	.900	.136	.098	.225	

Note: The statistical purist will point out that the correlations are, technically, not "independent." What we actually did was to correlate two variables made up of random numbers with eight other variables made up of random numbers. Thus, there is a lack of independence in the analyses. Given the low absolute values of the correlations, this fact is true and trivial. Listwise $N = 10{,}000$.
* Correlation is significant at the .05 level (two-tailed).

effect sizes in the population, we can then sample from that population repeatedly. Using these multiple samples of a specific sample size from the same universe, we can solve for the proportion of significance tests that are in the critical region of rejection. This proportion provides us with an unbiased estimate the power of a research design that has to detect the effect for a sample size of that size.

Consider the question raised above. What is the power of an experiment to detect a $.25z$ effect with $N = 100$ and $\alpha = .05$? The power formula said that power = .70. To satisfy the skeptic, we conducted a Monte Carlo power simulation. Using the 100,000 random numbers created above, we

- standardized each $N = 10{,}000$ variable of random numbers as follows: $[z = (X = \bar{X})/\text{sd}]$;
- added the $.25z$ effect (by adding .5 to one cell and .0 to the other cell);
- created 100 independent random samples of $N = 100$ from this population;
- conducted the ANOVA *F* ratios for the difference between two means;
- counted the number of *F* ratios that were $p \leq .05$.

There were, in our simulation, 73 out of 100 such significant *F* ratios. Thus, the Monte Carlo simulated power estimate was .73 compared to the formula-driven power of .70.

This evidence shows that power derived from this Monte Carlo simulation is consistent with this formula-driven power. These two techniques for establishing power provided, in this instance, roughly equal power estimates. But what would happen if we changed the parameters? Would the formula-driven power and the Monte Carlo simulated power be roughly equal if the effect sizes varied? ... if the sample size varied?

2.1. Varying sample sizes and effect sizes

Table 3 and Fig. 1 present power likelihoods when sample sizes and effect sizes vary. In Fig. 1, software power estimates are defined by lines with squares; Monte Carlo simulation power estimates are defined by lines with triangles. When the null hypothesis (e.g., H_0: $\mu_1 = \mu_2$) is true, the effect size is zero and "power" is equal to the α of .05. Thus, the a priori specified probability of making a Type I error, a false positive, when the null hypothesis is true 5 in 100. The power formula specifies this .05 a level in its calculations; the Monte Carlo simulation shows that this .05 α level is approximated with false positive rates of between .01 and .05. In this situation, there is no effect of sample size on the power analysis. Increasing the sample size does not alter the probability of a false positive.

When the null hypothesis (e.g., H_0: $\mu_1 \neq \mu_2$) is false, the effect size varies. SamplePower1.0 specifies that an effect size of .10*z* is a "small effect," an effect size of ".25*a*" is a "medium effect," and an effect size of .40*z* is a "large effect." Table 3 and Fig. 1 present the power likelihoods when sample sizes vary from 10 to 1000 and effect sizes vary from .10*z* to .40*z*. An examination of Table 3 and Fig. 1 shows that power, the likelihood of detecting an effect:

- increases as the effect size increases,
- increases as the sample size increases, and
- is estimated almost identically using formulas and simulations.

Let us discuss each of these patterns.

Table 3
Power analyses using software and Monte Carlo simulations

Effect	Type	Cell (*N*)						
		5 (10)	10 (20)	25 (50)	50 (100)	100 (200)	250 (500)	500 (1000)
.00	Software	.05	.05	.05	.05	.05	.05	.05
	Simulation	.04	.01	.05	.05	.05	.03	.05
.10	Software	.06	.07	.11	.17	.29	.61	.88
	Simulation	.04	.10	.11	.18	.30	.64	.91
.25	Software	.11	.19	.41	.70	.94	1.00	1.00
	Simulation	.08	.17	.38	.73	.92	.99	1.00
.40	Software	.20	.40	.79	.98	1.00	1.00	1.00
	Simulation	.11	.38	.78	.99	1.00	1.00	1.00

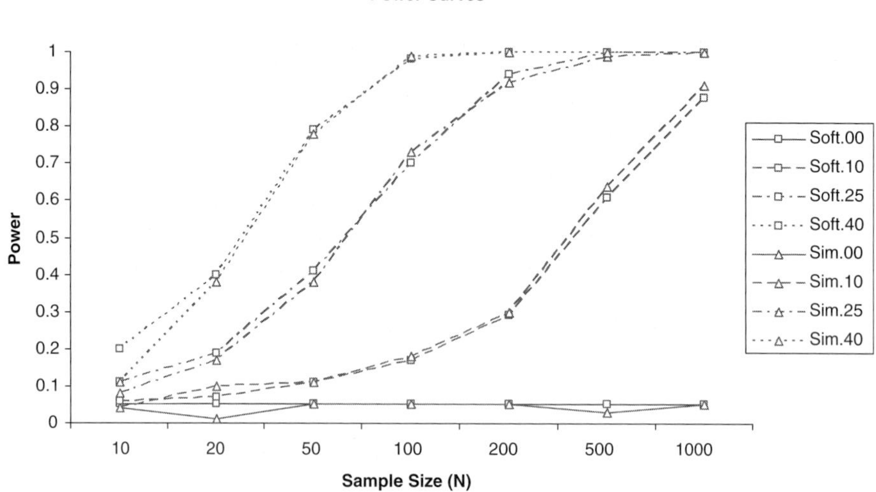

Fig. 1. Graphic plot of power curves from Table 3.

2.2. Power and effect size

As effect size increases, power increases. This principle is illustrated in Table 3 and Fig. 1. When $N = 50$, 25 per cell, the power to detect this effect is .11 for a .10z effect, .41 for a .25z effect, and .79z for a .40z effect. Thus, for a "small" effect size, the power of .11 is only a small amount higher than the .05 power when the null hypothesis is true. For a "large" effect size, the power of .79 is nearly the industry standard of .80.

For very small sample sizes, differences in power by effect size are minor. For example, when $N = 10$, 5 per cell, the power to detect this effect is .06 for a .10z effect, .11 for a .25z effect, and .20z for a .40z effect. A larger effect size increases power, but the odds are still strongly against discovery of the effect when the sample size is this small.

For very large sample sizes, differences in power by effect size are also minor. For example, when $N = 1000$, 500 per cell, the power to detect this effect is .88 for a .10z effect, 1.00 for a .25z effect, and 1.00z for a .40z effect. A larger effect size increases power, but the odds are still strongly in favor of discovery of the effect when the sample size is this large.

Table 3 presents an apparent contradiction. We know that the likelihood of detecting an effect is never a "sure thing." There is always the possibility, however remote, of conducting a study and failing to detect an effect. But some of the "power likelihoods" reported in Table 3 are "1.00." How could this be? Power formulas do not produce perfect powers, i.e., 1.00 powers. However, when power is $\geq .995$, power, rounded to two decimal places, is reported as 1.00. In Monte Carlo simulations, we conducted 100 simulations within each effect size – sample size condition. If all 100 tests were $p < .05$, we reported the simulated power to be 1.00.

2.3. *Power and sample size*

As sample size increases, power increases. This principle is illustrated in Table 3 and Fig. 1. Consider a .25*z* effect size. The power to detect this effect is .11 for $N = 10$, .41 when $N = 50$, .94 when $N = 200$, and 1.00 when $N = 1000$.

There is a diminishing marginal return on increasing sample size. In this example, it makes good cost-effective research design sense to increase the sample size from 10 to 50; this sample size increase results in an increase in power from .11 to .41 for a .25*z* effect. However, it makes only marginal sense to increase the sample size from 100 to 200; this sample size increase results in an increase in power from .70 to .94 for a .24*z* effect. Moreover, it makes no sense whatever to increase the sample size from 500 to 1000; this sample size increase results in an increase less than .005. Both power estimates are $\geq .995$.

3. Comparing simulation and software approaches to power

Table 3 and Fig. 1 present power derived from a software approach and from a simulation approach. Software based upon power formulas is the gold standard of power calculations. Given this,

- How does simulation validate software?
- In what power situations does software apply?
- In what power situations does simulation apply?

We now turn to these questions.

3.1. *How simulation validates software*

Probability is the likelihood of the occurrence of an event. Probability (p) is assessed on a scale from zero to one. A zero probability means that under no circumstances will that event occur. In fact, that circumstance is a "non-event" because it cannot happen. This "non-event" is symbolized: $p = 0$. A "perfect" probability is a "sure bet." "The sun rising tomorrow" is as close as we can get to an "always-event." This "always-event" is symbolized as $p = 1$. A common major league baseball batting average is $p = .250$. For every 4 "at bats," a batter will get one "hit." The probability that a baby is a boy is roughly 50–50; $p \cong .5$. (Note: We say "roughly" because, while the probability that a baby is a boy is close to .5, it is not .5 exactly.)

Statisticians construct theory about how probability operates. Probability theory makes assumptions and draws out the likelihood implications of those assumptions. Virtually all of inferential statistics is based on probability theory. Power analysis is an extension of probability theory. Beyond the assumptions of probability theory, the primary assumption of power analysis is effect size. Effect size is an assumption because, as we argued earlier, if the researcher knew the effect size, there would be no need for conducting the research.

But assumptions are tricky things. In some situations, the researcher can safely ignore an assumption. The statistical analysis will have the same inferential properties as if the assumption had been met. In other situations, the violation of an assumption can render the inferential properties moot.

A robust assumption is an assumption that, if violated, will not alter the inferential outcome of a statistical analysis. The effect size assumption that the size of the effect that the researcher assumes is, in fact, the effect size in the universe of all observations from which the sample is to be drawn. The effect size assumption is not robust! An error in an estimated effect size will result in an erroneous power probability. An over-estimation of the effect size will overstate the power; an under-estimation of the effect size will understate the power. Because an effect size error consistently biases power inferences, it must be taken very seriously.

The assumption that a variable is normally distributed is robust! Data drawn from an evenly distributed rectangular distribution will result in the same probability inferences as if the data were drawn from a normal distribution. This principle is illustrated above. All 2800 F ratios in Table 3 and Fig. 1 were drawn from such a rectangular distribution. Those 2800 F ratios behaved consistently with the normal distribution assumption required by such ANOVA tests.

The fact that the 2800 F ratios in Table 3 and Fig. 1 were drawn from rectangular, not normal, distributions supports not only the robustness of the normality assumption of ANOVA, it also provides application validity for the accuracy of the probability theory-derived formulas that produced those power values. The logic for this assertion is as follows: probability theory that assumed normal distributions was used to derive the formulas which were, in turn, used to program the software to produce power likelihoods with varying universe parameters. This was used for the "software" power calculations in Table 3 and Fig. 1.

These same universe parameters were used to create an $N = 10{,}000$ population, but the distributions were rectangular. The characteristics of this population were very similar to the universe parameters. Many repeated simple random samples were drawn from this $N = 10{,}000$ population. ANOVAs were calculated on each of these samples, and the proportion of them that rejected the null hypothesis was calculated. This was used for the "simulation" power calculations in Table 3 and Fig. 1.

The fact that the "software" and "simulation" power calculations produced nearly identical power probabilities, even in the face of different distributions, provides credibility for both of the techniques. Given that the probability-based software power calculations are the "gold standard," why do we need the simulations? In addition to providing validity for the probability-based software power calculations, the simulations can be applied to areas where the software formulations have not yet been applied. Before we turn to this matter, let us consider the variety of situations where software has been applied.

3.2. Use of software

There are a variety of commercially available software packages currently on the market. We recommend SamplePower1.0. SamplePower1.0 is a computer software package that allows the user to specify the sample size needed for a specific power given specified universe parameters of a research situation. SamplePower1.0 addresses questions of statistical power for means, proportions, correlations, ANOVA's, and regression equations. For example, if a researcher wants to conduct an ANOVA, the researcher will need to specify whether the ANOVA or ANCOVA has one or more factors.

The above sections of this chapter described power analysis software and simulation methods in social behavior research. For epidemiologists and medical statisticians, there are various software packages, SAS macros, R or S+ functions available for performing the power analysis and/or sample size calculations based on different research questions.

UnifyPow, developed by O'Brien (1998) in Cleveland Clinic Foundation, is a freeware SAS module/macro that performs statistical power analysis and sample size determination with a variety of test statistics. One-group tests include the t-test, Wilcoxon for single group or paired continuous data, the binomial and Z approximation for single proportion, McNemar's paired proportions, and Fisher's r-to-Z correlation coefficients. Two-group tests include t-test and Wilcoxon–Mann–Whitney for continuous data, chi-square, likelihood ratio (LR), Fisher's exact tests for proportions, and r-to-Z for correlation coefficients. K-group tests include ANOVA via the cell-means model with general linear contrasts, chi-square and LR tests for $2 \times K$ tables with general linear contrasts on K logits. Regression tests include the likelihood-based tests for a regression coefficient at a specified value in multiple linear regression model, logistic, log-linear, or Cox survival models.

PASS (power analysis and sample size) is a stand-alone commercial software that has the capacity similar to UnifyPow for power analysis and sample size determination related to the commonly used statistical tests. In addition, it includes more topics for specific research applications (e.g., cross-over, equivalences and non-inferiority, group sequential, two- or three-stage, post-marketing surveillance, etc.). Some clinical studies require power analysis and sample size determination specific to their circumstances. From time to time, when these new methods are developed, their authors often distribute the software through SAS macros, S+, or R routines.

In recent years, there are many new developments in sample size determination and power analysis, especially for correlated data. In this section, we review some of these new developments based on generalized estimating equations (GEEs) approach. Correlated data occurs frequently in clinical and epidemiological studies. Example included repeated measurements in longitudinal studies in which several observations are collected from each study subject, neighborhood studies in which observations of individuals from the same neighborhood are correlated, urological studies in which both kidneys from an individual patient share some similarities, and so on.

When research interest is marginal average, then the GEE developed by Liang and Zeger (1986) is the most widely used statistical method for data analysis. GEE accommodates both discrete and continuous outcomes, and even when working correlation matrix is misspecified, the regression coefficient estimator is still consistent and asymptotically normal, and the robust covariance estimator can be used to draw proper statistical inference. GEE-based sample size/power analysis methods include general approach that accommodates various types of outcome measurements, and specific approach that is applicable to a certain situation.

3.3. Theoretical developments in software

Liu and Liang (1997) extended work by Self and Mauritsen (1988) into correlated data setting. Let y_i be the $n_i \times 1$ vector of response $(y_{i1}, \ldots, y_{ini})'$ for ith cluster, $i = 1, 2, \ldots m$. Suppose the research questions can be formulated through a population average marginal model:

$$g(u_{ij}) = x'_{ij}\psi + z'_{ij}\lambda,$$

where $u_{ij} = E(y_{ij})$ and g is a link function relating the expectation of y_{ij} to vectors of covariates x_{ij} and z_{ij}. Here ψ is $p \times 1$ vector of parameters of interest and λ is $q \times 1$ vector of nuisance parameters. The hypothesis interested is H_0: $\psi = \psi_0$ vs. H_1: $\psi = \psi_1$.

For example, a cohort study is initiated to determine the relationship of four types of cancer (A–D) and development of disabilities. Each patient will be evaluated once every year for 4 years. Patients with no cancer serve as the reference group (E) and age is major confounding variable categorized into three groups (<65, 65–74, and 75+). The sample size determination aims to testing the null hypothesis that odds ratios of disability of patients A–D vs. referent patients E are equal to 1, i.e., OR(A vs. E) = OR(B vs. E) = OR(C vs. E) = OR(D vs. E) = 1 against the alternative hypothesis OR(A vs. E) = OR(B vs. E) = 2.5, OR(C vs. E) = OR(D vs. E) = 2, adjusting for confounding effect of age. Although the research interest is the effects of cancer type on the risk of disability and age effects are the nuisance parameters, we have to specify these parameter values under the alternative hypothesis, for example, with patients younger than 65 years old as the reference group, OR(65–74 vs. <65) is 1.5 and OR(75+ vs. <65) is 3.

$$H_0 : \psi = (0, 0, 0, 0) \text{ vs. } H_1 : \psi = (\log 2.5, \log 2.5, \log 2, \log 2).$$

They considered the following GEE quasi-score test statistic

$$T = S_\psi(\psi_0, \hat{\lambda}_0, \alpha)' \sum_0^{-1} S_\psi(\psi_0, \hat{\lambda}_0, \alpha),$$

where

$$S_\psi(\psi_0, \hat{\lambda}_0, \alpha) = \sum_{i=1}^{m} \left(\frac{\partial \mu_i}{\partial \psi}\right)' V_i^{-1}(y_i - \mu_i),$$

$$\sum\nolimits_0 = \text{cov}_{H_0}[S_\psi(\psi_0, \hat{\lambda}_0, \alpha)].$$

And $\hat{\lambda}_0$ is an estimator of λ under H_0: $\psi = \psi_0$ obtained by solving

$$S_\lambda(\psi_0, \lambda_0, \alpha) = \sum_{i=1}^{m} \left(\frac{\partial \mu_i}{\partial \lambda}\right)' V_i^{-1}(y_i - \mu_i) = 0.$$

Under H_0, T converges as $m \to \infty$ to a chi-square distribution with p degree of freedom; whereas under H_1: $\psi = \psi_1$ and $\lambda = \lambda_1$, T follows a non-central chi-square distribution asymptotically with the non-centrality parameter

$$v = \xi' \sum_{1}^{-1} \xi,$$

where ξ and Σ_1 are the expectation and covariance of $S_\psi(\psi_0, \hat{\lambda}_0, \alpha)$ under H_1. See Liu and Liang (1997) for detailed expressions of ξ and Σ_1. Therefore, the statistical power for testing H_0: $\psi = \psi_0$ vs. H_1: $\psi = \psi_1$ can be obtained from the non-central chi-square distribution. Specifically, let $F_{\chi_p^2(v)}$ is the cdf of $\chi_p^2(v)$, a chi-square random variable with degree of freedom p and a non-centrality parameter v. For a given level of Type I error α, let $d_{1-\alpha}$ be the $(1-\alpha)$th percentile of $\chi_p^2(0)$, then the power is given by $1 - F_{\chi_p^2(v)}(d_{1-\alpha})$.

To determine sample size, they assume that cluster size are identical across all clusters, i.e., $n_i = n$ for all i, and that covariates $\{(x_{ij}, z_{ij}), j = 1, \ldots, n\}$ are discrete with L distinct values. With these assumptions, they derived

$$\xi = m\tilde{\xi} \text{ and } \sum_1 = m \tilde{\sum_1},$$

where $\tilde{\xi}$ and $\tilde{\Sigma}_1$ contain the weights based on the probabilities of joint distribution of x and z with L distinct values. The non-centrality parameter v can be expressed as

$$v = m\tilde{\xi}' \tilde{\sum}_1^{-1} \tilde{\xi},$$

therefore, the sample size needed to achieve the nominal power is given by

$$m = \frac{v}{\tilde{\xi}' \tilde{\Sigma}_1^{-1} \tilde{\xi}}.$$

Note, v is a non-centrality parameter, which can be derived from a non-central chi-square distribution with degree of freedom of p – length of vector ψ given the nominal power and significant level of the test.

Using the quasi-score test statistic for power analysis and sample size determination provide a general approach for correlated data. There is no close form for this general approach, thus the numeric methods is needed. However, in some special cases, this approach leads to simple close expressions. For example, for a simple two-group comparison of n repeated continuous measurements, the sample size formula is

$$m = \frac{(z_{1-\alpha/2} + z_{1-\beta})^2 \sigma^2}{\pi_0 \pi_1 d^2 (\mathbf{1}'\mathbf{R}^{-1}\mathbf{1})},$$

where σ^2 is the variance of measurements assumed to be same in two groups, and π_0 and π_1 are the proportions of sample in groups A and B, respectively. d is the difference between the average response for groups A and B under the alternative hypothesis H_1. $\mathbf{R}$ is a correlation matrix for repeated measurements, and $\mathbf{1}$ is a $n \times 1$ vector of ones.

For a simple two-group comparison of n repeated binary measurements, the sample size formula is

$$m = \frac{(z_{1-\alpha/2} + z_{1-\beta})^2[\pi_1 p_0(1 - p_0) + \pi_0 p_1(1 - p_1)]}{\pi_0 \pi_1 (p_1 - p_0)^2(\mathbf{1}'\mathbf{R}^{-1}\mathbf{1})},$$

where p_0 and p_1 are the probabilities of outcome in groups A and B, respectively. Note, if one assumes exchangeable correlation matrix $\mathbf{R}$, i.e., 1 for diagonal elements and ρ otherwise, then

$$\mathbf{1}'\mathbf{R}^{-1}\mathbf{1} = \frac{n}{1 + (n-1)\rho}.$$

The quantity $(1+(n-1)\rho)$ is known as the design effect.

Another general approach for sample size calculations with GEE framework was based on Wald tests, developed by Rochon (1998). Assuming there are S subpopulations under consideration, indexed by letter s. The subpopulations could be treatment comparison groups only, or treatment comparison groups with stratifying variables. In a three-group clinical trial design, there are $S = 3$ subpopulations, corresponding to the three treatment groups. If we compare the three treatments within four different age strata, then we have $3 \times 4 = 12$ subpopulations.

In each S subpopulation, patients are scheduled for T times repeated measurements, with expected values across the T measurements $\mu_s = [\mu_{s1} \ldots \mu_{sT}]$. An appropriate link function $g(\mu_s)$ is chosen to link μ_s with linear predictors η_s, along with the variance function $v(\mu_s)$. With $v(\mu_s)$, $\mathbf{A_s}$, a diagonal matrix with $v(\mu_s)$ as the diagonal elements, is well defined; and together with the assumed correlation matrix $\mathbf{R_s}(\alpha)$, $\mathbf{V_s}$, the covariance matrix among the set of repeated measurements, is then well specified. Solving for $\hat{\boldsymbol{\beta}}$ by the weighted least squares estimator:

$$\hat{\boldsymbol{\beta}} = \left[\sum_s \mathbf{X}_s'\boldsymbol{\Delta}_s\mathbf{V}^{-1}\boldsymbol{\Delta}_s\mathbf{X}_s\right]^{-1}\left[\sum_s \mathbf{X}_s'\boldsymbol{\Delta}_s\mathbf{V}^{-1}\boldsymbol{\Delta}_s g(\mu_s)\right],$$

where $\boldsymbol{\Delta}_s = (\partial\mu_s/\partial\eta_s)$. The "model-based" covariance matrix of $\hat{\boldsymbol{\beta}}$ is obtained as

$$\text{cov}(\hat{\boldsymbol{\beta}}) = \left[n\sum_s \mathbf{D}_s'\mathbf{V}_s^{-1}\mathbf{D}_s\right]^{-1} = n^{-1}\boldsymbol{\Omega},$$

where $\mathbf{D}_s = \boldsymbol{\Delta}_s\mathbf{X}_s$.

For testing specific hypothesis:

$$H_0 : \mathbf{H}\beta = \mathbf{h}_0 \text{ vs. } H_1 : \mathbf{H}\beta \neq \mathbf{h}_0,$$

the Wald-type test statistic

$$T = n(\mathbf{H}\hat{\boldsymbol{\beta}} - \mathbf{h}_0)'[\mathbf{H}\boldsymbol{\Omega}\mathbf{H}']^{-1}(\mathbf{H}\hat{\boldsymbol{\beta}} - \mathbf{h}_0)$$

is asymptotically distributed as a chi-square distribution, with non-centrality parameter

$$v \approx n(\mathbf{H}\hat{\boldsymbol{\beta}} - \mathbf{h}_0)'[\mathbf{H}\boldsymbol{\Omega}\mathbf{H}']^{-1}(\mathbf{H}\hat{\boldsymbol{\beta}} - \mathbf{h}_0).$$

With the given Type I error and power, one can derive the non-centrality parameter, v. Therefore, one can derive the sample size n with the estimated $\hat{\boldsymbol{\beta}}$ and covariance matrix of $\hat{\boldsymbol{\beta}}$.

Kim et al. (2005) extended the Rochon's sample size method to ordinal response case. Suppose that a categorical random variable of value k ($k = 1, \ldots, K$) is being observed for each of repeated T measurements in ith subject ($i = 1, \ldots, N$), let $Z_{it} = k$ ($k = 1, \ldots, K$) denote the ordinal response measured at tth time for ith subject and $Y_{itk} = I(Z_{it} = k)$ be an indicator variable that takes a value of 1 if the response for the tth time of the ith subject is in kth category, and 0 otherwise. Denote the corresponding marginal probabilities by $\Pr[Z_{it} = k]$, and the corresponding marginal cumulative probabilities by $\Pr[Z_{it} \leqslant k]$. Under proportional odds model with the cumulative logit link, the marginal cumulative probabilities can be expressed as a lincr function of covariates. With the GEE method of Lipsitz et al. (1994), a set of regression coefficient estimates and their covariance matrix can be obtained. For sample size determination and power analysis, we need to specify the marginal probabilities $\Pr[Z_{it} - k]$, expected at the end of study, in each K categories of each measurement time in each s subpopulation. With the specification of design matrix for each s population, and common correlation structure, $\mathbf{D_s}$, $\mathbf{A_s}$, and $\mathbf{V_s}$ can be determined, therefore, the estimated $\hat{\boldsymbol{\beta}}$ and covariance matrix of $\hat{\boldsymbol{\beta}}$ can be obtained. Given the Type I and Type II error and the hypothesis matrix $\mathbf{H}$ and $\mathbf{h}_0$, the sample size can be determined.

Although Rochon's method can accommodate a wide variety of clinical research designs, it has to categorize continuous covariates to formulate subpopulations. Therefore, that approach does not effectively incorporate continuous covariates in the power analysis and sample size determination. Tu et al. (2004) proposed a method for extending the existing approach and rendering the limitation moot. For testing specific hypothesis:

$$H_0 : \mathbf{H}\beta = 0 \text{ vs. } H_1 : \mathbf{H}\beta = d,$$

the Wald-type test statistic

$$T = n(\mathbf{H}\hat{\boldsymbol{\beta}})'[\mathbf{H}\boldsymbol{\Omega}\mathbf{H}']^{-1}(\mathbf{H}\hat{\boldsymbol{\beta}})$$

is asymptotically distributed as a central chi-square distribution under H_0, and as a non-central chi-square distribution under H_1. The non-centrality parameter is

$$v = nd'[\mathbf{H}\boldsymbol{\Omega}\mathbf{H}']^{-1}d.$$

When the link function is identity link (i.e., normal outcome data), the GEE estimates $\hat{\boldsymbol{\beta}}$ can be expressed in a closed form; with assumed first two moments (expectation and variance of covariates, and the expectation of cross-product of covariates), the covariance of $\hat{\boldsymbol{\beta}}$ can be easily obtained. For non-linear links, covariance of $\hat{\boldsymbol{\beta}}$ is not in closed form, and does not depend on covariates through its first two moments. Therefore, the entire distribution of covariates has to be specified. Let $F(\gamma)$ denote the probability distribution function of covariates X, then,

$$\Omega = \left[\int D'(\gamma) V^{-1}(\gamma) D(\gamma) dF(\gamma) \right]^{-1}.$$

As Tu noted, for discrete X, the above quantity can be easily expressed in closed form. For continuous X, the quantity is generally not in the closed form; therefore, approximation through Monte Carlo simulation is needed. That is, by generating a sample of size M from the distribution of X, one can approximate Ω by the sample average:

$$\Omega \approx \frac{1}{M} \left[\sum_{k=1}^{m} D'_k V_k^{-1} D_k \right]^{-1}.$$

3.3.1. Specific approach based on robust variance estimator

Pan (2001) extends Shih's (1997) approach to derive the closed form expression for sample size determination for the repeated binary outcome of two-treatment comparison based on the robust variance estimator. He considers two scenarios: one is that the treatment is given at the cluster level. In this scenario, all cluster members receive the same treatment. Another scenario is that each cluster receives both treatments. The goal is to test the treatment effect, and the hypothesis of interest can be formulated as

$$H_0 : \beta = 0 \text{ vs. } H_1 : \beta = b > 0,$$

where β is the log-odds ratio. Since $\sqrt{N}(\hat{\beta} - \beta)$ has an approximately normal distribution $N(0, v)$, a z-statistic can be used to test the null hypothesis and power analysis. In the first scenario where a cluster is the unit of treatment allocation, the robust variance estimator of $\sqrt{N}(\hat{\beta} - \beta)$ is

$$v = N \frac{\mathbf{1}'_{n_i} \mathbf{R}_{\mathbf{w}}^{-1} \mathbf{R}_0 \mathbf{R}_{\mathbf{w}}^{-1} \mathbf{1}_{n_i}}{(\Sigma_{i=1}^{N} \mathbf{1}'_{n_i} \mathbf{R}_{\mathbf{w}}^{-1} \mathbf{1}_{n_i})^2} \times A,$$

where $\mathbf{R}_0$ and $\mathbf{R}_{\mathbf{w}}$ are true correlation and working correlation matrices, respectively. The term A only involves the proportion of patients in each study group and the assumed probabilities of the event in each group. For various cases with three commonly used correlation structures – the independence, compound symmetry(CS), and the first-order autoregressive (AR(1)) in assumed working/true correlation matrix – explicit formula are derived for the robust variance estimator v.

In the second scenario where a cluster member is the unit of treatment allocation, close formula for v in two special cases ($\mathbf{R}_w$ and $\mathbf{R}_0$ both with CS, or $\mathbf{R}_w$ with independence but $\mathbf{R}_0$ with CS) are derived.

3.3.2. Specific approach for comparing slopes

Jung and Ahn (2003, 2005) derived sample size formula for comparing slopes in repeated measurements of continuous and binary data. In continuous-data case, the model can be expressed as

$$y_{ij} = \beta_1 + \beta_2 r_i + \beta_3 t_{ij} + \beta_4 r_i t_{ij} + \varepsilon_{ij},$$

where r_i is the treatment indicator taking 0 for control group and 1 for treatment group. β_1 and β_2 are intercept and slope for the control group and β_3 and β_4 are differences between two treatment groups in intercept and slope, respectively. Here, β_4 is the parameter of interest. For easier calculation, the model can be reparameterized as

$$y_{ij} = b_1 + b_2(r_i - \bar{r}) + b_3 t_{ij} + b_4(r_i - \bar{r})t_{ij} + \varepsilon_{ij}.$$

With GEE method, parameter estimates of bs and their covariance matrix can be obtained. For testing hypothesis H_0: $b_4 = 0$ vs. H_1: $b_4 = b$, the test statistic $\sqrt{n}\hat{b}_4/\hat{\sigma}_4$ is used, where $\hat{\sigma}_4^2$ is the (4, 4)-component of the covariance matrix of regression parameter estimates. Given Type I and Type II errors (α, γ), the required sample size is

$$n = \frac{\sigma^2(z_{1-\alpha/2} + z_{1-\gamma})^2}{b^2}.$$

In order to obtain the estimate of σ^2, Jung and Ahn (2003, 2005). derived the closed form expression of the covariance matrix of regression parameter estimates. In their derivation, two missing patterns can be accommodated. One is the independent missing pattern, where missing at time t_j is independent of missing at $t_{j'}$. Another is the monotone missing pattern, where missing at time t_j imply missing at all times following t_j. Two "true" correlation structures – CS and the first-order autoregressive – can be incorporated in the closed form.

For repeated binary measurements, the marginal model for the expectation of binary response measured at jth time from ith subject in kth treatment group is

$$p_{kij}(a_k, b_k) = g^{-1}(a_k + b_k t_{kij}) = \frac{\exp(a_k + b_k t_{kij})}{1 + \exp(a_k + b_k t_{kij})},$$

where coefficient b_k represents the rate of change in log-odds per unit change in measurement time. To test the difference in the rate of change between two groups, they give the test statistic as follow,

$$\frac{\hat{b}_1 - \hat{b}_2}{\sqrt{\hat{v}_1/n_1 + \hat{v}_2/n_2}},$$

where v_k is the (2, 2) component of covariance matrix of GEE (a_k, b_k) estimates. Given Type I error α, in order to have a power of $1-\gamma$ for $H_1{:}|b_1-b_2|=d$, the required sample size is

$$n=\frac{(z_{1-\alpha/2}+z_{1-\gamma})^2(\hat{v}_1/r_1+\hat{v}_2/r_2)}{d^2},$$

where r_1 and r_2 are the proportion of patients allocated to groups 1 and 2, respectively. To estimate the sample size, Jung et al. derived explicit expression for estimate of v_k, which can accommodate the same missing pattern and correlation structures as in continuous outcome.

4. Using power to decrease sample size

As shown above, power analysis can be used to establish how many cases are needed so that a research design has sufficient power to detect an effect of specified size. Indeed, recent advances in software applications of the principles of probability have resulted substantial increases in the capability of establishing power probabilities for complex designs. The purpose of this section is to argue that power analyses can be used to decrease sample size requirements without information loss. Indeed, we seek to simultaneously increase information value-add and decrease sample size!

The search for efficient, powerful research designs with small sample sizes requires the comparison of simple and complex designs. This search complicates the challenge faced by the power analyst, for power analyses now need to be calculated for each research design under consideration. At the same time, as the design becomes more complex, the formulas and software designed to establish power probabilities become more opaque. Moreover, the more opaque the formulas and software designed to establish power probabilities, the more skeptical the skeptic becomes. The skeptic who needed satisfaction with the power analyses designed for the relatively simple research designs has an even greater need for satisfaction when the designs are complex. We now turn our attention to this important use of power analysis. There are many ways to credibly demonstrate a causal clinical effect. Let us compare the experimental design with the repeated measures experimental design.

Using the experimental design, subjects are randomly assigned to the "treatment" or "control" conditions. After the treatment is administered to the treatment group, the outcome is measured. If the outcome is significantly superior in the treatment group compared to the control group, the clinical researcher can credibly claim that the treatment has a beneficial effect. The strength of the experimental is that this design clearly satisfies the causal criteria of correlation, time ordering, and non-spuriousness. The weaknesses of the experimental design are the difficulty of making useful generalizations and implementing this design's protocols. Moreover, the experimental design demands a relatively large number of observations needed to have sufficient power to detect clinically important effects. That is, the experimental design lacks power.

The repeated measures experimental design adds one feature to the experimental design. This additional design feature is that subjects are measured before and after the treatment is administered to the treatment group. These are usually called the "pre-score" and "post-score" measures, respectively. Because of random assignment, the treatment and control "pre-score" means are approximately equal. If the "post-score" mean is significantly superior in the treatment group compared to the control group, the clinical researcher can credibly claim that the treatment has a beneficial effect. The repeated measures experimental design enjoys the same strengths and suffers from the same weaknesses as the experimental design except that the repeated measures experimental design

(1) measures change from "pre-score" to "post-score" and
(2) requires a relatively small number of observations to have sufficient power to detect clinically important effects.

That is, the repeated measures experimental design is powerful. The power of this design derives from the fact that the "pre-score" and the "post-score" are usually positively correlated. Often this positive correlation is substantial (e.g., $r = .7$). This positive correlation between "pre-score" and "post-score" results in a reduction in the within means variance. The reduction in the within means variance results in an increase in the F ratio. The most useful way to use power analysis to reduce sample size is to capitalize on the over-time non-zero correlations inherent in repeated measures designs. The formulas and software applications in Section 3 demonstrate this. For the skeptic, we now wish to provide a Monte Carlo simulation demonstrating how such designs work.

4.1. Creation of a non-zero correlation matrix

The random numbers that we created had universe inter-correlations of zero, as shown in Table 2. We now wish to create universe inter-correlations of non-zero values (e.g., $\rho^2 = .500$). To combine X and Y into a non-zero correlation, divide X^2 by the sum of a fraction of $(X+Y)^2$. For example, if X and Y are standardized random numbers, the universe correlation squared between X and $X+Y$ is

$$Y^2 = \frac{X^2}{(X+Y)^2} = \frac{X^2}{X^2 + 2XY + Y^2} = \frac{X^2}{X^2 + Y^2} = \frac{1}{2} = .5.$$

Because X and Y are random, the expected value of $2XY$ is zero. The logic of this formulation is that X and Y share half of their variance. The respective correlation is

$$\rho = \sqrt{.5} = .707.$$

Correlations ranging from 0 to 1 can be created by changing the mix of common and unique components of this formula. For example, a .8 universe squared correlation is

$$\rho^2 = \frac{X^2}{(X + .5Y)^2} = \frac{1}{1.25} = .8.$$

And a .2 universe squared correlation is

$$\rho^2 = \frac{X^2}{.5X^2 + Y^2} = \frac{1}{5} = .2.$$

Table 4 presents the universe and population correlations and correlations squared using various combinations of common and unique, random components. *With this capability, the power analyst can create a Monte Carlo simulation for repeated measures designs using any specified between-time correlation.* Thus, the Monte Carlo simulation becomes reasonable, useful, and productive for complex research designs. Specifically, using these statistical principles, clinical researchers can conduct power analyses for complex designs to satisfy the skeptic that the newly created formulas are properly specifying power probabilities. We now turn to the creation of a repeated measures Monte Carlo simulated power analyses.

4.2. Simulating power for repeated measures power analyses

Using the repeated measures design, subjects are observed before and after a treatment. If the outcome is significantly superior after the treatment compared to

Table 4
Correlations[a] created by random numbers

Correlation of X with		ρ		ρ^2		Universe ρ^2 Calculation
		Universe	Population	Universe	Population	
$Y.1$	$X+.1Y$	.995	.995	.990	.990	$X^2/(X^2+.1Y^2)$
$Y.2$	$X+.2Y$	.981	.980	.962	.960	$X^2/(X^2+.2Y^2)$
$Y.3$	$X+.3Y$	.958	.957	.917	.916	$X^2/(X^2+.3Y^2)$
$Y.4$	$X+.4Y$	.928	.928	.862	.861	$X^2/(X^2+.4Y^2)$
$Y.5$	$X+.5Y$	.894	.893	.800	.797	$X^2/(X^2+.5Y^2)$
$Y.6$	$X+.6Y$	.857	.856	.735	.733	$X^2/(X^2+.6Y^2)$
$Y.7$	$X+.7Y$	.819	.817	.671	.667	$X^2/(X^2+.7Y^2)$
$Y.8$	$X+.8Y$	.781	.778	.610	.605	$X^2/(X^2+.8Y^2)$
$Y.9$	$X+.9Y$	.743	.739	.552	.546	$X^2/(X^2+.9Y^2)$
XY	$X+Y$	.707	.702	.500	.493	$X^2/(X^2+Y^2)$
$X.9$	$.9X+Y$	.669	.664	.447	.441	$X^2/(.9X^2+Y^2)$
$X.8$	$.8X+Y$	.625	.618	.390	.382	$X^2/(.8X^2+Y^2)$
$X.7$	$.7X+Y$	.573	.566	.329	.320	$X^2/(.7X^2+Y^2)$
$X.6$	$.6X+Y$	.514	.506	.265	.256	$X^2/(.6X^2+Y^2)$
$X.5$	$.5X+Y$	.447	.438	.200	.192	$X^2/(.5X^2+Y^2)$
$X.4$	$.4X+Y$	.371	.361	.138	.130	$X^2/(.4X^2+Y^2)$
$X.3$	$.3X+Y$	.287	.276	.083	.076	$X^2/(.3X^2+Y^2)$
$X.2$	$.2X+Y$	.196	.184	.038	.034	$X^2/(.2X^2+Y^2)$
$X.1$	$.1X+Y$	.100	.087	.010	.008	$X^2/(.1X^2+Y^2)$

[a] Population $N = 10{,}000$.

before the treatment, the clinical researcher can credibly claim that the treatment has a beneficial effect. The strength of the repeated measures design derives from over-time within-subject correlations. When this major source of variation is removed from "error," the power to detect the effect increases dramatically.

However, the claim of a beneficial effect in a repeated measures design suffers from all the extraneous factors that are associated with time. Indeed, the good doctor allows the passage of time to be one of the "medicines" by which patients are treated, for the "wisdom of body" often makes the superior outcome occur if nothing were done! Therefore, the "credibility" of the repeated measures design outcome is called into question.

In order to quash the criticism of repeated measures designs, the clever researcher will combine the comparative design with the repeated measures design. In the tradition of the comparative design, the researcher will randomly assign subjects to the treatment or control conditions. Then this researcher will observe the outcome before and after the treatment group gets the treatment but the control group does not. This design assures that the treatment and control group are "identical" prior to the treatment, and that only subjects in the treatment group enjoy the improvement in the outcome that results from the treatment over any improvement in the outcome that results from the passage of time.

But this is a complex research design. In statistical terms, the researcher is primarily interested in the "treatment" by "time" interaction effect! This complex design requires the advanced software described above. In addition, the careful researcher designer is advised to conduct a Monte Carlo simulation.

Let us specify the parameters of such a random assignment clinical trials research design for burn itch reduction. Then we will conduct a power analysis using both the software and the simulation specifications as follows:

- The "pre-post" correlation is $\sqrt{.5} = .707$.
- The cell means and standard deviations are presented in Table 5.

The fact that subjects are randomly assigned means that the pre-scores will, within the limits of probability, be equal. If these scores are measured before treatment conditions are assigned, they can be constrained to be equal (Zeller et al., 1997).

Table 5
Universe and population means and standard deviations for simulation

	Group	Universe Mean	Universe Standard Deviation	Population Mean	Population Standard Deviation	Population N
Pre	Treatment	6	1	5.9927	1.00120	5000
	Control	6	1	6.0073	.99885	5000
	Total	6	1	6.0000	1.00000	10000
Post	Treatment	4	1	3.9983	1.00044	5000
	Control	5	1	5.0017	.99966	5000
	Total	4.5	1.11834	4.5000	1.11879	10000

A traditional approach to this question has the researcher conducting a between groups independent variables t-test comparing the treatment and control groups on the post-scores. However, a more powerful approach is to examine the pre–post by treatment–control interaction effect. The reason this latter approach is more powerful is that the variance within subjects is removed from the error term.

In the Monte Carlo simulation, we created a population of $N = 10{,}000$ consistent with the universe specifications above. The population correlation between the pre and post variables was .702, close to the universe specified correlation of .707. The pre- and post-scores were standardized and the effects were added as follows:

Pre-score = Pre-variable + 6
Post-score = Post-variable + 4[a]

[a] An additional 1 was added for subjects in the control group.

These transformations produced the descriptive statistics presented in Table 5. The observant reader will note that the population means and standard deviations are very good approximations or the universe specifications. As expected, the transformations inserting the effects reduced the pre–post correlation to .631.

A total of 100 samples of $N = 20$ were randomly drawn from this $N = 10{,}000$ population. A repeated measures ANOVA was conducted on each of these 100 samples. The results of this analysis showed the following statistically significant F ratios at the .05 level:

- 100 F ratios for the pre–post time main effect were significant;
- 79 of the 100 F ratios for the time by treatment group interaction effect were significant; and
- 19 of the 100 F ratios for the treatment group between subjects main effect were significant.

Thus, using 20 cases, the Monte Carlo simulation estimated the power of the group by time interaction effect to be .79 and the group effect to be .19. Because the substantively important null hypothesis was the group by time interaction effect, 20 cases was sufficient to establish the sample size needed for the research design with these specifications.

Baker et al. (2001) used a more complex 2×4 research design that randomly assigned subjects to treatment and control conditions. A Monte Carlo simulation provided Baker et al. (2001) with the needed power analysis. The Baker Monte Carlo simulation specified 20 cases. Baker et al. (2001) ran 17 cases, found a statistically significant interaction effect, declared the study to be done, and published the results. Now, fewer burn patients must tolerate a severe itch because we know which of two protocols reduces itch the most.

5. Discussion

Power analysis is a valuable tool for establishing an appropriate sample size. Traditional formula-driven power analyses and their software derivatives provide useful tools for simple null hypothesis testing power analyses. Important advances have been made in using software to solve for power likelihoods in relatively complex designs. The mathematical bases of these software power likelihoods are presented in this paper. These formula-driven power analysis are validated by Monte Carlo simulations. As the research design becomes complex, it becomes more difficult to apply the software. In these situations, and when clinical observations are difficult to get, the use of the more cumbersome but effective Monte Carlo simulations makes sense. Indeed, the analyses presented in this paper suggest that traditional advice may have greatly overstated the sample sizes needed for repeated measures analyses.

References

Baker, R.A.U., Zeller, R.A., Klein, R.L., Thornton, R.J., Shuber, J.H., Harshall, R.E., Leibfarth, A.G., Latko, J.A. (2001). Burn wound itch control using H_1 and H_2 antagonists. *Journal of Burn Care and Rehabilitation* **22**(4), 263–268.

Cohen, J. (1977). *Statistical Power Analysis for the Behavioral Sciences (Revised Edition)*. Academic Press, New York.

Cohen, J., Cohen, P. (1983). *Applied Multiple Regression/Correlation Analysis for the Behavioral Sciences*, 2nd ed. Lawrence Erlbaum Associates, Hillsdale, NJ, pp. 59–61.

Jung, S.H., Ahn, C.W. (2003). Sample size estimation for GEE for comparing slopes in repeated measurements data. *Statistics in Medicine* **22**, 1305–1315.

Jung, S.H., Ahn, C.W. (2005). Sample size for a two-group comparison of repeated binary measurements using GEE. *Statistics in Medicine* **24**, 2583–2596.

Kim, H.Y., Williamson, J.M., Lyles, C.M. (2005). Sample-size calculations for studies with correlated ordinal outcomes. *Statistics in Medicine* **24**, 2977–2987.

Liang, K.Y., Zeger, S.L. (1986). Longitudinal data analysis using generalized linear models. *Biometrika* **73**, 13–22.

Lipsitz, S.R., Kim, K., Zhao, L. (1994). Analysis of repeated categorical data using generalized estimating equations. *Statistics in Medicine* **13**, 1149–1163.

Liu, G., Liang, K.Y. (1997). Sample size calculations for studies with correlated observations. *Biometrics* **53**, 937–947.

O'Brien, R.G. (1998), A tour of UnifyPow: a SAS module/macro for sample-size analysis, Proceedings of the 23rd Annual SAS Users Group International Conference, SAS Institute Inc, Cary, NC, pp. 1346–1355.

Pan, W. (2001). Sample size and power calculations with correlated binary data. *Controlled Clinical Trials* **22**, 211–227.

PASS (Hintze, J. (2004). NCSS and PASS: number Cruncher Statistical Systems, Kaysville, Utah, WWW.NCSS.Com)

Rochon, J. (1998). Application of GEE procedures for sample size calculations in repeated measures experiments. *Statistics in Medicine* **17**, 1643–1658.

Self, S.G., Mauritsen, R.H. (1988). Power/sample size calculations for generalized linear models. *Biometrics* **44**, 79–86.

Shih, W.J. (1997). Sample size and power calculations for periodontal and other studies with clustered samples using the method of generalized estimating equations. *Biometrical Journal* **39**, 899–908.

Tu, X.M., Kowalski, J., Zhang, J., Lynch, K.G., Crits-Christoph, P. (2004). Power analyses for longitudinal trials and other cluster designs. *Statistics in Medicine* **23**, 2799–2815.

Zeller, R.A., Anderson, G., Good, M., Zeller, D.L. (1997). Strengthening experimental design by balancing potentially confounding variables across eight treatment groups. *Nursing Research* **46**(6), 345–349.

Handbook of Statistics, Vol. 27
ISSN: 0169-7161

DOI: 10.1016/S0169-7161(07)27023-3

23

Statistical Learning in Medical Data Analysis

Grace Wahba

Abstract

This article provides a tour of statistical learning regularization methods that have found application in a variety of medical data analysis problems. The uniting feature of these methods is that they involve an optimization problem which balances fidelity to the data with complexity of the model. The two settings for the optimization problems considered here are reproducing kernel Hilbert spaces (a brief tutorial is included) and ℓ_1 penalties, which involve constraints on absolute values of model coefficients. The tour begins with thin plate splines, smoothing spline ANOVA models, multicategory penalized likelihood estimates, and models for correlated Bernoulli data for regression, in these two settings. Leaving regression, the tour proceeds to the support vector machine, a modern and very popular tool for classification. Then classification based on dissimilarity information rather than direct attribute information is considered. All of the learning models discussed require dealing with the so-called bias-variance tradeoff, which means choosing the right balance between fidelity and complexity. Tuning methods for choosing the parameters governing this tradeoff are noted. The chapter ends with remarks relating empirical Bayes and Gaussian process priors to the regularization methods.

1. Introduction

In this article we will primarily describe regularization methods for statistical learning. In this class of methods a flexible, or nonparametric, statistical learning model is built as the solution to an optimization problem which typically has a term (or group of terms) that measures closeness of the model to the observations, balanced against another term or group of terms which penalizes complexity of the model. This class of methods encompasses the so-called "kernel methods" in the machine learning literature which are associated with support vector machines (SVMs) – SVMs are of primary importance for nonparametric classification and learning in biomedical data analysis. The classic penalized likelihood methods are also regularization/kernel methods, and between SVMs, penalized likelihood methods, and other regularization methods, a substantial part of statistical learning methodology is covered.

The general learning problem may be described as follows: we are given a labeled (or partly labeled) training set – $\{y_i, x(i), i = 1, \ldots, n\}$, where $x(i)$ is an attribute vector of the ith subject and y_i a response associated with it. We have $x \in \mathcal{X}$, $y \in \mathcal{Y}$, but we are deliberately not specifying the nature of either $\mathcal{X}$ or $\mathcal{Y}$ – they may be very simple or highly complex sets. The statistical learning problem is to obtain a map $f(x) \rightarrow y$ for $x \in \mathcal{X}$, so that, given a new subject with attribute vector $x_* \in \mathcal{X}, f(x)$, generalizes well. That is, $f(x_*)$ predicts $\hat{y}_* \in \mathcal{Y}$, such that, if y_* associated with x_* were observable, then $\hat{y}_*$ would be a good estimate of it. More generally, one may want to estimate a conditional probability distribution for $y|x$. The use to which the model f is put may simply be to classify, but in many interesting examples, x is initially a large vector, and it is of scientific interest to know how f or some functionals of f depend on components or groups of components of x – the sensitivity, interaction, or variable selection problem. A typical problem in demographic medical studies goes as follows: sets of $\{y_i, x(i)\}$ are collected in a defined population, where the attribute vectors are vectors of relevant medical variables such as age, gender, blood pressure, cholesterol, body mass index, smoking behavior, lifestyle factors, diet, and other variables of interest. A simple response might be whether or not the person exhibits a particular disease of interest ($y \in \{\text{yes, no}\}$). A major goal of evidence-based medicine is to be able to predict the likelihood of the disease for a new subject, based on its attribute vector. Frequently the nature of f (for example, which variables/patterns of variables most influence f) is to be used to understand disease processes and suggest directions for further biological research.

The statistical learning problem may be discussed from different points of view, which we will call "hard" and "soft" (Wahba, 2002). For hard classification, we would like to definitively assign an object with attribute x_* to one of the two or more classes. For example, given microarray data it is desired to classify leukemia patients into one of the four possible classes (Brown et al., 2000; Lee et al., 2004). In the examples in Lee et al. (2004) classification can be carried out nearly perfectly with a multicategory SVM (MSVM) (for other methods, see the references there). The difficulty comes about when the attribute vector is extremely large, the sample size is small, and the relationship between x and y is complex. The task is to mine the data for those important components or functionals of the entire attribute vector which can be used for the classification. Soft classification as used here is just a synonym for risk factor estimation where one desires to form an estimate of a probability measure on a set of outcomes – in typical demographic studies, if the outcome is to be a member of one of the several classes, the classes are generally not separable by attribute vector, since two people with the same attribute vector may well have different responses. It is just that the probability distribution of the responses is sensitive to the attribute vector. The granddaddy of penalized likelihood estimation for this problem (O'Sullivan et al., 1986) estimated the 19 year risk of a heart attack, given blood pressure and cholesterol at the start of the study. Classes of people who do and do not get heart attacks are generally far from separable on the basis of their risk factors – people with high blood pressure and high cholesterol can live a long life, but as a group their life expectancy is less than people without those risk factors. In both hard and soft classifications, frequently one of the major issues is to understand which attributes are important, and how changes in them affect the risk. For example, the results can be used by doctors to decide when to persuade patients to lower their cholesterol, or for epidemiologists to estimate disease rates and design public health strategies in the general population. In other problems, particularly involving genetic data, it is of particular interest to determine which components of the genome may be associated with a particular response, or phenotype.

In Section 2 we review soft classification, where the emphasis is on obtaining a variety of flexible, nonparametric models for risk factor estimation. Vector-valued observations of various types are considered. A brief review of reproducing kernel Hilbert spaces (RKHS) is included here. Section 3 describes recent developments in soft classification where individual variable selection and variable pattern selection are important. Section 4 goes on to classification with SVMs, including multiple categories and variable selection. Section 5 discusses data that are given as dissimilarities between pairs of subjects or objects, and Section 6 closes this article with an overview of some of the tuning methods for the models discussed.

2. Risk factor estimation: penalized likelihood estimates

2.1. Thin plate splines

The Western Electric Health Study followed 1665 men for 19 years and obtained data including men who were alive at the end of the follow-up period and those who had died from heart disease. Participants dying from other causes were excluded. Penalized likelihood estimation for members of the exponential family (McCullagh and Nelder, 1989), which includes Bernoulli data (i.e., zero–one, alive or dead, etc.), was first proposed in O'Sullivan et al. (1986). The authors used a penalized likelihood estimate with a thin plate spline (tps) penalty to get a flexible estimate of the 19 year risk of death by heart attack as a function of diastolic blood pressure and cholesterol. Figure 1 (O'Sullivan et al., 1986) gives a parametric (linear) and nonparametric tps fit to the estimated log odds ratio after transformation back to probability.

It can be seen that the nonparametric fit has a plateau, which cannot be captured by the parametric fit. We now describe penalized likelihood estimation for Bernoulli data, and how the tps is used in the estimate in O'Sullivan et al. (1986). Let x be a vector of attributes, and $y = 1$ if a subject with attribute x has the outcome of interest and 0 if they do not. Let the log odds ratio $f(x) = \log p(x)/(1 - p(x))$, where $p(x)$ is the probability that $y = 1$ given x. Then $p(x) = e^{f(x)}/(1 + e^{f(x)})$. f is the so-called canonical link for Bernoulli data (McCullagh and Nelder, 1989). Given data $\{y_i, x(i), i = 1, \ldots, n\}$, the likelihood function is

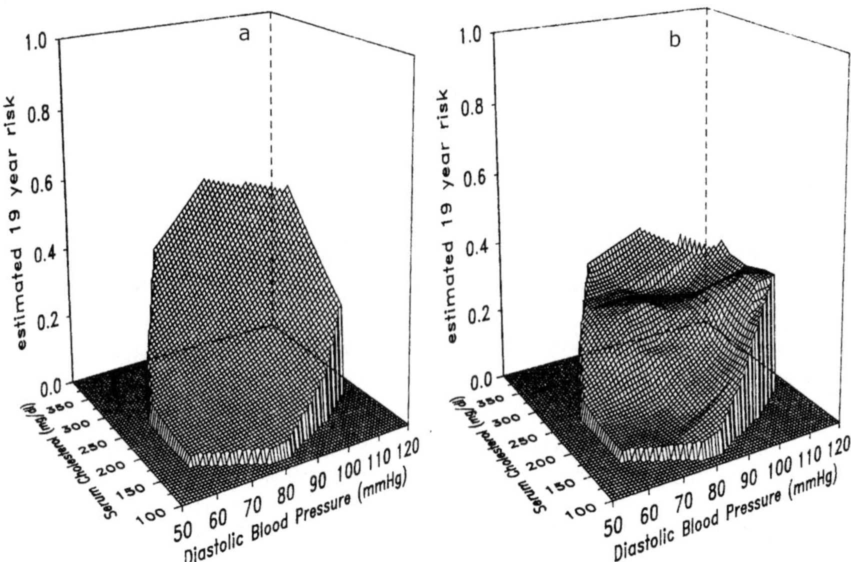

Fig. 1. Nineteen year risk of a heart attack given serum cholesterol and diastolic blood pressure. (Left) Linear model in the log odds ratio. (Right) tps estimate. (From O'Sullivan et al. (1986), ©*Journal of the American Statistical Association*, reprinted with permission.)

$\prod_{i=1}^{n} p(x(i))^{y_i}(1-p(x(i)))^{1-y_i}$, and the negative log likelihood can be expressed as a function of f:

$$\mathscr{L}(y,f) = \sum_{i=1}^{n} -y_i f(x(i)) + \log(1 + \mathrm{e}^{f(x(i))}). \tag{1}$$

Linear (parametric) logistic regression would assume that $f(x) = \Sigma_\ell c_\ell B_\ell(x)$, where the B_ℓ are a small, fixed number of basis functions appropriate to the problem, generally linear or low degree polynomials in the components of x.

The penalized likelihood estimate of f is a solution to an optimization problem of the form: find f in $\mathscr{H}$ to minimize

$$\mathscr{L}(y,f) + \lambda J(f). \tag{2}$$

Here $\mathscr{H}$ is a special kind of RKHS (Gu and Wahba, 1993a). For the Western Electric Study, $J(f)$ was chosen so that f is a tps. See Duchon (1977), Meinguet (1979), O'Sullivan et al. (1986), Wahba (1990), and Wahba and Wendelberger (1980) for technical details concerning the tps. For the Western Electric Study, the attribute vector $x = (x_1, x_2) =$ (cholesterol, diastolic blood pressure) was of dimension $d = 2$, and the two-dimensional tps penalty functional of order 2 (involving second derivatives) is

$$J(f) = J_{2,2}(f) = \int_{-\infty}^{\infty}\int_{-\infty}^{\infty} f_{x_1x_1}^2 + 2f_{x_1x_2}^2 + f_{x_2x_2}^2 \, dx_1\, dx_2, \tag{3}$$

where the subscript (2, 2) stands for (dimension, order). In this case f is known to have a representation

$$f(x) = d_0 + d_1 x_1 + d_2 x_2 + \sum_{i=1}^{n} c_i E(x, x(i)), \tag{4}$$

where

$$E(x, x(i)) = ||x - x(i)||^2 \log ||x - x(i)||, \tag{5}$$

where $||\cdot||$ is the Euclidean norm. There is no penalty on linear functions of the components (x_1, x_2) of the attribute vector (the "null space" of $J_{2,2}$). It is known that c_i for the solution satisfy $\Sigma_{i=1}^{n} c_i = 0$, $\Sigma_{i=1}^{n} c_i x_1(i) = 0$, and $\Sigma_{i=1}^{n} c_i x_2(i) = 0$, and furthermore

$$J(f) = \sum_{i,j=1,\ldots,n} c_i c_j E(x(i), x(j)). \tag{6}$$

Numerically, the problem is to minimize (2) under the stated conditions and using (6) to obtain $d_0, d_1, d_2, c = (c_1, \ldots, c_n)$.

We have described the penalty functional for the tps and something about what it looks like for the $d = 2, m = 2$ case in (3). However, the tps is available for general d and for any m with $2m - d > 0$. The general tps penalty functional in d dimensions and m derivatives is

$$J_{d,m} = \sum_{\alpha_1+\cdots+\alpha_d=m} \frac{m!}{\alpha_1!\cdots\alpha_d!} \int_{-\infty}^{\infty} \cdots \int_{-\infty}^{\infty} \left(\frac{\partial^m f}{\partial x_1^{\alpha_1} \cdots \partial x_d^{\alpha_d}} \right)^2 \prod_j dx_j. \tag{7}$$

See Wahba (1990). Note that there is no penalty on polynomials of degree less than m, so that the tps with d greater than 3 or 4 is rarely attempted because of the very high-dimensional null space of $J_{d,m}$.

The choice of the tuning parameter λ here governs the tradeoff between the goodness of fit to the data, as measured by the likelihood, and the complexity, or wiggliness, of the fit. Note that second derivative penalty functions limit curvature, and tend to agree with human perceptions of smoothness, or lack of wiggliness. When the data are Gaussian (as in Wahba and Wendelberger, 1980) rather than Bernoulli, the tuning (smoothing) parameter λ can be chosen by the generalized cross-validation (GCV) method; a related alternative method is generalized maximum likelihood (GML), also known as restricted maximum likelihood (REML). The order m of the tps may be chosen by minimizing with respect to λ for each value of m and then choosing m with the smallest minimum. See Craven and Wahba (1979), Golub et al. (1979), and Gu and Wahba (1991). As λ tends to infinity, the solution tends to its best fit in the unpenalized space, and as λ tends to 0, the solution attempts to interpolate the data. In the case of biomedical data it is sometimes the case that a simple parametric model (low degree polynomials, for example) is adequate to describe the data. The experimenter can design such a model to be in the null space of the penalty functional, and then a sufficiently large λ will produce the parametric model. Detailed discussion of tuning parameters for Bernoulli data is in Section 6.

A number of commercial as well as public codes exist for computing the tps, with the GCV or GML method of choosing the tuning parameters. Public codes in R (http://cran.r-project.org) include assist, fields, gss, and mgcv. The original Fortran tps code is found in netlib (www.netlib.org/gcv). Further details on the tps can be found in the historical papers (Duchon, 1977; Meinguet, 1979; Wahba, 1990; Wahba and Wendelberger, 1980), in the documentation for the fields code in R, and elsewhere. tps's are used in the "morphing" of medical images (Bookstein, 1997), and have been used to fit smooth surfaces to data that have been aggregated over irregular geometrical shapes such as counties (Wahba, 1981).

2.2. Positive definite functions and reproducing kernel Hilbert spaces

We will give a brief introduction to positive definite functions and RKHSs here, because all of the so-called "kernel methods" which we will be discussing have their foundation as optimization problems in these spaces. The reader who wishes to avoid this technicality may skip this subsection. Let $\mathscr{T}$ be *some* domain, emphasizing the generality of the domain. For concreteness you may think of $\mathscr{T}$ as Euclidean d-space. $K(\cdot,\cdot)$ is said to be positive definite if, for every n and any $t(1),\ldots,t(n) \in \mathscr{T}$ and $c_1,\ldots,c_n$

$$\sum_{i,j=1}^{n} c_i c_j K(t(i), t(j)) \geq 0. \tag{8}$$

In this article we denote the inner product in an RKHS by $\langle\cdot,\cdot\rangle$. To every positive definite function $K(\cdot,\cdot)$ there is associated an RKHS $\mathscr{H}_K$ (Aronszajn, 1950; Wahba, 1990) which can be constructed as a collection of all functions of the form

$$f_L^a(t) = \sum_{\ell=1}^{L} a_\ell K(t, t(\ell)) \tag{9}$$

with the inner product

$$\langle f_L^a, f_M^b \rangle = \sum_{\ell,m} a_\ell b_m K(t(\ell), t(m)) \tag{10}$$

and all functions that can be constructed as the limits of all Cauchy sequences in the norm induced by this inner product; these sequences can be shown to converge pointwise. What makes these spaces so useful is that in an RKHS $\mathscr{H}_K$ we can always write for any $f \in \mathscr{H}_K$

$$f(t_*) = \langle K_{t_*}, f \rangle, \tag{11}$$

where $K_{t_*}(\cdot)$ is the function of t given by $K(t_*, t)$ with t_* considered fixed. A trivial example is that $\mathscr{T}$ is the integers $1,\ldots,n$. There K is an $n \times n$ matrix, the elements of $\mathscr{H}_K$ are n-vectors, and the inner product is $\langle f, g\rangle = f'K^{-1}g$. Kernels with penalty functionals that involve derivatives are popular in applications. A simple example of a kernel whose square norm involves derivatives is the kernel K associated with the space of periodic functions on $[0, 1]$ which integrate to 0 and which have square integrable second derivative. It is $K(s, t) = B_2(s)B_2(t)/(2!)^2 - B_4(|s-t|)/4!$, where $s, t \in [0, 1]$ and B_m is the mth Bernoulli polynomial; see Wahba (1990). The square norm is known to be $\int_0^1 (f''(s))^2 ds$. The periodic and integration constraints are removed by adding linear functions to the space and the fitted functions can be shown to be cubic polynomial splines. For more on polynomial splines, see Craven and Wahba (1979), de Boor (1978), and Wahba (1990). Another popular kernel is the Gaussian kernel, $K(s, t) = exp(-(1/\sigma^2)||s-t||^2)$ defined for s, t in Euclidean d space, E^d, where the norm in the exponent is the Euclidean norm. Elements of this space are generated from functions of $s \in E^d$ of the form $K_{t_*}(s) = exp(-(1/\sigma^2)||s-t_*||^2)$, for $t_* \in E^d$. Kernels on E^d that depend only on the Euclidean distance between their two arguments are known as radial basis functions (rbf's). Another popular class of rbf's is the Matern class; see Stein (1999). Matern kernels have been used to model arterial blood velocity in Carew et al. (2004), after fitting the velocity measurements, estimates of the wall shear stress are obtained by differentiating the fitted velocity model.

We are now ready to write a (special case of) general theorem about optimization problems in RKHS.

The representer theorem (special case) (Kimeldorf and Wahba, 1971): Given observations $\{y_i, t(i), i = 1, 2, \ldots, n\}$, where y_i is a real number and $t(i) \in \mathcal{T}$, and given K and (possibly) some particular functions $\{\phi_1, \ldots, \phi_M\}$ on $\mathcal{T}$, find f of the form $f(s) = \Sigma_{v=1}^{M} d_v \phi_v(s) + h(s)$, where $h \in \mathcal{H}_K$, to minimize

$$I_\lambda\{y, f\} = \frac{1}{n}\sum_{i=1}^{n} \mathcal{C}(y_i, f(t(i))) + \lambda ||h||^2_{\mathcal{H}_K}, \tag{12}$$

where $\mathcal{C}$ is a convex function of f. It is assumed that the minimizer of $\Sigma_{i=1}^{n} \mathcal{C}(y_i, f(t(i)))$ in the span of the ϕ_v is unique. Then the minimizer of $I_\lambda\{y, f\}$ has a representation of the form:

$$f(s) = \sum_{v=1}^{M} d_v \phi_v(s) + \sum_{i=1}^{n} c_i K(t(i), s). \tag{13}$$

The coefficient vectors $d = (d_1, \ldots, d_M)'$ and $c = (c_1, \ldots, c_n)'$ are found by substituting (13) into the first term in (12), and using the fact that $||\Sigma_{i=1}^{n} c_i K_{t(i)}(\cdot)||^2_{\mathcal{H}_K} = c' K_n c$, where K_n is the $n \times n$ matrix with i, jth entry $K(t(i), t(j))$. The name "reproducing kernel (RK)" comes from the fact that $\langle K_{t_*}, K_{s_*} \rangle = K(t_*, s_*)$.

The minimization of (12) generally has to be done numerically by an iterative descent method, except in the case that $\mathcal{C}$ is quadratic in f, in which case a linear system has to be solved. When $K(\cdot, \cdot)$ is a smooth function of its arguments and n is large, it has been found that excellent approximations to the minimizer of (12) for various $\mathscr{C}$ can be found with functions of the form:

$$f(s) = \sum_{v=1}^{M} d_v \phi_v(s) + \sum_{j=1}^{L} c_{i_j} K(t(i_j), s), \tag{14}$$

where $t(i_1), \ldots, t(i_L)$ are a relatively small subset of $t(1), \ldots, t(n)$, thus reducing the computational load. $t(i_1), \ldots, t(i_L)$ may be chosen in various ways, as a random subset, by clustering $\{t(i)\}$ and selecting from each cluster (Xiang and Wahba, 1997), or by a greedy algorithm, as, for example, in Luo and Wahba (1997), depending on the problem.

2.3. Smoothing spline ANOVA models

Thin plate spline estimates and fits based on the Gaussian kernel and other rbf's are (in their standard form) rotation invariant in the sense that rotating the coordinate system, fitting the model, and rotating back do not change anything. Thus, they are not appropriate for additive models or for modeling interactions of different orders.

Smoothing spline ANOVA (SS-ANOVA) models provide fits to data of the form $f(t) = C + \Sigma_\alpha f_\alpha(t_\alpha) + \Sigma_{\alpha<\beta} f_{\alpha\beta}(t_\alpha, t_\beta) + \cdots$. Here f_α is in some RKHS $\mathscr{H}^\alpha$, $f_{\alpha\beta} \in \mathscr{H}^\alpha \otimes \mathscr{H}^\beta$, and so forth. The components of the decomposition satisfy side conditions which generalize the usual side conditions for parametric ANOVA which make the solutions unique. The f_α integrate to zero, the $f_{\alpha\beta}$ integrate to zero over both arguments, and so forth. f is obtained as the minimizer, in an appropriate function space, of

$$I_\lambda\{y, f\} = \mathscr{L}(y, f) + \sum_\alpha \lambda_\alpha J_\alpha(f_\alpha) + \sum_{\alpha<\beta} \lambda_{\alpha\beta} J_{\alpha\beta}(f_{\alpha\beta}) + \cdots, \tag{15}$$

where $\mathscr{L}(y, f)$ is the negative log likelihood of $y = (y_1, \ldots, y_n)$ given f, $J_\alpha, J_{\alpha\beta}, \ldots$ are quadratic penalty functionals in RKHS, the ANOVA decomposition is terminated in some manner, and the λ's are to be chosen. The "spline" in SS-ANOVA models is somewhat of a misnomer, since SS-ANOVA models do not have to consist of splines. The attribute vector $t = (t_1, \ldots, t_d)$, where $t_\alpha \in \mathscr{T}^{(\alpha)}$, is in $\mathscr{T} = \mathscr{T}^{(1)} \otimes \mathscr{T}^{(2)} \otimes \cdots \otimes \mathscr{T}^{(d)}$, where the $\mathscr{T}^{(\alpha)}$ may be quite general. The ingredients of the model are: for each α, there exists a probability measure $\mu_{(\alpha)}$ on $\mathscr{T}^{(\alpha)}$ and an RKHS of functions $\mathscr{H}^\alpha$ defined on $\mathscr{T}^{(\alpha)}$ such that the constant function is in $\mathscr{H}^\alpha$ and the averaging operator $\mathscr{E}_\alpha f = \int f_\alpha(t_\alpha) d\mu_\alpha$ is well defined for any $f_\alpha \in \mathscr{H}^\alpha$. Then f is in (a subspace of) $\mathscr{H} = \mathscr{H}^1 \otimes \mathscr{H}^2 \cdots \mathscr{H}^d$. The ANOVA decomposition generalizes the usual ANOVA taught in elementary statistics courses via the expansion

$$\begin{aligned} I = \prod_\alpha (\mathscr{E}_\alpha + (I - \mathscr{E}_\alpha)) &= \prod_\alpha \mathscr{E}_\alpha + \sum_\alpha (I - \mathscr{E}_\alpha) \prod_{\beta \neq \alpha} \mathscr{E}_\beta \\ &+ \sum_{\alpha<\beta} (I - \mathscr{E}_\alpha)(I - \mathscr{E}_\beta) \prod_{\gamma \neq \alpha,\beta} \mathscr{E}_\gamma + \cdots + \prod_\alpha (I - \mathscr{E}_\alpha). \end{aligned} \tag{16}$$

The components of this decomposition generate the ANOVA decomposition of f by

$$C = \left(\prod_{\alpha} \mathscr{E}_{\alpha}\right) f, \; f_{\alpha} = \left((I - \mathscr{E}_{\alpha}) \prod_{\beta \neq \alpha} \mathscr{E}_{\beta}\right) f,$$

$$f_{\alpha\beta} = \left((I - \mathscr{E}_{\alpha})(I - \mathscr{E}_{\beta}) \prod_{\gamma \neq \alpha,\beta} \mathscr{E}_{\gamma}\right) f, \quad \ldots, \tag{17}$$

and so forth. The spaces $\mathscr{H}^{\alpha}$ are decomposed into the one-dimensional spaces of constant functions, and $\mathscr{H}^{(\alpha)}$, whose elements satisfy $\mathscr{E}_{\alpha} f = 0$. $\mathscr{H}^{(\alpha)}$ may be further decomposed into low-dimensional unpenalized subspaces plus smooth subspaces that will be penalized. All this allows the exploitation of the geometry of RKHS to obtain the minimizer of $I_{\lambda}\{y,f\}$ of (15) in a convenient manner. RKs for the various subspaces are constructed from Kronecker products of the RKs for functions of one variable. SS-ANOVA models are studied in detail in Gu (2002). Other references include Davidson (2006), Gao et al. (2001), Gu and Wahba (1993b), Lin (2000), Wahba (1990), Wahba et al. (1995), Wang (1998), and Wang et al. (2003).

Figure 2 (Wahba et al., 1995) plots the four year probability of progression of diabetic retinopathy based on three predictor variables, dur = duration of diabetes, gly = glycosylated hemoglobin, and bmi = body mass index. An SS-ANOVA model based on cubic splines was fitted with the result

$$f(t) = C + f_1(\text{dur}) + a\,\text{gly} + f_3(\text{bmi}) + f_{13}(\text{dur}, \text{bmi}). \tag{18}$$

In the cubic spline fit, there is no penalty on linear functions. For the gly term, the estimated smoothing parameter was sufficiently large so that the fit in gly was indistinguishable from linear; thus f_2(gly) became a gly. For the plot, gly has been

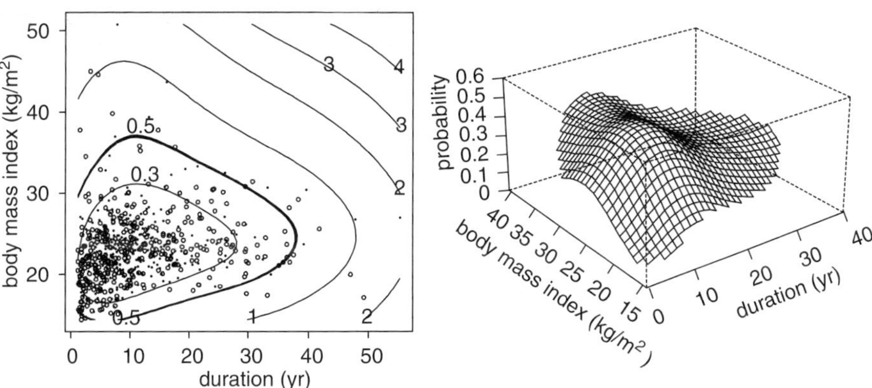

Fig. 2. Four year probability of progression of diabetic retinopathy as a function of duration of diabetes at baseline and body mass index, with glycosylated hemoglobin set at its median. (From Wahba et al. (1995), ©*Annals of Statistics*, reprinted with permission.)

set equal to its median. Software for SS-ANOVA models can be found in the R codes gss, which is keyed to Gu (2002), and assist. Software for main effects models is found in the R code gam, based on Hastie and Tibshirani (1986).

2.4. Multicategory penalized likelihood estimates

Multicategory penalized likelihood methods were first proposed in Lin (1998); see also Wahba (2002). In this setup, the endpoint is one of the several categories; in the works cited, the categories were "alive" or "deceased" by cause of death. Considering $K+1$ possible outcomes, with $K>1$, let $p_j(x), j=0,1,\ldots,K$, be the probability that a subject with attribute vector x is in category j, $\Sigma_{j=0}^{K} p_j(x)=1$. The following approach was proposed in Lin (1998): let $f_j(x)=log[p_j(x)/p_0(x)], j=1,\ldots,K$, where p_0 is assigned to a base class. Then

$$p_j(x)=\frac{e^{f_j(x)}}{1+\sum_{j=1}^{K} e^{f_j(x)}}, \quad j=1,\ldots,K,$$

$$p_0(x)=\frac{1}{1+\sum_{j=1}^{K} e^{f_j(x)}}. \tag{19}$$

The class label for the ith subject is coded as $y_i=(y_{i1},\ldots,y_{iK})$, where $y_{ij}=1$ if the ith subject is in class j and 0 otherwise. Letting $f=(f_1,\ldots,f_K)$, the negative log likelihood can be written as

$$\mathscr{L}(y,f)=\sum_{i=1}^{n}\left\{\sum_{j=1}^{K} -y_{ij}f_j(x(i))+\log\left(1+\sum_{j=1}^{K} e^{f_j(x(i))}\right)\right\}, \tag{20}$$

and an SS-ANOVA model was fitted as a special (main effects) case of (15) with cubic spline kernels.

Figure 3 (Lin, 1998) gives 10 year risk of mortality by cause as a function of age. The model included two other risk factors, glycosylated hemoglobin and systolic blood pressure at baseline, and they have been set equal at their medians for the plot. The differences between adjacent curves (from bottom to top) are probabilities for alive, diabetes, heart attack, and other causes. The data are plotted as triangles (alive, on the bottom), crosses (diabetes), diamonds (heart attack), and circles (other).

See also Zhu and Hastie (2003), who proposed a version of the multicategory penalized likelihood estimate for Bernoulli data that did not have a special base class. The model is

$$p_j(x)=\frac{e^{f_j(x)}}{\sum_{j=1}^{K} e^{f_j(x)}}, \quad j=1,\ldots,K. \tag{21}$$

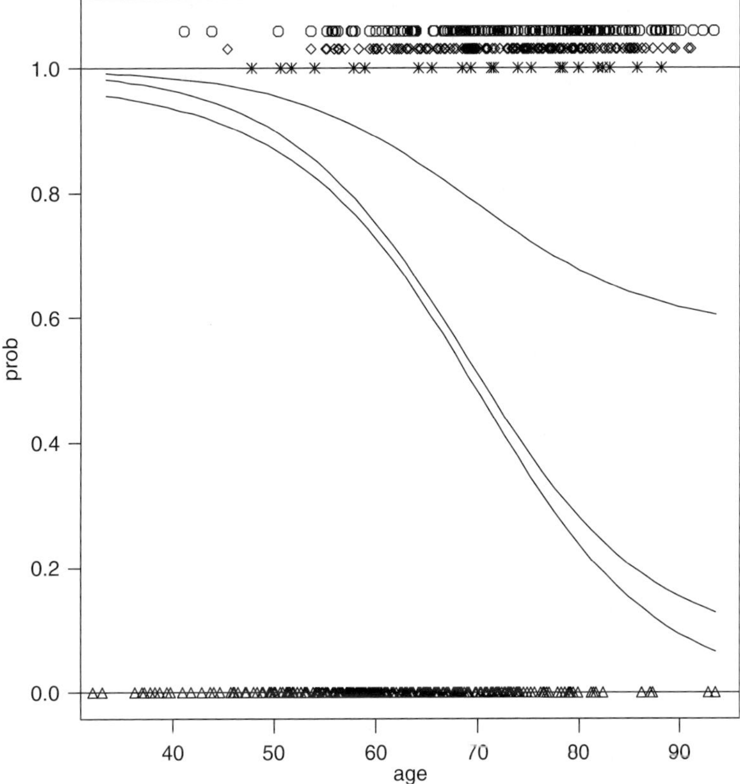

Fig. 3. Ten year risk of mortality, by cause. See text for explanation.

This model is overparameterized, but that can be handled by adding a sum-to-zero constraint $\Sigma_{j=1}^{K} f_j(x) = 0$, as was done in the multicategory SVM (Lee et al., 2004) discussed later. The authors show that this constraint is automatically satisfied in the optimization problem they propose.

2.5. Correlated Bernoulli data: the two-eye problem, the multiple sibs problem

In Gao et al. (2001), a general model including the following is considered: there are n units, each unit has K members, and there is a Bernoulli outcome that is 0 or 1, for each member. There may be member-specific risk factors and unit-specific risk factors. Thus, the responses are vectors $y_i = (y_{i1}, \ldots, y_{iK})$, where $y_{ij} \in \{0, 1\}$ is the response of the jth member of the ith unit. Allowing only first-order correlations, a general form of the negative log likelihood is

$$\mathscr{L}(y,f) = \sum_{i=1}^{n} \left\{ \sum_{j=1}^{K} -y_{ij} f_j(x(i)) - \sum_{j \neq k} \alpha_{jk} y_{ij} y_{ik} + b(f, \alpha) \right\}, \tag{22}$$

where (suppressing the dependence of f_j on $x(i)$), we have

$$b(f,\alpha) = \log\left(1 + \sum_{j=1}^{K} e^{f_j} + \sum_{j\neq k} e^{f_j+f_k+\alpha_{jk}} + \sum_{j\neq k\neq l} e^{f_j+f_k+f_l+\alpha_{jk}+\alpha_{jl}+\alpha_{kl}} + \cdots + e^{\sum_{j=1}^{K} f_j + \sum_{j\neq k}\alpha_{jk}}\right). \quad (23)$$

The α_{jk} are the log odds ratios (log OR) and are a measure of the correlation of the jth and kth outcomes when the other outcomes are 0:

$$\alpha_{jk} = \log \mathrm{OR}(j,k) = \left.\frac{Pr(y_j = 1, y_k = 1)Pr(y_j = 0, y_k = 0)}{Pr(y_j = 1, y_k = 0)Pr(y_j = 0, y_k = 1)}\right| y_r = 0, \quad r\neq j,k. \quad (24)$$

The two-eye problem was considered in detail in Gao et al. (2001) where the unit is a person and the members are the right eye and the left eye. The outcomes are pigmentary abnormality in each eye. There only person-specific predictor variables were considered, so that K is 2, $f_1(x) = f_2(x) = f(x)$, where $x(i)$ is the ith vector of person-specific risk factors, and there is a single $\alpha_{12} = \alpha$. In that work α was assumed to be a constant, f is an SS-ANOVA model, and $I_\lambda(y,f)$ of the form (15) is minimized with $\mathscr{L}(y,f)$ of the form (22). The cross-product ratio $\alpha_{12} = \log \mathrm{OR}(1,2)$ is a measure of the correlation between the two eyes, taking into account the person-specific risk factors. It may be used to estimate whether, e.g., the second eye is likely to have a bad outcome, given that the first eye already has. The case where the unit is a family and the members are a sibling pair within the family with person-specific attributes is considered in Chun (2006), where the dependence on person-specific attributes has the same functional form for each sibling. Then $K = 2$ and $f_j(x(i))$ becomes $f(x_j(i))$, where $x_j((i))$ is the attribute vector of the jth sibling, $j = 1, 2$ in the ith family. Again, an optimization problem of the form (15) is solved. If α is large, this indicates correlation within the family, taking account of person-specific risk factors, and may suggest looking for genetic components.

3. Risk factor estimation: likelihood basis pursuit and the LASSO

3.1. The l_1 penalty

In Section 2 the penalty functionals were all quadratic, being square norms or seminorms[1] in an RKHS. Generally if there are n observations there will be n

[1] A seminorm here is the norm of the projection of f onto a subspace with orthocomplement of low dimension. The orthocomplement is the null space of J. The thin plate penalty functionals are seminorms.

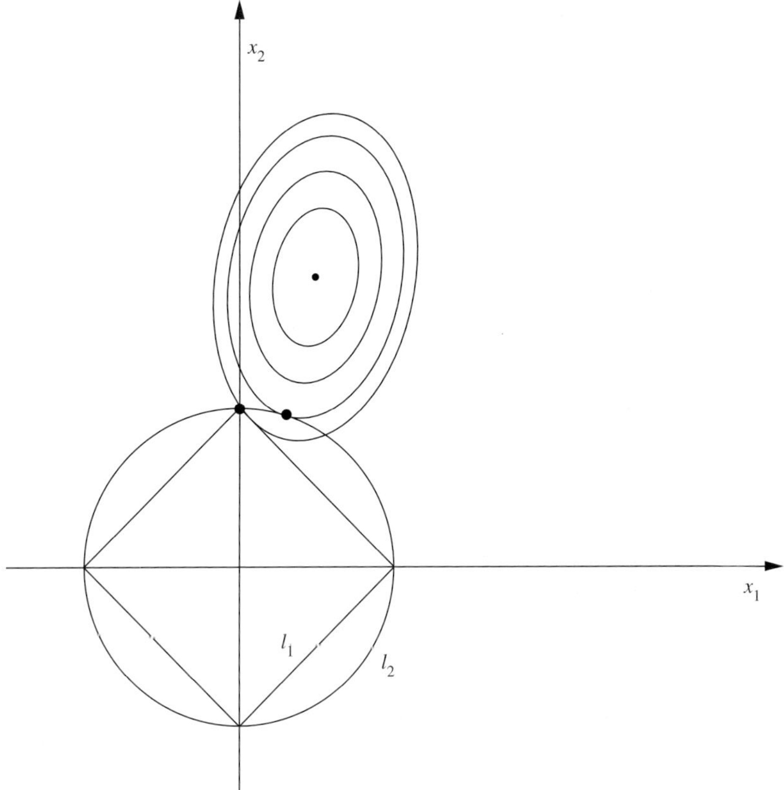

Fig. 4. Absolute value penalties lead to solutions at the extreme points of the diamond, which means sparsity in the solution vector.

representers in the solution; for very large n this is not desirable. This may be mitigated as in (14), but it is well known that imposing an absolute value penalty (l_1 penalty) on coefficients of the form $\Sigma_{i=1}^{n}|c_i|$ (as opposed to a quadratic form in the c's) will tend to provide a sparse solution, i.e., many c_i will be zero. Figure 4 suggests why. The concentric ellipses are meant to represent the level curves of a quadratic function $Q(x_1, x_2)$ in x_1 and x_2 (with the minimum in the middle) and the circle and inscribed diamond are level curves of $|x|_{l_2} = x_1^2 + x_2^2$ and $|x|_{l_1} = |x_1| + |x_2|$, respectively. If the problem is to minimize $Q(x) + |x|_{l_p}$ for $p = 1$ or 2, it can be seen that with the l_1 norm, the minimum is more likely to be at one of the corners of the diamond. The desirability of sparsity comes up in different contexts: to select a sparser number of basis functions given an overcomplete set of basis functions, or to select a smaller number of variables or clusters of variables out of a much larger set to be used for regression or classification. Likelihood basis pursuit (Chen et al., 1998) and the LASSO (Tibshirani, 1996) are two basic papers in the basis function context and variable selection context, respectively. There is a large literature in the context of variable selection in linear models, based on the LASSO, which in its simplest form imposes an l_1 penalty on the coefficients in a linear model; see Efron et al. (2004), Fan and Li (2001), Knight and Fu (2000), and others. An overcomplete set of basis functions in a wavelet context was generated in Chen et al. (1998), who then reduced the number of basis functions in their model via an l_1 penalty on the coefficients. In the spirit of Chen et al. (1998), Zhang et al. (2004) generated an overcomplete set of basis functions by the use of representers in an SS-ANOVA model to do model fitting and variable selection in a flexible way, similarly reducing the number of main effects or interactions by an l_1 penalty on basis function coefficients. The method was used to obtain flexible main effects models for risk factors for eye diseases based on data collected in the Beaver Dam Eye Study (Klein et al., 1991). Beginning with Gunn and Kandola (2002) various authors have simultaneously imposed l_1 and quadratic penalties in the context of flexible nonparametric regression/kernel methods; see Zhang and Lin (2006a, 2006b) and Zhang (2006) (who called it "COSSO"). Software for the COSSO may be found at http://www4.stat.ncsu.edu/~hzhang/software.html. Later Zou and Hastie (2005) (calling it "Elastic Net"), in the context of (linear) parametric regression, used the same idea of a two term penalty functional, one quadratic and the other l_1.

3.2. LASSO-Patternsearch

The LASSO-Patternsearch method of Shi et al. (2006) was designed with specially selected basis functions and tuning procedures to take advantage of the sparsity inducing properties of l_1 penalties to enable the detection of potentially important higher order variable interactions. Large and possibly very large attribute vectors $x = (x_1, \ldots, x_p)$ with entries 0 or 1 are considered, with Bernoulli outcomes. The log odds ratio $f(x) = \log[p(x)/(1 - p(x))]$ is modeled there as

$$f(x) = \mu + \sum_{\alpha=1}^{p} c_\alpha B_\alpha(x) + \sum_{\alpha<\beta} c_{\alpha\beta} B_{\alpha\beta}(x) + \sum_{\alpha<\beta<\gamma} c_{\alpha\beta\gamma} B_{\alpha\beta\gamma}(x) + \cdots + c_{123\cdots p} B_{123\cdots p}(x), \tag{25}$$

where $B_\alpha(x) = x_\alpha$, $B_{\alpha\beta}(x) = x_\alpha x_\beta$, and so forth, and the optimization problem to be solved is: find f of the form (25) to minimize

$$I_\lambda\{y, f\} = \sum_{i=1}^{n} -y_i f(x(i)) + \log(1 + e^{f(x(i))}) + \lambda \sum_{\text{all } c} |c|, \tag{26}$$

where the sum taken over all c means the sum of the absolute values of the coefficients (the l_1 penalty). For small p (say, $p = 8$), the series in (25) may be continued to the end, but for large p the series will be truncated. A special purpose numerical algorithm was proposed that can handle a very large number (at least 4000) of unknown coefficients, many of which will turn out to be 0. The "patterns" or basis functions in (25) follow naturally from the log linear representation of the multivariate Bernoulli distribution; see Shi et al. (2006) and Whittaker (1990). This approach is designed for the case when the directions of all or almost all of the "risky" variables are known and are coded as 1, since then the representation of (25) is most compact, although this is by no means necessary. When this and similar problems are tuned for predictive loss, there is a bias toward overestimating the number of basis functions and including some noise patterns. However, at the same time it insures a high probability of including all the important basis functions; see Leng et al. (2006) and Zou (2006). The LASSO-Patternsearch is a two-step approach, with the first step global, as opposed to a greedy approach. In the first step the model is fitted globally and tuned by a predictive loss criteria. Then a second step takes those patterns surviving the first step and enters them a parametric generalized linear model. Finally, all basis functions whose coefficients fail a significance test in this model at level q are deleted, where the value of q is treated as another tuning parameter. This method uncovered an interesting relation between smoking, vitamins and cataracts as risk factors in myopia data collected as part of the Beaver Dam Eye study (Klein et al., 1991). The method has also been successfully used to select patterns of single nucleotide polymorphisms (SNPs) in DNA data that can separate cases from controls with a high degree of accuracy. Pseudocode is found in Shi et al. (2006). Other approaches for finding clusters of important variables include Breiman (2001), Ruczinski et al. (2002), Yuan and Lin (2006), and Park and Hastie (2007). These methods rely on sequential, stepwise or greedy algorithms, and tend to work well in a broad range of scenarios, although stepwise algorithms are not guaranteed to always find the best subset. Some preliminary results suggest that under certain kinds of correlated scenarios the global aspects of the LASSO-Patternsearch may prove advantageous over stepwise approaches.

4. Classification: support vector machines and related estimates

SVMs were proposed by Vapnik and colleagues as a nonparametric classification method in the early 1990s; see Vapnik (1995) and references cited there, where it was obtained in an argument quite different than the description we give here. However, in the late 1990s (Evgeniou et al., 2000; Wahba, 1999) it was observed that SVMs could be obtained as the solution to an optimization problem in an RKHS. This made it easy to compare and contrast SVMs with other nonparametric methods involving optimization problems in an RKHS, to develop generalizations, and to examine its theoretical properties. In any case the efficiency of the SVM was quickly recognized in practice, and theory soon followed to explain just why SVMs worked so well. Before giving details, we note the following books: Cristianini and Shawe-Taylor (2000), Scholkopf et al. (1999, 2004), Scholkopf and Smola (2002), Shawe-Taylor and Cristianini (2004), and Smola et al. (2000).

4.1. Two-category support vector machines

Figure 5 illustrates the flexibility of a (two-category) SVM. The locations of the + and o "attribute vectors" were chosen according to a uniform distribution on the

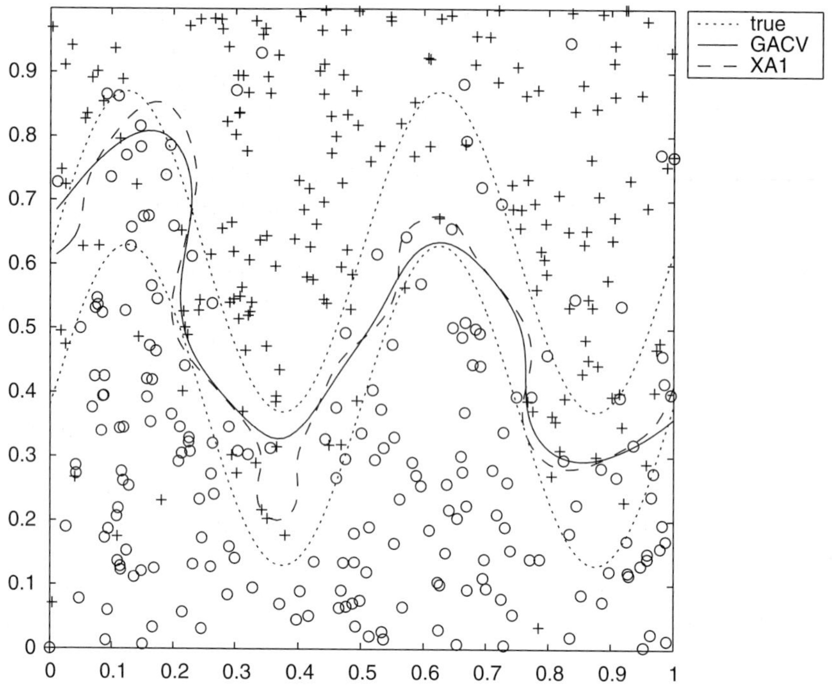

Fig. 5. SVM: toy problem, tuned by GACV and the XiAlpha method.

unit rectangle. Attribute vectors falling between the two dotted lines were assigned to be + or o with equal probability of .5. Points above the upper dotted (true) line were assigned + with .95 and o with probability .05, and below the lower dotted line the reverse: o with probability .95 and + with probability .05. Thus, any classifier whose boundary lies within the two dotted lines is satisfying the Bayes rule – that is, it will minimize the expected classification error from new observations drawn from the same distribution.

In the two-category SVM the training data is coded $y_i \pm 1$ according as the ith object is in the + class or the o class. The classifier f is assumed to be of the form $f(s) = d + h(s)$, where the constant d and $h \in \mathcal{H}_K$ are chosen to minimize

$$I_\lambda\{y,f\} = \frac{1}{n}\sum_{i=1}^{n} \mathcal{C}(y_i, f(t(i))) + \lambda |h|^2_{\mathcal{H}_K}, \tag{27}$$

where $\mathcal{C}$ is the so-called hinge function: $\mathcal{C}(y,f) = (1 - yf)_+$, where $(\tau)_+ = 1$ if $\tau > 0$ and 0 otherwise. A new object will be classified as in the + class if $f(x) > 0$ and in the o class if $f(x) < 0$. From the representer theorem, the minimizer of $I_\lambda\{y,f\}$ again has a representation of the form:

$$f(s) = d + \sum_{i=1}^{n} c_i K(t(i), s). \tag{28}$$

Using $||\Sigma_{i=1}^n c_i K_{t(i)}(\cdot)||^2_{\mathscr{H}_K} = c' K_n c$, where K_n is the $n \times n$ matrix with i, jth entry $K(t(i), t(j))$ is substituted into (27). The problem of finding d and $c_1, \ldots, c_n$ is solved numerically by transforming the problem to its dual problem, which results in the problem of minimizing a convex functional subject to a family of linear inequality constraints. Details of this transformation may be found in any of the books cited, in Evgeniou et al. (2000), Wahba et al. (2000), and elsewhere.

For the toy problem in Fig. 5, the RK $K(s, t)$ was taken as the Gaussian kernel $K(s, t) = \mathrm{e}^{-(1/2\sigma^2)||s-t||^2}$, so that the two tuning parameters λ and σ^2 have to be chosen. The solid line in Fig. 5 is the 0 level curve of f obtained by choosing λ and σ^2 by the generalized approximate cross-validation (GACV) method, and the dashed line by choosing λ and σ^2 by Joachim's XiAlpha method; see Section 6.4. The SVM^{light} software is popular code for computing the two-class SVM, and the XiAlpha method is implemented in it. See Joachims (1999), http://svmlight.joachims.org. Other codes and references can be found at http://www.kernel-machines.org.

Figure 6 is a toy example which demonstrates the difference between SVM and penalized likelihood estimates. The penalized likelihood method provides an estimate of the probability p that an object is in the "1" class. p is above or below .5 according as f is positive or negative. Therefore, a classification problem with a representative number of objects in each class in the training set and equal costs

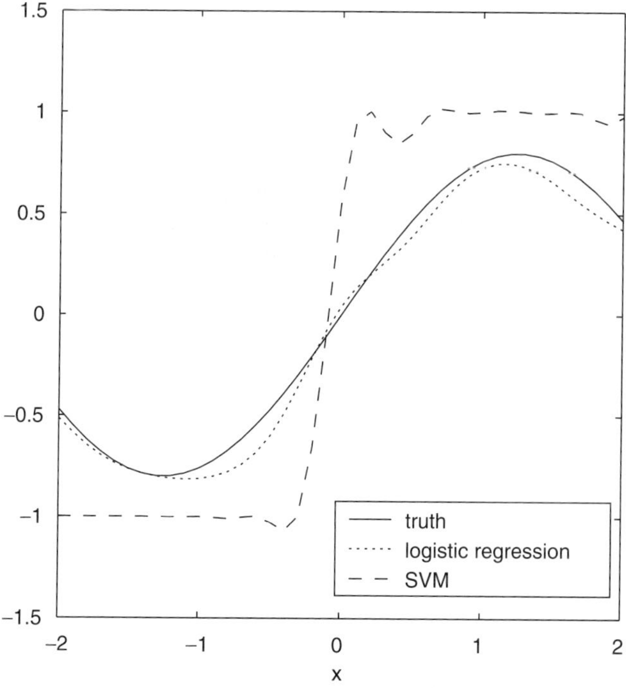

Fig. 6. Penalized likelihood and the support vector machine compared.

of misclassification can be solved by implementing the Bayes rule, which is equivalent to determining whether the log odds ratio f is positive or negative. The fundamental reason why the SVM works so well is that *it is estimating the sign of the log odds ratio*. See Lin (2001, 2002) and Lin et al. (2002) for proofs. This is demonstrated in Fig. 6. The vertical scale in Fig. 6 is $2p-1$. Three hundred equally spaced samples in x were selected and assigned the + class with probability p, given by the solid ("truth") line in Fig. 5. The dotted line (labeled "logistic regression") is the penalized likelihood estimate of $2p-1$ and is very close to the true $2p-1$. The dashed line is the SVM. The SVM is very close to -1 if $2p-1<0$, and close to $+1$ for $2p-1>0$. Note however that they result in almost exactly the same classifier. The SVM is just one member of the class of large margin classifiers. A large margin classifier is one where $\mathscr{C}(y,f)$ depends only on the product yf. When the data are coded as ± 1, then the negative log likelihood becomes $\log(1+e^{yf})$ and so it is also a large margin classifier. From Lin (2001, 2002) it can be seen that under very weak conditions on $\mathscr{C}(y,f) = \mathscr{C}(yf)$, large margin classifiers implement the Bayes rule, i.e., the sign of the estimate of f is an estimate of the sign of the log odds ratio. Among the special properties of the SVM, however, is that the hinge function is, in some sense, the closest convex upper bound to the misclassification counter $[-yf]^*$, where $[\tau]^*=1$ if $\tau>0$ and 0 otherwise. Furthermore, due to the nature of the dual optimization problem, the SVM estimate of f tends to have a sparse representation, i.e., many of the coefficients c_i are 0, a property not shared by the penalized likelihood estimate.

Regarding the form $f(s)=d+h(s)$ with $h\in\mathscr{H}_K$ of (27), frequently the kernel K is taken as a rbf. In some applications, particularly in variable selection problems as we shall see later, it is convenient to choose K as tensor sums and products of univariate rbf's, as in SS-ANOVA models, with one important difference: the null space of the penalty functional should only contain at most the constant function. For technical reasons, the SVM may fail to have a unique solution for larger null spaces.

4.2. Nonstandard support vector machines

The previous (standard) SVM, when appropriately tuned, asymptotically implements the Bayes rule, i.e., it minimizes the expected cost, when the training set is representative of the population to be classified in the future, and the costs of each kind of misclassification are the same. The nonstandard SVM of Lin et al. (2002) is a modification of the standard SVM which implements the Bayes rule when neither of these conditions hold. Let π^+ and $\pi^-=1-\pi^+$ be prior probabilities of + and − classes, and let π_s^+ and π_s^- be proportions of + and − classes in the training set, and c^+ and c^- be the costs for false + and false − classifications. Let $g^+(x)$ and $g^-(x)$ be the densities for x in the + class and the 1 class, respectively. Let $p(x)$ be $Pr[y=1|x]$ in the population to be classified. Then

$$p(x)=\frac{\pi^+g^+(x)}{\pi^+g^+(x)+\pi^-g^-(x)}. \tag{29}$$

Let $p_s(x)$ be $Pr[y=1|x]$ in a population distributed as the training sample. Then

$$p_s(x) = \frac{\pi_s^+ g^+(x)}{\pi_s^+ g^+(x) + \pi_s^- g^-(x)}. \tag{30}$$

Then the Bayes rule classifies as + when $p(x)/(1-p(x)) > c^+/c^-$ and – otherwise, equivalently when $p_s(x)/(1-p_s(x)) > (c^+/c^-)(\pi_s^+/\pi_s^-)(\pi^-/\pi^+)$. Letting $L(-1) = c^+\pi_s^+\pi^-$ and $L(1) = c^-\pi_s^-\pi^+$, the Bayes rule is then equivalent to classifying as + when $\text{sign}\{p_s - [L(-1)/(L(-1)+L(1))]\} > 0$ and – otherwise. The nonstandard SVM finds f of the form

$$\frac{1}{n}\sum_{i=1}^{n} L(y_i)[(1 - y_i f(x(i))]_+ + \lambda ||h||^2_{\mathcal{H}_K} \tag{31}$$

over functions of the form $f(x) = h(x) + b$. It is shown in Lin et al. (2002) that the nonstandard SVM of (31) is estimating sign $\{p_s - [L(-1)/(L(-1)+L(1))]\}$, again just what you need to implement the Bayes rule.

4.3. Multicategory support vector machines

Many approaches have been proposed to classify into one of the k possible classes by using SVMs. A Google search as of 2006 for "multiclass SVM" or "multicategory support vector machine" gives over 500 hits. For the moment, letting $y_j \in \{1, \ldots, k\}$ and considering the standard situation of equal misclassification costs and representative training sample, if $P(y=j|x) = p_j(x)$, then the Bayes rule assigns a new x to the class with the largest $p_j(x)$. Two kinds of strategies appear in the literature. The first solves the problem via solving several binary problems, one-vs.-rest, one-vs.-one, and various designs of several-vs.-several. See, for example, Allwein et al. (2000) and Dietterich and Bakiri (1995). The second considers all classes at once. Two examples of this are Crammer and Singer (2000) and Weston and Watkins (1999) with many variants in the recent literature. Many of these methods are highly successful in general practice, but, in general, situations can be found where they do not implement the Bayes rule; see Lee et al. (2004).

The MSVM of Lee and Lee (2003) and Lee et al. (2004) goes as follows: first, y_i is coded as a k-dimensional vector $(y_{i1}, \ldots, y_{ik})$ with 1 in the jth position if y_j is in class j, and $-1/(k-1)$ in the other positions; thus, $\Sigma_{r=1}^{k} y_{ir} = 0$, $i = 1, \ldots, n$. Let $L_{jr} = 1$ for $j \neq r$ and 0 otherwise. The MSVM solves for a vector of functions $f_\lambda = (f_\lambda^1, \ldots, f_\lambda^k)$, with $f^r(x) = d^r + h^r(x)$, each h^k in $\mathcal{H}_K$ satisfying the *sum-to-zero* constraint $\Sigma_{r=1}^{k} f^r(x) = 0$ all x, which minimizes

$$\frac{1}{n}\sum_{i=1}^{n}\sum_{r=1}^{k} L_{\text{cat}(i)r}(f^r(x(i)) - y_{ir})_+ + \lambda \sum_{j=1}^{k} ||h^j||^2_{\mathcal{H}_K}, \tag{32}$$

equivalently

$$\frac{1}{n}\sum_{i=1}^{n}\sum_{r\neq \mathrm{cat}(i)}\left(f^r(x(i))+\frac{1}{k-1}\right)_+ +\lambda\sum_{j=1}^{k}||h^j||^2_{\mathscr{H}_K}, \tag{33}$$

where cat(i) is the category of y_i.

It can be shown that $k = 2$ case reduces to the usual two-category SVM. The target for the MSVM is shown in Lee et al. (2004) to be $f(t) = (f^1(t), \ldots, f^k(t))$ with $f^j(t) = 1$ if $p_j(t)$ is bigger than the other $p_l(t)$ and $f^j(t) = -1/(k-1)$ otherwise, thus implementing an estimate of the Bayes rule. Similar to the two-class case, there is a nonstandard version of the MSVM. Suppose the sample is not representative, and misclassification costs are not equal. Let

$$L_{jr} = \left(\frac{\pi^j}{\pi^j_{\mathrm{s}}}\right)c_{jr}, \quad j\neq r, \tag{34}$$

where c_{jr} is the cost of misclassifying a j as an r and $c_{rr} = 0 = L_{rr}$. π^j is the prior probability of category j and π^j_{s} the fraction of samples from category j in the training set. Substituting (34) into (32) gives the nonstandard MSVM, and it is shown in Lee et al. (2004) that the nonstandard MSVM has as its target the Bayes rule. That is, the target is $f_j(x) = 1$ if j minimizes

$$\sum_{\ell=1}^{k} c_{\ell j}p_\ell(x),$$

equivalently

$$\sum_{\ell=1}^{k} L_{\ell j}p^{\mathrm{s}}_\ell(x),$$

and $f_j(x) = -1/(k-1)$ otherwise.

To illustrate the use of the MSVM, Lee et al. (2004) revisited the small round blue cell tumors (SRBCTs) of childhood data set in Khan et al. (2001). There are four classes: neuroblastoma (NB), rhabdomyosarcoma (RMS), non-Hodgkin lymphoma (NHL), and the Ewing family of tumors (EWS), and the data were cDNA gene expression profiles. There was a training set of 63 samples (NB: 12, RMS: 20, BL: 8, EWS: 23), and a test set of 20 SRBCT cases (NB: 6, RMS: 5, BL: 3, EWS: 6) and 5 non-SRBCTs. The gene expression profiles contained observations on 2308 genes; after several preprocessing steps the observations were reduced to those on 100 genes, and the final data set for classification consisted of a vector of three principal components based on the 100 gene observations for each profile. The principal components turned out to contain enough information for nearly perfect classification.

The four class labels are coded according as EWS: $(1, -1/3, -1/3, -1/3)$, BL: $(-1/3, 1, -1/3, -1/3)$, NB: $(-1/3, -1/3, 1, -1/3)$, and RMS: $(-1/3, -1/3, -1/3, 1)$.

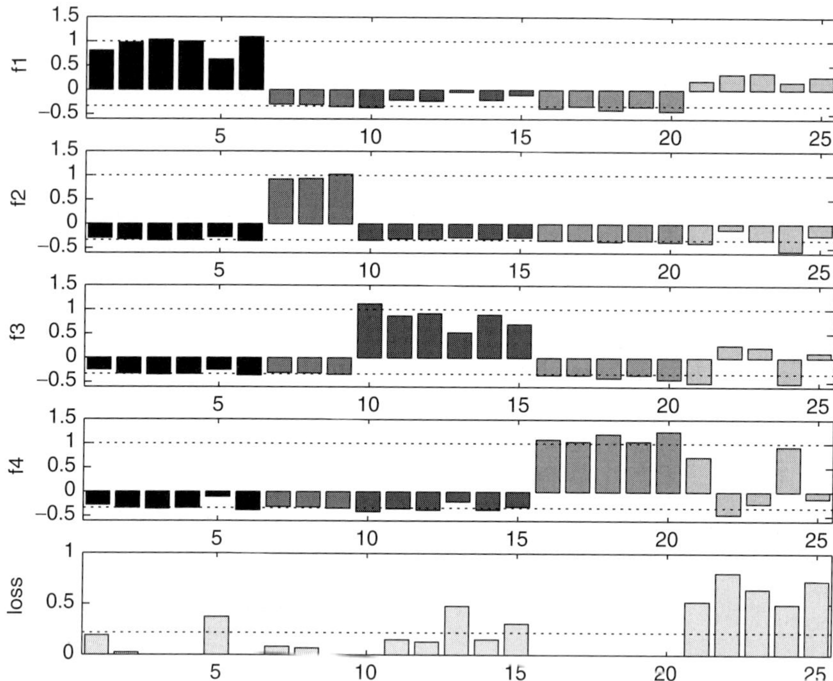

Fig. 7. Predicted four-dimensional decision vectors for 20 test samples in four classes and 5 test samples in "none of the above." (Adapted from Lee et al. (2004), © *Journal of the American Statistical Association*, reprinted with permission.)

The top four panels in Fig. 7 show the predicted decision vectors (f_1, f_2, f_3, f_4) at the test examples. The first six columns are the estimated class labels for the six EWS cases in the test set: ideally they will be $(1, -1/3, -1/3, -1/3)$. As can be seen, of these six cases the f_1 bars (top panel) are all close to 1, and in the three next lower panels, the f_2, f_3, and f_4 bars are all negative, so that these six members of the test set are all identified correctly. The next three columns are the three BL cases in the test set, ideally their estimates are $(-1/3, 1, -1/3, -1/3)$ – in the second panel they are all about 1, and in the first, third, and fourth panels they are all negative, so that these BL cases are all classified correctly. In the next six columns, the six members of the NB class are classified correctly, i.e., f_3 is close to 1 and the other components are negative, and the next five RMS cases are all classified correctly. The last five columns are the five non-SRBT cases, and with one exception none of the bars are close to one, with the exceptional case having both f_1 and f_4 positive, leading to a dubious classification ("none of the above"). The bottom panel gives a measure of the weakness of the classification, obtained from a bootstrap argument, and it is suggesting that the classification of all of the "none of the above" cases is weak. Software for the MSVM can be found at http://www.stat.ohio-state.edu/~yklee/software.html.

4.4. Support vector machines with variable selection

In dealing with classification problems with very large observation vectors such as occur, for example, in microarray (gene chip) or SNP data, classification is only part of the problem. It is typically of scientific interest to know which genes out of the thousands obtained from the gene chip data are important for the classification, or which SNPs from the thousands that are observed are important. Google provides thousands of hits for "Variable Selection" and SVM. Here we briefly provide the flavor of three recent papers appropriate to these situations. We describe only two-category SVMs, but most of the results generalized to the MSVM.

In Zhang (2006), f is modeled as a (low order) SS-ANOVA model which can be written:

$$f(x_1, \ldots, x_d) = d + \sum_{\alpha=1}^{d} h_\alpha(x_\alpha) + \sum_{\alpha<\beta} h_{\alpha\beta}(x_\alpha, x_\beta) + \cdots, \tag{35}$$

with $h_\alpha \in \mathscr{H}^\alpha$, $h_{\alpha\beta} \in \mathscr{H}^\alpha \otimes \mathscr{H}^\beta \cdots$, and so forth. The proposed SVM optimization problem becomes

$$\min_{f\in\mathscr{F}} \sum_{i=1}^{n} [1 - y_i f(x(i))]_+ + \tau \left[\sum_{\alpha=1}^{d} ||h_\alpha||_{\mathscr{H}^\alpha} + \sum_{\alpha<\beta} ||h_{\alpha\beta}||_{\mathscr{H}^\alpha\otimes\mathscr{H}^\beta} + \cdots \right], \tag{36}$$

where $x = (x_1, \ldots, x_d)$. Note that (36) uses norms rather than squared norms in the penalty functional. This formulation is shown to be equivalent to

$$\min_{f\in\mathscr{F}} \sum_{i=1}^{n} [1 - y_i f(x(i))]_+ + \left[\sum_{\alpha=1}^{d} \theta_\alpha^{-1} \|h_\alpha\|^2_{\mathscr{H}^\alpha} + \sum_{\alpha<\beta} \theta_{\alpha\beta}^{-1} ||h_{\alpha\beta}||^2_{\mathscr{H}^\alpha\otimes\mathscr{H}^\beta} + \cdots \right] + \lambda \left[\sum \theta_\alpha + \sum \theta_{\alpha\beta} + \cdots \right], \tag{37}$$

where θs are constrained to be nonnegative. Lee et al. (2006) also considered the approach of (37), in the context of the MSVM of Lee et al. (2004) and applied the method to the data of Khan et al. (2001) that were used there, to select influential genes. The home pages of both these first authors cited contain related software relevant to this problem.

Mukherjee and Wu (2006) performed variable selection via an algorithm which learns the gradient of the response with respect to each variable – if the gradient is small enough, then the variable is deemed not important. They applied their method to the same two-class leukemia data of Golub et al. (1999) that was analyzed in Lee and Lee (2003).

5. Dissimilarity data and kernel estimates

In many problems direct attribute vectors are not known, or are not convenient to deal with, while some sort of pairwise dissimilarity score between pairs of objects in a training set is known. Examples could be subjective pairwise differences between images as provided by human observers, pairwise differences between graphs, strings, sentences, microarray observations, protein sequences, etc. Given pairwise dissimilarity scores we describe two approaches to obtaining a kernel, which can then be used in an SVM for classifying protein sequence data.

5.1. Regularized kernel estimation

The regularized kernel estimation (RKE) method (Lu et al., 2005) goes as follows: given K, a nonnegative definite $n \times n$ matrix, the squared distance $\hat{d}_{ij}$ between the ith and jth objects in a set of n objects can be defined by $\hat{d}_{ij}(K) = K(i,i) + K(j,j) - 2K(i,j)$, where $K(i,j)$ is the (i,j) entry of K. Given a set of noisy, possibly incomplete, set of pairwise distances $\{d_{ij}\}$ between n objects, the RKE problem is to find an $n \times n$ nonnegative definite matrix which minimizes

$$\min_{K \succcurlyeq 0} \sum_{(i,j)\in\Omega} |d_{ij} - \hat{d}_{ij}(K)| + \lambda \operatorname{trace}(K). \tag{38}$$

Here Ω is a set of pairwise distances which forms a connected set, i.e., a graph connecting the included pairs is connected. This problem can be solved numerically for K by a convex cone algorithm; see Benson and Ye (2004), Lu et al. (2005), and (Tütüncü et al. (2003)).

Letting $K = K_\lambda$ be the minimizer of (38), the eigenvalues of K_λ are set to zero after the pth largest, resulting in $K_{\lambda,p}$, say. Pseudodata $z(i)$, $i = 1, \ldots, n$, for the n objects can be found by letting $z(i) = (z_1(i), \ldots, z_p(i))$, where $z_v(i) = \sqrt{\lambda_v}\phi_v(i)$, $v = 1, \ldots, p$, with λ_v and ϕ_v being the eigenvalues and eigenvectors of $K_{\lambda,p}$. Given labels on (a subset of) the n objects, a SVM can be built on the pseudodata. To classify a new object, a "newbie" algorithm is used to obtain the pseudodata $z(n+1)$ for the $n+1$st object. The newbie algorithm obtains an $(n+1) \times (n+1)$ kernel K_{n+1} of the form

$$\tilde{K}_{n+1} = \begin{bmatrix} K_n & b^{\mathrm{T}} \\ b & c \end{bmatrix} \succcurlyeq 0 \tag{39}$$

(where $b \in R^n$ and c is a scalar) that solves the following optimization problem:

$$\begin{aligned} &\min_{c \geq 0, b} \sum_{i\in\Psi} |d_{i,n+1} - \hat{d}_{i,n+1}(K_{n+1})| \\ &\text{such that } b \in \operatorname{range}(K_n), \quad c - b^{\mathrm{T}} K_n^{+} b \geq 0, \end{aligned} \tag{40}$$

where K_n^+ is the pseudoinverse of $K_n = K_{\lambda,p}$ and Ψ a suitably rich subset of $\{1, 2, \ldots, n\}$. Pseudodata $z(n+1)$ are found on observing that $z(i)^{\mathrm{T}} z(n+1) = K(i, n+1) = b_i$. Figure 8 (Lu et al., 2005) gives the 280 eigenvalues for K based on dissimilarity scores from protein sequence alignment scores from 280 protein sequences. The eigenvalues of K_λ were truncated after $p = 3$, and a three-dimensional black and white plot of the pseudodata is given in Fig. 9. The four classes can be seen, although the original color plot in Lu et al. (2005) is clearer.

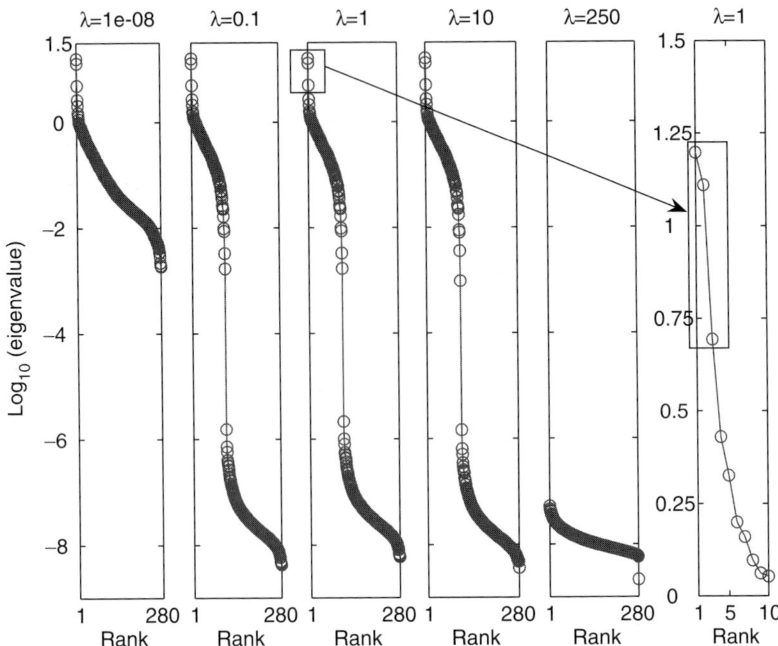

Fig. 8. (Left five panels) log scale eigensequence plots for five values of λ. As λ increases, smaller eigenvalues begin to shrink. (Right panel) First 10 eigenvalues of the $\lambda = 1$ case displayed on a larger scale. (From Lu et al. (2005), ©*Proceedings of the National Academy of Sciences of the United States of America*, reprinted with permission.)

This approach can easily tolerate missing data, in fact only about 36% of the pairs were used, and it is robust to very noisy or binned dissimilarity data, for example, dissimilarity information given on a scale of 1, 2, 3, 4, or 5.

The RKE can be used in the semisupervised situation, where the kernel is built on both labeled and unlabeled data, and then used to classify both the unlabeled data used to build it and new observations that were not.

Data from multiple sources, some of which may involve dissimilarity data and some direct attribute data, can be combined in an SVM once kernels are given for each source. Let z be a pseudoattribute vector of length p, obtained from the $n \times n$ kernel K_Z which was derived from dissimilarity data and then had its eigenvalues truncated after the pth, and let x be an attribute vector, with an associated kernel $K_X(x, x')$ to be chosen (for example, a Gaussian kernel). We can define a composite attribute vector as $t^{\mathrm{T}} = (z^{\mathrm{T}} : x^{\mathrm{T}})$ and build a SVM on the domain of the composite attribute vectors based on the kernel $K_\mu(t, t') = \mu_Z K_Z(z, z') + \mu_X K_X(x, x')$, where μ_Z and μ_X are nonnegative tuning parameters. $K_Z(z, z') = (z, z')$, the Euclidean inner product, from the way that z was obtained, but some other kernel, for example, a Gaussian or SS-ANOVA kernel could be built on top of the pseudodata. Then the (two-category) SVM finds d and $c = (c_1, \ldots, c_n)$ to

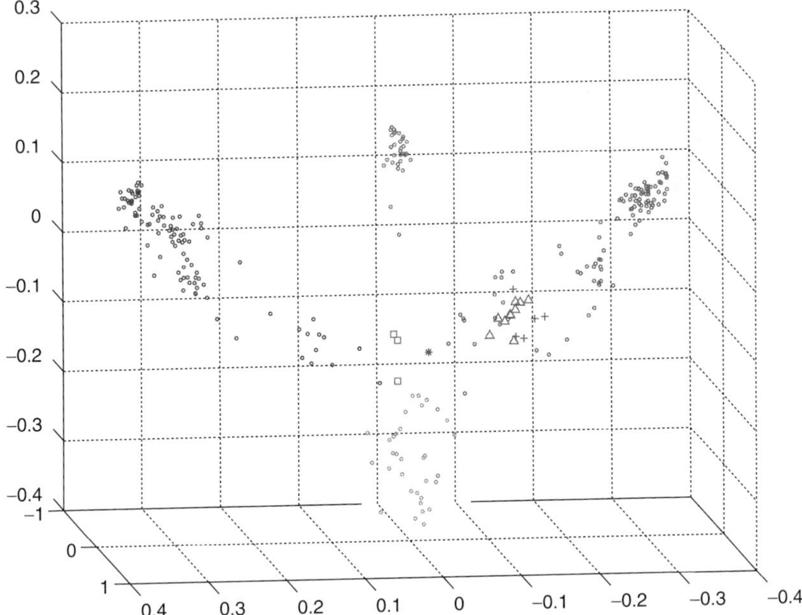

Fig. 9. 3D representation of the sequence space for 280 proteins from the globin family. (From Lu et al. (2005) ©*Proceedings of the National Academy of Sciences of the United States of America*, reprinted with permission.)

minimize

$$\sum_{i-1}^{n} [1 - y_i f(x(i))]_+ + \lambda c' K_\mu c, \tag{41}$$

as before where

$$f(t) = d + \sum_{i=1}^{n} c_i K_\mu(t(i), t), \tag{42}$$

and $\mu = (\mu_Z, \mu_X)$ are to be chosen. Generalizations to the MSVM can also be defined.

5.2. Kernels from constructed attribute vectors

In Lanckriet et al. (2004) a detailed study was carried out using data from several sources, including both direct data and dissimilarity data. For dissimilarity data they used a kernel constructed from n-dimensional attribute vectors whose components are themselves dissimilarity measures. The method is described in Liao and Noble (2003) and elsewhere. It goes as follows: the training set consists of n objects, with $\binom{n}{2}$ dissimilarity scores d_{ij} available between all pairs. The ith object is assigned an n-dimensional vector $x(i)$ whose rth component is d_{ir}. Then

$K(i,j)$ is defined as $(x(i), x(j))$, where the inner product is the Euclidean inner product.

6. Tuning methods

6.1. Generalized cross-validation

This article has concentrated on Bernoulli and categorical data, since this kind of data is typically assumed when "statistical learning" is the topic. However, to best explain several of the tuning methods used in conjunction with Bernoulli and categorical data, it is easiest to begin by describing tuning for nonparametric function estimation with Gaussian data. The model is

$$y_i = f(x(i)) + \varepsilon_i, \quad i = 1, \ldots, n, \tag{43}$$

where $x \in \mathcal{T}$ (some domain), $f \in \mathcal{H}_K$, and ε_i are i.i.d. Gaussian random variables with common unknown variance σ^2. The estimate f_λ is obtained as the solution to the problem: find $f \in \mathcal{H}_K$ to minimize

$$I_\lambda\{y, f\} = \frac{1}{n}\sum_{i=1}^{n}(y_i - f(x(i)))^2 + \lambda J(f), \tag{44}$$

where $J(f) = \|f\|^2_{\mathcal{H}_K}$ or a seminorm in $\mathcal{H}_K$. The target for choosing λ is to minimize

$$\frac{1}{n}\sum_{i=1}^{n}(f(x(i) - f_\lambda(x(i)))^2, \tag{45}$$

where f is the "true" f in the model. The GCV to be described (Craven and Wahba, 1979; Golub et al., 1979) is derived from a leaving-out-one estimate for λ which goes as follows: let $f_\lambda^{[-k]}(x(k))$ be the estimate of f based on the data omitting the kth data point. The leaving-out-one function $V_0(\lambda)$ is defined as

$$V_0(\lambda) = \frac{1}{n}\sum_{k=1}^{n}(y_k - f_\lambda^{[-k]}(x(k)))^2, \tag{46}$$

and the minimizer of V_0 is the leaving-out-one estimate. Let $A(\lambda)$ be the $n \times n$ influence matrix, which satisfies

$$(f_\lambda(x(1)), \ldots, f_\lambda(x(n)))^{\mathrm{T}} = A(\lambda)(y_1, \ldots, y_n)^{\mathrm{T}}, \tag{47}$$

which exists since the estimate is linear in the data. It is known from the leaving-out-one lemma (Craven and Wahba, 1979) that

$$V_0(\lambda) \equiv \frac{1}{n}\sum_{k=1}^{n}\frac{(y_k - f_\lambda(x(k)))^2}{(1 - a_{kk}(\lambda))^2}, \tag{48}$$

where $a_{kk} \in (0,1)$ are the diagonal elements of $A(\lambda)$. The GCV function $V(\lambda)$ is obtained by replacing each a_{kk} in (48) by their average, namely $(1/n)\text{trace}\,A(\lambda)$, to get

$$V(\lambda) = \frac{1}{n}\frac{\sum_{i=1}^{n}(y_i - f_\lambda(x(i)))^2}{(1-(1/n)\text{tr}\,A(\lambda))^2}, \tag{49}$$

and the estimate of λ is the minimizer of $V(\lambda)$. Theoretical properties are discussed in Li (1986), and the important randomized trace technique for calculating $\text{tr}\,A(\lambda)$ can be found in Girard (1989, 1995) and Hutchinson (1989). A different calculation method is found in Golub and vonMatt (1997). For comparison to the methods described below, we note that when $I_\lambda\{y,f\}$ is as in (44), i.e., J is a quadratic form in $(f_\lambda(x(i)),\ldots,f_\lambda(x(n)))$, then $A(\lambda)$ is the inverse Hessian of I_λ of (44) with respect to $f_i \equiv f_\lambda(x(i))$, $i = 1,\ldots,n$.

6.2. Generalized approximate cross-validation, Bernoulli data, and RKHS penalties

The GACV for Bernoulli data and RK squared norms or seminorms as penalties was provided in Xiang and Wahba (1996). As in Section 2 I_λ is of the form

$$I_\lambda\{y,f\} = \frac{1}{n}\sum_{i=1}^{n} -y_i f(x(i)) + \log(1+e^{f(x(i))}) + \lambda J(f), \tag{50}$$

where $J(f)$ is a squared norm or seminorm in an RKHS. The target for the GACV is the expected value of the so-called comparative Kullback Liebler distance (CKL) between the true and estimated probability distributions, and is

$$\text{CKL}(\lambda) = \frac{1}{n}\sum_{i=1}^{n} -p(x(i))f_\lambda(x(i)) + \log(1+e^{f_\lambda(x(i))}), \tag{51}$$

where $p(x)$ is the true but unknown probability that $y = 1|x$. The leaving-out-one estimate of the CKL is

$$V_0(\lambda) = \frac{1}{n}\sum_{k=1}^{n} -y_k f_\lambda^{[-k]}(x(k)) + \log(1+e^{f_\lambda(x(k))}). \tag{52}$$

The GACV is obtained from $V_0(\lambda)$ by a series of approximations followed by averaging over the diagonal elements of a matrix which plays the role of the influence matrix, and the result is

$$\text{GACV}(\lambda) = \frac{1}{n}\sum_{i=1}^{n} -y_i f_\lambda(x(i)) + \log(1+e^{f_\lambda(x(i))}) + \frac{1}{n}\text{tr}\,A(\lambda)\frac{\sum_{i=1}^{n} y_i(y_i - p_\lambda(x(i)))}{n - \text{tr}\,W^{1/2}A(\lambda)W^{1/2}}. \tag{53}$$

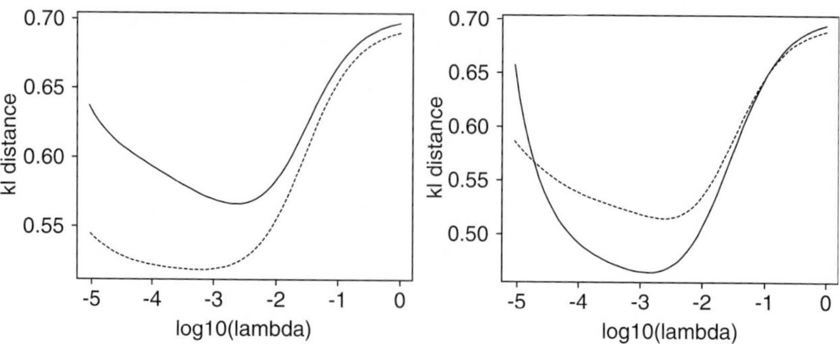

Fig. 10. Two GACV(λ) (solid lines) and CKL(λ) (dotted lines) curves. (From Xiang and Wahba (1996), ©*Statistica Sinica*, reprinted with permission.)

Here $A(\lambda) = A(\lambda, f_\lambda)$ is the inverse Hessian of $I_\lambda\{y,f\}$ with respect to $f_i \equiv f_\lambda(x(i))$, $i = 1,\ldots,n$, and $W = W(\lambda, f_\lambda)$ the diagonal matrix with iith entry $p_\lambda(x(i))(1 - p_\lambda(x(i)))$, which is the variance of the estimated Bernoulli distribution as well as the second derivative of $\log(1 + e^{f_\lambda(x(i))})$. Figure 10 (Xiang and Wahba, 1996) gives two plots comparing the true CKL(λ) with GACV(λ) in a simulation experiment where $p(x)$ is known. Numerous experimental works show that the minimizer of the GACV provides a good estimate of the minimizer of the CKL, but theoretical results analogous to those in Li (1986) for GCV remain to be found. A generalization of the GACV to the two-eye problem of Section 5 based on leaving-out-one-unit is found in Gao et al. (2001).

6.3. *Generalized approximate cross-validation, Bernoulli data, and l_1 penalties*

A general version of GACV targeted at the CKL adapted for LASSO-type optimization problems appears in Zhang et al. (2004). A special case, for optimization problems like that of the LASSO-Patternsearch (Shi et al., 2006), goes as follows. For each trial value of λ, there will be, say, $N = N(\lambda)$ basis functions in the model with nonzero coefficients. Let B be the $n \times N$ design matrix for the N basis functions and W be as before. Let $A(\lambda, f_\lambda) = B(B^{\mathrm{T}} WB)^{-1} B^{\mathrm{T}}$ and observe that $\mathrm{tr}\, W^{1/2} A(\lambda) W^{1/2} = N$. The GACV becomes

$$\mathrm{GACV}(\lambda) = \frac{1}{n}\sum_{i=1}^{n} -y_i f(x(i)) + \log(1 + e^{f(x(i))}) + \frac{1}{n}\mathrm{tr}\, A(\lambda) \frac{\sum_{i=1}^{n} y_i (y_i - p_\lambda(x(i)))}{n - N}. \tag{54}$$

6.4. *Support vector machines*

A large number of competing methods have been proposed for tuning SVMs. When sufficiently large data sets are available, a common practice is to divide the data into three parts: a training set, a tuning set for choosing λ and any other tuning parameters, and a test set for evaluating the results. Five-fold and 10-fold cross-validation are both popular. Several tuning methods related in some way to cross-validation ideas are described in Chapelle et al. (2002) and Gold and Sollich (2003). Tuning methods based on structural risk minimization appear in Lanckriet et al. (2004). A perturbation method which perturbs both inputs and outputs is proposed in Wang and Shen (2006). A popular method is Joachims' (2000) XiAlpha method, which is part of the SVM^{light} package at http://svmlight.joachims.org/. A GACV method was derived in Wahba (1999) by methods analogous to those in Section 2. The XiAlpha and GACV methods are seen to be related (Wahba et al., 2001), where a generalization of both methods to the nonstandard case is proposed. A GACV for the multicategory SVM of Lee, Lin, and Wahba is in Lee et al. (2004).

6.5. *Regularized kernel estimates*

A leaving out pairs algorithm can be obtained to choose λ in the RKE estimate, although K_λ appears to be insensitive to λ over a fairly broad range. To date the choice of p has been made visually by plotting eigenvalues, but when the pseudodata are used for classification one possibility is to choose it simultaneously with the SVM parameters. A definitive automatic procedure is yet to be obtained.

7. Regularization, empirical Bayes, Gaussian processes priors, and reproducing kernels

It is well known that there is a duality between zero mean Gaussian processes and RKHS: for every positive definite function K there is a unique RKHS with K as its RK, and for every positive definite function K there is an associated zero mean Gaussian process prior with K as its covariance; see Aronszajn (1950), Kimeldorf and Wahba (1971), Parzen (1970), and Wahba (1990). When the first term in the optimization problem is a negative log likelihood $\mathscr{L}\{y,f\}$ and the penalty term involves RKHS squared norms, then for fixed tuning parameters the estimate is a Bayes estimate with a Gaussian Process prior. These remarks extend to the case when the penalty term involves squared seminorms, which correspond to an improper prior; see Kimeldorf and Wahba (1971) and Wahba (1990). Similarly, in the LASSO class of estimates, the l_1 penalty corresponds to negative exponential priors on the coefficients. In typical regularization methods like those described here the tuning parameters are chosen by generalization and model selection arguments, in "frequentist" style. There is a large literature labeled empirical Bayes methods, as well as Gaussian process priors methods, and the discerning reader may consider the relationships between those and regularization methods.

Acknowledgements

Grace Wahba's research is at the time of this writing supported by NSF Grants 0505636 and 0604572, NIH Grant EY09946, and ONR Grant N00014-06-1-0095.

The author wishes to acknowledge her gratitude to her collaborators, former students, present students, and, in particular, David Callan. Former and present students are listed on her home page.

References

Allwein, E.L., Schapire, R.E., Singer, Y. (2000). Reducing multiclass to binary: A unifying approach for margin classifiers. In: *Proceedings of 17th International Conference on Machine Learning*, Morgan Kaufmann, San Francisco, CA, pp. 9–16.

Aronszajn, N. (1950). Theory of reproducing kernels. *Transactions of the American Mathematical Society* **68**, 337–404.

Benson, S., Ye, Y. (2004). DSDP5: A software package implementing the dual-scaling algorithm for semidefinite programming. Technical Report ANL/MCS-TM-255, Mathematics and Computer Science Division, Argonne National Laboratory, Argonne, IL, http://www-unix.mcs.anl.gov/~benson/dsdp/dsdp5userguide.pdf

Bookstein, F. (1997). *Morphometric Tools for Landmark Data: Geometry and Biology*. Cambridge University Press, Cambridge, England.

Breiman, L. (2001). Random forests. *Machine Learning* **45**, 5–32.

Brown, M., Grundy, W., Lin, D., Cristianini, N., Sugnet, C., Furey, T., Ares, M., Haussler, D. (2000). Knowledge-based analysis of microarray gene expression data by using support vector machines. *Proceedings of the National Academy of Sciences of the United States of America* **97**, 262–267.

Carew, J., Dalal, R., Wahba, G., Fain, S. (2004). A nonparametric method for estimation of arterial wall shear stress. In: *Proceedings of International Society of Magnetic Resonance in Medicine 12*. International Society for Magnetic Resonance in Medicine, Berkeley, CA, p. 1924.

Chapelle, O., Vapnik, V., Bousquet, O., Mukherjee, S. (2002). Choosing multiple parameters for support vector machines. *Machine Learning* **46**, 131–159.

Chen, S., Donoho, D., Saunders, M. (1998). Atomic decomposition by basis pursuit. *SIAM Journal on Scientific Computing* **20**, 33–61.

Chun, H. (2006). *Smoothing Spline ANOVA Model for Bivariate Bernoulli Observations*, Abstract, Program of the 2006 Joint Statistical Meetings, American Statistical Association, Arlington, VA.

Crammer, K., Singer, Y. (2000). On the learnability and design of output codes for multiclass problems. In: *Proceedings of the Thirteenth Annual Conference on Computational Learning Theory*, Stanford University, pp. 35–46.

Craven, P., Wahba, G. (1979). Smoothing noisy data with spline functions: Estimating the correct degree of smoothing by the method of generalized cross-validation. *Numerische Mathematik* **31**, 377–403.

Cristianini, N., Shawe-Taylor, J. (2000). *An Introduction to Support Vector Machines*. Cambridge University Press, Cambridge, England.

Davidson, L. (2006). Comparing tongue shapes from ultrasound imaging using smoothing spline analysis of variance. *The Journal of the Acoustical Society of America* **120**, 407–415.

de Boor, C. (1978). *A Practical Guide to Splines*. Springer-Verlag, New York.

Dietterich, T.G., Bakiri, G. (1995). Solving multiclass learning problems via error-correcting output codes. *Journal of Artificial Intelligence Research* **2**, 263–286.

Duchon, J. (1977). Splines minimizing rotation-invariant semi-norms in Sobolev spaces. In: *Constructive Theory of Functions of Several Variables*. Springer-Verlag, Berlin, pp. 85–100.

Efron, B., Hastie, T., Johnstone, I., Tibshirani, R. (2004). Least angle regression. *Annals of Statistics* **33**, 407–499.

Evgeniou, T., Pontil, M., Poggio, T. (2000). Regularization networks and support vector machines. *Advances in Computational Mathematics* **13**, 1–50.

Fan, J., Li, R. (2001). Variable selection via nonconcave penalized likelihood and its Oracle properties. *Journal of the American Statistical Association* **96**, 1348–1360.

Gao, F., Wahba, G., Klein, R., Klein, B. (2001). Smoothing spline ANOVA for multivariate Bernoulli observations, with applications to ophthalmology data, with discussion. *Journal of the American Statistical Association* **96**, 127–160.

Girard, D. (1989). A fast 'Monte-Carlo cross-validation' procedure for large least squares problems with noisy data. *Numerische Mathematik* **56**, 1–23.

Girard, D. (1995). The fast Monte-Carlo cross-validation and C_L procedures: Comments, new results and application to image recovery problems. *Computational Statistics* **10**, 205–231.

Gold, C., Sollich, P. (2003). Model selection for support vector machine classification. *Neurocomputing* **55**, 221–249.

Golub, G., Heath, M., Wahba, G. (1979). Generalized cross validation as a method for choosing a good ridge parameter. *Technometrics* **21**, 215–224.

Golub, G., vonMatt, U. (1997). Generalized cross-validation for large-scale problems. *Journal of Computational and Graphical Statistics* **6**, 1–34.

Golub, T., Slonim, D., Tamayo, P., Huard, C., Gaasenbeek, M., Mesirov, J., Coller, H., Loh, M., Downing, J., Caligiuri, M., Bloomfield, C., Lander, E. (1999). Molecular classification of cancer: Class discovery and class prediction by gene expression monitoring. *Science* **286**, 531–537.

Gu, C. (2002). *Smoothing Spline ANOVA Models*. Springer, New York, NY, USA.

Gu, C., Wahba, G. (1991). Minimizing GCV/GML scores with multiple smoothing parameters via the Newton method. *SIAM Journal on Scientific Computing* **12**, 383–398.

Gu, C., Wahba, G. (1993a). Semiparametric analysis of variance with tensor product thin plate splines. *Journal of the Royal Statistical Society. Series B* **55**, 353–368.

Gu, C., Wahba, G. (1993b). Smoothing spline ANOVA with component-wise Bayesian "confidence intervals". *Journal of Computational and Graphical Statistics* **2**, 97–117.

Gunn, S., Kandola, J. (2002). Structural modelling with sparse kernels. *Machine Learning* **48**, 137–163.

Hastie, T., Tibshirani, R. (1986). Generalized additive models. *Statistical Science* **1**, 297–318.

Hutchinson, M. (1989). A stochastic estimator for the trace of the influence matrix for Laplacian smoothing splines. *Communications in Statistics-Simulation* **18**, 1059–1076.

Joachims, T. (1999). Making large-scale svm learning practical. In: Scholkopf, B., Burges, C., Smola, A. (Eds.), *Advances in Kernel Methods – Support Vector Learning*. MIT Press, Cambridge, MA, USA, pp. 69–88.

Joachims, T. (2000). Estimating the generalization performance of an SVM efficiently. In: *Proceedings of the International Conference on Machine Learning*. Morgan Kaufman, San Francisco.

Khan, J., Wei, J., Ringner, M., Saal, L., Ladanyi, M., Westermann, F., Berthold, F., Schwab, M., Atonescu, C., Peterson, C., Meltzer, P. (2001). Classification and diagnostic prediction of cancers using gene expression profiling and artificial neural networks. *Nature Medicine* **7**, 673–679.

Kimeldorf, G., Wahba, G. (1971). Some results on Tchebycheffian spline functions. *Journal of Mathematical Analysis and Applications* **33**, 82–95.

Klein, R., Klein, B.E.K., Linton, K., DeMets, D. (1991). The Beaver Dam eye study: Visual acuity. *Ophthalmology* **98**, 1310–1315.

Knight, K., Fu, W. (2000). Asymptotics for LASSO-type estimators. *Annals of Statistics* **28**, 1356–1378.

Lanckriet, G., Cristianini, N., Bartlett, P., El Ghoui, L., Jordan, M. (2004). Learning the kernel matrix with semidefinite programming. *Journal of Machine Learning Research* **5**, 27–72.

Lee, Y., Kim, Y., Lee, S., Koo, J. (2006). Structured multicategory support vector machines with analysis of variance decomposition. *Biometrika* **93**, 555–571.

Lee, Y., Lee, C.-K. (2003). Classification of multiple cancer types by multicategory support vector machines using gene expression data. *Bioinformatics* **19**, 1132–1139.

Lee, Y., Lin, Y., Wahba, G. (2004). Multicategory support vector machines, theory, and application to the classification of microarray data and satellite radiance data. *Journal of the American Statistical Association* **99**, 67–81.

Leng, C., Lin, Y., Wahba, G. (2006). A note on the LASSO and related procedures in model selection. *Statistica Sinica* **16**, 1273–1284.

Li, K.C. (1986). Asymptotic optimality of C_L and generalized cross validation in ridge regression with application to spline smoothing. *Annals of Statistics* **14**, 1101–1112.

Liao, L., Noble, W. (2003). Combining pairwise sequence similarity and support vector machines for detecting remote protein evolutionary and structural relationships. *Journal of Computational Biology* **10**, 857–868.

Lin, X. (1998). Smoothing spline analysis of variance for polychotomous response data. Technical Report 1003, PhD thesis, Department of Statistics, University of Wisconsin, Madison, WI, available via G. Wahba's website.

Lin, Y. (2000). Tensor product space ANOVA models. *Annals of Statistics* **28**, 734–755.

Lin, Y. (2001). A note on margin-based loss functions in classification. *Statistics and Probability Letters* **68**, 73–82.

Lin, Y. (2002). Support vector machines and the Bayes rule in classification. *Data Mining and Knowledge Discovery* **6**, 259–275.

Lin, Y., Lee, Y., Wahba, G. (2002). Support vector machines for classification in nonstandard situations. *Machine Learning* **46**, 191–202.

Lin, Y., Wahba, G., Zhang, H., Lee, Y. (2002). Statistical properties and adaptive tuning of support vector machines. *Machine Learning* **48**, 115–136.

Lu, F., Keles, S., Wright, S., Wahba, G. (2005). A framework for kernel regularization with application to protein clustering. *Proceedings of the National Academy of Sciences of the United States of America* **102**, 12332–12337, open source at www.pnas.org/cgi/content/full/102/35/12332.

Luo, Z., Wahba, G. (1997). Hybrid adaptive splines. *Journal of the American Statistical Association* **92**, 107–114.

McCullagh, P., Nelder, J. (1989). *Generalized Linear Models*, 2nd ed. Chapman and Hall, Boca Raton, FL, USA.

Meinguet, J. (1979). Multivariate interpolation at arbitrary points made simple. *Journal of Applied Mathematics and Physics (ZAMP)* **30**, 292–304.

Mukherjee, S., Wu, Q. (2006). Estimation of gradients and coordinate covariation in classification. *Journal of Machine Learning Research* **7**, 2481–2514.

O'Sullivan, F., Yandell, B., Raynor, W. (1986). Automatic smoothing of regression functions in generalized linear models. *Journal of the American Statistical Association* **81**, 96–103.

Park, M., Hastie, T. (2007). *Penalized logistic regression for detecting gene interactions*, manuscript.

Parzen, E. (1970). Statistical inference on time series by RKHS methods. In: Pyke, R. (Ed.), *Proceedings 12th Biennial Seminar, Canadian Mathematical Congress*, Montreal. 1–37.

Ruczinski, I., Kooperberg, C., LeBlanc, M. (2002). Logic regression – Methods and software. In: Denison, D., Hansen, M., Holmes, C., Mallick, B., Yu, B. (Eds.), *Nonlinear Estimation and Classification*. Springer, New York, NY, USA, pp. 333–344.

Scholkopf, B., Burges, C., Smola, A. (1999). *Advances in Kernel Methods – Support Vector Learning*. Cambridge University Press, Cambridge, England.

Scholkopf, B., Smola, A. (2002). *Learning with Kernels Support Vector Machines, Regularization, Optimization and Beyond*. MIT Press, Cambridge, MA, USA.

Scholkopf, B., Tsuda, K., Vert, J.-P. (2004). *Kernel Methods in Computational Biology*. MIT Press, Cambridge, MA, USA.

Shawe-Taylor, J., Cristianini, N. (2004). *Kernel Methods for Pattern Analysis*. Cambridge University Press, Cambridge, England.

Shi, W., Wahba, G., Lee, K., Klein, R., Klein, B. (2006). LASSO-Patternsearch algorithm with application to ophthalmology data. Technical Report 1131, Department of Statistics, University of Wisconsin, Madison, WI.

Smola, A., Bartlett, P., Scholkopf, B., Schuurmans, D. (2000). *Advances in Large Margin Classifiers*. MIT Press, Cambridge, MA, USA.

Stein, M. (1999). *Interpolation of Spatial Data: Some Theory for Kriging*. Springer-Verlag, New York, NY, USA.

Tibshirani, R. (1996). Regression shrinkage and selection via the lasso. *Journal of the Royal Statistical Society. Series B* **58**, 267–288.

Tütüncü, R.H., Toh, K.C., Todd, M.J. (2003). Solving semidefinite-quadratic-linear programs using SDPT3. *Mathematical Programming* **95**(2), 189–217.

Vapnik, V. (1995). *The Nature of Statistical Learning Theory*. Springer, New York, NY, USA.
Wahba, G. (1981). Numerical experiments with the thin plate histospline. *Communications in Statistics-Theory and Methods* **A10**, 2475–2514.
Wahba, G. (1990). *Spline Models for Observational Data*, SIAM. CBMS-NSF Regional Conference Series in Applied Mathematics, v. 59.
Wahba, G. (1999). Support vector machines, reproducing kernel Hilbert spaces and the randomized GACV. In: Scholkopf, B., Burges, C., Smola, A. (Eds.), *Advances in Kernel Methods – Support Vector Learning*. MIT Press, Cambridge, MA, USA, pp. 69–88.
Wahba, G. (2002). Soft and hard classification by reproducing kernel Hilbert space methods. *Proceedings of the National Academy of Sciences of the United States of America* **99**, 16524–16530.
Wahba, G., Lin, Y., Lee, Y., Zhang, H. (2001). On the relation between the GACV and Joachims' $\xi\alpha$ method for tuning support vector machines, with extensions to the non-standard case. Technical Report 1039, Statistics Department University of Wisconsin, Madison, WI.
Wahba, G., Lin, Y., Zhang, H. (2000). Generalized approximate cross validation for support vector machines. In: Smola, A., Bartlett, P., Scholkopf, B., Schuurmans, D. (Eds.), *Advances in Large Margin Classifiers*. MIT Press, Cambridge, MA, USA, pp. 297–311.
Wahba, G., Wang, Y., Gu, C., Klein, R., Klein, B. (1995). Smoothing spline ANOVA for exponential families, with application to the Wisconsin Epidemiological Study of Diabetic Retinopathy. *Annals of Statistics* **23**, 1865–1895, Neyman Lecture.
Wahba, G., Wendelberger, J. (1980). Some new mathematical methods for variational objective analysis using splines and cross-validation. *Monthly Weather Review* **108**, 1122–1145.
Wang, J., Shen, X. (2006). Estimation of generalization error: Random and fixed inputs. *Statistica Sinica* **16**, 569–588.
Wang, Y. (1998) Mixed-effects smoothing spline ANOVA. *Journal of the Royal Statistical Society. Series B* **60**, 159–174.
Wang, Y., Ke, C., Brown, M. (2003). Shape-invariant modeling of circadian rhythms with random effects and smoothing spline ANOVA decompositions. *Biometrics* **59**, 241–262.
Weston, J., Watkins, C. (1999). Support vector machines for multiclass pattern recognition. In: *Proceedings of the Seventh European Symposium on Artificial Neural Networks*, citeseer.nj.nec.com/article/weston99support.html.
Whittaker, J. (1990). *Graphical Models in Applied Mathematical Multivariate Statistics*. Wiley, Hoboken, NJ, USA.
Xiang, D., Wahba, G. (1996). A generalized approximate cross validation for smoothing splines with non-Gaussian data. *Statistica Sinica* **6**, 675–692.
Xiang, D., Wahba, G. (1997). Approximate smoothing spline methods for large data sets in the binary case. Technical Report 982, Department of Statistics, University of Wisconsin, Madison, WI. Proceedings of the 1997 ASA Joint Statistical Meetings, Biometrics Section, pp. 94–98 (1998).
Yuan, M., Lin, Y. (2006). Model selection and estimation in regression with grouped variables. *Journal of the Royal Statistical Society. Series B* **68**, 49–67.
Zhang, H. (2006). Variable selection for SVM via smoothing spline ANOVA. *Statistica Sinica* **16**, 659–674.
Zhang, H., Lin, Y. (2006a). Component selection and smoothing for nonparametric regression in exponential families. *Statistica Sinica* **16**, 1021–1042.
Zhang, H., Lin, Y. (2006b). Component selection and smoothing in multivariate nonparametric regression. *Annals of Statistics* **34**, 2272–2297.
Zhang, H., Wahba, G., Lin, Y., Voelker, M., Ferris, M., Klein, R., Klein, B. (2004). Variable selection and model building via likelihood basis pursuit. *Journal of the American Statistical Association* **99**, 659–672.
Zhu, J., Hastie, T. (2003). Classification of gene microarrays by penalized logistic regression. *Biostatistics* **5**, 427–443.
Zou, H. (2006). The adaptive LASSO and its Oracle properties. *Journal of the American Statistical Association* **101**, 1418–1429.
Zou, H., Hastie, T. (2005). Regularization and variable selection via the elastic net. *Journal of the Royal Statistical Society. Series B* **67**(Part 2), 301–320.

Handbook of Statistics, Vol. 27
ISSN: 0169-7161

DOI: 10.1016/S0169-7161(07)27024-5

24

Evidence Based Medicine and Medical Decision Making

Dan Mayer, MD

Abstract

Evidence Based Medicine (EBM) is a movement within the field of medicine to assure that physicians use the best available evidence from well done clinical research studies in making the decisions regarding the types of therapies and diagnostic tests used for their patients. EBM uses many of the tools of "clinical epidemiology" to help physicians appraise the quality of scientific medical research studies. However, it is the blending of critical appraisal of the best evidence, patient preferences, the clinical predicament and clinical judgment that allow the best evidence to be used in patient care. The critical appraisal function of EBM becomes synonymous with improved critical thinking by physicians and other members of the health care team.

Writing about Evidence Based Medicine (EBM) and Medical Decision Making (MDM) for a textbook on medical statistics is not an easy task. I could simply write about the tools of EBM and MDM, which I shall do. However, this would not do justice to a concept that has swept over the practice and changed the culture of medicine since the early 1990s. What is EBM? Is it simply a repackaging of previously elucidated skill sets that formerly belonged to the realm of epidemiology? Is it simply the application of a hierarchy of study designs to rank the strength of results of those studies? Does it delineate the boundaries of the practice of medicine through the application of practice guidelines and clinical prediction rules? I will discuss the definitions of EBM and its history and then present some of the tools that are commonly used by EBM practitioners. I will then give a brief introduction to the field of MDM.

1. The definition and history of evidence based medicine

There are three main goals for physicians. The most obvious is to bring the best information from medical research (and some would argue, medical technology) to the patient's bedside. The second goal is to improve the health of the public through control of epidemic diseases (whether caused by microorganisms or environmental contaminants). Finally, the physician is charged with comforting the patient and their immediate social group in times of illness. Evidence-based medicine (EBM) has taken all of these physician roles and asked us to make them scientific. According to the on-line dictionary, Wikipedia, "EBM is a medical movement based upon the application of the scientific method to medical practice, recognizing that many long-established medical traditions are not yet subjected to adequate scientific scrutiny." (http://en.wikipedia.org/wiki/Evidence-based_medicine) According to the Centre for Evidence-Based Medicine, EBM "is the conscientious, explicit and judicious use of current best evidence in making decisions about the care of individual patients. The practice of evidence-based medicine means integrating individual clinical expertise with the best available external clinical evidence from systematic research." The centre also defines Evidence-Based Health Care as an extension of EBM "to all professions associated with health care, including purchasing and management". (http://www.cebm.net) The bottom line is that EBM is the application of the scientific method to medicine.

Physicians must make the correct diagnosis and choose the most appropriate treatment to return the patient to health or reduce the burden of their illness. This must be done under conditions that can only be described as extremely uncertain. There are an increasing number of sources of information that physicians and for that matter, patients, can access. The physician should want to find the most effective way to access current information from the medical literature and be able to critically evaluate this information. The scope and content of EBM is very complex and I will begin my discussion with a brief historical overview. Those readers interested in more detail about the history of EBM are referred to the excellent website at the James Lind Library (http://www.jameslindlibrary.org/index.html) and recent book by Jeanne Daly (Daly, 2005).

According to some, the elements of Evidence Based Medicine go back to the bible. In the Book of Daniel there is a description of a trial of diet in which the participants (Daniel's friends) were randomized to eat only vegetables or the king's food. Hippocrates often spoke about the need for the physician to observe his patient and to only perform those actions that could be helpful. His aphorism 'first do no harm' implies that the physician must be able to distinguish helpful from potentially harmful therapies. A brief discussion of the modern history of EBM will help to put this topic into perspective (Daly, 2005, Trohler, 2000).

The modern origins of EBM go back to the eighteenth century, when George Forsythe, a British physician first demanded that the medical profession provide better evidence for their therapies. Captain James Lind, a British naval surgeon performed the first "modern" randomized clinical trial on a dozen seamen with scurvy in a non-blinded but randomized manner. Each pair got a different experimental treatment, but were treated the same in all other respects. Even though the results very clearly showed that citrus was vastly superior to the other treatments, the fact that citrus cured scurvy didn't conform to the theory of scurvy prevalent at the time. It took another fifty years before citrus became standard issue for the Royal Navy. A French physician and statistician, Pierre Charles

Alexandre Louis was the first to apply the new science of statistics to show that a medical therapy was ineffective. In this case, he found that bloodletting was unlikely to benefit patients with typhoid fever (Trohler, 2000).

The most recent history of EBM can be traced to a 1947 editorial in the Lancet by Austin Bradford Hill in which he demanded that physicians study statistics and use statistical methods to evaluate their practice of medicine. (Hill, 1947) At this same time, John Paul in the USA coined the term, 'clinical epidemiology'. (Paul, 1966) However, neither concept was accepted by mainstream physicians at the time and languished in obscurity for another fifty years. The first modern randomized clinical trial was done in 1948 by the Medical Research Council of the National Health Service in the United Kingdom. It showed that streptomycin was beneficial for curing tuberculosis. (Medical Research Council, 1948) A subsequent review of perinatal interventions done in 1986 by Iain Chalmer's group at Oxford was the first modern systematic review placed on a computerized database. This led to the formation of the Cochrane Collaboration, named for Archie Cochrane, a British General Practitioner and epidemiologist who called attention to the need to develop large databases of studies so that bias could be eliminated from medical studies. The Cochrane Collaboration, founded in 1993, is currently composed of over six thousand people in sixty countries and has created over one thousand reviews. Cochrane work groups, linked electronically through the Internet all over the world are responsible for searching and reporting on the results of clinical trials and combining the results of those trials, wherever possible, into a single meta-analytic systematic review. There are over thirty thousand trials entered into the Cochrane Controlled Trials Registry (http://www.cochrane.org/index0.htm).

From the 1950s to the 1970s there was a rich development and debate into the nature of EBM in modern medicine. Dr. Alvan Feinstein differentiated the science of clinical epidemiology as distinct from the common public health definition of epidemiology. His work served as the basis for the statistical revolution in medicine that began in the 1960s. (Feinstein, 1967) Research by John Wennberg in the 1970s demonstrated a large degree of variation in the health care provided to populations living in a relatively small geographical area. (Wennberg and Gittelsohn, 1973) This time period also saw an explosion in the number of medical research articles published. Health outcomes and process research done at McMaster University led the way for dissemination of these subjects. The development of a unique curriculum at McMasters incorporated the new science of Clinical Epidemiology into the medical school curriculum and research institutes.

The new science of clinical epidemiology has become the vehicle for practicing physicians to learn the principles of critical appraisal of studies about their patients. EBM became the watch word for the explicit application of the results of research published in the medical literature to improve patient care. Is EBM the medical profession looking for a short-cut to find out what the best studies are for their patients? Has EBM become a substitute for the critical thinking skills that need to be practiced by all physicians? Feinstein believed that this dangerous direction could easily become the road taken by evidence based practitioners. He defined the role of clinical epidemiology as making physicians thought processes more transparent and explicit and improving the critical thinking required for modern scientific medical practice.

What began as a way of channeling the scientific method into the daily practice of medicine became a world wide movement that would redefine medical care. (Evidence-Based Medicine Working Group, 1992) Yet, health care workers are still not in agreement as to what proficiencies define EBM. If EBM is seen as a tool to improve the ability of any health care worker to become a better and more critical thinker, we can define those elements that must be taught. Through the 1990s, there has been an explosion in courses teaching physicians how to become more intelligent consumers of the medical literature through the use of EBM and statistical methods in medical decision making.

EBM has been said to lack the qualities of being the base or foundation principle for medicine (Upshur, 2002). Those who hold this philosophy look more at the specific tasks that were made part of this new paradigm of practice. I would propose that EBM is really a surrogate for critical thinking, which is the base of medicine as postulated by Feinstein. EBM can teach the application of critical thinking to all health care workers. It encompasses clinical epidemiology, research methodology, narrative based medicine, ethics, public health, health policy, social and community medicine and population medicine. EBM bridges the care for the individual with that of populations.

2. Sources and levels of evidence

With the rise of EBM, various groups have developed ways to package evidence to make it more useful to individual practitioners. This is the output of critical evaluation of clinical research studies. Physicians can access these pre-digested "EBM reviews" through various on-line databases around the world. A major center for the dissemination of these sources of best evidence has been in the United Kingdom through various contracts with the National Health Service. The Centre for Evidence Based Medicine of Oxford University is the home of several of these EBM sources. Bandolier is a (slightly irregular) biweekly-published summary of recent interesting evidence evaluated by the centre and found at http://www.jr2.ox.ac.uk/bandolier/ that is free to all. The centre has various other easily accessible and also free features related to the practice of EBM located on its main site found at http://cebm.jr2.ox.ac.uk. Every six months the British Medical Journal publishes an updated Clinical Evidence, a summary of critically evaluated topics in therapeutics. These are regularly updated and available on line.

There are also many commonly used forms of pre-prepared critical appraisals of various clinical questions. The Journal Club Bank (JCB) is the format for the Evidence Based Interest Group of the American College of Physicians (ACP) and the Evidence Based Emergency Medicine website (http://ebem.org/index.php). Critically Appraised Topics (CATs) are pre-appraised summaries of research studies that can be found on the Evidence Based Medicine Resource Center of the New York Academy of Medicine (http://www.ebmny.org/). Other organizations are beginning to use this format to disseminate critical reviews on the web. The CAT format developed by the Centre for Evidence Based Medicine is being made available on CD-ROM for use outside the centre. The University of Sheffield (UK) has an excellent resource listing most EBM related websites at www.shef.ac.uk/scharr/ir/netting/.

Disease Oriented Evidence (DOE) is not always the same as "Patient Oriented Evidence that Matters" (POEMs), which can be found on the InfoPOEMs website (www.infopoems.com). The DOEs and POEM format was developed by family physicians for the American Academy of Family Practice. A DOE suggests that there is a change in the disease status when a particular intervention is applied. However, this disease specific outcome may not make a difference to the outcome for an individual patient. For example, it is clear that certain drugs such as statins lower cholesterol. However, it is not necessarily true that the same drugs reduce mortality or improve life. Studies for some of these statin drugs have shown this correlation and therefore are POEMS. Another example is the PSA test for detecting prostate cancer. There is no question that the test can detect prostate cancer most of the time at an earlier stage than would be detected by a physician examination (positive DOE). However, it has yet to be shown that early detection using the PSA results in longer life span or an improved quality of life (negative POEM).

Attempting to evaluate the strength of evidence for a particular clinical query has led to several methods of rank-ordering different types of studies. These are ranked from most to least important in having the ability to determine causation for the question at hand. The Centre for Evidence Based Medicine of the National Health Service in the United Kingdom developed the most commonly used scheme of categorization. Their specific grading schemes vary depending on the nature of the clinical query and are listed in Table 1. (http://www.cebm.net)

Table 1
Levels of Evidence for studies of therapy

A1a. Systematic review of homogeneous randomized clinical trials (RCT)
A1b. Individual RCT with narrow confidence limits (usually seen in studies with large number of subjects)
A1c. All or none case series. In this case, there is a 100% change from previous experience. Either some patients live with the new treatment where they all died before or all patients now survive with the new treatment where some died before.
B2a. Systematic review of homogeneous cohort studies.
B2b. Individual well-done cohort study with good follow up or poorly done RCT with <80% follow up.
B2c. Cross sectional study
B3a. Systematic review of homogeneous case control studies.
B3b. Individual case control study.
C4. Case series or poor quality case control or cohort study
D5. Expert opinion without any critically appraised evidence. This includes opinion based upon bench research, physiological principles, or 'first principles' From: Ball C, Sackett D, Phillips, B, et. al. Levels of evidence and grades of recommendations. Centre for Evidence Based Medicine, http://cebm.jr2.ox.ac.uk/docs/levels.html, 1999. Last revised Nov. 18, 1999.

These have been challenged as being too doctrinaire and should be used in a flexible manner, without forgetting to be critical of each study evaluated, regardless of study design. There is some concern among EBM scholars that the research agenda has been hijacked by proprietary interests (pharmaceutical and technology companies). The studies sponsored by these groups are frequently high quality RCTs. However, they are also very likely to have built in biases that are designed to achieve results favorable to the sponsoring organization.

3. The five stage process of EBM

Because of the phenomenal growth in the amount of medical research information available, it is now more important that physicians have the tools to assess this information in the medical literature. Breakthroughs in information systems technology including Internet access to MEDLINE via Pub Med and other medical databases allow physician to obtain the most current information to answer educational needs more quickly and easily than in the past. EBM has been defined as a five step process. (Sackett et al., 2000) This is outlined in Table 2.

The first step in the EBM process is to recognize an educational need based on a real or hypothetical patient. The next step is to develop a clinical question that maximizes the likelihood of finding good quality evidence through a search of the literature. This is best done using a four part PICO question, which includes the following elements; Patient or Population (P), Intervention or Exposure to a risk factor (I), Comparator (C), and Outcome (O). Some schemes for searching add the dimension of Time (T) to the question. It is beyond the scope of this chapter to present the details for searching the medical literature for the sources most likely to give the answer to the clinical question (Mayer, 2004).

The next step is critical appraisal of the medical literature. This is the heart of EBM. The evaluation of the medical literature attempts to identify potential shortcomings of a research study. Is the study valid or are there sources of bias? The essence of the critical appraisal part of the EBM process is asking if there are other reasonable explanations for the results of the study. Finally, the reader must draw inferences and apply the results of the study to the care of their individual patient. While many physicians consider this to be a difficult challenge, it is the way that EBM is integrated into actual practice. The complete understanding of

Table 2
Five step EBM process (often with a sixth added step)

First you must recognize an educational need.
1. Ask a question using the PICO(T) format
2. Access studies that may answer that question (through appropriate searching)
3. Acquire the study (studies) that are most likely to answer the question.
4. Appraise the studies critically looking for validity, impact and applicability
5. Apply the results to your patient (if possible)

There is a sixth step, which is often considered part of Quality Assurance: Assess the outcome of that application sophisticated statistical testing is less important than the application of common sense and skeptical evaluation of what is read (Woolf, 1999).

When using this evidence, the practitioner must keep in mind that the results of clinical studies are for the average patient and may not apply to all patients. The individual practitioner must determine how to use the evidence in an individual patient and whether their patient is similar enough to the patients in a study. Issues of patient preferences must weigh heavily in their decision making. These can be quantified and will be discussed later.

The medical literature gives a rational basis for care provided to patients. Evidence-Based medical decisions maximize the probability that the patient has a good outcome and that this is done in the most efficient way. While clinicians do not have to be biostatistics experts in order to critically evaluate scientific papers, an understanding of research designs and basic statistical methods will allow the physician to critically evaluate most published clinical research and avoid most errors of interpretation. Evaluation of the methodology of a research study is the most important part of the critical evaluation of the literature process.

The first step in critically understanding study results is to determine the research study design. Understanding this will help identify most of the problems that can potentially influence the results of a poorly done research study. An understanding of the nature of causation will help the reader determine the strength of the evidence. To determine causation for diseases with multifactorial causes requires showing that the cause and effect are associated with each other more likely than by chance alone, that the cause precedes the effect, and that changing the cause changes the effect. These three conditions are known as contributory cause and all three are required to prove causation for a multifactorial disease.

4. The hierarchy of evidence: study design and minimizing bias

Research is done to answer questions about populations by studying samples of individuals who are part of a given population. Individuals in a population have variable characteristics that might affect outcomes of research. The design of a study will alert the critical reader to potential problems in the conclusions of a study.

The best research design is one that minimizes the chance of bias. It is the responsibility of the researcher to minimize bias in a study. Sometimes this cannot easily be done making it the responsibility of the reader to determine if biases that exist in a study, whether real or potential are enough to affect the outcome. The end result may not be compatible with the research hypothesis when there is a large degree of bias in the conditions of the research. Different research designs have different propensities for bias.

The researcher has the responsibility to ensure that as many of the population characteristics as possible are represented in the study sample. In most cases, the study sample is divided into two groups to test the hypothesis that the two groups are different in some important characteristic. If the two groups are not equivalent with regard to their baseline characteristics, confounding of the results can occur, leading to an incorrect conclusion. It might be erroneously concluded that a difference in the desired outcome between the groups occurred because of a presumed causative factor when in reality it was produced by a difference in the pre-study characteristics of the two groups. When the groups being studied are different enough that the results could be affected, bias is present.

The hierarchy of clinical research design is listed in Table 1. The highest type of study in this hierarchy is the Randomized Clinical Trial (RCT) because it is most likely to be able to prove causation, and least likely to contain biases that can lead to incorrect and misleading results.

In RCTs the study subjects are assigned to the treatment (exposed) or comparison (placebo or not exposed) group on the basis of chance. The researcher uses some technique that assures a random placement of each participant in one group or the other. This maximizes the probability that the two groups are equal with respect to characteristics that could affect the outcome under consideration at the outset of the study. If a large number of baseline characteristics could affect the outcome, more study subjects will be needed to insure that adequate randomization will result in two similar groups. RCTs generally identify the characteristics of the two study groups at the beginning of the study. They are the best design to minimize bias but are usually costly in money and time needed to do the study. If the outcome being studied is rare, an exceptionally large number of study subjects may be necessary to find any difference between the two groups, making this an unrealistic study design.

In a cohort study, as in an RCT, the subjects are identified on the basis of exposure or risk. However, in a cohort study the subjects are chosen either because they have been exposed or chose to expose themselves to the risk. For example, a researcher determining whether cigarette smoking causes brain tumors could take a sample of smokers and nonsmokers and follow them for a period of time to determine the numbers in each group who develop brain tumors. Since the subjects were not assigned to the exposed or not exposed groups, it is possible on the basis of chance alone that the two groups are not similar in all other important characteristics. Men who smoke may have a higher degree of exposure to other toxins than nonsmokers and these could be contributory causes of brain cancer. This is known as a confounding variable and is a relatively commonly found occurrence in cohort studies. Cohort studies usually cost less than RCTs and may allow for the study of issues for which randomization would be unethical or very difficult to perform with truly informed subjects.

In RCTs and cohort studies, the subjects are identified on the basis of risk or exposure and the incidence (rate of new outcomes over time) can be calculated. When incidence can be calculated one can calculate the Relative Risk, the incidence of the outcome in the exposed divided by that in the unexposed. This represents the relative benefit to the patient of using a therapy or modifying a risky behavior. If our researchers found that over a 20-year period, 4% of cigarette smokers and 1% of nonsmokers developed brain tumors, the Relative Risk of developing a brain tumor would be 4. Patients could be told that their risk of developing a brain tumor is four times greater if they smoke. Multivariate analysis can be used to minimize the effect of confounding variables, but must be done cautiously (Concato et al., 1993).

A more useful statistic is the Absolute Risk Increase or Reduction (ARI or ARR). This is simply the difference between the outcome rates in the experimental (exposed) or control (comparison or non-exposed) groups. This can then be used to calculate the Number Needed to Treat (NNT) or Number Needed to Harm (NNH). These represent the number of patients that must be treated (or exposed) in order for one additional patient to get benefit or be harmed.

Unlike RCTs and cohort studies, in a case-control study the subjects are identified by the presence or absence of the outcome. Researchers start with a group of individuals who have the outcome of interest (cases of disease) and match them to a group without the outcome that is similar to the case group in every way other than the characteristic under study. A researcher could study a group of 20 patients with brain tumors and 20 of similar age and gender without brain tumors to look at the proportion of cigarette smokers in each group. Because subjects are identified based on their outcome, incidence cannot be calculated. The Odds Ratio is used as a proxy for Relative Risk.

The Odds Ratio is the odds that a subject with the outcome has been exposed to the risk factor divided by the odds that a subject without the outcome has been exposed. This ratio is a good estimate of the Relative Risk when the outcome of interest is rare (Mayer, 2004). In the case-control study of 20 individuals with brain tumor, if 15 were smokers (exposed) and 5 were not, the odds of someone with a brain tumor being a smoker is 15 to 5 or 3. If among the 20 individuals without brain tumors, 4 were smokers and 16 were not, their odds of being a smoker are 4 to 16 or 0.25. The odds ratio, the ratio of the two odds is 3 divided by 0.025 or 12. The odds of a patient having the exposure is 12 times more if they have a brain tumor and for all practical purposes, this is equivalent to a Relative Risk of 12. Bias is more difficult to avoid in a case-control study but, the advantages are that a case-control study can be completed more quickly than a RCT or cohort study and is generally less costly. It is especially useful to study outcomes that are rare or uncommon.

In a case series, the author describes the experience of a set of individuals with a given exposure and generally describes their attainment of a certain outcome. A surgeon might describe her experience using a new operative technique for brain tumors and show the frequency with which the patients were cured or reached some defined outcome. The reader would like to know if the new procedure was better than existing operative technique. But without a comparison group of patients receiving the standard or no therapy, questions regarding the value of this new procedure cannot be answered. Case series are valuable for generating research hypotheses or suggesting necessary studies to the research community.

Cross-sectional studies measure the relationship between variables at one point in time. The frequency of a variable in a sample at a given point in time is its prevalence. They cannot prove the temporal relationship between cause and effect and are used to generate new research hypotheses.

5. Assessing the significance or impact of study results: Statistical significance and confidence intervals

The impact of a study tells the reader if there is likely to be an association between the outcomes of the two groups (treatment and comparator or exposed and non-exposed). Even with the best attention to study design it is possible that the study can get the wrong answer. It may demonstrate a difference between groups that is not really present in the larger population or no difference when one really exists (but was simply not found). Before beginning to test a hypothesis the researcher decides what level of uncertainty they will accept to indicate that a positive research finding was unlikely to be due to chance. This statistic, called alpha is generally set to be equal to 0.05. The findings of the study would be rejected as being indicative of a true difference in the population when the calculated probability of a chance association is greater than 5%. This is called the probability of making a Type I error and concluding that a difference found actually existed when in reality there is no difference.

Readers of the medical literature should be aware of those factors that can cause a Type I error in a study. Multiple comparisons done between two groups of patients are known as "dredging the data". It becomes more and more likely that one or more differences between groups that are found to be statistically significant actually occurred on the basis of chance, when in fact no such difference exists in the larger population. Composite outcomes can also cause a Type I error when several outcomes are put together creating a single composite outcome. This is more likely to be different between the two groups. The problem is that most of the time, the different outcomes do not have the same values (e.g., death, myocardial infarction and repeat admission for chest pain). Subgroup and post hoc analysis of the data are other ways in which a Type I error can occur (Mayer, 2004).

To protect against concluding that if no difference is found between the two groups there is truly no difference, the researcher sets another statistic known as beta. This is the probability of concluding that there is no difference between the findings of the two groups being studied when in fact there is. This is known as making a Type II error and beta is the probability of making that error. The beta statistic is usually set at 0.20. The power of the study is one minus β, which is the probability of finding a difference if one is really there. Power increases if there are more study subjects or a larger difference is considered to be clinically important. A smaller number of research subjects are needed to find a larger difference in outcomes.

Another way to assess how close the study results are to the actual estimate of a parameter is through calculating confidence intervals. These tell how much the estimate of any outcome may vary if the study is repeated with different samples from the same population. Usually a 95% confidence interval is calculated giving the range within which the result of the study would occur 95% of the time if the study was repeated. This can help the physician and patient make an informed decision when presenting estimates from sample populations.

6. Meta-analysis and systematic reviews

In the past, review articles summarized the literature on a topic in a subjective manner often including significant author biases. Systematic Reviews critically combine multiple studies that answer the same research question. The results of multiple studies can be combined statistically in a meta-analysis that "transcends" simple analysis. These can be done to reconcile studies with different results. When there are multiple negative studies a meta-analysis may uncover Type II errors due to an inadequate sample size of one or more of the studies to be combined. Meta-analysis can also help to identify a study that produced a Type I error or a study that has outlier results as part of a collection of many other studies. Meta-analyses can also be used to provide a rational synthesis of the existing literature on a given topic. By searching for evidence using a meta-analysis, the clinician can save hours of analysis to answer common problems.

The performance of a meta-analysis requires several steps and the critical reader of the literature should be able to determine their validity. There should be an exhaustive search for studies including not only Medline but also unpublished studies and dissertations. The studies included in the analysis should be critically reviewed and graded using a standardized grading scheme. The statistical results should be compared and presence of heterogeneity determined. If the studies are heterogeneous, they cannot be directly compared. However, this process may uncover one outlier among the studies and the reasons for this usually lie in the methodology of the studies. Finally, the summary statistics can be calculated and conclusions drawn about the bottom line. (Olson, 1994, Sacks et al., 1987) A technique known as cumulative meta-analysis can be done whenever a new study is reported on a given topic. The analysis will then determine when in time the intervention first showed statistically significant results (Lau et al., 1995).

7. The value of clinical information and assessing the usefulness of a diagnostic test

To accomplish the primary duty of the physician to help the patient return to health and have minimal suffering requires accurate diagnosis. Part of this duty is also to be a good steward of society's resources. A physician must always try to meet this duty using the least costly resource when faced with the possibility of using different strategies.

The two components of the diagnostic decision-making process at the patient's bedside are gathering useful information to create and refine the differential diagnosis and then sharing this information with the patient in a way that facilitates informed decision making. The physician must be able to critically assess the value of the information gathered to help their patient. However, while some of this information appears to be of value, it may not discriminate among diagnostic possibilities and be misleading. The patient's preferences must be added to the diagnostic process to assess the value of diagnostic information (Wulff and Gotzsche, 2000).

Two basic concepts that must be understood to judge the usefulness of a diagnostic clinical maneuver or test are reliability and validity. Reliability means that if a test is run more than once on the same specimen, the same result will occur. Reliable tests are reproducible. If the test result depends on who is performing it, interrater or interobserver reliability may suffer. Poor inter-rater reliability as measured by the kappa (or equivalent) statistic should lead the clinician to be cautious about using the result of the test in decision making. The same problem exists if the result varies when the same person does the test on the same specimen leading to poor intra-rater or intra-observer reliability. Test results should be precise or vary little from each other and accurate or vary little from the "true" value.

For diagnostic tests, validity is the test's ability to truly discriminate between patients with and without a given disease. Diagnostic tests are judged against a "gold standard" that conclusively defines the presence or absence of the disease. The gold standard for bacteremia is a positive blood culture and for a malignant tumor a tissue specimen containing malignant tumor cells. Figure 1 shows the distribution of test results in patients with and without a disease. Extreme test results can determine who has the disease and who does not. But, values near the middle (around the cutoff point between normal and abnormal) will show significant overlap for diseased and non-diseased individuals. Sensitivity and specificity are the mathematical descriptions of this degree of overlap. In the past, most studies of diagnostic tests reported the correlation between a diagnostic test result and the presence or absence of disease. This is not helpful to the clinician who needs to know the likelihood of the illness under consideration after application of a given test.

Most clinical laboratories present the results of diagnostic tests as dichotomous "normal" or "abnormal" values on the basis of the Gaussian or normal (bell-shaped) distribution. In this situation, 95% of all results lie within two standard

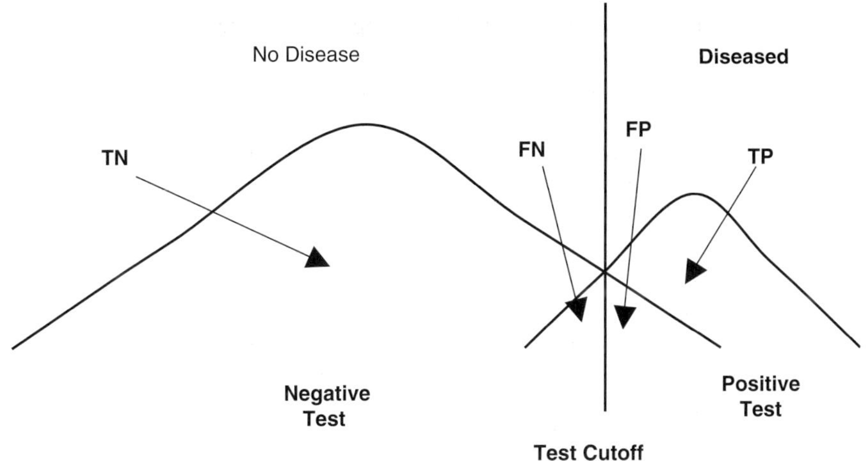

Fig. 1. Theoretical distribution of diagnostic test values for two populations.

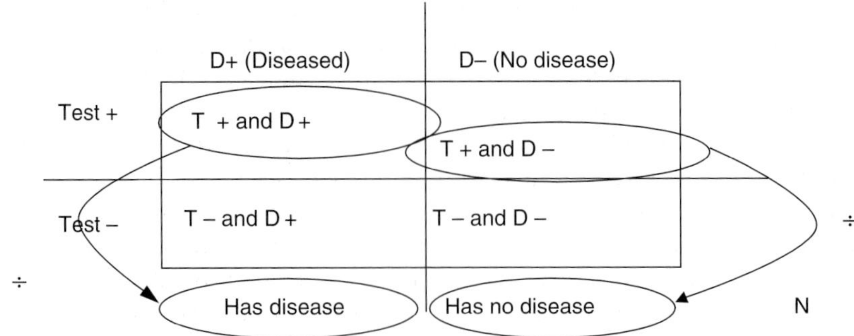

Fig. 2. Diagnostic test characteristics.

deviations (SD) of the mean. This information is not very useful to the clinician and sensitivity and specificity or likelihood ratios are a much more useful way to describe diagnostic test results.

The sensitivity of a test is the percentage of patients with the disease who will test positive. Also called the true positive rate (TPR) it is the ratio of subjects with the disease and a positive test (true positives, TP) to all subjects with the disease as shown in Figure 2. The specificity, also called the true negative rate (TNR) measures the percentage of people without the disease who test negative. It is the ratio of subjects without disease who test negative (true negatives, TN) to all those who don't have the disease.

The sensitivity and specificity are usually considered static characteristics of a test. For the purposes of decision making these usually won't change with the prevalence of disease in the patient. However, most diseases have varying levels of severity related to different stages of disease. This may lead a diagnostic test to demonstrate spectrum bias. In these cases, the test is usually more sensitive in patients with classical or severe disease and less sensitive in patients with mild or early disease. A test with high sensitivity is preferred for readily treated diseases with serious morbidity in order to minimize the number of missed cases (FN). The test will then rule out disease if it is negative. A test with high specificity is preferred for diseases that have minimal morbidity or in those for which there is either no effective or risky treatment. The test will rule in disease if it is positive. The critical reader of the medical literature will appreciate that published sensitivity and specificity values are point estimates and should always be accompanied by 95% confidence intervals. If these values come from large studies with sound methodology, the estimate will be more precise and accurate.

Knowing test sensitivity and specificity is not sufficient for the clinician at the bedside who needs to know the probability that their patient has the disease if the test is positive or negative. This probability is called the positive or negative predictive value or the posttest or posterior probability of disease given a positive or negative test. The Positive Predictive Value is the ratio of True Positive test results to all positive tests results or the fraction of patients with positive tests who really have the disease. The probability that a patient with a negative test result does not have disease, the Negative Predictive Value, is the ratio of true negative test results to all negative tests. One minus the Negative Predictive Value is called the False Reassurance Rate as we are falsely reassuring patients who have a negative test that they are disease free, when in fact they actually have the disease.

The predictive value of a test depends on three variables: the sensitivity, specificity, and the prevalence of disease in the population from which the patient comes. This pre-test prevalence is also referred to as the prior probability of disease. The prior probability must be determined from the clinical presentation of the patient or the baseline prevalence of the disease in the population. This is where clinical experience enters into the picture. Experienced clinicians are better able to recognize a pattern of disease in patients with atypical presentations.

Studies of diagnostic test results that only present predictive values are not helpful unless the prevalence of disease is also presented. For example, the Western blot analysis has a sensitivity and specificity of about 99% for human immunodeficiency virus (HIV). In some populations of intravenous drug abusers, the HIV prevalence can be as high as 33%. The positive predictive value is then 98% and the negative predictive value is 99.5%. (Table 3) However, if this test is used to screen a very low-risk population with a prevalence of 1 in 10,000, the positive predictive value falls to 1%. This means that there are 99 False Positives for every True Positive and using this test to screen this population for HIV would falsely label more than 99% of those with positive tests as having HIV. This is called the False Alarm Rate.

A more direct way to calculate the posttest probability of disease is using Bayes' Theorem and the likelihood ratio (LR). The LR combines sensitivity and specificity into one number and is a measure of the strength of a diagnostic test. The LR of a positive test (LR+) is equal to the sensitivity divided by one minus specificity. The LR of a negative test (LR-) is one minus sensitivity divided by the specificity. Figure 2 illustrates this. Tests that have a positive LR greater than 10 or a negative LR less than 0.1 are considered strong tests. Those with LR+ between 2 and 10 and LR- between 0.1 and 0.5 are fair tests. Those with an LR+ less than 2 or an LR- of greater than 0.5 are almost worthless. Bayes' Theorem uses LRs to revise disease probabilities using the formula; pretest odds x LR = posttest odds. The explanation of Bayes theorem is beyond the scope of this chapter. Bayes' Theorem is daunting to most physicians because it uses odds rather than probability. To convert the pretest probability to odds simply divide the probability by one minus the probability. To convert odds to probability divide the odds by the odds plus one. A nomogram is available to go from pretest to posttest probability using the LR without going through the odds conversion

Table 3
Use of diagnostic test characteristics for HIV test

Prevalence	Pretest odds	Posttest odds	Positive Predictive Value	False Reassurance Rate
0.33	0.5	(0.5×99) 49.5	(49.5/50.5) 0.98	$0.5 \times 0.01 = 0.005$
0.0001	0.0001	0.0099 (or 0.01)	0.01	$0.0001 \times 0.01 = 0.000001$

Sensitivity = 0.99 and Specificity = 0.99 LR+ = 99 and LR− = 0.01

(Fagan, 1975). In the case of continuous test results, for example the peripheral white blood cell count, the results can be broken into intervals. This preserves test information that would be lost in reducing the test to one single normal or abnormal cutoff. This will create multiple likelihood ratios (interval or iLRs) for each interval of test results.

Receiver operating characteristic (ROC) curves are a way to compare two or more tests or to select the best single cutoff for one diagnostic test. The ROC curve plots sensitivity on the y axis against one minus specificity, or the False Positive Rate on the x axis for all possible test cutoffs. A perfect test is at the 0,1 point in the upper left and represents 100% sensitivity and specificity and there are no False Positives or False Negatives. The 0,0 point at the lower left corresponds to 0% sensitivity and 100% specificity and here there are no False Positives and no True Positives. When looking for the best cutoff point or comparing two tests represented by curves that do not overlap, the best single cutoff point or test result is the one closest to the 0,1 point.

The area under the ROC curve (AUC) gives a mathematical description of the likelihood that one can identify a patient with the disease using that test alone. The diagonal line drawn from the lower left to the upper right corner of the ROC curve has an AUC of 0.5 meaning that the probability of identifying a diseased patient from one without the disease is 50% or no better than a coin toss. The AUC is useful for evaluating two tests whose ROC curves cross or a single test to determine its usefulness in general. Ideally an AUC should be as near to one as possible. However, before deciding which test to use the clinician must assess the trade-off of sensitivity for specificity for each test and cutoff point. The clinician must balance the harm of missing a patient with the disease and the risk of treating a patient without the disease.

8. Expected values decision making and the threshold approach to diagnostic testing

The most difficult part of medical decision making is combining the probability of an event with its value. This has been done 'by the seat of their pants' by physicians for generations. However, there is now a more advanced method of determining the optimal decision in medicine. This is called Expected Values Decision Making. It uses the concept of instrumental rationality to determine the optimal course of action based on the combination of probability of an event and the utility or value of the outcome. Instrumental rationality begins by using a schematic decision tree that shows all the possible actions that would be taken for a particular therapeutic or diagnostic decision. The starting point is a place where the physician must make a decision. From here, each outcome of the decision is followed to its logical conclusion. For example, if one choice is surgery, the outcomes could be death during the operation, complete cure, or some intermediate outcome such as relief from symptoms but shortened life. There is a probability and a value, or utility associated with each of these outcomes. After the tree has been constructed, the probability is multiplied by the utility for each branch until you get back to the starting point. A final expected value is obtained for each decision and the one with the highest value would be the preferred decision. Researchers should perform a sensitivity analysis for the tree, incorporating plausible ranges of values for probability and utility for each of the decisions. If the final outcomes are pretty much the same for these different values, the tree is said to be 'robust' and the results considered reasonable (Sox et al., 1988).

Pauker and Kassirer (Pauker 1980) introduced the concept of the threshold approach to diagnostic testing to help clinicians decide on whether to test or not. This method should maximize the effectiveness of diagnostic testing and limit unnecessary testing. Two pretest probabilities or thresholds are defined. If the clinician judges that the prior probability of disease is below the testing threshold then the patient is unlikely to have the disorder. A diagnostic test would not raise the probability sufficiently to change the decision not to treat for the disease. If the prior probability is below this level, the test should not be done. If the clinician judges the prior probability of disease to be above the treatment threshold then the patient most likely has the disorder. A diagnostic test would not lower the probability enough to change the decision to treat for the disease. If the prior probability is above this level the patient should be treated and the test should not be done. For prior probabilities between these two thresholds, the patient should be tested and treatment based on the test result. These thresholds are determined by balancing the benefits and risks of appropriate therapy, the risks of inappropriate therapy, the risks of the test, and the test sensitivity and specificity. They can be determined using formal decision analysis the details of which are beyond the scope of this chapter.

9. Summary

Evidence Based Medicine is a worldwide movement aimed at making medicine and health care more transparent. It has evolved from an amalgamation of biostatistics, epidemiology, research methodology and critical thinking to become a tool that is useful for physicians to understand the content of the medical literature. Understanding the principles of EBM is required for effective medical decision making. The methods of critical appraisal taught by EBM can be learned by all health care workers and be used to improve the way that uncertainty is handled in the health care system.

10. Basic principles

1. The clinician can reduce the risk of misinterpreting research studies by understanding basic research design.
2. The randomized controlled trial is the strongest design in clinical research because it minimizes the chance of bias.
3. In the randomized controlled trial and the cohort study, the subjects are identified on basis of risk or exposure. Case control studies begin with the outcome and are useful to study rare diseases.

4. Type I errors occur when a statistically significant difference is found when in fact the two groups are not different. Composite and multiple outcomes and sub group or post hoc analyses are a source of Type I errors.
5. Type II errors can occur when the study does not have enough subjects and the difference found is not statistically significance.
6. Clinicians can maximize the benefit of diagnostic testing by explicitly considering diagnostic test characteristics (reliability and validity).
7. Sensitivity and specificity are fixed properties of a diagnostic test and are, independent of the prevalence of disease when gold standards are consistent.
8. Predictive values are based on the sensitivity, specificity, and prevalence of the disease in the population of interest.
9. LRs are a summary of sensitivity and specificity and a nomogram can be used to determine posttest probability from the pretest probability and the LR.
10. ROC curves are useful in comparing two or more diagnostic tests.
11. Expected Values Decision Making is a useful tool in quantifying the outcomes for several choices in the medical decision making process.

References

Centre for Evidence Based Medicine http://www.cebm.net/

Cochrane Collaboration http://www.cochrane.org/index0.htm

Concato, J., Freinstein, A.R., Halford, T.S. (1993). The risk of determining risk with multivariate analysis. *Ann. Int. Med* **118**, 200–210.

Daly, J. (2005). *Evidence Based Medicine and the Search for a Science of Clinical Care*. University of California Press/Milbank Memorial Fund, Berkeley.

Evidence-Based Medicine Working Group (1992). Evidence-based medicine: a new approach to teaching the practice of medicine. *Lama* **268**, 2420–2425.

Fagan, T.J. (1975). Nomogram for Bayes' Theorem. *N Engl l Med* **293**, 25–27, (Letter).

Feinstein, A.R. (1967). *Clinical Judgment*. Robert E. Krieger Publishing, Malabar.

Hill, A.B. (1947). Statistics in the medical curriculum? British Medical Journal; ii, 366, September 6.

James Lind Library http://www.jameslindlibrary.org/index.html

Lau, J., Schmid, C.H., Chalmers, T.C. (1995). Cumulative meta-analyses of clinical trials builds evidence for exemplary medical care. *J Clin Epidemiol* **48**, 45–57.

Mayer, D. (2004). *Essential Evidence Based Medicine*. Cambridge University Press, Cambridge, UK.

Medical Research Council (1948). Streptomycin treatment of pulmonary tuberculosis. *British Medical Journal* **2**, 769–782.

Olson, C.M. (1994). Understanding and evaluating a meta-analysis. *Acad Emerg Med* **1**, 392–398.

Pauker, S.G., Kassirer, J.P. (1980). The threshold approach to clinical decision making. *N Engl J Med* **302**, 1109–1117.

Paul, J.R. (1966). *Clinical Epidemiology. Rev. ed.* University of Chicago Press, Chicago.

Sackett, D.L., Straus, S.E., Richardson, W.S., Rosenberg, W., Haynes, R.B. (2000). *Evidence Based Medicine: How to Practice and Teach EBM*. Churchill Livingstone, Edinburgh.

Sacks, H.S., Berrier, J., Reitman, D. et al. (1987). Meta-analyses of randomized clinical trials. *New Engl J Med* **316**, 450–455.

Sox, H.C., Blatt, M.A., Higgins, M.C., Marton, K.I. et al. (1988). *Medical Decision Making*. Butterworth Heinemann.

Trohler, U. (2000). *To Improve the Evidence of Medicine: The 18th Century British Origins of a Critical Approach*. Royal College of Physicians of Edinburgh, Edinburgh.

Upshur, R.E.G. (2002). If not evidence, then what? Or does medicine really need a base. *J. Eval Clin Prac* **8**, 113.

Wennberg, J.E., Gittelsohn, A.M. (1973). Small area variations in health care delivery. *Science* **182**, 1102–1108.

Wikipedia http://en.wikipedia.org/wiki/Evidence-based_medicine

Woolf, S.H. (1999). The need for perspective in evidence based medicine. *JAMA* **282**, 2358–2365.

Wulff, H.R., Gotzsche, P.C. (2000). *Rational Diagnosis and Treatment: Evidence-Based Clinical Decision Making*, 3rd ed. Blackwell Science Publications, Oxford.

Handbook of Statistics, Vol. 27
ISSN: 0169-7161

DOI: 10.1016/S0169-7161(07)27025-7

25

Estimation of Marginal Regression Models with Multiple Source Predictors

Heather J. Litman, Nicholas J. Horton, Bernardo Hernández and Nan M. Laird

Abstract

Researchers frequently use multiple informants to predict a single outcome and compare the marginal relationships of each informant with response; a common application is diagnostic testing where the goal is to determine which diagnostic test best predicts disease. We review generalized estimating equations (GEE) for marginal regression models using continuous multiple source predictors with a continuous outcome and introduce a new maximum likelihood (ML) approach. ML and GEE yield the same regression coefficient estimates when (1) allowing different regression coefficients for each informant report, (2) assuming equal variance for the two multiple informant reports and constraining the marginal regression coefficients to be equal and (3) including non-multiple informant covariates with cases 1 or 2. With the ML technique, likelihood ratio tests (LRTs) can be formed to easily compare regression models and a broader array of models can be fit. Using asymptotic relative efficiency (ARE), we show that a constrained model assuming equal variance is more efficient than an unconstrained model. We apply the methods to a study investigating the effect of vigorous exercise on body mass index (BMI) with measures of exercise collected on two informants: children and their mothers.

1. Introduction

Multiple informant data refer to information obtained from different individuals or sources used to measure a single construct. We use the term multiple informant data to describe data obtained from either multiple sources or multiple measures on a commensurate scale. Typically, researchers are interested in the relationship of each multiple informant predictor with response (Horton et al., 1999; Horton and Fitzmaurice, 2004). For example, Field et al. (2003) conducted a study to estimate the marginal correlation of different measures of body mass index (BMI) with a gold standard measurement of percentage body fat; the aim of the study is to find the best measure of BMI. Pepe et al. (1999) compared results from different informants to predict adult obesity from childhood obesity. We consider a validation study by Hernández et al. (1999) used to design a larger study of the relationship between physical activity/inactivity and obesity in children. Physical activity and inactivity in the validation study are reported by multiple informants: children and their mothers, but feasibility issues dictate that only children's responses will be used in the main study. Our goal is to compare the relationship of child's report of physical activity and BMI with the relationship of mother's report of physical activity and BMI in the context of study design. In some settings, if both informants yield similar results, it may be useful to obtain a more efficient and robust estimate of the effect by fitting a model with common slopes. For instance, Horton et al. (2001) predict mortality in a 16-year follow-up period of Stirling County Study subjects from multiple informants (self and physician report) about psychiatric disorders; their final model has a constrained estimate of the association between diagnosis and overall mortality (controlling for age and gender).

For simplicity, we define the response as $\mathbf{Y}$ and the two reports of physical activity measured by informants as $\mathbf{X}_1$ and $\mathbf{X}_2$, though extensions to more than two informants can be accommodated. In general, multiple informants can be used either as outcomes or as predictors in a standard regression model. Multiple informant outcomes have been considered by Fitzmaurice et al. (1995, 1996), Kuo et al. (2000) and Goldwasser and Fitzmaurice (2001). As described above, we instead consider the case where the multiple informants are predictors.

Over the years, researchers have developed many 'ad hoc' techniques to analyze multiple informants as predictors. One analysis method is to pool reports from the multiple informants (Offord et al., 1996). However, this method does not take into account the potential differences between the informants. Investigators also proposed models predicting $E(\mathbf{Y}|\mathbf{X}_1,\mathbf{X}_2)$ where all multiple informants are in the model simultaneously (Horton and Fitzmaurice, 2004). In this case, the regression coefficient for a given multiple informant covariate is conditional on all other multiple informants in the model. However, as in the Field et al. (2003) study, the objective is not to best predict percentage body fat using all multiple informants, but rather to find the single measure of BMI that best predicts body fat. Thus, rather than fitting a model with all the multiple informants where we obtain a regression coefficient for each covariate that is conditional on the others in the model, we model the univariate relationship between percentage body fat and one BMI measure by predicting $E(\mathbf{Y}|\mathbf{X}_1)$ and also model the relationship between percentage body fat and another BMI measure by predicting $E(\mathbf{Y}|\mathbf{X}_2)$ (Horton and Fitzmaurice, 2004). Performing separate analyses such as this (Gould et al., 1996) has been done, but because measures from the different informants are not independent of one another, separate analyses are not amenable to comparing coefficients from the two models and it is not clear how to interpret a combined analysis.

Pepe et al. (1999) and Horton et al. (1999) independently developed a nonstandard application of generalized estimating equations (GEE) (Liang and Zeger, 1986; Zeger and Liang, 1986) in regression analyses with multiple informants as predictors. The technique provides marginal estimates of the multiple informants while appropriately controlling for the outcomes being the same. Using GEE requires fewer assumptions than maximum likelihood (ML); in particular, it only assumes that the model for the mean is correctly specified. We review this approach in Section 2.

This paper describes a ML approach for analysis of multiple informants as predictors and introduces constrained models that can increase efficiency. For simplicity, only the complete-data case is considered here, although additional research has been performed considering missingness (Litman et al., 2007). ML has been previously used for analysis of multiple informants as covariates when the responses and multiple informants are discrete (O'Brien et al., 2006). This research showed no loss of efficiency associated with using GEE compared with ML when there are no shared parameters. With a common parameter for the association between outcome and two multiple informant predictors, efficiency loss is modest with the minimum asymptotic relative efficiency (ARE) over a range of conditional parameter values being approximately 0.90 (O'Brien et al., 2006). Our paper instead considers a continuous outcome and continuous predictors. For simplicity, we consider a model from the Hernández et al. (1999) dataset with one univariate response and one predictor measured by two informants. Section 3 describes our new ML technique. Simulations to compare GEE and ML variance estimates are presented in Section 4 and efficiency of a constrained model is discussed in Section 5. Application of ML to the Hernández et al. (1999) study is presented in Section 6.

2. Review of the generalized estimating equations approach

We briefly review the method introduced by Horton et al. (1999) and Pepe et al. (1999) that was originally presented for a binary response using a logit link function, but here we assume a linear model. We define an outcome $\mathbf{Y}$ and K multiple source predictors $\mathbf{X}_1, \ldots, \mathbf{X}_k$. The GEE approach models the marginal associations between $\mathbf{Y}$ and $\mathbf{X}_k$, defined as $E(\mathbf{Y}|\mathbf{X}_k)$ for $k = 1, \ldots, K$. In the simplest case with no covariates and distinct parameters for each informant, the model fit is

$$E(\mathbf{Y}|\mathbf{X}_k) = \alpha_k + \beta_k \mathbf{X}_k \quad \text{for } k = 1, \ldots, K, \tag{1}$$

where α_k and β_k are parameters in the kth regression. Defining

$$\tilde{\mathbf{Y}} = \begin{pmatrix} Y_i \\ Y_i \\ \vdots \\ Y_i \end{pmatrix}_{(K\times 1)} \quad \mathbf{X}_i = \begin{pmatrix} 1 & X_{i1} & 0 & 0 & \cdots & 0 & 0 \\ 0 & 0 & 1 & X_{i2} & \cdots & 0 & 0 \\ \vdots & & & & & & \\ 0 & 0 & 0 & 0 & \cdots & 1 & X_{iK} \end{pmatrix}_{(K\times 2K)} \quad \beta = \begin{pmatrix} \alpha_1 \\ \beta_1 \\ \alpha_2 \\ \beta_2 \\ \vdots \\ \alpha_K \\ \beta_K \end{pmatrix}_{(2K\times 1)},$$

the GEE equations assuming an identity link, constant variance and a working independence correlation matrix simplify to the ordinary least squares (OLS) equations:

$$\sum_{i=1}^{n} \mathbf{X}_i^T(\tilde{\mathbf{Y}}_i - \mathbf{X}_i\beta) = 0. \tag{2}$$

Note that each vector of responses, $\tilde{\mathbf{Y}}_i$, consists of the same response K times (Pepe et al., 1999). Also, the data records from each subject are treated as independent clusters. We assume an independence working correlation matrix as have previous papers developing GEE (Horton et al., 1999; Pepe et al., 1999); we show later that the use of this matrix is optimal under the likelihood model. Solving Eq. (2), we find that $\hat{\beta} = \Sigma_{i=1}^{n}(\mathbf{X}_i^T\mathbf{X}_i)^{-1}\mathbf{X}_i^T\tilde{\mathbf{Y}}_i$ where $\hat{\alpha}_k$ and $\hat{\beta}_k$ are the intercept and slope estimates from a univariate regression model with response $\mathbf{Y}$ and a single predictor $\mathbf{X}_k$. A strength of the GEE approach is that it provides a joint variance–covariance matrix for the $2K$ univariate parameter estimates (Pepe et al., 1999).

Estimates of var$(\hat{\beta})$ can be derived using empirical or model-based variance formulas. The empirical or 'sandwich' variance estimator has traditionally been used because it allows the variance of the response to depend on the design matrix while taking the correlation of the residuals into account (Huber, 1967). Using the empirical variance formula and assuming working independence,

$$\widehat{\mathrm{var}}(\hat{\beta}) = \left(\sum_{i=1}^{n} \mathbf{X}_i^T\mathbf{X}_i\right)^{-1} \left(\sum_{i=1}^{n} \mathbf{X}_i^T(\tilde{\mathbf{Y}}_i - \mathbf{X}_i\hat{\beta})(\tilde{\mathbf{Y}}_i - \mathbf{X}_i\hat{\beta})^T\mathbf{X}_i\right) \times \left(\sum_{i=1}^{n} \mathbf{X}_i^T\mathbf{X}_i\right)^{-1}. \tag{3}$$

Since the 'sandwich' variance makes no modeling assumptions, it provides a robust expression appropriate for many applications. Because ML assumes var$(\mathbf{Y}_i)$ does not depend on $\mathbf{X}_i$, to facilitate comparison of ML to GEE, we use a version of the model-based variance for the GEE estimator:

$$\widehat{\mathrm{var}}(\hat{\beta}) = \left(\sum_{i=1}^{n} \mathbf{X}_i^T\mathbf{X}_i\right)^{-1} \left(\sum_{i=1}^{n} \mathbf{X}_i^T\hat{\Sigma}\mathbf{X}_i\right) \left(\sum_{i=1}^{n} \mathbf{X}_i^T\mathbf{X}_i\right)^{-1}, \tag{4}$$

where

$$\hat{\Sigma} = \frac{\sum_{i=1}^{n}(\tilde{\mathbf{Y}}_i - \mathbf{X}_i\hat{\beta})(\tilde{\mathbf{Y}}_i - \mathbf{X}_i\hat{\beta})^T}{n}. \tag{5}$$

We define the diagonal elements of $\hat{\Sigma}$ as $\hat{\Sigma}_{11}, \ldots, \hat{\Sigma}_{KK}$ (estimated variances) and the off-diagonal elements as $\hat{\Sigma}_{12}, \ldots, \hat{\Sigma}_{(K-1)K}$ (estimated covariances). The variance in Eq. (4) is model-based since it assumes the same $\hat{\Sigma}$ for each individual and $\hat{\Sigma}$ does not depend on the design matrix. Using Eq. (4) and because $\Sigma_{i=1}^{n}\mathbf{X}_i^T\mathbf{X}_i$ is block diagonal, the estimated variance–covariance matrix for the slopes can be expressed as

$$\widehat{\text{var}}\begin{pmatrix}\hat{\beta}_1\\ \hat{\beta}_2\\ \vdots\\ \hat{\beta}_K\end{pmatrix} = \begin{pmatrix}\dfrac{\hat{\Sigma}_{11}}{\text{SS}_{X_1^2}} & \cdots & \dfrac{\text{SS}_{X_1,X_K}\hat{\Sigma}_{1K}}{\text{SS}_{X_1^2}\text{SS}_{X_K^2}}\\ \vdots & & \\ \dfrac{\text{SS}_{X_1,X_K}\hat{\Sigma}_{1K}}{\text{SS}_{X_1^2}\text{SS}_{X_K^2}} & \cdots & \dfrac{\hat{\Sigma}_{KK}}{\text{SS}_{X_K^2}}\end{pmatrix}, \tag{6}$$

where

$$\text{SS}_{X_k^2} = \sum_{i=1}^{n}(X_{ik} - \bar{X}_k)^2,$$

and

$$\text{SS}_{X_kX_l} = \sum_{i=1}^{n}(X_{ik} - \bar{X}_k)(X_{il} - \bar{X}_l).$$

We also consider a constrained model with $\beta_1 = \beta_2 = \ldots = \beta_K = \beta_C$ defined as

$$E(\mathbf{Y}|\mathbf{X}_k) = \alpha_k + \beta_C\mathbf{X}_k \qquad \text{for } k = 1,\ldots,K, \tag{7}$$

where $\tilde{\mathbf{Y}}_i$ remain the same as in the unconstrained model,

$$\mathbf{X}_i = \begin{pmatrix}1 & 0 & \ldots & 0 & X_{i1}\\ 0 & 1 & \ldots & 0 & X_{i2}\\ \vdots & & & & \\ 0 & 0 & \ldots & 1 & X_{iK}\end{pmatrix} \quad \text{and } \beta = (\alpha_1, \alpha_2, \ldots, \alpha_K, \beta_C)^T.$$

The same general expression for $\hat{\beta}$ holds and it is again straightforward to show that

$$\hat{\beta} = \left(\bar{Y} - \hat{\beta}_C\bar{X}_1, \ldots, \bar{Y} - \hat{\beta}_C\bar{X}_K, \right.$$
$$\left. \frac{\sum_{i=1}^{n}(X_{i1} - \bar{X}_1)(Y_i - \bar{Y}) + \cdots + \sum_{i=1}^{n}(X_{iK} - \bar{X}_K)(Y_i - \bar{Y})}{\sum_{i=1}^{n}(X_{i1} - \bar{X}_1)^2 + \cdots + \sum_{i=1}^{n}(X_{iK} - \bar{X}_K)^2}\right)^T,$$

and from Eq. (4),

$$\widehat{\text{var}}(\hat{\beta}_C) = \frac{\text{SS}_{X_1^2}\hat{\Sigma}_{11} + \cdots + \text{SS}_{X_K^2}\hat{\Sigma}_{KK} + \sum_{i>j}\text{SS}_{X_i,X_j}\hat{\Sigma}_{ij}}{(\text{SS}_{X_1^2} + \cdots + \text{SS}_{X_K^2})^2}. \tag{8}$$

We also extend the model to incorporate a vector of continuous or discrete covariates $\mathbf{Z}$ not measured by multiple informants. We predict $E(\mathbf{Y}|\mathbf{X}_k,\mathbf{Z})$ using the following model:

$$E(\mathbf{Y}|\mathbf{X}_k, \mathbf{Z}) = \alpha_k + \beta_k\mathbf{X}_k + \gamma_k\mathbf{Z} \quad \text{for } k = 1,\ldots,K. \tag{9}$$

This model is a simplification of a more general one that includes an interaction between each $\mathbf{X}_k$ and $\mathbf{Z}$. Our simplified model makes the standard regression assumption that the variance–covariance matrix of ($\mathbf{Y}$, $\mathbf{X}_1$, $\mathbf{X}_2$, ... , $\mathbf{X}_K$) is conditioned on $\mathbf{Z}$, but does not depend explicitly on $\mathbf{Z}$, e.g., is not a function of $\mathbf{Z}$. To implement the GEE approach we modify $\mathbf{X}_i$ and β as

$$\mathbf{X}_i = \begin{pmatrix} 1 & X_{i1} & Z_i & 0 & 0 & 0 & \cdots & 0 & 0 & 0 \\ 0 & 0 & 0 & 1 & X_{i2} & Z_i & \cdots & 0 & 0 & 0 \\ \vdots & & & & & & & & & \\ 0 & 0 & 0 & 0 & 0 & 0 & \cdots & 1 & X_{iK} & Z_i \end{pmatrix}$$

$$\beta = (\alpha_1, \beta_1, \gamma_1, \alpha_2, \beta_2, \gamma_2, \ldots, \alpha_K, \beta_K, \gamma_K)^T.$$

Similar to the case without covariates, $\hat{\alpha}_k, \hat{\beta}_k$ and $\hat{\gamma}_k$ are estimates from a univariate regression model with response $\mathbf{Y}$, multiple informant $\mathbf{X}_k$ and covariates $\mathbf{Z}$. Using Eq. (4), we can obtain variances as in the case without covariates.

3. Maximum likelihood estimation

To use ML we assume a joint multivariate distribution for the outcome and multiple informants. For simplicity, we consider only two predictors here but the model extends straightforwardly. For each of n observations, let $\mathbf{Q}_i = (Y_i, X_{1i}, X_{2i})^T$ and thus

$$\mathbf{Q}_i \sim MVN\left(\begin{pmatrix} \mu_Y \\ \mu_{X_1} \\ \mu_{X_2} \end{pmatrix}, \begin{pmatrix} \sigma_Y^2 & \sigma_{X_1,Y} & \sigma_{X_2,Y} \\ \sigma_{X_1,Y} & \sigma_{X_1}^2 & \sigma_{X_1,X_2} \\ \sigma_{X_2,Y} & \sigma_{X_1,X_2} & \sigma_{X_2}^2 \end{pmatrix} \right).$$

From this distribution, we find estimates for $\theta = (\mu_Y, \mu_{X_1}, \mu_{X_2}, \sigma_Y^2, \sigma_{X_1Y}, \sigma_{X_2,Y}, \sigma_{X_1,X_2}, \sigma_{X_1}^2, \sigma_{X_2}^2)^T$. However, we are interested in the regression parameter estimates from Eq. (1) with $K = 2$. Thus, we make a transformation from the original parameters, θ, to the parameters of interest $\tau = (\alpha_1, \beta_1, \alpha_2, \beta_2, V_{11}, V_{22}, V_{12})^T$. To make the transformation full rank, we include two parameters, μ_Y and σ_Y^2, from θ into τ. Using conditional mean formulas for the multivariate normal distribution, we find $E(\mathbf{Y}|\mathbf{X}_i) = \mu_Y + \sigma_{X_i,Y}(\mathbf{X}_i - \mu_{X_i})/\sigma_{X_i}^2$, where $i = 1, 2$. We define $\alpha_i = \mu_Y - \beta_i\mu_{X_i}$ and $\beta_i = \sigma_{X_i,Y}/\sigma_{X_i}^2$, where $i = 1, 2$ and thus Eq. (1) follows. We also define V_{11}, V_{22} and V_{12} in terms of θ by utilizing conditional variance formulas for the multivariate normal distribution, e.g., $V_{11} = \mathrm{var}(\mathbf{Y}|\mathbf{X}_1)$, $V_{22} = \mathrm{var}(\mathbf{Y}|\mathbf{X}_2)$ and $V_{12} = \mathrm{cov}(\mathbf{Y}|\mathbf{X}_1, \mathbf{Y}|\mathbf{X}_2)$.

From standard ML theory, $\hat{\theta}$ are sample means, variances and covariances with n in the denominators of the variances and covariances; we then make the full rank transformation to obtain $\hat{\tau}$ and find that the ML estimates of β are identical to the estimates found by GEE. Furthermore, using the multivariate normal model, we find $\text{var}(\hat{\beta}) = \mathbf{J}\text{var}(\hat{\theta})\mathbf{J}^T$, where $\mathbf{J}$ is the 9×9 Jacobian matrix for the transformation from $\boldsymbol{\theta}$ to τ. Thus, asymptotically

$$\text{var}\begin{pmatrix} \sqrt{n}\hat{\beta}_1 \\ \sqrt{n}\hat{\beta}_2 \end{pmatrix} \to \begin{pmatrix} \dfrac{\sigma_Y^2(1-\rho_{X_1,Y}^2)}{\sigma_{X_1}^2} & \dfrac{\sigma_Y^2(1-A)\sigma_{X_1,X_2}}{\sigma_{X_1}^2\sigma_{X_2}^2} \\ \dfrac{\sigma_Y^2(1-A)\sigma_{X_1,X_2}}{\sigma_{X_1}^2\sigma_{X_2}^2} & \dfrac{\sigma_Y^2(1-\rho_{X_2,Y}^2)}{\sigma_{X_2}^2} \end{pmatrix}, \tag{10}$$

where

$$A = 2(\rho_{X_1,Y}^2 + \rho_{X_2,Y}^2 - \rho_{X_1,Y}\rho_{X_2,Y}\rho_{X_1,X_2}) - \frac{\rho_{X_1,Y}\rho_{X_2,Y}}{\rho_{X_1,X_2}}.$$

If we estimate the asymptotic ML variance using the ML estimates of $\sigma_{X_1,Y}$, $\sigma_{X_2,Y}$, σ_{X_1,X_2}, the estimated variances of GEE and ML are the same; the estimated covariances given by GEE and ML are not identical but are quite similar in practice (results not presented).

We also consider the constrained model where $\beta_1 = \beta_2 = \beta_C$; one approach is to define

$$\sigma_{X_1,Y} = \beta_C\sigma_{X_1}^2, \sigma_{X_2,Y} = \beta_C\sigma_{X_2}^2 \tag{11}$$

and all other variance–covariance terms remain as in the unconstrained model. ML estimation assuming Eq. (11), where β_C is the common slope and no assumption is made regarding equality of the multiple informant variances, does not lead to closed form solutions. We find no obvious way to set up GEE to reproduce the model assuming Eq. (11). However, if we constrain the slopes to be equal and also assume equal multiple informant variances, we can derive the same estimates as obtained by fitting Eq. (7) using GEE when assuming

$$\sigma_{X_1,Y} = \sigma_{X_2,Y} = \sigma_{X,Y}, \sigma_{X_1}^2 = \sigma_{X_2}^2 = \sigma_X^2. \tag{12}$$

The model assuming Eq. (12) implies that $\beta_1 = \beta_2 = \beta_C$ when assuming the variances for the two covariates are equal and also implies equal correlation of each informant with the response. Similar to the unconstrained case, we define $\theta = (\mu_Y, \mu_{X_1}, \mu_{X_2}, \sigma_Y^2, \sigma_{X,Y}, \sigma_{X_1,X_2}, \sigma_X^2)^T$ and $\tau = (\alpha_1, \alpha_2, \beta_C, V_{11C}, V_{12C})^T$. Equation (7) follows directly with $\alpha_k = \mu_Y - \beta_C\mu_{X_k}$ for $k = 1$, 2 and $\beta_C = \sigma_{X,Y}/\sigma_X^2$. The ML estimates of θ under the constrained model are the same as in the unconstrained case except with $\hat{\sigma}_{X,Y} = (\Sigma_{i=1}^n(X_{i1} - \bar{X}_1)(Y_i - \bar{Y}) + \Sigma_{i=1}^n(X_{i2} - \bar{X}_2)(Y_i - \bar{Y}))/2n$ and $\hat{\sigma}_X^2 = (\Sigma_{i=1}^n(X_{i1} - \bar{X}_1)^2 + \Sigma_{i=1}^n(X_{i2} - \bar{X}_2)^2)/2n$; furthermore, we find that $\hat{\beta}_C$ is the same for GEE and ML. An expression for $\text{var}(\hat{\beta}_C)$ is derived; asymptotically

$$\text{var}(\sqrt{n}\hat{\beta}_C) \to \left(\frac{\sigma_Y^2(1+\rho_{X_1,X_2})(1-\rho_{Y|X_1,X_2}^{(C)^2})}{2\sigma_X^2}\right), \tag{13}$$

where

$$\rho^{(C)^2}_{Y|X_1,X_2} = \frac{2\rho^2_{X,Y}}{1+\rho_{X_1,X_2}}.$$

Next we incorporate a vector of covariates $\mathbf{Z}$ not measured by multiple informants using the model in Eq. (9) and find the same estimates as derived by the GEE approach. We assume that

$$\mathbf{Q}_i \sim MVN\left(\begin{pmatrix} \mu_0+\mu_1\mathbf{Z} \\ \delta_0+\delta_1\mathbf{Z} \\ v_0+v_1\mathbf{Z} \end{pmatrix}, \begin{pmatrix} \sigma^2_{Y|Z} & \sigma_{X_1,Y|Z} & \sigma_{X_2,Y|Z} \\ \sigma_{X_1,Y|Z} & \sigma^2_{X_1|Z} & \sigma_{X_1,X_2|Z} \\ \sigma_{X_2,Y|Z} & \sigma_{X_1,X_2|Z} & \sigma^2_{X_2|Z} \end{pmatrix}\right),$$

and make no distributional assumptions on $\mathbf{Z}$. As done previously, we obtain mean expressions for $\mathbf{Y}$ given ($\mathbf{X}_1$, $\mathbf{Z}$) and $\mathbf{Y}$ given ($\mathbf{X}_2$, $\mathbf{Z}$) and relate these to Eq. (9). Using the results of standard multivariate normal regression theory, estimates for θ are obtained from three separate regressions. In summary, (μ_0, μ_1) are regression coefficients from fitting $E(\mathbf{Y}|\mathbf{Z})$, (δ_0, δ_1) are from $E(\mathbf{X}_1|\mathbf{Z})$ and (v_0, v_1) are from $E(\mathbf{X}_2|\mathbf{Z})$. After obtaining these estimates, we make a transformation to τ; the vector consists of the regression coefficients from Eq. (9) (β), variance–covariance terms that condition on $\mathbf{Z}$ and values from θ that ensure a full rank transformation. We find that estimates of β obtained from ML are the same as those from GEE. We calculate var($\hat{\beta}$) using the same technique as without covariates.

In this section, we have found that ML and GEE give the same estimates under an unconstrained model, assuming a constrained model with equal variances and with inclusion of covariates not measured by multiple informants. To obtain ML estimates, we have assumed multivariate normality. However, in the situations where the ML and GEE estimates are identical, ML is clearly robust to the distributional assumptions on the multiple informants.

4. Simulations

We performed 10,000 simulations to compare the empirical GEE, model-based GEE and ML variances. We generate our first dataset from the trivariate normal distribution with response $\mathbf{Y}$ and multiple informants $\mathbf{X}_1$ and $\mathbf{X}_2$ for $i = 1, \ldots, 500$. For the subsequent 9999 draws, we generate each of the 500 $\mathbf{Y}$ values from a normal distribution with mean $E(\mathbf{Y}|\mathbf{X}_1,\mathbf{X}_2)$ and variance var($\mathbf{Y}|\mathbf{X}_1,\mathbf{X}_2$); thus $\mathbf{X}_1$ and $\mathbf{X}_2$ are fixed since each iteration has the same set of 500 $\mathbf{X}_1$, $\mathbf{X}_2$ values. We consider four scenarios assuming different unconstrained parameters; the first case we present, $\sigma_{X_1,Y} = -0.142$, $\sigma_{X_2,Y} = -0.156$ and $\sigma_{X_1,X_2} = 0.333$, are values from the illustration described in Section 6. Table 1 gives the slope variances from the simulations using Eqs (3) and (6) for the empirical GEE and model-based

Table 1
Variance simulation results – unconstrained model

			$\text{var}(\hat{\beta}_1)$			
$\sigma_{X_1,Y}$	$\sigma_{X_2,Y}$	σ_{X_1,X_2} [a]	Empirical	Model-Based	ML	Simulation
−0.142	−0.156	0.333	0.00229	0.00229	0.00229	0.00231
0.300	0.600	0.600	0.00327	0.00324	0.00324	0.00270
0.800	0.500	0.000	0.00459	0.00459	0.00459	0.00415
0.000	0.000	0.333	0.00171	0.00172	0.00172	0.00173

			$\text{cov}(\hat{\beta}_1, \hat{\beta}_2)$			
$\sigma_{X_1,Y}$	$\sigma_{X_2,Y}$	σ_{X_1,X_2} [a]	Empirical	Model-Based	ML	Simulation
−0.142	−0.156	0.333	0.00062	0.00061	0.00061	0.00061
0.300	0.600	0.600	0.00156	0.00161	0.00158	0.00162
0.800	0.500	0.000	0.00111	0.00032	0.00032	0.00028
0.000	0.000	0.333	0.00074	0.00074	0.00074	0.00078

[a] $\sigma_Y^2 = \sigma_{X_1}^2 = \sigma_{X_2}^2 = 1$.

GEE variances, respectively. We calculate the ML variance using

$$\widehat{\text{var}}\begin{pmatrix} \sqrt{n}\hat{\beta}_1 \\ \sqrt{n}\hat{\beta}_2 \end{pmatrix} = \begin{pmatrix} \dfrac{\hat{\sigma}^2_Y(1-\hat{\rho}^2_{X_1,Y})}{\hat{\sigma}^2_{X_1}} & \dfrac{\hat{\sigma}^2_Y(1-\hat{\rho}^2_{Y|X_1,X_2})\hat{\sigma}_{X_1,X_2}}{\hat{\sigma}^2_{X_1}\hat{\sigma}^2_{X_2}} \\ \dfrac{\hat{\sigma}^2_Y(1-\hat{\rho}^2_{Y|X_1,X_2})\hat{\sigma}_{X_1,X_2}}{\hat{\sigma}^2_{X_1}\hat{\sigma}^2_{X_2}} & \dfrac{\hat{\sigma}^2_Y(1-\hat{\rho}^2_{X_2,Y})}{\hat{\sigma}^2_{X_2}} \end{pmatrix}, \tag{14}$$

where

$$\hat{\rho}^2_{Y|X_1,X_2} = \frac{\hat{\sigma}^2_{X_2}\hat{\sigma}^2_{X_1,Y} - 2\hat{\sigma}_{X_1,Y}\hat{\sigma}_{X_1,X_2} + \hat{\sigma}^2_{X_1}\hat{\sigma}^2_{X_2,Y}}{(\hat{\sigma}^2_{X_1}\hat{\sigma}^2_{X_2} - \hat{\sigma}^2_{X_1,X_2})\hat{\sigma}^2_Y}.$$

We omit $\text{var}(\hat{\beta}_2)$ since its results are similar to $\text{var}(\hat{\beta}_1)$; we also present the covariance between the slopes, $\text{cov}(\hat{\beta}_1, \hat{\beta}_2)$.

We compare the variance using each of the three methods (empirical GEE and model-based GEE and ML) to the variance of the simulations (reported in the column of Table 1 entitled Simulation) calculated as

$$\text{var}(\hat{\beta}_1) = \frac{\sum_{i=1}^{m}(\hat{\beta}_{1i} - \overline{\hat{\beta}_1})^2}{m}, \tag{15}$$

where m is the number of simulations and $\overline{\hat{\beta}_1}$ is the average of the $\hat{\beta}^{(1)}_{1i}$ values over all simulations. We compare the covariance using a similar technique. Nonparametric 95% confidence intervals (not reported) for the empirical, model-based and ML variances illustrate that the estimated variances are similar and closely approximate the simulated variances in most cases. In general, we find that the empirical estimates are more variable than their model-based and ML counterparts. The largest difference occurred when $\sigma_{X_1,Y} = 0.8$, $\sigma_{X_2,Y} = 0.5$ and $\sigma_{X_1,X_2} = 0$, for example, the empirical covariance appears inconsistent with the simulated covariance, but its confidence interval (0.00054, 0.00174) nearly includes the simulated value. All other empirical values fell within the nonparametric confidence intervals, and hence were trivial differences. Table 2 presents results when assuming a constrained model with equal variances

Table 2
Variance simulation results – constrained model

			$\text{var}(\hat{\beta}_C)$			
$\sigma_{X_1,Y}$	$\sigma_{X_2,Y}$	σ_{X_1,X_2} [a]	Empirical	Model-Based	ML	Simulation
−0.149	−0.149	0.333	0.00125	0.00125	0.00124	0.00123
0.400	0.400	0.600	0.00206	0.00204	0.00201	0.00198
0.500	0.500	0.000	0.00217	0.00194	0.00169	0.00173

[a] $\sigma^2_Y = \sigma^2_{X_1} = \sigma^2_{X_2} = 1$.

(Eq. (12)) under three scenarios assuming different constrained parameters. As in the unconstrained case, the estimated variances from the GEE and ML techniques are similar and both are consistent with the true variance estimates for the constrained case.

5. Efficiency calculations

We now discuss when using a constrained model leads to efficiency gains by comparing the variances of the slope estimates under the unconstrained model and the constrained model assumed in Eq. (12) using ARE, defined as the ratio of two asymptotic variances. Specifically, ARE is the ratio of $\text{var}(\hat{\beta}_1)$ to $\text{var}(\hat{\beta}_C)$ assuming $\beta_1 = \beta_2 = \beta_C$ since $\text{var}(\hat{\beta}_1) = \text{var}(\hat{\beta}_2)$ under the constrained model. If the ARE is greater than 1, then the estimated slope variance of the constrained model is more efficient than the estimated slope of the unconstrained model; this leads to increased power for detecting associations between multiple informants and response.

Using the asymptotic ML variances derived in Section 3 and assuming $\sigma_{X_1,Y} = \sigma_{X_2,Y} = \sigma_{X,Y}$ and $\sigma^2_{X_1} = \sigma^2_{X_2} = \sigma^2_X$, we calculate

$$\text{ARE} = \frac{2(1 - \rho^2_{X,Y})}{(1 + \rho_{X_1,X_2})(1 - \rho^2_{Y|X_1,X_2})}.$$

Because $\rho^2_{Y|X_1,X_2} \geq \rho^2_{X,Y} \geq 0$ and $-1 \leq \rho_{X_1,X_2} \leq 1$ it follows that ARE$\geq$1 for all values of ρ_{X_1,X_2}, $\rho^2_{X,Y}$ and $\rho^2_{Y|X_1,X_2}$. Therefore, the slope estimate under the

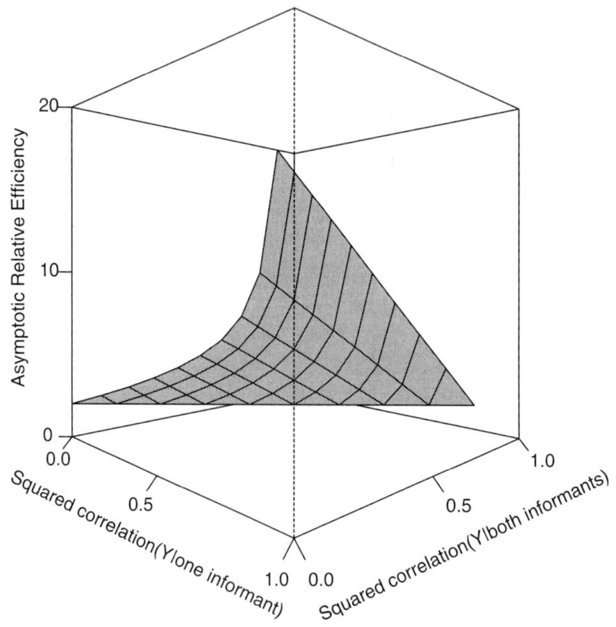

Fig. 1. Asymptotic relative efficiency ($\rho_{X_1,X_2} = 0$).

constrained model is always as efficient or more efficient than the unconstrained estimate when the constrained model holds. We consider ARE at particular values of ρ_{X_1,X_2}; for instance, with $\rho_{X_1,X_2} = 0$, ARE increases as the difference between $\rho^2_{Y|X_1,X_2}$ and $\rho^2_{X,Y}$ increases (Fig. 1). As ρ_{X_1,X_2} increases, the general shape of the ARE function remains the same but both the minimum and maximum ARE values decrease. In summary, if the slopes are similar, fitting a constrained model offers efficiency in the slope estimate over fitting an unconstrained model.

6. Illustration

In 1996, a study investigating the association between physical activity/inactivity and obesity was performed in two towns of Mexico City (Hernández et al., 1999, 2000, Hernández, 1998). Our goal is to compare the marginal relationship between BMI (**Y**) and vigorous exercise as reported by the child ($\mathbf{X}_1$) and the relationship between BMI and vigorous exercise reported by the child's mother ($\mathbf{X}_2$). We also fit a constrained model for increased efficiency. Although we could control for many covariates concerning the child (age, grade, gender, school, socioeconomic status, whether or not the child was sick on the evaluation day, nutritional status and whether or not the child was obese), for illustration we include only child's grade level in school. Grade is dichotomized with elementary school children of grades 5 and 6 in one category compared with secondary school children of grades 1 and 2. Complete information is available for 82 observations.

The raw summary measures for BMI and vigorous exercise are given in Table 3. Because the vigorous exercise measurements are highly skewed and the multiple informant variances are not equal, we convert the measurements to normal scores and then mean center and standardize these in order to compare the covariance of BMI and each covariate on the same scale. Grade is also mean centered and standardized for simplicity. Table 4 provides a summary of the estimates derived

Table 3
Estimated means and variance–covariance matrix for vigorous exercise

Variable	Estimated Mean
BMI (**Y**)	21.382
Vigorous exercise reported by child ($\mathbf{X}_1$)	0.986
Vigorous exercise reported by mother ($\mathbf{X}_2$)	0.786

Σ

	Y	$\mathbf{X}_1$	$\mathbf{X}_2$
Y	12.108	−0.374	−0.413
$\mathbf{X}_1$	−0.374	0.897	0.150
$\mathbf{X}_2$	−0.413	0.150	0.455

Table 4
Parameter estimates and standard errors for models using vigorous exercise to predict BMI

$\hat{\beta}_1$	Emp/ML[a] $\widehat{se}(\hat{\beta}_1)$	$\hat{\beta}_2$	Emp/ML[a] $\widehat{se}(\hat{\beta}_2)$	$\hat{\gamma}_1$	Emp/ML[a] $\widehat{se}(\hat{\gamma}_1)$	$\hat{\gamma}_2$	Emp/ML[a] $\widehat{se}(\hat{\gamma}_2)$
−0.511	0.341/0.380	−0.561	0.345/0.379				
−0.536[b]	0.249/0.308[b]						
−0.377	0.360/0.381	−0.514	0.353/0.372	−0.673	0.401/0.381	−0.714	0.369/0.372
−0.447[b]	0.264/0.305[b]			−0.659	0.384/0.378	−0.718	0.373/0.371

[a] Empirical GEE standard error/ML standard error.
[b] Constrained slope estimate.

Table 5
$-2\log$ likelihood values

Model	$-2\log$(Likelihood)
Unconstrained model	437.856
Constrained model	437.869
Unconstrained model with covariate	431.437
Constrained model with covariate	431.572

from GEE or ML and their standard errors (empirical GEE, model-based GEE/ML) for models of BMI and vigorous exercise fit using *R* (2004).

The marginal relationship between BMI and child's report of vigorous exercise, $\hat{\beta}_1$, and the marginal relationship between BMI and mother's report, $\hat{\beta}_2$, are not statistically significantly different; furthermore, both measures have a negative relationship with BMI and neither are statistically significant predictors of BMI. Thus, we fit a constrained model to gain efficiency (although physical activity is still not statistically significantly related to BMI); the constrained slope coefficient is -0.536, indicating that for every one unit increase in vigorous exercise a child receives, BMI decreases by over one half of a unit. In addition, fitting a constrained slope is more efficient than fitting two separate slopes ($\widehat{\text{ARE}} = 1.51$); the estimated variance of the constrained slope is approximately 50% smaller than when fitting an unconstrained model and provides more power to assess the association between vigorous exercise and BMI. We report $-2\log$(likelihood) values to compare models by constructing likelihood ratio tests (LRTs) in Table 5; according to a one degree of freedom LRT, fitting a constrained model as compared with the unconstrained model is appropriate. We also include grade in the models; according to a two degree of freedom LRT, adding grade is reasonable (p-value $= 0.04$). We also find that fitting a model where we constrain the slope to be equal in the presence of grade is appropriate according to a one degree of freedom LRT. Therefore, the relationship between vigorous exercise and BMI is similar regardless of respondent. Fitting a constrained model is simpler and more efficient; adding the covariate increases the predictive power. With regard to design issues, using either mother or child responses should yield similar results. Including both would increase power, although may not be feasible.

7. Conclusion

In this paper, we review a nonstandard application of GEE (Horton et al., 1999, Pepe et al., 1999) and introduce a novel ML method for modeling marginal regression models with multiple source predictors. ML and GEE yield the same estimates of the regression coefficients in the following situations: (1) unconstrained model, (2) constrained model with the multiple informants having equal variances (assuming Eq. (12)) and (3) including covariates not measured by multiple informants (assuming covariates have possibly different slopes). The model-based GEE and ML variances are similar; in practice, the covariances are as well. Our work also demonstrates that, at least in simple cases, the working correlation matrix recommended by Pepe et al. (1999) is optimal. The GEE empirical variance yields similar variance and covariance estimates as the model-based GEE and ML estimates, but the GEE empirical variance quantities are more variable than the former.

Throughout this paper, our goal has been to estimate the marginal relationship of each multiple informant covariate with response; we have presented two approaches to do so. Alternative techniques include use of latent variable or measurement error models; in both cases, the problem could be construed as each of the multiple informants being an imprecise surrogate for the true value (Horton and Fitzmaurice, 2004). However, when comparing diagnostic tests in practice researchers are interested in the actual reports and how they compare.

The ML technique can be extended to include more than two sets of multiple informants. For example, the Hernández et al. (1999) study had additional multiple informant measures including video viewing, moderate exercise and video-game playing. To implement ML in this setting, two equations with sets of regression slope coefficients for each additional multiple informant measure are necessary. This provides estimates of each multiple informant measure conditional on the other multiple informant measures in the model. If we take the case of two sets of multiple informants with $\mathbf{X}_{ij}$, where $i=$ set, $j=$ multiple informant, instead of using $E(\mathbf{Y}|\mathbf{X}_1)$ and $E(\mathbf{Y}|\mathbf{X}_2)$ to find the transformation from θ to τ, $E(\mathbf{Y}|\mathbf{X}_{11},\mathbf{X}_{21})$ and $\mathrm{E}(\mathbf{Y}|\mathbf{X}_{12},\mathbf{X}_{22})$ is used. Aside from the proliferation of parameters, solutions should extend from the existing methods.

Another extension is dealing with one construct measured with more than two multiple informants ($K>2$). In this situation, K separate regression equations are fit rather than 2. This may lead to estimation of a large number of parameters and a Jacobian matrix for the transformation from θ to τ of high dimension; e.g., with $K=3$, θ consists of 14 parameters. The models can also be extended to include a vector of covariates not measured by multiple informants. Rather than predicting $\mathbf{Y}$, $\mathbf{X}_1$, $\mathbf{X}_2$ from $\mathbf{Z}$ using an intercept and a slope, the model would be a multiple linear regression with an intercept and K slopes. Using a potentially cumbersome transformation from θ to τ, the $2(K+1)$ regression parameters are found as previously described. While extending the ML technique leads to additional parameters, ML can accommodate constrained models where the slope parameters are equal. In addition to providing efficiency gains, constraining coefficients also helps maintain parsimonious models.

Considering the advantages and disadvantages of using GEE and ML for analysis of multiple informants as predictors, GEE is more flexible than ML since it does not require a model for the multiple informants nor does it need normality of the multiple informants or the dependent variable. However, because ML and GEE yield the same solutions in most situations, ML does not require the multivariate normality assumption to be valid. In fact, the vigorous activity multiple informant measurements in the Hernández et al. (1999) dataset were skewed to the left; although we standardized this data, an analysis without standardization reveals that ML is still equivalent to GEE, thus confirming the robustness of ML to deviations from normality. A drawback of the GEE approach is that the independence working correlation structure must be assumed for the model to be valid (Pepe and Anderson, 1994). However, we have shown that the use of the independence working correlation matrix is optimal for certain models when assuming normality where the GEE and ML approaches yield identical estimates and standard errors.

An advantage of ML is the ability to fit a broader range of models than what can be fit using GEE; for example, ML can fit a model when a constrained effect is desired but the variance differs across levels of $\mathbf{X}_1$ and $\mathbf{X}_2$ (e.g. with large amounts of missing data on the multiple informants). Another positive aspect of the ML approach is that likelihood-based tests can be constructed to easily compare models; this is particularly helpful when considering many models. Perhaps the biggest advantage ML can offer is an efficiency gain compared with GEE when considering data with missingness (Litman et al., 2007).

Acknowledgement

We are gratcful for the support provided by the National Institute of Mental Health (NIMH) grant number MH54693 and National Institute of Health (NIH) grant number T32-MH017119.

References

Field, A.E., Laird, N.M., Steinberg, E., Fallon, E., Semega-Janneh, M., Yanovski, J.A. (2003). Which metric of relative weight best captures body fatness in children? *Obesity Research* **11**, 1345–1352.

Fitzmaurice, G.M., Laird, N.M., Zahner, G.E.P. (1996). Multivariate logistic models for incomplete binary responses. *Journal of the American Statistical Association* **91**(433), 99–108.

Fitzmaurice, G.M., Laird, N.M., Zahner, G.E.P., Daskalakis, C. (1995). Bivariate logistic regression analysis of child psychopathology ratings using multiple informants. *American Journal of Epidemiology* **142**(11), 1194–1203.

Goldwasser, M.A., Fitzmaurice, G.M. (2001). Multivariate linear regression of childhood psychopathology using multiple informant data. *International Journal of Methods in Psychiatric Research* **20**, 1–11.

Gould, M.S., Fisher, P., Parides, M., Flory, M., Shaffer, D. (1996). Psychosocial risk factors of child and adolescent completed suicide. *Archives of General Psychiatry* **53**, 1155–1162.

Hernández, B. (1998). *Diet, physical activity and obesity in Mexican children.* PhD thesis. Harvard School of Public Health, Boston, MA, USA.

Hernández, B., Gortmaker, S.L., Colditz, G.A., Peterson, K.E., Laird, N.M., Parra-Cabrera, S. (1999). Association of obesity with physical activity, television programs and other forms of video viewing among children in Mexico City. *International Journal of Obesity* **23**, 845–854.

Hernández, B., Gortmaker, S.L., Laird, N.M., Colditz, G.A., Parra-Cabrera, S., Peterson, K.E. (2000). Validity and reproducibility of a physical activity and inactivity questionnaire for Mexico City's schoolchildren. *Salud Publica de Mexico* **42**(4), 315–323.

Horton, N.J., Fitzmaurice, G.M. (2004). Tutorial in biostatistics: Regression analysis of multiple source and multiple informant data from complex survey samples. *Statistics in Medicine* **23**(18), 2911–2933.

Horton, N.J., Laird, N.M., Murphy, J.M., Monson, R.R., Sobol, A.M., Leighton, A.H. (2001). Multiple informants: Mortality associated with psychiatric disorders in the Stirling County Study. *American Journal of Epidemiology* **154**(7), 649–656.

Horton, N.J., Laird, N.M., Zahner, G.E.P. (1999). Use of multiple informant data as a predictor in psychiatric epidemiology. *International Journal of Methods in Psychiatric Research* **8**, 6–18.

Huber, P.J. (1967). The behaviour of maximum likelihood estimators under non-standard conditions. In: LeCam, L.M., Neyman, J. (Eds.),**Vol. 1** *Proceedings of the Fifth Berkeley Symposium on Mathematical Statistics and Probability*. University of California Press, pp. 221–233.

Kuo, M., Mohler, B., Raudenbush, S.L., Earls, F.J. (2000). Assessing exposure to violence using multiple informants: Application of hierarchical linear models. *Journal of Child Psychology and Psychiatry and Allied Disciplines* **41**, 1049–1056.

Liang, K., Zeger, S.L. (1986). Longitudinal data analysis using generalized linear models. *Biometrika* **73**(1), 13–22.

Litman, H.J., Horton, N.J., Hernández, B., Laird, N.M. (2007). Incorporating missingness for estimation of marginal regression models with multiple source predictors. *Statistics in Medicine* **26**, 1055–1068.

O'Brien, L.M., Fitzmaurice, G.M., Horton, N.J. (2006). Maximum likelihood estimation of marginal pairwise associations with multiple source predictors. *Biometrical Journal* **48**(5), 860–875.

Offord, D.R., Boyle, M.H., Racine, Y., Szatmari, P., Fleming, J.E., Sanford, M., Lipman, E.L. (1996). Integrating assessment data from multiple informants. *Journal of the American Academy of Child and Adolescent Psychiatry* **35**(8), 1078–1085.

Pepe, M.S., Anderson, G.L. (1994). A cautionary note on inference for marginal regression models with longitudinal data and general correlated response data. *Communications in Statistics* **23**(4), 939–951.

Pepe, M.S., Whitaker, R.C., Seidel, K. (1999). Estimating and comparing univariate associations with application to the prediction of adult obesity. *Statistics in Medicine* **18**, 163–173.

R Development Core Team (2004). *R: A language and environment for statistical computing*. R Foundation for Statistical Computing, Vienna, Austria.

Zeger, S.L., Liang, K. (1986). Longitudinal data analysis for discrete and continuous outcomes. *Biometrics* **42**, 121–130.

Handbook of Statistics, Vol. 27
ISSN: 0169-7161

DOI: 10.1016/S0169-7161(07)27026-9

26

Difference Equations with Public Health Applications

Asha Seth Kapadia and Lemuel A. Moyé

Abstract

The difference equation is a powerful tool for providing analytical solutions to probabilistic models of dynamic systems in health-related research. These applications include, but are not limited to, issues commonly encountered in stochastic processes, clinical research, and epidemiology. In practice, many important applications, such as the occurrence of a clinical event and patterns of missed clinic visits in randomized clinical trials as well as drought predictions, can be described in terms of recursive elements. In this chapter difference equations are motivated and are solved using the generating function approach.

1. Introduction

In its most general form a linear difference equation can be written as

$$p_0(k)y_{k+n} + p_1(k)y_{k+n-1} + p_2(k)y_{k+n-2} + \cdots + p_n(k)y_k = R(k). \tag{1}$$

It consists of terms involving members of the $\{y_k\}$ sequence, and, in addition, coefficients such as $p_j(k)$, of elements of the $\{y_k\}$ sequence in the equation. These coefficients may or may not be a function of k. When the coefficients are not functions of k, the difference equation has constant coefficients. Difference equations with coefficients that are functions of k are described as difference equations with variable coefficients. In general, difference equations with constant coefficients are easier to solve than those difference equations that have nonconstant coefficients.

If the term $R(k)$ on the right side of the equation is equal to zero, then the difference equation is *homogeneous*. If the right side of the equation is not zero, then Eq. (1) becomes a *nonhomogeneous* difference equation. For example, the family of difference equations

$$y_{k+2} = 6y_{k+1} - 3y_k \tag{2}$$

for k, an integer (from zero to infinity), is homogeneous since each term in the equation is a function of a member of the sequence $\{y_k\}$. The equation

$$y_{k+3} = 6y_{k+1} - 3y_k + 12, \quad k = 1, 2, \ldots, \tag{3}$$

is a nonhomogeneous one because of the inclusion of the term 12. The equation

$$3y_{k+4} + (k+3)y_{k+3} + 2^{k+2}y_{k+2} + (k+1)y_{k+1} + 4ky_k = (k+2)(k+1)$$

would be designated as a fourth-order, nonhomogeneous difference equation with variable coefficients.

Finally, the order of a family of difference equations is the difference between the largest index and the smallest index of the $\{y_1, y_2, y_3, \ldots, y_k, \ldots\}$ sequence in (1). Equation (2) is a second-order difference equation while Eq. (3) is a third-order one.

There are several approaches to the solutions of difference equations. However, two rather intuitive approaches are mentioned in passing. The first is the iterative approach and the second is the use of mathematical induction. Both are briefly discussed below.

Consider the simple first-order difference equation

$$y_{k+1} = ay_k.$$

The solution to the above equation using iterative reasoning assuming y_0 is known would result in the following solution:

$$y_k = a^k y_0.$$

Unfortunately, this intuitive approach to the solution, which is very useful for first-order difference equations, becomes somewhat complicated if the order is increased as, for example, in the second-order, nonhomogeneous family of difference equations

$$y_{k+2} = a_1 y_{k+1} + by_k + c.$$

Another way to solve simple equations is to guess the solution and then prove that the guessed solution is correct through the use of induction. Briefly, the induction argument outlines a simple sequence of the following three steps:

(1) Demonstrate the assertion is true for $k = 1$.
(2) Assume the assertion is true for k.
(3) Use (1) and (2) to prove that the assertion is true for $k+1$.

This method again has its limitations particularly when a good initial guess is not easily available. In this chapter we will be solving most of the difference equations using generating functions (Wilf, 1994) and wherever possible inverting them to obtain the exact solutions.

2. Generating functions

A generating function $G(s)$ is a function that contains the (Chiang, 1980) information necessary to produce or generate the sequence of y_k's. $G(s)$ is defined as

$$G(s) = \sum_{k=0}^{\infty} y_k s^k.$$

$G(s)$ provides the content of the sequence $\{y_k\}$ which will be the solution to the family of difference equations. Consider a simple first-order, homogeneous family of difference equations

$$y_{k+1} = 3y_k \tag{4}$$

for $k = 0, 1, 2, \ldots, \infty$, and y_0 is a known constant. Multiplying both sides of (4) by s^k we have

$$s^k y_{k+1} = 3s^k y_k.$$

The next step is to add these equations from $k = 0$ to ∞, recognizing that the sum of left side of these equations is equal to the sum of the right side of all of these equations, giving us

$$\begin{aligned} s^{-1}\sum_{k=0}^{\infty} s^{k+1} y_{k+1} &= s^{-1}\left[\sum_{k=0}^{\infty} s^{k+1} y_{k+1} + s^0 y_0 - s^0 y_0\right] \\ &= s^{-1}\left[\sum_{k=0}^{\infty} s^k y_k - y_0\right] \\ &= s^{-1}[G(s) - y_0] \end{aligned}$$

revealing

$$\begin{aligned} G(s) - y_0 &= 3sG(s), \\ G(s) &= \frac{y_0}{1-3s}. \end{aligned}$$

From the above simple generating function y_k can be easily obtained by inverting $G(s)$ as

$$y_k = y_0(3)^k,$$

assuming $|3s| < 1$.

The additive principle of generating functions states that for two sequences $\{y_{1k}\}$ and $\{y_{2k}\}$ and the corresponding generating functions $G_1(s)$ and $G_2(s)$, the generating function of the sequence $\{y_{1k} \pm y_{2k}\}$ is $G_1(s) \pm G_2(s)$. Similarly the scaling principle of generating functions states that if $G_1(s)$ is the generating function associated with the sequence $\{y_k\}$, then the generating function associated with the sequence $\{cy_k\}$ is $cG_1(s)$.

Unfortunately, the product of generating functions is not the product of the kth terms of each of the infinite series. Instead, for two generating functions, $G_1(s)$ and $G_2(s)$ associated with sequences $\{a_k\}$ and $\{b_k\}$

$$G_1(s)G_2(s) = (a_0 + a_1 s + a_2 s^2 + a_3 s^3 + \cdots)(b_0 + b_1 s + b_2 s^2 + b_3 s^3 + \cdots).$$

The coefficient of s^k is then $\sum_{j=0}^{k} a_j b_{k-j}$.

Here, we only need evaluate this product term by term and gather together those coefficients which are associated with like powers of s. The skillful use of generating functions is invaluable in solving families of difference equations. However, generating functions have been developed in certain specific circumstances. Consider the circumstance where the sequence $\{p_k\}$ are probabilities. Then, using our definition of $G(s)$ we see that $G(s) = \sum_{k=0}^{\infty} p_k s^k$, where $\sum_{k=0}^{\infty} p_k = 1$. In probability it is often useful to describe the relative frequency of an event in terms of an outcome of an experiment. Among the most useful of these experiments are those for which outcomes are discrete (the integers or some subset of the integers). These discrete models have many applications, and it is often helpful to recognize the generating function associated with the models. The generating function associated with such a model is described as the probability generating function. We will continue to refer to these probability generating functions using the nomenclature $G(s)$. Note that in this context of probability, the probability generating function can be considered an expectation, i.e., $G(s) = E[s^x]$.

3. Second-order nonhomogeneous equations and generating functions

A family of second-order, nonhomogeneous difference equation can be written as

$$ay_{k+2} + by_{k+1} + cy_k = d, \quad k = 0, 1, 2, \ldots, \infty,$$

where a, b, c, or d, are known, fixed, and not equal to zero. Assume that y_0, y_1, and y_2 are also known constants.

During this development the impact of the nonhomogeneous part of this family of difference equations will be noted. Multiply each term in the above equation by s^k, and sum over the range $0 \leqslant k < \infty$.

$$as^{-2}\sum_{k=0}^{\infty} s^{k+2} y_{k+2} + bs^{-1}\sum_{k=0}^{\infty} s^{k+1} y_{k+1} + c\sum_{k=0}^{\infty} s^k y_k = d\sum_{k=0}^{\infty} s^k. \tag{5}$$

The first three terms are easy to convert to expressions involving $G(s)$. The last term represents the nonhomogeneous component $d/(1-s)$. Converting each summation in the equation to a term involving $G(s)$, Eq. (5) becomes

$$as^{-2}[G(s) - y_0 - y_1 s - y_2 s^2] + bs^{-1}[G(s) - y_0 - y_1 s] + cG(s) = d\sum_{k=0}^{\infty} s^k,$$

or

$$G(s)[cs^2 + bs + a] = ay_0 + s(ay_1 + by_0) + s^2(ay_2 + by_1) + \frac{ds^2}{1-s}.$$

$G(s)$ is then obtained as

$$G(s) = \frac{ay_0}{cs^2 + bs + a} + \frac{s(ay_1 + by_0)}{cs^2 + bs + a} + \frac{s^2(ay_2 + by_1)}{cs^2 + bs + a} + \frac{ds^2}{(cs^2 + bs + a)(1-s)}. \tag{6}$$

The nonhomogeneous component of this family of difference equations has introduced the right most term on the right side of the above equation. In order to invert (6) note that each term in $G(s)$ involves inversion of $1/(a+bs+cs^2)$. We now proceed with the inversion by writing

$$\frac{1}{a+bs+cs^2}=\frac{1/a}{1-(-1)((b/a)+(c/a)s)s}, \tag{7}$$

recognizing that the expression on the right side of the above equation is the sum of the series whose kth term is $(1/a)(-1)^k((b/a)+(c/a)s)^k s^k$. Using the binomial theorem to reevaluate this expression we have

$$\frac{(-1)^k}{a}\left(\frac{b}{a}+\frac{c}{a}s\right)^k s^k=\frac{(-1)^k}{a^{k+1}}(b+cs)^k s^k=\frac{(-1)^k}{a^{k+1}}\sum_{j=0}^{k}\binom{k}{j}c^j b^{k-j}s^{k+j}.$$

Next we pull together the coefficients of s^k. Introducing the new index variables j and m such that $0\leqslant j\leqslant m\leqslant k$, observe that we must accumulate the coefficient

$$\binom{m}{j}c^j b^{m-j}$$

whenever $m+j=k$. Coefficient of s^k is

$$\left\{\frac{(-1)^k}{a^{k+1}}\sum_{m=0}^{k}\sum_{j=0}^{m}\binom{m}{j}c^j b^{m-j}I_{m+j=k}\right\}.$$

The indicator function $I_{m+j=k}$ in the above expression is defined as $I_{m+j=k}=1$ if $m+j=k$ and is 0 otherwise.

We are now in a position to completely invert $G(s)$, with repeated use of the scaling, addition, translation, and multiplication principles of generating functions.

Coefficient of s^k in $G(s)$ is

$$\begin{aligned}
&ay_0\frac{(-1)^k}{a^{k+1}}\sum_{m=0}^{k}\sum_{j=0}^{m}\binom{m}{j}c^j b^{m-j}I_{m+j=k}\\
&+(ay_1+by_0)\frac{(-1)^{k-1}}{a^k}\sum_{m=0}^{k-1}\sum_{j=0}^{m}\binom{m}{j}c^j b^{m-j}I_{m+j=k-1}\\
&+(ay_2+by_1)\frac{(-1)^{k-2}}{a^{k-1}}\sum_{m=0}^{k-2}\sum_{j=0}^{m}\binom{m}{j}c^j b^{m-j}I_{m+j=k-2}\\
&+d\sum_{h=0}^{k}\frac{(-1)^h}{a^{h+1}}\sum_{m=0}^{h}\sum_{j=0}^{m}\binom{m}{j}c^j b^{m-j}I_{m+j=h}.
\end{aligned}$$

4. Example in rhythm disturbances

We present here our ability to work with difference equations to an unusual problem in cardiology involving heart rhythms. Typically, the heart follows a regular rhythm, but occasionally, in normal hearts, that regular rhythm is interrupted.

Most everyone remembers when their "heart skips a beat." Children (and adults) do this to each other fairly easily by jumping out from a closet or a darkened hallway. The effect on the frightened person is immediate. The fright causes a series of nervous system and neuro-hormonal responses and aberrations. One of the most common is that the ventricles contract prematurely, before they are completely full. It is a fascinating observation that the off rhythm beat is so noticeable, especially when hundreds of thousands of regular beats go relatively unnoticed. Nevertheless, we can all recall the thud in our chest when so startled. For the majority of us, this one premature ventricular contraction (PVC) is at most a short-lived, unpleasant sensation. The sinoatrial node (SA node) quickly reasserts its predominance as the source of electrical activity of the heart, and the heart quickly returns to its normal sinus rhythm.

Occasionally, PVCs do not occur in isolation. They may however occur more frequently. This is seen in patients who have heart disease. For example, patients who have heart attacks, when a portion of heart muscle dies, may have the electrical conductivity system of the heart affected. As the SA node functions less and less efficiently, other parts of the electrical conducting system try to break through, attempting to exert their own control over the flow of electricity through the heart. PVCs begin to occur more and more frequently, finally occurring as couplets or two consecutive ones. The occurrence of such a couple is termed bigeminy. Trigeminy is the occurrence of three consecutive PVCs and quadgeminy defines the consecutive occurrence of four such PVCs.

These short bursts of ectopic ventricular activity can occur in the normal heart as well, as one of the authors can attest. On his first day as an intern, he was learning about his new responsibilities as a physician, while smoking a pipe and drinking coffee. The combination of stress from the new job, the nicotine from the pipe (a heart stimulant), and the caffeine (another heart stimulant) from the coffee produced a very memorable burst of trigeminy.

As the consecutive occurrence of PVCs becomes more frequent, even the runs of bigeminy, trigeminy, and quadgeminy begin to come together into a burst of ventricular tachycardia (VT, rapid heart rate). These episodes of VT (sometimes termed bouts of VT) are extremely dangerous. As we pointed out, when a PVC occurs in isolation, normal sinus rhythm is quickly restored, and the heart returns to its efficient filling mechanism. However, when many of these abnormal ventricular beats occur in a row, the movement of blood through the heart is profoundly disturbed. The ventricles contract rapidly, but they contract far too rapidly, well before the atria have the opportunity to fill the ventricles with blood. Thus, in VT, the ventricles contract to no good end, since they are not pumping blood at all. This condition, if not treated, can deteriorate to ventricular fibrillation (VF) where the complicated interrelated muscle system in the ventricles no longer contracts as a cohesive unit, and the ability to move blood out to the systemic circulation is effectively destroyed.

This destruction results in the sudden death of the individual. One moment the person appears fine – the next moment they are on the floor within seconds of death. In the case of drowning, even though there has been no breathing, the heart has continued to pump throughout the accident. Thus, even though the victim's brain is receiving only deoxygenated blood, they are still receiving blood, and survival is prolonged. However, in sudden death, the heart stops beating at once. The brain receives no blood, and brain cells die by the tens of millions in a matter of seconds. Certainly, sudden death syndrome must be avoided at all costs.

Cardiologists have long recognized the sudden death syndrome and have worked hard to identify both risk factors for the syndrome and a way to treat it. Over the past 30 years, many esteemed workers in cardiology have constructed a theory that has come to be known as the arrhythmia suppression hypothesis. This hypothesis states that the harbinger of sudden death was not the occurrence of "runs of VT" but the occurrence of bigeminy, trigeminy, and even PVCs. Since these relatively mild rhythm abnormalities sometimes deteriorate to runs of VT, and from VT to VF and death, preventing the mild ventricular rhythm disturbances would prevent sudden death. This hypothesis was put to test in a complicated experiment called Cardiac Arrhythmia Suppression Trial (CAST, Pratt and Moyé, 1995) by testing drugs known to reduce mild ventricular arrhythmias. However, the drugs that were tested produced even worse rhythms than the ones they were designed to reduce and the experiment had to be stopped. Many cardiologists still believe in the arrhythmia suppression hypothesis, and are waiting for the correct drug to be developed. For all computations in the cardiac rhythm domain, it will be assumed that each beat represents a Bernoulli trial. There are only two possibilities for the beat; it is either a normal sinus beat, which occurs with probability p, or a PVC (abnormal beat) which occurs with probability q. Thus, a failure is the occurrence of a premature, ventricular contraction. We may therefore think of a burst of bigeminy as a failure run of length 2, since bigeminy is two consecutive aberrant ventricular beats. Analogously, the occurrence of three successive irregular ventricular beats (trigeminy) will be considered as a failure run of length 3 and so on. We will explore several applications of the $T_{[K,L]}(n)$ probabilities below to model these occurrences.

Define:

$T_{[K,L]}(n) = P$ [the minimum and maximum failure run lengths is in the interval (K, L) when $K \leqslant L$ in n trials].

For example, $T_{[2,6]}(12)$ is the probability that in 12 Bernoulli trials all failure runs have lengths 2, 3, 4, 5, or 6, with all other failure run lengths excluded. Then:

$T_{[K,K]}(n) = P$ [all failure run lengths are exactly of length K];
$T_{[0,L]}(n) = P$ [all failure runs are $\leqslant L$ in length];
$1 - T_{[0,L]}(n) = P$ [at least one failure run length is greater than L].

If $M_F(n)$ is the maximum failure run length in n trials, then

$$E[M_F(n)] = \sum_{L=0}^{n} L[T_{[0,L]}(n) - T_{[0,L-1]}(n)],$$

$$\mathrm{Var}[M_F(n)] = \sum_{L=0}^{n} L^2[T_{[0,L]}(n) - T_{[0,L-1]}(n)] - E^2[M_F(n)].$$

Define:

$T_{0,[K,L]}(n) = P$ [that either the maximum failure run length is zero or the minimum failure run length and the maximum failure run length are each in $[K, L]$].

In this case $T_{0,[K,L]}(n)$ is simply $T_{[K,L]}(n) + p^n$. The boundary conditions for $T_{0,[K,L]}(n)$ are:

$T_{0,[K,L]}(n) = 0$ for all $n<0$;
$T_{0,[K,L]}(n) = 1$ for $n = 0$;
$T_{0,[K,L]}(n) = p^n$ for $0<n<K$.

Using the indicator function, we may write the recursive relationship for $T_{0,[K,L]}(n)$ for $0<K\leqslant\min(L, n)$ as

$$\begin{aligned} T_{0,[K,L]}(n) = {} & pT_{0,[K,L]}(n-1) + q^K pT_{0[K,L]}(n-K-1) \\ & + q^{K+1}pT_{0,[K,L]}(n-K-2) + q^{K+2}pT_{0,[K,L]}(n-K-3) \\ & + \cdots + q^L pT_{0,[K,L]}(n-L-1) + q^n I_{K\le n\le L}. \end{aligned}$$

$I_{x\in A} = 1$ if x is in the set A and 0 otherwise. This difference equation may be rewritten as $T_{0,[K,L]}(n) = pT_{0,[K,L]}(n-1) + \sum_{j=K}^{L} q^j pT_{0,[K,L]}(n-j-1) + q^n I_{K\le n\le L}$.

Assume that the run length interval bounds K and L and probability of failure q are known.

The plan will be to tailor the above equation to a model to predict runs of irregular ventricular beats. Let n be the total number of heartbeats that are observed. Begin by computing the probability that in a consecutive sequence of heartbeats, the only ectopy (i.e., abnormal heart rhythm) that occurs is an isolated PVC. An isolated PVC is a failure run of length 1. Converting this to model terminology, $K = L = 1$ we compute for $n>0$

$$T_{0,[1,1]}(n) = pT_{0,[1,1]}(n-1) + qpT_{0,[1,1]}(n-2) + qI_{n=1}. \tag{8}$$

The above equation provides for failure runs of length 0 or 1, and does not permit failure runs of length >1 for $n\geqslant 1$. From the boundary conditions we have defined $T_{0,[1,1]}(0) = 1$. We compute from this equation $T_{0,[1,1]}(1) = p + q$ and $T_{[1,1]}(1) = q$. Likewise we can compute

$$T_{0,[1,1]}(2) = p(p+q) + qp = p^2 + 2pq$$

and

$$T_{[1,1]}(2) = T_{0,[1,1]}(2) - p^2 = 2pq.$$

The goal is to solve Eq. (8) in its entirety, by finding a general solution for $T_{0,[1,1]}(n)$ using the generating function approach. Define

$$G(s) = \sum_{n=0}^{\infty} s^n T_{0,[1,1]}(n).$$

Proceed by multiplying each side of Eq. (8) by s^n and begin the conversion process

$$s^n T_{0,[1,1]}(n) = s^n p T_{0,[1,1]}(n-1) + s^n qp T_{0,[1,1]}(n-2) + s^n q I_{n=1},$$

$$\sum_{n=1}^{\infty} s^n T_{0,[1,1]}(n) = \sum_{n=1}^{\infty} s^n p T_{0,[1,1]}(n-1) + \sum_{n=1}^{\infty} s^n qp T_{0,[1,1]}(n-2) + \sum_{n=1}^{\infty} s^n q I_{n=1}. \quad (9)$$

The term on the left side of the equality in the above equation is $G(s)-1$. The last term on the right side of the equality is qs. Consider the first two terms on the RHS of (9)

$$\sum_{n=1}^{\infty} s^n p T_{0,[1,1]}(n-1) = ps \sum_{n=1}^{\infty} s^{n-1} T_{0,[1,1]}(n-1) = ps \sum_{n=0}^{\infty} s^n T_{0,[1,1]}(n) = psG(s)$$

and

$$\begin{aligned} \sum_{n=1}^{\infty} s^n qp T_{0,[1,1]}(n-2) &= qps^2 \sum_{n=1}^{\infty} s^{n-2} T_{0,[1,1]}(n-2) \\ &= qps^2 \sum_{n=0}^{\infty} s^n T_{0,[1,1]}(n) = qps^2 G(s). \end{aligned}$$

We may rewrite Eq. (9) in terms of $G(s)$ and simplify

$$\begin{aligned} G(s) - 1 &= psG(s) + qps^2 G(s) + qs \\ G(s)[1 - ps - qps^2] &= qs + 1 \\ G(s) &= \frac{qs+1}{1 - ps - qps^2} \end{aligned} \quad (10)$$

The above equation is a polynomial generating function with no helpful roots for the denominator, so we proceed with the inversion by first collecting coefficient of s^n in the denominator. The nth term of the series $[1-(1+qs)ps)]^{-1}$ is

$$p^n \sum_{j=0}^{n} \binom{n}{j} q^j s^{n+j}.$$

Now collecting coefficients we see that the coefficient of s^n in (10), i.e., $T_{0,[1,1]}(n)$ is

$$q \sum_{m=0}^{n-1} p^m \sum_{j=0}^{m} \binom{m}{j} q^j I_{m+j=n-1} + \sum_{m=0}^{n} p^m \sum_{j=0}^{m} \binom{m}{j} q^j I_{m+j=n}$$

and

$$T_{[1,1]}(n) = q\sum_{m=0}^{n-1} p^m \sum_{j=0}^{m}\binom{m}{j} q^j I_{m+j=n-1} + \sum_{m=0}^{n} p^m \sum_{j=0}^{m}\binom{m}{j} q^j I_{m+j=n} - p^n.$$

With the experience from the isolated PVC model, we can expand our application of the difference equation approach to arrhythmia occurrence. In this section, we will focus solely on failure runs of length 2, i.e., the $T_{0,[2,2]}(n)$ model. The family of difference equations for $n>0$ can be written as

$$T_{0,[2,2]}(n) = pT_{0,[2,2]}(n-1) + q^2 pT_{0,[2,2]}(n-3) + q^2 I_{n=2}. \tag{11}$$

We will proceed as we did in the previous section. Define

$$T_{0,[2,2]}(0) = 1, \quad T_{0,[2,2]}(1) = p, \quad T_{0,[2,2]}(2) = p(p) + q^2 = p^2 + q^2.$$

To find the general solution for the probability of bigeminy alone, define

$$G(s) = \sum_{n=0}^{\infty} s^n T_{0,[2,2]}(n),$$

and multiply each term in Eq. (11) by s^n; we find

$$s^n T_{0,[2,2]}(n) = s^n pT_{0,[2,2]}(n-1) + s^n q^2 pT_{0,[2,2]}(n-3) + s^n q^2 I_{n=2}.$$

The next step requires taking the sum from n equal to 1 to ∞ in each term of the above equation obtaining

$$\sum_{n=1}^{\infty} s^n T_{0,[2,2]}(n) = \sum_{n=1}^{\infty} s^n pT_{0,[2,2]}(n-1) + \sum_{n=1}^{\infty} s^n q^2 pT_{0,[2,2]}(n-3) + \sum_{n=1}^{\infty} s^n q^2 I_{n=2}. \tag{12}$$

The first term on the right side of the above equation may be written as

$$\sum_{n=1}^{\infty} s^n pT_{0,[2,2]}(n-1) = psG(s).$$

Rewriting Eq. (12) in terms of $G(s)$

$$G(s) - 1 = psG(s) + q^2 ps^3 G(s) + q^2 s^2.$$

A little simplification leads to

$$G(s) = \frac{1}{1 - ps - q^2 ps^3} + \frac{q^2 s^2}{1 - ps - q^2 ps^3}. \tag{13}$$

The coefficient of s^k in the above equation is

$$\left\{\sum_{m=0}^{n} p^m \sum_{j=0}^{m} \binom{m}{j} q^{2j} I_{m+2j=n} + q^2 \sum_{m=0}^{n-2} p^m \sum_{j=0}^{m} \binom{m}{j} q^{2j} I_{m+2j=n-2}\right\}.$$

Hence

$$T_{[2,2]}(n) = \sum_{m=0}^{n} p^m \sum_{j=0}^{m} \binom{m}{j} q^{2j} I_{m+2j=n} + q^2 \sum_{m=0}^{n-2} p^m \sum_{j=0}^{m} \binom{m}{j} q^{2j} I_{m+2j=n-2} - p^n.$$

With the experience of the isolated PVC and bigeminy problem, we are now in a position to provide a general solution for the probability of the occurrence of VT of runs of length k by solving the $T_{0,[K,K]}(n)$ model that will be the purpose of the next demonstration. The solution can be provided for bigeminy, trigeminy, quadgeminy, or any run of VT of length k. The solution derived is the probability for k-geminy only. As before begin with the $T_{0,[K,K]}(n)$ model ($n>0$)

$$T_{0,[K,K]}(n) = pT_{0,[K,K]}(n-1) + q^K pT_{0,[K,K]}(n-K-1) + q^K I_{n=K}. \tag{14}$$

Define $G(s)$ as

$$G(s) = \sum_{n=0}^{\infty} s^n T_{0,[K,K]}(n),$$

and proceed with conversion and consolidation. Begin by multiplying each term in Eq. (14) by s^n and after a little simplification obtain

$$G(s) - 1 = ps \sum_{n=1}^{\infty} s^{n-1} T_{0,[K,K]}(n-1) + q^K ps^{K+1} \sum_{n=1}^{\infty} s^{n-K-1} T_{0,[K,K]}(n-K-1) + s^K q^K.$$

We need to examine two of these terms in some detail. Begin with the first term on the right side of the above equation

$$ps \sum_{n=1}^{\infty} s^{n-1} T_{0,[K,K]}(n-1) = ps \sum_{n=0}^{\infty} s^n T_{0,[K,K]}(n) = psG(s).$$

Observe that

$$q^K ps^{K+1} \sum_{n=1}^{\infty} s^{n-K-1} T_{0,[K,K]}(n-K-1) = q^K ps^{K+1} G(s),$$

$$G(s) = \frac{1}{1 - ps - q^K ps^{K+1}} + \frac{s^K q^K}{1 - ps - q^K ps^{K+1}}.$$

The coefficient of s^k obtained on inversion of $G(s)$ is

$$\left\{\sum_{m=0}^{n} p^m \sum_{j=0}^{m} \binom{m}{j} q^{Kj} I_{m+Kj=n} + q^K \sum_{m=0}^{n-K} p^m \sum_{j=0}^{m} \binom{m}{j} q^{Kj} I_{m+Kj=n-K}\right\}.$$

5. Follow-up losses in clinical trials

Clinical experiments have evolved over hundreds of years. The current state-of-the-art clinical experiment is the randomized controlled clinical trial. These advanced experiments have been used to demonstrate important relationships in public health. Two examples are (1) the association between reductions in elevated levels of blood pressure and the reduced incidence of strokes, and (2) the reduction of blood cholesterol levels and the reduced occurrence of heart attacks. However, many patients who agree to participate in these trials often choose not to return to the clinical trial physician for regularly scheduled follow-up visits. Although this behavior is understandable, and is in no way unethical, the absence of these patients from all future participation in the trial can complicate the interpretation of the trial.

The use of randomized controlled clinical trials reflects the accumulated experience and methodological advances in the evolution of scientific, experimental design in medicine. These experiments are very complicated, involving the complexities of choosing patients from the population at large, choosing the type and concentration of the intervention, and deciding how long patients must stay in contact with the scientists who are controlling the trial (some trials take 1–2 days to complete, while others can take 5 years or more).

One of the crucial features of clinical trials is the occurrence of endpoints, the clinical events that will be used to determine the effectiveness of the intervention. For example, consider a trial designed to reduce the occurrence of death. By this we mean that the investigators believe at the trial's end, there will be more deaths that occurred in the placebo group than in the group receiving the active intervention (the active group). In this trial, death is the endpoint. A clinical trial that is designed to measure the effect of medication to reduce the total number of deaths from a disease during the next 5 years must follow every patient until the end of the trial to ensure that they know who died. Without following each individual patient, the scientists will be uncertain as to who died and who survived, and without a careful count of this number, these scientists will have difficulty in deciding the true reduction in the number of deaths to which the medication can be attributed.

This problem is sometimes complicated by the low frequency of the occurrence of endpoints in the study. In recent clinical trials (SHEP, 1991; Pfeffer et al., 1992; Sacks et al., 1991), the rates at which endpoints are predicted to occur are relatively small. In these trials, the measure of therapy effectiveness, i.e., measuring the difference in death rates between the intervention and the control group, depends on the occurrence of relatively infrequently occurring endpoints. The incomplete ascertainment of these endpoints would weaken the trial by making the final endpoint death rate unclear.

An important reason for incomplete endpoint ascertainment is the patient who is "lost to follow-up." This means that patients choose not to return to their clinical trial doctors for scheduled (i.e., required) visits. They are seen for the first visit (in fact, in many circumstances, the first visit is the visit at which the patient often enters the clinical trial, or is "randomized"). Such "follow-up losses" do not stay in contact with their doctors. These patients often will stop taking the medication they received in the study, and may refuse any attempt by the study to recontact them. They completely "drop out" of the study. There are many reasons for dropping out of a study. Divorce, changing city and state (or country) of residence, a life of crime, and joining reclusive cults are all reasons that are given for patients dropping out of a study. However, the occurrence of a drop out means that the study cannot determine if the patient is alive or dead at the trial's conclusion (i.e., it cannot determine the patient's vital status). Tremendous effort is required on the part of clinical trial workers to insure that the vital status of all trial participants is obtained. In fact, a major constraint to the execution of long-term follow-up studies is often the time, money, ingenuity, and perseverance required to successfully trace subjects.

Follow-up losses make the effect of the therapy difficult to determine by precluding an accurate computation of the total number of deaths experienced by patients treated with placebo and those treated with the intervention. Clinical trial workers labor intently to find patients who are lost to follow-up, often resorting to private investigating agencies after the patient has stopped attending the required clinic visits. The strengths and weaknesses of mailings to participants to remind them of missed visits have been described (Cutter et al., 1980; Austin et al., 1979) and the advantages and disadvantages of city directories, telephone contacts, and the use of postal services have been delineated (Boice, 1978). A National Death Index was established to promote statistical research in health care (Patterson, 1980), and search procedures using this index have been utilized to identify patients who have dropped out from clinical trials (Edlavitch et al., 1985; Williams et al., 1992; Stampfer et al., 1984; Davis et al., 1985; Curb et al., 1985); in addition, information from the Social Security Administration is also useful in ascertaining vital status (Wentworth et al., 1983). The hallmark of patients who are eventually lost to follow-up is that they miss scheduled visits. Many different patient visit patterns are often observed in clinical trials. A patient's attendance for scheduled visits may first be perfect. Over time, the visit pattern becomes sporadic as the patient gradually misses scheduled visits at a greater frequency until they no longer attend visits and are lost from the study. Other patients may have perfect attendance and then suddenly, inexplicably, and completely drop out of the study. However, missed visits is the common theme among these disparate visit patterns. Thus, one way to identify patients who are at risk of loss to follow-up is to examine their visit pattern.

The pattern of missed visits for patients who will eventually be lost to follow-up is the occurrence of consecutive missed visits. In fact, this is a necessary condition for the patient to be lost to follow-up. Our purpose here is to develop and explore a monitoring rule applicable to clinical trials to identify potential follow-up losses, based on the number of consecutive visits that have been missed. Once a candidate rule for identifying patients who are potentially lost to follow-up is identified, it is useful to know how likely a patient is to violate this rule by chance alone.

Over the course of the clinical trial, each patient is scheduled for a sequence of n consecutive visits. The total number of these visits is known in advance. We begin by denoting the probability that a patient will keep a scheduled visit by p and let this probability be a known constant, fixed over the entire sequence of n visits. Denote $q = 1-p$ as the probability that the patient misses a particular visit. Consider the following monitoring rule $V(L)$ for loss to follow-up patients:

$V(L) = 1$ if the patient has missed at least L consecutively scheduled visits (rule violator).
$V(L) = 0$ otherwise (nonviolator).

We need to compute $P(V(L) = 1)$, the probability that a patient has missed at least L consecutive visits as a function of q and n. Once this probability is estimated, its relationship with L can be used to identify the optimum value of L for the trial. Patients who then meet the criteria can be targeted for special attention in an attempt to get them back into the mainstream of the clinical trial and a more standard visit pattern.

The monitoring rule $V(L)$ is based on a string or run of consecutive failures. Thus, the monitoring rule is triggered when there is at least one run of failures of length L or greater. With this development, difference equations may be used to identify the crucial recursive relationships in the occurrence of failure runs of the required lengths.

Recall that $T_{[0,L-1]}(n)$ is the probability that in a collection of n consecutive Bernoulli trials, there are no failure runs of length L or greater. Thus, all failure runs must be of length $L-1$ or less. In this development, $1-T_{[0,L-1]}(n)$ is the probability that in n trials, there is at least one occurrence of a failure run of length greater than or equal to L, i.e., the monitoring rule is violated. Thus, $P(V(L) = 1) = 1-T_{[0,L-1]}(n)$.

To find $T_{[0,L]}(n)$, a recursive relationship for $n \geqslant 0$ is:

$$\begin{aligned} T_{[0,L]}(n) &= pT_{[0,L]}(n-1) + qpT_{[0,L]}(n-2) + q^2pT_{[0,L]}(n-3) \\ &\quad + q^3pT_{[0,L]}(n-4) + \cdots + q^LpT_{[0,L]}(n-L-1) \\ &\quad + q^nI_{0\le n\le L} = \sum_{j=0}^{L} q^jpT_{[0,L]}(n-j-1) + q^nI_{0\le n\le L}. \end{aligned}$$

The boundary conditions for the family of difference equations represented by the above equation are

$$T_{[0,L]}(n) = 0, \quad \text{for } n<0, \quad \text{and} \quad T_{[0,L]}(n) = 1, \quad \text{for } 0 \le n \le L.$$

$1-T_{[0,L-1]}(n)$ is the probability of at least one failure run of length L or greater in n trials. This is also the probability that the maximum failure run length is $\geqslant L$.

Similarly, $1-T_{[0,L]}(n)$ is the probability that there is at least one failure run of length $L+1$ or greater in n trials, or the probability that the maximum failure run length is $\geqslant L+1$. Thus

$$\begin{aligned} &P[\text{maximum failure run length} = L \text{ in } n \text{ trials}] \\ &= [1 - T_{[0,L-1]}(n)] - [1 - T_{[0,L]}(n)] = T_{[0,L]}(n) - T_{[0,L-]}(n). \end{aligned}$$

Using this probability, we can compute in n trials the expected maximum failure run length $E(n, q)$ and its standard deviation $\mathrm{SD}(n, q)$ in n trials as

$$E(n,q) = \sum_{L=0}^{n} L[T_{[0,L]}(n) - T_{[0,L-1]}(n)]$$

$$\mathrm{SD}(n,q) = \sqrt{\sum_{L=0}^{n} L^2[T_{[0,L]}(n) - T_{[0,L-1]}(n)] - E^2(n,q)}.$$

In the context of missed visits for a patient in a follow-up study, $E(n, q)$ is the expected maximum number of consecutive visits missed by chance alone, i.e., the expected worst visit pattern, and $\mathrm{SD}(n, q)$ its standard deviation.

5.1. $T_{[0,L]}(n)$ and missed visits

Define $G(s) = \sum_{n=0}^{\infty} s^n T_{[0,L]}(n)$.

Then

$$\sum_{n=0}^{\infty} s^n T_{[0,L]}(n) = \sum_{n=0}^{\infty} s^n \sum_{j=0}^{L} q^j p T_{[0,L]}(n-j-1) + \sum_{n=0}^{\infty} s^n q^n I_{0 \leq n \leq L}$$

$$G(s) = \sum_{n=0}^{\infty} s^n \sum_{j=0}^{L} q^j p T_{[0,L]}(n-j-1) + \sum_{n-0}^{L} s^n q^n,$$

and completing the consolidation process

$$G(s) = \frac{\sum_{n=0}^{L} s^n q^n}{1 - \sum_{j=0}^{L} q^j p s^{j+1}}.$$

The coefficient of s^n in $1/(1 - \sum_{j=0}^{L} q^j p s^{j+1})$ is

$$\left\{ \sum_{m=0}^{n} p^m \sum_{j_1=0}^{m} \sum_{j_2=0}^{m-j_1} \sum_{j_3=0}^{m-j_1-j_2} \cdots \sum_{j_L=0}^{m-\sum_{i=1}^{L-1} j_i} \binom{m}{j_1 j_2 \cdots j_L} q^{\sum_{i=1}^{L} i j_i} I_{m+\sum_{i=1}^{L} i j_i = n} \right\}.$$

The coefficient of s^n in $G(s)$ will be

$$\left\{ \sum_{h=0}^{\min(n,L)} q^h \sum_{m=0}^{n-h} p^m \sum_{j_1=0}^{m} \sum_{j_2=0}^{m-j_1} \sum_{j_3=0}^{m-j_1-j_2} \cdots \sum_{j_L=0}^{m-\sum_{i=1}^{L-1} j_i} \binom{m}{j_1 j_2 \cdots j_L} q^{\sum_{i=1}^{L} i j_i} I_{m+\sum_{i=1}^{L} i j_i = n-h} \right\}.$$

Thus, $T_{[0,L]}(n)$ is an explicit function of n, the total number of visits, q the probability of a missed visit, and L the monitoring rule.

Since the difference equations and their solutions are in terms of q, the probability of a missed clinic visit, n, the number of visits, and V_L, the vigilance rule, $T_{0,L-1}(n)$ can be examined as a function of these parameters. As a first example, the value of $1-T_{0,L-1}(n)$, the probability of L or more consecutive missed visits, was explored as a function of both q, the probability of a missed visit, and L for $n = 10$ visits. Table 1 displays the anticipated relationship between $1-T_{[0,L]}(n)$, and q for fixed L.

As the probability of a missed visit (q) increases, the probability of missing L or more consecutive visits also increases. For example, the probability of missing at least two consecutive visits increases from 0.021 for $q = 0.05$ to 0.504 for $q = 0.30$. The probability of missing at least k consecutive visits as a function of L can also be observed from Table 1. For each value of q examined, the probability of L or more consecutive missed visits decreases rapidly. For example, when the probability of a missed visit is 0.10, the probability that, out of 10 scheduled visits, a patient will miss at least 1 or more consecutive visits is 0.651. However, the probability that a patient will miss two or more consecutive visits decreases to 0.080 for the same value of q.

This phenomenon of rapid fall off in the probability of consecutive missed visits as L increases was observed for each value of q examined. This property of rapidly decreasing probability of greater run lengths suggests that a value of L may be readily identified that would trigger additional attention to the patient who misses this many consecutive visits.

The development of $T_{[0,L]}(n)$ also provides a direct computation of the expected maximum number of consecutive missed visits $E(n, q)$ a typical patient will experience, and its standard deviation $SD(n, q)$. Table 2 demonstrates the relationship between the expected worst visit performance and the probability of a missed visit q and n. Note that $E(n, q)$ increases as the total number of scheduled visits increases.

Table 1
Probability of at least L consecutive missed visits out of 10 scheduled visits as a function of the probability of a missed visit $a(q)$

	Probability of a Missed Visit					
	0.05	0.10	0.15	020	0.25	0.30
1	0.401	0.651	0.803	0.893	0.944	0.972
2	0.021	0.080	0.168	0.273	0.388	0.504
3	0.001	0.007	0.023	0.052	0.096	0.155
4	0.000	0.001	0.003	0.009	0.021	0.042
5	0.000	0.000	0.000	0.002	0.005	0.011
6	0.000	0.000	0.000	0.000	0.001	0.003
7	0.000	0.000	0.000	0.000	0.000	0.001
8	0.000	0.000	0.000	0.000	0.000	0.000
9	0.000	0.000	0.000	0.000	0.000	0.000
10	0.000	0.000	0.000	0.000	0.000	0.000

Table 2
Expected worst visit performance $E(n, q)$ as a function of n and q

n	q		
	0.10	0.20	0.30
10.00	0.7 (0.9)	1.2 (2.1)	1.7 (3.7)
20.00	1.1 (1.5)	1.6 (3.2)	2.2 (5.9)
30.00	1.2 (1.8)	1.8 (4.1)	3.0 (7.5)
40.00	1.3 (2.1)	2.0 (4.8)	2.8 (8.8)

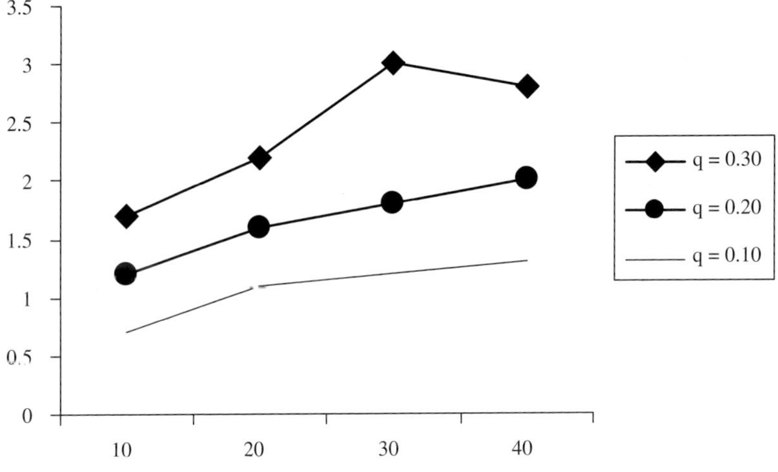

Fig. 1. Expected worst visit performance by n and q.

This satisfies intuition, since the more visits available, the greater the number of opportunities for missed consecutive visits. However, the increase in expected worst visit performance increases only gradually as the total number of scheduled visits is quadrupled from 10 to 40. In addition, Table 2 and Fig. 1 reveal the relationship between expected worst visit performances as a function of the probability of a missed visit, worst visit performance worsening as q increases.

The standard deviation of the maximum number of consecutive missed visits is more sensitive to changes in both the probability of a missed visit and the number of scheduled visits. This standard deviation increases from 0.9 to 3.7 as the probability of a missed visit increases from 0.10 to 0.30. In addition, this increased $SD(n, q)$ is a function of n, the total number of scheduled visits.

Figure 2 displays the relationship between the upper 5% tail of the worst visit performance (mean + 1.96SD) and the probability of a missed visit. Even though the increase in expected maximum as a function of n is modest, the upper 5% of the distribution of the maximum is more sensitive to increases in the probability of a missed visit. Thus, although in a clinical trial with 20 scheduled visits, if it is

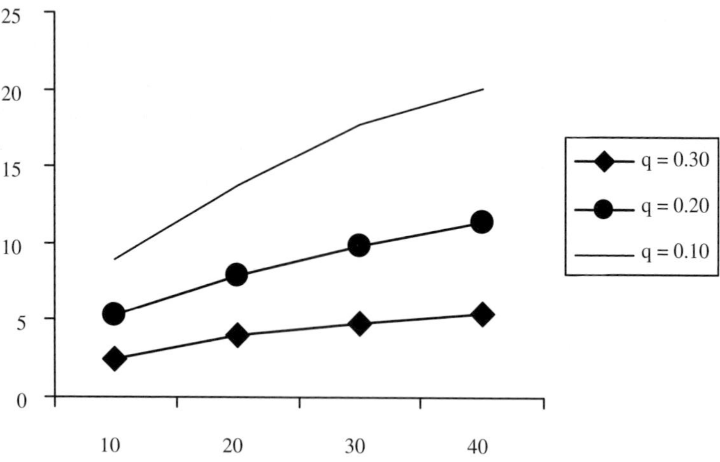

Fig. 2. Ninety-fifth percentile of expected worst visit performance by n and q.

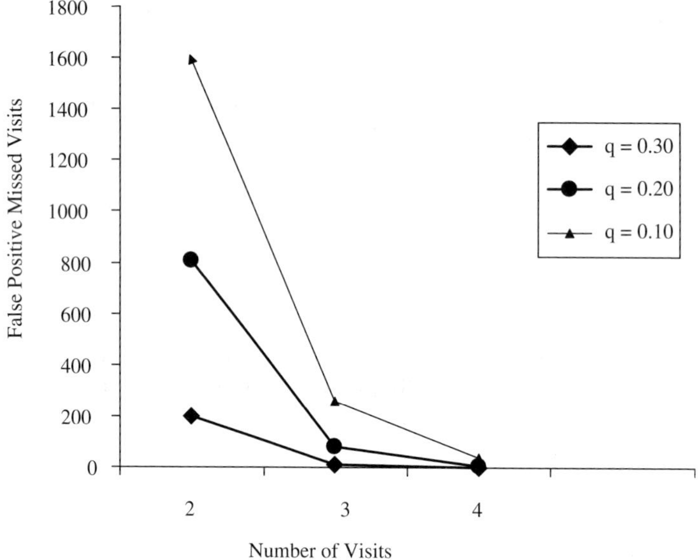

Fig. 3. False positive missed visit frequency by q and violator rule L.

anticipated that a typical patient will miss 1 in 5 scheduled visits, the expected maximum number of missed consecutive visits is 1.6. However, through the random mechanism of chance the distribution of the worst visit performance could be as large as 4 or 20% of scheduled visits.

Figure 3 depicts the relationship between the number of typical patients at risk for follow-up loss (false positives) in a 5000 patient trial as a function of both the probability of a missed visit and the vigilance rule V_L (i.e., they have missed at least L consecutive visits). The number of false positive patients at risk for a follow-up loss is the expected number of patients who violate the vigilance rule. We see that as the probability of a missed visit increases, the expected number of patients who violate this rule V_L (false positives) also increases. It is also clear that the expected number of false positives who violate V_L decreases as L increases. For each combination of q and V_L, the number of patients who require increased vigilance for follow-up loss can be determined.

6. Applications in epidemiology

Difference equation perspective may be used by epidemiologists as they work to understand the spread of a disease in a population. After a brief discussion of the purposes of epidemiology, we will develop both the nomenclature and the difference equations used to predict the number of patients with a disease under a mix of interesting and useful assumptions. These equations will be well recognized by the advanced worker as immigration models, emigration models, birth models, and death models, and will be so labeled in this chapter. In each of these developments, the focus here will be to elaborate the role of difference equations in providing solutions to these dynamic systems.

During this development, we will confront for the first time not just difference equations, but differential and partial differential equations as well. The reader with no background in differential equations need not be alarmed, however. Only the concepts of differential equations relevant to our immediate needs for this section discussions and absorption will be presented.

6.1. The immigration model

For this first model, the goal is to compute the number of patients who have a disease. The assumptions that the disease is not contagious and that no one in the population has the illness at the beginning of the process will be made. Since the disease does not spread from individual to individual, the only people who will have the illness are those that arrive with the disease.

Define $P_n(t)$ as the probability that there are n individuals in the system at time t. Assume that patients with the disease arrive at the rate of λ arrivals per unit of time. The rate of these arrivals is independent of the number of patients in the diseased population. If 10 diseased patients arrive per week, then, on average in 2 weeks we would expect 20 diseased patients, in 3 weeks, 30 diseased patients would be expected, etc. In general, in the short time interval Δt, we would expect $\lambda \Delta t$ arrivals. With neither deaths, cures, nor exits, cases can only accumulate in the system.

To develop the difference equation, consider how there may be n cases (diseased individuals) at time $t + \Delta t$. One possibility is that there are $n-1$ diseased individuals at time t, and there is exactly one arrival that occurs with probability $\lambda \Delta t$. The other possibility is that there are n patients with the disease at time t, and there is no arrival in the time interval Δt, an event that occurs with probability $1-\lambda\,\Delta t$. The Chapman–Kolmogorov forward equation for this model is

$$P_n(t+\Delta t) = \lambda\,\Delta t P_{n+1}(t) + P_n(t)(1-\lambda\,\Delta t), \quad n \geq 0.$$

For $n = 0$ the equation is

$$P_0(t+\Delta t) = P_0(t)(1-\lambda\,\Delta t),$$

which can be solved as (Feller, 1965)

$$P_n(t) = \frac{(\lambda t)^n}{n!} e^{-\lambda t}.$$

If there are a_0 cases in the system at time 0, then by the assumptions made for the immigration process (i.e., there are neither deaths nor exits of diseased patients), these patients are still available at time t and

$$P_n(t) = \frac{(\lambda t)^{n-a_0}}{(n-a_0)!} e^{-\lambda t} I_{n>a_0},$$

where $I_{n>a_0}$ represents the indicator function which takes value 1 when $n>a_0$ and 0 otherwise.

6.2. Emigration model

We will produce the Chapman–Kolmogorov forward equation for the emigration process paralleling the model used for the immigration process. As before, consider the dynamics of patients with the disease as time moves from t to $t+\Delta t$ when Δt is very small, allowing only a change in the number of diseased patients by 1. In this framework, the number of cases at time t can only be (1) reduced by 1 or (2) remain the same. The number of patients with disease is reduced by 1 with probability $\mu\,\Delta t$, or the number can stay the same with probability $1-\mu\,\Delta t$. Therefore, using the Chapman–Kolmogorov forward equation approach (Feller, 1965). Assuming a_0 patients at time $t = 0$

$$P_n(t) = \left\{ \frac{(\mu t)^{a_0-n}}{(a_0-n)!} e^{-\mu t} \right\}.$$

Thus, the probability that there are n subjects with the disease at time t is the probability that a_0-n diseased subjects have departed by time t.

6.3. Birth model

The immigration and emigration models served as useful tools for the introduction to the use of difference-differential equations in modeling the movement of patients with disease through a population. However, helpful as they have been, these models have not included an important naturally observed phenomenon of disease dynamics – that is the spread of the disease from one infected individual to another susceptible person. This section will examine this important concept.

Unfortunately, the inclusion of this component adds a new complication to the difference-differential equation required, namely the equation becomes a partial difference-differential equation (Moyé and Kapadia, 2000).

In this model new cases (i.e., patients with disease) are produced from established cases and their ability to spread depends on the number of patients with the disease. The larger the number of cases, the greater the spread of the disease will be. A small number of cases will diminish the rate at which the disease will spread throughout the population. The parameter associated with the spread of the disease is v. And if there are a_0 cases in the system at time $t = 0$

$$P_n(t) = \binom{n-1}{a_0 - 1} \mathrm{e}^{-a_0 vt}(1 - \mathrm{e}^{-vt})^{n-a_0}.$$

This distribution can be used to obtain the expected number of cases of disease at time t as $a_0\, \mathrm{e}^{vt}$.

6.4. The death process

Just as the birth model led to the propagation of new patients with disease in a way where the force of growth of the disease cases was related to the number of cases available, it stands to reason that there are circumstances where the number of cases will decline, the force of decline being related to the number of cases. This is called the death process. The plan here is to identify the probability distribution of the number of cases at time t when the number of cases cannot increase, but only decrease due to death. Just as in the birth model, we will need to develop and solve a family of partial differential equations.

As with the birth process, the force of death is related to the number of patients with disease. The larger the number of cases, the greater the likelihood of death. This relationship between the number of patients with the disease and the death rate is what distinguishes the death process from the emigration process. In the latter case the departure rate is independent of the number of patients with the disease.

Let the probability that a patient with disease who is alive at time t will die in time $t + \Delta t$ be $\omega\, \Delta t$. To construct appropriate equations, we will need to determine in what way the number of cases can change from time t to time $t + \Delta t$ if there are to be n cases at time $t + \Delta t$. Also, assume Δt is so small that the number of cases can only change by 1. In this short span of time only one of the two events can occur. There can be a death with probability $(n + 1)\omega\, \Delta t$ or there is no change, that occurs with probability $1 - n\omega\, \Delta t$. For $P_{a_0}(0) = 1$

$$P_n(t) = \binom{a_0}{n} \mathrm{e}^{-n\omega t}(1 - \mathrm{e}^{-\omega t})^{a_0 - n},$$

for $0 < n \leqslant a_0$. Note that the expected number of patients with disease in the system at time t is

$$E[X_t] = a_0\, \mathrm{e}^{-n\omega t},$$

and the variance of X_t is

$$\mathrm{Var}[X_t] = a_0\,\mathrm{e}^{-n\omega t}(1 - \mathrm{e}^{-\omega t}).$$

6.5. Immigration–birth–death–emigration model

The last model to be considered is a combination of the models developed in the previous sections. This model will be the most complicated representation of the spread of a contagious disease that will be considered. Patients are allowed to arrive into the population, and, once in the population, can spread the disease to other patients. In addition, patients are removed from the population either through death or through cure with subsequent immunity. In the derivation of $G_t(s)$ we will identify a partial differential equation in both t and s. Its solution will be straightforward, but there may be some complications in the final simplification of $G_t(s)$.

Begin the development of the family of difference equations which govern this process by using the parameters defined in the previous subsections. If time is slowed down sufficiently, how can we compute n cases in the population at time $t+\Delta t$ allowing only one event and one event only to occur in the time interval $(t, t+\Delta t)$? This can happen in one of the five ways: (1) if there are $n-1$ patients in the population at time t, and an arrival occurs with probability $\lambda\,\Delta t$; (2) if the population has $n-1$ patients in the system at time t and a "birth" occurs, with probability $(n-1)v\,\Delta t$; (3) if there are $n+1$ patients in the population at time t, there could be a death, an event which occurs with probability $(n+1)\omega\,\Delta t$; (4) if there are $n+1$ patients at time t, a patient leaves the system with probability $\mu\,\Delta t$; and (5) if there are n patients in the system with neither an arrival nor a birth, a death, or emigration occurs in time Δt. As in previous cases, we will assume that $P_0(t) = 0$ and $P_{a_0}(0) = 1$.

It is important to distinguish the immigration and emigration processes from the birth and death processes. Certainly both the immigration and birth processes lead to an increase in the number of diseased patients in the population. However, the increase from immigration is constant over time, independent of the population size. The birth process force is proportional to the population size. However, people emigrate independent of the population size.

Chapman–Kolmogorov equation for the immigration–birth–death–emigration process is

$$\begin{aligned}P_n(t + \Delta t) &= \lambda\,\Delta t P_{n-1}(t) + (n-1)v\,\Delta t P_{n-1}(t) + (n+1)\omega\,\Delta t P_{n+1}(t)\\ &\quad +\mu\,\Delta t P_{n+1}(t) + P_n(t)(1 - \lambda\,\Delta t - nv\,\Delta t - n\omega\,\Delta t - \mu\,\Delta t).\end{aligned}$$

We proceed with the development of the partial differential equation which represents this process by consolidating the terms involving Δt

$$\begin{aligned}\frac{P_n(t+\Delta t) - P_n(t)}{\Delta t} &= \lambda P_{n-1}(t) + (n-1)vP_{n-1}(t) + (n+1)\omega P_{n+1}(t)\\ &\quad +\mu P_{n+1}(t) - \lambda P_n(t) - nvP_n(t) - n\omega P_n(t) - \mu P_n(t).\end{aligned}$$

Then taking limits as $\Delta t \to 0$

$$\frac{dP_n(t)}{dt} = \lambda P_{n-1}(t) + vP_{n-1}(t)(n-1) + \omega(n+1)P_{n+1}(t) - \mu P_{n+1}(t)$$
$$-\lambda P_n(t) - nvP_n(t) - n\omega P_n(t) - \mu P_n(t). \tag{15}$$

Define

$$G_t(s) = \sum_{n=0}^{\infty} s^n P_n(t),$$

and move forward with the conversion and consolidation of Eq. (15). Multiplying each side of this equation by s^n we find

$$s^n \frac{dP_n(t)}{dt} = \lambda s^n P_{n-1}(t) + vs^n P_{n-1}(t)(n-1) + \omega s^n P_{n+1}(t)(n+1)$$
$$+\mu s^n P_{n+1}(t) - \lambda s^n P_n(t) - vns^n P_n(t) - \omega ns^n P_n(t) - \mu s^n P_n(t).$$

Summing for n from 1 to ∞

$$\sum_{n-0}^{\infty} s^n \frac{dP_n(t)}{dt} = \lambda \sum_{n=0}^{\infty} s^n P_{n-1}(t) + v \sum_{n=0}^{\infty} (n-1)s^n P_{n-1}(t)$$
$$+\omega \sum_{n=0}^{\infty} (n+1)s^n P_{n+1}(t) + \mu \sum_{n=0}^{\infty} s^n P_{n+1}(t)$$
$$-\lambda \sum_{n=0}^{\infty} s^n P_n(t) - v \sum_{n=0}^{\infty} ns^n P_n(t)$$
$$-\omega \sum_{n=0}^{\infty} ns^n P_n(t) - \mu \sum_{n=0}^{\infty} s^n P_n(t).$$

Interchanging the summation and differentiation procedures reveals

$$\frac{d \sum_{n=0}^{\infty} s^n P_n(t)}{dt} = \lambda s \sum_{n=0}^{\infty} s^{n-1} P_{n-1}(t) + vs^2 \sum_{n=0}^{\infty} (n-1)s^{n-2} P_{n-1}(t)$$
$$+\omega \sum_{n=0}^{\infty} (n+1)s^n P_{n+1}(t) + \mu \sum_{n=0}^{\infty} s^n P_{n+1}(t)$$
$$-\lambda \sum_{n=0}^{\infty} s^n P_n(t) - vs \sum_{n=0}^{\infty} ns^{n-1} P_n(t)$$
$$-\omega s \sum_{n=0}^{\infty} ns^{n-1} P_n(t) - \mu \sum_{n=0}^{\infty} s^n P_n(t).$$

We can now recognize these summands as functions of $G_t(s)$ and write

$$\frac{\partial G_t(s)}{\partial t} = \lambda s G_t(s) + vs^2 \frac{\partial G_t(s)}{\partial s} + \omega \frac{\partial G_t(s)}{\partial s} + \mu s^{-1} G_t(s) - \lambda G_t(s)$$
$$-vs \frac{\partial G_t(s)}{\partial s} - \omega s \frac{\partial G_t(s)}{\partial s} - \mu G_t(s),$$

which can be simplified as follows:

$$\frac{\partial G_t(s)}{\partial t} - (vs-\omega)(s-1)\frac{\partial G_t(s)}{\partial s} - [\lambda(s-1)+\mu(s^{-1}-1)]G_t(s) = 0.$$

Recognize that the above equation is a partial differential equation in t and s of the form which will allow us to find a general solution using a subsidiary set of equations. Write these equations as

$$\frac{dt}{1} = \frac{ds}{-(vs-\omega)(s-1)} = \frac{dG_t(s)}{-[\lambda(s-1)+\mu(s^{-1}-1)]G_t(s)}. \tag{16}$$

Continuing with the first two terms of the above equation, we evaluate these equalities in two combinations to provide information on the form of the generating function $G_t(s)$. From the second and third terms we have

$$\frac{ds}{-(vs-\omega)(s-1)} = \frac{dG_t(s)}{-[\lambda(s-1)+\mu(s^{-1}-1)]G_t(s)}$$

$$\frac{[\lambda(s-1)+\mu(s^{-1}-1)]ds}{(vs-\omega)(s-1)} = \frac{dG_t(s)}{G_t(s)}$$

$$\frac{\lambda\, ds}{vs-\omega} + \frac{\mu(s^{-1}-1)ds}{(vs-\omega)(s-1)} = \frac{dG_t(s)}{G_t(s)}$$

$$\frac{\lambda\, ds}{vs-\omega} + \frac{\mu(1-s)ds}{s(vs-\omega)(s-1)} = \frac{dG_t(s)}{G_t(s)}$$

$$\frac{\lambda\, ds}{vs-\omega} - \frac{\mu ds}{s(vs-\omega)} = \frac{dG_t(s)}{G_t(s)}$$

Using partial fractions

$$\frac{\mu}{s(vs-\omega)} = \frac{\mu v}{\omega}\left[\frac{1}{vs-\omega}\right] - \frac{\mu}{\omega}\left[\frac{1}{s}\right],$$

$$\frac{dG_t(s)}{G_t(s)} = \left(\frac{\lambda}{vs-\omega} + \frac{\mu v}{\omega}\left[\frac{1}{vs-\omega}\right] - \frac{\mu}{\omega}\left[\frac{1}{s}\right]\right)ds = \left(\frac{\lambda+(\mu v/\omega)}{vs-\omega} - \frac{\mu}{\omega}\left[\frac{1}{s}\right]\right)ds,$$

$$\int\frac{dG_t(s)}{G_t(s)} = \int\left(\frac{\lambda+(\mu v/\omega)}{vs-\omega} - \frac{\mu}{\omega}\left[\frac{1}{s}\right]\right)ds,$$

$$\begin{aligned}\ln G_t(s) &= \left(\frac{\lambda}{v}+\frac{\mu}{\omega}\right)\ln(vs-\omega) - \frac{\mu}{\omega}\ln(s) + C\\ &= \frac{\lambda}{v}\ln(vs-\omega) + \frac{\mu}{\omega}\ln\left[\frac{vs-\omega}{s}\right] + C\\ &= \ln(vs-\omega)^{\lambda/v} + \ln\left[\frac{vs-\omega}{s}\right]^{\mu/\omega} + C,\end{aligned}$$

$$G_t(s) = (vs-\omega)^{\lambda/v}\left[\frac{vs-\omega}{s}\right]^{\mu/\omega} C.$$

This development provides $G_t(s) = (vs-\omega)^{(\lambda/v)+(\mu/\omega)}s^{-\mu/\omega}C$ which can be written in the form

$$G_t(s) = (vs-\omega)^{(\lambda/v)+(\mu/\omega)}s^{-(\mu/\omega)}\Phi(C_2).$$

The remaining task is to identify the function $\Phi(C_2)$. Using the first and second terms from Eq. (16) write

$$\frac{dt}{1} = \frac{ds}{-(vs-\omega)(s-1)}. \tag{17}$$

Using partial fractions

$$\frac{1}{(vs-\omega)(s-1)} = \frac{1/(v-\omega)}{s-1} + \frac{-v/(v-\omega)}{vs-\omega}.$$

Equation (17) may be written as

$$-dt = \frac{1/(v-\omega)}{s-1} - \frac{v/(v-\omega)}{vs-\omega},$$

$$dt = \frac{v/(v-\omega)}{vs-\omega} - \frac{1/(v-\omega)}{s-1},$$

$$\int dt = \int\left[\frac{v/(v-\omega)}{vs-\omega} - \frac{1/(v-\omega)}{s-1}\right]ds,$$

$$t + C = \frac{1}{v-\omega}\ln(vs-\omega) - \frac{1}{v-\omega}\ln(s-1) = \frac{1}{v-\omega}\ln\left(\frac{vs-\omega}{s-1}\right),$$

$$(v-\omega)t + C_2 = \ln\left(\frac{vs-\omega}{s-1}\right),$$

$$C_2 = -(v-\omega)t + \ln\left(\frac{vs-\omega}{s-1}\right),$$

$$C_2 = \mathrm{e}^{-(v-\omega)t}\left(\frac{vs-\omega}{s-1}\right),$$

from which

$$C_1 = \Phi(C_2) = \Phi\left[\mathrm{e}^{-(v-\omega)t}\left(\frac{vs-\omega}{s-1}\right)\right].$$

Combining the above expressions

$$G_t(s) = (vs-\omega)^{(\lambda/v)+(\mu/\omega)}s^{-(\mu/\omega)}\Phi\left(\mathrm{e}^{-(v-\omega)t}\left(\frac{vs-\omega}{s-1}\right)\right).$$

Having identified $G_t(s) = (vs-\omega)^{(\lambda/v)+(\mu/\omega)}s^{-(\mu/\omega)}\Phi[\mathrm{e}^{-(v-\omega)t}((vs-\omega)/(s-1))]$ we can now pursue a specific solution, beginning with the boundary conditions. At $t=0$, there are a_0 patients in the population; therefore

$$G_0(s) = s^{a_0} = (vs-\omega)^{(\lambda/v)+(\mu/\omega)}s^{-(\mu/\omega)}\Phi\left(\frac{vs-\omega}{s-1}\right). \tag{18}$$

Now, let $z = (\nu s - \omega)/(s-1)$, then $s = (z-\omega)/(z-\nu)$ and substituting this result into Eq. (18), we obtain

$$\left(\frac{z-\omega}{z-\nu}\right)^{a_0} = \left(\nu\frac{z-\omega}{z-\nu} - \omega\right)^{(\lambda/\nu)+(\mu/\omega)}\left[\frac{z-\omega}{z-\nu}\right]^{-(\mu/\omega)}\Phi(z)$$

or

$$\Phi(z) = \left(\frac{z-\omega}{z-\nu}\right)^{a_0}\left(\nu\frac{z-\omega}{z-\nu} - \omega\right)^{-[(\lambda/\nu)+(\mu/\omega)]}\left[\frac{z-\omega}{z-\nu}\right]^{\mu/\omega},$$

allowing us to write

$$\begin{aligned} G_t(s) &= (\nu s-\omega)^{(\lambda/\nu)+(\mu/\omega)}s^{-(\mu/\omega)}\Phi\left(e^{-(\nu-\omega)t}\left(\frac{\nu s-\omega}{s-1}\right)\right) \\ &= (\nu s-\omega)^{(\lambda/\nu)+(\mu/\omega)}s^{-(\mu/\omega)}\left[\frac{(\nu e^{-(\nu-\omega)t}-\omega)s+\omega(1-e^{-(\nu-\omega)t})}{\nu(e^{-(\nu-\omega)t}-1)s+(\nu-\omega e^{-(\nu-\omega)t})}\right]^{a_0+(\mu/\omega)} \\ &\times\left(\nu\frac{e^{-(\nu-\omega)t}[(\nu s-\omega)/(s-1)]-\omega}{e^{-(\nu-\omega)t}[(\nu s-\omega)/(s-1)]-\nu} - \omega\right)^{-[(\lambda/\nu)+(\mu/\omega)]}. \end{aligned} \tag{19}$$

The inversion of $G_t(s)$ is straightforward, requiring only some algebra to complete. Begin by rewriting the last term on the right hand side of Eq. (19) as

$$\begin{aligned} &\left(\nu\frac{e^{-(\nu-\omega)t}[(\nu s-\omega)/(s-1)]-\omega}{e^{-(\nu-\omega)t}[(\nu s-\omega)/(s-1)]-\nu} - \omega\right)^{-[(\lambda/\nu)+(\mu/\omega)]} \\ &= \left[\frac{e^{-(\nu-\omega)t}(\nu-\omega)(\nu s-\omega)}{\nu(e^{-(\nu-\omega)t}-1)s+(\nu-\omega e^{-(\nu-\omega)t})}\right]^{-[(\lambda/\nu)+(\mu/\omega)]}. \end{aligned} \tag{20}$$

Substituting the above equation into Eq. (19) and simplifying we obtain

$$G_t(s) = s^{-(\mu/\omega)}[e^{-(\nu-\omega)t}(\nu-\omega)]^{-[(\lambda/\nu)+(\mu/\omega)]}\frac{[(\nu e^{-(\nu-\omega)t}-\omega)s+\omega(1-e^{-(\nu-\omega)t})]^{a_0+(\mu/\omega)}}{[\nu(e^{-(\nu-\omega)t}-1)s+(\nu-\omega e^{-(\nu-\omega)t})]^{a_0-(\lambda/\nu)}}.$$

The expression $[e^{-(\nu-\omega)t}(\nu-\omega)]^{-[(\lambda/\nu)+(\mu/\omega)]}$ is a constant with respect to s, and the final term $[(\nu e^{-(\nu-\omega)t}-\omega)s+\omega(1-e^{-(\nu-\omega)t})]^{a_0+(\mu/\omega)}/[\nu(e^{-(\nu-\omega)t}-1)s+(\nu-\omega e^{-(\nu-\omega)t})]^{a_0-(\lambda/\nu)}$ is of the form $[as+b]^{n_1}/[c+ds]^{n_2}$. It can be shown that the coefficient of s^n in $[as+b]^{n_1}/[c+ds]^{n_2}$ is

$$\left[\frac{1}{c}\right]^{n_2}\sum_{j=0}^{\min(k,n_1)}\binom{n_2+j-1}{j}\left[\frac{d}{c}\right]^{j}\binom{n_1}{k-j}b^{k-j}a^{n_1-k+j}.$$

Applying this result to the last expression in the above equation reveals that the coefficient of s^k in

$$\frac{[(\nu e^{-(\nu-\omega)t}-\omega)s+\omega(1-e^{-(\nu-\omega)t})]^{a_0+(\mu/\omega)}}{[(\nu-\omega e^{-(\nu-\omega)t})+\nu(e^{-(\nu-\omega)t}-1)s+]^{a_0-(\lambda/\nu)}}$$

is

$$\left[\frac{1}{v-\omega\,\mathrm{e}^{-(v-\omega)t}}\right]^{a_0-(\lambda/v)}\sum_{j=0}^{\min(k,a_0+(\mu/\omega))}\begin{pmatrix}a_0-\frac{\lambda}{v}+j-1\\ j\end{pmatrix}\times\left[\frac{(v-\omega\,\mathrm{e}^{-(v-\omega)t})}{v(\mathrm{e}^{-(v-\omega)t}-1)}\right]^{-j}\times\begin{pmatrix}a_0+\frac{\mu}{\omega}\\ k-j\end{pmatrix}\frac{[\omega(1-\mathrm{e}^{-(v-\omega)t})]^{k-j}}{[(v\,\mathrm{e}^{-(v-\omega)t}-\omega)]^{-[a_0+(\mu/\omega)-k+j]}},$$

and the final solution then is:

$$P_k(t)=[\mathrm{e}^{-(v-\omega)t}(v-\omega)]^{-[(\lambda/v)+(\mu/\omega)]}\left[\frac{1}{v-\omega\,\mathrm{e}^{-(v-\omega)t}}\right]^{a_0-(\lambda/v)}$$
$$\times\sum_{j=0}^{\min(k+(\mu/\omega),a_0+(\mu/\omega))}\begin{pmatrix}a_0-\frac{\lambda}{v}+j-1\\ j\end{pmatrix}\left[\frac{v-\omega\,\mathrm{e}^{-(v-\omega)t}}{v(\mathrm{e}^{-(v-\omega)t}-1)}\right]^{-j}\begin{pmatrix}a_0+\frac{\mu}{\omega}\\ k+\frac{\mu}{\omega}-j\end{pmatrix}$$
$$\times\frac{[\omega(1-\mathrm{e}^{-(v-\omega)t})]^{k+(\mu/\omega)-j}}{[(v\,\mathrm{e}^{-(v-\omega)t}-\omega)]^{-[a_0-k+j]}}.$$

References

Austin, M.A., Berrcysea, E., Elliott, J.L., Wallace, R.B., Barrett-Connor, E., Criqui, M.H. (1979). Methods for determining long-term survival in a population based study. *American Journal of Epidemiology* **110**, 747–752.

Boice, J.D. (1978). Follow-up methods to trace women treated for pulmonary tuberculosis, 1930–1954. *American Journal of Epidemiology* **107**, 127–138.

Chiang, C.L. (1980). *An Introduction to Stochastic Processes and their Applications.* Robert E. Krieger Publishing Company, Huntington, New York.

Curb, J.D., Ford, C.E., Pressel, S., Palmer, M., Babcock, C., Hawkins, C.M. (1985). Ascertainment of the vital status through the National Death Index and the social security administration. *American Journal of Epidemiology* **121**, 754–766.

Cutter, G., Siegfried, H., Kastler, J., Draus, J.F., Less, E.S., Shipley, T., Stromer, M. (1980). Mortality surveillance in collaborative trials. *American Journal of Public Health* **70**, 394–400.

Davis, K.B., Fisher, L., Gillespie, M.J., Pettinger, M. (1985). A test of the National Death Index using the coronary artery surgery study (CASS). *Contemporary Clinical Trials* **6**, 179–191.

Edlavitch, S.A., Feinleib, M., Anello, C. (1985). A potential use of the National Death Index for post marketing drug surveillance. *JAMA* **253**, 1292–1295.

Feller, W. (1965). *An Introduction to Probability Theory and its Applications.* Wiley, New York.

Moyé, L.A., Kapadia, A.S. (2000). *Difference Equations with Public Health Applications.* Marcel-Dekker, New York.

Patterson, J.E. (1980). The establishment of a National Death Index in United States. Banbury Report 4: Cancer Incidence in Defined Populations. Cold Spring Harbor Laboratory, New York, pp. 443–447.

Pfeffer, M.A., Brauwald, E., Moyé, L.A., Basta, L., Brown, E.J., Cuddy, T.E., Davis, B.R., Geltman, E.M., Goldman, S., Flaker, G.C., Klein, M., Lamas, G.A., Packer, M., Roleau, J., Routeau, J., Rutherford, J., Wertheimer, J.H., Hawkins, C.M. (1992). Effect of captopril on mortality and morbidity in patients with left ventricular dysfunction after myocardial infarction – Results of the Survival and Ventricular Enlargement Trial. *The New England Journal of Medicine* **327**, 669–677.

Pratt, C.M., Moyé, L.A. (1995). The cardiac arrhythmia suppression trial (CAST). Casting suppression in a different light. *Circulation* **95**(1), 245–247.

Sacks, F.M., Pfeffer, M.A., Moyé, L.A. et al. (1991). The cholesterol and recurrent events trial (CARE): Rationale, design and baseline characteristics of secondary prevention trial of lowering serum cholesterol and myocardial infarction. *The American Journal of Cardiology* **68**(15), 1436–1446.

Stampfer, M.J., Willett, W.C., Speizer, F.E., Dysert, D.C., Lipnick, R., Rosner, B., Hennekens, C.H. (1984). Test of the national death index. *American Journal of Epidemiology* **119**, 837–839.

The SHEP Cooperative Research Group (1991). Prevention of stroke by antihypertensive drug therapy in older persons with isolated systolic hypertension: Final results of the systolic hypertension in the elderly program (SHEP). *JAMA* **265**, 3255–3264.

Wentworth, D.N., Neaton, J.D., Rasmusen, W.L. (1983). An evaluation of the social security administration master beneficiary record file and the National Death Index in the ascertainment of vital status. *American Journal of Public Health* **73**, 1270–1274.

Wilf, H.S. (1994). *Generating Functionology*, 2nd ed. Academic Press, New York.

Williams, B.C., Bemitrack, L.B., Bries, B.E. (1992). The accuracy of the National Death Index when personal identifiers other than social security number are used. *American Journal of Public Health* **82**, 1145–1146.

Handbook of Statistics, Vol. 27
ISSN: 0169-7161

DOI: 10.1016/S0169-7161(07)27027-0

27

The Bayesian Approach to Experimental Data Analysis

Bruno Lecoutre

Abstract

This chapter introduces the conceptual basis of the objective Bayesian approach to experimental data analysis and reviews some of its methodological improvements. The presentation is essentially non-technical and, within this perspective, restricted to relatively simple situations of inference about proportions. Bayesian computations and softwares are also briefly reviewed and some further topics are introduced.

> It is their straightforward, natural approach to inference that makes them [Bayesian methods] so attractive.
>
> (Schmitt, 1969, preface)

Preamble: and if you were a Bayesian without knowing it?

In a popular statistical textbook that claims the goal of "understanding statistics," Pagano (1990, p. 288) describes a 95% confidence interval as

> an interval such that the probability is 0.95 that the interval contains the population value.

If you agree with this statement, or if you feel that it is not the correct interpretation but that it is desirable, you should ask yourselves: "and if I was a Bayesian without knowing it?"

The *correct* frequentist interpretation of a 95% confidence interval involves a long-run repetition of the same experiment: in the long run 95% of computed confidence intervals will contain the "true value" of the parameter; each interval in isolation has either a 0 or 100% probability of containing it. Unfortunately, treating the data as random *even after observation* is so strange that this "correct" interpretation does not make sense for most users. Actually, virtually all users interpret frequentist confidence intervals in terms of "a *fixed* interval having a 95% chance of including the true value of interest."

In the same way, many statistical users misinterpret the p-values of null hypothesis significance tests as "inverse" probabilities: $1-p$ is "the probability that the alternative hypothesis is true." Even experienced users and experts in statistics (Neyman himself) are not immune from *conceptual* confusions.

> In these conditions [a p-value of 1/15], the odds of 14 to 1 that this loss was caused by seeding [of clouds] do not appear negligible to us. (Battan et al., 1969)

After many attempts to rectify these (Bayesian) interpretations of frequentist procedures, I completely agree with Freeman (1993, p. 1446) that in these attempts "we are fighting a losing battle."

> It would not be scientifically sound to justify a procedure by frequentist arguments and to interpret it in Bayesian terms. (Rouanet, 2000b, p. 54)

We then naturally have to ask ourselves whether the "Bayesian choice" will not, sooner or later, be unavoidable (Lecoutre et al., 2001).

1. Introduction

Efron (1998, p. 106) wrote

> A widely accepted objective Bayes theory, which fiducial inference was intended to be, would be of immense theoretical and practical importance. A successful objective Bayes theory would have to provide good frequentist properties in familiar situations, for instance, reasonable coverage probabilities for whatever replaces confidence intervals.

I suggest that such a theory is by no means a speculative viewpoint but, on the contrary, is perfectly feasible (see especially, Berger, 2004). It is better suited to the needs of users than frequentist approach and provides scientists with relevant answers to essential questions raised by experimental data analysis.

1.1. *What is Bayesian inference for experimental data analysis?*

One of the most important objective of controlled clinical trials is to impact on public health, so that their results need to be accepted by a large community of scientists and physicians. For this purpose, null hypothesis significance testing (NHST) has been long conventionally required in most scientific publications for analyzing experimental data. This publication practice dichotomizes each experimental result (significant vs. non-significant) according to the NHST outcome.

But scientists cannot in this way find all the answers to the precise questions posed in experimental investigations, especially in terms of effect size evaluation.

> But the primary aim of a scientific experiment is not to precipitate decisions, but to make an appropriate adjustment in the degree to which one accepts, or believes, the hypothesis or hypotheses being tested. (Rozeboom, 1960)

By their insistence on the decision-theoretic elements of the Bayesian approach, many authors have obscured the contribution of Bayesian inference to experimental data analysis and scientific reporting. Within this context, many Bayesians place emphasis on a *subjective* perspective. This can be the reasons why until now scientists have been reluctant to use Bayesian inferential procedures in practice for analyzing their data. It is not surprising that the most common (and easy) criticism of the Bayesian approach by frequentists is the need for prior probabilities. Without dismissing the merits of the decision-theoretic viewpoint, it must be recognized that there is another approach that is just as Bayesian, which was developed by Jeffreys in 1930s (Jeffreys, 1961/1939). Following the lead of Laplace (1986/1825), this approach aimed at assigning the prior probability when nothing was known about the value of the parameter. In practice, these *non-informative* prior probabilities are vague distributions that, a priori, do not favor any particular value. Consequently, they let the data "speak for themselves" (Box and Tiao, 1973, p. 2). In this form, the Bayesian paradigm provides, if not objective methods, at least *reference* methods appropriate for situations involving scientific reporting. This approach of Bayesian inference is now recognized as a standard.

> A common misconception is that Bayesian analysis is a subjective theory; this is neither true historically nor in practice. The first Bayesians, Bayes (see Bayes (1763)) and Laplace (see Laplace (1812)) performed Bayesian analysis using a constant prior distribution for unknown parameters ... (Berger, 2004, p. 3)

1.2. Routine Bayesian methods for experimental data analysis

For more than 30 years now, with other colleagues in France we have worked in order to develop routine Bayesian methods for the most familiar situations encountered in experimental data analysis. These methods can be learned and used as easily, if not more, as the t, F or χ^2 tests. We argued that they offer promising new ways in statistical methodology (Rouanet et al., 2000).

We have especially developed methods based on non-informative priors. In order to promote them, it seemed important to us to give them a more explicit name than "standard," "non-informative" or "reference." Recently, Berger (2004) proposed the name *objective Bayesian analysis*.

> The statistics profession, in general, hurts itself by not using attractive names for its methodologies, and we should start systematically accepting the 'objective Bayes' name before it is co-opted by others. (Berger, 2004, p. 3)

With the same incentive, we argued for the name *fiducial Bayesian* (Lecoutre, 2000; Lecoutre et al., 2001). This deliberately provocative name pays tribute to Fisher's work on scientific inference for research workers (Fisher, 1990/1925). It indicates their specificity and their aim to let the statistical analysis express *what the data have to say* independently of any outside information.

An objective (or fiducial) Bayesian analysis has a privileged status in order to gain public use statements. However, this does not preclude using other Bayesian techniques when appropriate.

1.3. The aim of this chapter

The aim of this chapter is to introduce the conceptual basis of objective Bayesian analysis and to illustrate some of its methodological improvements. The presentation will be essentially non-technical and, within this perspective, restricted to simple situations of inference about proportions. A similar presentation for inferences about means in the analysis of variance framework is available elsewhere (Lecoutre, 2006a).

The chapter is divided into four sections. (1) I briefly discuss the frequentist and Bayesian approaches to statistical inference and show the difficulties of the frequentist conception. I conclude that the Bayesian approach is highly desirable, if not unavoidable. (2) Its feasibility is illustrated in detail from a simple illustrative example of inference about a proportion in a clinical trial; basic Bayesian procedures are contrasted with usual frequentist techniques and their advantages are outlined. (3) Other examples of inferences about proportions serve me to show that these basic Bayesian procedures can be straightforward extended to deal with more complex situations. (4) The concluding remarks summarize the main advantages of the Bayesian methodology for experimental data analysis. Bayesian computations and softwares are also briefly reviewed. At last, some further topics are introduced.

The reader interested in more advanced aspects of Bayesian inference, with an emphasis on modeling and computation, is especially referred to the Volume 25 of this series (Dey and Rao, 2005).

2. Frequentist and Bayesian inference

2.1. Two conceptions of probabilities

Nowadays, probability has at least two main definitions (Jaynes, 2003). (1) Probability is the long-run frequency of occurrence of an event, either in a sequence of repeated trials or in an ensemble of "identically" prepared systems. This is the "frequentist" conception of probability, which seems to make probability an observable ("objective") property, existing in the nature independently of us, that should be based on empirical frequencies. (2) Probability is a measure of the degree of belief (or confidence) in the occurrence of an event or in a proposition. This is the "Bayesian" conception of probability.

This dualistic conception was already present in Bernoulli (1713), who clearly recognized the distinction between probability ("degree of certainty") and frequency, deriving the relationship between probability of occurrence in a single trial and frequency of occurrence in a large number of independent trials.

Assigning a frequentist probability to a single-case event is often not obvious, since it requires imagining a reference set of events or a series of repeated experiments in order to get empirical frequencies. Unfortunately, such sets are seldom available for assignment of probabilities in real problems. By contrast, the Bayesian definition is more general: it is not conceptually problematic to assign a probability to a unique event (Savage, 1954; de Finetti, 1974).

> It is beyond any reasonable doubt that for most people, probabilities about single events do make sense even though this sense may be naive and fall short from numerical accuracy. (Rouanet, 2000a, p. 26)

The Bayesian definition fits the meaning of the term probability in everyday language, and so the Bayesian probability theory appears to be much more closely related to how people intuitively reason in the presence of uncertainty.

2.2. *Two approaches to statistical inference*

The frequentist approach to statistical inference is self-proclaimed *objective* contrary to the Bayesian conception that should be necessary *subjective*. However, the Bayesian definition can clearly serve to describe "objective knowledge," in particular based on symmetry arguments or on frequency data. So Bayesian statistical inference is no less objective than frequentist inference. It is even the contrary in many contexts.

Statistical inference is typically concerned with both known quantities – the observed data – and unknown quantities – the parameters and the data that have not been observed. In the frequentist inference, all probabilities are conditional on parameters that are assumed known. This leads in particular to

- significance tests, where the parameter value of at least one parameter is fixed by hypothesis;
- confidence intervals.

In the Bayesian inference, parameters can also be probabilized. This results in distributions of probabilities that express our uncertainty:

- before observations (they do not depend on data): *prior* probabilities;
- after observations (conditional on data): *posterior* (or *revised*) probabilities;
- about future data: *predictive* probabilities.

As a simple illustration let us consider a finite population of size 20 with a dichotomous variable success/failure and a proportion φ (the *unknown parameter*) of success. A sample of size 5 has been observed, hence these *known data:*

$$0 \quad 0 \quad 0 \quad 1 \quad 0 \qquad f = 1/5$$

The inductive reasoning is fundamentally a generalization from a known quantity (here the data $f = 1/5$) to an unknown quantity (here the parameter φ).

2.3. *The frequentist approach: from unknown to known*

In the frequentist framework, we have no probabilities and consequently no possible inference. The situation must be reversed, but we have no more probabilities … unless we fix a parameter value. Let us assume, for instance, $\varphi = 0.75$.

Then we get sampling probabilities $\Pr(f|\varphi = 0.75)$ – that is frequencies – involving *imaginary repetitions* of the observations. They can be obtained by simulating repeated drawing of samples of 5 marbles (without replacement) from a box that contains 15 black and 5 white marbles. Alternatively, they can be (exactly) computed from a hypergeometric distribution. These sampling probabilities serve to define a null hypothesis significance test. If the null hypothesis is true ($\varphi = 0.75$), one find in 99.5% of the repetitions a value $f > 1/5$ (the proportion of black marbles in the sample), greater than the observation in hand: the null hypothesis $\varphi = 0.75$ is rejected ("significant test": $p = 0.005$). Note that I do not enter here in the one-sided/two-sided test discussion, which is irrelevant for my purpose.

However, this conclusion is based on the probability of the samples *that have not been observed*, what Jeffreys (1961, Section 7.2) ironically expressed in the following terms:

> If P is small, that means that there have been unexpectedly large departures from prediction. But why should these be stated in terms of P? The latter gives the probability of departures, measured in a particular way, equal to or greater than the observed set, and the contribution from the actual value is nearly always negligible. What the use of P implies, therefore, is that a hypothesis that may be true may be rejected because it has not predicted observable results that have not occurred. This seems a remarkable procedure.

As another example of null hypothesis, let us assume $\varphi = 0.50$. In this case, if the null hypothesis is true ($\varphi = 0.50$), one find in 84.8% of the repetitions a value $f > 1/5$, greater than the observation: the null hypothesis $\varphi = 0.50$ is not rejected by the data in hand. Obviously, *this does not prove that* $\varphi = 0.50$!

Now a frequentist confidence interval can be constructed as the set of possible parameter values that are not rejected by the data. Given the data in hand we get the following 95% confidence interval: [0.05, 0.60]. How to interpret the confidence 95%? The frequentist interpretation is based on the universal statement:

> whatever the fixed value of the parameter is, in 95% (at least) of the repetitions the interval that should be computed includes this value.

But this interpretation is very strange since *it does not involve the data in hand*! It is at least unrealistic, as outlined by Fisher (1990/1973, p. 71):

> Objection has sometimes been made that the method of calculating Confidence Limits by setting an assigned value such as 1% on the frequency of observing 3

or less (or at the other end of observing 3 or more) is unrealistic in treating the values less than 3, which have not been observed, in exactly the same manner as the value 3, which is the one that has been observed. This feature is indeed not very defensible save as an approximation.

2.4. The Bayesian approach: from known to unknown

As long as we are uncertain about values of parameters, we will fall into the Bayesian camp. (Iversen, 2000)

Let us return to the inductive reasoning, starting from the known data, and adopting a Bayesian viewpoint. We can now use, in addition to sampling probabilities, probabilities that express our uncertainty about all possible values of the parameter. In the Bayesian inference, we consider, not the frequentist probabilities of imaginary samples but the frequentist probabilities of *the observed data* $\Pr(f = 1/5|\varphi)$ for all possible values of the parameter. This is the *likelihood* function that is denoted by

$$\ell(\varphi|\text{data}).$$

We assume prior probabilities $\Pr(\varphi)$ before observations. Then, by a simple product, we get the joint probabilities of the parameter values and the data:

$$\Pr\left(\varphi \text{ and } f = \frac{1}{5}\right) = \Pr\left(f = \frac{1}{5}\middle|\varphi\right) \times \Pr(\varphi) = \ell(\varphi|\text{data}) \times \Pr(\varphi).$$

The sum of the joint probabilities gives the marginal predictive probability of the data, before observation:

$$\Pr\left(f = \frac{1}{5}\right) = \sum_{\varphi} \Pr\left(\varphi \text{ and } f = \frac{1}{5}\right).$$

The result is very intuitive since the predictive probability is a weighted average of the likelihood function, the weights being the prior probabilities.

Finally, we compute the posterior probabilities after observation, by application of the definition of conditional probabilities. The posterior distribution (given by Bayes' theorem) is simply the normalized product of the prior and the likelihood:

$$\Pr\left(\varphi\middle|f = \frac{1}{5}\right) \propto \ell(\varphi|\text{data}) \times \Pr(\varphi) = \frac{\Pr(\varphi \text{ and } f = 1/5)}{\Pr(f = 1/5)}.$$

2.5. The desirability of the Bayesian alternative

We can conclude with Berry (1997):

Bayesian statistics is difficult in the sense that thinking is difficult.

In fact, it is the frequentist approach that involves considerable difficulties due to the mysterious and unrealistic use of the sampling distribution for justifying null hypothesis significance tests and confidence intervals. As a consequence, even experts in statistics are not immune from *conceptual* confusions about frequentist confidence intervals.

For instance, in a methodological paper, Rosnow and Rosenthal (1996, p. 336) take the example of an observed difference between two means $d = +0.266$. They consider the interval $[0, +0.532]$ whose bounds are the "null hypothesis" (0) and what they call the "counternull value" ($2d = +0.532$), computed as the symmetrical value of 0 with regard to d. They interpret this specific interval $[0, +0.532]$ as "a 77% confidence interval" ($0.77 = 1-2 \times 0.115$, where 0.115 is the one-sided p-value for the usual t-test). If we repeat the experience, the counternull value and the p-value will be different, and, in a long-run repetition, the proportion of null–counternull intervals that contain the true value of the difference δ will not be 77%. Clearly, 0.77 is here a *data-dependent* probability, which needs a Bayesian approach to be correctly interpreted. Such difficulties are not encountered with the Bayesian inference: the posterior distribution, being conditional on data, only involves the sampling probability of the data *in hand*, via the likelihood function $\ell(\varphi|\text{data})$ that writes the sampling distribution in the *natural order:* "from unknown to known."

Moreover, since most people use "inverse probability" statements to interpret NHST and confidence intervals, the Bayesian definition of probability, conditional probabilities and Bayes' formula are already – at least implicitly – involved in the use of frequentist methods. Which is simply required by the Bayesian approach is a very natural shift of emphasis about these concepts, showing that they can be used consistently and appropriately in statistical analysis. This makes this approach highly desirable, if not unavoidable.

With the Bayesian inference, intuitive justifications and interpretations of procedures can be given. Moreover, an empirical understanding of probability concepts is gained by applying Bayesian procedures, especially with the help of computer programs.

2.6. *Training strategy*

The reality of the current use of statistical inference in experimental research cannot be ignored. On the one hand, experimental publications are full of significance tests and students and researchers are (and will be again in the future) constantly confronted to their use. My opinion is that NHST is an inadequate method for experimental data analysis (which has been denounced by the most eminent and most experienced scientists), not because it is an incorrect normative model, just because it does not address the questions that scientific research requires (Lecoutre et al., 2003; Lecoutre, 2006a, 2006b). However, NHST is such an integral part of experimental teaching and scientists' behavior that its misuses and abuses should not be discontinued by flinging it out of the window.

On the one hand, confidence intervals could quickly become a compulsory norm in experimental publications. On the other hand, for many reasons due to their frequentist conception, confidence intervals can hardly be viewed as the ultimate method. In practice, two probabilities can be routinely associated with a specific interval estimate computed from a particular sample.

- The first probability is "the proportion of repeated intervals that contain the parameter." It is usually termed the coverage probability.
- The second probability is the Bayesian "posterior probability that this interval contains the parameter," assuming a non-informative prior distribution.

In the frequentist approach, it is forbidden to use the second probability. On the contrary, in the Bayesian approach, the two probabilities are valid. Moreover, an objective Bayes interval is often "a great frequentist procedure" (Berger, 2004).

As a consequence, it is a challenge for statistical instructors to introduce Bayesian inference without discarding either NHST or the "official guidelines" that tend to supplant it by confidence intervals. I argue that the sole effective strategy is *a smooth transition towards the Bayesian paradigm* (Lecoutre et al., 2001).

The suggested training strategy is to introduce Bayesian methods as follows: (1) to present natural *Bayesian interpretations* of NHST outcomes to call attention about their shortcomings. (2) To create as a result of this the need for *a change of emphasis in the presentation and interpretation* of results. (3) Finally, to equip users with a real possibility of *thinking sensibly about statistical inference* problems and behaving in a more reasonable manner.

3. An illustrative example

My first example of application will concern the inference about a proportion in a clinical trial (Lecoutre et al., 1995). The patients under study were post-myocardial infarction patients, treated with a low-molecular-weight heparin as a prophylaxis of an intra-cardial left ventricular thrombosis. Because of the limited knowledge available on drug potential efficacy, the trial aimed at abandoning further development as early as possible if the drug was likely to be not effective, and at estimating its efficacy if it turned out to be promising. It was considered that 0.85 was the success rate (no thrombosis) above which the drug would be attractive, and that 0.70 was the success rate below which the drug would be of no interest.

The trial was initially designed within the traditional Neyman–Pearson framework. Considering the null hypothesis H_0: $\varphi = 0.70$, the investigators planned a one-sided fixed sample Binomial test with specified respective Type I and Type II error probabilities $\alpha = 0.05$ and $\beta = 0.20$, hence a power $1-\beta = 0.80$ at the alternative H_a: $\varphi = 0.85$ (the hypothesis that they wish to accept!). The associated sample size was $n = 59$, for which the Binomial test rejects H_0 at level 0.05 if the observed number of success a is greater than 47. Indeed, for a sample of size n, the probability of observing a successes is given by the Binomial distribution

$$a|\varphi \sim \mathrm{Bin}(\varphi, n),$$

$$\Pr(a|\varphi) = \binom{n}{a}\varphi^a(1-\varphi)^{n-a},$$

hence the likelihood function

$$\ell(\varphi|\text{data}) \sim \varphi^a(1-\varphi)^{n-a}.$$

For $n = 59$ (which can be found by successive iterations), we get:

$$\Pr(a > 47|H_0 : \varphi = 0.70) = 0.035 < 0.05\ (\alpha)$$
$$\Pr(a > 47|H_a : \varphi = 0.85) = 0.834 > 0.80\ (1-\beta).$$

Note that, due to the discreteness of the distribution, the actual Type I error rate and the actual power differ from α and $1-\beta$.

Since it would be preferable to stop the experiment as early as possible if the drug was likely to be ineffective, the investigators planned an interim analysis after 20 patients have been included. Since the traditional Neyman–Pearson framework requires specification of all possibilities in advance, they designed a stochastically curtailed test. Stochastic curtailment suggests that an experiment be stopped at an interim stage when the available information determines the outcome of the experiment with high probability under either H_0 or H_a. The notations are summarized in Table 1.

3.1. *Stochastically curtailed testing and conditional power*

Stochastically curtailed testing uses the "conditional power" at interim analysis, which is defined as the probability, given φ and the available data, that the test rejects H_0 at the planned termination. At interim analysis, termination occurs to reject H_0 if the conditional power at the null hypothesis value is high, say greater than 0.80. In our example, even if after 20 observations 20 successes have been observed, we do not stop the trial.

Similarly, early termination may be allowed to accept H_0 if the conditional power at the alternative hypothesis value is weak, say smaller than 0.20. For instance, if 12 successes have been observed after 20 observations this rule suggests stopping and accepting the null hypothesis. A criticism addressed to this procedure is that there seems little point in considering a prediction that is based on hypotheses that may be no longer fairly plausible given the available data. In fact, the procedure ignores the knowledge about the parameter accumulated by the time of the interim analysis.

Table 1
Summary of the notations for the inference about a proportion

	Number of Successes	Number of Errors	Sample Size
Current data at interim stage	a_1	n_1-a_1	$n_1 = 20$
Future data	a_2	n_2-a_2	$n_1 = 39$
Complete data	$a = a_1 + a_2$	$n-a$	$n = 59$

3.2. An hybrid solution: the predictive power

Many authors have advocated calculating the "predictive power," averaging conditional power over values of the parameter in a Bayesian calculation. We are led to a Bayesian approach, but still with a frequentist test in mind. Formally, the prediction uses the posterior distribution of φ given a prior and the data available at the interim analysis. For the inference about a proportion, the calculations are particularly simple if we choose a conjugate Beta prior distribution

$$\varphi \sim \text{Beta}(a_0, b_0),$$

with density

$$p(\varphi) = \frac{1}{\text{B}(a_0, b_0)} \varphi^{a_0-1}(1-\varphi)^{b_0-1}.$$

The advantage is that the posterior is also a Beta distribution (hence the name conjugate), with density

$$p(\varphi|\text{data}) \propto \ell(\varphi|\text{data}) \times p(\varphi) \propto \varphi^{a_0+a-1}(1-\varphi)^{b_0+b-1}.$$

The prior weights a_0 and b_0 are added to the observed counts a_1 and b_1, so that at the interim analysis

$$\varphi|\text{data} \sim \varphi|a_1 \sim \text{Beta}(a_1 + a_0, b_1 + b_0).$$

The predictive distribution, which is a mixture of Binomial distributions, is naturally called a Beta–Binomial distribution

$$a_2|a_1 \sim \text{Beta-Bin}(a_1 + a_0, b_1 + b_0; n_2).$$

A vague or *non-informative* prior is generally considered. It is typically defined by small weights a_0 and b_0, included between 0 and 1. Here, I have retained a Beta prior with parameters 0 and 1

$$\varphi \sim \text{Beta}(0, 1).$$

This choice is consistent with the test procedure. I shall address this issue in greater detail later on.

In the example above with $n_1 = 20$ and $a_1 = 20$, the predictive probability of rejecting H_0 at the planned termination ($n = 59$) explicitly takes into account the available data (no failure has been observed). It is with no surprise largely greater than the probability conditional on the null hypothesis value

$$\Pr(a{>}47|a_1 = 20) = \Pr(a_2{>}27|a_1 = 20) = 0.997{>}0.80,$$

hence the decision to stop and reject H_0.

This predictive probability is a weighted average of the probabilities conditional to φ, the weights being given by the posterior distribution

$$\Pr(a{>}47|a_1 = 20 \text{ and } \varphi) = \Pr(a_2{>}27|a_1 = 20 \text{ and } \varphi),$$

some examples of which being

φ	$\mapsto$	$\Pr(a>47 \mid a_1 = 20 \text{ and } \varphi)$
1		1
0.95		0.9999997
0.85		0.990
0.70		0.482

Since the predictive power approach is a hybrid one, it is most unsatisfactory. In particular, it does not give us direct Bayesian information about φ. The trouble is that a decision (to accept H_0 or to accept H_a) is taken at the final analysis (or eventually at an interim analysis), even if the observed proportion falls in the no-decision region [0.70, 0.85], in which case *nothing has been proved.*

What the investigators need is to evaluate at any stage of the experiment the probability of some specified regions of interest and the ability of a future sample to support and corroborate findings already obtained. The Bayesian analysis addresses these issues.

3.3. The Bayesian solution

Bayesian methodology enables the probabilities of the pre-specified regions of interest to be obtained. Such statements give straight answers to the question of effect sizes and have no frequentist counterpart. Consider the following example of Bayesian interim analysis, with 10 observed successes ($n_1 = 20$ and $a_1 = 10$).

3.3.1. Evaluating the probability of specified regions

Let us assume the Jeffreys prior Beta(1/2, 1/2) – hence the posterior Beta(10.5, 10.5) shown in Fig. 1 – that will give the privileged non-informative solution (I shall also address this issue later on).

In this case it is very likely that the drug is ineffective ($\varphi<0.70$), as indicated by the following statements

$$\Pr(\varphi<0.70 \mid a_1 = 10) = 0.971$$

$$\Pr(0.70<\varphi<0.85 \mid a_1 = 10) = 0.029 \quad \Pr(\varphi>0.85 \mid a_1 = 10) = 0.0001.$$

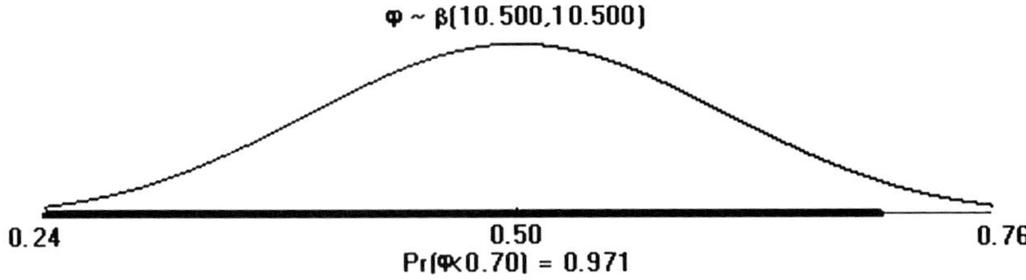

Fig. 1. Example of interim analysis ($n_1 = 20$ and $a_1 = 10$). Density of the posterior distribution Beta(10.5, 10.5) associated with the prior Beta(1/2, 1/2).

Note that in this case, the Bayesian inference about φ at the interim analysis does not explicitly integrate the stopping rule (which is nevertheless taken into account in the predictive probability). In the frequentist framework, the interim inferences are usually modified according to the stopping rule. This issue – that could appear as an area of disagreement between the frequentist and Bayesian approaches – will be considered later on. Resorting to computers solves the technical problems involved in the use of Bayesian distributions. This gives the users an attractive and intuitive way of understanding the impact of sample sizes, data and prior distributions. The posterior distribution can be investigated by means of visual display.

3.3.2. Evaluating the ability of a future sample to corroborate the available results
As a summary to help in the decision whether to continue or to terminate the trial, it is useful to assess the predictive probability of confirming the conclusion of ineffectiveness. If a guarantee of at least 0.95 for the final conclusion is wanted, that is $\Pr(\varphi < 0.70|a) > 0.95$, the total number of successes a must be less than 36 out of 59. Since $a_1 = 10$ successes have been obtained, we must compute the predictive probability of observing $0 \le a_2 \le 25$ successes in the future data. Here, given the current data, there is about 87% chance that the conclusion of ineffectiveness will be confirmed. Table 2 gives a summary of the analyses for the previous example and for another example more favorable to the new drug.

3.3.3. Determining the sample size
Predictive procedures are also useful tools to help in the choice of the sample size Suppose that in order to plan a trial to demonstrate the effectiveness of the drug, we have realized a pilot study: for instance, with $n_0 = 10$ patients, we have observed zero failure. In this case, the posterior probability from the pilot

Table 2
Summary of the Bayesian interim analyses

	Prior Distribution Beta(1/2, 1/2)	
	Example 1: $n_1 = 20$ and $a_1 = 10$	
Inference about φ		Predictive probability ($n = 59$)
Posterior probability		Conclusion with guarantee$\ge$0.95
$\Pr(\varphi < 0.70 \mid a_1 = 10)$		$\varphi < 0.70$
0.971		0.873 ($a < 36$)
$\Pr(\varphi < 0.85 \mid a_1 = 10)$		$\varphi < 0.85$
0.9999		0.9998 ($a < 46$)
	Example 2: $n_1 = 20$ and $a_1 = 18$	
Inference about φ		Predictive probability ($n = 59$)
Posterior probability		Conclusion with guarantee$\ge$0.95
$\Pr(\varphi < 0.70 \mid a_1 = 10)$		$\varphi > 0.70$
0.982		0.939 ($a > 46$)
$\Pr(\varphi < 0.85 \mid a_1 = 10)$		$\varphi > 0.85$
0.717		0.301 ($a > 54$)

experiment (starting with the Jeffreys prior) is used as prior distribution. Here, for this prior, $\Pr(\varphi > 0.85) = 0.932$. If the preliminary data of the pilot study are integrated in the analysis ("full Bayesian" approach), the procedure is exactly the same as that of the interim analysis. However, in most experimental devices, the preliminary data are not included, and the analysis is conducted using a non-informative prior, here Beta(1/2, 1/2).

The procedure remains analogous: we compute the predictive probability that in the future sample of size n (not in the whole data), the conclusion of effectiveness ($\varphi > 0.85$) will be reached with a given guarantee γ. Hence, for instance, the following predictive probabilities for $\gamma = 0.95$

$$\begin{array}{ll} n = 20 \mapsto 0.582 \ (a > 19) & n = 30 \mapsto 0.696 \ (a > 28) \\ n = 40 \mapsto 0.744 \ (a > 37) & n = 50 \mapsto 0.770 \ (a > 46) \\ n = 60 \mapsto 0.787 \ (a > 55) & n = 70 \mapsto 0.696 \ (a > 64) \\ n = 71 \mapsto 0.795 \ (a > 65) & n = 72 \mapsto 0.829 \ (a > 65). \end{array}$$

Values within parentheses indicate those values of a that satisfy the condition

$$\Pr(\varphi > 0.85 | a) \geq 0.95.$$

Based on the preliminary data, there are 80% chances to demonstrate effectiveness with a sample size about 70. Note that it is not surprising that the probabilities can be non-increasing: this results in the discreteness of the variable (it is the same for power).

3.4. A comment about the choice of the prior distribution: Bayesian procedures are no more arbitrary than frequentist ones

Many potential users of Bayesian methods continue to think that they are too subjective to be scientifically acceptable. However, frequentist methods are full of more or less ad hoc conventions. Thus, the p-value is traditionally based on the samples that are "more extreme" than the observed data (under the null hypothesis). But, for discrete data, it depends on whether the observed data are included or not in the critical region. So, for the usual Binomial one-tailed test for the null hypothesis, $\varphi = \varphi_0$ against the alternative $\varphi > \varphi_0$, this test is *conservative*, but if the observed data are excluded, it becomes *liberal*. A typical solution to overcome this problem consists in considering a mid-p-value, but it has only ad hoc justifications.

In our example, suppose that 47 successes are observed at the final analysis ($n = 59$ and $a = 47$), that is the value above which the Binomial test rejects $H_0{:}\varphi = 0.70$. The p-value can then be computed according to the three following possibilities:

(1) $p_{\text{inc}} = \Pr(a \geq 47 | H_0{:}\ \varphi = 0.70) = 0.066$ ["including" solution]
  $\Rightarrow H_0$ is not rejected at level $\alpha = 0.05$ (conservative test)
(2) $p_{\text{exc}} = \Pr(a > 47 | H_0{:}\ \varphi = 0.70) = 0.035$ ["excluding" solution]
  $\Rightarrow H_0$ is rejected at level $\alpha = 0.05$ (liberal test)
(3) $p_{\text{mid}} = 1/2(p_{\text{inc}} + p_{\text{exc}}) = 0.051$ [mid-p-value]

Obviously, in this case the choice of a non-informative prior distribution cannot avoid conventions. But the particular choice of such a prior is an exact counterpart of the arbitrariness involved within the frequentist approach. For Binomial sampling, different non-informative priors have been proposed (for a discussion, see, e.g., Lee, 2004, pp. 79–81). In fact, there exist two extreme non-informative priors that are, respectively, the most unfavorable and the most favorable priors with respect to the null hypothesis. They are respectively the Beta distribution of parameters 1 and 0 and the Beta distribution of parameters 0 and 1. These priors lead to the Bayesian interpretation of the Binomial test: the observed significance levels of the inclusive and exclusive conventions are exactly the posterior Bayesian probabilities that φ is greater than φ_0, respectively, associated with these two extreme priors. Note that these two priors constitute an a priori "ignorance zone" (Bernard, 1996), which is related to the notion of imprecise probability (see Walley, 1996).

(1) $\Pr(\varphi < 0.70 | a = 47) = 0.066 = p_{\text{inc}}$
for the prior $\varphi \sim \text{Beta}(0, 1)$ (the most favorable to H_0)
hence the posterior $\varphi | \text{a} \sim \text{Beta}(47, 13)$

(2) $\Pr(\varphi < 0.70 | a = 47) = 0.035 = p_{\text{exc}}$
for the prior $\varphi \sim \text{Beta}(1, 0)$ (the most unfavorable to H_0)
hence the posterior $\varphi | \text{a} \sim \text{Beta}(48, 12)$

(3) $\Pr(\varphi < 0.70 | a = 47) = 0.049 \approx p_{\text{mid}}$
for the prior $\varphi \sim \text{Beta}(1/2, 1/2)$
hence the posterior $\varphi | \text{a} \sim \text{Beta}(47.5, 12.5)$

Then the usual criticism of frequentists towards the divergence of Bayesians with respect to the choice of a non-informative prior can be easily reversed. Furthermore, the Jeffreys prior, which is very naturally the intermediate Beta distribution of parameters 1/2 and 1/2, gives a posterior probability, fully justified, close to the observed mid-p-value. The Bayesian response should not be to underestimate the impact of the choice of a particular non-informative prior, as it is often done,

> In fact, the [different non informative priors] do not differ enough to make much difference with even a fairly small amount of data. (Lee, 2004, p. 81)

but on the contrary to assume it.

3.5. Bayesian credible intervals and frequentist coverage probabilities

In other situations, where there is no particular value of interest for the proportion, we may consider an interval (or more generally a region) estimate for φ. In the Bayesian framework, such an interval is usually termed a *credible interval* (or *credibility interval*), which explicitly accounts for the difference in interpretation with the frequentist confidence interval.

3.5.1. Equal-tails intervals

Table 3 gives 95% equal-tails credible intervals for the following two examples, assuming different non-informative priors.

The prior Beta(1, 0), which gives the largest limits, has the following frequentist properties: the proportion of samples for which the upper limit is less than φ is smaller than $\alpha/2$ and the proportion of samples for which the lower limit is more than φ is larger than $\alpha/2$. The prior Beta(0, 1), which gives the smallest limits, has the reverse properties. Consequently, simultaneously considering the limits of these two intervals protects the user both from erroneous acceptation and rejection of hypotheses about φ. This is undoubtedly an objective Bayesian analysis. If a single limit is wanted for summarizing and reporting results, these properties lead to retain the *intermediate* symmetrical prior Beta(1/2, 1/2) (which is the Jeffreys prior). Actually, the Jeffreys credible interval has remarkable frequentist properties. Its coverage probability is very close to the nominal level, even for small-size samples, and it can be favorably compared to most frequentist intervals (Brown et al., 2001; Agresti and Min, 2005).

> We revisit the problem of interval estimation of a Binomial proportion ... We begin by showing that the chaotic coverage properties of the Wald interval are far more persistent than is appreciated ... We recommend the Wilson interval or the equal-tailed Jeffreys prior interval for small *n*. (Brown et al., 2001, p. 101)

Note that similar results are obtained for *negative*-Binomial (or *Pascal*) sampling, in which we observe the number of patients n until a *fixed number of successes* a is obtained. In this case, the observed significance levels of the inclusive and exclusive conventions are exactly the posterior Bayesian probabilities associated with the two respective priors Beta(0, 0) and Beta(0, 1). This suggests privileging the intermediate Beta distribution of parameters 0 and 1/2, which is precisely the Jeffreys prior. This result concerns an important issue related to the "likelihood principle." I shall address it in greater detail further on.

3.5.2. Highest posterior density intervals

A frequently recommended alternative approach is to consider the *highest posterior density* (HPD) credible interval. For such an interval, which can be in fact an union of disjoint intervals (if the distribution is not unimodal), every point included has higher probability density than every point excluded. The aim is to

Table 3
Example of 95% credible intervals assuming different non-informative priors

Beta(0, 1)	Beta(1, 1)	Beta(1/2, 1/2)	Beta(0, 0)	Beta(1, 0)
$n_1 = 20$, $a_1 = 19$				
[0.7513, 0.9877]	[0.7618, 0.9883]	[0.7892, 0.9946]	[0.8235, 0.9987]	[0.8316, 0.9987]
$n_1 = 59$, $a_1 = 32$				
[0.4075, 0.6570]	[0.4161, 0.6633]	[0.4158, 0.6649]	[0.4240, 0.6728]	[0.4240, 0.6728]

get the shortest possible interval. However, except for a symmetric distribution, each of the two one-sided probabilities is different from $\alpha/2$. This property is generally undesirable in experimental data analysis, since more questions are "one-sided" as in the present example.

Moreover, such an interval is not invariant under transformation (except for a linear transformation), which can be considered with Agresti and Min (2005, p. 3) as "a fatal disadvantage." So, for the data $n = 59$, $a = 32$ and the prior Beta(1/2, 1/2), we get the HPD intervals

$$[0.4167, 0.6658] \text{ for } \varphi \text{ and } [0.7481, 2.1594] \quad \text{for} \quad \frac{\varphi}{1-\varphi},$$

with the one-sided probabilities

$$\Pr(\varphi < 0.4167) = 0.026 \text{ and } \Pr\left(\frac{\varphi}{1-\varphi} < 0.7481\right) = 0.039,$$

$$\Pr(\varphi < 0.6658) = 0.024 \text{ and } \Pr\left(\frac{\varphi}{1-\varphi} < 2.1594\right) = 0.011.$$

It must be emphasized, from this example, that the posterior distribution of $\varphi/(1-\varphi)$ is easily obtained: it is a Fisher–Snedecor F distribution. We find the 95% equal-tails interval [0.712, 1.984].

3.6. The contribution of informative priors

When an objective Bayesian analysis suggests a given conclusion, various prior distributions expressing results from other experiments or subjective opinions from specific, well-informed individuals ("experts"), whether *skeptical* or *convinced* (*enthusiastic*), can be investigated to assess the robustness of conclusions (see, in particular, Spiegelhalter et al., 1994).

The elicitation of a prior distribution from the opinions of "experts" in the field can be useful in some studies, but it must be emphasized that this needs appropriate techniques (see for an example in clinical trials Tan et al., 2003) and should be used with caution. The following examples are provided to understand how the Bayesian inference combines information, and are not intended to correspond to a realistic situation (in the current situation, no good prior information was available). I leave the reader the task to appreciate the potential contribution of these methods.

3.6.1. Skeptical and convinced priors

Consider again the example of data $n = 59$, $a = 32$, for which the objective Bayesian procedure concludes to inefficiency ($\varphi < 0.70$). For the purpose of illustration, let us assume the two priors, a priori, respectively, very skeptical and very convinced about the drug:

$$\varphi \sim \text{Beta}(20, 80) \quad \text{with mean } 0.200 \quad \text{for which } \Pr(\varphi < 0.70) \approx 1,$$

$$\varphi \sim \text{Beta}(98, 2) \quad \text{with mean } 0.980 \quad \text{for which } \Pr(\varphi > 0.85) = 0.999998.$$

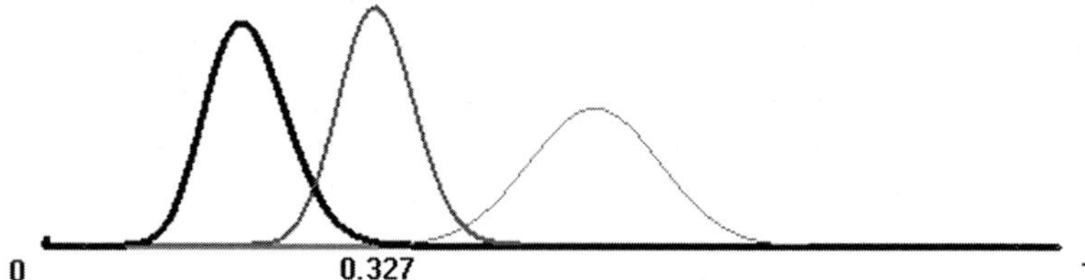

Fig. 2. Example of skeptical prior for the data $n = 59$ and $a = 32$. Densities of the prior Beta(20, 80) (thick line) and of the posterior distributions associated with this prior (medium line) and with the prior Beta(1/2, 1/2) (thin line).

The respective posteriors are

$$\varphi \sim \text{Beta}(52, 107) \quad \text{with mean } 0.327 \quad \text{for which } \Pr(\varphi < 0.70) \approx 1,$$
$$\varphi \sim \text{Beta}(130, 29) \quad \text{with mean } 0.818 \quad \text{for which } \Pr(\varphi > 0.85) = 0.143.$$

Of course the first prior reinforces the conclusion of inefficiency. Figure 2 shows this prior density (thick line) and the posterior (medium line), which can be compared to the objective posterior for the prior Beta(1/2, 1/2) (thin line). However, for the planned sample size, this prior opinion does not have any chance of being infirmed by the data. Even if 59 successes and 0 error had been observed, one would have $\Pr(\varphi < 0.70)|a = 59) = 0.99999995$.

The second prior allows a clearly less unfavorable conclusion. However, the efficiency of the drug cannot be asserted:

$$\Pr(\varphi > 0.70 | a = 32) = 0.997 \quad \text{but} \quad \Pr(\varphi > 0.85 | a = 32) = 0.143.$$

It is enlightening to examine the impact of the prior Beta(a_0, b_0) on the posterior mean. Letting $n_0 = a_0 + b_0$, the ratios $n_0/(n_0 + n)$ and $n/(n_0 + n)$ represent the relative weights of the prior and of the data. The posterior mean can be written

$$\frac{a_0 + a}{n_0 + n} = \frac{n_0}{n_0 + n} \frac{a_0}{n_0} + \frac{n}{n_0 + n} \frac{a}{n},$$

and is consequently equal to

prior relative weight × prior mean + data relative weight × observed mean.

The posterior means are as follows:

$$100/159 \times 0.200 + 59/159 \times 0.542 = 0.327 \text{ for the prior } \varphi \sim \text{Beta}(20, 80),$$

$$100/159 \times 0.980 + 59/159 \times 0.542 = 0.818 \text{ for the prior } \varphi \sim \text{Beta}(98, 2).$$

3.6.2. Mixtures of Beta densities

A technique that remains simple to manage is to use a prior with a density defined as a mixture of prior densities of Beta distributions. The posterior is again such a mixture. This prior has two main interests, on the one hand to approximate any arbitrary complex prior that otherwise would need numerical integration methods, and on the other hand to combine several pieces of information (or different opinions). As an illustration, let us consider for the same data a mixture of the two previous distributions with equal weights, that is

$$\varphi \sim \frac{1}{2}\text{Beta}(20, 80) \oplus \frac{1}{2}\text{Beta}(98, 2),$$

where $\oplus$ refers to a mixture of densities, that is symbolically written

$$p(\varphi) = \frac{1}{2}p(\text{Beta}(20, 80)) + \frac{1}{2}p(\text{Beta}(98, 2)).$$

Note that this distribution must not be confounded with the distribution of the linear combination of two variables with independent Beta distributions (that would have a much more complex density).

Figure 3 shows the prior density (thick line), which is bimodal, the corresponding posterior (medium line) and the Jeffreys posterior (thin line). In fact, in this case, the data $n = 59$, $a = 32$ allow us, in some sense, to discriminate between the two distributions of the mixture, as the posterior distribution is

$$0.999999903\text{Beta}(52, 107) \oplus 0.000000097\text{Beta}(130, 29),$$

so that it is virtually confounded with the distribution Beta(52, 107) associated with the prior Beta(20, 80).

It is enlightening to note that the weight associated with each Beta distribution of the posterior mixture is proportional to the product of the prior weight times the predictive probability of the data associated with the corresponding Beta prior.

If the number of patients is multiplied by 10, with the same proportion of successes ($n = 590$, $a = 320$), the posterior density, shown in Fig. 4, is virtually confounded with the posterior Beta(340, 350) associated with the prior Beta(20, 80). Of course, it is closer to the Jeffreys solution.

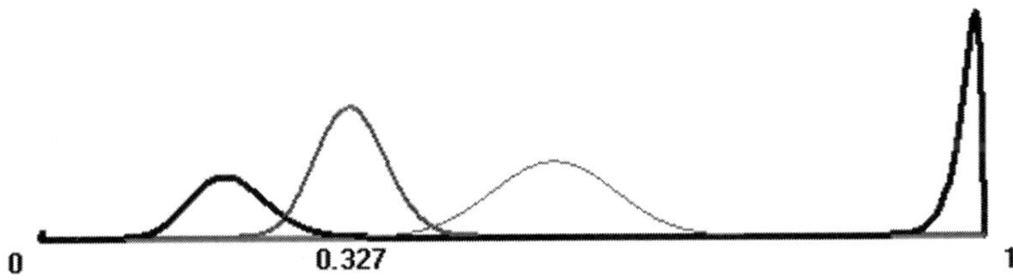

Fig. 3. Example of mixture prior for the data $n = 59$ and $a = 32$. Densities of the bimodal prior (1/2)Beta(20, 80)$\oplus$(1/2)Beta(98, 2) (thick line) and of the posterior distributions associated with this prior (medium line) and with the prior Beta(1/2, 1/2) (thin line).

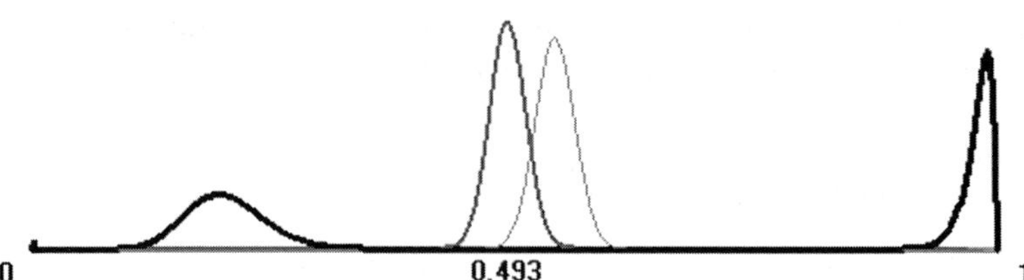

Fig. 4. Example of mixture prior for the data $n = 590$ and $a = 320$. Densities of the bimodal prior (1/2)Beta(20, 80)⊕(1/2)Beta(98, 2) (thick line) and of the posterior distributions associated with this prior (medium line) and with the prior Beta(1/2, 1/2) (thin line).

3.7. The Bayes factor

In order to complete the presentation of the Bayesian tools, I shall present the *Bayes factor*. Consider again the example of data $n = 59$, $a = 32$, with the convinced prior $\varphi \sim$ Beta(98, 2) and the corresponding a priori probabilities $\Pr(\varphi > 0.85) = 0.99999810$ (that will be denoted π_a), and consequently $\Pr(\varphi < 0.85) = 0.00000190$ (π_0). The notations π_0 and π_a are usual, since the Bayes factor is generally presented as a Bayesian approach to classical hypothesis testing; in this framework, π_0 and π_a are the respective prior probabilities of the null H_0 and alternative H_a hypotheses.

It is then quite natural to consider:

- the ratio of these two prior probabilities, hence

$$\frac{\pi_0}{\pi_a} = \frac{\Pr(\varphi < 0.85)}{\Pr(\varphi > 0.85)} = 0.0000019,$$

  which here is of course very small,
- and their posterior ratio, hence

$$\frac{p_0}{p_a} = \frac{\Pr(\varphi < 0.85 | a = 32)}{\Pr(\varphi > 0.85 | a = 32)} = \frac{0.8570}{0.1430} = 5.99,$$

  which is now distinctly larger than 1.

The Bayes factor (associated with the observation a) is then defined as the ratio of these two ratios

$$B(a) = \frac{p_0/p_a}{\pi_0/\pi_a} = \frac{p_0\pi_a}{p_a\pi_0} = 3154986,$$

which evaluates the modification of the relative likelihood of the null hypothesis due to the observation. However, the Bayes factor is only an incomplete summary, which cannot replace the information given by the posterior probabilities.

The Bayes factor applies in the same way to non-complementary hypotheses H_0 and H_a, for instance, here $\varphi < 0.70$ and $\varphi > 0.85$. However, in this case the interpretation is again more problematic, since the “no-decision” region $0.70 < \varphi < 0.85$ is ignored.

In the particular case of two simple hypotheses H_0: $\varphi = \varphi_o$ and H_a: $\varphi = \varphi_a$, the Bayes factor is simply the classical *likelihood ratio*

$$B(a) = \frac{p(\varphi_0|a)p(\varphi_a)}{p(\varphi_a|a)p(\varphi_0)} = \frac{p(a|\varphi_0)}{p(a|\varphi_a)},$$

since $p(\varphi_0|a) \propto p(a|\varphi_0)p(\varphi_0)$ and $p(\varphi_a|a) \propto p(a|\varphi_a)p(\varphi_a)$.

Note again that when H_0 and H_a are complementary hypotheses (hence $p_a = 1-p_0$), as in the example above, their posterior probabilities can be computed from the prior probabilities ($\pi_a = 1-\pi_0$) and the Bayes ratio. Indeed, it can be easily verified that

$$\frac{1}{p_0} = 1 + \frac{1-\pi_0}{\pi_0}\frac{1}{B(a)}.$$

4. Other examples of inferences about proportions

4.1. Comparison of two independent proportions

Conceptually, all the Bayesian procedures for a proportion can be easily extended to two Binomial independent samples, assuming two independent priors (see Lecoutre et al., 1995). In order to illustrate the conceptual simplicity and the flexibility of Bayesian inference, I give in the subsequent subsection an application of these procedures for a different sampling model.

4.2. Comparison of two proportions for the play-the-winner rule

From ethical point of view, adaptative designs can be desirable. In such designs subjects are assumed to arrive sequentially and they are assigned to a treatment with a probability that is updated as a function of the previous events. The intent is to favor the "most effective treatment" given available information. The *play-the-winner* allocation rule is designed for two treatments t^1 and t^2 with a dichotomous (e.g., success/failure) outcome (Zelen, 1969). It involves an "all-or-none" process: if subject $k-1$ is assigned to treatment t (t^1 or t^2) and if the outcome is a success (with probability φ_t), subject k is assigned to the same treatment; if, on the contrary, the outcome is a failure (with probability $1-\varphi_t$), subject k is assigned to the other treatment.

For simplicity, it is assumed here that the outcome of subject $k-1$ is known when subject k is included.

For a fixed number n of subjects, the sequel of treatment allocations (t_1, $t_2, \ldots,$ t_k, t_{k+1}, ..., t_{n+1}) contains all the information in the data. Indeed, $t_k = t_{k+1}$ implies that a success to t_k has been observed and $t_k \neq t_{k+1}$ implies that a failure to t_k has been observed. Moreover, the likelihood function is simply

$$\ell(\varphi_1, \varphi_2)|(t_1, \ldots, t_{n+1}) = \frac{1}{2}\varphi_1^{n_{11}}(1-\varphi_1)^{n_{10}}\varphi_2^{n_{21}}(1-\varphi_2)^{n_{20}},$$

where n_{ij} is the number of pairs (t_k, t_{k+1}) equal to (t^i, t^j), so that n_{11} and n_{21} are the respective numbers of success to treatments t^1 and t^2, and n_{10} and n_{20} are the numbers of failure (1/2 is the probability of t_1).

Since Bayesian methods only involve the likelihood function, they are immediately available. Moreover, since the likelihood function is identical (up to a multiplicative constant) with the likelihood function associated with the comparison of two independent binomial proportions, the same Bayesian procedures apply here, even if the sampling probabilities are very different. On the contrary, with the frequentist approach, specific procedures must be developed. Due to the complexity of the sampling distribution, only asymptotic solutions are easily available. Of course, except for large samples, they are not satisfactory.

4.2.1. Numerical example

Let us consider for illustration the results of a trial with $n = 150$ subjects. The observed rates of success are, respectively, 74 out of 94 attributions for treatment t^1 and 35 out of 56 attributions for treatment t^2. Note that, from the definition of the rule, the numbers of failures (here 20 and 21) can differ at most by 1. A joint probability statement is, in a way, the best summary of the posterior distribution. For instance, if we assume the Jeffreys prior, that is two independent Beta(1/2, 1/2) distributions for φ_1 and φ_2, the marginal posteriors Beta(74.5, 20.5) and Beta(35.5, 21.5) are again independent, so that a joint probability statement can be immediately obtained. We get, for instance,

$$\Pr(\varphi_1 > 0.697 \text{ and } \varphi_2 < 0.743 | \text{data}) = 0.95$$

which is deduced from $\Pr(\varphi_1 > 0.697) = \Pr(\varphi_2 > 0.743) = \sqrt{0.95} = 0.9747$, obtained as in the case of the inference about a single proportion.

It is, in a way, the best summary of the posterior distribution. However, a statement that deals with the comparison of the two treatments directly would be preferable. So we have a probability 0.984 that $\varphi_2 > \varphi_1$. Furthermore, the distribution of any derived parameter of interest can be easily obtained from the joint posterior distribution using numerical methods. We find the 95% equal-tails credible intervals:

$$[+0.013, +0.312] \text{ for } \varphi_1 - \varphi_2 [1.02, 1.62] \text{ for } \frac{\varphi_1}{\varphi_2} [1.07, 4.64] \text{ for } \frac{\varphi_1/(1-\varphi_1)}{\varphi_2/(1-\varphi_2)}.$$

For the Jeffreys prior, Bayesian methods have fairly good frequentist coverage properties for interval estimates (Lecoutre and ElQasyr, 2005).

4.2.2. The reference prior approach

For multidimensional parameter problems, the *reference prior* approach introduced by Bernardo (1979) (see also Berger and Bernardo, 1992) can constitute a successful refinement of the Jeffreys prior. This approach presupposes that we are interested in a particular derived parameter θ. It aims at finding the optimal objective prior, given that θ is the parameter of interest and the resulting prior is consequently dependent on this parameter. An objection can be raised against this approach in the context of experimental data analysis. Even when a particular parameter is privileged to summarize the findings, we are also interested in other parameters, so that joint prior and posterior distributions are generally wanted.

4.3. A generalization with three proportions: medical diagnosis

Berger (2004, p. 5) considered the following situation (Mossman and Berger, 2001; see also in a different context Zaykin et al., 2004).

> Within a population for which $\varphi_0 = \Pr(\text{Disease } D)$, a diagnostic test results in either a Positive (+) or Negative (−) reading. Let $\varphi_1 = \Pr(+|\text{patient has } D)$ and ($\varphi_2 = \Pr(+|\text{patient does not have } D)$. [the authors notations p_i have been changed to φ_i]

By Bayes' theorem, one get the probability θ that the patient has the disease given a positive diagnostic test

$$\theta = \Pr(D|+) = \frac{\Pr(+|D)\Pr(D)}{\Pr(+|D)\Pr(D) + \Pr(+|-D)\Pr(-D)} = \frac{\varphi_1\varphi_0}{\varphi_1\varphi_0 + \varphi_2(1-\varphi_0)}.$$

It is assumed that for $i = 0, 1, 2$ there are available (independent) data a_i, having Binomial distributions

$$a_i|\varphi_i \sim \text{Bin}(\varphi_i, n_i),$$

hence a straightforward generalization of the inference about two independent proportions. Note that, conditionally to φ_0, the situation is that of inference about the ratio of two independent Binomial proportions, since for instance

$$\Pr(\theta < u|\varphi_0) = \Pr\left(\frac{\varphi_2}{\varphi_1} > \frac{1-\varphi_0}{\varphi_0}\frac{1-u}{u}\right).$$

The marginal probability is a mixture of these conditional probabilities.

It results "a simple and easy to use procedure, routinely usable on a host of applications," which, from a frequentist perspective "has better performance [...] than any of the classically derived confidence intervals" (Berger, 2004, pp. 6–7).

Another situation that involves a different sampling model but leads to the same structure is presented in greater detail hereafter.

4.4. Logical models in a contingency table

Let us consider a group of n patients, with two sets of binary attributes, respectively, $V = \{v1, v0\}$ and $W = \{w1, w0\}$. To fix ideas, let us suppose that W is cardiac mortality (yes/no) and that V is myocardial infarction (yes/no). Let us consider the following example of logical model (Lecoutre and Charron, 2000).

An absolute (or logical) *implication* $v1 \Rightarrow w1$ (for instance) exists if all the patient having the modality v_1 also have the modality $w1$, whereas the converse is not necessarily true.

However, the hypothesis of an absolute implication (here "myocardial infarction implies cardiac mortality") is of little practical interest, since a single observation of the event $(v1, w0)$ is sufficient to falsify it.

Consequently, we have to consider the weaker hypothesis "$v1$ implies in most cases $w0$" ($v1 \hookrightarrow w1$).

The issue is to evaluate the departure from the logical model "the cell $(v1, w0)$ should be empty." A departure index $\eta_{v1 \hookrightarrow w1}$ can be defined from the cell proportions

	$W1$	$w0$	
$v1$	φ_{11}	φ_{10}	$\varphi_{1.}$
$v0$	φ_{01}	φ_{00}	$\varphi_{0.}$
	$\varphi_{.1}$	$\varphi_{.0}$	1

as

$$\eta_{v1 \hookrightarrow w1} = 1 - \frac{\varphi_{10}}{\varphi_{1.}\varphi_{.0}} \quad (-\infty < \eta_{v1 \hookrightarrow w1} < +1).$$

This index has been actually considered in various frameworks, with different approaches. It can be viewed as a measure of *predictive efficiency* of the model when predicting the outcome of W given $v1$.

- The prediction is perfect (there is an absolute implication) when $\eta_{v1 \hookrightarrow w1} = +1$.
- The closer to 1 $\eta_{v1 \hookrightarrow w1}$ is, the more efficient the prediction.
- In case of independence, $\eta_{v1 \hookrightarrow w1} = 0$.
- A null or negative value means that the model is a prediction failure.

Consequently, in order to investigate the predictive efficiency of the model, we have to demonstrate that $\eta_{v1 \hookrightarrow w1}$ has a value close to $+1$. Of course, one can define in the same way the indexes $\eta_{v1 \hookrightarrow w0}$, $\eta_{w1 \hookrightarrow v1}$, and $\eta_{w0 \hookrightarrow v0}$ One can, again, characterize the *equivalence* between two modalities. An absolute equivalence between $v1$ and $w1$ (for instance) exists if $\eta_{v1 \hookrightarrow w1} = +1$ and $\eta_{v0 \hookrightarrow w0} = +1$ (the two cells $[v1, w0]$ and $[v0, w1]$ are empty). Consequently, the minimum of these two indexes is an index of departure from equivalence.

Let us assume a multinomial sampling model, hence for a sample of size n, the probability of observing the cell counts n_{ij}

$$\Pr(n_{11}, n_{10}, n_{01}, n_{00} | \varphi_{11}, \varphi_{10}, \varphi_{01}, \varphi_{00}) = \frac{n!}{n_{11}!n_{10}!n_{01}!n_{00}!} \varphi_{11}^{n_{11}} \varphi_{10}^{n_{10}} \varphi_{01}^{n_{01}} \varphi_{00}^{n_{00}}.$$

4.5. Frequentist solutions

Asymptotic procedures (see, e.g., Fleiss, 1981) are clearly inappropriate for small samples. Alternative procedures based on Fisher's conditional test (Copas and Loeber, 1990; Lecoutre and Charron, 2000) have been proposed. This test involves the sampling distribution of n_{11} (for instance). A classical result is that this distribution, given fixed observed margins, only depends on the cross product $\rho = \varphi_{11}\varphi_{00}/\varphi_{10}\varphi_{01}$ (Cox, 1970, p. 4). The null hypothesis $\rho = \rho_0$ can be tested against the alternative $\rho < \rho_0$ (or against $\rho > \rho_0$), by using the probability that n_{11} exceeds the observed value in the appropriate direction.

Consequently, the procedure is analogous to the Binomial test considered for the inference about a proportion. We can define in the same way an "including" solution and an "excluding" solution.

In the particular case $\rho_0 = 0$, this test is the Fisher's randomization test of the null hypothesis $\rho = 1$ (i.e., $\eta_{v1 \hookrightarrow w1} = 0$) against $\rho < 1$ ($\eta_{v1 \hookrightarrow w1} < 0$).

By inverting this conditional test, confidence intervals can be computed for the cross product ρ. An interval for $\eta_{v1 \hookrightarrow w1}$ is then deduced by replacing ρ by its confidence limits in the following expression that gives $\eta_{v1 \hookrightarrow w1}$ as a function of ρ

$$\eta_{v1 \hookrightarrow w1} = \frac{1 + (\rho - 1)(\varphi_{1.} + \varphi_{.1} - \varphi_{1.}\varphi_{.1} - [(1 + (\varphi_{1.} + \varphi_{.1})(\rho - 1))^2 - 4\varphi_{1.}\varphi_{.1}\rho(\rho - 1)]^{1/2}}{2(\rho - 1)\varphi_{.1}(1 - \varphi_{1.})}.$$

Unfortunately, these limits depend on the true margin values $\varphi_{.1}$ and $\varphi_{1.}$. The most common procedure consists in simply replacing these *nuisance parameters* by their estimates $f_{.1}$ and $f_{1.}$. It is much more performing than asymptotic solutions, but is unsatisfactory for extreme parameter values. More efficient principles for dealing with nuisance parameters exist (for instance, Toecher, 1950; Rice, 1988). However, one comes up against a problem that is eternal within the frequentist inference, and that is of course entirely avoided in the Bayesian approach. In any case, Bayesian inference copes with the problem of nuisance parameters. Moreover, it explicitly handles the problems of discreteness and unobserved events (null counts) by way of the prior distribution.

4.6. The Bayesian solution

The Bayesian solution is a direct generalization of the Binomial case. Let us assume a joint (conjugate) *Dirichlet* prior distribution, which is a multidimensional extension of the Beta distribution

$$(\varphi_{11}, \varphi_{10}, \varphi_{01}, \varphi_{00}) \sim \text{Dirichlet}(\nu_{11}, \nu_{10}, \nu_{01}, \nu_{00}).$$

The posterior distribution is also a Dirichlet in which the prior weights are simply added to the observed cell counts.

$$(\varphi_{11}, \varphi_{10}, \varphi_{01}, \varphi_{00})|\text{data} \sim \text{Dirichlet}(n_{11} + \nu_{11}, n_{10} + \nu_{10}, n_{01} + \nu_{01}, n_{00} + \nu_{00}).$$

From the basic properties of the Dirichlet distribution (see, e.g., Bernardo and Smith, 1994, p. 135), the marginal posterior distribution for the derived parameter

η_{11} can be characterized as a function of three independent Beta distributions

$$X = \varphi_{10}|\text{data} \sim \text{Beta}(n_{10} + \nu_{10}, n_{11} + \nu_{11} + \eta_{01} + \upsilon_{01} + \eta_{00} + \upsilon_{00}),$$
$$Y = \frac{\varphi_{00}}{1 - \varphi_{10}} = \frac{\varphi_{00}}{1 - X}|\text{data} \sim \text{Beta}(n_{00} + \upsilon_{00}, n_{11} + \nu_{11}, n_{01} + \upsilon_{01}),$$
$$Z = \frac{\varphi_{11}}{1 - \varphi_{10} - \varphi_{00}} = \frac{\varphi_{11}}{(1 - Y)(1 - X)}|\text{data} \sim \text{Beta}(n_{11} + \upsilon_{11}, n_{01} + \upsilon_{01}),$$

since

$$\eta_{v1 \hookrightarrow w1} = 1 - \frac{X}{(X + Z(1 - Y)(1 - X))(X + Y(1 - X))}$$

This leads to straightforward numerical methods.

4.7. *Numerical example: mortality study*

4.7.1. *Non-treated patients*

The data in Table 4 were obtained for 340 high-risk patients who received no medical treatment. Let us consider the implication "Myocardial infarction $\hookrightarrow$ Cardiac mortality within 2 years."

The observed values of the index are

- for the implication "Infarction $\hookrightarrow$ Decease" (cell [yes,no] empty): $H_{v1 \hookrightarrow w1} = 0.12$,
- for the implication "Decease $\hookrightarrow$ Infarction" (cell [no,yes] empty): $H_{v1 \hookrightarrow w1} = 0.37$.

The marginal proportions of decease are (fortunately!) rather small – respectively, 0.22 after infarction and 0.07 without infarction – so that the count 72 in the cell [yes,no] is proportionally large. Consequently, relatively small values of the index are here "clinically significant." Assuming the Jeffreys prior Dirichlet(1/2, 1/2, 1/2, 1/2), we get the posterior

$$\Phi = (\varphi_{11}, \varphi_{10}, \varphi_{01}, \varphi_{00})|\text{data} \sim \text{Dirichlet}(20.5, 72.5, 17.5, 231.5).$$

from which we derive the marginal posteriors. Figure 5 shows the decreasing distribution function of the posterior of $\eta_{v1 \hookrightarrow w1}$ and its associated 90% credible interval.

Table 4
Mortality data for 340 high-risk patients who received no medical treatment

		Decease			
		Yes	No		
Myocardial infarction	Yes	20	72	92	[20/92 = 0.22]
	No	17	231	248	[17/248 = 0.07]
		37	303	340	

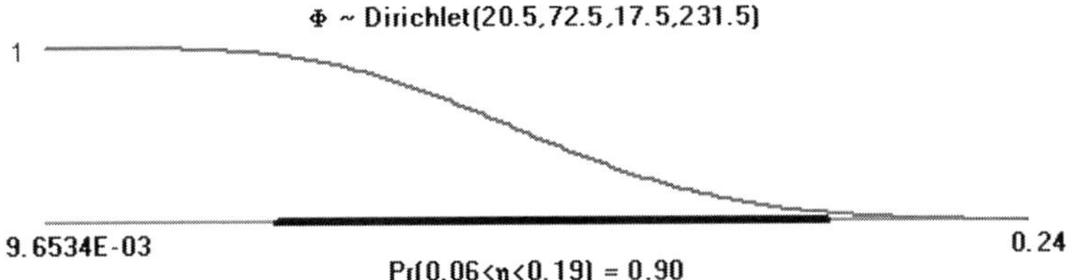

Fig. 5. Implication "Infarction ↪ Decease" (non-treated patients). Decreasing distribution function for $\eta_{v1 \hookrightarrow w1}$ [$\Pr(\eta_{v1 \hookrightarrow w1} < x)$] associated with the prior Dirichlet(1/2, 1/2, 1/2, 1/2).

Table 5
Mortality data for 357 high-risk patients who received a preventive treatment

		Decease			
		Yes	No		
Myocardial infarction	Yes	1	78	79	[1/79 = 0.01]
	No	13	265	278	[13/278 = 0.05]
		14	343	357	

From the two credible intervals,

- "Infarction ↪ Decease": $\Pr(+0.06 < \eta_{v1 \hookrightarrow w1} < +0.19) = 0.90$
- "Decease ↪ Infarction": $\Pr(+0.20 < \eta_{w1 \hookrightarrow v1} < +0.54) = 0.90$.

we can assert an implication of limited importance. In fact, it appears that decease is a better prognostic factor for infarction than the reverse.

4.7.2. Treated patients

Other data reported in Table 5 were obtained for 357 high-risk patients who received a preventive treatment.

Here, it is, of course, expected that the treatment would reduce the number of deceases after infarction. Ideally, if there was no cardiac decease among the treated patients after infarction (cell [yes,yes] empty), there would be an absolute implication "Infarction ⇒ No decease." We get the following results for this implication:

"Infarction ↪ No decease" : $H_{v1 \hookrightarrow w0} = +0.68$ and $\Pr(-0.10 < \eta_{v1 \hookrightarrow w0} < +0.94) = 0.90$.

Here, in spite of a distinctly higher observed value, it cannot be concluded to the existence of an implication. The width of the credible interval shows a poor precision. This is a consequence of the very small observed proportions of decease. Of course, it cannot be concluded that there is no implication or that the implication is small. This illustrate the abuse of interpreting the non-significant result of usual "tests of independence" (chi-square for instance) in favor of the null hypothesis.

4.8. *Non-informative priors and interpretation of the observed level of Fisher's permutation tests*

The Bayesian interpretation of the permutation test (conditional to margins) generalizes the interpretation of the Binomial test. For the usual one-sided test (including solution), the null hypothesis H_0: $\eta_{v1 \hookrightarrow w0} = 0$ is not rejected ($p_{\text{inc}} = 0.145$). It is well known that this test is conservative, but if we consider the excluding solution, we get a definitely smaller p-value $p_{\text{exc}} = 0.028$. This results from the poor experimental accuracy. As in the case of a single proportion, there exist two extreme non-informative priors, Dirichlet(1, 0, 0, 1) and Dirichlet(0, 1, 1, 0) that constitute the ignorance zone. They give an enlightening interpretation of these two p-values, together with an objective Bayesian analysis.

(1) $\Pr(\eta_{v1 \hookrightarrow w0} < 0) = 0.145 = p_{\text{inc}}$
for the prior Dirichlet(1, 0, 0, 1) (the most favorable to H_0)
hence the posterior Dirichlet(2, 78, 13, 266)
(2) $\Pr(\eta_{v1 \hookrightarrow w0} < 0) = 0.028 = p_{\text{exc}}$
for the prior Dirichlet(0, 1, 1, 0) (the most unfavorable to H_0)
hence the posterior Dirichlet(1, 79, 14, 265)
(3)$\Pr(\eta_{v1 \hookrightarrow w0} < 0) = 0.072 \approx (p_{\text{inc}} + p_{\text{exc}})/2 = 0.086$
for the prior Dirichlet(1/2, 1/2, 1/2, 1/2)
hence the posterior Dirichlet(1.5, 78.5, 13.5, 265.5)

4.8.1. *The choice of a non-informative prior*

As for a single proportion, the choice of a non-informative prior is no more arbitrary or subjective than the conventions of frequentist procedures. Moreover, simulation studies of frequentist coverage probabilities favorably compare Bayesian credible intervals with conditional confidence intervals (Lecoutre and Charron, 2000). For each lower and upper limits of the $1-\alpha$ credible interval, the frequentist error rates associated with the two *extreme* priors always include $\alpha/2$. Moreover, if a single limit is wanted for summarizing and reporting results, the symmetrical *intermediate* prior Dirichlet(1/2, 1/2, 1/2, 1/2) has fairly good coverage properties, including the cases of moderate sample sizes and small parameter values. Of course the differences between the different priors in the ignorance zone is less for small or medium values of $\eta_{v1 \hookrightarrow w1}$ and vanishes as the sample size increases.

4.9. *Further analyses*

There is no difficulty in extending the Bayesian procedures to any situation involving the multinomial sampling model, for instance, the comparison of two proportions based on paired data. Here, in particular, the distribution of the minimum of the two indexes for asserting equivalence is easily obtained by simulation. Moreover, the procedures can be extended to compare the indexes associated with two independent groups (for instance, here treated and non-treated patients).

Of course, in all these situations, informative priors and predictive probabilities can be used in the same way as for a single proportion.

Note again that binary and polychotomous response data can also be analyzed by Bayesian regression methods. Relevant references are Albert and Chib (1993) and Congdon (2005).

5. Concluding remarks and some further topics

Time's up to come to a positive agreement for procedures of experimental data analysis that bypass the common misuses of NHST. This agreement should fills up its role of "an aid to judgment," which "should not be confused with automatic acceptance tests, or 'decision functions'" (Fisher, 1990/1925, p. 128). Undoubtedly, there is an increasing acceptance that Bayesian inference can be ideally suited for this purpose. It fulfills the requirements of scientists: objective procedures (including traditional p-values), procedures about effect sizes (beyond p-values) and procedures for designing and monitoring experiments. Then, why scientists, and in particular experimental investigators, really appear to want a different kind of inference but seem reluctant to use Bayesian inferential procedures in practice? In a very lucid paper, Winkler (1974, p. 129) answered that "this state of affairs appears to be due to a combination of factors including philosophical conviction, tradition, statistical training, lack of 'availability', computational difficulties, reporting difficulties, and perceived resistance by journal editors." He concluded that if we leave to one side the choice of philosophical approach, none of the mentioned arguments are entirely convincing. Although Winkler's paper was written more than 30 years ago, it appears as if it had been written today.

> We [statisticians] will all be Bayesians in 2020, and then we can be a united profession. (Lindley, in Smith, 1995, p. 317)

In fact the times we are living in at the moment appear to be crucial. On the one hand, an important practical obstacle is that the standard statistical packages that are nowadays extensively used do not include Bayesian methods. On the other hand, one of the decisive factors could be the recent "draft guidance document" of the US Food and Drug Administration (FDA, 2006). This document reviews "the least burdensome way of addressing the relevant issues related to the use of Bayesian statistics in medical device clinical trials." It opens the possibility for experimental investigators to really be Bayesian in practice.

5.1. Some advantages of Bayesian inference

5.1.1. A better understanding of frequentist procedures

> Students [exposed to a Bayesian approach] come to understand the frequentist concepts of confidence intervals and P values better than do students exposed only to a frequentist approach. (Berry, 1997)

To take another illustration, let us consider the basic situation of the inference about the difference δ between two normal means. It is especially illustrative of how the Bayesian procedures combine descriptive statistics and significance tests.

Let us denote by d (assuming $d \neq 0$) the observed difference and by t the value of the Student's test statistic. Assuming the usual non-informative prior, the posterior for δ is a generalized (or scaled) t distribution (with the same degrees of freedom as the t-test), centered on d and with scale factor the ratio $e = d/t$ (see, e.g., Lecoutre, 2006a).

From this *technical* link with the t statistic, it results *conceptual* links. The one-sided p-value of the t-test is exactly the posterior Bayesian probability that the difference δ has the opposite sign of the observed difference. Given the data, if for instance $d > 0$, there is a p posterior probability of a negative difference and a $1-p$ complementary probability of a positive difference. In the Bayesian framework these statements are *statistically correct*. Another important feature is the interpretation of the usual confidence interval in natural terms. It becomes correct to say that "there is a 95% [for instance] probability of δ being included between the fixed bounds of the interval" (conditionally on the data).

In this way, Bayesian methods allow users to overcome usual difficulties encountered with the frequentist approach. In particular, using the Bayesian interpretations of significance tests and confidence intervals in the language of probabilities about unknown parameters is quite natural for the users. In return, the common misuses and abuses of NHST are more clearly understood. In particular, users of Bayesian methods become quickly alerted that non-significant results cannot be interpreted as "proof of no effect."

5.1.2. Combining information from several sources

An analysis of experimental data should always include an objective Bayesian analysis in order to express *what the data have to say* independently of any outside information. However, informative Bayesian priors also have an important role to play in experimental investigations. They may help refining inference and investigating the sensitivity of conclusions to the choice of the prior. With regard to scientists' need for objectivity, it could be argued with Dickey (1986, p. 135) that

> an objective scientific report is a report of the whole prior-to-posterior mapping of a relevant range of prior probability distributions, keyed to meaningful uncertainty interpretations.

Informative Bayesian techniques are ideally suited for *combining information* from the data in hand and from other studies, and therefore planning a series of experiments. More or less realistic and convincing uses have been proposed (for a discussion of how to introduce these techniques in medical trials, see, e.g., Irony and Pennello, 2001). Ideally, when "good prior information is available," it could (should) be used to reach the same conclusion that an "objective Bayesian analysis," but with a smaller sample size. Of course, they should integrate a real knowledge based on data rather than expert opinions, which are generally controversial. However, in my opinion, the use of these techniques must be more extensively explored before appreciating their precise contribution to experimental data analysis.

5.1.3. The predictive probabilities: a very appealing tool

> An essential aspect of the process of evaluating design strategies is the ability to calculate predictive probabilities of potential results. (Berry, 1991, p. 81)

A major strength of the Bayesian paradigm is the ease with which one can make predictions about future observations. The predictive idea is central in experimental investigations, as "the essence of science is replication: a scientist should always be concerned about what would happen if he or another scientist were to repeat his experiment" (Guttman, 1983). Bayesian predictive procedures give users a very appealing method to answer essential questions such as: "how big should be the experiment to have a reasonable chance of demonstrating a given conclusion?" "given the current data, what is the chance that the final result will be in some sense conclusive, or on the contrary inconclusive?" These questions are unconditional in that they require consideration of all possible values of parameters. Whereas traditional frequentist practice does not address these questions, predictive probabilities give them direct and natural answer.

In particular, from a pilot study, the predictive probabilities on credible limits give a useful summary to help in the choice of the sample size of an experiment (for parallels between Bayesian and frequentist methods, see Inoue et al., 2005).

The predictive approach is a very appealing method (Baum et al., 1989) to aid the decision to stop an experiment at an interim stage. On the one hand, if the predictive probability that it will be successful appears poor, it can be used as a rule to abandon the experiment for futility. On the other hand, if the predictive probability is sufficiently high, this suggests to early stop the experiment and conclude success.

Predictive probabilities are also a valuable tool for missing data imputation. Note that interim analyses are a kind of such imputation. The case of censored survival data is particularly illustrative. At the time of interim analysis, available data are divided into three categories: (1) included patients for whom the event of interest has been observed, (2) included patients definitely censored and (3) included patients under current observation for whom the maximum observation period has not ended. Consequently, the missing data to be predicted are respectively related to these last patients for which we have partial information and to the new patients planned to be included for which we have no direct information. The Bayesian approach gives us straightforward and effective ways to deal with this situation (Lecoutre et al., 2002).

It can again be outlined that the predictive distributions are also a useful tool for constructing a subjective prior, as it is often easier to express an opinion relative to expected data.

5.2. Bayesian computations and statistical packages

There is currently increasingly widespread application of Bayesian inference for experimental data analysis. However, an obstacle to the routine use of objective Bayesian methods is the lack of user-friendly general purpose software that would be a counterpart to the standard frequentist software. This obstacle may be expected to be removed in the future. Some packages have been designed to learn elementary Bayesian inference: see, for example, First Bayes (O'Hagan, 1996) and a package of Minitab macros (Albert, 1996). With a more ambitious perspective, we have developed a statistical software for Bayesian analysis of variance (Lecoutre and Poitevineau, 1992; Lecoutre, 1996). It incorporates both traditional frequentist practices (significance tests, confidence intervals) and routine Bayesian procedures (non-informative and conjugate priors). These procedures are applicable to general experimental designs (in particular, repeated measures designs), balanced or not balanced, with univariate or multivariate data, and covariables. This software also includes the basic Bayesian procedures for inference about proportions presented in this chapter.

At a more advanced level, the privileged tool for the Bayesian analysis of complex models is a method called Markov Chain Monte Carlo (MCMC). The principle of MCMC techniques (Gilks et al., 1996; Gamerman, 1997) is to simulate, and consequently approximate, the posterior and predictive distributions (when they cannot be determined analytically). This can be done for virtually any Bayesian analysis. WinBUGS (a part of the BUGS project) is an any general purpose flexible and efficient Bayesian software. It "aims to make practical MCMC methods available to applied statisticians" and largely contributes to the increasing use of Bayesian methods. It can be freely downloaded from the web site: http://www.mrc-bsu.cam.ac.uk/bugs/welcome.shtml. However, it can hardly be recommended to beginners unless they are highly motivated.

Very recently, Bayesian analysis has been added in some procedures of the SAS/STAT software. In addition to the full functionality of the original ones, the new procedures produce Bayesian modeling and inference capability in generalized linear models, accelerated life failure models, Cox regression models, and piecewise constant baseline hazard models (SAS Institute Inc., 2006).

5.3. Some further topics

I do not intend to give here an exhaustive selection of topics, but rather to simply outline some areas of research that seems to me particularly important for the methodological development of objective Bayesian analysis for experimental data.

5.3.1. The interplay of frequentist and Bayesian inference

Bayarri and Berger (2004) gave an interesting view of the interplay of frequentist and Bayesian inference. They argued that the traditional frequentist argument, involving "repetitions of the same problem with different data" is not what is done in practice. Consequently, it is "a joint frequentist–Bayesian principle" that is practically relevant: a given procedure (for instance, a 95% confidence interval for a normal mean) is in practice used "on a series of different problems involving a series of different normal means with a corresponding series of data" (p. 60). More generally, they reviewed current issues in the Bayesian–frequentist synthesis from a methodological perspective. It seems a reasonable conclusion to hope a methodological unification, but not a philosophical unification.

> Philosophical unification of the Bayesian and frequentist positions is not likely, nor desirable, since each illuminates a different aspect of statistical inference. We can hope, however, that we will eventually have a general methodological unification, with both Bayesians and frequentists agreeing on a body of standard statistical procedures for general use. (Bayarri and Berger, 2004, p. 78)

In this perspective, an active area of research aims at finding "probability matching priors" for which the posterior probabilities of certain specified sets are equal (at least approximately) to their coverage probabilities: see Fraser et al. (2003) and Sweeting (2005).

5.3.2. Exchangeability and hierarchical models

Roughly speaking, random events are *exchangeable* "if we attribute the same probability to an assertion about any given number of them" (de Finetti, 1972, p. 213). This is a key notion in statistical inference. For instance, future patients must be assumed to be exchangeable with the patients who have already been observed in order to make predictive probabilities reasonable. In the same way, similar experiments must be assumed to be exchangeable for a coherent integration of the information.

The notion of exchangeability is very important and useful in the Bayesian framework. Using multilevel prior specifications, it allows a flexible modeling of related experimental devices by means of *hierarchical models* (Bernardo, 1996).

> If a sequence of observations is judged to be exchangeable, then any subset of them must be regarded as a random sample from some model, and there exist a prior distribution on the parameter of such model, hence requiring a Bayesian approach. (Bernardo, 1996, p. 5)

Hierarchical models are important to make full use of the data from a multicenter experiment. They are also particularly suitable for meta-analysis in which we have data from a number of relevant studies that may be exchangeable on some levels but not on others (Dumouchel, 1990). In all cases, the problem can be decomposed into a series of simpler conditional models, using the hierarchical Bayesian methodology (Good, 1980).

5.3.3. The stopping rule principle: a need to rethink

Experimental designs often involve interim looks at the data for the purpose of possibly stopping the experiment before its planned termination. Most experimental investigators feel that the possibility of early stopping cannot be ignored, since it may induce a bias on the inference that must be explicitly corrected.

Consequently, they regret the fact that the Bayesian methods, unlike the frequentist practice, generally ignore this specificity of the design. Bayarri and Berger (2004) considered this desideratum as an area of current disagreement between the frequentist and Bayesian approaches. This is due to the compliance of most Bayesians with the *likelihood principle* (a consequence of Bayes' theorem), which implies the *stopping rule principle* in interim analysis:

> Once the data have been obtained, the reasons for stopping experimentation should have no bearing on the evidence reported about unknown model parameters. (Bayarri and Berger, 2004, p. 81)

Would the fact that "people resist an idea so patently right" (Savage, 1954) be fatal to the claim that "they are Bayesian without knowing it?" This is not so sure, experimental investigators could well be right! They feel that the experimental design (incorporating the stopping rule) is prior to the sampling information and that *the information on the design is one part of the evidence.* It is precisely the point of view developed by de Cristofaro (1996, 2004, 2006), who persuasively argued that the correct version of Bayes' formula must integrate the parameter θ, the design d, the initial evidence (prior to designing) e_0, and the statistical information i. Consequently, it must be written in the following form:

$$p(\theta|i, e_0, d) \propto (\theta|e_0, d)p(i|\theta, e_0, d).$$

It becomes evident that the *prior depends on d.* With this formulation, both the likelihood principle and the stopping rule principle are no longer automatic consequences. It is not true that, under the same likelihood, the inference about θ is the same, irrespective of d. Note that the role of the sampling model in the derivation of the Jeffreys prior in Bernoulli sampling for the Binomial and the *Pascal* models was previously discussed by Box and Tiao (1973, pp. 45–46), who stated that the Jeffreys priors are different as the two sampling models are also different. In both cases, the resulting posterior distribution have remarkable frequentist properties (i.e., coverage probabilities of credible intervals).

This result can be extended to general stopping rules (Bunouf, 2006). The basic principle is that the design information, which is ignored in the likelihood function, *can be recovered in the Fisher's information.* Within this framework, we can get a coherent and fully justified Bayesian answer to the issue of sequential analysis, which furthermore satisfy the experimental investigators desideratum (Bunouf and Lecoutre, 2006).

References

Agresti, A., Min, Y. (2005). Frequentist performance of Bayesian confidence intervals for comparing proportions in 2×2 contingency tables. *Biometrics* **61**, 515–523.

Albert, J. (1996). *Bayesian Computation Using Minitab.* Wadsworth Publishing Company, Belmont.

Albert, J., Chib, S. (1993). Bayesian analysis of binary and polychotomous response data. *Journal of the American Statistical Association* **88**, 669–679.

Battan, L.J., Neyman, J., Scott, E.L., Smith, J.A. (1969). Whitetop experiment. *Science* **165**, 618.

Baum, M., Houghton, J., Abrams, K.R. (1989). Early stopping rules: clinical perspectives and ethical considerations. *Statistics in Medicine* **13**, 1459–1469.

Bayarri, M.J., Berger, J.O. (2004). The interplay of Bayesian and frequentist analysis. *Statistical Science* **19**, 58–80.

Berger, J. (2004). The case for objective Bayesian analysis. *Bayesian Analysis* **1**, 1–17.

Berger, J.O., Bernardo, J.M. (1992). On the development of reference priors (with discussion). In: Bernardo, J.M., Berger, J.O., Dawid, A.P., Smith, A.F.M. (Eds.), *Bayesian Statistics 4. Proceedings of the Fourth Valencia International Meeting*. Oxford University Press, Oxford, pp. 35–60.

Bernard, J.-M. (1996). Bayesian interpretation of frequentist procedures for a Bernoulli process. *The American Statistician* **50**, 7–13.

Bernardo, J.M. (1979). Reference posterior distributions for Bayesian inference (with discussion). *Journal of the Royal Statistical Society, Series B, Methodological* **41**, 113–147.

Bernardo, J.M. (1996). The concept of exchangeability and its applications. *Far East Journal of Mathematical Sciences* **4**, 111–121.

Bernardo, J., Smith, A.F.M. (1994). *Bayesian Theory*. Wiley, New York.

Bernoulli, J. (1713). *Ars Conjectandi* (English translation by Bing Sung as Technical report No. 2 of the Department of Statistics of Harvard University, February 12, 1966), Basel, Switzerland.

Berry, D.A. (1991). Experimental design for drug development: a Bayesian approach. *Journal of Biopharmaceutical Statistics* **1**, 81–101.

Berry, D.A. (1997). Teaching elementary Bayesian statistics with real applications in science. *The American Statistician* **51**, 241–246.

Box, G.E.P., Tiao, G.C. (1973). *Bayesian Inference in Statistical Analysis*. Addison Wesley, Reading, MA.

Brown, L.D., Cai, T., DasGupta, A. (2001). Interval estimation for a binomial proportion (with discussion). *Statistical Science* **16**, 101–133.

Bunouf, P. (2006). *Lois Bayesiennes a priori dans un Plan Binomial Sequentiel*. Unpublished Doctoral Thesis in Mathematics, Université de Rouen, France.

Bunouf, P., Lecoutre, B. (2006). Bayesian priors in sequential binomial design. *Comptes Rendus de L'Academie des Sciences Paris, Série I* **343**, 339–344.

Congdon, P. (2005). *Bayesian Models for Categorical Data*. Wiley, Chichester.

Copas, J.B., Loeber, R. (1990). Relative improvement over chance (RIOC) for 2×2 tables. *British Journal of Mathematical and Statistical Psychology* **43**, 293–307.

Cox, D.R. (1970). *The Analysis of Binary Data*. Methuen, London.

de Cristofaro, R. (1996). L'influence du plan d'echantillonnage dans inférence statistique. *Journal de la Société Statistique de Paris* **137**, 23–34.

de Cristofaro, R. (2004). On the foundations of likelihood principle. *Journal of Statistical Planning and Inference* **126**, 401–411.

de Cristofaro, R. (2006). Foundations of the 'objective Bayesian inference'. In: *First Symposium on Philosophy, History and Methodology of ERROR*. Virginia Tech., Blacksburg, VA.

de Finetti, B. (1972). *Probability, Induction and Statistics: The Art of Guessing*. Wiley, London.

de Finetti, B. (1974). *Theory of Probability* Vol. 1, Wiley, New York.

Dey, D., Rao, C.R. (eds.) (2005). Handbook of Statistics, 25, Bayesian Thinking, Modeling and Computation. Elsevier, North Holland.

Dickey, J.M. (1986). Discussion of Racine, A., Grieve, A. P., Fliihler, H. and Smith, A. F. M., Bayesian methods in practice: experiences in the pharmaceutical industry. *Applied Statistics* **35**, 93–150.

Dumouchel, W. (1990). Bayesian meta-analysis. In: Berry, D. (Ed.), *Statistical Methodology in Pharmaceutical Science*. Marcel-Dekker, New York, pp. 509–529.

Efron, B. (1998). R.A. Fisher in the 21st century [with discussion]. *Statistical Science* **13**, 95–122.

FDA. (2006). *Guidance for the Use of Bayesian Statistics in Medical Device, Draft Guidance for Industry and FDA Staff.* U.S. Department of Health and Human Services, Food and Drug Administration, Center for Devices and Radiological Health, Rockville MD.

Fisher, R.A. (1990/1925). *Statistical Methods for Research Workers* (Reprint, 14th ed., 1925, edited by J.H. Bennett). Oxford University Press, Oxford.

Fisher, R.A. (1990/1973). *Statistical Methods and Scientific Inference* (Reprint, 3rd ed., 1973, edited by J.H. Bennett). Oxford University Press, Oxford.

Fleiss, J.L. (1981). *Statistical Methods for Rates and Proportions*, 2nd ed. Wiley, New York.

Fraser, D.A.S., Reid, N., Wong, A., Yi, G.Y. (2003). Direct Bayes for interest parameters. In: Bernardo, J.M., Bayarri, M.J., Berger, J.O., Dawid, A.P., Heckerman, D., Smith, A.F.M., West, M. (Eds.), *Bayesian Statistics 7*. Oxford University Press, Oxford, pp. 529–534.

Freeman, P.R. (1993). The role of *p*-values in analysing trial results. *Statistics in Medicine* **12**, 1443–1452.

Gamerman, D. (1997). *Markov chain Monte Carlo: stochastic simulation for Bayesian inference*. Chapman & Hall, London.

Gilks, W.R., Richardson, S., Spiegelhalter, D.J. (1996). *Markov Chain Monte Carlo in Practice*. Chapman & Hall, London.

Good, I.J. (1980). Some history of the hierarchical Bayesian methodology. In: Bernardo, J.M., DeGroot, M.H., Lindley, D.V., Smith, A.F.M. (Eds.), *Bayesian Statistics*. Valencia University Press, Valencia, pp. 489–519.

Guttman, L. (1983). What is not what in statistics? *The Statistician* **26**, 81–107.

Inoue, L.Y.T., Berry, D.A., Parmigiani, G. (2005). Relationship between Bayesian and frequentist sample size determination. *The American Statistician* **59**, 79–87.

Irony, T.Z., Pennello, G.A. (2001). Choosing an appropriate prior for Bayesian medical device trials in the regulatory setting. In: *American Statistical Association 2001 Proceedings of the Biopharmaceutical Section*. American Statistical Association, Alexandria, VA.

Iversen, G.R. (2000). Why should we even teach statistics? A Bayesian perspective. In: *Proceedings of the IASE Round Table Conference on Training Researchers in the Use of Statistics*, The Institute of Statistical Mathematics, Tokyo, Japan.

Jaynes, E.T. (2003). In: Bretthorst, G.L. (Ed.), *Probability Theory: The Logic of Science*. Cambridge University Press, Cambridge.

Jeffreys, H. (1961). *Theory of Probability*, 3rd ed. Clarendon, Oxford (1st ed.: 1939).

Laplace, P.-S. (1986/1825). *Essai Philosophique sur les Probabilités* (Reprint, 5th ed., 1825). Christian Bourgois, Paris (English translation: *A Philosophical Essay on Probability*, 1952, Dover, New York).

Lecoutre, B. (1996). *Traitement statistique des donnees experimentales: des pratiques traditionnelles aux pratiques bayésiennes* [*Statistical Analysis of Experimental Data: From Traditional to Bayesian Procedures*]. DECISIA, Levallois-Perret, FR (with Windows Bayesian programs by B. Lecoutre and J. Poitevineau, freely available from the web site: http://www.univ-rouen.fr/LMRS/Persopage/Lecoutre/Eris).

Lecoutre, B. (2000). From significance tests to fiducial Bayesian inference. In: Rouanet, H., Bernard, J.-M., Bert, M.-C., Lecoutre, B., Lecoutre, M.-P., Le Roux, B. (Eds.), *New ways in statistical methodology: from significance tests to Bayesian inference (2nd ed.)*. Peter Lang, Bern, pp. 123–157.

Lecoutre, B. (2006a). Training students and researchers in Bayesian methods for experimental data analysis. *Journal of Data Science* **4**, 207–232.

Lecoutre, B. (2006b). And if you were a Bayesian without knowing it? In: Mohammad-Djafari, A. (Ed.), *26th Workshop on Bayesian Inference and Maximum Entropy Methods in Science and Engineering. AIP Conference Proceedings Vol. 872*, Melville, pp. 15–22.

Lecoutre, B., Charron, C. (2006b). Bayesian procedures for prediction analysis of implication hypotheses in 2×2 contingency tables. *Journal of Educational and Behavioral Statistics* **25**, 185–201.

Lecoutre, B., Derzko, G., Grouin, J.-M. (1995). Bayesian predictive approach for inference about proportions. *Statistics in Medicine* **14**, 1057–1063.

Lecoutre, B., ElQasyr, K. (2005). Play-the-winner rule in clinical trials: models for adaptative designs and Bayesian methods. In: Janssen, J., Lenca, P. (Eds.), *Applied Stochastic Models and*

Data Analysis Conference 2005 Proceedings, Part X. Health. ENST Bretagne, Brest, France, pp. 1039–1050.

Lecoutre, B., Lecoutre, M.-P., Poitevineau, J. (2001). Uses, abuses and misuses of significance tests in the scientific community: won't the Bayesian choice be unavoidable? *International Statistical Review* **69**, 399–418.

Lecoutre, B., Mabika, B., Derzko, G. (2002). Assessment and monitoring in clinical trials when survival curves have distinct shapes in two groups: a Bayesian approach with Weibull modeling. *Statistics in Medicine* **21**, 663–674.

Lecoutre, B., Poitevineau, J. (1992). *PAC (Programme d Analyse des Comparaisons): Guide d'utilisation et manuel de reference*. CISIA-CERESTA, Montreuil, France.

Lecoutre, M.-P., Poitevineau, J., Lecoutre, B. (2003). Even statisticians are not immune to misinterpretations of null hypothesis significance tests. *International Journal of Psychology* **38**, 37–45.

Lee, P. (2004). *Bayesian Statistics: An Introduction*, 3rd ed. Oxford University Press, New York.

Mossman, D., Berger, J. (2001). Intervals for post-test probabilities: a comparison of five methods. *Medical Decision Making* **21**, 498–507.

O'Hagan, A. (1996). *First Bayes* [Teaching Package for Elementary Bayesian Statistics]. Retrieved January 10, 2007, from http://www.tonyohagan.co.uk/1b/.

Pagano, R.R. (1990). *Understanding Statistics in the Behavioral Sciences*, 3rd ed. West, St. Paul, MN.

Rice, W.R. (1988). A new probability model for determining exact *P* value for 2×2 contingency tables. *Biometrics* **44**, 1–22.

Rosnow, R.L., Rosenthal, R. (1996). Computing contrasts, effect sizes, and counternulls on other people's published data: general procedures for research consumers. *Psychological Methods* **1**, 331–340.

Rouanet, H. (2000a). Statistics for researchers. In: Rouanet, H., Bernard, J.-M., Bert, M.-C., Lecoutre, B., Lecoutre, M.-P., Le Roux, B. (Eds.), *New Ways in Statistical Methodology: From Significance Tests to Bayesian Inference (2nd ed.)*. Peter Lang, Bern, pp. 1–27.

Rouanet, H. (2000b). Statistical practice revisited. In: Rouanet, H., Bernard, J.-M., Bert, M.-C., Lecoutre, B., Lecoutre, M.-P., Le Roux, B. (Eds.), *New Ways in Statistical Methodology: From Significance Tests to Bayesian Inference (2nd ed.)*. Peter Lang, Bern, pp. 29–64.

Rouanet, H., Bernard, J.-M., Bert, M.-C., Lecoutre, B., Lecoutre, M.-P., Le Roux, B. (2000). *New Ways in Statistical Methodology: From Significance Tests to Bayesian Inference*, 2nd ed. Peter Lang, Bern.

Rozeboom, W.W. (1960). The fallacy of the null hypothesis significance test. *Psychological Bulletin* **57**, 416–428.

SAS Institute Inc. (2006). *Preliminary Capabilities for Bayesian Analysis in SAS/STAT® Software*. SAS Institute Inc, Cary, NC.

Savage, L. (1954). *The Foundations of Statistical Inference*. Wiley, New York.

Schmitt, S.A. (1969). *Measuring Uncertainty: An Elementary Introduction to Bayesian Statistics*. Addison Wesley, Reading, MA.

Smith, A. (1995). A conversation with Dennis Lindley. *Statistical Science* **10**, 305–319.

Spiegelhalter, D.J., Freedman, L.S., Parmar, M.K.B. (1994). Bayesian approaches to randomized trials. *Journal of the Royal Statistical Society, Series A* **157**, 357–416.

Sweeting, T.J. (2005). On the implementation of local probability matching priors for interest parameters. *Biometrika* **92**, 47–57.

Tan, S.B., Chung, Y.F.A., Tai, B.C., Cheung, Y.B., Machin, D. (2003). Elicitation of prior distributions for a phase III randomized controlled trial of adjuvant therapy with surgery for hepatocellular carcinoma. *Controlled Clinical Trials* **24**, 110–121.

Toecher, K.D. (1950). Extension of the Neyman–Pearson theory of tests to discontinuous variables. *Biometrika* **37**, 130–144.

Walley, P. (1996). Inferences from multinomial data: learning about a bag of marbles [with discussion]. *Journal of the Royal Statistical Society B* **58**, 3–57.

Winkler, R.L. (1974). Statistical analysis: theory versus practice. In: Stael Von Holstein, C.-A.S. (Ed.), *The Concept of Probability in Psychological Experiments*. D. Reidel, Dordrecht, pp. 127–140.

Zaykin, D.V., Meng, Z., Ghosh, S.K. (2004). Interval estimation of genetic susceptibility for retrospective case–control studies. *BMC Genetics* **5**(9), 1–11.

Zelen, M. (1969). Play the winner rule and the controlled clinical trial. *Journal of the American Statistical Association* **64**, 131–146.

Subject Index

accelerated failure time model 5, 169, 309, 325
Accelerated titration designs 514, 519
Adaptive randomization 69, 526, 550
additivity 42–43
affinely invariant matching methods 46
AIDS 82, 268, 373, 586
alpha spending function 493, 496–497
analysis of variance (ANOVA), 66, 134, 161, 431, 434–437, 442, 445, 448, 456, 625, 656, 660, 664–665, 676, 679, 686–688, 690, 692, 696, 700, 702, 778, 806
approximate Bayesian bootstrap imputation 576
approximately unbiased estimates 570
assignment mechanism 28, 34–48, 54, 66, 68
Assignment-based modes 41, 45
– of inference 45
assumed
– linear relationship 53
– normality 53–54, 269
assumption-free causal inference 33
asymptotic normality of the likelihood 583
asymptotic test 131
available-case analysis 570, 573, 587

bacterial pathogens 585
balanced repeated replication 575
baselines 472–474, 476
– analysis under ignorability 582
Bayes factor 794–795
Bayes' theorem 725, 728, 781, 797, 808
Bayesian
– analyses 57, 67, 440, 467, 557–558, 570, 583, 777–778, 786, 790–791, 802, 804, 806
– approach 55–56, 267–268, 415, 501, 534, 557, 775, 777–779, 781–783, 785, 787, 789, 791, 793–795, 797, 799, 801, 803, 805, 807–808
– conception of probability 778
– inference 40, 47–48, 572, 583, 776–779, 781–783, 787, 791, 795, 799, 803, 806
– interim analysis 786
– interpretation of the Binomial test 789
– interpretation of the permutation test 802
– iterative simulation methods 583
– modeling 57, 514, 806
– monitoring 501
– perspective 55–56, 583
– posterior predictive inference 28
– posterior simulation 582
– procedure 117, 778, 782, 788, 791, 795–796, 802, 804, 806
Bentler–Weeks model 396
Beta prior 785, 793
Beta–Binomial distribution 785
biased sampling variance 580
bias-variance tradeoff 679
binomial
– proportion 129, 131, 555, 790, 796–797
– random variable 111
bioequivalence 464, 487
biologic variation 65
biomarker 9, 11, 19–20, 22, 109–113, 115–121, 123–129, 131, 133–144, 526
bivariate
– normal 142, 355, 381, 452
– predictive mean matching imputation 577
Bland-Altman method 119, 120, 123
Bonferroni 626–627, 629–631, 638–639
bootstrap 117, 120, 163, 166, 168, 182, 404–406, 482, 499, 570, 575–577, 699
bounds 55, 188, 328, 488, 530–531, 536–537, 754, 782, 804
box plot 127
Box-Cox
– family 128
– transformation 128, 269, 270
breast cancer 9, 15–16, 21–22, 47, 533, 547
Breslow–Day 605–606

cancer mortality and survival rates 586
carry-over effects 464, 476–477, 480
case-cohort 85, 87, 97–99, 101, 323
– studies 97
case-control study 7, 22, 64–65, 73, 83–91, 93–97, 99–101, 103–104, 207, 209, 586, 606–607, 720

case-crossover study 102
causal effect 28–43, 45–49, 51, 53–57, 176–177, 492
Causal models 148, 176
censored data 151, 232–233, 235, 282, 285–286, 288, 291, 299, 303, 305, 307, 325, 587
choice of the sample size 787, 805
Classical
– design 434, 507
– experiment design 55
classification and regression trees (CART), 10, 151, 173–174, 182
clinical epidemiology 712, 714–715, 728
clinically relevant 121, 174, 522, 627, 635, 640
closed population 75
Cluster
– Analysis 342–345, 347–351, 353, 355, 357, 359, 361, 363–365
– randomized trials 72
clustering in design 57
Cochran Q test 111–113, 118
Cochran-Armitage (C-A) test 130, 131
Cochrane Collaboration 602, 609, 614, 714, 728
Cochran–Mantel–Haenszel 604–609
coefficient of concordance 119–120, 191–192, 195
Cohen's kappa 114–115, 118
cohort study 3, 6–7, 9–10, 12, 65, 73–75, 82–88, 90, 91, 96–100, 103, 606, 666, 716, 719–720, 727
Combining rules for proper multiple imputation 579
community intervention trial 64–65, 67, 72
competing risks 74–75, 99, 281–282, 287–288, 292, 294, 308, 310–311, 313, 316, 321–329, 331, 333, 335, 337, 339
complementary log-log 207, 313, 317
complete-case analysis 570, 573–574, 587
completed data
– estimated variance 579
– methods of analysis 587
– methods 180, 570, 574, 587
– sufficient statistics 583
completely randomized experiment 39–41, 43, 45
complex sample survey 580
Complications 28, 47, 55, 57, 71, 95, 238, 643, 768
conditional
– approach 129, 130
– null distribution 130
– permutation distribution 133
– power 19, 492, 500, 506, 559, 560, 561, 784, 785
confidence
– limits 115–116, 190, 199–202, 205, 208, 488, 606, 608, 613, 716, 780, 799
– proper 576, 580
confirmatory factor analysis 367–368, 375, 396, 398
confounded assignment mechanism 39–40
confounders 34, 68, 78, 96, 102, 164, 176
confounding 7–8, 10, 13, 15, 21, 66, 68, 84, 102, 150, 162, 164, 465, 534, 538, 666, 719–720
congenial 580
conservative 130, 157, 227, 371, 460, 495, 505, 554, 559–560, 629–630, 643, 788, 802
conservativeness 130
constant bias 123, 126
– proportional bias 123
constant variance 123, 151, 153, 155–157, 733
contingency table 132–133, 195, 345, 383, 474–475, 555, 797
Continuous reassessment method 514, 520
convergence 179, 197, 261, 405, 414, 418, 450, 457, 578, 582–583
correlation
– coefficient tests 127
– coefficient 119–120, 127, 133, 138–140, 142, 267, 553, 570, 632, 665
Correspondence analysis 361–362
count response 210–211, 213, 215, 217, 219, 221, 223, 225, 227, 229, 231, 233, 235, 237, 239, 241, 243, 245, 247, 249–251
counterfactual world 30–32
covariance adjustment 38
covariate-adjusted designs 533
credible interval 789–790, 796, 800–802, 808
cross
– classified categorical data 129
– over trial 464–467, 469, 471–473, 475, 477–479, 481, 483, 485–488
– product ratio 88, 690
– sectional studies 65, 429, 720
– sectional survey data 586
– validation 156, 163, 174, 266, 368, 410, 683, 695, 704–707
cumulative incidence function 282, 287–289, 292–293, 295, 310–311, 313, 322–326, 328, 333, 335, 338–339
curves 11, 175, 192, 194, 295, 300, 317, 339, 412, 444, 498–499, 555, 662, 688, 691, 706, 726, 728

Dangers of model-based extrapolations 53
data augmentation 56
– algorithm 578
de Finetti's theorem 44, 49
degree of agreement 114–115
degrees of freedom in the MI analysis 579
Deming regression 119, 122–123, 125
demographic 585–586, 644, 646, 680

designed missing data 587
designed-based 42
detection limits 142
diagnostic test characteristics 724–725, 728
dichotomous biomarkers 113–114, 116, 118
direct analyses 570, 581, 584, 587
Direct and indirect causal effects 56
Dirichlet 524, 799–802
discarding irrelevant units 47
discriminant analysis 45, 343
discriminant mixtures of ellipsoidal distributions 46
Disease
– prevention 2–3, 15, 17
– screening 2, 10
– surveillance system 585
– treatment epidemiology
distance measures 344–348, 364
distributional assumptions 126, 134, 151, 153, 174, 243, 249, 255, 259, 268, 381, 403, 406, 481, 502, 737
distribution-free 109, 128, 134–135, 403
– test 128, 135
domain indicators 580
Dose
– escalation with overdose control 514, 522
– response relationships 130
– response shape 131
toxicity function 520–521
double-blind 69, 467, 479, 547, 551, 602, 637
drop out 169, 255, 271, 569, 577, 759
Dunnett's
– C 137–138
T3, 137 138
dynamic population 74

E-step 163, 179–180, 416, 582
ECM 583
ECME 583
ecologic studies 65
economic impact of that event 32
economics 35, 46–47, 56, 322
effect
– of vaccination 33
– size 166, 272, 507, 552–553, 604, 613, 618–619, 623, 641, 646, 649, 656–664, 777, 786, 803
ellipsoidal distributions 46
EM 56, 179, 261, 357, 360, 414–415, 439, 455, 578, 582–583, 587
– algorithm 56, 179, 261, 414–415, 439, 455, 582–583
empirical Bayes 259, 261, 263, 269, 679, 707
endpoints 84, 325, 502, 504, 514, 522, 524, 529–530, 532, 535, 538–541, 552, 554, 556, 616–617, 619–624, 631–632, 635–641, 643, 649, 758–759
enumeration 133, 135, 528
environmental exposure data 143
epidemiological databases 571, 584, 587
Equal Percent Bias Reducing 46
equal-tails credible intervals 790, 796
(equal-variance) t-test 134, 136–137, 188, 219, 244, 272, 347, 436, 456, 471, 474, 555, 651, 665, 676, 782, 804
equipoise 67–68
error variance 123–125, 269, 368
estimated
– standard errors 575
– variance 43, 286, 290, 329, 481, 579, 733, 736, 739–740, 743
ethical considerations 67, 629
Evidence Based Medicine 712–713, 715–717, 719, 721, 723, 725, 727–729
Exact
– distribution 129, 133, 135, 272, 481
– inference 129, 133
– logistic regression 182, 187, 196, 198–201
– test 129–131, 198–199, 201, 475, 498–499, 665
exchangeability 807
expectation-maximization algorithm 578
Expected Values Decision Making 726, 728
explicit or implicit 515, 580
Exploratory factor analysis 368, 396, 407–408, 417
explosion of potential outcomes 32
external information 53

F-test 134, 136, 154, 262–263, 435–436, 456, 480, 555
factor analysis 367–369, 371, 373, 375, 377, 379, 381, 383, 385, 387, 389, 396–398, 403, 407–408, 412, 417
factorial designs 42, 478
factorization 49
fiducial Bayesian 778
Field trials 64–65, 67, 71–72
final point estimate 579
Fisher exact test 198–199, 201
Fisher's
– conditional test 799
– exact test 129–131, 475, 498–499, 665
– z transformation 133, 140
– z-transforms 141
Fisherian
– perspective 43
– randomization distribution 45
– randomization-based inference 41
fit indices 378, 381, 395, 406–408, 410

fixed
– cohorts 75
– effects 158, 244, 246–248, 256, 258–264, 266, 268–269, 272, 275, 439–440, 443, 481–482, 605, 607–610
forest plot 602, 609–612
formal notation for potential outcomes 34
fraction of information 579
frequentist
– confidence interval 776, 780, 782, 789
– conception of probability 778
full matching 46
functional errors-in-variables model 123
funnel plot 613

Gaussian process 283, 679, 707
Generalized
– additive models (GAMs), 151, 173
– approximate cross-validation 695, 705–706
– cross-validation 683, 704
– linear mixed model 273–274, 276, 450, 452–453, 484
– linear models 148, 151, 156, 170, 172–173, 177, 182, 249, 274, 446–447, 496, 806
– maximum likelihood 683
generating function 747–751, 755, 770
Gibbs
– sample 56, 578, 583
– sampler 56, 578, 583
gold standard 110, 114–116, 119, 492, 550, 565, 603, 663–664, 723, 728, 730
"Gompertz" function 207
goodness of fit 195–196, 207, 218, 407–408, 683
graphical 10, 28, 126–127, 196, 268, 418, 501–502, 528, 532, 613
– methods 126
– technique 127, 268, 613
Group
– comparisons 19, 136, 142
– Sequential Designs 491, 493, 495, 497, 499, 501, 503, 505, 507
growth curve SEM 395, 412

heterogeneity 2, 20, 109, 136–137, 154, 224–225, 227, 230, 243–244, 246, 250–251, 325, 446, 451, 514, 522, 524, 529, 533–534, 607–609, 612, 722
hierarchical
– Bayesian model 584
– clustering 342, 344, 349–352, 354–356, 362, 364
– models 253, 807
highest posterior density (HPD) credible interval 790–791
histogram 127, 221–222, 230
history of the potential outcomes 34
homogeneity 2, 111, 123, 125, 136, 170, 174, 416, 482, 606, 636–637
hormone replacement therapy 32, 57
Horvitz–Thompson 45
Hosmer-Lemeshow test 195, 196
hypergeometric 129–130, 198, 780
– distribution 130, 780

ignorability 46, 48, 571–572, 574–576, 582, 588
ignorable 39–41, 44, 48, 54–55, 178, 181, 271, 415, 453–454, 572, 574, 579, 582, 588
– and nonignorable models 579, 588
– assignment mechanisms 39–40
– missing data 178, 582, 588
– treatment assignment 41, 48, 54
"ignorance zone", 789, 802
ignoring the missing-data mechanism 572, 582
imbalanced assignment 69
Immortal person-time 80–81
improper 31, 109, 292, 377, 387–389, 418, 576, 642–643, 707
"Imputation and Variance Estimation" software 581
Imputation 56, 142, 180, 271, 569–570, 574–581, 584–587, 805
– based procedures 570
– model is proper or confidence proper 580
impute 37, 48, 50–53, 141, 576–578, 581, 584–585
impute the missing potential outcome 37
imputing missing values 578
Index of Crude Agreement 114–115
induction time 76–80, 82, 100, 102
inference in surveys 42
inflation 16, 19, 154, 177, 230, 235, 238–239, 241, 251, 493, 496–497
– factor 154, 493, 496–497
Information-based design 507
informed consent 68
intent-to-treat 70, 549
intermediate potential outcomes 57
International Conference on Survey Nonresponse 570
interplay of frequentist and Bayesian inference 806
"interrater bias"
inter-rater reliability 110, 113, 115, 723
Interval
– estimates 42, 459, 570, 579, 796
– estimation 569, 575, 790

interventions 1–2, 5, 13–16, 18, 20–21, 28, 37, 65, 71–73, 494, 508, 546–547, 550, 565, 627–628, 714
intra-class correlation 120
Intra-rater reliability 110
invariance 411
inverse probabilities 45
Item nonresponse 570, 574
iterative computational methods 577
IV clinical trial 546–547, 549, 551, 553, 555, 557, 559, 561, 563

jackknife 163, 182, 326, 570, 575

k-Means clustering 350, 356, 364
Known propensity scores 45–46
Kolmogorov-Smirnov test 136
Kruskal-Wallis (K-W) test 126, 134–135

lagged 75, 382, 524
Lagrange Multiplier 216, 395, 409
large databases 569, 714
LASSO 163, 690–693, 706–707
– Patternsearch 692–693, 706
last observation carried forward 587
latent variable 367–368, 375–376, 381, 395–399, 410–411, 413–414, 417, 744
least squares regression 479, 577
left-censored 141
likelihood
– based analyses 583
– basis pursuit 690–691
– function 4–5, 142, 152, 214, 223, 225, 232, 238–239, 241, 246–247, 260–261, 265, 270, 357, 363, 372, 433, 449, 572, 582, 681, 781–782, 784, 795–796, 808
– or Bayesian inferences 572
– principle 557, 790, 808
– ratio chi-square 188, 191, 194, 202, 204, 206, 207, 297
– ratio statistics 580
– ratios 724, 726
limit of detection (LOD), 141–142
limits of agreement 121
Lin's coefficient 119–120, 126
linear model 53–54, 148–151, 153–157, 159, 164, 166–175, 177–178, 182, 214, 218–219, 224, 226, 246–247, 249, 254–255, 266–268, 270, 272–274, 277, 308, 397, 413, 415, 417, 436–437, 446–447, 449, 465–466, 468, 476, 482, 484, 496, 682, 691–693, 732, 806
linear-by-linear
– association 132–133
– association test 132–133
– test 133
Lisrel model 396
listwise deletion 383, 415, 570, 573
log-likelihood 152, 154, 156, 160, 170, 178–179, 191, 214, 216, 218, 221, 223, 231, 236–239, 241, 246–247, 260–261, 265, 363, 582
log-transformed data 128, 135
logistic
– regression 7, 11, 14, 45, 150, 157, 172, 182, 187–209, 273, 446, 523, 555, 576–577, 682, 695–696
– regression models 187, 523, 576
logit function 189, 206, 483
longitudinal
– data 103, 160, 253–255, 259–262, 268–273, 429, 431–432, 434–437, 446–448, 451, 453, 455–456, 553
– studies 254, 272, 429–431, 434, 436, 446, 453, 456, 459–460, 586–587, 665
– surveys 577
Lord's Paradox 35, 37, 41

Mahalanobis metric 46
– matching within propensity score calipers 46
Mann-Whitney-Wilcoxon (M-W-W) test 134, 135, 136, 142
marginal homogeneity 111
Markov Chain Monte Carlo 57, 382, 416, 578, 806
– methods 578
Markov Chain 57, 382, 416, 446, 578, 806
matched
– on the propensity scores 45
– sampling 45
matching 7, 46–47, 53–54, 86, 91–93, 95, 97, 204, 209, 345–346, 376, 467, 574–577, 807
– methods 46
matrix sampling designs 587
Maximum likelihood estimates 143, 261, 263, 269, 433, 438, 440, 449–450, 735–737, 744
Maximum likelihood estimation 45, 161, 169, 190–191, 197, 202, 205, 208, 214, 218–219, 356–357, 401, 522, 582–583, 735
MCMC methods 416, 583, 806
McNemar's test 111, 113
mean and covariance structures 395
measurement error 8–9, 82, 96, 148, 151, 177, 182, 379, 435, 439, 456, 744
medical
– decision making 712–713, 715, 717, 719, 721, 723, 725–729
– literature 606–607, 713–715, 717–718, 721, 724, 727

meta-analysis 602–614, 722, 728, 807
method comparison studies 119–120
Metropolis–Hastings algorithm 578, 583
MI in practice 580
mid p-value 130, 788, 789
midrank 134, 142
minimax design 528–529
MINISNAP 123, 125
missing at random (MAR), 178–181, 271, 415–416, 453–455, 571–572, 574, 582
missing completely at random (MCAR), 178, 181, 271, 415–416, 453–455, 571–574, 581, 587
missing covariates in propensity score analyses 57
missing data mechanism 142, 178–180, 415, 453
Missing data 35, 40, 48, 55–57, 141–142, 148, 178–182, 253, 255, 270–272, 390, 395, 411, 415–416, 438, 453–455, 460, 557–558, 569–582, 584–588, 702, 745, 805
– problem 35, 40, 48, 148, 415
missing outcomes with noncompliance 57
"missing" due to death 569
missing-data mechanism 571–572, 576, 582
Missing-data mechanisms 571
missing-data pattern 577–578, 585
missing potential outcomes 48–49, 51–53
misspecified models 395, 405
MIX 485, 581, 606, 673, 765
mixture of prior densities 792
Model selection 162, 166, 253–254, 262, 264–268, 277, 299, 384, 707
– identification 376, 398–399
– is the science 48
Model-based
– clustering 355–356, 358, 363
– extrapolation 53
– perspective 47
– procedures 581
modeling assumptions 9, 17, 45–46, 587–588, 733
monitoring boundaries 496, 506
monotone 170, 206, 305, 495, 539, 577, 581, 584–586, 671
– missing data 584–585
– missingness 577–578
– pattern 577, 581, 585
– transformation 135, 154
Monte Carlo simulation 494, 656, 659, 661–662, 670, 673–677
more unusual 42–43
MSVM 680, 697–700, 703
MTD 514–523, 525–526, 539
Multicategory
– penalized likelihood 679, 688
– support vector machines 697
– SVM 680, 689, 707
Multi-dimensional scaling 358, 360
Multi-group SEM 410–411
multi-level SEM 395, 414
Multinomial logistic regression 202, 204, 206, 555
Multiple
– imputation 56, 142, 180, 569–570, 576, 578–579, 581, 586–587
– informant 730–732, 734–737, 740–741, 743–745
– treatments 42, 55, 525
multiply impute 48, 579–581
multivariate X 46, 54
myocardial infarction 68, 71, 102, 505–506, 549, 557, 564, 611–613, 637, 721, 783, 797–798, 800–801

Nagelkerke R2, 191
National Health Interview Survey 574
negligence 31
Nested case-control studies 97
network algorithms 135
Neymanian
– confidence interval 44
– evaluations 55
– perspective 43, 45
– randomization-based inference 42
– variance 45
Neyman–Pearson framework 783–784
No contamination of imputations across treatments 50
no interference between units 33
no versions of treatments
non-detects 141
non-informative 52, 282, 777, 783, 785–786, 789–790, 802, 804, 806
non-parametric test 142
Noncompliance 40, 56–57, 66, 70
nonexperimental 64–67, 73, 104
– studies 64–65, 73, 104
nonhomogeneous 747–748, 750–751
nonignorable 37, 41–42, 54–55, 572, 579, 582, 588
– assignment mechanism 37
– designs 55
– missing data 582, 588
– missingness 582
– treatment assignment mechanism 41, 54
nonmonotone missingness 578
nonparametric 17, 126, 142, 156, 322, 324–325, 327, 332, 339, 576, 679, 681, 692–693, 704, 739
– statistical methods 126
nonprobabilistic assignment mechanism 41, 46
nonstandard SVM 696–697

normal
– approximation 135, 405, 537
– density plot 127
not missing at random (NMAR), 415–416, 454, 571–572
"nuisance" null hypotheses 42
null hypothesis significance test 776, 780, 782

objective Bayesian analysis 777–778, 790–791, 802, 804, 806
observational
– data set 44
– nonrandomized studies 40
– studies 6–7, 10–11, 13, 28, 34–35, 46–47, 54, 68, 177, 456, 620–622, 644
observed-data
– likelihood 582
– posterior distribution 583
Odds Ratio 7, 9, 13–14, 85–88, 96, 99, 101, 103–104, 130, 172, 190, 197–202, 205–209, 307, 448, 451–452, 604–610, 612–613, 621, 666, 670, 681–682, 690, 692, 696, 720
open cohort 75
optimal
– design 459–460, 479, 528–531, 537
– matching 46
Ordinal logistic regression 201, 204, 206, 555
Ordinary least squares 153, 187, 226, 467, 481, 733
Ordination (scaling), 342–344, 347–350, 358, 360–361, 364, 402, 749, 751
ordination or scaling 342–343, 358
outcome data 9, 13, 18, 47, 172, 253, 273, 277, 504, 584, 670
overdispersion 210, 219, 223–226, 229–230, 243, 247
overlap
– in multivariate X distributions 54
– in the distributions of the estimated propensity scores in the treatment and control groups 46
– in the estimated propensity scores 45

P-step 583
Pneg, 116–118
ppos, 116–117
Prevalence – adjusted and bias – adjusted kappa (PABAK) 115–118
pairwise comparisons 137, 433, 477–478
PAN 581, 670
Panel on Incomplete Data 570
paradox 35, 37–39, 41, 54, 604
Parametric irrelevance of marginal distribution of X 49
partial differential equations 765, 767
partitioning 174, 342–344, 350, 355, 357, 364, 371, 632, 638
patient dropout 577
pattern-mixture models 455, 581–582
Pearson 119–120, 128, 133, 138, 218, 223, 380, 384, 603–604, 608, 610–611, 783–784
– correlation coefficient 120, 133, 138
– family 128
Pearson's correlation coefficient r 119
penalized likelihood 679–682, 688, 695–696
perfect
– agreement 117, 120, 122, 125
– disagreement 120
permutation
– approach 16, 113
– argument 135
– test 130–131, 182, 802
person-time 74–77, 79–83, 86–87, 90–91, 97–100
Phase I designs 514–515, 524
Phase II designs 514, 526, 529, 531, 535–538, 541
phase III 17, 166, 485–486, 513–514, 534–535, 538, 546–547, 549–551, 553, 555, 557, 559, 561, 563
phase IV 513, 546–549, 551, 553, 555, 557, 559, 561, 563
physical randomization of treatments to units 35
placebo 4, 67, 69, 71, 433–434, 458, 467, 474, 479, 505–506, 548–549, 555–556, 584, 620, 637, 644, 649, 719, 758–759
– patients 584
– response 69
plausibility 41–42, 621
point estimates 55, 157, 502, 575, 579–580, 724
pooled OR 607–609, 612–613
population-based 7, 88, 97, 585
positive definite functions 684
– and reproducing kernel Hilbert spaces 684
posterior
– distribution 48, 50–52, 440, 501, 522, 524, 558, 576–577, 581, 583–584, 781–782, 785–787, 791–794, 796–797, 799, 808
– predictive causal inference 47
– predictive distribution of Ymis 48, 50, 578
– predictive distribution 48, 50–51, 576, 578
– probabilities 526, 781, 794–795, 807
– variance 53
potential outcomes 28–42, 48–49, 51–55, 57, 66
– framework 34–36
potentially incompatible Gibbs sampler 578
prediction error 162–163, 167

predictive 28, 47–48, 50–51, 266, 268, 501, 526, 549, 574–578, 693, 724–725, 728, 743, 779, 781, 785–788, 793, 798, 803, 805–807
– mean matching imputation 575, 577
– power 743, 785–786
– probability 501, 781, 785, 787–788, 793, 805
prevalence-adjusted and bias-adjusted kappa (PABAK), 115–118
Principal
– of maximum likelihood 187, 190
– stratification 57
prior distribution 49–50, 52, 54–55, 67, 101, 501, 526, 557–558, 576, 583–584, 777, 783, 785, 787–789, 791, 799, 807
prior probabilities 696, 727, 777, 779, 781, 794–795
probabilistic 34–36, 39–40, 173, 501, 747
probability plot 126–127
probit regression 45, 187, 206
PROC MI 262, 266, 276, 433–436, 442–443, 445, 581
PROC MIANALYZE 581
profile likelihood 143, 305
prognostic factors 324, 534, 586
propensity
– score matching 47
– scores 44–46, 176
proper 81, 104, 109–110, 134, 139, 143, 215, 259, 263, 265, 285, 323, 377, 400, 494, 531, 536, 550, 576–580, 641–643, 646, 666
– imputation 576–579
– MIs
Properly
– drawing imputations 577–578
– drawn single imputations 576
proportional
– bias 123, 126
– Odds Assumption 202, 204, 206
pseudo-rates 87–88
pseudo-risks 98–99
publication bias 602, 610, 612–613
public-use data 580

quadratic trend 584
quantile-quantile (Q-Q) plot 126–127, 156
quasi-complete separation 197, 199

random
– allocation 65–66, 68, 550
– digit dialing 92
– effects models 160, 246–247, 437–439, 446, 448, 464, 602, 607
– effects 158, 160–161, 173, 244, 246–249, 254–255, 257, 259–260, 263, 266, 269–270, 273–275, 437–446, 448, 452–453, 457, 464, 481, 602, 605, 607–612
Randomization 13–15, 17, 35, 41–43, 45, 47, 52, 64, 66–69, 72–73, 149, 158, 433–434, 465, 470, 475, 498, 505, 508, 526, 546–547, 550, 554, 603, 643, 719, 799
– distribution 42–43, 45
randomization-based 35, 41–42, 45, 47
– methods
– perspective 35, 47
randomized
– and nonrandomized data 28
– clinical trial 433, 492, 549–550, 556, 565, 584, 614, 624, 713–714, 716, 719, 728, 747
– controlled trials 1, 8, 10–12, 547, 602, 611, 614
– experiment 28, 34–35, 37, 39–41, 43, 45–47, 54, 57, 164
– phase II trials 514, 534
ratio-adjusted versions 45
receiver operating characteristic (ROC) curve 11, 192, 496, 726, 728
reference
– distribution 112, 154, 579
– laboratories 586
– method 123, 777
– prior 796
– set 130, 133, 779
regression
– adjustment 38, 176
– imputation methods 578
– imputation 575, 578
regular 10, 44–46, 53, 80, 89, 110, 297, 492, 752
– design 44–46, 53
Regularized kernel estimation 701
"related" correlation coefficients 139–140
relative
– frequency 115, 750
– Risk 4, 172, 209, 295–299, 306, 555, 579, 606, 624, 719–720
reliability 9, 11, 110–111, 113, 115–116, 322, 368, 379, 723, 728
repeated
– measures 150, 154–155, 158, 161, 255, 260, 266, 272–273, 412, 431–432, 434–438, 440, 448, 450–451, 456, 459–460, 552–553, 584, 651, 656, 672–677, 806
– treatments in time 55
replicates 9, 124, 294
Replication 32–33, 232, 368, 487, 575–576, 805
– technique 575
Representativeness 2, 94–95
reproducing kernel Hilbert spaces 679, 681, 684
Resampling methods 570

retrospective cohort studies 83
risk factor 2, 6–7, 11, 15–16, 20, 22, 34, 71, 138, 202, 207–209, 255, 326–327, 430, 441, 443–444, 549, 586, 644, 680–681, 688–690, 692–693, 717, 720, 753
risk-set sampling 99–100
robust
– estimation 226, 270
– methods 109, 128, 482
row scores 132
Rubin's Causal Model 28

sample size calculation 139–140, 144, 273, 470, 493, 496, 498, 554, 665, 668
sampling zero 198
sandwich variance estimators 160
Satorra–Bentler correction 380–381
Satterthwaite approximation 136
scalar estimand 579
scatterplot 121–123, 125, 613
Science 10, 34, 46, 48, 54, 714
scientific
– model 37
– values 33
scores 38, 44–46, 131–132, 176, 372, 412, 605, 675–676, 701, 703, 741
second control group 55
secondary
– analysts 580
– base 88–89, 91
segmented regression models 173
selection
– design 534–535
– model 180–181, 210, 239, 241, 243, 245, 581–582
sensitivity 11, 13, 47, 55–56, 67, 101, 116, 153, 156, 161, 166, 192, 455, 472, 519, 582, 587–588, 640, 680, 723–728, 804
– analyses 47, 55, 582, 587–588
– of inference 56
sequential
– designs 40, 55, 491, 493, 495, 497, 499, 501–503, 505, 507, 535
– regression multivariate 586
serially associated
serotyping 586
Shapiro-Wilk (S-W) test 127–128
"sharp" null hypotheses 42
shift alternatives 135
significance
– level 20, 41–42, 130, 140, 161, 433, 456, 459, 472, 495, 497–499, 502, 505, 507–508, 533, 580, 627, 629–630, 656–658, 789–790
– tests 124, 222, 368, 372, 379, 381, 494, 605, 631, 660, 776, 779, 782, 804, 806
Simple
– imputation methods 574
– normal example 51–52
– normal example with covariate 52
Simpson's Paradox 54, 604
smoking prevention program 33
smoking-related expenditures 31
smoothing spline ANOVA 679, 686
single imputation 574–576, 578–579
Software
– for multiple imputation 581
– packages 181, 226, 249, 251, 253, 276, 326–328, 365, 383, 450, 467, 491, 573, 581, 587, 664–665
source population 65, 73, 85–101, 103–104
Spearman's
– coefficient 133
– correlation coefficient 133
– correlation 132–133
– rs 138, 142
specificity 1, 11, 20, 116, 192, 723–728, 778, 808
split questionnaire designs 587
stable unit 32–33
– treatment value assumption 32–33
staggered enrollment 584
– significance 164, 604, 618, 623, 647, 721
– software 110, 131, 181, 190, 207, 211, 249–250, 276, 328, 365, 450, 499, 502, 569, 581, 587, 604, 806
StatXact 110, 113, 128–129, 131, 133, 135–136, 144, 250
Stochastic
– curtailment 492, 500, 784
– regression imputation 575
stopping rule principle 807–808
stratified phase II trials 533
strongly ignorable 39–41, 44
– assignment mechanisms 39–40
Structural zeros 198
Student's t
– distribution 137
– reference distribution 579
Studentized
– maximum modulus 138
– range 138
subclasses of propensity scores 45
subclassification 46–47, 53
sub-distribution functions 325
sufficient statistic 129, 179, 583
support vector machine 343, 679, 693, 695–697, 700, 706

surveillance
– areas 586
– systems 586
surveys 42, 380, 429, 569, 574, 577
survival
– analysis 281, 283, 285, 287, 289, 291, 293, 295, 297, 299, 301, 303, 305, 307, 309, 311, 313, 315, 323, 325
– data 57, 169, 275–276, 283, 285, 288, 299, 305, 308, 323, 325–326, 333, 805
susceptibility testing 586
synthetic enzyme 584
systematic
– review 602, 614, 714, 716, 722
– variation 66

test
– for interaction 194–195
– for trend 130–131
– for symmetry of the funnel plot 613
– of significance 570
– of unconfoundedness 55
– statistics 16, 19, 43, 109, 155, 161, 188, 191, 291, 294, 297, 300–301, 328, 400–401, 405–407, 411, 414–415, 496–497, 501, 665
– threshold 727
therapeutic cancer vaccines 539–541
Thin plate splin 679, 681, 686
tranexamic acid 47
transform the imputations 48
Translational clinical trials 539–541
– threshold 727
"treatment-trial" confounding 534, 538
trim and fill 613
triple-blind 69, 551
truncation 56, 230–232, 234, 281–282, 286, 299, 303
– of outcomes due to death 56
t-test 134, 136–137, 188, 219, 244, 272, 347, 436, 456, 471, 474, 555, 651, 665, 676, 782, 804
Tukey
– ladder of powers 128
– method 137
Tuning methods 679, 681, 704, 707
two part models 211, 230, 239, 241
Type I error 13, 18, 21, 70, 261–262, 472, 494–496, 503, 527, 531, 534–535, 552, 559–560, 616, 622–628, 630–633, 638–639, 646, 651, 656–658, 661, 667, 669, 672, 721–722, 728, 784
Type II error 500, 527, 531, 552–553, 646, 656–657, 669, 671, 721–722, 728, 783
typhoid fever 603, 714

unbiased point estimates 575
uncertainty due to the process of imputation 578
Unconditional mean imputation 574
unconfounded
– assignment mechanism 39–40
– but nonprobabilistic assignment mechanism 41
under dispersion 219, 224
unequal variance t-test 136–137
Unintended missing data 55
– nonresponse 570, 574
univariate prediction models 577
Unknown propensity scores 45–46
unmatchable 47
unobserved covariate 47, 55
unusual 42–43, 158, 247, 384, 482, 752
Up-and-down designs 514, 518–519

valid inferences 272, 569–570, 572, 578
variables
– used in the design of the data collection 580
– used to derive sampling weights 580
vector-valued estimates 580

Wald test 154, 262–263, 296–298, 395, 409–410, 432, 668
Wald-type confidence interval 143
"weighted Deming regression", 125
Weighting
– adjustments 574
– procedures 570, 574
Welch test 136
within
– imputation variance 579
– subject repeatability 121

X-linked recessive genetic disorder 584

Zero inflation 230, 235, 238–239, 241, 251

Handbook of Statistics
Contents of Previous Volumes

Volume 1. Analysis of Variance
Edited by P.R. Krishnaiah
1980 xviii + 1002 pp.

1. Estimation of Variance Components by C.R. Rao and J. Kleffe
2. Multivariate Analysis of Variance of Repeated Measurements by N.H. Timm
3. Growth Curve Analysis by S. Geisser
4. Bayesian Inference in MANOVA by S.J. Press
5. Graphical Methods for Internal Comparisons in ANOVA and MANOVA by R. Gnanadesikan
6. Monotonicity and Unbiasedness Properties of ANOVA and MANOVA Tests by S. Das Gupta
7. Robustness of ANOVA and MANOVA Test Procedures by P.K. Ito
8. Analysis of Variance and Problems under Time Series Models by D.R. Brillinger
9. Tests of Univariate and Multivariate Normality by K.V. Mardia
10. Transformations to Normality by G. Kaskey, B. Kolman, P.R. Krishnaiah and L. Steinberg
11. ANOVA and MANOVA: Models for Categorical Data by V.P. Bhapkar
12. Inference and the Structural Model for ANOVA and MANOVA by D.A.S. Fraser
13. Inference Based on Conditionally Specified ANOVA Models Incorporating Preliminary Testing by T.A. Bancroft and C.-P. Han
14. Quadratic Forms in Normal Variables by C.G. Khatri
15. Generalized Inverse of Matrices and Applications to Linear Models by S.K. Mitra
16. Likelihood Ratio Tests for Mean Vectors and Covariance Matrices by P.R. Krishnaiah and J.C. Lee
17. Assessing Dimensionality in Multivariate Regression by A.J. Izenman
18. Parameter Estimation in Nonlinear Regression Models by H. Bunke
19. Early History of Multiple Comparison Tests by H.L. Harter
20. Representations of Simultaneous Pairwise Comparisons by A.R. Sampson
21. Simultaneous Test Procedures for Mean Vectors and Covariance Matrices by P.R. Krishnaiah, G.S. Mudholkar and P. Subbaiah

22. Nonparametric Simultaneous Inference for Some MANOVA Models by P.K. Sen
23. Comparison of Some Computer Programs for Univariate and Multivariate Analysis of Variance by R.D. Bock and D. Brandt
24. Computations of Some Multivariate Distributions by P.R. Krishnaiah
25. Inference on the Structure of Interaction Two-Way Classification Model by P.R. Krishnaiah and M. Yochmowitz

Volume 2. Classification, Pattern Recognition and Reduction of Dimensionality
Edited by P.R. Krishnaiah and L.N. Kanal
1982 xxii + 903 pp.

1. Discriminant Analysis for Time Series by R.H. Shumway
2. Optimum Rules for Classification into Two Multivariate Normal Populations with the Same Covariance Matrix by S. Das Gupta
3. Large Sample Approximations and Asymptotic Expansions of Classification Statistics by M. Siotani
4. Bayesian Discrimination by S. Geisser
5. Classification of Growth Curves by J.C. Lee
6. Nonparametric Classification by J.D. Broffitt
7. Logistic Discrimination by J.A. Anderson
8. Nearest Neighbor Methods in Discrimination by L. Devroye and T.J. Wagner
9. The Classification and Mixture Maximum Likelihood Approaches to Cluster Analysis by G.J. McLachlan
10. Graphical Techniques for Multivariate Data and for Clustering by J.M. Chambers and B. Kleiner
11. Cluster Analysis Software by R.K. Blashfield, M.S. Aldenderfer and L.C. Morey
12. Single-link Clustering Algorithms by F.J. Rohlf
13. Theory of Multidimensional Scaling by J. de Leeuw and W. Heiser
14. Multidimensional Scaling and its Application by M. Wish and J.D. Carroll
15. Intrinsic Dimensionality Extraction by K. Fukunaga
16. Structural Methods in Image Analysis and Recognition by L.N. Kanal, B.A. Lambird and D. Lavine
17. Image Models by N. Ahuja and A. Rosenfield
18. Image Texture Survey by R.M. Haralick
19. Applications of Stochastic Languages by K.S. Fu
20. A Unifying Viewpoint on Pattern Recognition by J.C. Simon, E. Backer and J. Sallentin
21. Logical Functions in the Problems of Empirical Prediction by G.S. Lbov

22. Inference and Data Tables and Missing Values by N.G. Zagoruiko and V.N. Yolkina
23. Recognition of Electrocardiographic Patterns by J.H. van Bemmel
24. Waveform Parsing Systems by G.C. Stockman
25. Continuous Speech Recognition: Statistical Methods by F. Jelinek, R.L. Mercer and L.R. Bahl
26. Applications of Pattern Recognition in Radar by A.A. Grometstein and W.H. Schoendorf
27. White Blood Cell Recognition by F.S. Gelsema and G.H. Landweerd
28. Pattern Recognition Techniques for Remote Sensing Applications by P.H. Swain
29. Optical Character Recognition – Theory and Practice by G. Nagy
30. Computer and Statistical Considerations for Oil Spill Identification by Y.T. Chien and T.J. Killeen
31. Pattern Recognition in Chemistry by B.R. Kowalski and S. Wold
32. Covariance Matrix Representation and Object-Predicate Symmetry by T. Kaminuma, S. Tomita and S. Watanabe
33. Multivariate Morphometrics by R.A. Reyment
34. Multivariate Analysis with Latent Variables by P.M. Bentler and D.G. Weeks
35. Use of Distance Measures, Information Measures and Error Bounds in Feature Evaluation by M. Ben-Bassat
36. Topics in Measurement Selection by J.M. Van Campenhout
37. Selection of Variables Under Univariate Regression Models by P.R. Krishnaiah
38. On the Selection of Variables Under Regression Models Using Krishnaiah's Finite Intersection Tests by J.L. Schmidhammer
39. Dimensionality and Sample Size Considerations in Pattern Recognition Practice by A.K. Jain and B. Chandrasekaran
40. Selecting Variables in Discriminant Analysis for Improving upon Classical Procedures by W. Schaafsma
41. Selection of Variables in Discriminant Analysis by P.R. Krishnaiah

Volume 3. Time Series in the Frequency Domain
Edited by D.R. Brillinger and P.R. Krishnaiah
1983 xiv+485 pp.

1. Wiener Filtering (with emphasis on frequency-domain approaches) by R.J. Bhansali and D. Karavellas
2. The Finite Fourier Transform of a Stationary Process by D.R. Brillinger
3. Seasonal and Calendar Adjustment by W.S. Cleveland
4. Optimal Inference in the Frequency Domain by R.B. Davies

5. Applications of Spectral Analysis in Econometrics by C.W.J. Granger and R. Engle
6. Signal Estimation by E.J. Hannan
7. Complex Demodulation: Some Theory and Applications by T. Hasan
8. Estimating the Gain of a Linear Filter from Noisy Data by M.J. Hinich
9. A Spectral Analysis Primer by L.H. Koopmans
10. Robust-Resistant Spectral Analysis by R.D. Martin
11. Autoregressive Spectral Estimation by E. Parzen
12. Threshold Autoregression and Some Frequency-Domain Characteristics by J. Pemberton and H. Tong
13. The Frequency-Domain Approach to the Analysis of Closed-Loop Systems by M.B. Priestley
14. The Bispectral Analysis of Nonlinear Stationary Time Series with Reference to Bilinear Time-Series Models by T. Subba Rao
15. Frequency-Domain Analysis of Multidimensional Time-Series Data by E.A. Robinson
16. Review of Various Approaches to Power Spectrum Estimation by P.M. Robinson
17. Cumulants and Cumulant Spectra by M. Rosenblatt
18. Replicated Time-Series Regression: An Approach to Signal Estimation and Detection by R.H. Shumway
19. Computer Programming of Spectrum Estimation by T. Thrall
20. Likelihood Ratio Tests on Covariance Matrices and Mean Vectors of Complex Multivariate Normal Populations and their Applications in Time Series by P.R. Krishnaiah, J.C. Lee and T.C. Chang

Volume 4. Nonparametric Methods
Edited by P.R. Krishnaiah and P.K. Sen
1984 xx + 968 pp.

1. Randomization Procedures by C.B. Bell and P.K. Sen
2. Univariate and Multivariate Multisample Location and Scale Tests by V.P. Bhapkar
3. Hypothesis of Symmetry by M. Hušková
4. Measures of Dependence by K. Joag-Dev
5. Tests of Randomness against Trend or Serial Correlations by G.K. Bhattacharyya
6. Combination of Independent Tests by J.L. Folks
7. Combinatorics by L. Takács
8. Rank Statistics and Limit Theorems by M. Ghosh
9. Asymptotic Comparison of Tests – A Review by K. Singh
10. Nonparametric Methods in Two-Way Layouts by D. Quade
11. Rank Tests in Linear Models by J.N. Adichie

12. On the Use of Rank Tests and Estimates in the Linear Model by J.C. Aubuchon and T.P. Hettmansperger
13. Nonparametric Preliminary Test Inference by A.K.Md.E. Saleh and P.K. Sen
14. Paired Comparisons: Some Basic Procedures and Examples by R.A. Bradley
15. Restricted Alternatives by S.K. Chatterjee
16. Adaptive Methods by M. Hušková
17. Order Statistics by J. Galambos
18. Induced Order Statistics: Theory and Applications by P.K. Bhattacharya
19. Empirical Distribution Function by F. Csáki
20. Invariance Principles for Empirical Processes by M. Csörgő
21. M-, L- and R-estimators by J. Jurečková
22. Nonparametric Sequential Estimation by P.K. Sen
23. Stochastic Approximation by V. Dupač
24. Density Estimation by P. Révész
25. Censored Data by A.P. Basu
26. Tests for Exponentiality by K.A. Doksum and B.S. Yandell
27. Nonparametric Concepts and Methods in Reliability by M. Hollander and F. Proschan
28. Sequential Nonparametric Tests by U. Müller-Funk
29. Nonparametric Procedures for some Miscellaneous Problems by P.K. Sen
30. Minimum Distance Procedures by R. Beran
31. Nonparametric Methods in Directional Data Analysis by S.R. Jammalamadaka
32. Application of Nonparametric Statistics to Cancer Data by H.S. Wieand
33. Nonparametric Frequentist Proposals for Monitoring Comparative Survival Studies by M. Gail
34. Meteorological Applications of Permutation Techniques Based on Distance Functions by P.W. Mielke Jr
35. Categorical Data Problems Using Information Theoretic Approach by S. Kullback and J.C. Keegel
36. Tables for Order Statistics by P.R. Krishnaiah and P.K. Sen
37. Selected Tables for Nonparametric Statistics by P.K. Sen and P.R. Krishnaiah

Volume 5. Time Series in the Time Domain
Edited by E.J. Hannan, P.R. Krishnaiah and M.M. Rao
1985 xiv + 490 pp.

1. Nonstationary Autoregressive Time Series by W.A. Fuller
2. Non-Linear Time Series Models and Dynamical Systems by T. Ozaki
3. Autoregressive Moving Average Models, Intervention Problems and Outlier Detection in Time Series by G.C. Tiao

4. Robustness in Time Series and Estimating ARMA Models by R.D. Martin and V.J. Yohai
5. Time Series Analysis with Unequally Spaced Data by R.H. Jones
6. Various Model Selection Techniques in Time Series Analysis by R. Shibata
7. Estimation of Parameters in Dynamical Systems by L. Ljung
8. Recursive Identification, Estimation and Control by P. Young
9. General Structure and Parametrization of ARMA and State-Space Systems and its Relation to Statistical Problems by M. Deistler
10. Harmonizable, Cramér, and Karhunen Classes of Processes by M.M. Rao
11. On Non-Stationary Time Series by C.S.K. Bhagavan
12. Harmonizable Filtering and Sampling of Time Series by D.K. Chang
13. Sampling Designs for Time Series by S. Cambanis
14. Measuring Attenuation by M.A. Cameron and P.J. Thomson
15. Speech Recognition Using LPC Distance Measures by P.J. Thomson and P. de Souza
16. Varying Coefficient Regression by D.F. Nicholls and A.R. Pagan
17. Small Samples and Large Equations Systems by H. Theil and D.G. Fiebig

Volume 6. Sampling
Edited by P.R. Krishnaiah and C.R. Rao
1988 xvi + 594 pp.

1. A Brief History of Random Sampling Methods by D.R. Bellhouse
2. First Course in Survey Sampling by T. Dalenius
3. Optimality of Sampling Strategies by A. Chaudhuri
4. Simple Random Sampling by P.K. Pathak
5. On Single Stage Unequal Probability Sampling by V.P. Godambe and M.E. Thompson
6. Systematic Sampling by D.R. Bellhouse
7. Systematic Sampling with Illustrative Examples by M.N. Murthy and T.J. Rao
8. Sampling in Time by D.A. Binder and M.A. Hidiroglou
9. Bayesian Inference in Finite Populations by W.A. Ericson
10. Inference Based on Data from Complex Sample Designs by G. Nathan
11. Inference for Finite Population Quantiles by J. Sedransk and P.J. Smith
12. Asymptotics in Finite Population Sampling by P.K. Sen
13. The Technique of Replicated or Interpenetrating Samples by J.C. Koop
14. On the Use of Models in Sampling from Finite Populations by I. Thomsen and D. Tesfu
15. The Prediction Approach to Sampling Theory by R.M. Royall
16. Sample Survey Analysis: Analysis of Variance and Contingency Tables by D.H.Freeman Jr
17. Variance Estimation in Sample Surveys by J.N.K. Rao

18. Ratio and Regression Estimators by P.S.R.S. Rao
19. Role and Use of Composite Sampling and Capture-Recapture Sampling in Ecological Studies by M.T. Boswell, K.P. Burnham and G.P. Patil
20. Data-based Sampling and Model-based Estimation for Environmental Resources by G.P. Patil, G.J. Babu, R.C. Hennemuth, W.L. Meyers, M.B. Rajarshi and C. Taillie
21. On Transect Sampling to Assess Wildlife Populations and Marine Resources by F.L. Ramsey, C.E. Gates, G.P. Patil and C. Taillie
22. A Review of Current Survey Sampling Methods in Marketing Research (Telephone, Mall Intercept and Panel Surveys) by R. Velu and G.M. Naidu
23. Observational Errors in Behavioural Traits of Man and their Implications for Genetics by P.V. Sukhatme
24. Designs in Survey Sampling Avoiding Contiguous Units by A.S. Hedayat, C.R. Rao and J. Stufken

Volume 7. Quality Control and Reliability
Edited by P.R. Krishnaiah and C.R. Rao
1988 xiv + 503 pp.

1. Transformation of Western Style of Management by W. Edwards Deming
2. Software Reliability by F.B. Bastani and C.V. Ramamoorthy
3. Stress–Strength Models for Reliability by R.A. Johnson
4. Approximate Computation of Power Generating System Reliability Indexes by M. Mazumdar
5. Software Reliability Models by T.A. Mazzuchi and N.D. Singpurwalla
6. Dependence Notions in Reliability Theory by N.R. Chaganty and K. Joagdev
7. Application of Goodness-of-Fit Tests in Reliability by B.W. Woodruff and A.H. Moore
8. Multivariate Nonparametric Classes in Reliability by H.W. Block and T.H. Savits
9. Selection and Ranking Procedures in Reliability Models by S.S. Gupta and S. Panchapakesan
10. The Impact of Reliability Theory on Some Branches of Mathematics and Statistics by P.J. Boland and F. Proschan
11. Reliability Ideas and Applications in Economics and Social Sciences by M.C. Bhattacharjee
12. Mean Residual Life: Theory and Applications by F. Guess and F. Proschan
13. Life Distribution Models and Incomplete Data by R.E. Barlow and F. Proschan
14. Piecewise Geometric Estimation of a Survival Function by G.M. Mimmack and F. Proschan
15. Applications of Pattern Recognition in Failure Diagnosis and Quality Control by L.F. Pau

16. Nonparametric Estimation of Density and Hazard Rate Functions when Samples are Censored by W.J. Padgett
17. Multivariate Process Control by F.B. Alt and N.D. Smith
18. QMP/USP – A Modern Approach to Statistical Quality Auditing by B. Hoadley
19. Review About Estimation of Change Points by P.R. Krishnaiah and B.Q. Miao
20. Nonparametric Methods for Changepoint Problems by M. Csörgő and L. Horváth
21. Optimal Allocation of Multistate Components by E. El-Neweihi, F. Proschan and J. Sethuraman
22. Weibull, Log-Weibull and Gamma Order Statistics by H.L. Herter
23. Multivariate Exponential Distributions and their Applications in Reliability by A.P. Basu
24. Recent Developments in the Inverse Gaussian Distribution by S. Iyengar and G. Patwardhan

Volume 8. Statistical Methods in Biological and Medical Sciences
Edited by C.R. Rao and R. Chakraborty
1991 xvi + 554 pp.

1. Methods for the Inheritance of Qualitative Traits by J. Rice, R. Neuman and S.O. Moldin
2. Ascertainment Biases and their Resolution in Biological Surveys by W.J. Ewens
3. Statistical Considerations in Applications of Path Analytical in Genetic Epidemiology by D.C. Rao
4. Statistical Methods for Linkage Analysis by G.M. Lathrop and J.M. Lalouel
5. Statistical Design and Analysis of Epidemiologic Studies: Some Directions of Current Research by N. Breslow
6. Robust Classification Procedures and their Applications to Anthropometry by N. Balakrishnan and R.S. Ambagaspitiya
7. Analysis of Population Structure: A Comparative Analysis of Different Estimators of Wright's Fixation Indices by R. Chakraborty and H. Danker-Hopfe
8. Estimation of Relationships from Genetic Data by E.A. Thompson
9. Measurement of Genetic Variation for Evolutionary Studies by R. Chakraborty and C.R. Rao
10. Statistical Methods for Phylogenetic Tree Reconstruction by N. Saitou
11. Statistical Models for Sex-Ratio Evolution by S. Lessard
12. Stochastic Models of Carcinogenesis by S.H. Moolgavkar
13. An Application of Score Methodology: Confidence Intervals and Tests of Fit for One-Hit-Curves by J.J. Gart

14. Kidney-Survival Analysis of IgA Nephropathy Patients: A Case Study by O.J.W.F.Kardaun
15. Confidence Bands and the Relation with Decision Analysis: Theory by O.J.W.F.Kardaun
16. Sample Size Determination in Clinical Research by J. Bock and H. Toutenburg

Volume 9. Computational Statistics
Edited by C.R. Rao
1993 xix + 1045 pp.

1. Algorithms by B. Kalyanasundaram
2. Steady State Analysis of Stochastic Systems by K. Kant
3. Parallel Computer Architectures by R. Krishnamurti and B. Narahari
4. Database Systems by S. Lanka and S. Pal
5. Programming Languages and Systems by S. Purushothaman and J. Seaman
6. Algorithms and Complexity for Markov Processes by R. Varadarajan
7. Mathematical Programming: A Computational Perspective by W.W. Hager, R. Horst and P.M. Pardalos
8. Integer Programming by P.M. Pardalos and Y. Li
9. Numerical Aspects of Solving Linear Least Squares Problems by J.L. Barlow
10. The Total Least Squares Problem by S. van Huffel and H. Zha
11. Construction of Reliable Maximum-Likelihood-Algorithms with Applications to Logistic and Cox Regression by D. Böhning
12. Nonparametric Function Estimation by T. Gasser, J. Engel and B. Seifert
13. Computation Using the OR Decomposition by C.R. Goodall
14. The EM Algorithm by N. Laird
15. Analysis of Ordered Categorial Data through Appropriate Scaling by C.R. Rao and P.M. Caligiuri
16. Statistical Applications of Artificial Intelligence by W.A. Gale, D.J. Hand and A.E. Kelly
17. Some Aspects of Natural Language Processes by A.K. Joshi
18. Gibbs Sampling by S.F. Arnold
19. Bootstrap Methodology by G.J. Babu and C.R. Rao
20. The Art of Computer Generation of Random Variables by M.T. Boswell, S.D. Gore, G.P. Patil and C. Taillie
21. Jackknife Variance Estimation and Bias Reduction by S. Das Peddada
22. Designing Effective Statistical Graphs by D.A. Burn
23. Graphical Methods for Linear Models by A.S. Hadi
24. Graphics for Time Series Analysis by H.J. Newton
25. Graphics as Visual Language by T. Selkar and A. Appel
26. Statistical Graphics and Visualization by E.J. Wegman and D.B. Carr

27. Multivariate Statistical Visualization by F.W. Young, R.A. Faldowski and M.M. McFarlane
28. Graphical Methods for Process Control by T.L. Ziemer

Volume 10. Signal Processing and its Applications
Edited by N.K. Bose and C.R. Rao
1993 xvii + 992 pp.

1. Signal Processing for Linear Instrumental Systems with Noise: A General Theory with Illustrations from Optical Imaging and Light Scattering Problems by M. Bertero and E.R. Pike
2. Boundary Implication Results in Parameter Space by N.K. Bose
3. Sampling of Bandlimited Signals: Fundamental Results and Some Extensions by J.L. Brown Jr
4. Localization of Sources in a Sector: Algorithms and Statistical Analysis by K. Buckley and X.-L. Xu
5. The Signal Subspace Direction-of-Arrival Algorithm by J.A. Cadzow
6. Digital Differentiators by S.C. Dutta Roy and B. Kumar
7. Orthogonal Decompositions of 2D Random Fields and their Applications for 2D Spectral Estimation by J.M. Francos
8. VLSI in Signal Processing by A. Ghouse
9. Constrained Beamforming and Adaptive Algorithms by L.C. Godara
10. Bispectral Speckle Interferometry to Reconstruct Extended Objects from Turbulence-Degraded Telescope Images by D.M. Goodman, T.W. Lawrence, E.M. Johansson and J.P. Fitch
11. Multi-Dimensional Signal Processing by K. Hirano and T. Nomura
12. On the Assessment of Visual Communication by F.O. Huck, C.L. Fales, R. Alter-Gartenberg and Z. Rahman
13. VLSI Implementations of Number Theoretic Concepts with Applications in Signal Processing by G.A. Jullien, N.M. Wigley and J. Reilly
14. Decision-level Neural Net Sensor Fusion by R.Y. Levine and T.S. Khuon
15. Statistical Algorithms for Noncausal Gauss Markov Fields by J.M.F. Moura and N. Balram
16. Subspace Methods for Directions-of-Arrival Estimation by A. Paulraj, B. Ottersten, R. Roy, A. Swindlehurst, G. Xu and T. Kailath
17. Closed Form Solution to the Estimates of Directions of Arrival Using Data from an Array of Sensors by C.R. Rao and B. Zhou
18. High-Resolution Direction Finding by S.V. Schell and W.A. Gardner
19. Multiscale Signal Processing Techniques: A Review by A.H. Tewfik, M. Kim and M. Deriche
20. Sampling Theorems and Wavelets by G.G. Walter
21. Image and Video Coding Research by J.W. Woods
22. Fast Algorithms for Structured Matrices in Signal Processing by A.E. Yagle

Volume 11. Econometrics
Edited by G.S. Maddala, C.R. Rao and H.D. Vinod
1993 xx + 783 pp.

1. Estimation from Endogenously Stratified Samples by S.R. Cosslett
2. Semiparametric and Nonparametric Estimation of Quantal Response Models by J.L. Horowitz
3. The Selection Problem in Econometrics and Statistics by C.F. Manski
4. General Nonparametric Regression Estimation and Testing in Econometrics by A. Ullah and H.D. Vinod
5. Simultaneous Microeconometric Models with Censored or Qualitative Dependent Variables by R. Blundell and R.J. Smith
6. Multivariate Tobit Models in Econometrics by L.-F. Lee
7. Estimation of Limited Dependent Variable Models under Rational Expectations by G.S. Maddala
8. Nonlinear Time Series and Macroeconometrics by W.A. Brock and S.M. Potter
9. Estimation, Inference and Forecasting of Time Series Subject to Changes in Time by J.D. Hamilton
10. Structural Time Series Models by A.C. Harvey and N. Shephard
11. Bayesian Testing and Testing Bayesians by J.-P. Florens and M. Mouchart
12. Pseudo-Likelihood Methods by C. Gourieroux and A. Monfort
13. Rao's Score Test: Recent Asymptotic Results by R. Mukerjee
14. On the Strong Consistency of M-Estimates in Linear Models under a General Discrepancy Function by Z.D. Bai, Z.J. Liu and C.R. Rao
15. Some Aspects of Generalized Method of Moments Estimation by A. Hall
16. Efficient Estimation of Models with Conditional Moment Restrictions by W.K. Newey
17. Generalized Method of Moments: Econometric Applications by M. Ogaki
18. Testing for Heteroscedasticity by A.R. Pagan and Y. Pak
19. Simulation Estimation Methods for Limited Dependent Variable Models by V.A.Hajivassiliou
20. Simulation Estimation for Panel Data Models with Limited Dependent Variable by M.P. Keane
21. A Perspective Application of Bootstrap Methods in Econometrics by J. Jeong and G.S.Maddala
22. Stochastic Simulations for Inference in Nonlinear Errors-in-Variables Models by R.S. Mariano and B.W. Brown
23. Bootstrap Methods: Applications in Econometrics by H.D. Vinod
24. Identifying Outliers and Influential Observations in Econometric Models by S.G. Donald and G.S. Maddala
25. Statistical Aspects of Calibration in Macroeconomics by A.W. Gregory and G.W. Smith
26. Panel Data Models with Rational Expectations by K. Lahiri
27. Continuous Time Financial Models: Statistical Applications of Stochastic Processes by K.R. Sawyer

Volume 12. Environmental Statistics
Edited by G.P. Patil and C.R. Rao
1994 xix + 927 pp.

1. Environmetrics: An Emerging Science by J.S. Hunter
2. A National Center for Statistical Ecology and Environmental Statistics: A Center Without Walls by G.P. Patil
3. Replicate Measurements for Data Quality and Environmental Modeling by W. Liggett
4. Design and Analysis of Composite Sampling Procedures: A Review by G. Lovison, S.D. Gore and G.P. Patil
5. Ranked Set Sampling by G.P. Patil, A.K. Sinha and C. Taillie
6. Environmental Adaptive Sampling by G.A.F. Seber and S.K. Thompson
7. Statistical Analysis of Censored Environmental Data by M. Akritas, T. Ruscitti and G.P. Patil
8. Biological Monitoring: Statistical Issues and Models by E.P. Smith
9. Environmental Sampling and Monitoring by S.V. Stehman and W. Scott Overton
10. Ecological Statistics by B.F.J. Manly
11. Forest Biometrics by H.E. Burkhart and T.G. Gregoire
12. Ecological Diversity and Forest Management by J.H. Gove, G.P. Patil, B.F. Swindel and C. Taillie
13. Ornithological Statistics by P.M. North
14. Statistical Methods in Developmental Toxicology by P.J. Catalano and L.M. Ryan
15. Environmental Biometry: Assessing Impacts of Environmental Stimuli Via Animal and Microbial Laboratory Studies by W.W. Piegorsch
16. Stochasticity in Deterministic Models by J.J.M. Bedaux and S.A.L.M. Kooijman
17. Compartmental Models of Ecological and Environmental Systems by J.H. Matis and T.E. Wehrly
18. Environmental Remote Sensing and Geographic Information Systems-Based Modeling by W.L. Myers
19. Regression Analysis of Spatially Correlated Data: The Kanawha County Health Study by C.A. Donnelly, J.H. Ware and N.M. Laird
20. Methods for Estimating Heterogeneous Spatial Covariance Functions with Environmental Applications by P. Guttorp and P.D. Sampson
21. Meta-analysis in Environmental Statistics by V. Hasselblad
22. Statistical Methods in Atmospheric Science by A.R. Solow
23. Statistics with Agricultural Pests and Environmental Impacts by L.J. Young and J.H. Young
24. A Crystal Cube for Coastal and Estuarine Degradation: Selection of Endpoints and Development of Indices for Use in Decision Making by M.T. Boswell, J.S.O'Connor and G.P. Patil

25. How Does Scientific Information in General and Statistical Information in Particular Input to the Environmental Regulatory Process? by C.R. Cothern
26. Environmental Regulatory Statistics by C.B. Davis
27. An Overview of Statistical Issues Related to Environmental Cleanup by R. Gilbert
28. Environmental Risk Estimation and Policy Decisions by H. Lacayo Jr

Volume 13. Design and Analysis of Experiments
Edited by S. Ghosh and C.R. Rao
1996 xviii + 1230 pp.

1. The Design and Analysis of Clinical Trials by P. Armitage
2. Clinical Trials in Drug Development: Some Statistical Issues by H.I. Patel
3. Optimal Crossover Designs by J. Stufken
4. Design and Analysis of Experiments: Nonparametric Methods with Applications to Clinical Trials by P.K. Sen
5. Adaptive Designs for Parametric Models by S. Zacks
6. Observational Studies and Nonrandomized Experiments by P.R. Rosenbaum
7. Robust Design: Experiments for Improving Quality by D.M. Steinberg
8. Analysis of Location and Dispersion Effects from Factorial Experiments with a Circular Response by C.M. Anderson
9. Computer Experiments by J.R. Koehler and A.B. Owen
10. A Critique of Some Aspects of Experimental Design by J.N. Srivastava
11. Response Surface Designs by N.R. Draper and D.K.J. Lin
12. Multiresponse Surface Methodology by A.I. Khuri
13. Sequential Assembly of Fractions in Factorial Experiments by S. Ghosh
14. Designs for Nonlinear and Generalized Linear Models by A.C. Atkinson and L.M. Haines
15. Spatial Experimental Design by R.J. Martin
16. Design of Spatial Experiments: Model Fitting and Prediction by V.V. Fedorov
17. Design of Experiments with Selection and Ranking Goals by S.S. Gupta and S. Panchapakesan
18. Multiple Comparisons by A.C. Tamhane
19. Nonparametric Methods in Design and Analysis of Experiments by E. Brunner and M.L. Puri
20. Nonparametric Analysis of Experiments by A.M. Dean and D.A. Wolfe
21. Block and Other Designs in Agriculture by D.J. Street
22. Block Designs: Their Combinatorial and Statistical Properties by T. Calinski and S. Kageyama
23. Developments in Incomplete Block Designs for Parallel Line Bioassays by S. Gupta and R. Mukerjee

24. Row-Column Designs by K.R. Shah and B.K. Sinha
25. Nested Designs by J.P. Morgan
26. Optimal Design: Exact Theory by C.S. Cheng
27. Optimal and Efficient Treatment – Control Designs by D. Majumdar
28. Model Robust Designs by Y.-J. Chang and W.I. Notz
29. Review of Optimal Bayes Designs by A. DasGupta
30. Approximate Designs for Polynomial Regression: Invariance, Admissibility, and Optimality by N. Gaffke and B. Heiligers

Volume 14. Statistical Methods in Finance
Edited by G.S. Maddala and C.R. Rao
1996 xvi + 733 pp.

1. Econometric Evaluation of Asset Pricing Models by W.E. Person and R. Jegannathan
2 Instrumental Variables Estimation of Conditional Beta Pricing Models by C.R. Harvey and C.M. Kirby
3. Semiparametric Methods for Asset Pricing Models by B.N. Lehmann
4. Modeling the Term Structure by A.R. Pagan, A.D. Hall and V. Martin
5. Stochastic Volatility by E. Ghysels, A.C. Harvey and E. Renault
6. Stock Price Volatility by S.F. LeRoy
7. GARCH Models of Volatility by F.C. Palm
8. Forecast Evaluation and Combination by F.X. Diebold and J.A. Lopez
9. Predictable Components in Stock Returns by G. Kaul
10. Interset Rate Spreads as Predictors of Business Cycles by K. Lahiri and J.G. Wang
11. Nonlinear Time Series, Complexity Theory, and Finance by W.A. Brock and P.J.F. deLima
12. Count Data Models for Financial Data by A.C. Cameron and P.K. Trivedi
13. Financial Applications of Stable Distributions by J.H. McCulloch
14. Probability Distributions for Financial Models by J.B. McDonald
15. Bootstrap Based Tests in Financial Models by G.S. Maddala and H. Li
16. Principal Component and Factor Analyses by C.R. Rao
17. Errors in Variables Problems in Finance by G.S. Maddala and M. Nimalendran
18. Financial Applications of Artificial Neural Networks by M. Qi
19. Applications of Limited Dependent Variable Models in Finance by G.S. Maddala
20. Testing Option Pricing Models by D.S. Bates
21. Peso Problems: Their Theoretical and Empirical Implications by M.D.D. Evans

22. Modeling Market Microstructure Time Series by J. Hasbrouck
23. Statistical Methods in Tests of Portfolio Efficiency: A Synthesis by J. Shanken

Volume 15. Robust Inference
Edited by G.S. Maddala and C.R. Rao
1997 xviii + 698 pp.

1. Robust Inference in Multivariate Linear Regression Using Difference of Two Convex Functions as the Discrepancy Measure by Z.D. Bai, C.R. Rao and Y.H. Wu
2. Minimum Distance Estimation: The Approach Using Density-Based Distances by A. Basu, I.R. Harris and S. Basu
3. Robust Inference: The Approach Based on Influence Functions by M. Markatou and E. Ronchetti
4. Practical Applications of Bounded-Influence Tests by S. Heritier and M.-P. Victoria-Feser
5. Introduction to Positive-Breakdown Methods by P.J. Rousseeuw
6. Outlier Identification and Robust Methods by U. Gather and C. Becker
7. Rank-Based Analysis of Linear Models by T.P. Hettmansperger, J.W. McKean and S.J. Sheather
8. Rank Tests for Linear Models by R. Koenker
9. Some Extensions in the Robust Estimation of Parameters of Exponential and Double Exponential Distributions in the Presence of Multiple Outliers by A. Childs and N. Balakrishnan
10. Outliers, Unit Roots and Robust Estimation of Nonstationary Time Series by G.S. Maddala and Y. Yin
11. Autocorrelation-Robust Inference by P.M. Robinson and C. Velasco
12. A Practitioner's Guide to Robust Covariance Matrix Estimation by W.J. den Haan and A. Levin
13. Approaches to the Robust Estimation of Mixed Models by A.H. Welsh and A.M. Richardson
14. Nonparametric Maximum Likelihood Methods by S.R. Cosslett
15. A Guide to Censored Quantile Regressions by B. Fitzenberger
16. What Can Be Learned About Population Parameters When the Data Are Contaminated by J.L. Horowitz and C.F. Manski
17. Asymptotic Representations and Interrelations of Robust Estimators and Their Applications by J. Jurecková and P.K. Sen
18. Small Sample Asymptotics: Applications in Robustness by C.A. Field and M.A. Tingley
19. On the Fundamentals of Data Robustness by G. Maguluri and K. Singh

20. Statistical Analysis With Incomplete Data: A Selective Review by M.G. Akritas and M.P. La Valley
21. On Contamination Level and Sensitivity of Robust Tests by J.Á. Vissšek
22. Finite Sample Robustness of Tests: An Overview by T. Kariya and P. Kim
23. Future Directions by G.S. Maddala and C.R. Rao

Volume 16. Order Statistics – Theory and Methods
Edited by N. Balakrishnan and C.R. Rao
1997 xix + 688 pp.

1. Order Statistics: An Introduction by N. Balakrishnan and C.R. Rao
2. Order Statistics: A Historical Perspective by H. Leon Harter and N. Balakrishnan
3. Computer Simulation of Order Statistics by Pandu R. Tadikamalla and N. Balakrishnan
4. Lorenz Ordering of Order Statistics and Record Values by Barry C. Arnold and Jose A. Villasenor
5. Stochastic Ordering of Order Statistics by Philip J. Boland, Moshe Shaked and J. George Shanthikumar
6. Bounds for Expectations of L-Estimates by T. Rychlik
7. Recurrence Relations and Identities for Moments of Order Statistics by N. Balakrishnan and K.S. Sultan
8. Recent Approaches to Characterizations Based on Order Statistics and Record Values by C.R. Rao and D.N. Shanbhag
9. Characterizations of Distributions via Identically Distributed Functions of Order Statistics by Ursula Gather, Udo Kamps and Nicole Schweitzer
10. Characterizations of Distributions by Recurrence Relations and Identities for Moments of Order Statistics by Udo Kamps
11. Univariate Extreme Value Theory and Applications by Janos Galambos
12. Order Statistics: Asymptotics in Applications by Pranab Kumar Sen
13. Zero-One Laws for Large Order Statistics by R.J. Tomkins and Hong Wang
14. Some Exact Properties of Cook's D_I by D.R. Jensen and D.E. Ramirez
15. Generalized Recurrence Relations for Moments of Order Statistics from Non-Identical Pareto and Truncated Pareto Random Variables with Applications to Robustness by Aaron Childs and N. Balakrishnan
16. A Semiparametric Bootstrap for Simulating Extreme Order Statistics by Robert L.Strawderman and Daniel Zelterman
17. Approximations to Distributions of Sample Quantiles by Chunsheng Ma and John Robinson
18. Concomitants of Order Statistics by H.A. David and H.N. Nagaraja
19. A Record of Records by Valery B. Nevzorov and N. Balakrishnan
20. Weighted Sequential Empirical Type Processes with Applications to Change-Point Problems by Barbara Szyszkowicz

21. Sequential Quantile and Bahadur–Kiefer Processes by Miklós Csörgő and Barbara Szyszkowicz

Volume 17. Order Statistics: Applications
Edited by N. Balakrishnan and C.R. Rao
1998 xviii + 712 pp.

1. Order Statistics in Exponential Distribution by Asit P. Basu and Bahadur Singh
2. Higher Order Moments of Order Statistics from Exponential and Right-truncated Exponential Distributions and Applications to Life-testing Problems by N. Balakrishnan and Shanti S. Gupta
3. Log-gamma Order Statistics and Linear Estimation of Parameters by N. Balakrishnan and P.S. Chan
4. Recurrence Relations for Single and Product Moments of Order Statistics from a Generalized Logistic Distribution with Applications to Inference and Generalizations to Double Truncation by N. Balakrishnan and Rita Aggarwala
5. Order Statistics from the Type III Generalized Logistic Distribution and Applications by N. Balakrishnan and S.K. Lee
6. Estimation of Scale Parameter Based on a Fixed Set of Order Statistics by Sanat K.Sarkar and Wenjin Wang
7. Optimal Linear Inference Using Selected Order Statistics in Location-Scale Models by M. Masoom Ali and Dale Umbach
8. *L*-Estimation by J.R.M. Hosking
9. On Some *L*-estimation in Linear Regression Models by Soroush Alimoradi and A.K.Md. Ehsancs Saleh
10. The Role of Order Statistics in Estimating Threshold Parameters by A. Clifford Cohen
11. Parameter Estimation under Multiply Type-II Censoring by Fanhui Kong
12. On Some Aspects of Ranked Set Sampling in Parametric Estimation by Nora Ni Chuiv and Bimal K. Sinha
13. Some Uses of Order Statistics in Bayesian Analysis by Seymour Geisser
14. Inverse Sampling Procedures to Test for Homogeneity in a Multinomial Distribution by S. Panchapakesan, Aaron Childs, B.H. Humphrey and N. Balakrishnan
15. Prediction of Order Statistics by Kenneth S. Kaminsky and Paul I. Nelson
16. The Probability Plot: Tests of Fit Based on the Correlation Coefficient by R.A. Lockhart and M.A. Stephens
17. Distribution Assessment by Samuel Shapiro
18. Application of Order Statistics to Sampling Plans for Inspection by Variables by Helmut Schneider and Frances Barbera

19. Linear Combinations of Ordered Symmetric Observations with Applications to Visual Acuity by Marios Viana
20. Order-Statistic Filtering and Smoothing of Time-Series: Part I by Gonzalo R. Arce, Yeong-Taeg Kim and Kenneth E. Barner
21. Order-Statistic Filtering and Smoothing of Time-Series: Part II by Kenneth E.Barner and Gonzalo R. Arce
22. Order Statistics in Image Processing by Scott T. Acton and Alan C. Bovik
23. Order Statistics Application to CFAR Radar Target Detection by R. Viswanathan

Volume 18. Bioenvironmental and Public Health Statistics
Edited by P.K. Sen and C.R. Rao
2000 xxiv + 1105 pp.

1. Bioenvironment and Public Health: Statistical Perspectives by Pranab K. Sen
2. Some Examples of Random Process Environmental Data Analysis by David R.Brillinger
3. Modeling Infectious Diseases – Aids by L. Billard
4. On Some Multiplicity Problems and Multiple Comparison Procedures in Biostatistics by Yosef Hochberg and Peter H. Westfall
5. Analysis of Longitudinal Data by Julio M. Singer and Dalton F. Andrade
6. Regression Models for Survival Data by Richard A. Johnson and John P. Klein
7. Generalised Linear Models for Independent and Dependent Responses by Bahjat F.Qaqish and John S. Preisser
8. Hierarchial and Empirical Bayes Methods for Environmental Risk Assessment by Gauri Datta, Malay Ghosh and Lance A. Waller
9. Non-parametrics in Bioenvironmental and Public Health Statistics by Pranab Kumar Sen
10. Estimation and Comparison of Growth and Dose-Response Curves in the Presence of Purposeful Censoring by Paul W. Stewart
11. Spatial Statistical Methods for Environmental Epidemiology by Andrew B. Lawson and Noel Cressie
12. Evaluating Diagnostic Tests in Public Health by Margaret Pepe, Wendy Leisenring and Carolyn Rutter
13. Statistical Issues in Inhalation Toxicology by E. Weller, L. Ryan and D. Dockery
14. Quantitative Potency Estimation to Measure Risk with Bioenvironmental Hazards by A. John Bailer and Walter W. Piegorsch
15. The Analysis of Case-Control Data: Epidemiologic Studies of Familial Aggregation by Nan M. Laird, Garrett M. Fitzmaurice and Ann G. Schwartz

16. Cochran–Mantel–Haenszel Techniques: Applications Involving Epidemiologic Survey Data by Daniel B. Hall, Robert F. Woolson, William R. Clarke and Martha F.Jones
17. Measurement Error Models for Environmental and Occupational Health Applications by Robert H. Lyles and Lawrence L. Kupper
18. Statistical Perspectives in Clinical Epidemiology by Shrikant I. Bangdiwala and Sergio R. Muñoz
19. ANOVA and ANOCOVA for Two-Period Crossover Trial Data: New vs. Standard by Subir Ghosh and Lisa D. Fairchild
20. Statistical Methods for Crossover Designs in Bioenvironmental and Public Health Studies by Gail E. Tudor, Gary G. Koch and Diane Catellier
21. Statistical Models for Human Reproduction by C.M. Suchindran and Helen P. Koo
22. Statistical Methods for Reproductive Risk Assessment by Sati Mazumdar, Yikang Xu, Donald R. Mattison, Nancy B. Sussman and Vincent C. Arena
23. Selection Biases of Samples and their Resolutions by Ranajit Chakraborty and C. Radhakrishna Rao
24. Genomic Sequences and Quasi-Multivariate CATANOVA by Hildete Prisco Pinheiro, Françoise Seillier-Moiseiwitsch, Pranab Kumar Sen and Joseph Eron Jr
25. Statistical Methods for Multivariate Failure Time Data and Competing Risks by Ralph A. DeMasi
26. Bounds on Joint Survival Probabilities with Positively Dependent Competing Risks by Sanat K. Sarkar and Kalyan Ghosh
27. Modeling Multivariate Failure Time Data by Limin X. Clegg, Jianwen Cai and Pranab K. Sen
28. The Cost–Effectiveness Ratio in the Analysis of Health Care Programs by JosephC. Gardiner, Cathy J. Bradley and Marianne Huebner
29. Quality-of-Life: Statistical Validation and Analysis An Example from a Clinical Trial by Balakrishna Hosmane, Clement Maurath and Richard Manski
30. Carcinogenic Potency: Statistical Perspectives by Anup Dewanji
31. Statistical Applications in Cardiovascular Disease by Elizabeth R. DeLong and David M. DeLong
32. Medical Informatics and Health Care Systems: Biostatistical and Epidemiologic Perspectives by J. Zvárová
33. Methods of Establishing In Vitro–In Vivo Relationships for Modified Release Drug Products by David T. Mauger and Vernon M. Chinchilli
34. Statistics in Psychiatric Research by Sati Mazumdar, Patricia R. Houck and Charles F. Reynolds III
35. Bridging the Biostatistics–Epidemiology Gap by Lloyd J. Edwards
36. Biodiversity – Measurement and Analysis by S.P. Mukherjee

Volume 19. Stochastic Processes: Theory and Methods
Edited by D.N. Shanbhag and C.R. Rao
2001 xiv + 967 pp.

1. Pareto Processes by Barry C. Arnold
2. Branching Processes by K.B. Athreya and A.N. Vidyashankar
3. Inference in Stochastic Processes by I.V. Basawa
4. Topics in Poisson Approximation by A.D. Barbour
5. Some Elements on Lévy Processes by Jean Bertoin
6. Iterated Random Maps and Some Classes of Markov Processes by Rabi Bhattacharya and Edward C. Waymire
7. Random Walk and Fluctuation Theory by N.H. Bingham
8. A Semigroup Representation and Asymptotic Behavior of Certain Statistics of the Fisher–Wright–Moran Coalescent by Adam Bobrowski, Marek Kimmel, Ovide Arino and Ranajit Chakraborty
9. Continuous-Time ARMA Processes by P.J. Brockwell
10. Record Sequences and their Applications by John Bunge and Charles M. Goldie
11. Stochastic Networks with Product Form Equilibrium by Hans Daduna
12. Stochastic Processes in Insurance and Finance by Paul Embrechts, Rüdiger Frey and Hansjörg Furrer
13. Renewal Theory by D.R. Grey
14. The Kolmogorov Isomorphism Theorem and Extensions to some Nonstationary Processes by Yûichirô Kakihara
15. Stochastic Processes in Reliability by Masaaki Kijima, Haijun Li and Moshe Shaked
16. On the supports of Stochastic Processes of Multiplicity One by A. Kłopotowski and M.G. Nadkarni
17. Gaussian Processes: Inequalities, Small Ball Probabilities and Applications by W.V. Li and Q.-M. Shao
18. Point Processes and Some Related Processes by Robin K. Milne
19. Characterization and Identifiability for Stochastic Processes by B.L.S. Prakasa Rao
20. Associated Sequences and Related Inference Problems by B.L.S. Prakasa Rao and Isha Dewan
21. Exchangeability, Functional Equations, and Characterizations by C.R. Rao and D.N.Shanbhag
22. Martingales and Some Applications by M.M. Rao
23. Markov Chains: Structure and Applications by R.L. Tweedie
24. Diffusion Processes by S.R.S. Varadhan
25. Itô's Stochastic Calculus and Its Applications by S. Watanabe

Volume 20. Advances in Reliability
Edited by N. Balakrishnan and C.R. Rao
2001 xxii + 860 pp.

1. Basic Probabilistic Models in Reliability by N. Balakrishnan, N. Limnios and C. Papadopoulos
2. The Weibull Nonhomogeneous Poisson Process by A.P Basu and S.E. Rigdon
3. Bathtub-Shaped Failure Rate Life Distributions by C.D. Lai, M. Xie and D.N.P. Murthy
4. Equilibrium Distribution – its Role in Reliability Theory by A. Chatterjee and S.P. Mukherjee
5. Reliability and Hazard Based on Finite Mixture Models by E.K. Al-Hussaini and K.S. Sultan
6. Mixtures and Monotonicity of Failure Rate Functions by M. Shaked and F. Spizzichino
7. Hazard Measure and Mean Residual Life Orderings: A Unified Approach by M. Asadi and D.N. Shanbhag
8. Some Comparison Results of the Reliability Functions of Some Coherent Systems by J. Mi
9. On the Reliability of Hierarchical Structures by L.B. Klebanov and G.J. Szekely
10. Consecutive k-out-of n Systems by N.A. Mokhlis
11. Exact Reliability and Lifetime of Consecutive Systems by S. Aki
12. Sequential k-out-of-n Systems by E. Cramer and U. Kamps
13. Progressive Censoring: A Review by R. Aggarwala
14. Point and Interval Estimation for Parameters of the Logistic Distribution Based on Progressively Type-II Censored Samples by N. Balakrishnan and N. Kannan
15. Progressively Censored Variables-Sampling Plans for Life Testing by U. Balasooriya
16. Graphical Techniques for Analysis of Data From Repairable Systems by P.A. Akersten, B. Klefsjö and B. Bergman
17. A Bayes Approach to the Problem of Making Repairs by G.C. McDonald
18. Statistical Analysis for Masked Data by B.J. Flehinger[†], B. Reiser and E. Yashchin
19. Analysis of Masked Failure Data under Competing Risks by A. Sen, S. Basu and M. Banerjee
20. Warranty and Reliability by D.N.P. Murthy and W.R. Blischke
21. Statistical Analysis of Reliability Warranty Data by K. Suzuki, Md. Rezaul Karim and L. Wang
22. Prediction of Field Reliability of Units, Each under Differing Dynamic Stresses, from Accelerated Test Data by W. Nelson
23. Step-Stress Accelerated Life Test by E. Gouno and N. Balakrishnan

24. Estimation of Correlation under Destructive Testing by R. Johnson and W. Lu
25. System-Based Component Test Plans for Reliability Demonstration: A Review and Survey of the State-of-the-Art by J. Rajgopal and M. Mazumdar
26. Life-Test Planning for Preliminary Screening of Materials: A Case Study by J. Stein and N. Doganaksoy
27. Analysis of Reliability Data from In-House Audit Laboratory Testing by R. Agrawal and N. Doganaksoy
28. Software Reliability Modeling, Estimation and Analysis by M. Xie and G.Y. Hong
29. Bayesian Analysis for Software Reliability Data by J.A. Achcar
30. Direct Graphical Estimation for the Parameters in a Three-Parameter Weibull Distribution by P.R. Nelson and K.B. Kulasekera
31. Bayesian and Frequentist Methods in Change-Point Problems by N. Ebrahimi and S.K. Ghosh
32. The Operating Characteristics of Sequential Procedures in Reliability by S. Zacks
33. Simultaneous Selection of Extreme Populations from a Set of Two-Parameter Exponential Populations by K. Hussein and S. Panchapakesan

Volume 21. Stochastic Processes: Modelling and Simulation
Edited by D.N. Shanbhag and C.R. Rao
2003 xxviii + 1002 pp.

1. Modelling and Numerical Methods in Manufacturing System Using Control Theory by E.K. Boukas and Z.K. Liu
2. Models of Random Graphs and their Applications by C. Cannings and D.B. Penman
3. Locally Self-Similar Processes and their Wavelet Analysis by J.E. Cavanaugh, Y. Wang and J.W. Davis
4. Stochastic Models for DNA Replication by R. Cowan
5. An Empirical Process with Applications to Testing the Exponential and Geometric Models by J.A. Ferreira
6. Patterns in Sequences of Random Events by J. Gani
7. Stochastic Models in Telecommunications for Optimal Design, Control and Performance Evaluation by N. Gautam
8. Stochastic Processes in Epidemic Modelling and Simulation by D. Greenhalgh
9. Empirical Estimators Based on MCMC Data by P.E. Greenwood and W. Wefelmeyer
10. Fractals and the Modelling of Self-Similarity by B.M. Hambly
11. Numerical Methods in Queueing Theory by D. Heyman
12. Applications of Markov Chains to the Distribution Theory of Runs and Patterns by M.V. Koutras

13. Modelling Image Analysis Problems Using Markov Random Fields by S.Z. Li
14. An Introduction to Semi-Markov Processes with Application to Reliability by N. Limnios and G. Oprişan
15. Departures and Related Characteristics in Queueing Models by M. Manoharan, M.H. Alamatsaz and D.N. Shanbhag
16. Discrete Variate Time Series by E. McKenzie
17. Extreme Value Theory, Models and Simulation by S. Nadarajah
18. Biological Applications of Branching Processes by A.G. Pakes
19. Markov Chain Approaches to Damage Models by C.R. Rao, M. Albassam, M.B. Rao and D.N. Shanbhag
20. Point Processes in Astronomy: Exciting Events in the Universe by J.D. Scargle and G.J. Babu
21. On the Theory of Discrete and Continuous Bilinear Time Series Models by T. Subba Rao and Gy. Terdik
22. Nonlinear and Non-Gaussian State-Space Modeling with Monte Carlo Techniques: A Survey and Comparative Study by H. Tanizaki
23. Markov Modelling of Burst Behaviour in Ion Channels by G.F. Yeo, R.K. Milne, B.W. Madsen, Y. Li and R.O. Edeson

Volume 22. Statistics in Industry
Edited by R. Khattree and C.R. Rao
2003 xxi + 1150 pp.

1. Guidelines for Selecting Factors and Factor Levels for an Industrial Designed Experiment by V. Czitrom
2. Industrial Experimentation for Screening by D.K.J. Lin
3. The Planning and Analysis of Industrial Selection and Screening Experiments by G. Pan, T.J. Santner and D.M. Goldsman
4. Uniform Experimental Designs and their Applications in Industry by K.-T. Fang and D.K.J. Lin
5. Mixed Models and Repeated Measures: Some Illustrative Industrial Examples by G.A. Milliken
6. Current Modeling and Design Issues in Response Surface Methodology: GLMs and Models with Block Effects by A.I. Khuri
7. A Review of Design and Modeling in Computer Experiments by V.C.P. Chen, K.-L. Tsui, R.R. Barton and J.K. Allen
8. Quality Improvement and Robustness via Design of Experiments by B.E. Ankenman and A.M. Dean
9. Software to Support Manufacturing Experiments by J.E. Reece
10. Statistics in the Semiconductor Industry by V. Czitrom
11. PREDICT: A New Approach to Product Development and Lifetime Assessment Using Information Integration Technology by J.M. Booker, T.R. Bement, M.A. Meyerand W.J. Kerscher III

12. The Promise and Challenge of Mining Web Transaction Data by S.R. Dalal, D. Egan, Y. Ho and M. Rosenstein
13. Control Chart Schemes for Monitoring the Mean and Variance of Processes Subject to Sustained Shifts and Drifts by Z.G. Stoumbos, M.R. Reynolds Jr and W.H.Woodall
14. Multivariate Control Charts: Hotelling T^2, Data Depth and Beyond by R.Y. Liu
15. Effective Sample Sizes for T^2 Control Charts by R.L. Mason, Y.-M. Chou and J.C.Young
16. Multidimensional Scaling in Process Control by T.F. Cox
17. Quantifying the Capability of Industrial Processes by A.M. Polansky and S.N.U.A. Kirmani
18. Taguchi's Approach to On-line Control Procedure by M.S. Srivastava and Y. Wu
19. Dead-Band Adjustment Schemes for On-line Feedback Quality Control by A. Luceño
20. Statistical Calibration and Measurements by H. Iyer
21. Subsampling Designs in Industry: Statistical Inference for Variance Components by R. Khattree
22. Repeatability, Reproducibility and Interlaboratory Studies by R. Khattree
23. Tolerancing – Approaches and Related Issues in Industry by T.S. Arthanari
24. Goodness-of-fit Tests for Univariate and Multivariate Normal Models by D.K. Srivastava and G.S. Mudholkar
25. Normal Theory Methods and their Simple Robust Analogs for Univariate and Multivariate Linear Models by D.K. Srivastava and G.S. Mudholkar
26. Diagnostic Methods for Univariate and Multivariate Normal Data by D.N. Naik
27. Dimension Reduction Methods Used in Industry by G. Merola and B. Abraham
28. Growth and Wear Curves by A.M. Kshirsagar
29. Time Series in Industry and Business by B. Abraham and N. Balakrishna
30. Stochastic Process Models for Reliability in Dynamic Environments by N.D. Singpurwalla, T.A. Mazzuchi, S. Özekici and R. Soyer
31. Bayesian Inference for the Number of Undetected Errors by S. Basu

Volume 23. Advances in Survival Analysis
Edited by N. Balakrishnan and C.R. Rao
2003 xxv + 795 pp.

1. Evaluation of the Performance of Survival Analysis Models: Discrimination and Calibration Measures by R.B. D'Agostino and B.-H. Nam
2. Discretizing a Continuous Covariate in Survival Studies by J.P. Klein and J.-T. Wu

3. On Comparison of Two Classification Methods with Survival Endpoints by Y. Lu, H. Jin and J. Mi
4. Time-Varying Effects in Survival Analysis by T.H. Scheike
5. Kaplan–Meier Integrals by W. Stute
6. Statistical Analysis of Doubly Interval-Censored Failure Time Data by J. Sun
7. The Missing Censoring-Indicator Model of Random Censorship by S. Subramanian
8. Estimation of the Bivariate Survival Function with Generalized Bivariate Right Censored Data Structures by S. Keleş, M.J. van der Laan and J.M. Robins
9. Estimation of Semi-Markov Models with Right-Censored Data by O. Pons
10. Nonparametric Bivariate Estimation with Randomly Truncated Observations by Ü. Gürler
11. Lower Bounds for Estimating a Hazard by C. Huber and B. MacGibbon
12. Non-Parametric Hazard Rate Estimation under Progressive Type-II Censoring by N. Balakrishnan and L. Bordes
13. Statistical Tests of the Equality of Survival Curves: Reconsidering the Options by G.P. Suciu, S. Lemeshow and M. Moeschberger
14. Testing Equality of Survival Functions with Bivariate Censored Data: A Review by P.V. Rao
15. Statistical Methods for the Comparison of Crossing Survival Curves by C.T. Le
16. Inference for Competing Risks by J.P. Klein and R. Bajorunaite
17. Analysis of Cause-Specific Events in Competing Risks Survival Data by J. Dignam, J. Bryant and H.S. Wieand
18. Analysis of Progressively Censored Competing Risks Data by D. Kundu, N. Kannan and N. Balakrishnan
19. Marginal Analysis of Point Processes with Competing Risks by R.J. Cook, B. Chen and P. Major
20. Categorical Auxiliary Data in the Discrete Time Proportional Hazards Model by P. Slasor and N. Laird
21. Hosmer and Lemeshow type Goodness-of-Fit Statistics for the Cox Proportional Hazards Model by S. May and D.W. Hosmer
22. The Effects of Misspecifying Cox's Regression Model on Randomized Treatment Group Comparisons by A.G. DiRienzo and S.W. Lagakos
23. Statistical Modeling in Survival Analysis and Its Influence on the Duration Analysis by V. Bagdonavičius and M. Nikulin
24. Accelerated Hazards Model: Method, Theory and Applications by Y.Q. Chen, N.P. Jewell and J. Yang
25. Diagnostics for the Accelerated Life Time Model of Survival Data by D. Zelterman and H. Lin
26. Cumulative Damage Approaches Leading to Inverse Gaussian Accelerated Test Models by A. Onar and W.J. Padgett
27. On Estimating the Gamma Accelerated Failure-Time Models by K.M. Koti
28. Frailty Model and its Application to Seizure Data by N. Ebrahimi, X. Zhang, A. Berg and S. Shinnar
29. State Space Models for Survival Analysis by W.Y. Tan and W. Ke

30. First Hitting Time Models for Lifetime Data by M.-L.T. Lee and G.A. Whitmore
31. An Increasing Hazard Cure Model by Y. Peng and K.B.G. Dear
32. Marginal Analyses of Multistage Data by G.A. Satten and S. Datta
33. The Matrix-Valued Counting Process Model with Proportional Hazards for Sequential Survival Data by K.L. Kesler and P.K. Sen
34. Analysis of Recurrent Event Data by J. Cai and D.E. Schaubel
35. Current Status Data: Review, Recent Developments and Open Problems by N.P. Jewell and M. van der Laan
36. Appraisal of Models for the Study of Disease Progression in Psoriatic Arthritis by R. Aguirre-Hernández and V.T. Farewell
37. Survival Analysis with Gene Expression Arrays by D.K. Pauler, J. Hardin, J.R. Faulkner, M. LeBlanc and J.J. Crowley
38. Joint Analysis of Longitudinal Quality of Life and Survival Processes by M. Mesbah, J.-F. Dupuy, N. Heutte and L. Awad
39. Modelling Survival Data using Flowgraph Models by A.V. Huzurbazar
40. Nonparametric Methods for Repair Models by M. Hollander and J. Sethuraman

Volume 24. Data Mining and Data Visualization
Edited by C.R. Rao, E.J. Wegman and J.L. Solka
2005 xiv + 643 pp.

1. Statistical Data Mining by E.J. Wegman and J.L. Solka
2. From Data Mining to Knowledge Mining by K.A. Kaufman and R.S. Michalski
3. Mining Computer Security Data by D.J. Marchette
4. Data Mining of Text Files by A.R. Martinez
5. Text Data Mining with Minimal Spanning Trees by J.L. Solka, A.C. Bryant and E.J. Wegman
6. Information Hiding: Steganography and Steganalysis by Z. Duric, M. Jacobs and S. Jajodia
7. Canonical Variate Analysis and Related Methods for Reduction of Dimensionality and Graphical Representation by C.R. Rao
8. Pattern Recognition by D.J. Hand
9. Multidimensional Density Estimation by D.W. Scott and S.R. Sain
10. Multivariate Outlier Detection and Robustness by M. Hubert, P.J. Rousseeuw and S. Van Aelst
11. Classification and Regression Trees, Bagging, and Boosting by C.D. Sutton
12. Fast Algorithms for Classification Using Class Cover Catch Digraphs by D.J. Marchette, E.J. Wegman and C.E. Priebe
13. On Genetic Algorithms and their Applications by Y.H. Said

14. Computational Methods for High-Dimensional Rotations in Data Visualization by A. Buja, D. Cook, D. Asimov and C. Hurley
15. Some Recent Graphics Templates and Software for Showing Statistical Summaries by D. B. Carr
16. Interactive Statistical Graphics: the Paradigm of Linked Views by A. Wilhelm
17. Data Visualization and Virtual Reality by J.X. Chen

Volume 25. Bayesian Thinking: Modeling and Computation
Edited by D.K. Dey and C.R. Rao
2005 xx + 1041 pp.

1. Bayesian Inference for Causal Effects by D.B. Rubin
2. Reference Analysis by J.M. Bernardo
3. Probability Matching Priors by G.S. Datta and T.J. Sweeting
4. Model Selection and Hypothesis Testing based on Objective Probabilities and Bayes Factors by L.R. Pericchi
5. Role of P-values and other Measures of Evidence in Bayesian Analysis by J. Ghosh, S. Purkayastha and T. Samanta
6. Bayesian Model Checking and Model Diagnostics by H.S. Stern and S. Sinharay
7. The Elimination of Nuisance Parameters by B. Liseo
8. Bayesian Estimation of Multivariate Location Parameters by A.C. Brandwein and W.E. Strawderman
9. Bayesian Nonparametric Modeling and Data Analysis: An Introduction by T.E. Hanson, A.J. Branscum and W.O. Johnson
10. Some Bayesian Nonparametric Models by P. Damien
11. Bayesian Modeling in the Wavelet Domain by F. Ruggeri and B. Vidakovic
12. Bayesian Nonparametric Inference by S. Walker
13. Bayesian Methods for Function Estimation by N. Choudhuri, S. Ghosal and A. Roy
14. MCMC Methods to Estimate Bayesian Parametric Models by A. Mira
15. Bayesian Computation: From Posterior Densities to Bayes Factors, Marginal Likelihoods, and Posterior Model Probabilities by M.-H. Chen
16. Bayesian Modelling and Inference on Mixtures of Distributions by J.-M. Marin, K. Mengersen and C.P Robert
17. Simulation Based Optimal Design by P. Müller
18. Variable Selection and Covariance Selection in Multivariate Regression Models by E. Cripps, C. Carter and R. Kohn
19. Dynamic Models by H.S. Migon, D. Gamerman, H.F. Lopes and M.A.R. Ferreira
20. Bayesian Thinking in Spatial Statistics by L.A. Waller
21. Robust Bayesian Analysis by F. Ruggeri, D. Ríos Insua and Jacinto Martín
22. Elliptical Measurement Error Models – A Bayesian Approach by H. Bolfarine and R.B. Arellano-Valle

23. Bayesian Sensitivity Analysis in Skew-elliptical Models by I. Vidal, P. Iglesias and M.D. Branco
24. Bayesian Methods for DNA Microarray Data Analysis by V. Baladandayuthapani, S. Ray and B.K. Mallick
25. Bayesian Biostatistics by D.B. Dunson
26. Innovative Bayesian Methods for Biostatistics and Epidemiology by P. Gustafson, S. Hossain and L. McCandless
27. Bayesian Analysis of Case-Control Studies by B. Mukherjee, S. Sinha and M. Ghosh
28. Bayesian Analysis of ROC Data by V.E. Johnson and T.D. Johnson
29. Modeling and Analysis for Categorical Response Data by S. Chib
30. Bayesian Methods and Simulation-Based Computation for Contingency Tables by J.H. Albert
31. Multiple Events Time Data: A Bayesian Recourse by D. Sinha and S.K. Ghosh
32. Bayesian Survival Analysis for Discrete Data with Left-Truncation and Interval Censoring by C.Z. He and D. Sun
33. Software Reliability by L. Kuo
34. Bayesian Aspects of Small Area Estimation by T. Maiti
35. Teaching Bayesian Thought to Nonstatisticians by D.K. Stangl

Volume 26. Psychometrics
Edited by C.R. Rao and S. Sinharay
2007 xx + 1169 pp.

1. A History and Overview of Psychometrics by Lyle V. Jones and David Thissen
2. Selected Topics in Classical Test Theory by Charles Lewis
3. Validity: Foundational Issues and Statistical Methodology by Bruno D. Zumbo
4. Reliability Coefficients and Generalizability Theory by Noreen M. Webb, Richard J. Shavelson and Edward H. Haertel
5. Differential Item Functioning and Item Bias by Randall D. Penfield and Gregory Camilli
6. Equating Test Scores by Paul W. Holland, Neil J. Dorans and Nancy S. Petersen
7. Electronic Essay Grading by Shelby J. Haberman
8. Some Matrix Results Useful in Psychometric Research by C. Radhakrishna Rao
9. Factor Analysis by Haruo Yanai and Masanori Ichikawa
10. Structural Equation Modeling by Ke-Hai Yuan and Peter M. Bentler
11. Applications of Multidimensional Scaling in Psychometrics by Yoshio Takane

12. Multilevel Models in Psychometrics by Fiona Steele and Harvey Goldstein
13. Latent Class Analysis in Psychometrics by C. Mitchell Dayton and George B. Macready
14. Random-Effects Models for Preference Data by Ulf Böckenholt and Rung-Ching Tsai
15. Item Response Theory in a General Framework by R. Darrell Bock and Irini Moustaki
16. Rasch Models by Gerhard H. Fischer
17. Hierarchical Item Response Theory Models by Matthew S. Johnson, Sandip Sinharay and Eric T. Bradlow
18. Multidimensional Item Response Theory by Mark D. Reckase
19. Mixture Distribution Item Response Models by Matthias von Davier and Jürgen Rost
20. Scoring Open Ended Questions by Gunter Maris and Timo Bechger
21. Assessing the Fit of Item Response Theory Models by Hariharan Swaminathan, Ronald K. Hambleton and H. Jane Rogers
22. Nonparametric Item Response Theory and Special Topics by Klaas Sijtsma and Rob R. Meijer
23. Automatic Item Generation and Cognitive Psychology by Susan Embretson and Xiangdong Yang
24. Statistical Inference for Causal Effects, with Emphasis on Applications in Psychometrics and Education by Donald B.Rubin
25. Statistical Aspects of Adaptive Testing by Wim J. van der Linden and Cees A. W. Glas
26. Bayesian Psychometric Modeling From An Evidence-Centered Design Perspective by Robert J. Mislevy and Roy Levy
27. Value-Added Modeling by Henry Braun and Howard Wainer
28. Three Statistical Paradoxes in the Interpretation of Group Differences: Illustrated with Medical School Admission and Licensing Data by Howard Wainer and Lisa M. Brown
29. Meta-Analysis by Larry V. Hedges
30. Vertical Scaling: Statistical Models for Measuring Growth and Achievement by Richard J. Patz and Lihua Yao
31. COGNITIVE DIAGNOSIS
    a. Review of Cognitively Diagnostic Assessment and a Summary of Psychometric Models by Louis V. DiBello, Louis A. Roussos and William Stout
    b. Some Notes on Models for Cognitively Based Skills Diagnosis by Shelby J. Haberman and Matthias von Davier
32. The Statistical Procedures Used in National Assessment of Educational Progress: Recent Developments and Future Directions by Matthias von Davier, Sandip Sinharay, Andreas Oranje and Albert Beaton
33. Statistical Procedures Used in College Admissions Testing by Jinghua Liu, Deborah J. Harris and Amy Schmidt

34. FUTURE CHALLENGES IN PSYCHOMETRICS
a. Integration of Models by Robert L. Brennan
b. Linking Scores Across Computer and Paper-Based Modes of Test Administration by Daniel R. Eignor
c. Linking Cognitively-Based Models and Psychometric Methods by Mark J. Gierl and Jacqueline P. Leighton
d. Technical Considerations in Equating Complex Assessments by Ida Lawrence
e. Future Challenges to Psychometrics: Validity, Validity, Validity by Neal Kingston
f. Testing with and without Computers by Piet Sanders
g. Practical Challenges to Psychometrics Driven by Increased Visibility of Assessment by Cynthia Board Schmeiser